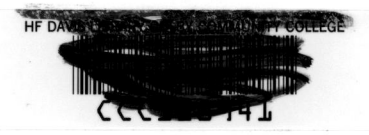

```
636.7    DeBartola, Stephen P
D543f    Fluid therapy in
2000     small animal
         practice.
```

Fluid Therapy in Small Animal Practice

2ND EDITION

Stephen P. DiBartola, DVM, Dipl. ACVIM

Professor of Medicine, Department of Veterinary Clinical Sciences
College of Veterinary Medicine
Ohio State University
Columbus, Ohio

W.B. SAUNDERS COMPANY
A Harcourt Health Sciences Company
Philadelphia   London   New York   St. Louis   Sydney   Toronto

W.B. SAUNDERS COMPANY
A Harcourt Health Sciences Company

The Curtis Center
Independence Square West
Philadelphia, Pennsylvania 19106

Library of Congress Cataloging-in-Publication Data

DiBartola, Stephen P.

Fluid therapy in small animal practice / Stephen P. DiBartola.—2nd ed.

p.   cm.

ISBN 0–7216–7739–8

1. Dogs—Diseases—Treatment.   2. Cats—Diseases—Treatment.
3. Veterinary fluid therapy.   I. Title.

SF991.D53 2000   636.7′08963992—dc21

DNLM/DLC   99-046857

Editor: Raymond R. Kersey
Production Manager: Denise LeMelledo
Project Editor: Lee Ann Draud
Illustration Coordinator: Robert Quinn

FLUID THERAPY IN SMALL ANIMAL PRACTICE   ISBN 0–7216–7739–8

Copyright © 2000, 1992 by W.B. Saunders Company

All rights reserved. No part of this publication may be reproduced or transmitted in any form or by any means, electronic or mechanical, including photocopy, recording, or any information storage and retrieval system, without permission in writing from the publisher.

Printed in the United States of America.

Last digit is the print number: 9   8   7   6   5   4   3   2   1

*To my parents, Martha Weimann and Philip DiBartola,
for insisting that I acquire the formal education
they could not;
To my wife, Maxey Wellman, for standing by me
despite my imperfections;
To my children, Matthew, Michael, Alex, and
Stephanie, for teaching me about unconditional love;
To my childhood friend, Pudge Albao,
for teaching me about loyalty; and,
To my colleague, Dennis Chew, for teaching me
enthusiasm for clinical medicine and
compassion for pet owners.*

Contributors

Nichole Birnbaum, DVM
Internist, Small Animal Internal Medicine, Manassas, Virginia
Fluid and Electrolyte Disturbances in Gastrointestinal, Pancreatic, and Hepatic Disease

John D. Bonagura, DVM, Dipl. ACVIM
Gilbreath-McLorn Professor of Cardiology, Department of Veterinary Medicine and Surgery, College of Veterinary Medicine, University of Missouri, Columbia, Missouri
Fluid and Diuretic Therapy in Heart Failure

Sharon A. Center, DVM, Dipl. ACVIM
Professor of Medicine, College of Veterinary Medicine, Cornell University, Ithaca, New York
Fluid and Electrolyte Disturbances in Gastrointestinal, Pancreatic, and Hepatic Disease

Dennis J. Chew, DVM, Dipl. ACVIM
Professor of Medicine, Department of Clinical Sciences, College of Veterinary Medicine, Ohio State University, Columbus, Ohio
Disorders of Calcium: Hypercalcemia and Hypocalcemia; Fluid Therapy During Intrinsic Renal Failure; Peritoneal Dialysis

Larry D. Cowgill, DVM, PhD, Dipl. ACVIM
Professor, Department of Medicine and Epidemiology, School of Veterinary Medicine, University of California, Davis; Director, Companion Animal Hemodialysis Unit, Veterinary Medical Teaching Hospital, Davis, California
Hemodialysis

M. Susan Crisp, DVM, Dipl. ACVIM
Internist, Small Animal Internal Medicine, Columbus, Ohio
Peritoneal Dialysis

Thomas K. Day, DVM, Dipl. ACVA, Dipl. ACVECC
Emergency and Critical Care Veterinarian, Louisville Veterinary Specialty and Emergency Services, Louisville, Kentucky
Shock Syndromes in Veterinary Medicine: Pathophysiology, Clinical Recognition, and Treatment

Helio Autran de Morais, DVM, PhD, Dipl. ACVIM
Associate Professor and Department Chair, Departamento de Clínicas Veterinárias, Universidade Estadual de Londrina; Internist/Cardiologist, Hospital Veterinário, Universidade Estadual de Londrina, Londrina, Paraná, Brazil
Appendix; Disorders of Chloride: Hyperchloremia and Hypochloremia; Disorders of Potassium: Hypokalemia and Hyperkalemia; Fluid and Diuretic Therapy in Heart Failure; Mixed Acid-Base Disorders; Respiratory Acid-Base Disorders

Stephen P. DiBartola, DVM, Dipl. ACVIM
Professor of Medicine, Department of Veterinary Clinical Sciences, College of Veterinary Medicine, Ohio State University, Columbus, Ohio
Appendix; Composition and Distribution of Body Fluids in Dogs and Cats; Disorders of Phosphorus: Hypophosphatemia and Hyperphosphatemia; Disorders of Potassium: Hypokalemia and Hyperkalemia; Disorders of Sodium and Water: Hypernatremia and Hyponatremia; Introduction to Acid-Base Disorders; Introduction to Fluid Therapy; Metabolic Acid-Base Disorders; Peritoneal Dialysis; Renal Physiology; Respiratory Acid-Base Disorders

Denise A. Elliott, BVSc, Dipl. ACVIM
Hills Fellow in Clinical Nutrition, Department of Molecular Biosciences, School of Veterinary Medicine, University of California, Davis; Companion Animal Hemodialysis Unit, Veterinary Medical Teaching Hospital, Davis, California
Hemodialysis

Amy M. Grooters, DVM, Dipl. ACVIM
Chief, Companion Animal Medicine, School of Veterinary Medicine, Louisiana State University, Baton Rouge, Louisiana
Fluid Therapy in Endocrine and Metabolic Disorders

Bernie Hansen, DVM, Dipl. ACVIM, Dipl. ACVECC
Assistant Professor, College of Veterinary Medicine, North Carolina State University, Raleigh, North Carolina
Disorders of Magnesium; Technical Aspects of Fluid Therapy: Catheters and Monitoring of Fluid Therapy

Ann E. Hohenhaus, DVM, Dipl. ACVIM
Chairman, Department of Medicine, and Head, George Jaqua Transfusion Medicine Service, The Animal Medical Center, New York, New York
Blood Transfusions and Blood Substitutes

Dez Hughes, BVSc, Dipl. ACVECC
Senior Lecturer, Section of Critical Care, School of Veterinary Medicine, University of Pennsylvania, Philadelphia, Pennsylvania
Fluid Therapy with Macromolecular Plasma Volume Expanders

Catherine W. Kohn, VMD, Dipl. ACVIM
Professor of Medicine, Department of Veterinary Clinical Sciences, College of Veterinary Medicine, Ohio State University, Columbus, Ohio
Composition and Distribution of Body Fluids in Dogs and Cats

Linda B. Lehmkuhl, DVM, Dipl. ACVIM
Cardiologist, Small Animal Internal Medicine, MedVet Associates, Inc., Columbus, Ohio
Fluid and Diuretic Therapy in Heart Failure

Larry A. Nagode, DVM, PhD
Associate Professor, Department of Veterinary Biosciences, College of Veterinary Medicine, Ohio State University, Columbus, Ohio
Disorders of Calcium: Hypercalcemia and Hypocalcemia

Peter J. Pascoe, BVSc, Dipl. ACVA
Professor of Veterinary Anesthesiology, Department of Surgical and Radiological Sciences, School of Veterinary Medicine, University of California, Davis; Anesthesiologist, Veterinary Medical Teaching Hospital, Davis, California
Perioperative Management of Fluid Therapy

Rebecca L. Remillard, PhD, DVM, Dipl. ACVN
Staff Nutritionist, Angell Memorial Animal Hospital, Boston, Massachusetts
Parenteral Nutrition

Virginia Rentko, VMD, Dipl. ACVIM
Clinical Assistant Professor, Department of Clinical Studies, School of Veterinary Medicine, Tufts University, North Grafton; Vice President, Veterinary Medicine, Biopure Corporation, Medway, Massachusetts
Blood Transfusions and Blood Substitutes

Thomas J. Rosol, DVM, PhD, Dipl. ACVP
Professor, Department of Veterinary Biosciences, College of Veterinary Medicine, Ohio State University, Columbus, Ohio
Disorders of Calcium: Hypercalcemia and Hypocalcemia

Patricia Schenck, DVM, PhD
Veterinary Nutritionist, Buckeye Nutrition, Dalton, Ohio
Disorders of Calcium: Hypercalcemia and Hypocalcemia

Eric R. Schertel, DVM, PhD, Dipl. ACVS
Staff Surgeon, MedVet Associates, Inc., Columbus, Ohio
Hypertonic Fluid Therapy

Kenneth W. Simpson, BVM&S, PhD, Dipl. ACVIM
Assistant Professor of Medicine, College of Veterinary Medicine, Cornell University, Ithaca, New York
Fluid and Electrolyte Disturbances in Gastrointestinal, Pancreatic, and Hepatic Disease

Todd A. Tobias, DVM, Dipl. ACVS
Adjunct Professor, Mississippi State University, Starkville, Mississippi; Staff Surgeon, MedVet Memphis, Cordova, Tennessee
Hypertonic Fluid Therapy

M. D. Willard, DVM, Dipl. ACVIM
Professor of Small Animal Medicine and Surgery, College of Veterinary Medicine, Texas A&M University, College Station, Texas
Disorders of Phosphorus: Hypophosphatemia and Hyperphosphatemia

Preface

The purpose of the second edition of *Fluid Therapy in Small Animal Practice* remains the same as that of the first edition, namely, "to bring together in one place information about fluid, electrolyte, and acid-base physiology and fluid therapy as they apply to small animal practice." I remain convinced that a good grounding in physiology and pathophysiology is an essential part of veterinary education and enhances the clinician's approach to the patient. Thoughtful evaluation of laboratory results provides valuable insight into the fluid, electrolyte, and acid-base status of the animal and can only improve the veterinary care provided.

I was gratified that the first edition of the book was well received by clinicians-in-training and their institutional mentors. Its value seems to have extended beyond internists to include veterinarians in clinical pathology and critical care. The in-depth approach of the first edition has been retained in the second edition. The book now is divided into five sections: applied physiology, electrolyte disorders, acid-base disorders, fluid therapy, and special therapy. The first sections of the book on fluid, electrolyte, and acid base physiology and disorders have been changed and updated. Many of the figures in these sections have been redrawn for clarity and visual appeal by Mr. Tim Vojt, artist and computer graphics specialist in our Biomedical Media section at the College of Veterinary Medicine at Ohio State University. New chapters on disorders of magnesium (Chapter 8, by Dr. Bernie Hansen) and chloride (Chapter 4, by Dr. Helio Autran de Morais) have been added. The importance of magnesium deficiency in critically ill patients has been increasingly recognized in recent years, and the crucial role of chloride in the metabolic regulation of acid-base balance was felt sufficient to warrant a separate chapter on this anion. Drs. Tom Rosol, Dennis Chew, Larry Nagode, and Pat Schenck have extensively revised and updated the chapter on calcium, and Dr. Mike Willard has condensed and updated the material on phosphorus. The section on acid-base chemistry has been condensed. Material on the nontraditional approach to acid-base chemistry has been summarized in Chapter 9, along with the traditional approach to this subject, and metabolic acidosis and metabolic alkalosis have been combined into a single chapter on metabolic acid-base disorders (Chapter 10).

Some chapters in the fluid therapy section have been completely rewritten (e.g., Chapters 15, 16, and 20). One constructive criticism about the first edition of the book was its relative lack of material on colloid therapy. This deficiency has been corrected in the second edition by the inclusion of an entire chapter on plasma expanders (Chapter 23), by Dr. Dez Hughes from the University of Pennsylvania's Critical Care program. Also new in this section is the chapter on fluid therapy in endocrine and metabolic disorders (Chapter 17), by Dr. Amy Grooters. This chapter focuses on the important electrolyte and acid-base disturbances encountered in diabetic ketoacidosis, hypoadrenocorticism, and heatstroke. Drs. John Bonagura, Linda Lehmkuhl, and Helio Autran de Morais have extensively revised and updated the chapter on fluid therapy in heart disease.

The section on special therapy contains completely rewritten chapters on blood transfusions and blood substitutes (Chapter 21) and total parenteral nutrition (Chapter 22). Material from the first edition on enteral nutrition was not included in the second edition, whereas the chapter on hemodialysis (Chapter 26) is an entirely new chapter.

The number of clinical cases has been reduced to 34 to focus on problems most relevant to acid-base and electrolyte disturbances. Almost exclusively, the cases in the appendix describe clinical patients evaluated at the Ohio State University Veterinary Teaching Hospital. The excellent work of the clinicians (residents and faculty) who managed these animals while they were hospitalized is recognized and appreciated. Some of these cases have appeared in the veterinary literature, and the appropriate citations are noted.

I encourage those who read and use this book to write to me or send an e-mail message *(dibartola.1@osu.edu)* about errors, controversial issues, and suggestions for improvement. The use of textbooks should be supplemented by reading the current veterinary and human medical literature. Such an approach allows clinicians to maintain both a historical perspective and a contemporary view of medicine. Considerable effort has been expended to ensure the accuracy of information provided here, but drug dosages always should be verified.

Acknowledgments

I am grateful to many people for help in completing the second edition of this book. The concept of a book on disturbances of fluid, electrolyte, and acid-base balance for veterinarians originated in discussions with Dr. Dennis Chew, and this book represents the evolution of material taught to second-year veterinary students at the College of Veterinary Medicine and the approach to fluid therapy used in treating small animal patients at the Ohio State University Veterinary Teaching Hospital. I am indebted to Dr. Helio Autran de Morais for encouraging me to undertake revision of the first edition and for his support throughout the process. Warm thanks and sincere appreciation go to all contributors who have shared their expertise in specific areas and provided comprehensive chapters on clinically relevant topics. Tim Vojt of our Biomedical Media Department provided original artwork for several chapters. Tim has a natural talent for taking a clinician's scribbled ideas and turning them into logical and visually pleasing line drawings. Thanks also go to my editor at W.B. Saunders, Ray Kersey, and his editorial assistant, Cass Stamato. Ray encouraged me to undertake a second edition of the book and gently prodded me when necessary. Others at W.B. Saunders who contributed to the production of the second edition are Lee Ann Draud (project editor), Denise LeMelledo (production manager), and Robert Quinn (illustration specialist). I thank all of them for their contributions. Lastly, I must once again thank my family for putting up with me as I try to juggle all aspects of my personal and professional life.

NOTICE

Veterinary Medicine is an ever-changing field. Standard safety precautions must be followed, but as new research and clinical experience broaden our knowledge, changes in treatment and drug therapy become necessary or appropriate. Readers are advised to check the product information currently provided by the manufacturer of each drug to be administered to verify the recommended dose, the method and duration of administration, and contraindications. It is the responsibility of the treating veterinarian, relying on experience and the knowledge of the animal, to determine dosages and the best treatment for the animal. Neither the publisher nor the editor assumes any responsibility for any injury and/or damage to animals or property.

THE PUBLISHER

Contents

SECTION 1
Applied Physiology

1 ▶ Composition and Distribution of Body Fluids in Dogs and Cats — 3
Catherine W. Kohn   Stephen P. DiBartola

2 ▶ Renal Physiology — 26
Stephen P. DiBartola

SECTION 2
Electrolyte Disorders

3 ▶ Disorders of Sodium and Water
HYPERNATREMIA AND HYPONATREMIA — 45
Stephen P. DiBartola

4 ▶ Disorders of Chloride
HYPERCHLOREMIA AND HYPOCHLOREMIA — 73
Helio Autran de Morais

5 ▶ Disorders of Potassium
HYPOKALEMIA AND HYPERKALEMIA — 83
Stephen P. DiBartola
Helio Autran de Morais

6 ▶ Disorders of Calcium
HYPERCALCEMIA AND HYPOCALCEMIA — 108
Thomas J. Rosol   Dennis J. Chew
Larry A. Nagode   Patricia Schenck

7 ▶ Disorders of Phosphorus
HYPOPHOSPHATEMIA AND HYPERPHOSPHATEMIA — 163
M. D. Willard   Stephen P. DiBartola

8 ▶ Disorders of Magnesium — 175
Bernie Hansen

SECTION 3
Acid-Base Disorders

9 ▶ Introduction to Acid-Base Disorders — 189
Stephen P. DiBartola

10 ▶ Metabolic Acid-Base Disorders — 211
Stephen P. DiBartola

11 ▶ Respiratory Acid-Base Disorders — 241
Helio Autran de Morais
Stephen P. DiBartola

12 ▶ Mixed Acid-Base Disorders — 251
Helio Autran de Morais

SECTION 4
Fluid Therapy

13 ▶ Introduction to Fluid Therapy — 265
Stephen P. DiBartola

14 ▶ Technical Aspects of Fluid Therapy
CATHETERS AND MONITORING OF FLUID THERAPY — 281
Bernie Hansen

15 ▶ Perioperative Management of Fluid Therapy — 307
Peter J. Pascoe

16 ▶ Fluid and Electrolyte Disturbances in Gastrointestinal, Pancreatic, and Hepatic Disease — 330
Kenneth W. Simpson   Sharon A. Center
Nichole Birnbaum

17 ▶ Fluid Therapy in Endocrine and Metabolic Disorders 375
Amy M. Grooters

18 ▶ Fluid and Diuretic Therapy in Heart Failure 387
John D. Bonagura   Linda B. Lehmkuhl
Helio Autran de Morais

19 ▶ Fluid Therapy During Intrinsic Renal Failure 410
Dennis J. Chew

20 ▶ Shock Syndromes in Veterinary Medicine
PATHOPHYSIOLOGY, CLINICAL RECOGNITION, AND TREATMENT 428
Thomas K. Day

SECTION 5
Special Therapy

21 ▶ Blood Transfusions and Blood Substitutes 451
Ann E. Hohenhaus   Virginia Rentko

22 ▶ Parenteral Nutrition 465
Rebecca L. Remillard

23 ▶ Fluid Therapy with Macromolecular Plasma Volume Expanders 483
Dez Hughes

24 ▶ Hypertonic Fluid Therapy 496
Eric R. Schertel   Todd A. Tobias

25 ▶ Peritoneal Dialysis 507
Dennis J. Chew   Stephen P. DiBartola
M. Susan Crisp

26 ▶ Hemodialysis 528
Larry D. Cowgill   Denise A. Elliott

APPENDIX

Clinical Cases 548
Stephen P. DiBartola   Helio Autran de Morais

Index 589

SECTION 1

Applied Physiology

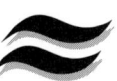

CHAPTER 1

Composition and Distribution of Body Fluids in Dogs and Cats

CATHERINE W. KOHN   STEPHEN P. DiBARTOLA

Treatment of abnormalities of water and electrolyte balance is best approached in the context of a basic understanding of the physiology of fluid balance. The purpose of this chapter is to provide an overview of the principles of body fluid homeostasis from a clinician's perspective, focusing on fluid homeostasis in adult dogs and cats. A short review of the units of measurement of solutes in body fluids is followed by a discussion of body fluid compartments. The concepts of anion gap, osmolal gap, and zero balance are also introduced.

▶ Units of Measure

The atomic weight of any element is the weight of that element relative to the weight of the ^{12}C isotope of carbon, which is defined as 12.000. The atomic weight of any element may be found in a periodic table of the elements. The atomic weights of elements are of less physiologic importance than the gram molecular (or formula) weights of the compounds they form. The molecular weight of a compound is defined as the sum of the atomic weights of all elements specified in the chemical formula of that compound. One mole (mol) of any substance is the molecular (or atomic) weight of the substance in grams. One millimole (mmol) is 10^{-3} mol, or the molecular weight of a substance expressed in milligrams (mg). Biological solutions are relatively dilute, and concentrations of charged solutes are usually expressed in millimoles per liter (mmol/L). Uncharged solutes (e.g., glucose, urea) are usually measured in mg/dL. The atomic weights of some biologically important elements and the molecular weights of important compounds in body fluids are given in Table 1–1.

Ions in biologic solutions combine according to their valence (charge) rather than according to their weights; thus, the number of cations (positively charged ions) in solution is always equal to the number of anions (negatively charged ions), and electroneutrality is maintained. Rose (1989) defines electrochemical equivalence as follows:

One equivalent is defined as the weight in grams of an element that combines with or replaces 1 gram of hydrogen ion (H^+). Since 1 g of H^+ is equal to 1 mole of H^+ (containing approximately 6.02×10^{23} particles), 1 mole of any univalent anion (charge equals 1^-) will combine with this H^+ and is equal to 1 equivalent (Eq).

For example, one atom of Ca^{2+} combines with two atoms of Cl^- to form $CaCl_2$. It is therefore useful to express

TABLE 1–1. Atomic and Molecular Weights of Physiologically Important Substances

Substance	Symbol or Formula	Atomic and Molecular Weight	Valence
Calcium ion	Ca	40.1	+2
Carbon	C	12.0	0
Chloride ion	Cl	35.5	−1
Hydrogen ion	H	1.0	+1
Magnesium ion	Mg	24.3	+2
Nitrogen	N	14.0	0
Oxygen	O	16.0	0
Phosphorus	P	31.0	0
Potassium ion	K	39.1	+1
Sodium ion	Na	23.0	+1
Sulfur	S	32.1	0
Ammonia	NH_3	17.0	0
Ammonium ion	NH_4	18.0	+1
Bicarbonate ion	HCO_3	61.0	−1
Carbon dioxide	CO_2	44.0	0
Glucose	$C_6H_{12}O_6$	180.0	0
Lactate ion	$C_3H_5O_3$	89.0	−1
Phosphate ion	PO_4	95.0	−3
	HPO_4	96.0	−2
	H_2PO_4	97.0	−1
Sulfate ion	SO_4	96.1	−2
Urea	NH_2CONH_2	60.0	0
Water	H_2O	18.0	0

Source: Adapted from Rose BD: *Clinical Physiology of Acid-Base and Electrolyte Disorders*, 3rd ed. New York, McGraw-Hill Book Co., 1989, with permission of the McGraw-Hill Companies.

concentrations of solutes in body fluids in equivalents per liter (Eq/L), thus reflecting the charge or valence of the solute. The equivalent weight of a substance is the atomic or molecular weight divided by the valence. The milliequivalent (mEq) weight is 10^{-3} the equivalent weight. The milliequivalent weight of Na^+ is equal to its atomic weight because the valence of this ion is +1. Therefore, each millimole of Na^+ provides 1 mEq. In contrast, the milliequivalent weight of Ca^{2+} is one-half its atomic weight because its valence is +2 and each millimole of Ca^{+2} provides 2 mEq. These relationships may be summarized as

Millimoles × valence = milliequivalents
Millimolecular weight/valence = milliequivalent weight

To convert concentrations:

$$mEq/L = mmol/L \times valence$$
$$mEq/L = \frac{mg/dL \times 10}{molecular\ weight} \times valence$$

Phosphate can exist in body fluids in three different ionic forms: $H_2PO_4^{1-}$, HPO_4^{2-}, and PO_4^{3-} (see Chapter 7 for more information). At the normal pH of extracellular fluid, approximately 80% of phosphate is in the HPO_4^{2-} form and 20% is in the $H_2PO_4^{1-}$ form. Therefore, the average valence of phosphate in extracellular fluid is $0.8 \times (-2) + 0.2 \times (-1) = -1.8$. At a normal plasma phosphate concentration of 4 mg/dL:

$$4\ mg/dL = \frac{4 \times 10}{31} \times 1.8 = 2.3\ mEq/L$$

Regardless of its weight, one mole of any substance contains the same number of particles (6.023×10^{23}) (Avogadro's law). Solutes exert an osmotic effect in solution that is dependent only on the number of particles in solution and not on their chemical formula, weight, or valence. One osmole (Osm) is defined as 1 gram molecular weight of any nondissociable substance; therefore, each osmole also contains 6.023×10^{23} molecules. If a compound in solution dissociates into two or three particles, the number of osmoles in solution is increased two or three times, respectively. For example, assuming that NaCl completely dissociates in solution, each millimole of NaCl provides 2 milliosmoles (mOsm): 1 mOsm of Na^+ and 1 mOsm of Cl^-. The milliosmolar concentration of a solution may be expressed as the solution's milliosmolarity or milliosmolality. *Osmolality* refers to the number of osmoles per kilogram of solvent. An aqueous solution with an osmolality of 1.0 results when 1 Osm of a solute is added to 1 kg of water. The volume of the resulting solution exceeds 1 L by the relatively small volume of the solute. On the other hand, *osmolarity* refers to the number of osmoles per liter of solution. If 1 Osm of a solute is placed in a beaker and enough water is added to make the total volume 1 L, the osmolarity of the resulting solution is 1. In biologic fluids, there is a negligible difference between osmolality and osmolarity, and the term osmolality is used in this discussion.

Serum or plasma osmolality may be measured by freezing-point depression. One osmole of a solute in 1 kg of water depresses the freezing point of the water by 1.86°C (Smithline and Gardner 1976). Average values for measured serum osmolality in the dog and cat are 300 and 310 mOsm/kg, respectively (Hardy and Osborne 1979; Chew et al. 1991).

In any fluid compartment, the osmotic effect of a solute is in part dependent on the permeability characteristics of the membranes surrounding the compartment. Consider the two fluid compartments in a rigid box in Figure 1–1. Assume that the membrane dividing the two compartments is freely permeable to urea and water but is impermeable to glucose. When urea is added to the left compartment (top panel), it moves down its concentration gradient from left to right, and water moves down its concentration gradient from right to left until there are equal concentrations of urea and water on both sides of the membrane. No fluid rises in the column attached to the left fluid compartment because urea is an *ineffective osmole* and does not generate osmotic pressure. When glucose is added to the left compartment (bottom panel), water moves down its concentration gradient from right to left but glucose cannot move across the membrane. This movement of water is called *osmosis*. The left fluid compartment cannot expand in size, and the influx of water resulting from the osmotic effect of glucose causes the solution to rise in the column. The height of fluid in the column is proportional to the osmotic pressure generated by glucose. In this example, glucose is an *effective osmole* because it generates osmotic pressure by causing

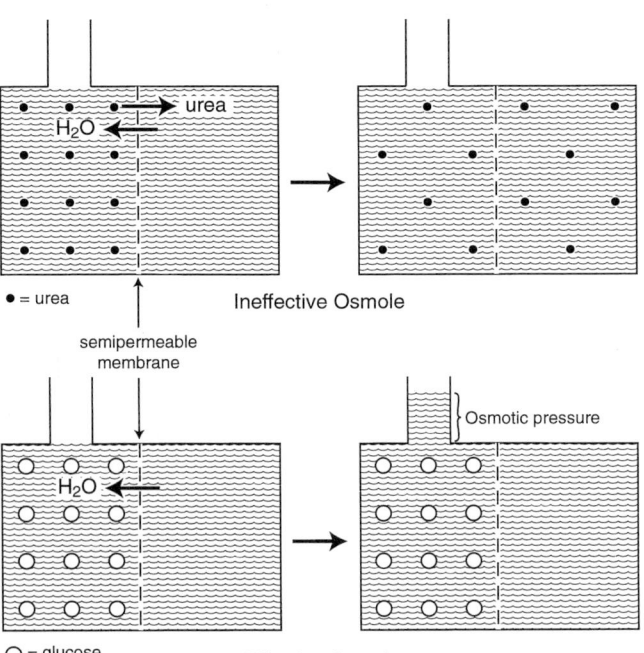

FIGURE 1–1. Effective and ineffective osmoles. *(Top)* Effect of adding a permeable solute such as urea (small closed circles) to the fluid on one side of a membrane. In this setting, equilibrium is reached by urea equilibration across the membrane rather than water movement into the urea compartment. Consequently, no osmotic pressure is generated. *(Bottom)* Effect of adding an impermeable solute such as glucose (large open circles) to the fluid on one side of a membrane. As water moves into the glucose compartment, hydraulic pressure is generated (measured by the height of the column of water above the glucose compartment), which at equilibrium equals the osmotic pressure of the solution.

a shift of water across the boundary membrane. Glucose is an effective osmole in this setting because the boundary membrane is impermeable to glucose but permeable to water.

The effective osmolality of a solution is referred to as the *tonicity* of the solution. A freezing-point depression osmometer measures all osmotically active particles in the solution. The measured osmolality of a solution thus includes both effective and ineffective osmoles. The tonicity of a solution may be less than the measured osmolality if both effective and ineffective osmoles are present. Thus, the tonicity and osmolality of a solution are not necessarily equal—a circumstance that often is true in biologic solutions.

▶ Volume Measurements for Body Fluid Spaces

Body fluids are distributed intracellularly and extracellularly. Extracellular fluid (ECF) comprises blood and interstitial fluid, the latter being outside the vascular compartment. Cerebrospinal fluid, gastrointestinal fluid, lymph, bile, glandular and respiratory secretions, and synovial fluid are in equilibrium with other extracellular fluids but are contained in specialized compartments such as the lumen of the gastrointestinal tract or the joint spaces. These fluids are not transudates of plasma but are produced by the action of specific cells and consequently are called *transcellular fluids* (Edelman et al. 1952). Water, Na^+, K^+, and Cl^- in the transcellular fluids studied (e.g., gastrointestinal fluid) are readily exchangeable with ECF (Edelman and Sweet 1956; Nadell et al. 1956). Thus, body fluid spaces are traditionally conceptualized anatomically with the capillary endothelium and cell membrane as boundaries of the vascular space and ECF compartment, respectively. Functionally, body fluid spaces are more correctly conceptualized as volumes of water and electrolytes in dynamic equilibrium because fluids and ions shift across these semipermeable boundary membranes.

The approximate sizes of the total body water (TBW), ECF, and intracellular fluid (ICF) spaces in health and disease reflect the partitioning of body fluids and solutes. Loss or gain of fluids or solutes from one of these compartments may result in alterations of the volumes of other compartments. The ability to predict relative changes in fluid compartment size is important in understanding the pathophysiology of disease processes and in formulating a fluid therapy regimen. Fluids administered parenterally initially enter the ECF. In most disease states, loss of fluids occurs initially from the ECF (for example, in diarrhea when a large volume of transcellular enteric fluid is lost or in polyuric renal failure when the urine volume is excessively large). It is therefore important to estimate the size of the ECF space.

The volume of a body fluid compartment may be assessed in two ways: by direct examination of cadavers (desiccation) or by dye or isotope dilution in an intact subject. The dilution technique is based on the principle that the volume of distribution of the indicator in the animal may be calculated if the concentration of the indicator after homogeneous mixing in the fluid space and the dose of the indicator are known:

$$V_d = \frac{\text{total dose of indicator}}{\text{concentration of indicator after mixing}}$$

where V_d represents the volume of distribution.

The ideal indicator for determining the volume of a particular fluid compartment must distribute rapidly and homogeneously within the space to be measured and must remain within that space. The indicator should not be metabolized or bound to protein or lipid, and its concentration in body fluid and elimination from the body must be easily measured. The indicator should not be toxic (Zweens et al. 1975). In dogs and cats, various indicator substances have been used to measure plasma volume (T-1824 [Evans' blue], ^{131}I, and $^{125}RISA$ [radioactive iodinated serum albumin]; Table 1-2), erythrocyte volume (^{51}Cr, ^{59}Fe, and ^{55}Fe; see Table 1-2), ECF volume (inulin, ferrocyanide, ^{23}Br, ^{22}Na, ^{24}Na, thiocyanate, thiosulfate, sucrose, $^{35}SO_4$, ^{38}Cl, ^{36}Cl, and mannitol; Table 1-3), and TBW (tritiated water, deuterium oxide, urea, and antipyrine; Table 1-4). After measurement of plasma volume (PV), erythrocyte volume, ECF, and TBW by indicator dilution, the interstitial fluid volume is derived by subtracting the calculated blood volume from the ECF volume. The ICF volume is the difference between the volumes of the TBW and ECF. The volume of the complex transcellular fluid compartment is difficult to measure in the living animal, but a limited number of estimates of transcellular fluid volumes have been made from human and canine cadavers (Harrison et al. 1936; Edelman and Leibman 1959).

In healthy animals and humans, estimates of PV, blood volume, and TBW vary slightly depending on the indicator used, but estimates of ECF volume vary dramatically with the indicator used. In adult dogs, PV estimates range from 42 to 58 mL/kg, erythrocyte volumes from 24 to 45 mL/kg, and TBW estimates from 534 to 660 mL/kg in animals that are neither very thin nor obese. Few data for cats are available. Estimates of erythrocyte volume (12–20 mL/kg), PV (37–49 mL/kg) and total blood volume (43–67 mL/kg) have been reported (see Table 1-2 for references). Jain (1986) noted that blood volume is a function of lean body mass and estimated blood volume in the cat as 62 to 66 mL/kg (6–7% of body weight) and in the dog as 77 to 78 mL/kg (8–9% of body weight).

Specific characteristics of the biologic behavior of each indicator affect its equilibration in body fluids and must be considered when describing physiologic body fluid spaces by indicator volumes of distribution. Dilution studies with T-1824 tend to overestimate PV because of trapping of plasma by packed erythrocytes and because of the varying optical densities of plasma samples collected at different times (Jain 1986). The erythrocyte volume of distribution determined by the ^{51}Cr method overestimates erythrocyte mass (and derived blood volumes) because ^{51}Cr-labeled erythrocytes may be sequestered in the spleen (Jain 1986).

Studies of fluid spaces are often performed in experimental animals that have been splenectomized, nephrectomized, or anesthetized for these experiments. Blood volume and erythrocyte mass are smaller in splenecto-

TABLE 1-2. **Estimates of Erythrocyte, Plasma, and Whole-Blood Volumes in Dogs and Cats**

Species	N	Erythrocyte Volume		Plasma Volume		Whole-Blood Volume		Reference
		Method	mL/kg	Method	mL/kg	Method	mL/kg	
Canine	17	^{51}Cr	36.1*	T-1824	48.5*	$V_P + V_{RBC}$	84.6	Hoff et al. 1966
	9			T-1824	56.2			Gregersen and Stewart 1939
	NR§	NR	38–43	NR	42–58	NR	83–101	Altman and Dittmer, 1974
	NR	^{51}Cr	34.1	T-1824	52.8			Baker and Remington 1960
	10	^{51}Cr	26.4*‡	T-1824	48.3*‡			Baker 1963
				^{131}I	41.6*‡			Baker 1963
	NR	^{51}Cr		T-1824			81	Clark and Woodley 1959
	NR	^{51}Cr	43	^{131}I	51.4		94.4	Parkinson and Dougherty 1958
	100	^{51}Cr	33.5*	T-1824	50.2*			Deavers et al. 1960
	NR			T-1824	54		79	Courtice 1943
	NR			NR	52.7 (35.0–70.4)			Spector, 1956
	5			T-1824	44*†			Swan and Pitts 1955
	4	^{51}Cr	31.4	^{125}RISA‖	52.4*			Bauer et al. 1975
	40	^{55}Fe, ^{59}Fe	38.8	T-1824	53.8			Gibson et al. 1946
	8	^{32}P	41	T-1824	51		92.0	Reeve 1953
	5	^{32}P	34.8*	T-1824	52.2*		87.0	Reeve 1953
	16	^{32}P	30.9‡	T-1824	46.9‡		77.8	Reeve 1953
	153	^{59}Fe	44.6 ± 7.7		58.0 ± 7.0		102.6 ± 12.0	Woodward 1968
	30	^{51}Cr	42.0 ± 6.7		56.7 ± 8.2		98.7 ± 12.0	Woodward 1968
	10		41.3 ± 4.5	^{131}I	43.4 ± 4.4		84.9 ± 8.1	Dellenback 1969
	25	^{51}Cr	24.0 ± 5.0*	^{131}I	51.0 ± 5.0*		75.0 ± 6.0	Lombardi 1972
	39		39.4 ± 5.8	^{131}I	52.1 ± 6.6		98.1 ± 8.9	Sabourin 1975
	NR	^{59}Fe	45.0 ± 2.0	T-1824	49.0 ± 4.0		94.0 ± 3.0	Lee 1976
	5			^{131}I	55.1 ± 4.1			Hood and Hightower 1976
Feline	7	^{51}Cr	17.0				56.3	Breznock and Strack 1982a
	10	^{51}Cr	12.2‡				43.4§	Breznock and Strack 1982a
	7			T-1824	37.4		67.1	DaSilva 1955
	10	^{51}Cr	19.9		46.8		66.7 ± 3.5	Spink 1966
	2	^{51}Cr	19.0		48.8		67.2	Reed 1970

Source: Partially adapted from Jain NC (ed): *Schalm's Veterinary Hematology*, 4th ed. Philadelphia, Lea & Febiger, pp. 87–102, 1986.
* Anesthetized.
† Nephrectomized.
‡ Splenectomized.
§ NR: not reported.
‖ ^{125}RISA, Radioiodinated serum albumin.
± SD, Standard deviation.

mized dogs and cats than in those with intact spleens (Breznock and Strack 1982a; Jain 1986). In both species, the spleen may act as a reservoir for erythrocytes, which may be released when splenic contraction is stimulated (e.g., during stress). Cats may sequester 20% of their red cell mass in the spleen (Breznock and Strack 1982b). The splanchnic vascular beds may also act as a reservoir for erythrocytes and, when contracted, may increase circulating blood volume by 20 to 30% (Jain 1986). Many studies of body fluid spaces have been performed in anesthetized animals. Pentobarbital anesthesia had no effect on deuterium oxide estimates of TBW in dogs (Zweens et al. 1980) but resulted in substantially decreased estimates of ECF volume as determined by ferrocyanide (9% reduction) and inulin (14% reduction) dilution (Zweens et al. 1978). It had no effect, however, on the thiocyanate volume of distribution. Fluid volume data from experiments using anesthetized dogs and cats thus provide only approximations of fluid compartment sizes in healthy awake animals.

Total body water volume is often defined as 60% of body weight, but there is considerable individual variation in this value. In humans, TBW declines with age and is lower in women than in men (Edelman and Leibman 1959). Total body water decreases during the first year of life in children because of a decrease in plasma and interstitial fluid volume (Edelman and Leibman 1959). The percentage of body water in puppies and kittens exclusive of fat has been measured and shown to decrease over the first 6 months of life (Moulton 1923). The decline in TBW over time in humans and the lower TBW in women than in men are most likely explained by differences in body composition (i.e., fat is lower in water content than is lean tissue) (Edelman and Leibman 1959). Thus, TBW constitutes about 60% of body weight in adult mammals that are not obese.

The fact that fat has a low water content suggests that fluid needs for patients should be estimated on the basis of lean body mass in order to avoid overhydration, especially in patients with cardiac or renal insufficiency or in those with hypoproteinemia. The following formulas are proposed for estimating lean body mass on the basis of the assumptions that (1) approximately 20% of body weight is due to fat in normal small animal patients, (2) morbid obesity represents an increase in body fat to at

TABLE 1-3. Estimates of Extracellular Fluid Volume in Dogs and Cats

Species	N	Method	ECF (mL/kg)	Reference
Feline		Thiocyanate	288	Spector 1956
Canine	9	Inulin	189	Gaudino and Levitt 1949
	6	Inulin	186	Soberman et al. 1951
	10	Inulin	216	Gaudino et al. 1948
	NR§	Inulin	198 (145–251)*	Spector 1956
	5	Inulin	167	Swan et al. 1954
	10	Inulin	204	Becker and Joseph 1955
	4	Inulin	172	Raisz et al. 1953
	6	Inulin†	230	Bowsher et al. 1984
	6	Ferrocyanide*†	224	Zweens et al. 1975
	14	Ferrocyanide†	237	Zweens et al. 1975
	4	^{36}Cl*†	273	Swan et al. 1954
	7	^{36}Cl‡	149	Hankes et al. 1973
	5	^{36}Cl†	346 (324–380)	Burch et al. 1950
	5	^{22}Na, ^{24}Na	305	Guadino et al. 1948
	NR	^{24}Na	299 (240–360)	Spector 1956
	3	^{23}Br	308	Guadino et al. 1948
	4	$^{35}SO_4$†	197	Bauer et al. 1975
	4	$^{35}SO_4$†	215	Bauer et al. 1975
	8	$^{35}SO_4$†‡	255	Vineyard and Osborne 1967
	5	$^{35}SO_4$*†	237	Swan and Pitts 1955
	12	$^{35}SO_4$*†	225	Swan et al. 1954
	16	$^{35}SO_4$	201	Walser et al. 1953
	9	Thiocyanate	307	Gregersen and Stewart 1939
	8	Thiocyanate	313	Guadino et al. 1948
	NR	Thiocyanate	320 (239–408)	Spector 1956
	9	Thiosulfate*†	224	Swan et al. 1954
	10	Thiosulfate	246	Becker and Joseph 1955
	7	Thiosulfate	244	Cardozo and Edelman 1952
	NR	Mannitol	216 (166–214)	Spector 1956
	13	Mannitol*†	226 (187–272)	Swan et al. 1954

* Nephrectomized.
† Anesthetized.
‡ Splenectomized.
§ NR, Not reported.

least 30% of body weight, and (3) body weight is a reasonable estimate of lean body mass in thin patients:

Obese   Body weight × 0.7 = lean body mass
Normal   Body weight × 0.8 = lean body mass
Thin   Body weight × 1.0 = lean body mass

An estimate of ECF volume expressed as a percentage of body weight is useful for clinical assessment of fluid shifts that occur during dehydration, for assessment of changes in hydration status, and as a basis for prescribing and monitoring fluid therapy. Unfortunately, data from dye dilution studies of ECF volume are difficult to interpret. Extracellular fluid volumes reported for adult, healthy dogs and cats vary between 15 and 30% of body weight, and many clinicians use 20% of body weight to estimate ECF volume. This wide range in estimates of ECF volume results from the variety of indicators used to measure this fluid space. Some indicators probably have a volume of distribution larger than the ECF volume. Relatively small, charged indicators (^{23}Br, $^{35}SO_4$) may penetrate cells. Radiosulfate ($^{35}SO_4$) enters erythrocytes freely and is found in bile, indicating that this ion penetrates some cells (Murphy et al. 1963). Seventeen percent of the body sulfate (with which $^{35}SO_4$ equilibrates) is not in the extracellular space (Barratt and Walser 1969). In addition, $^{35}SO_4$ is incorporated into albumin by the liver (Schloerb et al. 1967) and possibly into other organic compounds in the body (Hankes et al. 1973). Therefore, the volume of distribution of $^{35}SO_4$ is larger than the ECF volume. Thiocyanate and thiosulfate penetrate cells rapidly (Cardozo and Edelman 1952; Walser et al. 1953). Thiocyanate may also bind to plasma proteins (Lavietes et al. 1936). Thiocyanate and thiosulfate thus also overestimate the ECF volume.

Inulin and ferrocyanide do not penetrate intracellular water (Edelman and Leibman 1959; deGraaf et al. 1986). Inulin is a large, uncharged, biologically inert molecule unsuited for penetration of cell membranes. Neither inulin nor ferrocyanide penetrates transcellular fluids (Edelman and Leibman 1959; Zweens et al. 1975), which are an important component of ECF, especially in disease. Transcellular fluid losses in diarrhea, for example, may be life threatening. Inulin does not penetrate (or equilibrates very slowly with) 75% of the water in bone and dense connective tissue (Edelman and Leibman 1959). The ability of ferrocyanide to enter water in bone and dense connective tissue has not been reported. Both inulin and ferrocyanide dilution studies underestimate ECF volume.

TABLE 1-4. **Estimates of Total Body Water in Dogs and Cats**

Species	N	Method	Total Body Water (mL/kg)	Reference
Feline	1	Deuterium oxide	615†	Edelman 1952; Altman and Dittmer 1974
	1	Desiccation	580	Voit 1866
	3	Desiccation	677 (642–724)	Moulton 1923; Skelton 1927; Hatai 1917; Aron 1915
	8*	Sodium chloride	500 (420–560)	Eggleton 1951
	11	Urea	630 (565–715)	Eggleton 1951
	NR§	NR§	580	Spector 1956
	10	Tritiated water	580–600	Seefeldt and Chapman 1979
Canine				
Adult	8*	Antipyrine	599 (539–679)	Herrold and Sapirstein 1952
	40	Deuterium oxide	589 (350–900)†‡	Edelman 1952; Fogelman et al. 1952; Schwartz 1952; Guadino and Levitt 1949
	33	Deuterium oxide	619 (525–713)	Guadino and Levitt 1949
	16	Deuterium oxide	626 ± 28	Zweens et al. 1980
	6	Desiccation	628 (550–662)	Engels 1904; Harrison et al. 1936; Painter 1940
Lean	7	Antipyrine	734 (639–795)	Herrold and Sapirstein 1952; Soberman 1950
	4	Desiccation	700 (619–756)	Pfeiffer 1887; Weigert 1905
Obese	14	Desiccation	596 (503–690)	Painter 1940; Pfeiffer 1887; Weigert 1905
	7	Tritiated water	534†	Bauer et al. 1975
	7	Tritiated water	567†	Bauer et al. 1975
	5	Tritiated water	660	Richmond et al. 1962

* Numbers of observations.
† Anesthetized.
‡ Splenectomized.
§ NR, Not reported.

The mean inulin volume of distribution in data from four studies (involving at least 35 dogs) was 190 mL/kg or 19.0% of body weight (Guadino and Levitt 1948; Raisz et al. 1953; Swan et al. 1954; Becker and Joseph 1955; Spector 1956). The average ferrocyanide volume of distribution from data reported in two studies (20 dogs) was 230 mL/kg or 23% of body weight (Zweens et al. 1975).

Of the physiologic compounds available for use in dilution studies, ^{24}Na and ^{36}Cl probably have volumes of distribution that most closely approximate the physiologic ECF volume. In humans, 35 to 40% of body Na$^+$ is contained in bone and about 30% of bone Na$^+$ is nonexchangeable (Edelman and Leibman 1959). Total bone Na$^+$ in dogs has been estimated as 40 to 50 mEq/kg of body weight, and 55% of canine bone Na$^+$ is nonexchangeable (Edelman et al. 1954; Edelman and Leibman 1959). Therefore, in dogs, 45% of bone Na$^+$ (18–22 mEq/kg) is readily exchangeable with the ECF. This exchangeable Na$^+$ may be free in bone ECF or adsorbed to the surface of bone crystals, whereas nonexchangeable bone Na$^+$ is trapped within the crystalline portion of bone (Edelman and Leibman 1959). Sodium 24 equilibrates in the exchangeable Na$^+$ space within 24 h in humans (Edelman and Leibman 1959). Because of the large amount of exchangeable Na$^+$ in bone, the ^{24}Na volume of distribution overestimates the ECF volume. The mean ^{24}Na volume of distribution in five dogs in one study was 299 mL/kg or about 30% of body weight.

Approximately 12% of total body Cl$^-$ in humans is intracellular (erythrocytes, testis, and gastric mucosa) (Edelman and Leibman 1959). Concentrations of Cl$^-$ in some extracellular tissues, such as tendons, may be greater than the concentration of Cl$^-$ in plasma (Nichols et al. 1953; Edelman and Leibman 1959). Chloride may bind to albumin and possibly to other extracellular proteins in connective tissue (Edelman and Leibman 1959). Therefore, ^{36}Cl dilution studies also overestimate the ECF volume. The average ^{36}Cl volume of distribution in two studies (nine dogs) was 310 mL/kg of body weight or 31% of body weight (Burch et al. 1950; Swan et al. 1954).

It is unlikely that the ECF volume can be accurately estimated with any one indicator dye or radioisotope, because the space itself is heterogeneous (Edelman and Leibman 1959). Edelman and Leibman (1959) defined four subcompartments of the ECF: plasma; interstitial lymph; dense connective tissue, cartilage, and bone; and transcellular compartments. Although estimates of the size of the interstitial-lymph compartment in dogs and cats have not been reported, estimates for PV and TBW are available. On the basis of these values and values for ECF compartment sizes from studies in humans, estimates of the percentage of body weight for fluid in each subcompartment of the ECF can be derived (Fig. 1–2). Extracellular water contained in the PV, interstitial-lymph fluid, transcellular fluid, and 25% of the bone water compartments constitutes approximately 18% of body weight—a value close to the figure of 20% favored by many clinicians as an estimate of ECF volume. However, if the rest of the water contained in bone and dense connective tissue (about 9% of body weight) is included in the ECF, the ECF volume is approximately 27% of body weight.

Water lost during dehydration or fluid gained during therapy may equilibrate more slowly with some subcompartments of the ECF, such as bone and dense connective tissue water. Studies with deuterium oxide (D$_2$O) in dogs

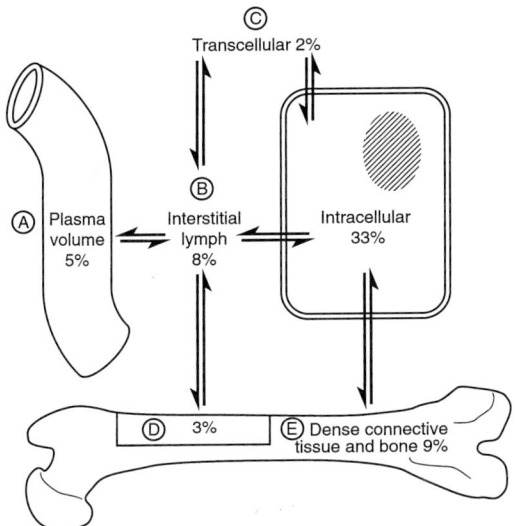

FIGURE 1–2. Compartments of total body water expressed as percentage of body weight. A + B + C + D = 18% body weight = rapidly equilibrating (inulin); A + B + C + D + E = 27% body weight = total extracellular fluid volume.

and in one cat indicated that D_2O equilibrates throughout plasma and interstitial lymph fluid in less than 1 min (Edelman 1952). Deuterium oxide distribution equilibrium is reached in 2 to 4 h and includes equilibration with bone water in the dog (Edelman et al. 1954). The volume and rate of distribution of dilute D_2O solutions used in these studies reflect the volume and rate of distribution of water itself with reasonable accuracy (Edelman 1952). The rate-limiting step in D_2O distribution appears to be transfer across cell membranes. The model assumes that water distribution is diffusion limited. Erythrocytes, cerebral cortex, and visceral tissue cells exchange water with ECF more rapidly than do cells of supporting structures (e.g., skeletal muscle, skin, connective tissue, and bone) (Edelman 1952). Nevertheless, "no regions of nonexchangeable water are known to exist" (Edelman and Leibman 1959) and, on the basis of D_2O studies, water equilibration in the entire ECF should be rapid (about 4 h). From a physiologic perspective and for the purpose of determining the fluid needs of adult small animal patients, ECF should therefore be estimated as about 27% of lean body weight.

▶ Distribution of Body Solutes

Total body content of solutes may be measured by cadaver analysis (desiccation) or by dilution studies utilizing the same principle previously described for estimating the volumes of body fluid spaces. Every solute has a space or apparent volume of distribution. Dilution studies of body solute content yield variable results depending on the volume of distribution of the particular tracer used to estimate the solute space. There are limited data in the literature from cadaver and isotope dilution studies of body solute content in small animals, and most of the following discussion is based on data from studies in humans (Edelman and Leibman 1959; Rose 1984).

Body solutes are not distributed homogeneously throughout TBW. Vascular endothelium and cell membranes have different permeabilities for different solutes. Healthy vascular endothelium is relatively impermeable to the cellular components of blood and to plasma proteins. Consequently, the volume of distribution of cells and proteins is the plasma space itself. The vascular endothelium, however, is freely permeable to ionic solutes, and the concentration of these ions is almost the same in interstitial as in plasma fluid. Concentrations of solutes in plasma and in interstitial and intracellular fluids are listed in Table 1–5, and the compositions of ECF and ICF are compared in Figure 1–3. The slightly increased concentration of anions and decreased concentration of cations in interstitial fluid as compared with plasma occur primarily because of the presence of negatively charged plasma proteins in plasma. The equilibrium concentrations of permeable anions and cations across the vascular endothelium are determined by the Gibbs-Donnan equilibrium. In clinical practice, the difference in concentrations of anions and cations across the vascular endothelium is negligible and the effects of the Gibbs-Donnan equilibrium are usually ignored. Thus, in clinical practice, the plasma concentrations of solutes are considered to reflect solute concentrations throughout the ECF. Average values for ECF concentrations of important solutes in dogs and cats are given in Table 1–6. Normal values may vary among laboratories.

Table 1–5 shows that the solute compositions of ICF and ECF are quite different, but the total numbers of cations and anions in all body fluids are equal. Electroneutrality must be maintained at all times. The most abundant positively charged ion in the ECF is Na^+. Most of the body Na^+ is in the extracellular space. Approximately 70% of body Na^+ in humans is exchangeable, and

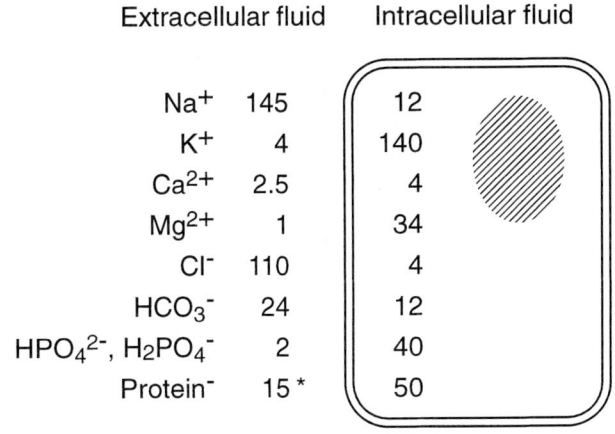

mEq/L

*0 in interstitial fluid, 15 in plasma

FIGURE 1–3. Average values for electrolyte concentrations in extracellular and intracellular fluid. Note marked concentration differences for many electrolytes.

TABLE 1-5. Approximate Ionic Composition of the Body Water Compartments

Ion	Plasma (mEq/L)	Plasma Water* (mEq/L)	Interstitial Fluid† (mEq/L)	Skeletal Muscle Cell (mEq/L)
Cations				
Na^+	142	152.7	145.1	12.0
K^+	4.3	4.6	4.4	140
Ca^{2+} (ionized)	2.5	2.7	2.4	4.0
Mg^{2+} (ionized)	1.1	1.2	1.1	34
Total	149.9	161.2	153	190
Anions				
Cl^-	104	111.9	117.4	4
HCO_3^-	24	25.8	27.1	12
$HPO_4^{2-}, H_2PO_4^{1-}$	2	2.2	2.3	40
Proteins	14	15	0	50
Other	5.9	6.3	6.2	84‡
Total	149.9	161.2	153	190

Source: Adapted from Woodbury DM. In Ruch TC and Patton HD (eds): *Physiology and Biophysics*, 20th ed. Philadelphia, WB Saunders, 1974; from Rose BD: *Clinical Physiology of Acid-Base and Electrolytes*, 3rd ed. New York, McGraw-Hill Book Co., 1989, with permission of the McGraw-Hill Companies.
* Plasma water content is assumed to be 93% of plasma volume.
† Gibbs-Donnan factors used as multipliers are 0.95 for univalent cations, 0.90 for divalent cations, 1.05 for univalent anions, and 1.10 for divalent anions.
‡ This largely represents organic phosphates such as ATP.

30% is bound to bone (Rose 1984). The percentage of exchangeable sodium is important because only exchangeable solutes are osmotically active. Cell membranes are permeable to Na^+, which tends to diffuse into cells. In health, however, the cell membrane Na^+,K^+-adenosinetriphosphatase (Na^+,K^+-ATPase) actively removes Na^+ from cells, thus maintaining a steep extracellular-to-intracellular concentration gradient for Na^+. The most abundant anions in ECF are Cl^- and HCO_3^-. The volume of distribution of Cl^- is primarily the ECF volume. Bicarbonate is present in all body fluids and can be generated from CO_2 and H_2O in the presence of carbonic anhydrase. The ECF contains a small but physiologically significant concentration of K^+. For example, alterations in ECF K^+ concentrations may result in muscle weakness (hypokalemia) or cardiotoxicity (hyperkalemia).

In contrast, the primary cations in ICF are K^+ and Mg^{2+}. Most of the body K^+ is stored in the ICF, where K^+ is the most abundant cation. Cell membranes are permeable to K^+. The K^+ concentration gradient between intracellular and extracellular fluid is maintained by cell membrane Na^+,K^+-ATPase, which moves K^+ into cells against a concentration gradient. The ratio of intracellular to extracellular K^+ concentration is important in generating and maintaining the cell membrane potential at approximately -70 mV (see Appendix). Almost 100% of body K^+ in humans is exchangeable (Rose 1984). Unfortunately, a reliable, practical method for measuring the intracellular K^+ concentration is not available, and changes in serum K^+ concentration may not reflect changes in total body K^+ stores (see Chapter 5). The predominant anions in the ICF are organic phosphates and proteins.

Intracellular water is often assumed to be a homogeneous pool. In reality, however, concentrations of solutes vary in different subcellular compartments as well as in different cell types. From a clinical perspective, these differences are usually ignored. It is important to remember, however, that the heterogeneity of the solute distribution in ICF or ECF may play an important role in some disease processes.

Transcellular fluid composition varies according to the cells that form the fluid and is not considered further here. Transcellular fluids are usually not simply transudates of plasma. Concentrations of solutes in specific transcellular fluids will be mentioned when specific alterations in fluid balance involving transcellular fluids, such as enteric fluids (e.g., in diarrhea), are reviewed in later chapters.

TABLE 1-6. Average Plasma Concentrations of Electrolytes in Dogs and Cats

Substance	Units	Dog	Cat
Sodium	mEq/L	145	155
Potassium	mEq/L	4	4
Ionized calcium	mg/dL	5.4	5.1
Total calcium	mg/dL	10	9
Total magnesium	mg/dL	3	2.5
Chloride	mEq/L	110	120
Bicarbonate	mEq/L	21	20
Phosphate	mg/dL	4	4
Proteins	g/dL	7	7
Lactate	mg/dL	15	15

▶ Exchange of Water Between Intracellular and Extracellular Fluid Spaces

The volume of the intracellular and extracellular fluid compartments is determined by the number of osmotically active particles in each space. Sodium is the most abundant cation in the ECF. Consequently, Na^+ and its associated anions account for most of the osmotically active particles in the ECF. The other osmotically active compounds that make a significant contribution to ECF osmolality are glucose and urea. The ECF osmolality may be estimated from the following formula (Rose 1984):

ECF osmolality (mOsm/kg) =
$$2(Na^+ + K^+) + \frac{glucose}{18} + \frac{BUN}{2.8}$$

where BUN is blood urea nitrogen.

Several other formulas have been suggested (Green 1978) for estimation of serum osmolality:

$$2.1 \times Na^+$$

$$2(Na^+ + K^+)$$

$$1.86 \times Na^+ + \frac{glucose}{18} + \frac{BUN}{2.8}$$

$$1.86(Na^+ + K^+) + \frac{glucose}{18} + \frac{BUN}{2.8}$$

$$1.86(Na^+ + K^+) + \frac{glucose}{18} + \frac{BUN}{2.8} + 9$$

$$2 \times Na^+ + \frac{glucose}{18} + \frac{BUN}{2.8}$$

Cell membranes are permeable to urea and K^+; therefore, these solutes are ineffective osmoles. Effective osmolality is calculated as (Rose 1984)

$$\text{Effective ECF osmolality} = 2 \times Na^+ + \frac{glucose}{18}$$

In healthy dogs and cats, the contribution of glucose to the effective osmolality of the ECF is small (about 4–6 mOsm/kg) based on blood glucose concentrations of 70 to 110 mg/dL. Therefore, $2 \times [Na^+]$ is a good approximation of the ECF effective osmolality.

All body fluid spaces are isotonic with one another. Thus, the effective osmolality of the ICF may also be estimated by doubling the ECF Na^+ concentration, $[Na^+]$, even though the Na^+ concentration in ICF is small. All body fluid spaces are isotonic, and the tonicity of the TBW may also be approximated by doubling the plasma $[Na^+]$. The tonicity of TBW may also be expressed as the ratio of the sum of all exchangeable cations and all exchangeable anions to the volume of TBW. The total number of milliosmoles of exchangeable cations and anions may be estimated from the expression

$$2[Na^+]_e + 2[K^+]_e$$

Therefore:

$$2 \times \text{plasma} [Na^+] \approx \frac{2[Na^+]_e + 2[K^+]_e}{TBW}$$

and

$$\text{Plasma} [Na^+] \approx \frac{[Na^+]_e + [K^+]_e}{TBW}$$

This relationship is represented graphically in Figure 1–4 (Edelman et al. 1958; Rose 1989). Examination of Figure 1–4 shows that when the total exchangeable Na^+ increases, the plasma sodium concentration also increases (Rose 1989), and these changes are usually associated with body fluid hypertonicity. A decrease in total ex-

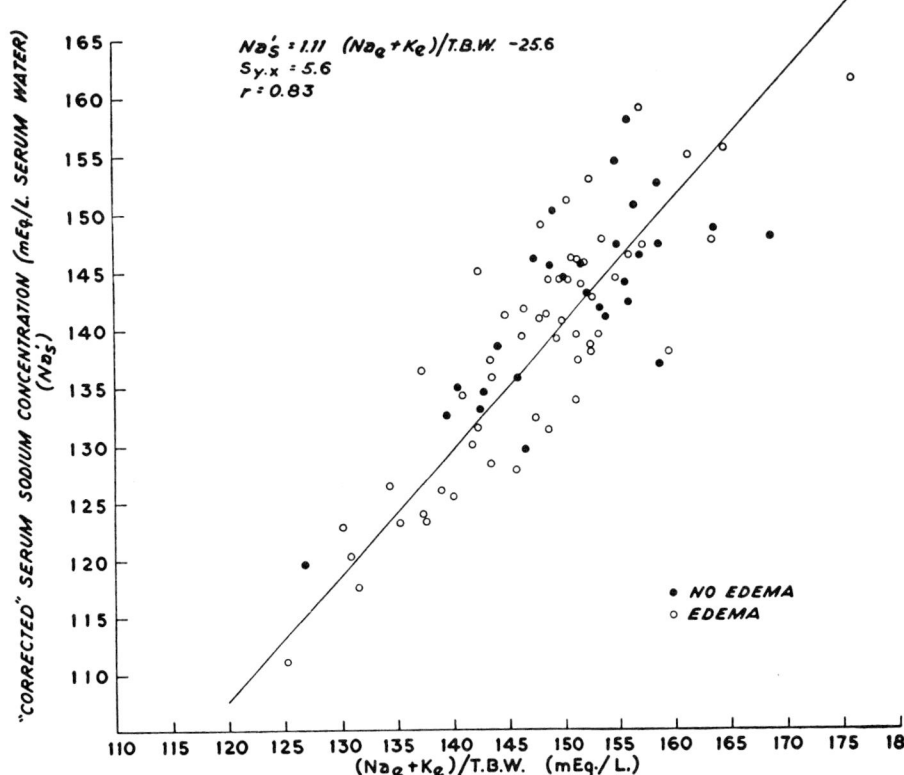

FIGURE 1–4. Relationship of plasma $[Na^+]$ to $([Na^+]_e + [K^+]_e)/TBW$ ($[Na^+]_e$ = total exchangeable Na^+; $[K^+]_e$ = total exchangeable K^+; TBW = total body water). (From Edelman IS, Leibman J, O'Meara MP, et al.: Interrelations between serum sodium concentration, serum osmolarity and total exchangeable sodium, total exchangeable potassium, and total body water. *J Clin Invest* 37:1236–1256, 1958.)

changeable Na^+ or K^+ is associated with hyponatremia, a decrease in plasma osmolality, and hypotonicity. The effect of a decrease in total exchangeable K^+ on the plasma $[Na^+]$ is not intuitively obvious but is clinically important. Rose (1989) explained that a decrease in serum $[K^+]$ results in a shift of K^+ out of cells. To maintain electroneutrality, Na^+ shifts into cells, thus causing hyponatremia.

Plasma (and therefore ECF) osmolality in dogs is approximately 300 mOsm/kg, and fluids with effective osmolalities greater than 300 mOsm/kg are hypertonic to plasma, whereas those with effective osmolalities less than 300 mOsm/kg are hypotonic to plasma. Those with effective osmolalities of 300 mOsm/kg are isotonic to plasma. In health, addition or loss of fluid or solute to or from the body results in alterations in body fluid space volumes and tonicity. These alterations elicit homeostatic shifts of fluid between compartments so that fluid spaces return to isotonicity (see Chapter 3).

In most disease states, fluid and solutes are initially lost from the ECF. Three basic types of fluid and solute loss may occur: solute in excess of water, isotonic loss, or water in excess of solute (Table 1–7) (Leaf 1962). Solute and water losses may theoretically occur in any proportion along the continuum between solute loss with no water loss (e.g., peritoneal dialysis with a salt-poor solution) and water loss with no solute loss (e.g., water deprivation). During water deprivation, the tonicity of ECF increases relative to that of ICF. Water shifts out of cells and into ECF until the osmolalities of the two compartments are equal, and the osmolalities in both are greater than during the state of normal hydration. This water shift augments the ECF volume, thus helping to preserve the effective circulating blood volume and protecting against the development of shock. When solute is lost in the absence of water loss, the osmolality of the ECF decreases relative to that of the ICF. Water passes through the cell membrane, thus diluting ICF solute until the effective osmolalities of ECF and ICF are again equal. The osmolalities of both ICF and ECF decrease. This homeostatic fluid shift decreases ECF volume. When hypertonic fluid is lost from the ECF and volume depletion occurs, homeostatic water shifts further compromise the ECF volume and effective circulating blood volume, thus compounding fluid losses. Loss or gain of isotonic fluid from the ECF results in no change in ECF osmolality, and no osmotically mediated water shifts between the ICF and ECF occur. Loss of isotonic fluid results in a decrease in ECF volume, whereas gain of isotonic fluid increases the ECF volume. Isotonic fluid loss, if of sufficient magnitude, results in hypovolemia and shock. Clinical signs of salt depletion are compared with those in water deprivation in Table 1–8. These concepts are discussed further in Chapter 3.

Although homeostatic fluid shifts in response to loss of salt or water from the ECF affect ECF and effective circulating blood volumes similarly, expansion of the ECF volume may be the consequence of expansion of the interstitial fluid at a time when PV and effective circulating blood volume are decreased. For example, edema in hypoproteinemic states increases ECF volume, but effective circulating blood volume is decreased. Thus, the effective circulating blood volume and interstitial volume may be altered differently by disease.

▶ Exchange of Water Between Plasma and Interstitial Spaces

The partitioning of fluid between plasma and interstitial fluid spaces is critically important for maintenance of the effective circulating blood volume. The effective blood volume has been defined as "the component of blood volume to which the volume-regulatory system responds by causing renal sodium and water retention in the setting of cardiac and hepatic failure even though measured total blood and plasma volume may be increased" (Peters 1948; Schrier 1988). Approximately 18% of the ECF (5%/27%) (see Fig. 1–2) is contained in the PV. Exchange of solutes and fluid between plasma and interstitial spaces occurs at the capillary level. The volume of the vascular space is controlled by a balance between forces that favor filtration of fluid through the vascular endothelium (capillary hydrostatic pressure and tissue oncotic pressure) and forces that tend to retain fluid within the vascular space (plasma oncotic pressure and tissue hydrostatic pressure). *Oncotic pressure* is the osmotic pressure generated by plasma proteins in the vascular space. These relationships are described by Starling's law (Fig. 1–5):

$$\text{Net filtration} = K_f [(P_{cap} - P_{if}) - (\pi_p - \pi_{if})]$$

TABLE 1–8. **Clinical Signs of Water versus Salt Depletion**

Clinical Features	Salt Depletion	Water Lack
Physical findings		
Thirst	Normal	Increased
Skin turgor	Decreased	Normal
Pulse	Rapid	Normal
Blood pressure	Low	Normal
Laboratory findings		
Urine volume	Normal	Decreased
Urine concentration	Normal	Increased
Serum proteins	Increased	Normal
Hemoglobin and hematocrit	Increased	Normal
Blood urea nitrogen	Increased	High normal
Serum sodium and chloride	Decreased	Increased
Treatment	Salt	Water

TABLE 1–7. **Effect of Water and Solute Losses from Body Fluids**

Loss	ECF	Theoretical Replacement Fluid
Hypotonic	Hypertonic	Hypotonic
Isotonic	Isotonic	Isotonic
Hypertonic	Hypotonic	Isotonic/hypertonic

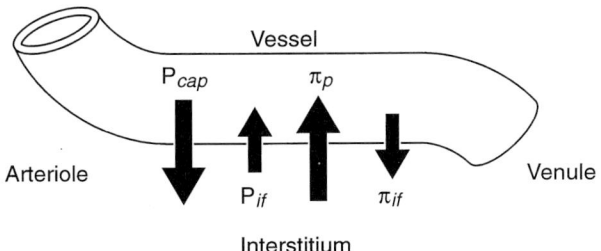

FIGURE 1-5. Factors affecting fluid movement at the level of the capillary. P_{cap} = capillary hydrostatic pressure; P_{if} = interstitial hydrostatic pressure, π_p = capillary oncotic pressure, π_{if} = interstitial oncotic pressure.

where K_f represents the net permeability of the capillary wall, P represents the hydrostatic pressure generated by the heart (P_{cap}) or tissues (P_{if}), and π represents the oncotic pressure generated by plasma proteins (π_p) or filtered proteins and mucopolysaccharides in the interstitium (π_{if}).

The net filtration pressure in healthy capillaries is about 0.3 to 0.5 mm Hg at the proximal (arteriolar) end of the capillary (Rose 1984). Near the venule, the forces favoring filtration are less than the forces favoring reabsorption of fluid into the vascular space because capillary hydrostatic pressure decreases along the length of the capillary but capillary oncotic pressure remains the same (Rose 1984). Some of the fluid that is filtered into the interstitium at the proximal end of the capillary is reabsorbed distally; the remainder of the filtered fluid is transported by lymphatics in the interstitium. The hydrostatic pressure transferred from arterioles to the capillaries is controlled by autoregulation of the precapillary sphincter. Autoregulation protects the capillary from increases in hydrostatic pressure caused by systemic hypertension, which might cause a dangerous loss of vascular fluid into the interstitial fluid by filtration.

During water depletion, capillary oncotic pressure increases and hydrostatic pressure may decrease if depletion is severe enough to cause hypovolemia. These alterations in Starling's forces favor a decrease in net filtration of fluid into the interstitium at the level of the capillary. Increased reabsorption of interstitial fluid augments effective circulating blood volume, thus decreasing plasma protein concentration and increasing hydrostatic pressure. Conversely, loss of plasma protein decreases plasma oncotic pressure and increases the net force favoring filtration of fluid out of the capillary. Loss of intravascular fluid increases plasma oncotic pressure, but filtration of fluid into the interstitium produces the edema observed in hypoproteinemic states. Thus, in the healthy animal, maintenance of PV depends on a fine balance between the forces favoring filtration and those favoring reabsorption in the capillary.

▶ Electroneutrality and the Anion Gap

In body fluids, the sum of all cations must equal the sum of all anions to fulfill the law of electroneutrality. In the clinical setting, however, all anions and cations in body fluids are usually not measured. Figure 1-6 compares the concentrations of the commonly measured anions and the commonly measured cations in a gamblegram. The commonly measured cations are Na^+ and K^+ and the commonly measured anions are Cl^- and HCO_3^-. The sum of the concentrations of commonly measured anions is less than the sum of the concentrations of commonly measured cations; therefore, there are more unmeasured anions than cations. From this observation, the concept of the anion gap was developed. It is important to remember that there is no real difference between the total number of anions and the total number of cations in the body.

The anion gap is defined as the difference between the unmeasured anions (UA) and the unmeasured cations (UC). According to the law of electroneutrality,

$$Na^+ + K^+ + UC = Cl^- + HCO_3^- + UA$$

Rearranging this equation,

$$(Na^+ + K^+) - (Cl^- + HCO_3^-) = UA - UC$$
$$= \text{anion gap}$$

The range for the normal anion gap varies by species and is approximately 12 to 24 mEq/L in the dog and 13 to 27 mEq/L in the cat (see Chapter 9). The anion gap may also vary with the age of the animal. Relative hyperphosphatemia and hypocalcemia decreased the anion gap in foals (Gossett 1983). Little information on variations in anion gap in pediatric small animal patients is available. In 3-day-old puppies, however, anion gap values were reported to be approximately 16 mEq/L in one study (Nattie et al. 1984), suggesting that anion gaps in neonatal puppies are within the reference ranges for adults. The primary usefulness of the anion gap is as an aid in diagnosis of metabolic acidosis. The derivation and clinical application of the principle of the anion gap are discussed further in Chapters 9 and 10.

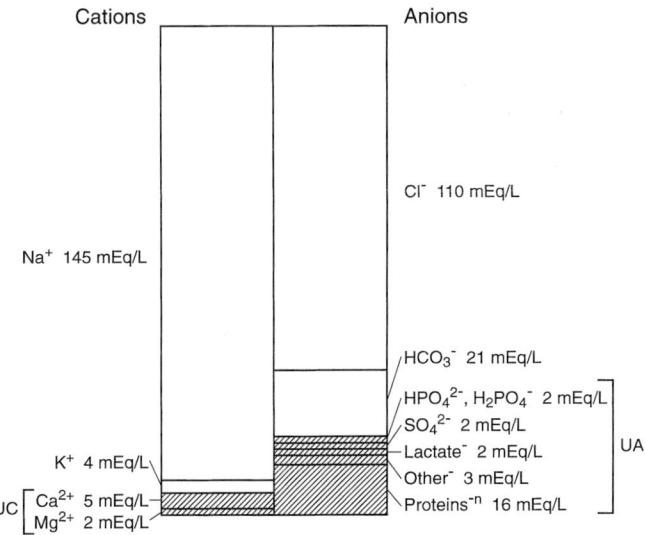

FIGURE 1-6. Relative concentrations of unmeasured anions (UA) and cations (UC) in ECF.

▶ The Osmolal Gap

The *osmolal gap* is defined as the difference between the measured and the calculated serum osmolalities. Reference values for osmolal gaps in dogs are given in Table 1–9. Data for osmolal gaps in cats are not reported in the literature. Attempts to derive osmolal gaps from published data on measured serum osmolalities and electrolyte concentrations in cats yield confusing results (see footnote to Table 1–9). Values for the osmolal gap vary with the formula used to calculate osmolality. Numerous formulas have been derived to calculate serum osmolality (see earlier section on exchange of water between intracellular and extracellular fluid spaces, above). We prefer to use the formula

$$2(Na^+ + K^+) + \frac{glucose}{18} + \frac{BUN}{2.8}$$

Calculation of the osmolal gap is most helpful when unsuspected osmoles are present in ECF, thus increasing the osmolal gap as a result of an increase in the measured but not the calculated osmolality (e.g., ethylene glycol poisoning), and when assessing the significance of the serum Na^+ concentration (see Chapter 3). Hyponatremia with a normal osmolal gap suggests dilutional hyponatremia (e.g., overhydration) and rules out the presence of abnormal osmotically active particles that could cause a shift of water from ICF to ECF, thus decreasing the serum sodium concentration. The osmolal gap is discussed further in Chapter 3.

▶ Homeostasis: Zero Balance

In the healthy adult animal at rest in a thermoneutral environment, daily intake of water, nutrients, and minerals is exactly balanced by daily excretion of these substances or their metabolic by-products. Thus, the animal does not experience a net gain or loss of water, nutrients, or minerals and is said to be in *zero balance*. In a sedentary dog or cat in a thermoneutral environment there are obligatory daily losses of water (Fig. 1–7). Input is equal to output in zero balance, and the volume of water added to body fluids by food and water consumption and by metabolism is equal to the volume of water lost by sensible (i.e., urine, feces, saliva) and insensible (i.e., evaporation from cutaneous and respiratory epithelia) routes

TABLE 1–9. **Reference Ranges for Osmolal Gap**

Species	Osmolal Gap (mOsm/kg)	Reference
Dog	10 ± 6	Grauer 1984
Dog	10.1 ± 5.9	Hauptman 1986
Dog	0–10	Shull 1978

Serum osmolality values in normal cats were reported to be approximately 308 ± 5 mOsm/kg (Chew et al. 1991). When mean values for serum Na (155 mEq/L), K (4 mEq/L), glucose (120 mg/dL), and BUN (24 mg/dL) are substituted into the equation 2(Na + K) + glucose/18 + BUN/2.8, a value of 333 mOsm/kg is obtained for cats. Calculated plasma osmolality values greater than measured values have generally been attributed to laboratory error. Why calculated plasma osmolality exceeds measured plasma osmolality using mean values from normal cats is unclear.

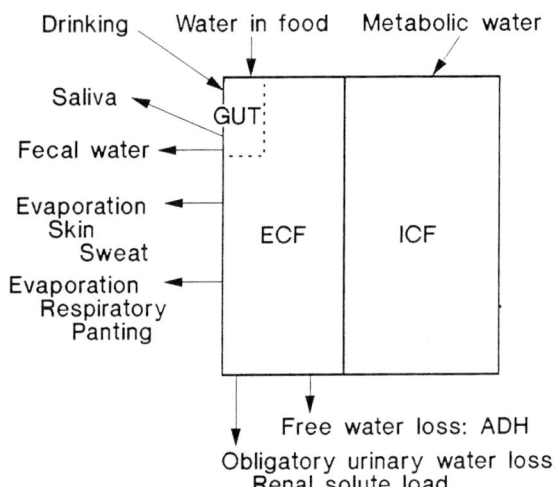

FIGURE 1–7. Total body water: Daily input and obligatory losses. (Adapted from Chew RW: Water metabolism of mammals. In: Mayer WW and Van Gelder RG (eds): *Physiologic Mammalogy: Vol. II Mammalian Reaction to Stressful Environments*. New York, Academic Press, pp. 43–177, 1965.)

(Maxwell et al. 1987). Although the classical definition of insensible water loss in healthy animals is water lost via the lung or the skin, in clinical veterinary medicine water lost in the feces and saliva is included in insensible losses. This approach is used because it is usually impractical to measure fecal and salivary water losses, which are small under normal conditions. This chapter uses the clinical definition of insensible water loss. Although evaporative losses may be great in heat-stressed, exercising, or active animals, the most important and predictable obligatory daily loss of water in healthy, sedentary dogs and cats in a thermoneutral environment occurs via the urine. Values for water input by drinking and water loss via urine, feces, or total insensible avenues in healthy dogs and cats have been variously estimated in the literature (Table 1–10).

Maintenance fluid need may be defined as the volume of fluid required daily to maintain the animal in zero fluid balance. Maintenance needs are thus determined by daily sensible and insensible losses, by ambient temperature and humidity, by the animal's voluntary or forced activity, and by disease. A high ambient temperature, especially with low humidity, results in increased insensible evaporative losses and therefore in increased maintenance fluid requirements. Similarly, fever and increased metabolic rate associated with disease may increase fluid requirements. Estimates of maintenance fluid needs during thermal stress or disease are usually based on empirical adjustments of the estimated basal fluid requirements. Maintenance fluid requirements are also determined partially by the composition of the diet. In dogs and cats, most absorbed dietary nitrogen and minerals not required to maintain zero balance or to provide for growth or tissue repair are excreted daily in the urine. The volume of urine required for solute excretion is thus a function of both the amount of solute in the diet and the osmolality of the urine. Diets with higher solute contents require a greater total water intake than diets of relatively lower solute content. Most small animals have free access to

TABLE 1-10. Measurements of Daily Water Intake and Output in Sedentary Dogs and Cats

Measurement	Species	mL/kg/day*	Condition or Diet	Reference
Input				
Water drunk	Feline	71.3		Chew 1965
	Feline	50.6		Thrall and Miller 1976
	Canine	56.1–70.8		Chew 1965
	Canine	38.9 (19.5–84)		O'Connor 1969
Output				
Urine volume	Canine	13.3 (10.5–17.9)	Caged	O'Connor 1969
Fecal water	Feline	25–29 g/day	Caged	Jackson and Tovey 1977
	Feline	56 g/day	Caged	Thrall 1976
Insensible loss	Canine	20.5	69% H_2O diet	Smith et al. 1964
	Feline	12.42	70% H_2O diet	Hamlin and Tashjian 1964
	Feline	29.0	Dry ration	Thrall and Miller 1976
	Canine	26.2 (8.1–70.7)	Beef and biscuit	O'Connor 1969

*Except as noted in table.

water and therefore ingest sufficient water to support urinary excretion of dietary solutes. Sick animals are often inactive and have a poor appetite or are anorexic. Water requirements to replace insensible losses related to activity and to support renal solute excretion are thus decreased and maintenance water requirements are presumably lower than in healthy individuals. Increased insensible water losses caused by fever or increased metabolic rate during disease may offset this decrease in water requirement. It is important to define basal needs accurately if water requirements during disease are to be estimated using increments of basal requirements. To address this issue, the following discussion focuses on the relationship between basal water requirements and dietary solute in sedentary small animals in a thermoneutral environment.

▶ Water Losses

Urinary and Fecal Water Loss

Daily urinary water losses may be divided into obligatory water loss (i.e., water needed to excrete the daily renal solute load) and free water loss (i.e., water excreted unaccompanied by solute under the control of antidiuretic hormone [ADH]). Clearance of free water increases during relative water excess, thus protecting the animal from the overhydration and hypotonicity that would result from retention of water in excess of solutes. Obligatory renal water loss must occur even in states of relative water deficit so that solute may be eliminated from the body. Similarly, a small daily, obligatory fecal water loss is required for fecal excretion of solute. Obligatory fecal water loss may increase if fecal solute increases (e.g., addition of $CaCl_2$ or $MgCl_2$ to the diet). These ions increase fecal solute, because Ca^{2+} and Mg^{2+} are poorly absorbed from the gastrointestinal tract. Maintenance water requirements must include at least enough water to allow renal and fecal solute excretion.

Obligatory Urinary and Fecal Water Losses

The amount of water required for elimination of the urinary solute load in theory depends on the maximal urine osmolality that can be achieved by the animal (Table 1–11). However, solute is usually not excreted at maximal urine osmolality, especially when water is readily available for voluntary consumption. Urinary osmolalities in experiments on dogs at rest and in water balance ranged from 1000 to 2000 mOsm/kg (Hardy and Osborne 1979). In a later study of client-owned dogs, urine osmolality ranged from 161 to 2830 mOsm/kg, and urine osmolality was greater in the morning (mean, 1541 ± 527 mOsm/kg; range, 273–2620 mOsm/kg) than in the evening (mean, 1400 ± 586 mOsm/kg; range, 161–2830 mOsm/kg) (van Vonderen et al. 1997). There was no effect of gender on urine osmolality, but urine osmolality decreased significantly with age.

Figure 1–8 depicts urine volume and urine osmolality plotted as a function of urine solute in a dog fed varying quantities of food (O'Connor and Potts 1969). Increased intake produced increased renal solute and increased urine volume; however, urine osmolality remained approximately 1600 mOsm/kg (1200–2000 mOsm/kg) (O'Connor and Potts 1988). Urine osmolalities did not, as might be expected, increase toward the maximum attainable (2400–2800 mOsm/kg) in water-deprived dogs (Chew 1965; Hardy and Osborne 1979). Thus, urine os-

TABLE 1-11. Maximal Urine Osmolalities (mOsm/kg)

Species	mOsm/kg	Reference
Dog	2425	Chew 1965
Dog	2791	Hardy and Osborne 1979*
Cat	3200	Chew 1965
Cat	3420–4980	Thrall and Miller 1976
Cat	2984	Ross and Finco 1981*

*Values obtained after dehydration resulting in 5% body weight loss.

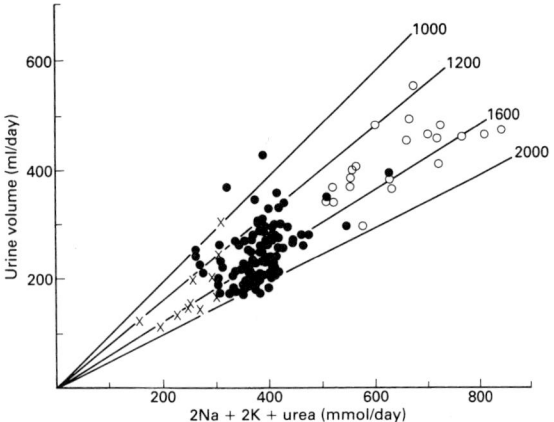

FIGURE 1-8. Urine volume of a dog plotted against urinary excretion of solute (2Na + 2K + urea) during consumption of 320 (×), 385 (●), and 770 (○) grams of food. Each symbol represents data from one day. The lines labeled 1000, 1200, 1600, and 2000 indicate urine osmolality (mOsm/kg). (From O'Connor WJ, Potts DJ: Kidneys and drinking in dogs. In Michell AR (ed): *Renal Disease in Dogs and Cats: Comparative and Clinical Aspects.* Oxford, Blackwell Scientific Publications, p. 35, 1988.)

molality is conserved in the presence of increased urine solute load by an increase in urine volume. The physiologic mechanisms that conserve urine osmolality as renal solute load varies are not well defined.

The renal solute load is derived from dietary sources of protein and minerals and comprises urea, Na^+, K^+, Ca^{2+}, Mg^{2+}, NH_4^+, and other cations and PO_4^{3-}, Cl^-, SO_4^{2-}, and other anions. When estimating solute load from diet for an animal in zero balance, all nitrogen is assumed to form urea. Urea constitutes two-thirds of the urinary solute load in dogs (O'Connor and Potts 1969). The amount of solute in the diet is determined by the composition as well as the quantity of food and minerals ingested. Increasing dietary protein results in increased urea production. Metabolism of carbohydrates and fats yields only CO_2 and H_2O and does not produce urea or other solutes that must be excreted in the urine. Diets high in minerals that are well absorbed from the gut (usually NaCl) provide more solute for excretion.

Not all solute produced by metabolism of ingested and absorbed food is necessarily excreted in the urine. Fecal excretion of solutes does occur. In most healthy dogs, however, daily fecal Na^+, K^+, and Cl^- excretion is substantially lower than urinary mineral excretion. The daily renal solute load is thus a function of the quantity of food ingested as well as of diet composition. Assuming a range of urine osmolalities in healthy dogs between 1000 and 2000 mOsm/kg and a urine solute load of approximately 400 mOsm in a 10-kg dog, the range of urine output would be 200 to 400 mL or 20 to 40 mL/kg/day. Urine volume is thus a function of renal solute load. Another important factor that determines urine volume is the total quantity of water ingested per day. Total water consumption depends both on water in the diet and on water voluntarily consumed by drinking.

Urinary Free Water

Excretion of urinary free water is controlled by stimulation or inhibition of secretion of ADH and by thirst. Urinary free water increases when enough water has been ingested to dilute body solute and result in hypotonicity. A 1 to 2% decrease in serum osmolality inhibits secretion of ADH and abolishes thirst in humans (Robertson et al. 1976; Robertson 1983). During water depletion, body water osmolality increases and ADH secretion is stimulated. An increase in serum osmolality of 1 to 2% is sufficient to provoke maximal ADH secretion in humans (Robertson et al. 1976; Robertson 1983). In dogs, osmolality increases of 1 to 3% stimulate thirst (O'Connor 1975; O'Connor and Potts 1988). A water loss of 5 mL/kg of body weight provoked drinking in experimental dogs (Robinson and Adolph 1943). Daily urinary free water losses, therefore, are very small during water deficiency in otherwise healthy dogs and cats.

Respiratory and Cutaneous Evaporative Losses

Cutaneous evaporative water losses are usually small in the dog and the cat. Cats in hot environments are reported to lick themselves with saliva to promote evaporative cooling (Chew 1965). This phenomenon is rarely observed in clinical practice but, if it occurs, salivary water losses could significantly increase water need. Evaporative water loss from the skin is minimal in dogs and cats, because eccrine sweat glands (which are limited in distribution to the foot pads) do not participate in thermoregulation in these species. Evaporative water losses are usually less in the healthy, sedentary cat in a thermoneutral environment than in the dog (see Table 1–10), probably because cats rarely pant. Evaporative losses in caged, sedentary laboratory dogs are quite variable from dog to dog, and some individuals experience significant daily losses via this route (Table 1–12). Dogs in the study summarized in Table 1–12 fell into two categories: those that remained quiet in their cages all the time and those that ran in circles, barking for several hours each day. The mean evaporative loss for all dogs was 27 mL/kg/day. This value overestimates evaporative loss in quiet dogs. For dogs at rest, evaporative losses were usually less than 1 mL/kg/h. During periods of activity, evaporative losses were estimated at almost 7 mL/kg/h (O'Connor and Potts 1969).

The total water intake per day of the dogs in Table 1–12 was quite variable from dog to dog, ranging from approximately 20 to 91 mL/kg/day. If the insensible loss (primarily composed of respiratory evaporative loss) for each dog is subtracted from its total daily water intake, the range of water intake unrelated to insensible losses is narrower (11–20 mL/kg/day) than the range for total water intake. This emphasizes the profound effect that insensible losses may have on daily water balance in the dog.

Increases in ambient temperature, especially in association with low relative humidity, may result in marked increases in respiratory water evaporation in dogs. The panting response to heat is more efficient in dogs than in cats. At an ambient temperature of 40°C, cats increase their respiratory rate 4.5 times, whereas dogs can increase their respiratory rate 12 to 20 times (Chew 1965). The estimated respiratory water loss in a panting dog at 41°C

TABLE 1-12. Water Intake and Urinary Losses of Solute and Water in Six Sedentary Experimental Dogs Receiving the Same Diet

Dog	Average Wt. (kg)	Water Intake				Water Loss						Urine Solute/Day (mOsm)
		Food and Metabolic (mL/day)	Drunk (mL/day)	Average Total Water		Evaporation		Urine				
				(mL/day)	(mL/kg/day)	(mL/day)	Average (mL/kg/day)	(mL/day)	Average (mL/kg/day)	Total H$_2$O Evaporated (mL/kg/day)	Urine (mOsm/kg)	
Titch	12.7	300	854 ± 465	1154	90.9	961 ± 358	75.7	243 ± 41	19.1	15.2	1706 ± 441	415
Lassie	15.2	300	291 ± 102	691	45.5	386 ± 115	25.4	204 ± 71	13.4	20.1	1836 ± 139	375
Kim	20.5	363	482 ± 188	842	41.1	545 ± 176	26.6	292 ± 50	14.2	14.5	1519 ± 211	444
Gina	10.7	187	135 ± 53	322	30.1	209 ± 49	19.5	123 ± 16	11.5	10.6	2016 ± 216	248
Blackie	20.7	250	153 ± 80	403	19.5	167 ± 54	8.1	217 ± 29	10.5	11.4	1652 ± 305	359
Sandy	19.8	250	151 ± 62	401	20.3	165 ± 50	8.3	258 ± 31	13	12	1079 ± 124	278
Mean		275	344.3	635.5	41.2	405.5	27.3	222.8	13.6	14	1634.7	353

Source: Adapted from O'Connor WJ and Potts DJ: The external water exchanges of normal laboratory dogs. *Q J Exp Physiol* 54:244-265, 1969.

TABLE 1-13. **Respiratory Water Losses of Panting Mammals***

Species	Weight (kg)	Respiratory Water Loss		Percentage Heat Production Lost
		(g/min)	(g/day)	
Dog	16	0.326	469	57
Cat	3.5	0.029	41.2	9.4

Source: Data from Chew RM: Water metabolism of mammals. In Mayer WW and Van Gelder RG (eds): *Physiologic Mammalogy: Vol II Mammalian Reaction to Stressful Environments.* New York, Academic Press, pp. 43–177, 1965.
* Temperature: 41°C; relative humidity: 32%.

was 469 mL/day, whereas that for a cat under the same conditions was 41 mL/day (Table 1–13).

▶ Water Intake

Water in Food

The percentage of water in pet foods is variable. In general, canned foods are more than 70% water, semimoist foods 20 to 40% water, and dry foods less than 10% water (Lewis and Morris 1987). Two representative cat diets are described in Table 1–14. Water in food, therefore, makes up a variable proportion of the total daily water consumption, depending on which diet is fed (Figs. 1–9 and 1–10). Cats can exist without drinking water if fed a diet of cod, salmon, or beefsteak (Prentiss et al. 1959). If the beefsteak or salmon was partially desiccated, cats became hydropenic (increased serum osmolality and serum sodium concentration), anorexic, and cachectic. Thus, cats may meet their water needs solely from the water in some foods.

Drinking

The volume of water voluntarily ingested each day by healthy, sedentary dogs and cats in a thermoneutral environment depends on the composition and the quantity of the diet ingested. Water intake decreases in experimental dogs if food intake is limited (Fig. 1–11) (Cizek 1959; Chew 1965; Morris and Collins 1967a and b). After a 1-day fast, drinking decreased to 25 to 50% of the normal volume in dogs. After a 14- to 18-day fast, drinking was

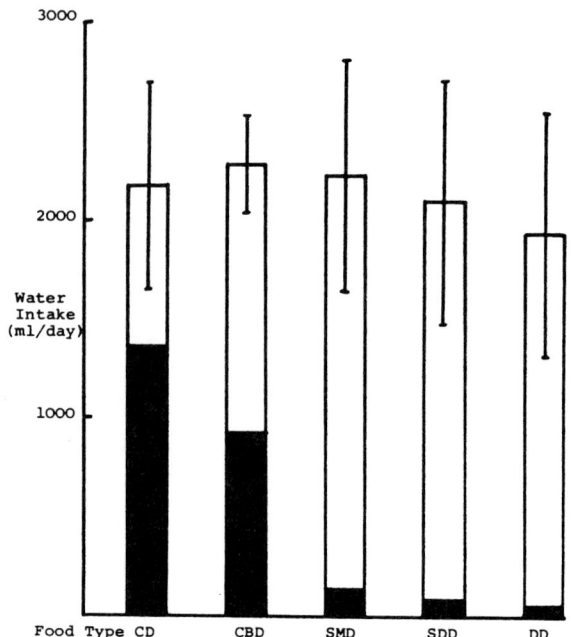

FIGURE 1-9. Effect of food type on water intake in dogs. Each column represents the total daily water intake (mean ± SD) for four dogs fed different diets. The solid area shows the amount of endogenous food water; the clear area shows water drunk. CD = canned; CBD = canned meat and biscuit mixture; SMD, SDD = intermediate moisture foods; DD = dry. (From Burger IH, Anderson RS, Holme DW: Nutritional factors affecting water balance in the dog and cat. In Anderson RS (ed): *Nutrition of the Dog and Cat.* Oxford, Pergamon Press, p. 149, 1980.)

45% of the normal volume in dogs (Chew 1965). Conversely, if water intake is limited, food intake decreases in dogs and cats (Prentiss et al. 1959). As mentioned earlier, cats continue to eat and survive on some diets without drinking water. In dogs that are chronically deprived of food, a basal level of drinking is maintained (Adolph 1939). In sick, anorexic small animal patients, drinking may decrease, and because they do not have access to water from food, total water intake may decrease drastically. However, the water requirement of such animals is probably quite low. In quiet, sick animals the major obligatory water loss occurs via the urine (assuming no other major contemporary fluid loss such as in diarrhea or vomitus). The renal solute load and obligatory renal water loss decrease because the animal is not eating.

TABLE 1-14. **Effect of Diet on Water Intake in Cats**

Food	Dry Matter Intake (g/day)	Food Water* (g/day)	Water Drunk† (mL/day)	Total Water Intake (mL/day)	Ratio of Total Water to Dry Matter
Dry	76.9 ± 17.4	7.4 ± 1.7 (8.8)	167.2 ± 40.1 (>90)	174.6 ± 41.6	2.3 ± 0.2
Canned	35.2 ± 7.2	116 ± 23.6 (76.8)	22.8 ± 12.8 (14)	139.0 ± 31.4	3.9 ± 0.3

Source: Seefeldt SL and Chapman TE: Body water content and turnover in cats fed dry and canned rations. *Am J Vet Res* 40:183–185, 1979.
* Figures in parentheses represent approximate percentage of diet that was water.
† Figures in parentheses represent approximate percentage of total water intake that was drunk.

experiencing abnormal losses, such as in vomitus or diarrhea. These contemporary water needs are in addition to the *maintenance* water required to maintain zero balance during inanition and inactivity in the presence of diminished but still present obligatory urinary water losses.

The volume of water drunk increases as the water in the diet decreases (see Table 1–14). The dog maintains a uniform total water intake when food water is decreased by commensurately increasing drinking (see Fig. 1–9). The cat, however, may not increase drinking enough to maintain total water intake when consuming a diet low in water (see Fig. 1–10). Cats receiving dry food diets may ingest insufficient water. This issue has been investigated extensively in cats as a contributing factor in the development of idiopathic feline lower urinary tract disease (FLUTD). Some investigators believe that a low ratio of total water intake to dry matter in the diet predisposes a cat to this disorder. Diets with a ratio of total water to dry matter greater than 3 have been suggested as an aid in prevention of FLUTD (Holme 1977; Anderson 1983). The ratio of total water to dry matter is an index of the moisture content of the food and of the cat's drinking response to that diet. As predicted, canned foods have higher ratios than do dry foods (Table 1–15). Although cats drink more when consuming dry instead of canned foods, their total water intakes are usually lower with dry than with canned foods.

Water drinking is also influenced by the solute load of the diet. Approximately two-thirds of the renal solute load is urea, an end product of protein metabolism, and increasing the protein content of the diet increases the renal solute load. Diets higher in protein are also associated with greater total water intakes. The ions Na^+, K^+, Ca^{2+}, Mg^{2+}, PO_4^{3-}, Cl^-, and SO_4^{2-} also contribute to dietary solute. Increasing percentages of salt in foods are associated with increased water intake in both cats and dogs (Holme 1977; Burger et al. 1980). This principle has been exploited to increase voluntary water consumption in cats that are fed dry food diets and are at risk for developing FLUTD. The protein content of the diet may significantly affect renal solute load and urine volume. Increased renal solute load supplied by a higher protein diet may provoke increased water consumption.

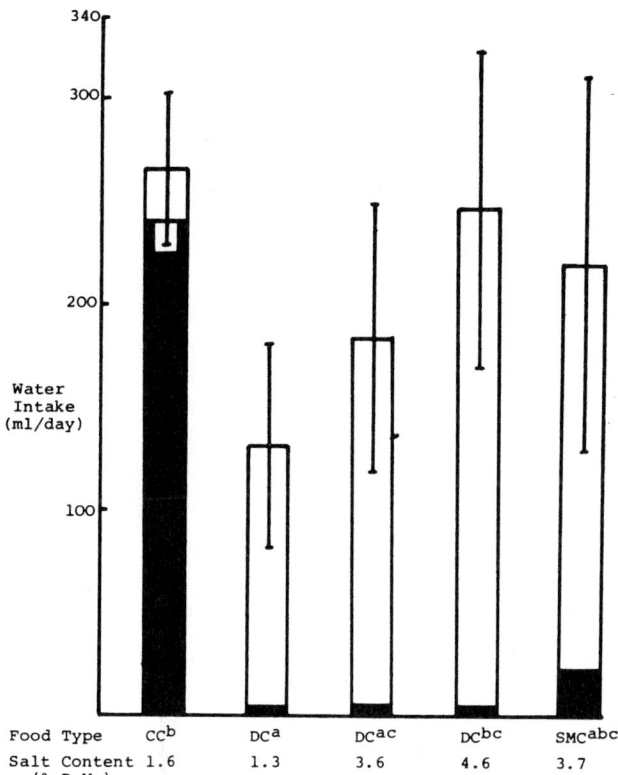

FIGURE 1-10. Effect of food type and salt content on water intake in cats. Each column represents the total daily water intake (mean ± SD) for cats on various diets. The same group of 6 cats was used for all foods except DC diet 4.6% salt, data for which were obtained from a different experiment using another group of 12 cats. The solid area shows food water, the clear area water drunk. Total water intake for foods bearing different superscript letters are significantly different ($p < 0.05$, Student's t test). CC = canned; DC = dry; SMC = intermediate moisture food. (From Burger IH, Anderson RS, Holme DW: Nutritional factors affecting water balance in the dog and cat. In Anderson RS (ed): *Nutrition of the Dog and Cat*. Oxford, Pergamon Press, p. 151, 1980.)

Animals in a catabolic state, however, obviously do produce urea and ions for excretion as a result of catabolism of lean body mass. Figures for renal solute loads generated from endogenous sources are not readily available in the literature. Water requirements of a sick animal may be increased if the animal is febrile, having seizures, or

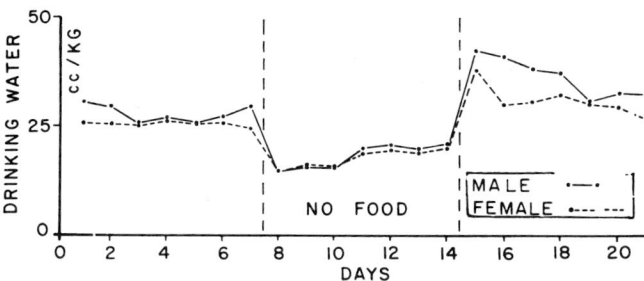

FIGURE 1-11. Comparison of composite drinking curves of male and female dogs during alimentation and food deprivation. Each curve is the composite of 10 experiments. (From Cizek LJ: Long-term observations on the relationship between food and water consumption in the dog. *Am J Physiol* 197:342–346, 1959.)

TABLE 1-15. **Ratios of Total Water to Dry Matter in Cat Foods**

Investigator	Canned Cat Foods	Semimoist Cat Foods	Dry Cat Foods
Thrall and Miller 1976	3.7		2.0–2.4
Jackson and Tovey 1977	3.2		2.8*, 2.3†
Holme 1977	5.6	2.8	2.4
Seefeldt and Chapman 1979	3.9		2.3
Jenkins and Coulter 1981	2.9	1.8	1.8

Source: Data from DiBartola SP and Buffington CA: Feline urologic syndrome. In Slatter D: *Textbook of Small Animal Surgery*. Philadelphia, WB Saunders Co., 1993, pp. 1473–1487.
*Expanded.
†Nonexpanded.

TABLE 1-16. **Metabolic Water per Gram of Nutrient**

Nutrient	Grams Metabolic Water per Gram of Nutrient
Carbohydrate	0.6
Protein	0.41
Fat	1.07

Source: Data from Davidson S, Passmore R, Brock JR, et al.: Water and electrolytes. In Davidson S (ed): *Human Nutrition and Dietetics.* Edinburgh, Churchill Livingstone, pp. 81–89, 1979.

Metabolic Water

Metabolic water contributes approximately 10 to 15% of total water intake in dogs and cats, depending on the diet (Anderson 1983). Nutrients differ in their yield of metabolic water (Table 1–16). Although fats provide the most water per gram, carbohydrates provide the most water per calorie and per liter of oxygen (Chew 1965; Anderson 1982). Therefore, high-carbohydrate diets spare the water requirement by providing more metabolic water per calorie. Carbohydrates and fats also spare water loss because they do not generate renal solute (Anderson 1982). The volume of metabolic water generated per day in humans, and by inference in dogs and cats, is relatively small compared with the total daily water intake (Davidson et al. 1979). Metabolic water is difficult to quantitate in the clinical setting and many studies ignore its contribution to water homeostasis. Definitive water balance studies should include evaluation of metabolic water (Seefeldt and Chapman 1979).

▶ Water Requirements

Maintenance

Water balance is complex, and there is no single maintenance water requirement for each animal. In healthy, sedentary dogs and cats in a thermoneutral environment, water intake is largely dependent on diet. Water requirement is a function of the renal solute load in the diet and the associated obligatory renal water losses for urinary solute excretion. In clinical practice, maintenance fluid needs in small animal patients are often empirically defined as 60 mL/kg/day for smaller dogs and 40 mL/kg/day for larger dogs (Muir and DiBartola 1983). Alternatively, maintenance needs have been assessed on the basis of caloric needs: 1 mL of water per kcal of energy required (Harrison et al. 1960; Haskins 1984). Early studies of water balance in healthy, caged dogs documented that mean water intake was approximately 1 mL/kcal ingested (Adolph 1939). Normal maintenance energy requirement is defined as the number of calories required to sustain the basal metabolic rate; to provide energy for digestion, absorption, and assimilation of nutrients (thermal effect of feeding); to maintain body temperature in a nonthermoneutral environment; and for normal activity (Kleiber 1975). Maintenance energy expenditure may be calculated from the following formula (Brody et al. 1934):

$$140 \text{ kcal} \times \text{body weight}^{0.73}$$

A 10-kg dog would require 750 kcal of energy per day or 75 kcal/kg/day. Following the rule of 1 mL/kcal, the water requirement would be 75 mL/kg/day.

Opinions vary on the formula for calculating maintenance caloric needs (Nutrient Requirements of Dogs, 1985). Basal energy requirements may be calculated and then multiplied by a factor of approximately 2 (Nutrient Requirements of Dogs, 1985) to obtain maintenance needs. The basal energy requirement is defined as the caloric need of a resting, healthy dog in a postabsorptive state (i.e., renal solute load has been excreted) about 18 h after feeding (Kleiber 1975) and in a thermoneutral environment. Basal energy requirement has been variously calculated from the following formulas (Brody et al. 1934; Abrams 1977):

Basal energy requirement = $70 \times \text{body weight (kg)}^{0.73}$ (a)

Basal energy requirement = $97 \times \text{body weight (kg)}^{0.655}$ (b)

There has been considerable debate over the most appropriate exponent to use to relate body weight to metabolic size in the dog (Abrams 1977; Rivers and Burger 1989; Kronfeld 1991). We prefer the exponent 0.655 and use formula (b), which has been supported in the veterinary literature (Rivers and Burger 1989; Kronfeld 1991).

Maintenance energy requirements are higher than basal needs primarily to provide calories for the normal activity of a healthy dog. On the basis of formula (b), a 10-kg dog has a basal energy requirement of 44 kcal/kg/day and a maintenance requirement of 88 kcal/kg/day. Assuming 1 mL of water required per kcal of energy need, the maintenance water requirement for this dog would be approximately 88 mL/kg/day. A 50-kg dog would require 25 mL/kg/day for basal water needs and 50 mL/kg/day for maintenance. If basal water requirements are estimated from formula (a), a 10-kg dog would have a basal daily water requirement of 38 mL/kg and a maintenance requirement of 76 mL/kg.

Estimates of maintenance water needs based on caloric requirements are similar to the empirical values for maintenance needs used by some clinicians. It is important to remember, however, that caloric needs are a logarithmic function of body weight, and larger dogs require less fluid per kilogram of body weight than do smaller dogs.

The physiologic reason for the correlation between caloric and water needs is not well documented. The relationship may, in fact, be indirect. Water requirements and caloric needs may be related because water intake is in part a function of renal solute load, which is related to diet: both to the quantity of food ingested and to the composition of the food. However, the renal solute load per calorie in the diet varies with the composition of the diet. Diets vary in water content (dry versus canned) and in nutrient composition and hence in renal solute load per calorie. Fats provide more kilocalories per gram (9 kcal/g) than do carbohydrates or proteins (4 kcal/g). Fats provide more milliliters of water per gram (1.07) than do carbohydrates (0.56) or proteins (0.40) (Anderson 1982). High-protein diets increase renal solute load, whereas fats and carbohydrates do not contribute to it. The mineral content of diets also varies. Therefore, the animal's water requirement may be viewed more accurately as a function

TABLE 1–17. Water Consumption in Food-Deprived Dogs and Cats

n	Body Weight (kg)	Days Starvation	Average Water Consumption (mL/kg)	Reference
10 dogs*	NR†	7	17.6 ± 2.2	Cizek 1959
5 dogs	8–11	15	4.0	Morris and Collins 1967a
2 dogs	9.47 / 11.71	4	4.1 (3.2–5.0)	Prentiss et al. 1959
2 dogs	11.71 / 9.47	9	5.4 (3.0–7.7)	Prentiss et al. 1959
2 cats	3.59	7	5.2 (3.7–6.7)	Prentiss et al. 1959

*Beagle or hound type of dogs.
†NR, Not reported.

of total water content and renal solute load of the diet rather than strictly as a function of calories ingested. Thus, the relationship 1 mL of water per 1 kcal of energy may be fortuitous.

Basal

Fluid requirements for sick, inappetent small animals have not been well documented. Decreased food intake or anorexia reduces renal solute load and hence water requirements. However, clinicians frequently base estimates of water requirements for patients on tables derived from the formula for maintenance energy requirements: $140 \times$ body weight $(kg)^{0.73}$ (Haskins 1984). Haskins (1984) commented that the use of tables for water intake based on this formula may overestimate the water requirements of sick patients. In fact, the water requirement of an inappetent, sedentary sick animal in a thermoneutral environment might approach basal water need. The basal water requirement for a healthy animal might be defined, analogously to the basal energy need, as water required when the animal is resting, is in a postabsorptive state (i.e., the renal solute load has been excreted), and is not exposed to thermal stress.

Basal water needs of dogs and cats have not been well studied. Water intake of healthy dogs and cats in a thermoneutral environment and deprived of food has been measured in a few experiments (Table 1–17). Two investigators found that quiet, food-deprived dogs (body weights 8–15 kg) or cats (approximately 3.5 kg) confined to metabolism cages drank about 5 mL/kg of water daily. A third investigator found that intake was considerably higher (17.6 ± 2.2 mL/kg/day) in dogs of about the same body weight. The dogs in the latter experiment may have been more active and may have had larger evaporative losses and greater compensatory drinking than dogs or cats in the previous experiments. If basal water need is estimated by determining the basal energy requirement, utilizing the preceding formula (Abrams 1977), the water requirement of a 10-kg dog would be 40 mL/kg/day, assuming 1 mL of water per kilocalorie of energy required. Data for dogs deprived of food suggest that basal water requirements may be much lower. This fact is not surprising if we consider that when water intakes of dogs in the study by O'Connor and Potts (1969) (see Table 1–12) were corrected for water intake that balanced evaporative losses, total water intakes were 11 to 20 mL/kg/day. This value approximates the accepted general range for daily urine production in dogs. Thus, if dogs are deprived of food and urine volumes decrease substantially (renal solute load decreases), the water need may be small.

Water requirements of sick animals may be increased over basal requirements owing to increased contemporary fluid losses with such causes as evaporation (through panting), diarrhea, vomiting, or dilute urine. Clinicians must estimate how much water needs increase by assessing the volume of these additional fluid losses. Fluid needs, however, still may not approach 40 to 60 mL/kg/day.

Assessing the basal water need of dogs and cats from the basal energy requirement provides a high estimate for water compared with the minimal requirement documented in experiments with dogs and cats deprived of food. This disparity makes estimating basal water needs of inappetent, quiet dogs problematic. Data on basal water needs of small animals would help clinicians to devise appropriate strategies for fluid therapy in inappetent, sick animals by providing a baseline assessment from which maintenance or replacement fluid needs may be estimated by use of a multiplication factor (i.e., maintenance = 2 × basal water need). Current methods for assessing fluid needs may overestimate the patient's actual requirements because sick patients are inappetent and inactive. Administration of an excessive volume of fluid could be detrimental, especially to patients with heart failure or oliguric renal failure. Most patients respond satisfactorily to currently employed standard fluid-replacement regimens, because excess fluid and solute are readily excreted by the kidneys. When calculating water needs, however, it would be prudent to consider that inactive, sick animals with decreased or no food intake may well require less water than usual empirical estimates may indicate.

REFERENCES

Abrams JT: The nutrition of the dog. In Rechcigl M (ed): *CRC Handbook Series in Nutrition and Food. Section G: Diets, Culture Media, and Food Supplements.* Boca Raton, FL, CRC Press, p. 1, 1977.

Adolph EF: Measurements of water drinking in dogs. *Am J Physiol* 125:75, 1939.

Altman PL and Dittmer DS (eds): *Biology Data Book*, 2nd ed. Bethesda, Maryland, Federation of American Societies for Experimental Biology, pp. 1846–1992, 1974.

Anderson RS: Water balance in the dog and cat. *J Small Anim Pract* 23:588, 1982.

Anderson RS: Fluid balance and diet. *Proceedings of the Seventh Kal Kan Symposium*, Columbus, p. 19, 1983.

Aron H: Biochemie des Wachstums des Menschen und der höheren Thiere. *Oppenheimer's Handbuch der Biochemie des Menschen und der Tiere*. Ergänzungsband, Jena, Gustav Fischer, 610, 1915.

Baker CH: Cr^{51}-labeled red cell, I^{131}-fibrinogen, and T-1824 dilution spaces. *Am J Physiol* 204:176–180, 1963.

Baker CH and Remington JW: Role of the spleen in determining total body hematocrit. *Am J Physiol* 198:906, 1960.

Barratt TM and Walser M: Extracellular fluid in individual tissues and in whole animals: The distribution of radiosulfate and radiobromide. *J Clin Invest* 48:56, 1969.

Bauer JH, Willis LR, Burt RW, et al.: Volume studies. II. Simultaneous determination of plasma volume, red cell mass, extracellular fluid, and total body water before and after volume expansion in dog and man. *J Lab Clin Med* 86:1009, 1975.

Becker EL and Joseph BJ: Measurement of extracellular fluid volumes in normal dogs. *Am J Physiol* 183:314, 1955.

Bowsher DJ, Avram MJ, Frederiksen MC, et al.: Urea distribution kinetics analyzed by simultaneous injection of urea and insulin: Demonstration that transcapillary exchange is rate limiting. *J Pharmacol Exp Ther* 230:269, 1984.

Breznock EM and Strack D: Blood volume of nonsplenectomized and splenectomized cats before and after acute hemorrhage. *Am J Vet Res* 43:1811, 1982a.

Breznock EM and Strack D: Effects of the spleen, epinephrine, and splenectomy on determination of blood volume in cats. *Am J Vet Res* 43:2062, 1982b.

Brody S, Proctor RC, and Ashworth US: Growth and development with special reference to domestic animals. XXXIV. Basal metabolism, endogenous nitrogen, creatinine and neutral sulphur excretions as functions of body weights. Columbia, University of Missouri, 1934.

Burch GE, Threefoot SA, and Ray CT: Rates of turnover and biologic decay of chloride and chloride space in the dog determined with the long-life isotope, ^{36}Cl. *J Lab Clin Med* 35:331, 1950.

Burger IH, Anderson RS, and Holme DW: Nutritional factors affecting water balance in the dog and cat. In Anderson RS (ed): *Nutrition of the Dog and Cat*. Oxford, Pergamon Press, p. 145, 1980.

Cardozo RH and Edelman IS: The volume of distribution of sodium thiosulfate as a measure of the extracellular fluid space. *J Clin Invest* 31:280, 1952.

Chew DJ, Leonard M, and Muir WW: Effect of sodium bicarbonate infusion on serum osmolality, electrolyte concentrations, and blood gas tensions in cats. *Am J Vet Res* 52:12, 1991.

Chew RM: Water metabolism of mammals. In Mayer WW and Van Gelder RG (eds): *Physiologic Mammalogy: Vol II: Mammalian Reaction to Stressful Environments*. New York, Academic Press, p. 43, 1965.

Cizek LJ: Longterm observations on relationship between food and water ingestion in the dog. *Am J Physiol* 197:342, 1959.

Clark CH, Woodley CH: A comparison of blood volumes as measured by rose bengal, T-1824 (Evans Blue), radiochromium-tagged erythrocytes, and a combination of the latter two. *Am J Vet Res* 20:1067, 1959.

Courtice FC: The blood volume of normal animals. *J Physiol* 102:290, 1943.

Da Silva AC, DeAngelis RC, Pontes MA, et al.: The domestic cat as a laboratory animal for experimental nutrition studies. IV. Folic acid deficiency. *J Nutr* 56:199, 1955.

Davidson S, Passmore R, Brock JF, et al.: Water and electrolytes. In Davidson S (ed): *Human Nutrition and Dietetics*. Edinburgh, Churchill Livingstone, p. 81, 1979.

Deavers S, Smith EL, and Huggins RA: Control circulatory values of morphine-pentobarbitalized dogs. *Am J Physiol* 5:797, 1960.

deGraaf SSN, deVries JA, and Zijlstra WG: Influence of high-dose methotrexate on the distribution of body fluid volumes in the dog. *Cancer Chemother Pharmacol* 17:227, 1986.

Dellenback RJ, Usami S, Chien S, et al.: Effects of splenectomy on blood picture, blood volume, and plasma proteins in beagles. *Am J Physiol* 217:891, 1969.

Edelman IS: Exchange of water between blood and tissues: Characteristics of deuterium oxide equilibration in body water. *Am J Physiol* 171:279, 1952.

Edelman IS and Leibman J: Review: Anatomy of body water and electrolytes. *Am J Med* 27:256, 1959.

Edelman IS and Sweet NJ: Gastrointestinal water and electrolytes. I. The equilibration of radiosodium in gastrointestinal contents and in the proportion of exchangeable sodium in the gastrointestinal tract. *J Clin Invest* 35:502, 1956.

Edelman IS, Olney JM, James AH, et al.: Body composition: Studies in the human being by the dilution principle. *Science* 115:447, 1952.

Edelman IS, James AH, Baden H, et al.: Electrolyte composition of bone and the penetration of radiosodium and deuterium oxide into dog and human bone. *J Clin Invest* 33:122, 1954.

Edelman IS, Leibman J, O'Meara MP, et al.: Interrelations between serum sodium concentration, serum osmolarity and total exchangeable sodium, total exchangeable potassium and total body water. *J Clin Invest* 37:1236, 1958.

Eggleton MG: The state of body water in the cat. *J Physiol* (London) 115:482, 1951.

Gibson JG, Peacock WC, Seligman AM, et al.: Circulating red cell volume measured simultaneously by the radioactive iron and dye methods. *J Clin Invest* 25:838, 1946.

Gossett KA: Effect of age on anion gap in clinically healthy normal Quarterhorses. *Am J Vet Res* 44:1744, 1983.

Green RA: Perspectives of clinical osmometry. *Vet Clin North Am* 8:287, 1978.

Gregersen MI and Stewart JD: Simultaneous determination of the plasma volume with T-1824, and the "available fluid" volume with sodium thiocyanate. *Am J Physiol* 125:142, 1939.

Guadino M and Levitt MF: Influence of the adrenal cortex on body water distribution and renal function. *J Clin Invest* 28:1487, 1949.

Guadino M and Levitt MF: Inulin volume of distribution as a measure of extracellular fluid in dog and man. *Proc Soc Exp Biol Med* 68:507, 1948.

Hamlin and Tashjian: Water and electrolyte intake and output and quantity of feces in healthy cats. *Vet Med/Small Animal Clin* 59:746, 1964.

Hankes GH, Nelson AW, and Swan H: Chlorine-36 as a continuing indicator of extracellular fluid volume in the dog. *Am J Vet Res* 34:221, 1973.

Hardy RM and Osborne CA: Water deprivation test in the dog: Maximal normal values. *J Am Vet Med Assoc* 174:479, 1979.

Harrison HE, Darrow DC, and Yannet H: The total electrolyte content of animals and its probable relation to the distribution of body water. *J Biol Chem* 113:515, 1936.

Harrison JB, Sussman HH, and Pickering DE: Fluid and electrolyte therapy in small animals. *J Am Vet Med Assoc* 137:637, 1960.

Haskins SC: Fluid and electrolyte therapy. *Compend Contin Educ Pract Vet* 6:244, 1984.

Hatai S: Changes in the composition of the entire body of the albino rat during the life span. *Am J Anat* 21:23, 1917.

Herrold M and Sapirstein LA: Measurement of total body water in the dog with antipyrine. *Proc Soc Exp Biol Med* 79:419, 1952.

Hoff HE, Deavers S, and Huggins RA: Effects of hypertonic glucose and mannitol on plasma volume. *Proc Soc Exp Biol Med* 122:630, 1966.

Holme DW: Research into the feline urological syndrome. *Proceedings of the Kal Kan Symposium for Treatment of Dog and Cat Diseases*, Columbus, p. 40, 1977.

Hood DM and Hightower D: Evaluation of radioiodinated human serum albumin in the dog for assessment of hemodynamic function. *Am J Vet Res* 37:227, 1976.

Jackson OF and Tovey JD: Water balance studies in domestic cats. *Feline Pract* 7:30, 1977.

Jain NC: *Schalm's Veterinary Hematology*. Philadelphia, Lea & Febiger, 1986.

Kleiber M: *The Fire of Life*. Huntington, NY, Robert E. Krieger Publishing Co., 1975.

Kronfeld DS: Protein and energy estimates for hospitalized dogs and cats. *Proceedings of Purina International Nutrition Symposium*, Orlando, FL, p. 5, 1991.

Lavietes PH, Bourdillon J, and Klinghoffer KA: The volume of the extracellular fluids of the body. *J Clin Invest* 15:261, 1936.

Leaf A: The clinical and physiologic significance of the serum sodium concentration. *N Engl J Med* 267:24, 1962.

Lee P, Brown ME, Hutzler PT: Blood volume changes and production and destruction of erythrocytes in newborn dogs. *Am J Vet Res* 37:561, 1976.

Lewis LD and Morris ML: *Small Animal Clinical Nutrition*. Topeka, KS, Mark Morris Associates, 1987.

Lombardi MH: Radioisotopic blood volume and cardiac output in dogs. *Am J Vet Res* 33:1825, 1972.

Maxwell MH, Kleeman CR, and Narins RG: *Clinical Disorders of Fluid and Electrolyte Metabolism*. New York, McGraw-Hill Book Co., 1987.

Morris ML and Collins DR: Anorexia in the dog. *Vet Med Small Anim Clin* 62:753, 1967a.

Morris ML and Collins DR: A new solution to the problem of anorexia. *Vet Med Small Anim Clin* 62:1075, 1967b.

Moulton CR: Age and chemical development in mammals. *J Biol Chem* 57:79, 1923.

Muir WW and DiBartola SP: Fluid therapy. In Kirk RW (ed): *Current Veterinary Therapy VIII*. Philadelphia, WB Saunders Co., p. 28, 1983.

Murphy B, Dossetor JB, and Beck JC: Serial determinations of extracellular fluid volume using the radiosulphate space method. *Can J Biochem Physiol* 41:497, 1963.

Nadell J, Sweet NJ, and Edelman IS: Gastrointestinal water and electrolytes. II. The equilibration of radiopotassium in gastrointestinal contents and the proportion of exchangeable potassium in the gastrointestinal tract. *J Clin Invest* 35:512, 1956.

Nattie EE, Edwards WH, and Marin-Padilla M: Newborn puppy cerebral acid-base regulation in experimental asphyxia and recovery. *J Appl Physiol* 56:1178, 1984.

Nichols G, Nichols N, Weil WB, et al.: The direct measurement of the extracellular phase of tissues. *J Clin Invest* 32:1299, 1953.

Nutrient Requirements of Dogs. Washington, DC, National Academy Press, 1985.

O'Connor WJ: Drinking by dogs during and after running. *J Physiol* 250:247, 1975.

O'Connor WJ and Potts DJ: The external water exchanges of normal laboratory dogs. *Q J Exp Physiol* 54:244, 1969.

O'Connor WJ and Potts DJ: Kidneys and drinking in dogs. In Michell AR (ed): *Renal Disease in Dogs and Cats: Comparative and Clinical Aspects*. Oxford, Blackwell Scientific Publications, p. 30, 1988.

Parkinson JE and Dougherty JH: Effect of internal emitters on red cell plasma volumes of beagle dogs. *Proc Soc Exp Biol Med* 97:722, 1958.

Peters JP: The role of sodium in the production of edema. *N Engl J Med* 239:353, 1948.

Pfeiffer L: Über den Fettgehalt des Körpers und verschiedener Theile desselben bei mageren und fetten Thieren. *Z Biol* (Munich) 23:340, 1887.

Prentiss PG, Wolf AV, and Eddy HA: Hydropenia in cat and dog. Ability of the cat to meet its water requirements solely from a diet of fish or meat. *Am J Physiol* 196:625, 1959.

Raisz LG, Young MK Jr, and Stinson IT: Comparison of the volumes of distribution of inulin, sucrose, and thiosulfate in normal and nephrectomized dogs. *Am J Physiol* 174:72, 1953.

Reed C, Ling GV, Gould D, et al.: Polycythemia vera in a cat. *J Am Vet Med Assoc* 157:85, 1970.

Reeve EB, Gregersen MI, Allen TH, et al.: Distribution of cells and plasma in the normal and splenectomized dog and its influence on blood volume estimates with ^{32}P and T-1824. *Am J Physiol* 175:195, 1953.

Richmond CR, Langham WH, and Trujillo TT: Comparative metabolism of tritiated water by mammals. *J Cell Comp Physiol* 59:45, 1962.

Rivers JPW and Burger LH: Allometry in dog nutrition. In *Nutrition of the Dog and Cat, Waltham Symposium No. 7*. Cambridge, Cambridge University Press, p. 67, 1989.

Robertson GL: Thirst and vasopressin function in normal and disordered states of water balance. *J Lab Clin Med* 101:351, 1983.

Robertson GL, Shelton RL, and Athar S: The osmoregulation of vasopressin. *Kidney Int* 10:25, 1976.

Robinson EA and Adolph EF: Pattern of normal water drinking in dogs. *Am J Physiol* 139:39, 1943.

Rose BD: *Clinical Physiology of Acid-Base and Electrolytes*. New York, McGraw-Hill Book Co., 1984.

Rose BD: *Clinical Physiology of Acid-Base and Electrolyte Disorders*. New York, McGraw-Hill, p. 5, 1989.

Ross LA and Finco DR: Relationship of selected clinical renal function tests to glomerular filtration rate and renal blood flow in cats. *Am J Vet Res* 42:1704, 1981.

Sabourin S, Stanley P, Chartrand C: Normogramme hematologique et biochemique et variations quotidiennes des parametres de base chez le chien normal. *Can J Comp Med* 39:397, 1975.

Schloerb PR, Peters CE, Cage GK, et al.: Evaluation of the sulfate space as a measure of extracellular fluid. *Surg Forum* 18:39, 1967.

Schrier RW: Pathogenesis of sodium and water retention in high-output and low-output cardiac failure, nephrotic syndrome, cirrhosis, and pregnancy. *N Engl J Med* 319:1065, 1988.

Seefeldt SL and Chapman TE: Body water content and turnover in cats fed dry and canned rations. *Am J Vet Res* 40:183, 1979.

Skelton H: The storage of water by various tissues of the body. *Arch Intern Med* 40:140, 1927.

Smith RC, Haschen T, Hamlin RL, et al.: Water and electrolyte intake and output and quantity of feces in the healthy dog. *Vet Med* 59:743, 1964.

Smithline N and Gardner KD: Gaps—Anionic and osmolal. *JAMA* 236:1594, 1976.

Soberman RJ, Keating RP, and Maxwell RD: Effect of acute whole-body x-irradiation upon water and electrolyte balance. *Am J Physiol* 164:450, 1951.

Spector WS: *Handbook of Biological Data*. Philadelphia, WB Saunders Co., p. 340, 1956.

Spink RR, Malvin RL, Cohen BJ: Determinations of erythrocyte half-life and blood volume in cats. *Am J Vet Res* 27:1041, 1966.

Swan RC, Madisso H, and Pitts RF: Measurement of extracellular fluid volume in nephrectomized dogs. *J Clin Invest* 33:1447, 1954.

Swan RC and Pitts RF: Neutralization of infused acid by nephrectomized dogs. *J Clin Invest* 34:205, 1955.

Thrall BE and Miller LG: Water turnover in cats fed dry rations. *Feline Pract* 6:10, 1976.

van Vonderen IK, Kooistra HS, and Rijnberk A: Intra- and interindividual variation in urine osmolality and urine specific gravity in healthy pet dogs of various ages. *J Vet Intern Med* 11:30, 1997.

Vineyard GC and Osborne DP Jr: Simultaneous determination of extracellular water by 35-sulfate and 82-bromide in dogs, with a note on the acute effects of hypotensive shock. *Surg Forum* 18:37, 1967.

von Voit C: Über die Verschiedenheiten der Eiweisszersetzung beim Hungern. *Z Biol* (Munich) 2:307, 1866.

Walser M, Seldin DW, and Grollman A: An evaluation of radiosulfate for the determination of the volume of extracellular fluid in man and dogs. *J Clin Invest* 32:299, 1953.

Weigert R: Jahrb Kinderheilk 61:178, 1905.

Woodward KT, Berman AR, Michaelson SM, et al.: Plasma, erythrocyte, and whole blood volume in the normal beagle. *Am J Vet Res* 29:1935, 1968.

Zweens J, Frankena H, Rispens P, et al.: Determination of extracellular fluid volume in the dog with ferrocyanide. *Pflugers Arch* 357:275, 1975.

Zweens J, Frankena H, and Zijlstra WG: The effect of pentobarbital anaesthesia upon the extracellular fluid volume in the dog, study by continuous infusion and single injection methods. *Pflugers Arch* 376:131, 1978.

Zweens J, Frankena H, Reicher A, et al.: Infrared-spectrometric determination of D$_2$O in biological fluids. *Pflugers Arch* 385:71, 1980.

APPENDIX TO CHAPTER 1

The cell membrane is composed of a hydrophobic lipid bilayer with embedded protein molecules that play structural and functional roles. This configuration allows the cell membrane to act as an electrical capacitor that stores energy. Some of the embedded proteins act as hydrophilic pores in the membrane. One embedded functional protein is Na$^+$, K$^+$-ATPase, which pumps sodium out of and potassium into the cell in an Na/K ratio of 3:2. In this model, the cell membrane acts as a capacitor, the hydrophilic protein pores provide resistance, and the Na$^+$, K$^+$-ATPase provides energy.

The intracellular concentration of potassium (140 mEq/L) is much higher than its extracellular concentration (4 mEq/L). Consequently, potassium diffuses out of the cell down its concentration gradient. The cell membrane, however, is impermeable to most intracellular anions (e.g., proteins, organic phosphates). A net negative charge develops inside the cell as potassium ions diffuse out of the cell, and a net positive charge accumulates outside the cell. As a result, a potential difference is generated across the cell membrane. The principal extracellular cation is sodium, which enters the cell relatively slowly down its concentration and electrical gradients because the cell membrane is much less permeable to sodium than to potassium. Diffusion of potassium from the cell continues until the ECF acquires sufficient positive charge to prevent further diffusion of potassium ions out of the cell.

The ratio of intracellular and extracellular concentrations of potassium ($[K^+]_I/[K^+]_O$) is the major determinant of the resting cell membrane potential difference. This potential difference is demonstrated by the Nernst equation, which is derived from the general equation for free-energy change (ΔG^C):

$$\Delta G^C = RT \times \ln\left(\frac{[c^+]_I}{[c^+]_O}\right) + z\mathscr{F} E_m \tag{1}$$

where R is the gas constant (8.314 J/K/mol), T is the absolute temperature in K (°C + 273), $[c^+]_I$ is the concentration of cation inside the cell, $[c^+]_O$ is the concentration of cation outside the cell, z is the valence, $\mathscr{F}$ is the Faraday constant (96,484 C/Eq), and E_m is the membrane potential in volts.

The first term on the right side of this equation represents the osmotic work required to transport 1 mol of particles across the membrane against a concentration gradient of $[c^+]_I/[c^+]_O$, and the second term represents the electrical work required to transport the same number of particles across the membrane against an electrical gradient.

At equilibrium, $\Delta G^C = 0$, and solving the equation for E_m yields

$$E_m = -\left(\frac{RT}{z\mathscr{F}}\right)\ln\left(\frac{[c^+]_I}{[c^+]_O}\right) \tag{2}$$

At 37°C and with a monovalent ion (e.g., K$^+$), the term $RT/z\mathscr{F} = 26.67$ mV. Converting to the base 10 logarithm and specifying potassium as the cation:

$$E_m = -26.67(2.303)\log_{10}\left(\frac{[K^+]_I}{[K^+]_O}\right)$$

$$E_m = -61\log_{10}\left(\frac{[K^+]_I}{[K^+]_O}\right) \tag{3}$$

The Nernst equation is valid only when there is no net current flow.

The Goldman-Hodgkin-Katz constant-field equation is a modification of the Nernst equation used to calculate the membrane potential on the basis of the membrane permeability ratio for sodium and potassium (P_{Na}/P_K). This equation allows determination of the individual ionic contributions to E_m by summing the individual concentrations and permeability effects:

$$E_m = -61\log_{10}\frac{P_K[K^+]_I + P_{Na}[Na^+]_I}{P_K[K^+]_O + P_{Na}[Na^+]_O} \tag{4}$$

where P_{Na} and P_K are the membrane permeabilities for sodium and potassium.

A term r is included in the constant-field equation to take into account the effect of the electrogenic Na$^+$,K$^+$-ATPase pump under steady-state conditions. This term is usually assigned the Na/K transport ratio of the Na$^+$, K$^+$-ATPase ($r = 3/2 = 1.5$). If the membrane permeability of potassium is assigned a value of 1.0 and the cell membrane is known to be 100 times more permeable to potassium than to sodium,

$$E_m = -61 \log_{10} \frac{rP_K [K^+]_I + P_{Na} [Na^+]_I}{rP_K [K^+]_O + P_{Na} [Na^+]_O}$$

$$E_m = -61 \log_{10} \frac{1.5P_K [K^+_I] + 0.01 P_{Na} [Na^+]_I}{1.5P_K [K^+]_O + 0.01 P_{Na} [Na^+]_O} \quad (5)$$

Any ion that is not actively transported across the membrane cannot contribute to the membrane potential, and the transmembrane distribution of such an ion must follow the resting potential. Chloride is not considered in the Goldman-Hodgkin-Katz equation because chloride is usually passively distributed across the cell membrane according to the prevailing E_m.

CHAPTER 2

Renal Physiology

STEPHEN P. DiBARTOLA

> *Superficially it might be said that the function of the kidneys is to make urine; but in a more considered view one can say that the kidneys make the stuff of philosophy itself.*
>
> Homer W. Smith

Each day, the glomeruli of the kidneys filter an enormous volume of plasma water and the tubules must reabsorb the vast majority of this water along with vital solutes so that only a small volume of water and unneeded solutes are excreted as urine. For example, a normal 10-kg dog might have a GFR of 4 mL/min/kg. In the course of 1 day, this dog would filter 57.6 L of plasma water in its kidneys. If 60% of body weight is water, this volume represents almost 10 times the dog's total body water. The same dog might have a urine output of 33 mL/kg/day. Thus, more than 99% of plasma water filtered by the glomeruli is reabsorbed by the tubules. The proximal tubules and loops of Henle reabsorb approximately 85% of the filtered water and solutes, whereas the collecting ducts adjust the final composition of urine to compensate for fluctuations in intake and prevent changes in the composition of extracellular fluid. The major functions of the various segments of the nephron are depicted in Figure 2–1.

▶ Concept of Renal Clearance

An appreciation of the concept of clearance is crucial to understanding how renal function is evaluated clinically.

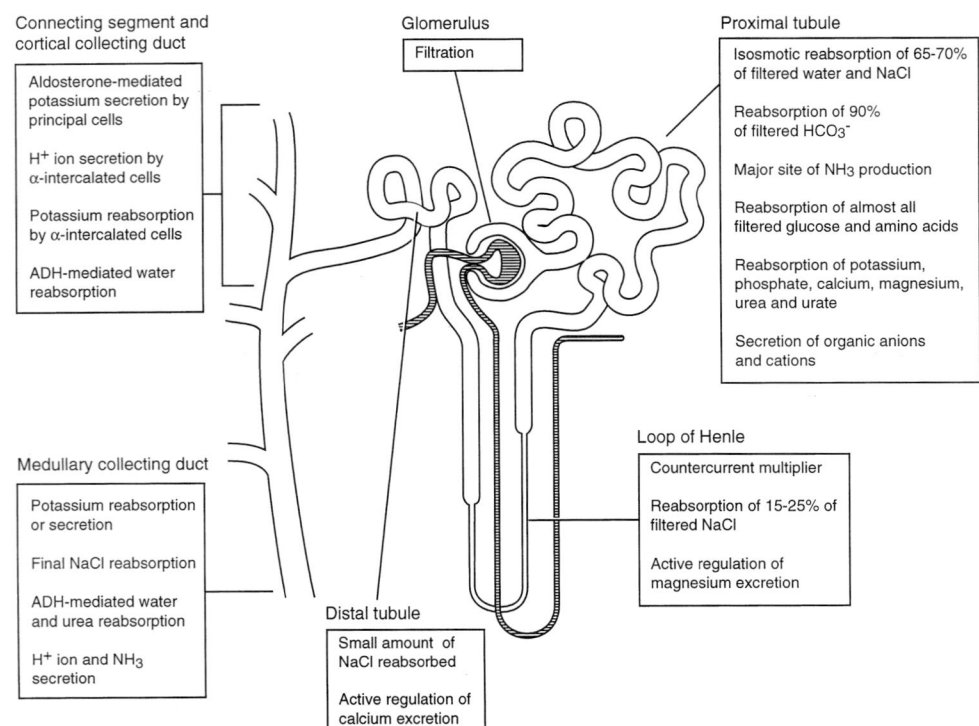

FIGURE 2–1. Major functions of each portion of the nephron. (Drawing by Tim Vojt.)

The renal clearance of a substance is the volume of plasma that contains the amount of the substance excreted in the urine in 1 min. It is the volume of plasma that must be filtered each minute to account for the amount of the substance appearing in the urine each minute under steady-state conditions. If the concentration of the substance in urine is U_x and the urine flow rate is V, the amount of the substance excreted in the urine per minute is U_xV. If the concentration of the substance in plasma is P_x, the volume of plasma that contains the same quantity of that substance or the volume of plasma that must be filtered per minute to account for that amount in the urine is U_xV/P_x, the standard clearance formula. The clearance of any substance may be calculated, but the clearance of certain substances (e.g., inulin, p-aminohippuric acid, creatinine) provides important information about renal function (see later).

▶ Glomerular Filtration

Glomerular Morphology

The glomerular capillary wall or filtration barrier consists of three components: the capillary endothelium, basement membrane, and visceral epithelium (see Fig. 2–2). The glomerulus is a unique vascular structure consisting of a capillary bed interposed between two arterioles, the afferent and efferent arterioles. The glomerular capillary divides into several branches, each of which forms a lobule of the glomerulus. The *capillary endothelium* of the glomerulus is fenestrated by openings 50 to 100 nm in diameter. These openings exclude cells from the ultrafiltrate, but macromolecules are not restricted on the basis of size. The luminal surface of the endothelium is covered by negatively charged sialoglycoproteins that contribute to the charge selectivity of the filtration barrier.

The *glomerular basement membrane* is composed of the lamina rara interna on the endothelial side, the central lamina densa, and the lamina rara externa on the epithelial side. The lamina rara interna and lamina rara externa contain polar noncollagenous proteins that contribute to the negative charge of the filtration barrier. The lamina densa contains nonpolar collagenous proteins that contribute primarily to the size selectivity of the filtration barrier. The filtration barrier is permeable to molecules with effective molecular radii less than 2 nm and impermeable to those with radii greater than 4 nm.

The *visceral epithelial cells* or *podocytes* constitute

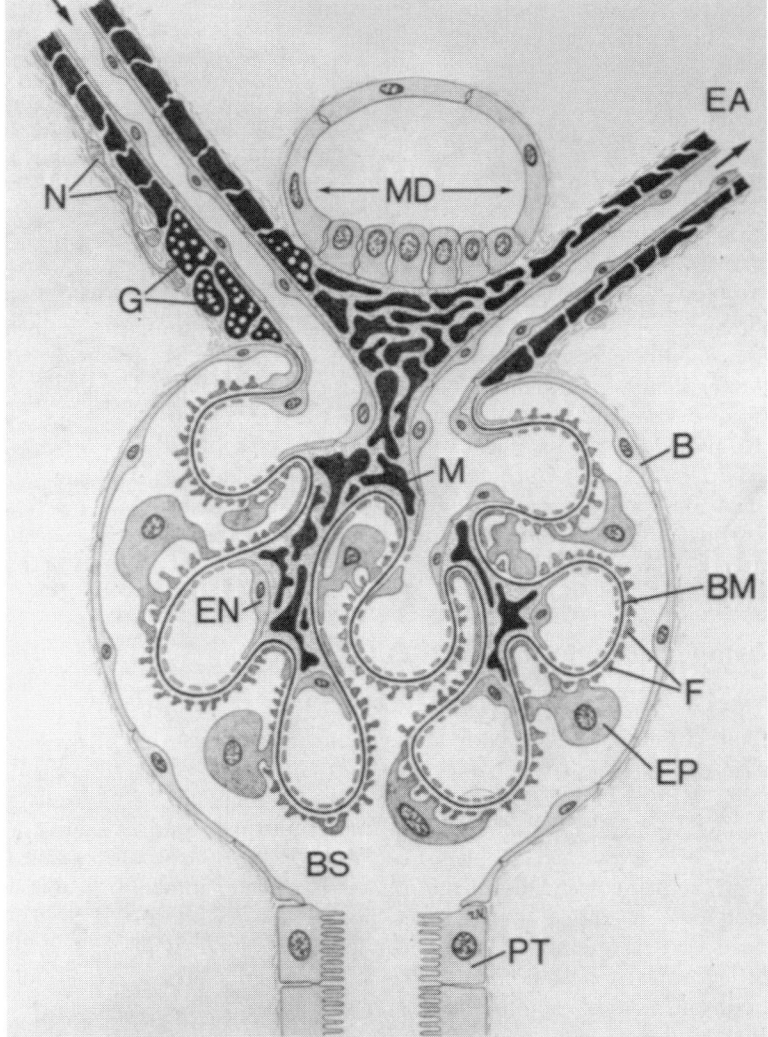

FIGURE 2–2. Schematic representation of the glomerulus demonstrating the afferent and efferent arterioles, juxtaglomerular apparatus, and glomerular capillary loops. At the vascular pole an afferent arteriole enters and an efferent arteriole (EA) leaves the glomerulus. At the urinary pole Bowman's space (BS) becomes the tubular lumen of the proximal tubule (PT). The epithelial cells composing Bowman's capsule (B) enclose Bowman's space. Smooth muscle cells proper of the arterioles and all cells derived from smooth muscle are shown in black, including the granular cells (G). The afferent arteriole is innervated by sympathetic nerve terminals (N). The extraglomerular mesangial cells are located at the angle between AA and EA and continue into the mesangial cells (M) of the glomerular tuft. The glomerular capillaries are outlined by fenestrated endothelial cells (EN) and covered from the outside by the epithelial cells (EP) with foot processes (F). The glomerular basement membrane (BM) is continuous throughout the glomerulus. At the vascular pole, the thick ascending limb touches with the macula densa (MD), the extraglomerular mesangium. (From Koushanpour E and Kriz W: *Renal Physiology: Principles, Structure, and Function*, 2nd ed. New York, Springer-Verlag, p. 55, 1986.)

the outermost portion of the filtration barrier. They cover the glomerular basement membrane and glomerular capillaries on the urinary side of the barrier with their primary and interdigitating secondary foot processes. Filtration slits, 10 to 30 nm in width, are located between the secondary foot processes. The podocytes are phagocytic and may engulf macromolecules trapped by the filtration slits. They are invested with a negatively charged sialoglycoprotein coat that contributes to the charge selectivity of the filtration barrier. The glomerular basement membrane is thought to be synthesized by the visceral epithelial cells.

The *mesangium* is not a part of the filtration barrier but a stabilizing core of tissue forming an anchor for the glomerulus at the vascular pole and along the axes of the capillary lobules. The mesangial cells are in contact with the basement membrane in areas where there is no capillary endothelium. The extraglomerular mesangium fills the space between the macula densa and the glomerular arterioles and constitutes part of the juxtaglomerular apparatus (JGA). The mesangial cells contain microfilaments and can contract in response to specific hormones (e.g., angiotensin II), thus altering the surface area available for filtration. They also synthesize prostaglandins that contribute to renal vasodilatation. The mesangium also contains macrophages that can clear filtration residues from the mesangial space by phagocytosis.

The glomerular capillary wall is both a size- and a charge-selective barrier to filtration. Its *size selectivity* resides primarily in the lamina densa of the glomerular basement membrane. The glomerulus generally excludes molecules with of radii greater than 4 nm. Inulin, with a molecular mass of 5200 daltons and radius of 1.4 nm permeates freely, whereas serum albumin, with a molecular mass of 69,000 daltons and radius of 3.6 nm, permeates minimally.

The *charge selectivity* of the glomerulus resides in the negatively charged sialoglycoproteins (e.g., laminin, fibronectin) and peptidoglycans (e.g., heparan sulfate) of the capillary endothelium, lamina rara interna, lamina rara externa, and visceral epithelium. At any given effective molecular radius, negatively charged macromolecules experience greater restriction to filtration than do neutral ones. Positively charged macromolecules experience less restriction to filtration than do neutral ones of the same size (Fig. 2–3).

Determinants of Glomerular Filtration

The term *glomerular filtration rate* (GFR) refers to the total filtration rate of both kidneys and represents the sum of the *single-nephron glomerular filtration rates* (SNGFRs) of all nephrons. The SNGFR may differ among some groups of nephrons under normal conditions, and additional changes may occur in response to such factors as water deprivation, increased water intake, increased salt intake, or increased protein intake. Superficial cortical nephrons have short loops of Henle with little or no penetration into the renal medulla. These nephrons tend to excrete relatively more solute and water. Juxtamedullary nephrons have long loops of Henle that

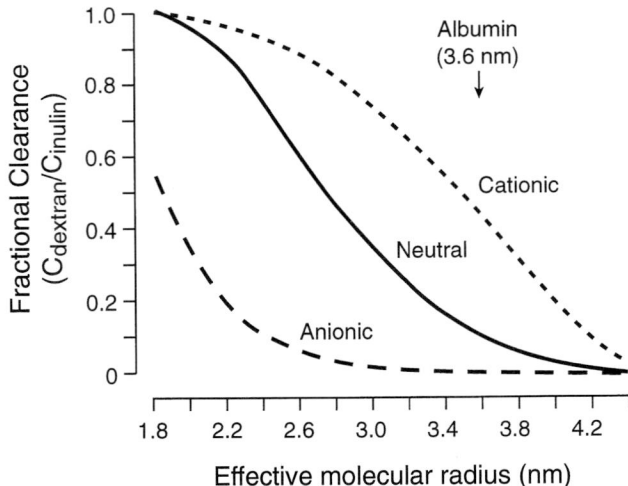

FIGURE 2–3. Effect of electrostatic charge on filtration of macromolecules across the glomerular capillary wall. (Drawing by Tim Vojt.)

penetrate the inner medulla, and these nephrons tend to conserve solute and water.

The glomerular ultrafiltrate is a protein-free ultrafiltrate of plasma containing water and all the crystalloids of plasma in concentrations similar to those in plasma. The concentrations are not exactly the same because of the Gibbs-Donnan effect. The SNGFR is determined by the same Starling forces that govern the movement of fluid across other capillaries in the body, but there are some important differences in the glomerulus that account for the relatively high rate of filtration:

$$\text{SNGFR} = K_f[(P_{GC} - P_T) - (\pi_{GC} - \pi_T)]$$

where P_{GC} is the hydrostatic pressure in the glomerular capillary, which falls slightly along the length of the glomerular capillary, averaging 55 mm Hg; P_T is the hydrostatic pressure in Bowman's space which is higher than systemic interstitial pressure, averaging 20 mm Hg; π_{GC} is the oncotic pressure in the glomerular capillary, which increases along the length of the capillary because of loss of protein-free ultrafiltrate into Bowman's space, averaging 20 mm Hg; and π_T is the oncotic pressure in Bowman's space and is negligible because the ultrafiltrate is nearly protein free. If π_T is neglected, the formula for SNGFR simplifies to

$$\text{SNGFR} = K_f(P_{GC} - P_T - \pi_{GC})$$

These relationships are depicted in Figure 2–4, in which average pressure values are those reported for dogs (Navar et al. 1977) and cats (Brown 1993). If the average pressures just described are considered alone, it can be seen that the net filtration pressure in the glomerulus is approximately 15 mm Hg, which is similar to values obtained for systemic capillaries. The fact that GFR is so much higher than the movement of fluid across systemic capillaries is explained by different values for K_f.

The ultrafiltration constant, K_f, is dependent on the surface area available for filtration and the permeability per unit area of capillary to crystalloids and water. The morphology of the glomerulus is such that the surface area available for filtration is greater than that found

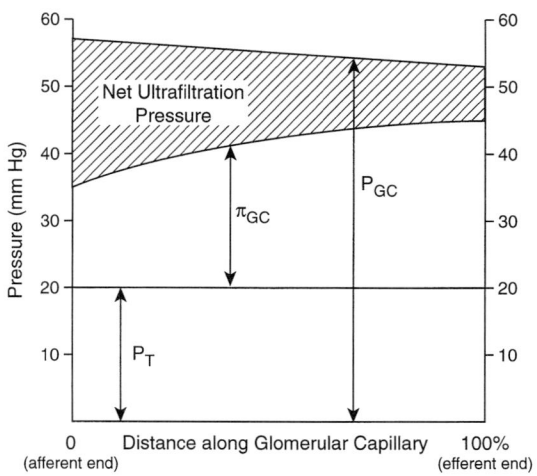

		Mean values for Dog and Cat	
P_{GC}	Hydrostatic pressure in glomerular capillary	52	58
π_{GC}	Plasma oncotic pressure in glomerular capillary	20	22
P_T	Hydrostatic pressure in Bowman's Space	20	18
π_T	Oncotic pressure in Bowman's Space	0	0
	Net ultrafiltration pressure	12	18

FIGURE 2-4. Graphic representation of the generation of net filtration pressure in the glomerulus as governed by Starling forces. (Drawing by Tim Vojt.)

in the capillary beds of skeletal muscle and the unit permeability of the glomerular endothelium is more than 100 times that of skeletal muscle capillaries. This much higher value for K_f in glomerular capillaries than in systemic capillaries accounts for the much higher rate of filtration. The ultrafiltration coefficient, K_f, is not constant and can change as a result of disease and in response to hormones that cause mesangial cells to contract (e.g., angiotensin II).

Changes in the resistance of the afferent (preglomerular) and efferent (postglomerular) arterioles may have a marked effect on GFR. Alterations in resistance in the afferent arterioles lead to parallel changes in GFR and renal blood flow (RBF), but changes in resistance in the efferent arterioles lead to divergent changes in GFR and RBF (Fig. 2-5). The interplay of the effects of neural and hormonal factors on vascular tone in the kidney is complex, but the main purpose of these effects is to minimize even slight changes in GFR that could have drastic adverse effects on the volume and composition of the extracellular fluid.

The resistance of these arterioles is regulated by the autonomic nervous system and by numerous vasoactive mediators (Table 2-1). Stimulation of the sympathetic nervous system results in release of norepinephrine from nerves terminating on the afferent and efferent arterioles. Norepinephrine can cause both afferent and efferent vasoconstriction, but efferent arteriolar constriction usually predominates. As a result, RBF decreases with minimal changes in GFR (i.e., filtration fraction increases). Angiotensin II also causes efferent more than afferent vasoconstriction and has similar effects on RBF and GFR. Stimulation of dopaminergic receptors causes afferent

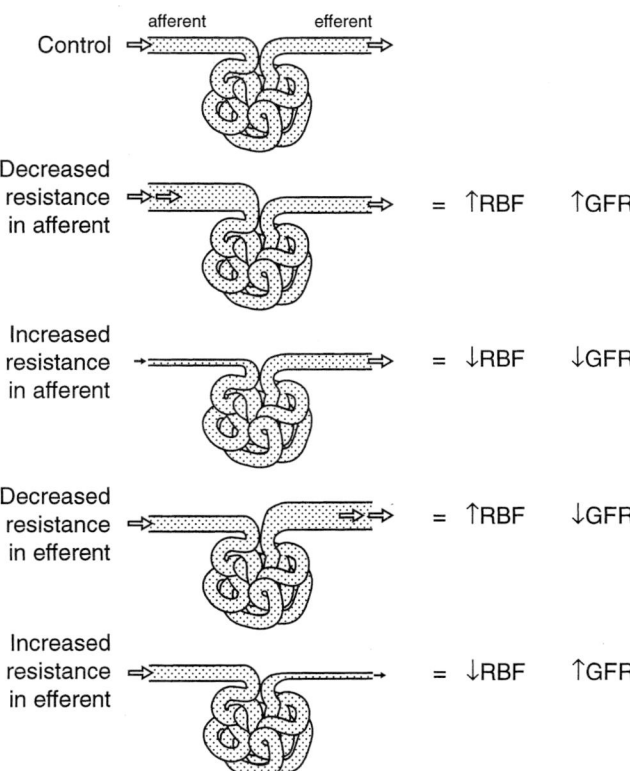

FIGURE 2-5. Effects of alterations in afferent and efferent arteriolar tone on renal blood flow and glomerular filtration rate. (Drawing by Tim Vojt.)

and efferent vasodilatation and increased RBF with little change in GFR at low concentrations of dopamine. Norepinephrine, angiotensin II, and antidiuretic hormone (ADH, vasopressin) cause vasoconstriction while at the same time promoting the production of prostaglandins that cause vasodilatation. These prostaglandins (PGE_2 and PGI_2) play an important role in maintaining renal blood

TABLE 2-1. Effects of Selected Vasoactive Mediators on Glomerular Hemodynamics

Substance	Afferent Arteriole	Efferent Arteriole
Vasodilators		
Acetylcholine	Relax	Relax
Nitric oxide	Relax	Relax
Dopamine	Relax	Relax
Bradykinin	Relax	Relax
Prostacyclin	Relax	Relax
Prostaglandin E_2	Relax	No effect
Prostaglandin I_2	Relax	Relax
Vasoconstrictors		
Norepinephrine	Constrict	Constrict
Angiotensin II	Constrict	Constrict
Endothelin	Constrict	Constrict
Thromboxane	Constrict	Constrict
Vasopressin	No effect	Constrict

Source: From Valtin H and Schafer JA: *Renal Function*. Boston, Little, Brown and Co., p. 107, 1995.

flow in hypovolemic states when angiotensin II and norepinephrine concentrations are increased. The effects of these prostaglandins are limited to the kidney, because they are rapidly metabolized in the pulmonary circulation. Nonsteroidal anti-inflammatory drugs that inhibit generation of prostaglandins by the cyclooxygenase pathway may cause renal ischemia and acute renal insufficiency in hypovolemic patients (Clive and Stoff 1984; Dunn 1984). Locally produced kinins also cause vasodilatation and favor redistribution of RBF to inner cortical nephrons. Mediators produced locally by the vascular endothelium also contribute to afferent and efferent vasoconstriction (e.g., endothelin, thromboxane) and vasodilatation (e.g., nitric oxide, prostacyclin).

Measurement of Glomerular Filtration Rate

Consider a substance that is filtered by the glomeruli but neither reabsorbed nor secreted by the tubules. Under steady-state conditions, the following mass balance equation may be written:

$$\text{Amount filtered} = \text{amount excreted}$$
$$P_x \times \text{GFR} = U_x \times V$$

where P_x is the plasma concentration of x (mg/mL), U_x is the urine concentration of x (mg/mL), V is the urine flow rate (mL/min), and GFR is the glomerular filtration rate (mL/min). Dividing both sides of the equation by P_x:

$$\text{GFR} = U_x V / P_x$$

Note that this equation is the same as the formula for clearance presented before. Thus, the renal clearance of a substance that is neither reabsorbed nor secreted is equal to GFR. Inulin is a polymer of fructose with a molecular mass of 5200 daltons. It is not bound to plasma proteins and is freely filtered by the glomeruli. It is neither reabsorbed nor secreted by the tubules. It is not metabolized by the kidney or any other organ. It is uncharged and not subject to the Gibbs-Donnan effect. In summary, inulin is an ideal substance for the measurement of GFR, and inulin clearance is the laboratory standard for GFR determination. Normal values for GFR as measured by inulin clearance are 3 to 5 mL/min/kg in the dog (Finco et al. 1981; Fettman et al. 1985) and 2.5 to 3.5 mL/min/kg in the cat (Ross and Finco 1981; Fettman et al. 1985).

Inulin clearance is not used clinically because it requires intravenous infusion of inulin and an assay that is not routinely available in most clinical pathology laboratories. Creatinine is produced endogenously in the body and excreted primarily by glomerular filtration, so its clearance can be used to estimate GFR in the steady state. The only requirements for determination of *endogenous* creatinine clearance are an accurately timed urine sample (usually 24 h), determination of the patient's body weight, and measurement of serum and urine creatinine concentrations.

In the dog and cat, creatinine is filtered by the glomeruli and is neither reabsorbed nor secreted by the tubules (Finco et al. 1981, 1991, 1993; Finco and Barsanti 1982). In most clinical pathology laboratories, creatinine is measured by the alkaline picrate reaction. This reaction is not entirely specific for creatinine and measures another group of substances collectively known as noncreatinine chromagens. These substances are found in plasma, where they may constitute up to 50% of the measured creatinine at normal serum creatinine concentrations, but only small amounts appear in urine (Finco and Duncan 1976; Finco et al. 1993). When the creatinine concentration is determined using the alkaline picrate reaction, the presence of noncreatinine chromagens causes endogenous creatinine clearance to underestimate GFR. This problem may be avoided by using more accurate methods (e.g., peroxidase-antiperoxidase) to measure the creatinine concentration (Finco et al. 1993). Values for endogenous creatinine clearance in the dog and cat are approximately 2 to 5 mL/min/kg (Finco 1971; Bovee and Joyce 1979; Finco et al. 1993).

To circumvent the problem of noncreatinine chromagens and improve accuracy, some investigators have advocated determination of *exogenous* creatinine clearance. In this test, which is somewhat more cumbersome, creatinine is administered subcutaneously to the animal to increase the serum creatinine concentration and reduce the relative effect of the noncreatinine chromagens. For example, a normal dog might have a serum creatinine concentration of 1.0 mg/dL, of which 0.5 mg/dL represents noncreatinine chromagens. This measurement represents a 50% error. If, however, the dog's serum creatinine concentration is increased to 10 mg/dL by subcutaneous administration of creatinine, the noncreatinine chromagens still represent only 0.5 mg/dL and the error is reduced to 5%. Exogenous creatinine clearance exceeds endogenous creatinine clearance and more closely approximates inulin clearance in the dog (Finco et al. 1981).

The amount of any substance excreted by the kidneys is the algebraic sum of the amount filtered and the amount handled by the tubules:

$$U_x V = P_x \text{GFR} + T_x$$

where T_x is the amount handled by tubules (mg/min).

The term T_x is a positive number if the substance experiences net secretion and a negative number if it experiences net reabsorption. Dividing both sides of the equation by P_x yields the familiar clearance formula:

$$C_x = \text{GFR} + T_x / P_x$$

Thus, the clearance of a substance experiencing net reabsorption is less than GFR (T_x is negative) and the clearance of a substance experiencing net secretion is greater than GFR (T_x is positive). The ratio of the clearance of a substance to inulin clearance gives an indication of the net handling of that substance by the kidney. If the ratio is less than 1.0, the substance experiences net reabsorption; if it is greater than 1.0, it experiences net secretion.

▶ Renal Blood Flow and Renal Plasma Flow

The kidneys receive 25% or more of cardiac output. The major sites of resistance within the kidney are the afferent and efferent arterioles, with an approximately 80 to 90%

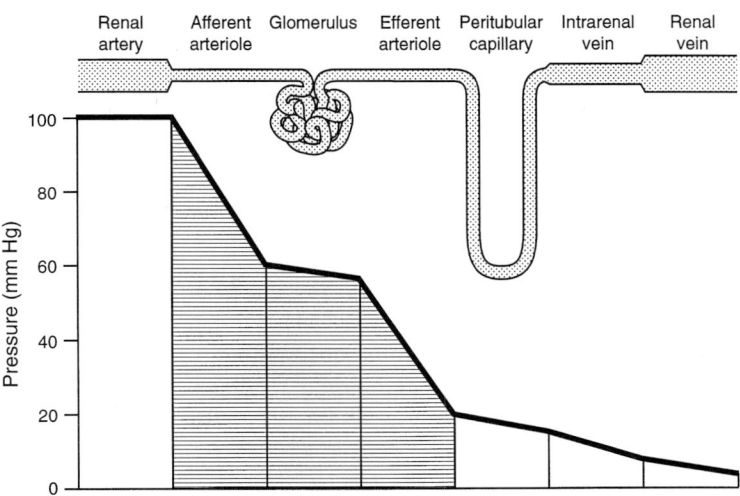

FIGURE 2-6. Pattern of hydrostatic pressure and vascular resistance in the renal circulation. (Drawing by Tim Vojt.)

drop in perfusion pressure across this region of the renal vasculature (Fig. 2–6). Blood flow is not uniform throughout the kidney. In dogs, more than 90% of RBF is normally directed to the renal cortex, less than 10% to the outer medulla, and only 2 to 3% to the inner medulla (Valtin and Schafer 1995a). The actual rate of flow to the renal cortex is approximately 100 times that of resting muscle and is required for glomerular filtration. Blood flow to the medulla is similar to that of resting muscle, and this reduced flow is necessary for normal function of the urinary concentrating mechanism.

Autoregulation

Autoregulation refers to the intrinsic ability of an organ to maintain blood flow at a nearly constant rate despite changes in arterial perfusion pressure. In the kidney, between perfusion pressures of 80 and 180 mm Hg, GFR and RBF vary less than 10% (Fig. 2–7). Flow (Q) is equal to pressure (P) divided by resistance (R). As pressure increases, flow can remain constant only if resistance increases proportionately. The site of this resistance change in the kidney is the afferent arteriole. Autoregulation is intrinsic to the kidney and occurs in the isolated, denervated kidney and in the adrenalectomized animal. It is, however, impaired by anesthesia in proportion to the depth of anesthesia. The afferent arterioles are maximally dilated at mean arterial pressures of 70 to 80 mm Hg and, at lower pressures, GFR declines linearly with RBF (i.e., autoregulation is lost). It is likely that autoregulation of RBF is a consequence of the need to regulate GFR closely and thus maintain tight control over water and salt balance.

Two physiologic mechanisms contribute to autoregulation. The *myogenic mechanism* is based on the principle that smooth muscle tends to contract when stretched and relax when shortened. Thus, as the afferent arteriole is stretched by increased perfusion pressure, it constricts, thus limiting transmission of this increased pressure to the glomerulus and minimizing any change in glomerular capillary hydrostatic pressure and SNGFR. The myogenic mechanism represents a coarse control that operates with a delay of 1 to 2 s.

Tubuloglomerular feedback represents a local intrarenal negative feedback mechanism for individual nephrons. The morphologic basis for this physiologic mechanism

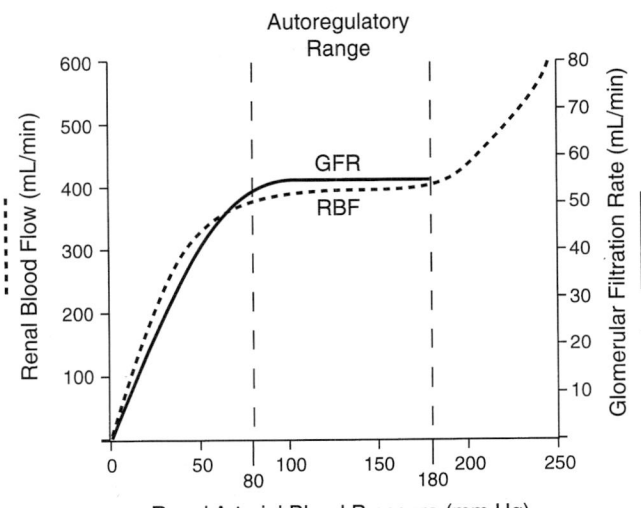

FIGURE 2-7. Autoregulation of renal blood flow and glomerular filtration rate. (Drawing by Tim Vojt.)

is the JGA. Increased sodium chloride concentration or transport in the distal tubule is sensed by the extraglomerular mesangial cells of the JGA as they monitor sodium chloride transport across the tubular cells of the macula densa. This results in afferent arteriolar constriction and possibly decreased capillary permeability in the parent glomerulus. The local mediator of this afferent arteriolar constriction is unknown. It may be adenosine, or it may result from increased interstitial chloride concentration or osmolality in the region of the JGA. Whatever the cause of the afferent arteriolar constriction, SNGFR is decreased, thus reducing filtration and minimizing NaCl loss in that nephron. Tubuloglomerular feedback represents a fine control that operates with a 10- to 12-s delay.

Measurement of Renal Blood Flow and Renal Plasma Flow

Consider the following mass balance equation (Valtin and Schafer 1995b):

Amount entering the kidney = amount leaving the kidney

$$P_{AX} \times RPF_A = P_{VX} \times RPF_V + U_XV$$
$$P_{AX} \times RPF_A - P_{VX} \times RPF_V = U_XV$$

where P_{AX} is the renal arterial plasma concentration of x, RPF_A is the arterial renal plasma flow, P_{VX} is the renal venous plasma concentration of x, RPF_V is the venous renal plasma flow, U_X is the urine concentration of x, and V is the urine flow.

If we ignore the slight difference between renal arterial and venous plasma flow (with probably less than 1% error), the equation simplifies to

$$(P_{AX} - P_{VX}) RPF = U_XV$$
$$RPF = U_XV/(P_{AX} - P_{VX})$$

If we choose a substance that is completely removed from the blood in one pass through the kidney, P_{VX} is zero and $RPF = U_X V/P_{AX}$. If the substance x is not metabolized and is not excreted by any organ other than the kidney, its concentration in any peripheral vessel equals P_{AX}. Thus, $RPF = U_XV/P_X$.

P-Aminohippuric acid (PAH) is filtered by the glomeruli and secreted by the peritubular capillaries into the tubules so that approximately 90% of it is removed in one pass through the kidney. It is not metabolized or excreted by any other organ. Thus, it approximately meets the preceding assumptions and $RPF = U_{PAH}V/P_{PAH}$. Now, it can be seen that the clearance of PAH is an estimate of RPF. When PAH is infused during a clearance study, it is essential that P_{PAH} be maintained at a concentration much below the tubular transport maximum (T_{max}) for PAH. If not, P_{VX} cannot be neglected.

Some blood flows through regions of the kidney that do not remove PAH (e.g., renal capsule, perirenal fat, renal pelvis) and, as a result, P_{VX} is not really zero. Thus, the term *effective* renal plasma flow is more appropriately used when speaking of PAH clearance. Furthermore, only 90% of PAH is removed from the blood during a single pass through the kidney. This also contributes to the fact that P_{VX} for PAH is not really zero. A closer approximation of RPF can be determined by sampling renal arterial and venous blood and measuring their respective PAH concentrations. The *extraction ratio* for PAH is then determined:

$$E_X = (P_{AX} - P_{VX})/P_{AX}$$

A more accurate calculation of RPF is then

$$RPF = C_{PAH}/E_{PAH}$$
$$RPF = U_{PAH}V/P_{PAH}E_{PAH}$$

The extraction ratio for PAH is 0.9 because approximately 90% of it is removed from the blood in a single pass through the kidney. Notice that if we substitute the equation for E_X into the preceding equation we get $RPF = U_XV/(P_{AX} - P_{VX})$, which is the same equation as derived before for RPF.

Another way to determine RPF is by use of the Fick principle, which states that the amount of a substance (V) removed by an organ is equal to the blood flow to the organ (Q) times the arteriovenous concentration difference of the substance in question ($C_A - C_V$):

$$V = Q(C_A - C_V)$$
$$Q = V/(C_A - C_V)$$

Using the kidney as an example and equating the amount of the substance removed to the amount excreted (U_XV):

$$RPF = U_XV/(P_{AX} - P_{VX})$$

Note that this equation is identical to that derived before using the mass balance principle.

If the hematocrit is known, RBF can be calculated from the RPF by using the following equation:

$$RBF = \frac{RPF}{(1 - hematocrit)}$$

In the dog and cat, normal values for RPF are 7 to 20 mL/min/kg and 8 to 22 mL/min/kg, respectively (Osbaldiston and Fuhrman 1970; Powers et al. 1977; Ross and Finco 1981).

If all of the plasma were filtered in one pass of blood through the glomeruli, an immovable mass of red blood cells would be all that remained behind at the efferent arteriole of the glomerular capillary. This does not occur because π_{GC} increases along the length of the capillary and, in conjunction with P_T, effectively opposes further filtration. The *filtration fraction* is the fraction of plasma flowing through the kidneys that is filtered into Bowman's space. It is determined by the following equation:

$$\text{Filtration fraction (FF)} = GFR/RPF$$

In the dog and cat, values for FF are 0.32 to 0.36 and 0.33 to 0.41, respectively. These values are higher than those observed in humans, in whom FF is approximately 0.20.

▶ Renal Tubular Function

The terms reabsorption and secretion refer to the direction of transport across an epithelium. In the kidney, *reabsorption* refers to movement of water and solutes from the tubular lumen to the peritubular interstitium. *Secretion* refers to movement of water and solutes from the peritubular interstitium to the tubular lumen. Some substances experience reabsorption in one part of the nephron and secretion in another part (e.g., urate, potassium). Often, the term reabsorption is used to denote net reabsorption, which is the algebraic sum of the fluxes in both directions across the renal tubular epithelium.

The *luminal* membranes separate the cytoplasm of the tubular cell from the tubular fluid. The *basolateral* membranes separate the cytoplasm of the tubular cell from the lateral intercellular spaces and the peritubular interstitium. The *transmembrane* potential difference (PD) refers to the electrical PD between the outside and inside of the cell. The *transepithelial* or *transtubular* PD is the electrical PD between the tubular lumen and the peritubular interstitium and is the algebraic sum of the transmembrane PD between the tubular lumen and cell cytoplasm and the transmembrane PD between the peritubular interstitium and cell cytoplasm. These relationships are depicted in Figure 2–8. Transmembrane PD is usually −60 to −70 mV (cell interior negative), whereas transepithelial PD is only a few mV. In the early proximal tubule, the tubular lumen is a few mV negative relative to the peritubular interstitium, whereas in the later proximal tubule the tubular lumen is a few mV positive relative to the peritubular interstitium. In the thick ascending limb of Henle's loop the transepithelial PD is lumen positive, but in the distal tubule the transepithelial PD is lumen negative. The transepithelial PD affects movement of charged solutes across the renal tubular epithelium and contributes to the electrochemical gradient for such solutes.

The *paracellular* route refers to movement of solutes and water between cells (i.e., from the tubular lumen to the lateral intercellular space across tight junctions connecting epithelial cells). The *transcellular* route refers to movement of solutes and water through the cytoplasm of the tubular cells. Tight junctions between renal epithelial cells at the luminal surface are classified as *leaky* (proximal tubules) or *tight* (distal convoluted tubules, collecting ducts). Leaky epithelia do not generate large transepithelial concentration gradients, exhibit a small transepithelial PD, and have high water permeability, whereas tight epithelia can generate large transepithelial concentration gradients, exhibit a large transepithelial PD, and have low basal water permeability. The paracellular route allows movement of ions (e.g., potassium, chloride) and large, nonpolar solutes by passive diffusion and solvent drag. Electrochemical, hydrostatic, and oncotic gradients are important driving forces for reabsorption by the paracellular route. The paracellular route accounts for only 1% of the surface area available for reabsorption and 5 to 10% of water transport, whereas the transcellular route accounts for 99% of the available surface area and 90 to 95% of water transport. Both passive and active transport processes occur by the transcellular route, and all active transport processes must occur by this route.

That renal tubular reabsorption occurs may be recognized intuitively by considering the composition of normal urine. Many low-molecular-weight solutes essential to normal physiological function (e.g., glucose, amino acids, bicarbonate) are freely filtered at the glomerulus but do

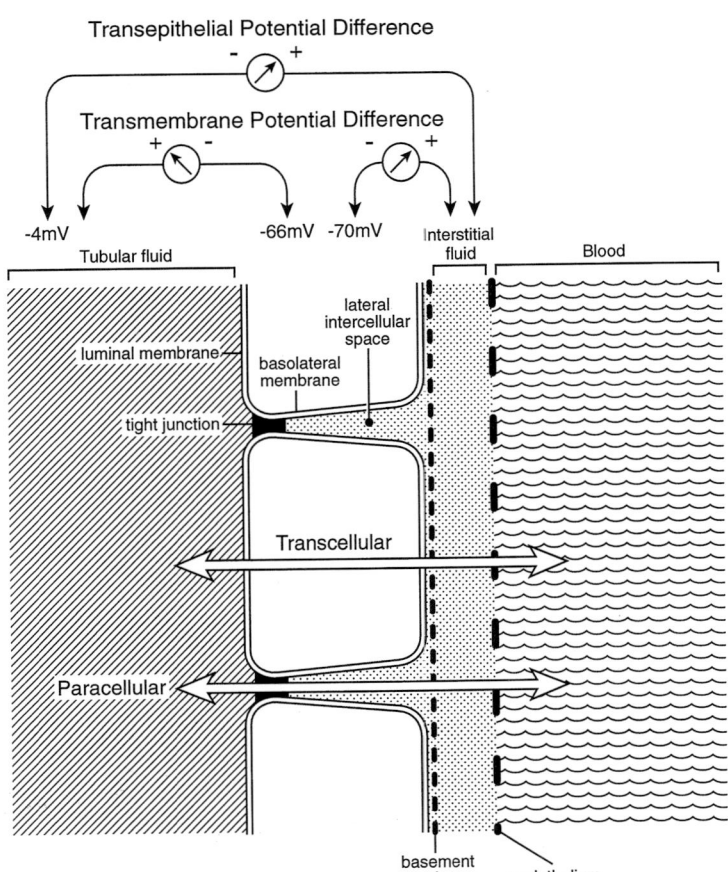

FIGURE 2–8. Diagram demonstrating selected terminology as applied to the renal tubular epithelium: luminal versus basolateral membranes, transmembrane versus transepithelial potential difference, transcellular versus paracellular transport. (Drawing by Tim Vojt.)

not normally appear in urine. Thus, they must have been reabsorbed along the course of the renal tubule. In the proximal tubule, water follows solute reabsorption osmotically and solute reabsorption is said to occur isosmotically (i.e., the reabsorbed fluid has the same osmolality as extracellular fluid). Approximately two-thirds of all water and solute reabsorption occurs in the proximal tubules. Almost 99% of glucose and amino acids and 90% or more of bicarbonate are reabsorbed in the early proximal tubules (Fig. 2–9). The reabsorption of bicarbonate occurs as a consequence of the tubular secretion of hydrogen ions and is crucial to renal regulation of acid-base balance (see Chapter 9).

Renal Transport Processes

Four types of transport processes contribute to renal tubular reabsorption: passive diffusion, facilitated diffusion, primary active transport, and secondary active transport.

Passive diffusion is the movement of a substance across a membrane as a result of random molecular motion. Simple diffusion can take place directly through the lipid bilayer of the cell membrane, which occurs for substances with high lipid solubility. Simple diffusion can also occur through hydrophilic protein channels embedded in the cell membrane. Simple diffusion requires no expenditure of metabolic energy. The rate of transfer of solute is dependent on the permeability characteristics of the membrane, the electrochemical gradient (i.e., the combination of the electrical PD and chemical concentration difference across the membrane), and the hydrostatic pressure across the membrane. The rate of diffusion is linearly related to the concentration of the diffusing solute and there is no maximal rate of transfer (V_{max}). Passive diffusion is not a saturable process because a carrier is not involved.

Facilitated diffusion is the movement of a substance across a membrane down its electrochemical gradient after binding with a specific carrier protein in the membrane. The carrier protein binds the substance to be transported at one side of the cell membrane. The occupied carrier then undergoes a conformational change that causes translocation of the substance across the cell membrane. The substance is then released from the carrier on the other side of the membrane. Unlike simple diffusion, facilitated diffusion is a saturable process characterized by a maximal rate of transfer (V_{max}) because a carrier is involved. The carrier has structural specificity and affinity for the substance transported, and the process is subject to competitive inhibition. Facilitated diffusion does not directly require metabolic energy, and transfer may occur in either direction across the membrane depending on the prevailing electrochemical gradient. Examples of facilitated diffusion in the proximal tubule include the transport of glucose and amino acids at the basolateral membrane.

Primary active transport is the movement of a substance across a membrane in combination with a carrier protein but against an electrochemical gradient. Active transport requires metabolic energy, which is supplied by the hydrolysis of ATP. It is a saturable process characterized by a V_{max} and is subject to metabolic (e.g., cellular oxidative poisons) and competitive (e.g., competition for the carrier by a structurally similar compound) inhibition. Examples of primary active transporters include Na^+,K^+-adenosinetriphosphatase (Na^+,K^+-ATPase) in basolateral membranes and H^+-ATPase in luminal membranes of tubular cells throughout the nephron and H^+,K^+-ATPase in luminal membranes of α-intercalated cells in the collecting ducts.

Secondary active transport is the movement of two substances across a membrane after combination with a single carrier protein. The process is called *cotransport* if the transported substances are moving in the same direction across the membrane (e.g., glucose, amino acids, or phosphate with sodium at the luminal membrane of the proximal tubular cell) and *countertransport* if the transported substances are moving in opposite directions across the membrane (e.g., sodium and hydrogen ions at the luminal membrane of the proximal tubular cell). The "uphill" (i.e., against a concentration gradient) transport of one substance (e.g., glucose) is linked to the "downhill" (i.e., down an electrochemical gradient) transport of another substance (e.g., sodium). When the carrier is occupied by only one of the substances it is not mobile in the cell membrane, whereas an unoccupied carrier or one that is occupied by both of the substances is mobile in the membrane. This process is saturable, demonstrates structural specificity and affinity of the carrier for the substances transported, and may be competitively inhibited. The uphill transport occurs without direct input of metabolic energy and the substance transported uphill is said to experience secondary active transport. The metabolic energy for secondary active transport at the luminal membranes comes from the primary active transport of sodium out of the tubular cell at the basolateral mem-

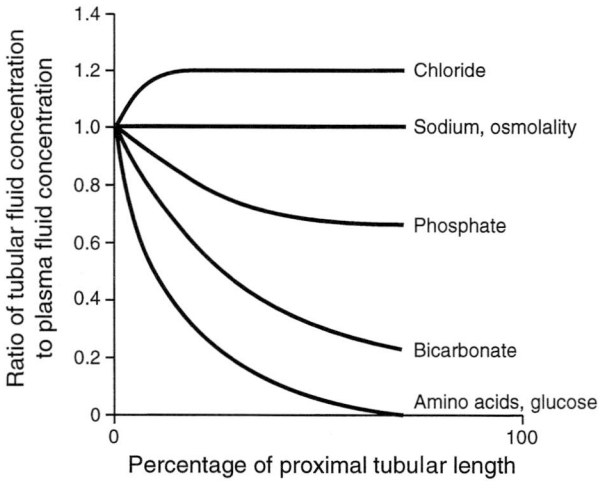

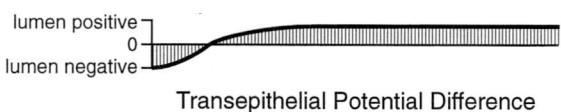

FIGURE 2–9. Changes in the solute composition and transepithelial potential difference along the length of the proximal nephron. (Drawing by Tim Vojt.)

brane by Na^+,K^+-ATPase, a process that maintains a low intracellular sodium concentration.

Pinocytosis refers to the uptake by cells of particles too large to diffuse through the cell membrane. Filtered proteins are reabsorbed in the proximal tubule by this mechanism (see later).

Solvent drag refers to the process whereby water (the solvent) moving across an epithelium by osmosis can drag dissolved solutes along with it.

Morphology of the Proximal Tubule

Several morphologic features of proximal tubular cells suggest their primary role in the reabsorption of solutes and water. The brush border of the luminal surface of the proximal tubular cells consists of microvilli, which increase surface area, and lateral cellular interdigitations, which increase the surface area of the basolateral membranes (Fig. 2–10). Abundant mitochondria supply energy in the form of ATP required for active transport.

The proximal tubule exhibits intrasegmental axial heterogeneity with the most proximal segments being ultrastructurally the most complex and suited for the mechanisms of solute transport described earlier (Koushanpour and Kriz 1986). This morphologic complexity decreases along the length of the proximal tubule. In the first segment of the proximal tubule (P1 or S1), sodium, water, bicarbonate, amino acids, glucose, and phosphate are transported. In the second segment (P2 or S2), sodium, water, and chloride are reabsorbed and organic acids and bases may be transported (Rose 1994a). Organic acids and bases may also be secreted in the third segment (P3 or S3) (Koushanpour and Kriz 1986). The low-specificity transport system for organic anions and cations in the proximal tubule allows elimination of many drugs and other foreign organic compounds from the body.

Sodium Transport

Sodium may enter tubular cells at their luminal surface by several different mechanisms. In the proximal tubule, sodium may be cotransported across the luminal membranes of the cell with glucose, amino acids, or phosphate or may experience countertransport with hydrogen ions secreted into the tubular lumen by the Na^+-H^+ antiporter that facilitates bicarbonate reabsorption. In the loop of Henle, sodium enters via an Na^+-K^+-$2Cl^-$ carrier that is competitively inhibited by furosemide (O'Grady et al. 1987), and in the distal convoluted tubule, sodium enters via an Na^+-Cl^- cotransporter that is inhibited by thiazide diuretics. In the collecting duct, sodium enters via a luminal sodium channel that generates a lumen-negative PD favoring chloride reabsorption.

Thus, in most segments of the nephron, sodium enters the tubular cell at the luminal membrane down an electrochemical gradient that favors sodium entry into the cell (i.e., the interior of the cell has a low sodium concentration and is negative with respect to the exterior). Sodium then experiences primary active transport out of the cell and into the lateral intercellular spaces and peritubular interstitium by the Na^+,K^+-ATPase located in the basolateral cell membranes. This enzyme hydrolyzes ATP and translocates two potassium ions into the cell and three sodium ions out of the cell (Avison et al. 1987). It is located only in the basolateral membranes and functions to maintain a favorable electrochemical gradient for the passive entry of sodium into the tubular cells across their luminal membranes. Thus, sodium is reabsorbed in conjunction with glucose, amino acids, phosphate, and bicarbonate in the proximal tubule and with chloride in the loop of Henle and distal tubule. The different mechanisms for sodium reabsorption in the nephron and the regulation of sodium reabsorption in the kidney are discussed in Chapter 3.

Glucose Transport

Sodium attaches to a carrier in the luminal membrane of the proximal tubular cell, and this step is followed by attachment of glucose to the carrier. Translocation of the carrier occurs and glucose is released to the interior of the cell while sodium enters down its electrochemical gradient (the interior of the cell is negative and its sodium concentration is low). As the intracellular glucose concentration increases, glucose leaves the cell by facilitated diffusion across the basolateral cell membranes. The Na^+,K^+-ATPase in the basolateral membranes continues to remove sodium from the cell, thus maintaining a favorable electrochemical gradient for sodium entry and expending the metabolic energy required for glucose transport.

Glucose transport meets the criteria for carrier-mediated transport in that it is a saturable process. Plotting the amount filtered ($P_x \times$ GFR), the amount excreted ($U_x \times V$), and the amount handled by the tubules (T_x) for a substance against the plasma concentration of that substance (P_x) yields a renal titration curve and allows determination of the *renal threshold* (plasma concentration at which the substance first appears in the urine) and *tubular transport maximum* (maximal amount of the substance that can be transported by the tubules, T_{max} or T_M). A renal titration curve for glucose is depicted in Figure 2–11. The T_{max} for glucose is constant and relatively high, so it is usually not exceeded in health. Consequently, the kidney does not regulate plasma glucose concentration. In human beings, the T_{max} for glucose is

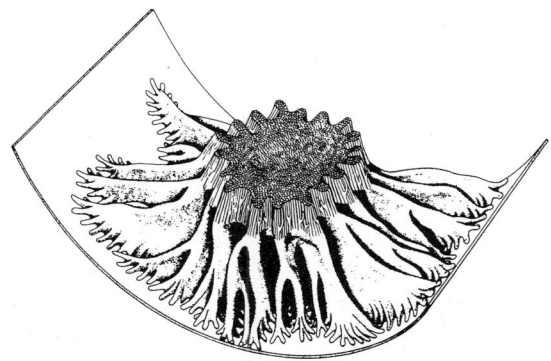

FIGURE 2–10. Three-dimensional model of a proximal tubular cell showing microvilli and lateral cellular interdigitations. (From Koushanpour E and Kriz W: *Renal Physiology: Principles, Structure, and Function*, 2nd ed. New York, Springer-Verlag, p. 141, 1986.)

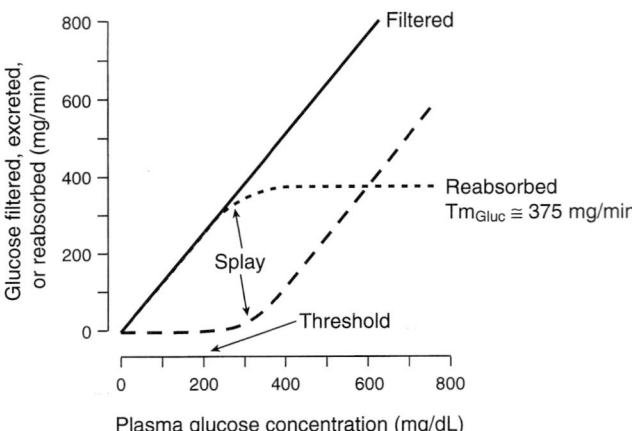

FIGURE 2-11. Glucose titration curve showing filtration, reabsorption, and urinary excretion of glucose at increasing plasma glucose concentrations. Tm_{Gluc} refers to the maximal amount of glucose that can be transported per minute. (Drawing by Tim Vojt.)

approximately 375 mg/min. In the dog, it is approximately 100 mg/min (Shannon et al. 1941; Keyes and Swanson 1971), and in the cat, 50 mg/min (Kruth and Cowgill 1982). In the renal titration curve, the T_{max} for glucose is approached somewhat gradually. This characteristic is called *splay* and is thought to be due to nephron heterogeneity. Some nephrons excrete glucose before the average T_{max} is reached, whereas others continue to reabsorb glucose after the average T_{max} has been reached (i.e., the T_{max} for glucose differs slightly among nephrons).

Phosphate

The uptake of phosphate into the proximal tubular cell is similar to that of glucose in that it is coupled to sodium entry at the luminal membrane. An important distinction from glucose transport, however, is that the T_{max} for phosphate is low and readily exceeded as plasma phosphate concentration increases. The T_{max} for phosphate is also altered by hormones, notably parathyroid hormone (PTH). Parathyroid hormone decreases the T_{max} for phosphate and increases renal phosphate excretion. Thus, the kidney, acting in concert with PTH, serves as a regulator of the plasma phosphate concentration.

Amino Acids

The proximal tubular reabsorption of amino acids is also coupled to luminal sodium uptake. The T_{max} values for the different groups of amino acids are very high and 99% of the filtered load of amino acids is reabsorbed in the proximal tubule. Thus, the kidney is not a regulator of plasma amino acid concentrations. There are at least four carrier systems for amino acids: one each for neutral, basic, acidic, and the iminoglycine (i.e., proline and hydroxyproline) amino acids.

Pinocytosis

Low-molecular-weight proteins (including several hormones and immunoglobulin light chains) are filtered at the glomerulus and reabsorbed by the proximal tubular cells, where they are hydrolyzed to their constituent amino acids, and these are returned to the circulation. Filtered proteins of small molecular mass may be hydrolyzed to amino acids by brush border enzymes at the luminal surface of the proximal tubular cell and their amino acids taken into the cell by cotransport with sodium. Alternatively, filtered proteins of larger molecular mass may attach to endocytic sites on the luminal cell membrane. These sites invaginate to form endosomes, which then fuse with lysosomes to form endolysosomes, in which digestion of the proteins occurs. The amino acids leave the endolysosomes and cross the basolateral membranes of the tubular cells by facilitated diffusion. This endocytic mechanism has a very high capacity, which is not normally exceeded in health.

Urea

Urea is passively reabsorbed in the proximal tubules. This passive reabsorption is dependent on the tubular flow rate. Increased tubular flow, as occurs during diuresis, is the result of decreased reabsorption of water from the tubular fluid. This decreases the tubular fluid urea concentration and decreases the concentration gradient of urea across the tubular epithelium. Thus, less urea is reabsorbed at higher tubular flow rates.

With decreased tubular flow, as occurs during dehydration, there is increased reabsorption of water from the tubular fluid. This increases the concentration gradient of urea across the tubular epithelium and increases passive urea reabsorption. In dehydrated patients, increased reabsorption of urea may lead to an increase in blood urea nitrogen (BUN) even before GFR is decreased. This contributes to the observation that the BUN/creatinine ratio tends to be higher in patients with prerenal azotemia than in hydrated patients with primary renal azotemia. The tubular handling of urea in other segments of the nephron plays an important role in the urinary concentrating mechanism.

▶ The Urinary Concentrating Mechanism

Urinary concentration is a function of the juxtamedullary nephrons with long loops of Henle that penetrate deep into the renal medulla. There are two main steps in this process. First, transport of sodium chloride without water from the ascending limb of Henle's loop renders the medullary interstitium hyperosmotic. Second, ADH (vasopressin) increases the water permeability of the collecting duct and tubular fluid traversing this segment of the nephron equilibrates osmotically with the hyperosmotic interstitium.

Strikingly different transport properties of various portions of the nephron form the basis for understanding the urinary concentrating mechanism (Table 2–2). The hairpin configuration of Henle's loop is the anatomic basis for countercurrent multiplication and allows a single osmotic effect to be multiplied over the length of the loop. The vessels accompanying the loops of Henle into the

TABLE 2–2. **Differential Permeability Characteristics of Nephron Segments**

Portion of Nephron	NaCl	Urea	Water (ADH)	Water (No ADH)
Descending limb of Henle's loop*	Passive	Passive†	Passive	Passive
Thin ascending limb of Henle's loop*	Passive	Passive†	0	0
Thick ascending limb of Henle's loop	Active	0	0	0
Distal convoluted tubule	Active	0	0	0
Cortical collecting duct	Active‡	0	Passive	0
Outer medullary collecting duct	0	0	Passive	0
Inner medullary collecting duct	Active	Passive	Passive§	0

Source: Modified from Rose BD: *Clinical Physiology of Acid-Base and Electrolyte Disorders.* New York, McGraw-Hill, p. 112, 1994, with permission of the McGraw-Hill Companies.
*Permeability to NaCl exceeds permeability to urea in these segments.
†Passive reabsorption in these segments constitutes urea recycling.
‡Responsive to aldosterone.
§Permeable to urea in the basal state and permeability increased by ADH.

medulla are called vasa recta. They prevent dissipation of the medullary osmotic gradient by a process called countercurrent exchange (see later). The countercurrent multiplier concept was first applied to urine concentration by W. Kuhn, a physical chemist, in 1942 (Berliner 1982; Jamison 1987) As early as 1909, however, K. Peter had noted a correlation between the length of the Henle's loop and the ability of a given species to concentrate its urine.

Role of the Ascending Limb of Henle's Loop

The ascending limb of Henle's loop is impermeable to water. Sodium chloride is actively transported from the thick portion of the ascending limb without accompanying water so that an osmotic gradient of approximately 200 mOsm/kg is generated. This active transport of sodium chloride is the primary energy-requiring step of the urinary concentrating mechanism.

Active sodium transport is accomplished by the Na^+,K^+-ATPase located in the basolateral membranes of the tubular cells. This enzyme maintains a low intracellular concentration of sodium and promotes passive entry of sodium at the luminal membrane down a concentration gradient. The luminal carrier binds one sodium ion, one potassium ion, and two chloride ions (O'Grady et al. 1987). Chloride delivery is the rate-limiting step in this transport process, and loop diuretics such as furosemide impair distal sodium reabsorption by competing with chloride for the luminal carrier (O'Grady et al. 1987).

Fluid reaching the distal convoluted tubule is hyposmotic (100 mOsm/kg) compared with the fluid entering the descending limb of Henle's loop (300 mOsm/kg). If fluid in the loops were stationary, the active transport of sodium chloride out of the thick ascending limb without water would increase the interstitial osmolality to 400 mOsm/kg and decrease the osmolality of the fluid within the ascending limb to 200 mOsm/kg. The descending limb of Henle's loop is highly permeable to water and water would be extracted from this site, increasing the osmolality of the tubular fluid in this segment of the nephron to 400 mOsm/kg.

The fluid within Henle's loops, however, is not stationary. New tubular fluid with an osmolality of 300 mOsm/kg is constantly entering the descending limb of Henle's loop from the proximal tubule. As fluid continues to move through the loops and an osmotic gradient of 200 mOsm/kg is generated, this single osmotic effect is multiplied over the length of Henle's loop (Fig. 2–12). The magnitude of the gradient from the beginning of the loop to its hairpin turn is a function of the length of the loop itself. Thus, the vertical osmotic gradient greatly exceeds the horizontal gradient at any given level. This is the countercurrent multiplier concept of urinary concentration.

Role of the Collecting Ducts and Antidiuretic Hormone

The collecting duct is divided into three segments: the cortical collecting duct, outer medullary collecting duct, and inner medullary collecting duct. These segments differ in their permeability to sodium and urea (see Table 2–2). The main role of the cortical collecting duct is delivery of fluid with a very high urea concentration to the outer medullary collecting duct. This occurs because sodium chloride and water are removed from this segment of the nephron but urea is not. The main functions of the inner medullary collecting duct are to add urea to the inner medullary interstitium and to produce maximally concentrated urine by osmotic equilibration of tubular fluid with the hyperosmotic interstitium under the influence of ADH (Chandhoke et al. 1985; Kokko 1987). This segment of the nephron is permeable to urea and its urea permeability is increased by ADH.

As just described, fluid entering the distal tubule is hyposmotic to plasma (approximately 100 mOsm/kg). Without the collecting duct, the so-called countercurrent multiplier would dilute tubular fluid. In the presence of ADH, this hyposmotic fluid equilibrates osmotically with the cortical interstitium (osmolality 300 mOsm/kg) as the tubular fluid flows through the cortical collecting duct. By this process, approximately two-thirds of the tubular water is removed before delivery to the medullary collecting duct. For example, 100 mOsm of solute in 1 L of tubular fluid is reduced to 100 mOsm of solute in 0.33 L of tubular fluid (300 mOsm/kg) with 0.67 L of water reabsorbed. Actually, even more water can be reabsorbed,

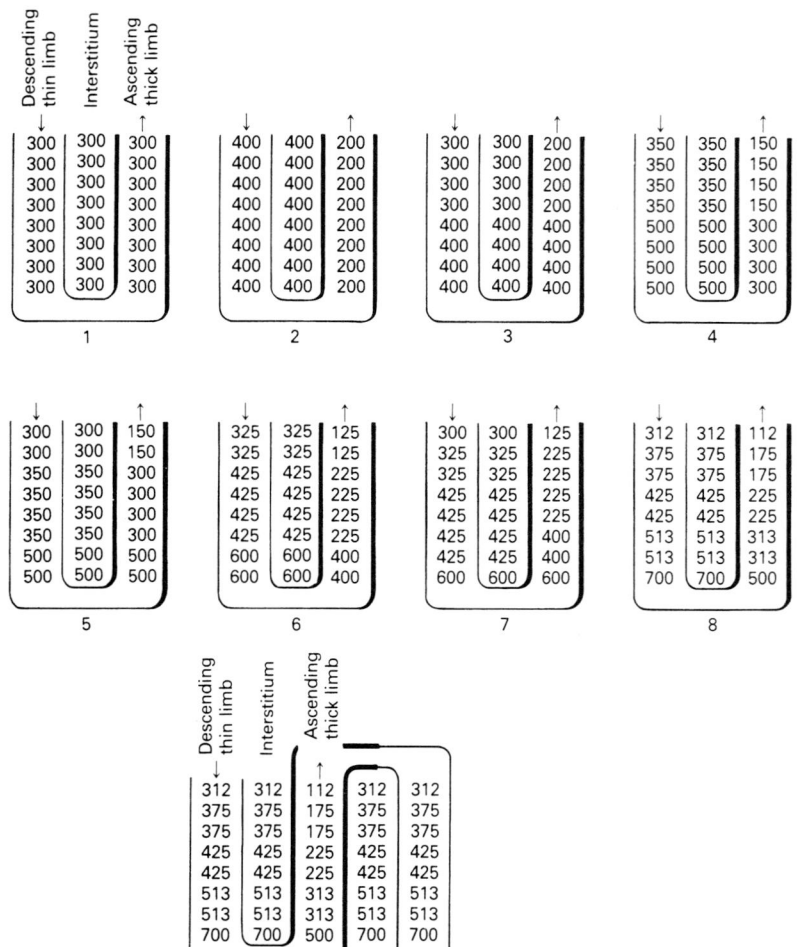

FIGURE 2-12. Stepwise operation of the countercurrent multiplier mechanism of urinary concentration. Numbers refer to osmolalities (mOsm/kg H₂O) of tubular fluid and interstitium. (Reprinted with permission from Valtin H: *Renal Function: Mechanisms Preserving Fluid and Solute Balance in Health*. 2nd ed. Boston, Little, Brown, p. 166, 1983.)

depending on how much active sodium reabsorption occurs in the cortical collecting duct in response to aldosterone stimulation. These effects markedly reduce fluid delivery to the medullary collecting duct. Tubular fluid entering the medullary collecting duct is thus isosmotic with plasma but much reduced in volume. It is in the medullary collecting duct that the final concentration of urine occurs.

The water permeability of the epithelium of the collecting duct is dependent on the action of ADH. In the presence of ADH, water is removed from the collecting duct as the fluid osmotically equilibrates with a progressively hyperosmotic medullary interstitium and the final osmolality of the urine may approximate that of the papillary interstitium. In human beings, this maximal urine osmolality is 900 to 1400 mOsm/kg (Rose 1994b). In dogs and cats, however, urine osmolality can approach 2800 and 3000 mOsm/kg, respectively (Hardy and Osborne 1979; Ross and Finco 1981). Water reabsorption in the distal convoluted tubule and connecting tubule is minimal because of their relative impermeability to water, regardless of the presence or absence of ADH. Thus, water reabsorption in the cortical collecting duct under the influence of ADH is important in reducing the fluid load delivered to the medullary collecting duct.

In the absence of ADH, the collecting duct is impermeable to water. The fluid entering this portion of the nephron has an osmolality of approximately 100 mOsm/kg. Under these conditions, additional sodium chloride without water is removed from the tubular fluid during its course through the cortical collecting duct and inner medullary collecting duct so that the final urine osmolality can be as low as 50 mOsm/kg. The outer medullary collecting duct, however, is impermeable to sodium.

Even in the absence of ADH, urine osmolality may be greater than 50 mOsm/kg if the animal is dehydrated. The GFR is decreased by dehydration, and there is an increase in the proximal tubular reabsorption of sodium chloride and water. Less tubular fluid reaches the distal nephron and urine osmolality can approach 400 mOsm/kg (Valtin and Edwards 1987).

Role of the Vasa Recta

If the water removed from the medullary collecting duct in the presence of ADH were allowed to remain in the medullary interstitium, the hyperosmotic gradient would dissipate rapidly. This does not occur, however, because of the countercurrent exchange function of the vasa recta. Plasma in the vasa recta entering the medulla from the cortex encounters an increasingly hyperosmotic medullary interstitium. As a result, water is removed from the vessels and solutes (e.g., sodium chloride, urea) enter the vessels. After passing the hairpin turn of the loop, the vasa recta climb back toward the renal cortex. Now, they encounter a medullary interstitium of progressively decreasing osmolality so that water enters the vessels and solutes are removed. In this way, water is removed from and solutes are recycled back into the medullary interstitium, thus preventing dissipation of the osmotic gradient. This process is known as countercurrent exchange. That the vasa recta can effectively remove water and recycle solute may be appreciated by considering the different flow rates in the vasa recta and medullary collecting duct. Although only 5% of RPF goes to the renal medulla, this flow is much greater than the approximately 3% of GFR that enters the medullary collecting ducts. Consider, for example, a 10-kg dog with a GFR of 4 mL/min/kg and RPF of 12 mL/min/kg. Renal plasma flow in the medulla would be 6 mL/min (5% of 120) and tubular fluid flow in the renal medulla would be 1.2 mL/min (3% of 40), a fivefold difference. These factors contribute to the effective removal of water from the medullary interstitium and prevent dissipation of the osmotic gradient in this region of the kidney.

Role of Urea

Although there is evidence for active transport of sodium chloride from the thick ascending limb of Henle's loop, active transport has not been demonstrated in the thin descending and ascending limbs. A two-solute model of the urinary concentrating mechanism was developed simultaneously in 1972 by Stephenson and by Kokko and Rector (Kokko and Rector 1972; Stephenson 1972; Jamison and Maffly 1976). This model requires an important contribution by urea as the second solute.

The thin descending limb of Henle's loop has a low passive permeability for sodium chloride and an even lower permeability for urea but it is highly permeable to water. The resting permeability of the inner medullary collecting duct to urea is enhanced by ADH. The distal convoluted tubule, cortical collecting duct, and outer medullary collecting duct are relatively impermeable to urea, even in the presence of ADH. Thus, the urea concentration of tubular fluid increases markedly in this portion of the nephron.

During a state of water conservation (i.e., antidiuresis), the plasma ADH concentration is high. More urea is passively removed from the inner medullary collecting duct and enters the medullary interstitium. In dogs, urea constitutes more than 40% of the total medullary solute concentration during antidiuresis (after 24 h of water deprivation) but less than 10% during water diuresis (Levitin et al. 1962; Bulger 1987).

Urea increases medullary interstitial osmolality without a change in the sodium concentration in this region. Water is thus removed osmotically from the thin descending limb of Henle's loop by the high concentration of urea in the medullary interstitium. The sodium concentration of the tubular fluid in the descending limb of Henle's loop eventually exceeds the medullary interstitial sodium concentration because the thin descending limb of Henle's loop has a low permeability for sodium. The sodium permeability of the thin ascending limb of Henle's loop is high and, as the tubular fluid rounds the hairpin turn and enters this portion of the nephron, sodium can be removed passively into the medullary interstitium down a concentration gradient (Figure 2–13).

▶ Endocrine Functions of the Kidney

The kidney is responsible for endocrine functions that play essential roles in the regulation of red cell production

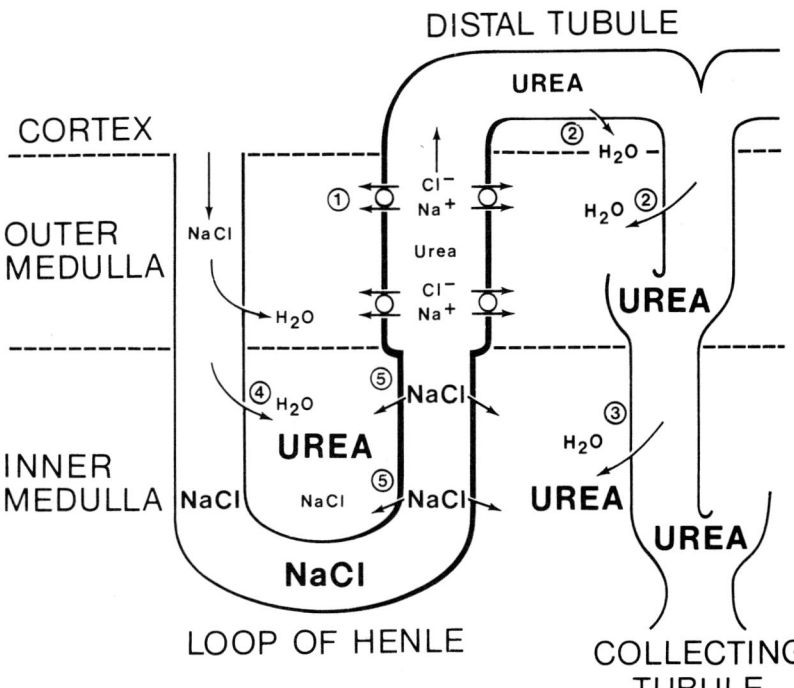

FIGURE 2–13. Role of urea in the urinary concentrating mechanism. (Reprinted by permission of the New England Journal of Medicine, Vol 295, pp. 1059–1067, 1976.)

by the bone marrow, defense of the extracellular fluid volume, and maintenance of calcium homeostasis. Gradual loss of these endocrine functions occurs during the progression of chronic renal disease and contributes to specific manifestations of the uremic syndrome such as nonregenerative anemia, systemic hypertension, and renal secondary hyperparathyroidism.

Erythropoietin Production

Erythropoietin (EPO) is glycoprotein hormone with a molecular mass of 35,000 to 40,000 daltons that stimulates red blood cell production by the bone marrow. The kidney is the major source of EPO in the adult animal, but the liver may also produce a small amount. Most EPO is metabolized in the liver. Decreased oxygen delivery to the kidney is the major stimulus for EPO production. The primary site of EPO synthesis in the kidney appears to be peritubular fibroblasts in the renal cortex and outer medulla (Maxwell et al. 1997). Erythropoietin stimulates erythroid precursors in the bone marrow to differentiate into mature red blood cells.

Renin-Angiotensin System

The main role of the renin-angiotensin system (RAS) is defense of the extracellular fluid volume (ECFV) via sodium homeostasis. The role of the kidney in maintenance of sodium balance is discussed further in Chapter 3.

Renin is an enzyme synthesized and stored in the granular cells of the JGA (specialized smooth muscle cells in the afferent arterioles). The kidney is the most important source of renin, but renin is also found in many other tissues (e.g., vascular endothelium, adrenal gland, brain). Local production of angiotensin II in some tissues may be important in the regulation of local processes without having a systemic effect. The RAS of the brain may be involved in control of systemic blood pressure, secretion of ADH, catecholamine release, and thirst.

There are three major stimuli for renin release. Decreased renal perfusion pressure caused by systemic hypotension (pressure below 80 to 90 mm Hg) or ECFV depletion is sensed in the afferent arterioles by the granular cells, which increase their secretion of renin. Stimulation of cardiac and arterial baroreceptors by systemic hypotension leads to increased sympathetic neural activity and increased concentrations of circulating catecholamines, which in turn stimulate renin release via β_1-adrenergic receptors on granular cells. Lastly, changes in distal tubular flow and delivery of chloride affect renin release. Decreased ECFV or chronic NaCl depletion decreases distal tubular flow and delivery of chloride to the macula densa (partly as a consequence of enhanced proximal reabsorption of water and NaCl), which in turn stimulates renin release. Expansion of the ECFV or NaCl loading increases distal tubular flow and delivery of chloride to the macula densa, which inhibits renin release. The release of renin is inhibited by a direct effect of angiotensin II on the granular cells, which constitutes a negative feedback loop.

Renin converts the α_2-globulin angiotensinogen (which is synthesized and released by the liver) to angiotensin I, and this is the rate-limiting step of the RAS cascade. Angiotensin-converting enzyme is found in vascular endothelium and cleaves the carboxyl-terminal (C-terminal) two amino acids from the inactive decapeptide angiotensin I to yield the active octapeptide angiotensin II. This step in the RAS cascade is not rate limiting, and most of the angiotensin I is rapidly converted to angiotensin II.

The effects of angiotensin II restore ECFV. Angiotensin II causes arteriolar vasoconstriction in many organs (renal, splanchnic, and cutaneous vascular beds are most sensitive), which increases systemic blood pressure. It enhances the sensitivity of vascular smooth muscle to and facilitates the release of norepinephrine from the adrenal medulla and sympathetic nerve terminals, thus secondarily affecting systemic blood pressure. Angiotensin II causes increased proximal tubular reabsorption of sodium by stimulating the Na^+-H^+ antiporter in luminal membranes of proximal tubular cells. It causes increased secretion of aldosterone from the zona glomerulosa of the adrenal cortex, and aldosterone in turn causes increased reabsorption of sodium chloride in the cortical collecting duct. Lastly, angiotensin II causes alterations in glomerular and postglomerular hemodynamics that enhance sodium and water reabsorption. Angiotensin II causes constriction of the efferent and afferent arterioles, an effect thought to be mediated by thromboxane A_2. The efferent arteriole constricts more than the afferent so that the filtration fraction increases (i.e., RPF decreases more than GFR). Renal hemodynamic changes favoring salt and water reabsorption occur in the postglomerular capillary beds secondary to these glomerular hemodynamic changes. These changes include decreased peritubular capillary hydrostatic pressure and increased peritubular capillary oncotic pressure. Angiotensin II can cause glomerular mesangial cells to contract, potentially reducing the surface area for filtration and decreasing the ultrafiltration coefficient, K_f. Angiotensin II stimulates release of vasodilator prostaglandins (e.g., PGE_2, PGI_2) from glomeruli. By this mechanism, the potentially harmful vasoconstrictive effects of angiotensin II on the kidney are be minimized.

Activation of Vitamin D

Vitamin D_3 (cholecalciferol) is obtained in the diet or by ultraviolet irradiation of the compound 7-dehydrocholesterol in skin. The liver hydroxylates cholecalciferol to 25-hydroxycholecalciferol, which is the predominant form of vitamin D_3 in plasma. In the kidney, 25-hydroxycholecalciferol is converted to the active form of vitamin D_3, 1,25-dihydroxycholecalciferol (calcitriol), by the enzyme 25-hydroxycholecalciferol-1α-hydroxylase, which is found in the mitochondria of the proximal tubular cells.

The activity of the 1α-hydroxylase system is closely regulated. It is inhibited by 1,25-dihydroxycholecalciferol (calcitriol). There is an inverse relationship between dietary calcium intake and the activity of the enzyme system. This may arise from a direct effect of dietary calcium or may be secondary to changes in the secretion of PTH in response to alterations in serum calcium concentration.

The enzyme system is stimulated by PTH and by hypophosphatemia.

The major effects of 1,25-dihydroxycholecalciferol (calcitriol) are increased intestinal absorption of calcium, a permissive effect on PTH-mediated bone resorption of calcium and phosphate, and negative feedback control on PTH secretion by the parathyroid glands. The actions of vitamin D are discussed further in Chapter 6.

REFERENCES

Avison MJ, Gullans SR, Ogino T, et al.: Measurement of Na-K coupling ratio of Na-K ATPase in rabbit proximal tubules. *Am J Physiol* 253:C126, 1987.

Berliner RW: Mechanisms of urine concentration. *Kidney Int* 22:202, 1982.

Bovee KC and Joyce T: Clinical evaluation of glomerular function: 24-hour creatinine clearance in dogs. *J Am Vet Med Assoc* 174:488, 1979.

Brown SA: Determinants of glomerular ultrafiltration in cats. *Am J Vet Res* 54:970, 1993.

Bulger RE: Composition of renal medullary tissue. *Kidney Int* 31:557, 1987.

Chandhoke PS, Saidel CM, and Knepper MA: Role of inner medullary collecting duct NaCl transport in urinary concentration. *Am J Physiol* 249:F688, 1985.

Clive DM and Stoff JS: Renal syndromes associated with nonsteroidal antiinflammatory drugs. *N Engl J Med* 310:563, 1984.

Dunn MJ: Nonsteroidal antiinflammatory drugs and renal function. *Annu Rev Med* 35:411, 1984.

Fettman MJ, Allen TA, Wilke WL, et al.: Single-injection method for evaluation of renal function with ^{14}C-inulin and ^{3}H-tetraethylammonium bromide in dogs and cats. *Am J Vet Res* 46:482, 1985.

Finco DR: Simultaneous determination of phenolsulfonphthalein excretion and endogenous creatinine clearance in the normal dog. *J Am Vet Med Assoc* 159:336, 1971.

Finco DR and Barsanti JA: Mechanism of urinary excretion of creatinine by the cat. *Am J Vet Res* 43:2207, 1982.

Finco DR and Duncan JR: Evaluation of blood urea nitrogen and serum creatinine concentrations as indicators of renal dysfunction: A study of 111 cases and a review of related literature. *J Am Vet Med Assoc* 168:593, 1976.

Finco DR, Coulter DB, and Barsanti JA: Simple, accurate method for clinical estimation of glomerular filtration rate in the dog. *Am J Vet Res* 42:1874, 1981.

Finco DR, Brown SA, Crowell WA, et al.: Exogenous creatinine clearance as a measure of glomerular filtration rate in dogs with reduced renal mass. *Am J Vet Res* 52:1029, 1991.

Finco DR, Tabaru H, Brown SA, et al.: Endogenous creatinine clearance measurement of glomerular filtration rate in dogs. *Am J Vet Res* 54:1575, 1993.

Hardy RM and Osborne CA: Water deprivation test in the dog: Maximal normal values. *J Am Vet Med Assoc* 174:479, 1979.

Jamison RJ: The renal concentrating mechanism. *Kidney Int* 32(suppl 21):S43, 1987.

Jamison RL and Maffly RH: The urinary concentrating mechanism. *N Engl J Med* 295:1059, 1976.

Keyes JL and Swanson RE: Dependence of glucose Tm on GFR and tubular volume. *Am J Physiol* 221:1, 1971.

Kokko JP: The role of the collecting duct in urinary concentration. *Kidney Int* 31:606, 1987.

Kokko JP and Rector FC Jr: Countercurrent multiplication system without active transport in inner medulla. *Kidney Int* 2:214, 1972.

Koushanpour E and Kriz W: *Renal Physiology: Principles, Structure, and Function.* New York, Springer-Verlag, 1986.

Kruth SA and Cowgill LD: Renal glucose transport in the cat (abstract). Proc Am Coll Vet Intern Med, p. 78, 1982.

Levitin H, Goodman A, Pigeon G, et al.: Composition of the renal medullar during water diuresis. *J Clin Invest* 41:1145, 1962.

Maxwell PH, Ferguson DJP, Nicholls LG, et al.: Sites of erythropoietin production. *Kidney Int* 51:393, 1997.

Navar LG, Bell PD, Crowell WA, et al.: Evaluation of the single nephron glomerular filtration coefficient in the dog. *Kidney Int* 12:137, 1977.

O'Grady SM, Palfrey HC, and Field M: Characteristics and function of Na-K-2Cl cotransport in epithelial tissues. *Am J Physiol* 253:C177, 1987.

Osbaldiston GW and Fuhrman W: The clearance of creatinine, inulin, *para*-aminohippurate and phenolsulfonphthalein in the cat. *Can J Comp Med* 34:138, 1970.

Powers TE, Powers JD, and Garg RC: Study of the double isotope single-injection method for estimating renal function in purebred beagle dogs. *Am J Vet Res* 38:1933, 1977.

Rose BD: *Clinical Physiology of Acid-Base and Electrolyte Disorders.* New York; McGraw-Hill, p. 94, 1994a.

Rose BD: *Clinical Physiology of Acid-Base and Electrolyte Disorders.* New York, McGraw-Hill, p. 115, 1994b.

Ross LA and Finco DR: Relationship of selected clinical renal function tests to glomerular filtration rate and renal blood flow in cats. *Am J Vet Res* 42:1704, 1981.

Shannon J, Farber S, and Troast L: The measurement of glucose Tm in the normal dog. *Am J Physiol* 133:752, 1941.

Stephenson JL: Concentration of urine in a central core model of the renal counterflow system. *Kidney Int* 2:85, 1972.

Valtin H and Edwards BR: GFR and the concentration of urine in the absence of vasopressin, Berliner-Davidson re-explored. *Kidney Int* 31:634, 1987.

Valtin H and Schafer JA: *Renal Function.* Boston; Little, Brown and Co., p. 98, 1995a.

Valtin H and Schafer JA: *Renal Function.* Boston; Little, Brown and Co., p. 90, 1995b.

… SECTION 2

Electrolyte Disorders

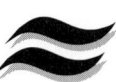

CHAPTER 3

Disorders of Sodium and Water

HYPERNATREMIA AND HYPONATREMIA

STEPHEN P. DiBARTOLA

The volume and tonicity of body fluids are maintained within a narrow normal range by regulation of sodium and water balance. The volume of extracellular fluid (ECF) is determined by the total body sodium content, whereas the osmolality and sodium concentration of ECF are determined by water balance. The kidney plays a crucial role in these processes by balancing the excretion of salt and water with their intake and by avidly conserving them when intake is restricted (Table 3–1).

▶ Terminology

Osmolality

The *osmolality* of a solution refers to the concentration of osmotically active particles in that solution. Osmolality is a function only of the number of particles and is not related to their molecular weight, size, shape, or charge. One mole of a nondissociating substance (e.g., glucose, urea) dissolved in 1 kg of water decreases the freezing point of the resultant solution by 1.86°C. Such a solution has an osmolality of 1 Osm/kg or 1000 mOsm/kg.

The term *osmolarity* refers to the number of particles of solute per liter of solution, whereas the term *osmolality* refers to the number of particles of solute per kilogram of solvent. When considering the physiology of body fluids, the difference between osmolality and osmolarity is negligible because body fluids are typically dilute aqueous solutions. In clinical medicine, the term osmolality is used, and the osmolality of body fluids is usually measured by freezing-point depression osmometry. A solution is said to be *hyperosmotic* if its osmolality is greater than that of the reference solution (often plasma) and *hyposmotic* if its osmolality is less than that of the reference solution. An *isosmotic* solution has an osmolality identical to that of the reference solution.

The normal plasma osmolality of dogs and cats is slightly higher than that of human beings and ranges from 290 to 310 mOsm/kg in dogs and from 290 to 330 mOsm/kg in cats. In one study, 20 dogs under resting conditions had plasma osmolality values of 292 to 308 mOsm/kg with a mean value of 301 mOsm/kg (Hardy and Osborne 1979). In a study of the effects of sodium bicarbonate infusion in cats, baseline serum osmolality ranged from 290 to 330 mOsm/kg (Chew et al. 1991). Plasma osmolality can be estimated from the equation

$$\text{Calculated plasma osmolality} = 2\text{Na} + \frac{\text{BUN}}{2.8} + \frac{\text{glucose}}{18}$$

where BUN is blood urea nitrogen. In this equation, the concentrations of urea and glucose in milligrams per deciliter are converted to millimoles per liter by the conversion factors 2.8 and 18. The *measured* osmolality should not exceed the *calculated* osmolality by more than 10 mOsm/kg (Shull 1978; Feldman and Rosenberg 1981). If it does, an abnormal *osmolal gap* is said to be present. This occurs when an unmeasured solute (i.e., one not accounted for in the equation) is present in large quantity in plasma (e.g., mannitol, metabolites of ethylene glycol) or when hyperlipemia or hyperproteinemia results in pseudohyponatremia (see later) (Feldman and Rosenberg 1981; Grauer and Grauer 1983; Gennari 1984).

TABLE 3–1. **Renal Regulation of Sodium and Water Balance**

	Osmoregulation	Volume Regulation
What is sensed	Plasma osmolality	Effective circulating volume
Sensors	Hypothalamic osmoreceptors	Carotid sinus
		Aortic arch
		Glomerular afferent arterioles
		Cardiac atria
		Large pulmonary vessels
Effectors	Vasopressin	Renin-angiotensin-aldosterone system
	Thirst	Sympathetic nervous system
		Atrial natriuretic peptide
		"Pressure natriuresis"
		Antidiuretic hormone
What is affected	Water excretion	Urine sodium excretion
	Water intake	

Modified from Rose BD: *Clinical Physiology of Acid Base and Electrolyte Disorders*, 4th ed. New York, McGraw-Hill Co., p. 256, 1994, with permission of the McGraw-Hill Companies.

Specific Gravity

The term *specific gravity* refers to the ratio of the weight of a volume of liquid to the weight of an equal volume of distilled water. Specific gravity depends not only on the number of particles present in the solution but also on their molecular weight. Specific gravity can be measured easily by the clinician with a handheld refractometer. Multiplying the last two digits of the urine specific gravity by 36 gives an rough estimate of urine osmolality in dogs (Hendriks et al. 1978). This rule may be misleading if the urine sample contains a large amount of high-molecular-weight solute, because substances with high molecular weights have a greater effect on specific gravity than on osmolality. The effects on urine osmolality of some solutes are shown in Table 3–2.

Tonicity or Effective Osmolality

Changes in the osmolality of ECF may or may not initiate movement of water between intracellular and extracellular compartments. A change in the concentration of *permeant* solutes (e.g., urea, ethanol) does not cause movement of water because these solutes are distributed equally throughout total body water. A change in the concentration of *impermeant* solutes (e.g., glucose, sodium) does cause movement of water because such solutes do not readily cross cell membranes. *Tonicity* refers to the ability of a solution to initiate water movement and is dependent on the presence of impermeant solutes in the solution (Feig and McCurdy 1977) Thus, tonicity may be thought of as *effective osmolality*. A solution is *hypertonic* to a reference solution from which it is separated by a semipermeable membrane if its concentration of impermeant solutes is greater than that of the reference solution. A solution is *hypotonic* to the reference solution if its concentration of impermeant solutes is less than that of the reference solution. A solution is *isotonic* to the reference solution if its concentration of impermeant solutes equals that of the reference solution.

Tonicity or effective osmolality may be estimated as $P_{osm} - BUN/2.8$. Consider a dog with the following laboratory values: serum sodium 125 mEq/L, BUN 280 mg/dL, glucose 90 mg/dL. This patient is hyponatremic and azotemic and has plasma hyperosmolality (calculated plasma osmolality = 355 mOsm/kg) but hypotonicity (effective plasma osmolality = 255 mOsm/kg). Clinical measurement of osmolality by freezing-point depression osmometry does not distinguish between permeant and impermeant solutes and thus does not provide direct information about the tonicity of a solution.

Diuresis

The term *diuresis* refers to urine flow that is greater than normal (i.e., >1–2 mL/kg/h in dogs and cats). The term *solute*, or *osmotic*, diuresis refers to increased urine flow caused by excessive amounts of nonreabsorbed solute within the renal tubules (e.g., polyuria associated with diabetes mellitus, administration of mannitol). During osmotic diuresis, urine osmolality approaches plasma osmolality. The term *water* diuresis refers to increased urine flow caused by decreased reabsorption of solute-free water in the collecting ducts (e.g., polyuria associated with psychogenic polydipsia or diabetes insipidus). During water diuresis, urine osmolality is less than plasma osmolality.

The term *isosthenuria* refers to urine with an osmolality equal to that of plasma, and *hyposthenuria* refers to urine with an osmolality less than that of plasma. The term *hypersthenuria*, or *baruria*, refers to urine with an osmolality greater than that of plasma, but this term is used rarely and only to describe urine that is very concentrated.

Types of Dehydration

Dehydration occurs when fluid loss from the body exceeds fluid intake. Dehydration may be classified according to the type of fluid lost from the body and the tonicity of the remaining body fluids. Pure water loss and loss of hypotonic fluid result in *hypertonic* dehydration because the tonicity of the remaining body fluids is increased. Loss of fluid with the same osmolality as that of ECF results in *isotonic* dehydration because there is no osmotic stimulus for water movement and the remaining body fluids are unchanged in tonicity. Loss of hypertonic fluid or loss of isotonic fluid with water replacement results in *hypotonic* dehydration because the remaining body fluids become hypotonic. The types of dehydration and their relative effects on the volume and tonicity of the intracellular and extracellular compartments are shown in Figure 3–1.

Serum Sodium Concentration

The serum sodium concentration is an indication of the amount of sodium relative to the amount of water in the ECF and provides no direct information about total body sodium content. Patients with hyponatremia or hypernatremia may have a decreased, normal, or increased total body sodium content. An increased serum sodium concentration (hypernatremia; >155 mEq/L in dogs or >162 mEq/L in cats) implies hyperosmolality, whereas a decreased serum sodium concentration (hyponatremia; <140 mEq/L in dogs or <149 mEq/L in cats) usually, but not always, implies hyposmolality. Hyponatremia develops when the patient is unable to excrete ingested water or when urinary and insensible fluid losses have a combined osmolality greater than that of ingested or parenterally

TABLE 3–2. **Effect of Selected Solutes on Urine Osmolality***

Substance	Molecular Mass (daltons)	Contribution to Osmolality (mOsm/kg)
Albumin	69,000	0.144
Diatrizoate ion	613	16.313
Glucose	180	55.555

*1.0 g/dL of each of the listed solutes added to distilled water would increase specific gravity by 0.010 but would have the effects on osmolality shown in the table.

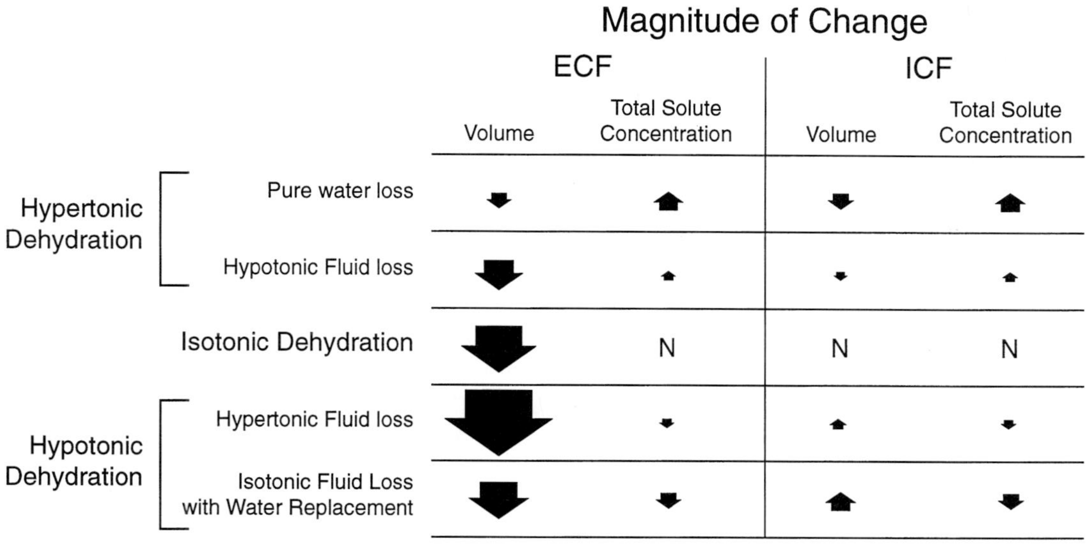

Magnitude of Change

		ECF		ICF	
		Volume	Total Solute Concentration	Volume	Total Solute Concentration
Hypertonic Dehydration	Pure water loss	↓	↑	↓	↑
	Hypotonic Fluid loss	↓↓	↑ (small)	↓ (small)	↑ (small)
Isotonic Dehydration		↓↓	N	N	N
Hypotonic Dehydration	Hypertonic Fluid loss	↓↓↓	↓ (small)	↑ (small)	↓ (small)
	Isotonic Fluid Loss with Water Replacement	↓↓	↓	↑	↓

FIGURE 3–1. Types of dehydration. ECF = extracellular fluid; ICF = intracellular fluid; N = normal. (Drawing by Tim Vojt.)

administered fluids. Hypernatremia develops when water intake has been inadequate, when the lost fluid is hypotonic to extracellular fluid, or when an excessive amount of sodium has been ingested or administered parenterally.

▶ Normal Physiology
Renal Handling of Sodium

Sodium is filtered by the glomeruli and reabsorbed by the renal tubules. The metabolic energy (i.e., ATP) for sodium transport in the kidney is required by Na^+,K^+-adenosinetriphosphatase (Na^+,K^+-ATPase) in the basolateral membranes of the tubular cells. This enzyme translocates sodium from the cytoplasm of the tubular cells to the peritubular interstitium and maintains a low intracellular concentration of sodium, which promotes sodium entry into the cell at the luminal surface.

Approximately 67% of the filtered load of sodium is reabsorbed isosmotically with water in the proximal tubules. In the early proximal tubule, sodium crosses the luminal membrane by cotransport with glucose, amino acids, and phosphate and in exchange for H^+ ions via the luminal Na^+-H^+ antiporter (during the latter process HCO_3^- is reabsorbed). Reabsorption of water and sodium with HCO_3^- and other solutes in this segment of the nephron increases the Cl^- concentration in tubular fluid and facilitates Cl^- reabsorption later in the proximal tubule. In the late proximal tubule, sodium is reabsorbed primarily with Cl^-. In this region, the luminal Na^+-H^+ antiporter works in parallel with a luminal Cl^--anion$^-$ antiporter, and the net effect is NaCl reabsorption (H^+ anion$^-$ is recycled back and forth across the membrane).

Approximately 25% of the filtered load of sodium is reabsorbed in the loop of Henle, primarily in the thick ascending limb. In the thin descending and ascending limbs of Henle's loop, sodium and Cl^- are passively reabsorbed. In the thick ascending limb, sodium crosses the luminal membranes via the Na^+-H^+ antiporter and by an Na^+-K^+-$2Cl^-$ cotransporter (O'Grady et al. 1987). This Na^+-K^+-$2Cl^-$ cotransporter is the site of action of the loop diuretics *furosemide* and *bumetanide*. There is a strong electrochemical gradient for Na^+ entry across the luminal membrane in this region (i.e., strongly lumen-positive transepithelial potential difference and high luminal sodium concentration).

Approximately 5% of the filtered load of sodium is reabsorbed in the distal convoluted tubule and connecting segment. In the early distal tubule (up to the connecting segment), sodium crosses the luminal membrane by means of an Na^+-Cl^- cotransporter. This cotransporter is inhibited by the *thiazide* diuretics (Ellison and Velazquez 1987).

Approximately 3% of the filtered load of sodium is reabsorbed in the collecting ducts, and this segment of the nephron is responsible for altering sodium reabsorption in response to dietary fluctuations. In the late distal tubule (so-called connecting segment) and collecting ducts, sodium enters passively through Na^+ channels in the luminal membranes of the principal cells (Palmer and Frindt 1986; Schuster and Stokes 1987). This movement of Na^+ generates a lumen-negative transepithelial potential difference that facilitates Cl^- reabsorption. The Na^+ channel in the principal cells is blocked by the diuretics *amiloride* and *triamterene*. One of the main effects of aldosterone is to increase the number of open luminal Na^+ channels in the cortical collecting ducts, thus altering sodium reabsorption in response to changes in dietary sodium intake. The renal tubular mechanisms for sodium reabsorption are summarized in Figure 3–2.

Renal Regulation of Sodium Balance

Extracellular fluid volume is directly dependent on body sodium content. The body is able to sense and respond to very small changes in sodium content. The adequacy of body sodium content is perceived as the fullness of the circulating blood volume. The term *effective circulating volume* has been used to refer to the relative fullness of

48 DISORDERS OF SODIUM AND WATER

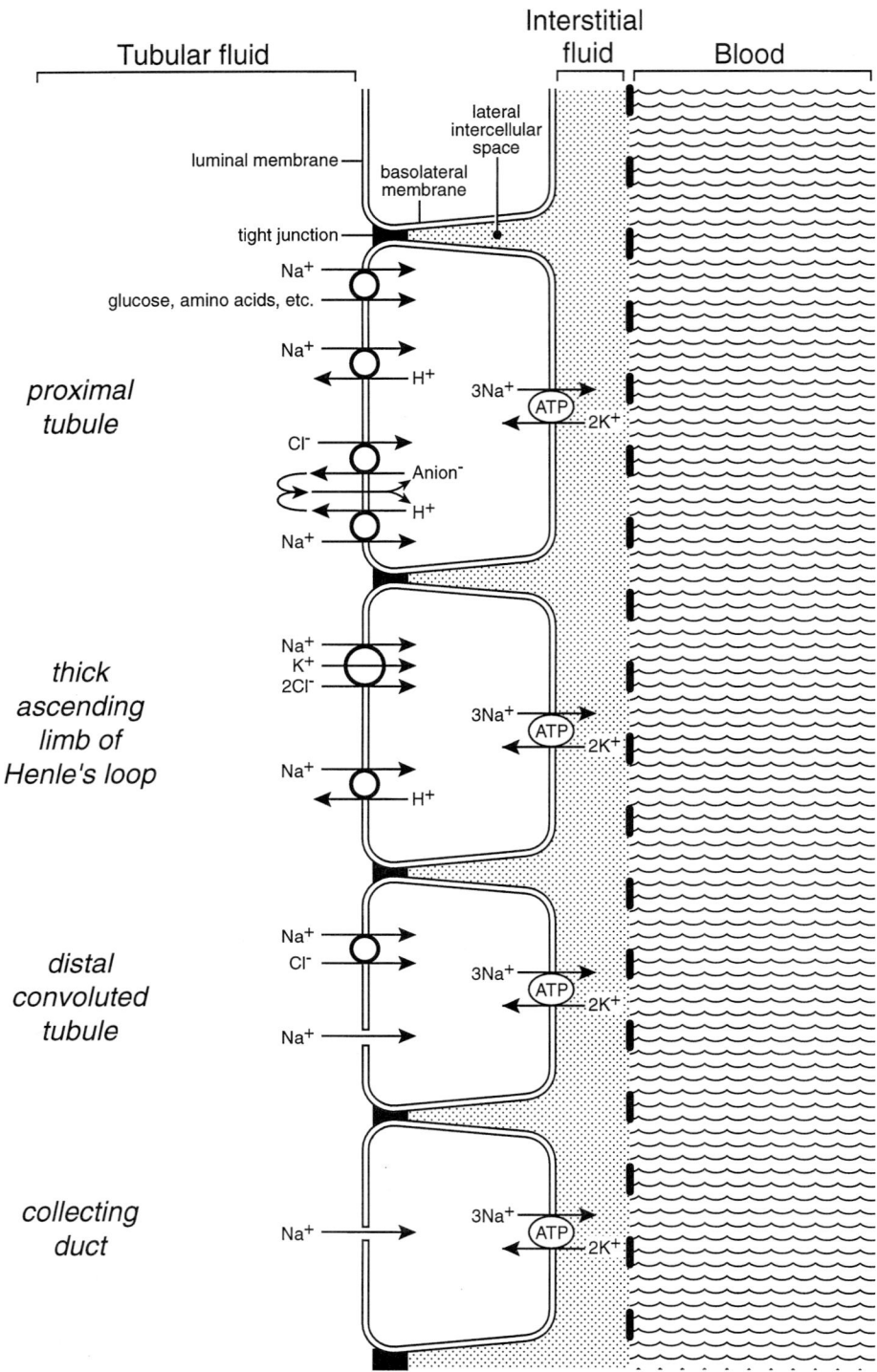

FIGURE 3-2. Renal tubular mechanisms for the reabsorption of sodium along the length of the nephron. (Drawing by Tim Vojt.)

the extracellular compartment as perceived by the body. There are several sensors in the afferent limb of the body's regulatory system for control of sodium balance (see Table 3–1). Low-pressure mechanoreceptors (i.e., volume receptors) in the cardiac atria and pulmonary vessels and high-pressure baroreceptors (i.e., pressure receptors) in the aortic arch and carotid sinus play a primary role in the body's ability to sense the adequacy of the circulating volume. Within the kidney, the juxtaglomerular apparatus responds to changes in perfusion pressure with changes in renin production and release. Less well characterized are receptors in the liver and the central nervous system that may contribute to sodium homeostasis.

The kidney constitutes the primary efferent limb of sodium control and regulates sodium balance by excreting an amount of sodium each day equal to that ingested. There are several overlapping control mechanisms for regulation of renal handling of sodium. This redundancy of controls serves to protect against sodium imbalance should one control mechanism fail. The two points of control for sodium balance in the kidney are glomerular filtration and tubular reabsorption. Autoregulation maintains renal blood flow and glomerular filtration rate (GFR) relatively constant despite fluctuations in systemic arterial pressure; thus, the filtered load of sodium is also kept relatively constant (see Chapter 2).

GLOMERULOTUBULAR BALANCE

Even slight changes in GFR have the potential to have drastic effects on sodium balance if the absolute amount of sodium reabsorbed by the tubules remains constant. Consider a normal 10-kg dog in sodium balance with a serum sodium concentration of 145 mEq/L and GFR of 4 mL/min/kg. The daily filtered load of sodium in this dog would be 57.6 L/day × 145 mEq/L = 8352 mEq/day. If the kidneys reabsorb 99.5% of the filtered load of sodium (8310 mEq/day), the amount excreted in the urine is 42 mEq/day. Consider what would happen if there was a *primary* (i.e., *spontaneous*) increase in GFR of only 1% but the absolute amount of sodium reabsorbed remained unchanged. The filtered load of sodium would be 58.2 L/day × 145 mEq/L = 8439 mEq/day but the amount reabsorbed would remain 8310 mEq/day. This would result in the excretion of 129 mEq/day, an amount three times that normally excreted. Under these conditions, the dog would develop negative sodium balance. Glomerulotubular balance prevents this scheme of events from occurring.

As spontaneous (primary) fluctuations in GFR occur, the absolute tubular reabsorption of filtered solutes changes in a similar direction. Thus, the fraction of the filtered load that is reabsorbed remains relatively constant despite spontaneous changes in GFR. This principle is called *glomerulotubular balance,* and its mechanisms are incompletely understood.

One mechanism is related to the fact that much of the sodium in the proximal tubules is reabsorbed along with several other solutes (e.g., glucose, amino acids, phosphate, bicarbonate). A spontaneous increase in GFR increases the filtered load of all of these solutes, and their increased concentration in the proximal tubule enhances sodium reabsorption. Changes in peritubular capillary hydrostatic and oncotic pressures probably also play an important role in glomerulotubular balance. If GFR spontaneously increases without a change in renal plasma flow (RPF) (i.e., the filtration fraction increases), the blood leaving the efferent arterioles has lower hydrostatic and higher oncotic pressures, thus favoring water and solute reabsorption in the proximal tubules. Autoregulation (see Chapter 2) also contributes to glomerulotubular balance. When renal perfusion pressure is increased, afferent arteriolar constriction prevents transmission of the increased hydrostatic pressure to the glomerular capillaries and minimizes any increase in GFR and filtered solute load.

Ingestion of a sodium load causes thirst, water consumption, and expansion of ECF volume. These events lead to a *compensatory (secondary)* increase in GFR by increasing hydrostatic pressure and decreasing oncotic pressure in the glomerular capillaries. Increased stretching of the afferent arterioles decreases renin secretion (and ultimately angiotensin II production). Volume expansion also causes increased atrial stretch, release of atrial natriuretic peptide, and natriuresis.

There is a paradox here. How can an increase in GFR in one situation cause an increase in the tubular reabsorption of sodium and in another situation cause a decrease in the tubular reabsorption of sodium? The answer to the paradox lies in the fundamental difference between the kidney's reaction to a spontaneous (primary) increase and its reaction to a compensatory (secondary) increase in GFR. Glomerulotubular balance is evoked in the former but not the latter situation.

ALDOSTERONE

Changes in renal reabsorption of sodium in response to dietary fluctuations in sodium intake are mediated by the hormone aldosterone, which is synthesized in the zona glomerulosa of the adrenal cortex. The production and release of aldosterone are stimulated by angiotensin II, hyperkalemia, and adrenocorticotropic hormone (ACTH). Its release is inhibited by dopamine and atrial natriuretic peptide. Aldosterone increases sodium reabsorption by increasing the number and activity of open sodium channels in the luminal membranes of the principal cells in the collecting ducts.

PERITUBULAR CAPILLARY FACTORS (STARLING FORCES)

Increased sodium intake leads to expansion of the ECF volume and compensatory increases in both GFR and RPF (i.e., the filtration fraction remains unchanged). This increases hydrostatic pressure and decreases oncotic pressure in the peritubular capillaries, thus reducing sodium and water reabsorption in the proximal tubules. Decreased sodium intake leads to volume contraction. In this setting, RPF decreases more than GFR (i.e., the filtration fraction increases). This results in decreased hydrostatic and increased oncotic pressures in the peritubular capillaries and enhanced proximal tubular reabsorption of sodium and water.

CATECHOLAMINES

Catecholamine-induced vasoconstriction usually affects the efferent more than the afferent arterioles. The resultant increase in filtration fraction alters peritubular capillary hemodynamics so as to favor water and sodium reabsorption (i.e., decreased hydrostatic pressure, increased oncotic pressure). Catecholamines also directly stimulate proximal tubular sodium reabsorption through an α_1-adrenergic effect and stimulate renin release from the granular cells of the juxtaglomerular apparatus through a β_1-adrenergic effect. The angiotensin II ultimately produced also stimulates proximal tubular sodium reabsorption. The direct effects of catecholamines on proximal tubular sodium reabsorption are important because they offset the tendency of the increase in systemic arterial pressure to cause pressure natriuresis (see later).

ANGIOTENSIN II

Decreased perfusion pressure in the afferent arterioles increases renin release from the granular cells of the juxtaglomerular apparatus and initiates the cascade of events leading to production of angiotensin II. Angiotensin II–induced vasoconstriction causes efferent more than afferent arteriolar constriction, which results in an in-

50 DISORDERS OF SODIUM AND WATER

TABLE 3-3. **Effectors of Sodium Balance**

Effector	Stimuli for Release	Inhibitors of Release	Major Effects
Aldosterone	Angiotensin II Hyperkalemia Adrenocorticotropic hormone	Dopamine ANP	Increased number and activity of luminal Na^+ channels and basolateral Na^+,K^+ATPase in principal cells of cortical collecting ducts
Angiotensin II	↓ Renal perfusion pressure*	↑ Renal perfusion pressure*	Systemic vasoconstriction Glomerular arteriolar vasoconstriction (efferent > afferent) Stimulates proximal Na^+ reabsorption Stimulates aldosterone secretion
Atrial natriuretic peptide (ANP)	↑ Atrial stretch	↓ Atrial stretch	Inhibits Na^+ reabsorption in parts of collecting duct Directly increases glomerular filtration rate
Catecholamines	↓ Effective circulating volume	↑ Effective circulating volume	Vasoconstriction Glomerular arteriolar vasoconstriction (efferent > afferent) Increase proximal tubular Na^+ reabsorption (α_1 effect) Stimulate renin release (β_1 effect)
Renin	↓ Perfusion pressure in juxtaglomerular apparatus Sympathetic nervous system activity Decreased Cl^- delivery to macula densa	Angiotensin II ANP Antidiuretic hormone	Not an "effector"—an enzyme that converts angiotensinogen to angiotensin I

*Via release and action of renin.

crease in filtration fraction and changes in peritubular capillary Starling forces (decreased hydrostatic pressure, increased oncotic pressure) that facilitate proximal tubular reabsorption of sodium and water. Angiotensin II also directly stimulates the Na^+-H^+ antiporter in the proximal tubules, which facilitates sodium reabsorption and stimulates secretion of aldosterone from the adrenal gland.

ATRIAL NATRIURETIC PEPTIDE

Atrial natriuretic peptide is synthesized and stored in atrial myocytes until it is released in response to atrial distention caused by volume expansion. It has a number of effects that facilitate renal excretion of sodium. Atrial natriuretic factor directly increases GFR, inhibits sodium reabsorption in the cortical and inner medullary collecting ducts, and inhibits renin secretion, thereby decreasing production of angiotensin II and limiting the effects of angiotensin II on proximal tubular sodium reabsorption. Finally, it inhibits aldosterone secretion by adrenal zona glomerulosa.

PRESSURE NATRIURESIS

Renal sodium excretion and water excretion are markedly increased when renal arterial pressure increases even slightly without a change in GFR. The mechanism for pressure natriuresis appears to be entirely intrarenal and does not require neural or endocrine input (i.e., occurs in the isolated denervated kidney). The effectors of sodium balance are summarized in Table 3–3.

Regulation of Water Balance

The osmolality of ECF and serum sodium concentration are regulated by adjusting water balance. Osmoreceptors in the hypothalamus constitute the afferent limb (sensors) for regulation of water balance. Vasopressin release is stimulated when the osmoreceptors shrink in response to plasma hyperosmolality and is inhibited when they swell in response to plasma hypoosmolality. Vasopressin (water output) and thirst (water input) constitute the efferent limb (effectors) for the regulation of water balance (see Table 3–1).

VASOPRESSIN

Vasopressin is a nine-amino-acid peptide synthesized in neurons of the supraoptic and paraventricular nuclei in the hypothalamus (Fig. 3–3). It travels down the axons of these neurons and is released into the circulation at the level of the neurohypophysis.

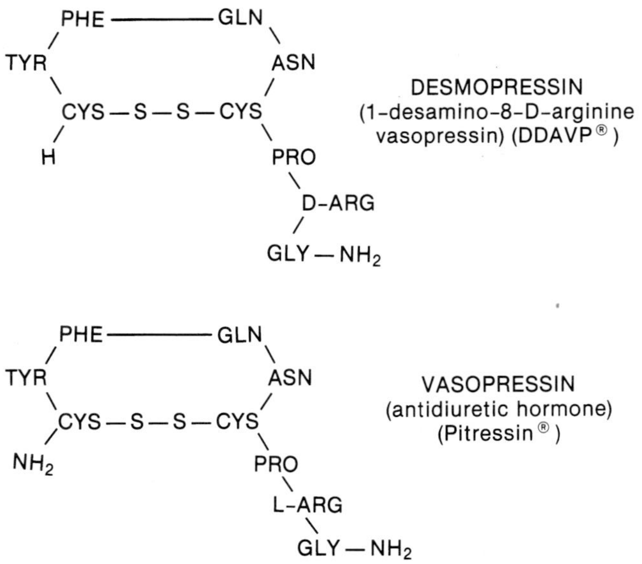

```
        PHE ——— GLN
       /           \
    TYR             ASN
       \           /
        CYS—S—S—CYS       DESMOPRESSIN
       /           \      (1-desamino-8-D-arginine
       H            PRO   vasopressin) (DDAVP®)
                    \
                    D-ARG
                    /
                 GLY—NH2


        PHE ——— GLN
       /           \
    TYR             ASN
       \           /
        CYS—S—S—CYS       VASOPRESSIN
       /           \      (antidiuretic hormone)
      NH2           PRO   (Pitressin®)
                    \
                    L-ARG
                    /
                 GLY—NH2
```

FIGURE 3–3. Comparison of the chemical structures of desmopressin and vasopressin. PHE = phenylalanine; TYR = tyrosine; GLN = glutamine; ASN = asparagine; CYS = cysteine; PRO = proline; ARG = arginine; GLY = glycine.

Vasopressin increases the reabsorption of water in the collecting ducts of the kidney and increases the permeability of the medullary collecting ducts to urea (Abramov et al. 1987). Vasopressin attaches to V_2 receptors on the basolateral membranes of the principal cells of the cortical and medullary collecting ducts. The hormone-receptor complex activates a guanine nucleotide regulatory protein, which in turn stimulates the activity of adenyl cyclase in the cell membrane. Formation of cyclic AMP initiates a series of intracellular events that lead to insertion of water channels in the luminal membranes of the tubular cells. When vasopressin is absent or in low concentration, these water channels are removed from the luminal membrane by endocytosis. In the absence of vasopressin, urine osmolality can be decreased to as low as 50 mOsm/kg by continued reabsorption of sodium without water as tubular fluid passes down the collecting ducts.

The effect of vasopressin on urea reabsorption may be important in the pathogenesis of medullary washout of solute in chronic polyuric states. Chronic diuresis can lead to depletion of urea from the medullary interstitium by suppression of vasopressin release and impaired urea reabsorption in the medullary collecting ducts. During antidiuresis, urea may constitute more than 40% of the medullary solute. During diuresis, however, it may constitute less than 10% of the medullary solute (Levitin et al. 1962; Bulger 1987). The urinary concentrating mechanism is discussed in Chapter 2.

STIMULI FOR VASOPRESSIN RELEASE

The major stimulus for vasopressin release is hypertonicity of plasma reaching the osmoreceptors of the hypothalamus. The threshold for vasopressin release in humans corresponds to a plasma osmolality of 280 mOsm/kg (Robertson 1983), and similar (Rijnberk et al. 1988) or slightly higher (DiBartola et al. 1994) threshold values have been observed in healthy experimental dogs. Below this osmolality, vasopressin release is suppressed and urine is maximally dilute. One hour after oral administration of water at 40 mL/kg, normal dogs developed a mean urine osmolality of 132 mOsm/kg (range 68–244) (Hardy and Osborne 1979). In humans, the release of vasopressin is maximal at a plasma osmolality of 294 mOsm/kg, and at this plasma osmolality the thirst mechanism becomes operative (Robertson 1983). Thus, changes in plasma osmolality as small as 1 to 2% above normal lead to maximal vasopressin release. The gain of the system is such that a 1 mOsm/kg increase in plasma osmolality leads to an almost 100 mOsm/kg increase in urine osmolality. The vasopressin system curtails water excretion, but further defense against hypertonicity of the ECF requires a normal thirst mechanism and access to water. The thirst mechanism has both osmoreceptors and volume receptors. The volume receptors for the thirst mechanism are stimulated by angiotensin II and may be under control of the renin-angiotensin system (Mann et al. 1987).

The next most important stimulus for vasopressin release is volume depletion sensed by baroreceptors in the left atrium, aortic sinus, and carotid sinuses. A decrease in blood volume of 5 to 10% lowers the threshold for vasopressin release and increases the sensitivity of the osmoregulatory mechanism (Fig. 3–4) (Robertson 1983;

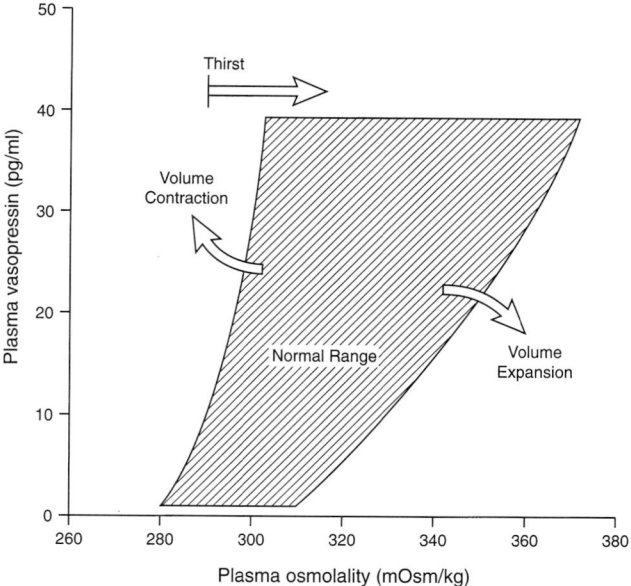

FIGURE 3–4. Relationship between plasma osmolality and plasma vasopressin concentration. Volume depletion lowers the threshold for vasopressin release and increases the sensitivity of the osmoregulatory system, whereas volume expansion has the opposite effect. (Drawing by Tim Vojt.)

Gross et al. 1987). Nonosmotic stimulation of vasopressin by actual or perceived volume depletion plays a major role in the generation and perpetuation of hyponatremia in states of true volume depletion and in edematous states associated with hypervolemia (see later).

Other stimuli for vasopressin release include nausea, pain, and emotional anxiety. Many drugs and some electrolyte disturbances affect the release and renal action of vasopressin. The effects of some of these are depicted in Figure 3–5.

ROLE OF THE KIDNEY IN WATER BALANCE

Three conditions must be met for the kidneys to excrete a water load normally. First, there must be adequate delivery of tubular fluid to distal diluting sites (ascending limb of Henle's loop) where NaCl is removed without water, rendering the tubular fluid hypotonic to the medullary interstitium. Adequate distal delivery requires normal RPF, normal GFR, and normal isosmotic reabsorption of sodium and water from the proximal tubules. In the presence of volume depletion, RPF is usually decreased more than GFR, and enhanced proximal tubular reabsorption of sodium and water may result from changes in postglomerular hemodynamics (see earlier). These factors may prevent adequate distal delivery of tubular fluid for dilution.

Second, the ascending limb of Henle's loop must function normally. That is, NaCl must be removed from this segment of the nephron without water. Loop diuretics (e.g., furosemide, ethacrynic acid) impair NaCl removal from this portion of the nephron, and some interstitial renal diseases may disrupt the normal architecture of this region, leading to impaired dilution of tubular fluid in the ascending limbs of Henle's loops.

Last, in the absence of vasopressin, the collecting ducts must remain impermeable to water throughout

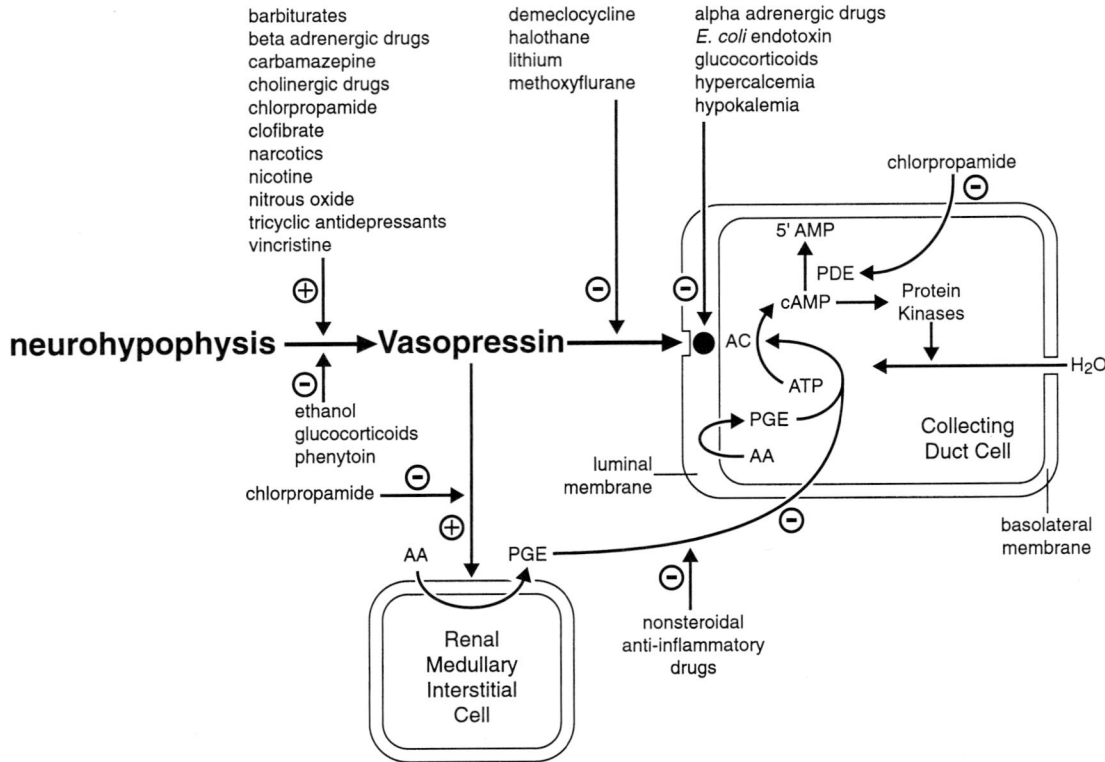

FIGURE 3-5. Effects of selected drugs and electrolytes on vasopressin release and action. AA = arachidonic acid; AC = adenyl cyclase; PGE = prostaglandin E; ATP = adenosine triphosphate; cAMP = cyclic adenosine monophosphate; PDE = phosphodiesterase; 5'-AMP = 5'-adenosine monophosphate.

their course. If any of these conditions is not met, a disorder of water excretion and a state of extracellular fluid hypotonicity and hyponatremia may result.

In the absence of vasopressin, the collecting ducts remain impermeable to water, the urine becomes maximally dilute, and polyuria develops. Hypertonicity and hypernatremia occur if the animal is unable to drink enough water to balance the tremendous loss of water in the urine. Hypertonicity and hypernatremia may also develop in states of osmotic diuresis (e.g., diabetes mellitus, mannitol administration, chronic renal failure, postobstructive diuresis). Urine osmolality approaches plasma osmolality during osmotic diuresis and the solute responsible for the diuresis displaces sodium and other electrolytes in the urine (Gennari and Kassirer 1974). Hypertonicity develops to the extent that displaced sodium remains in the ECF.

DEFENSE AGAINST HYPOTONICITY
It is crucial to the survival of the animal that the brain be protected against changes in plasma tonicity because an increase in brain water content of more than 10% is incompatible with life (Sterns et al. 1994). The fact that animals with chronic hyponatremia may have serum sodium concentrations 10% or more below normal attests to the brain's ability to adapt to hypotonicity. For example, on the basis of osmotic considerations alone, a decrease in serum sodium concentration from 145 to 132 mEq/L would correspond to an increase in intracellular water of 10%. During acute hypotonicity, water moves into the brain. The rise in hydrostatic pressure in the interstitial compartment of the brain immediately forces sodium-containing ECF into the cerebrospinal fluid. This movement of fluid out of the brain occurs within minutes and limits the change in brain water content to much less than would be anticipated on the basis of osmotic considerations alone (Sterns et al. 1994) During the first 24 h of hypotonicity, movement of potassium out of cells also contributes substantially to the protection of the brain from an acute decrease in plasma osmolality. After 24 to 48 h, a reduction in the cellular content of organic solutes contributes to the brain's defense against hypotonicity. These organic osmolytes are substances that can be used by cells to maintain intracellular tonicity without having adverse effects on cellular metabolism and include amino acids (e.g., taurine, glutamate, glutamine), methylamines (e.g., phosphocreatine), and polyols (e.g., *myo*-inositol). The very devices that protect the brain against plasma hypotonicity predispose it to injury when hyponatremia is corrected. Solutes lost during adaptation must be recovered, and this process requires several days. If correction of hyponatremia proceeds more quickly than recovery of lost solutes can occur, a devastating complication of treatment called osmotic demyelination syndrome may occur (see Treatment of Hyponatremia).

▶ Clinical Approach to the Patient with Hypernatremia
All clinical conditions associated with hypernatremia reflect hyperosmolality and hypertonicity of the ECF if the

solute in question is impermeant. Hypertonicity of the ECF and hypernatremia can be caused by a deficit of pure water, loss of hypotonic fluids, or gain of sodium. The causes of hypernatremia are listed in Table 3–4, and the clinical approach to the patient with hypernatremia is outlined in Figure 3–6.

Pure Water Loss

When a deficit of pure water develops, the ECF becomes hypertonic in relation to the intracellular fluid (ICF) and osmotic forces cause movement of water from the intracellular to the extracellular compartment. The end result is that the volume loss is shared proportionately between the extracellular and intracellular compartments. Approximately two-thirds of the volume loss comes from the intracellular compartment and one-third from the extracellular compartment. Plasma volume is one-fourth of the ECF, and thus 1/12 of the volume loss (1/4 × 1/3) is derived from the intravascular space. Actually, the oncotic pressure generated by plasma proteins favors retention of water within vessels, and the plasma compartment may not share proportionately in the volume loss (Feig and McCurdy 1977). As a result of these factors, volume depletion is usually not a clinical feature of pure water loss. It is almost impossible for a conscious animal with an intact thirst mechanism and access to water to develop hypertonicity caused by pure water loss. Thus, hypertonicity associated with pure water loss usually implies that water intake has been defective.

Consider a normal 10-kg dog with a serum osmolality of 300 mOsm/kg. We assume that total body water is 60% of body weight, with 40% being intracellular and 20% extracellular, and that the major extracellular (i.e., NaCl) and intracellular (i.e., KCl) solutes are impermeant. The number of osmoles of solute in ECF would be 2 L × 300 mOsm/kg = 600 mOsm and the number in ICF would be 4 L × 300 mOsm/kg = 1200 mOsm. Without access to drinking water, a loss of 1 L of pure water from ECF would cause water to move from ICF to ECF so as to equalize osmolality between the compartments according to the following equation:

$$\text{New ECF osmolality} = \text{new ICF osmolality}$$
$$600 \text{ mOsm}/(1 + x) \text{ L} = 1200 \text{ mOsm}/(4 - x) \text{ L}$$

where x is the volume of water moving between compartments:

$$600(4 - x) = 1200(1 + x)$$
$$x = 0.67 \text{ L}$$

The new volumes and osmolalities are

ECF: 600 mOsm/1.67 L = 360 mOsm/kg
ICF: 1200 mOsm/3.33 L = 360 mOsm/kg

Note that the intracellular compartment has lost an amount equal to two-thirds of the water deficit (0.67 L) and that the final ECF volume (1.67 L) is lower than the original volume (2 L) by an amount equal to one-third of the total water deficit (0.33 L). Thus, the two compartments have shared proportionately in the water loss. These changes are depicted in Figure 3–7.

Development of a pure water deficit is uncommon in small animal medicine. The main causes of hypertonicity related to pure water deficit are hypodipsia caused by neurologic disease and diabetes insipidus, which can be considered abnormal renal loss of water. Other causes of pure water deficit include respiratory losses during exposure to high environmental temperature (e.g., panting), fever, and inadequate access to water (e.g., frozen water bowl, inattentive owner).

Rarely, chronic hypernatremia may occur in fully conscious animals that have access to water. In these cases, abnormal osmoregulation of antidiuretic hormone (ADH) release caused by underlying hypothalamic lesions results in hypodipsia. Animals that are unable to obtain water because central nervous system disease has resulted in an altered sensorium may also be hypernatremic, but in these instances, the hypernatremia is simply a result of water deprivation. Hypodipsic hypernatremia related to defective osmoregulation of ADH has been reported in a dog with hydrocephalus and normal pituitary function (DiBartola et al. 1994). In normal individuals, administration of hypertonic saline increases plasma osmolality and simultaneously causes volume expansion. Osmoreceptors are stimulated by hyperosmolality but inhibited by vol-

TABLE 3–4. Causes of Hypernatremia

Pure Water Deficit
Primary hypodipsia (e.g., in miniature schnauzers)
Diabetes insipidus
   Central
   Nephrogenic
High environmental temperature
Fever
Inadequate access to water

Hypotonic Fluid Loss
Extrarenal
   Gastrointestinal
      Vomiting
      Diarrhea
      Small intestinal obstruction
   Third-space loss
      Peritonitis
      Pancreatitis
   Cutaneous
      Burns
Renal
   Osmotic diuresis
      Diabetes mellitus
      Mannitol infusion
   Chemical diuretics
   Chronic renal failure
   Nonoliguric acute renal failure
   Postobstructive diuresis

Impermeant Solute Gain
Salt poisoning
Hypertonic fluid administration
   Hypertonic saline
   Sodium bicarbonate
   Parenteral nutrition
   Sodium phosphate enema
Hyperaldosteronism
Hyperadrenocorticism

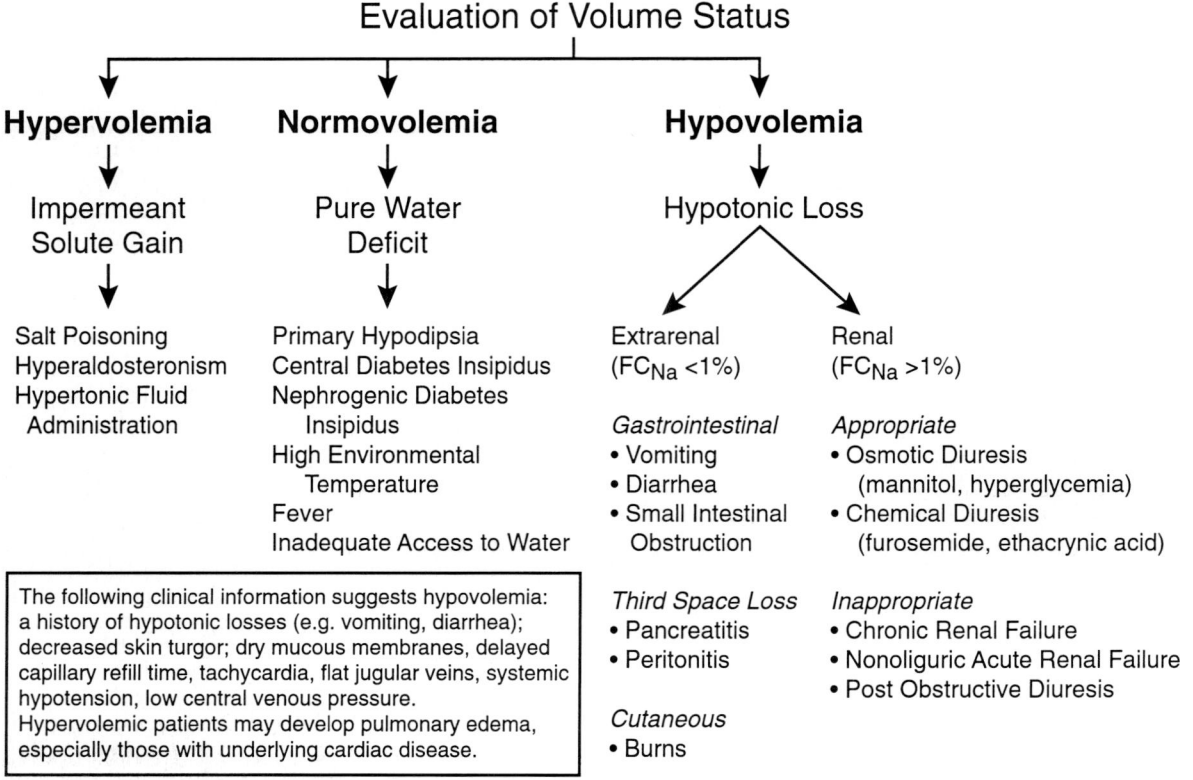

FIGURE 3–6. Clinical approach to the patient with hypernatremia. FC_{Na} = fractional clearance of sodium.

ume expansion. Normally, the response to hyperosmolality takes precedence and ADH secretion increases, resulting in decreased urine volume and increased urine osmolality. The affected dog experiences increased urine volume and decreased urine osmolality in response to an infusion of hypertonic saline, indicating defective osmoreceptor function as observed in human patients with hypodipsic hypernatremia. Weakness and polymyopathy have been reported in a young cat with hypodipsia, hypernatremia, and hypertonicity associated with hydrocephalus and hypopituitarism (Dow et al. 1987), and hypernatremia, adipsia, and diabetes insipidus have been observed in a young dalmatian dog with dysplasia of the rostral diencephalon (Bagley et al. 1993).

Hypodipsia, hypernatremia, and hypertonicity caused by an abnormal thirst mechanism have been reported in young female miniature schnauzers (Crawford et al. 1984; Hoskins and Rothschmitt 1984; Van Heerden et al. 1992) and in a young Great Dane (Hawks et al. 1991). These dogs appear to have a form of congenital adipsic hypernatremia. In one case, an infusion of hypertonic saline led to an increase in urine volume and decrease in urine osmolality compatible with defective osmoregulation of ADH (Crawford et al. 1984). Clinical signs in affected dogs are associated with hypertonicity and include anorexia, lethargy, weakness, disorientation, ataxia, and seizures. These dogs can be managed clinically by addition of water to their food, but hypernatremia and neurologic dysfunction recur whenever water supplementation is discontinued. In a Norwegian elkhound with adipsic hypernatremia, the adipsia resolved spontaneously at 2 years of age (Hall 1984).

Central or pituitary diabetes insipidus (CDI) is due to a partial or complete lack of vasopressin production and release from the neurohypophysis (Harb et al. 1996). It may result from trauma (Henry and Sieber 1965; Rogers et al. 1977; Authement et al. 1989) or neoplasia (Madewell et al. 1975; Neer and Reavis 1983; Davenport et al. 1986; Ferguson and Biery 1988) or may be idiopathic (Green and Farrow 1974; Burnie and Dunn 1979; Greene et al. 1979; Reidarson et al. 1990; Pittari 1996) in dogs and cats. Visceral larva migrans has also been reported to cause CDI in a dog (Lieberman et al. 1979). In one dog with hypernatremia, hypertonicity, and gastric dilatation-volvulus, CDI was present and caused by neurohypophyseal atrophy secondary to a cystic craniopharyngeal duct (Edwards et al. 1983). Congenital CDI is rare (Greene et al. 1979; Winterbotham and Mason 1983; Kraus 1987) but has been reported in two sibling Afghan pups (Post et al. 1989). Traumatic CDI may be transient in nature. Hypophysectomy for treatment of hyperadrenocorticism results in transient CDI that may take several weeks to resolve (Lubberink 1980). The transient nature of CDI in this setting may result from the fact that some of the vasopressin-producing neurons from the hypothalamus terminate in the median eminence.

DISORDERS OF SODIUM AND WATER

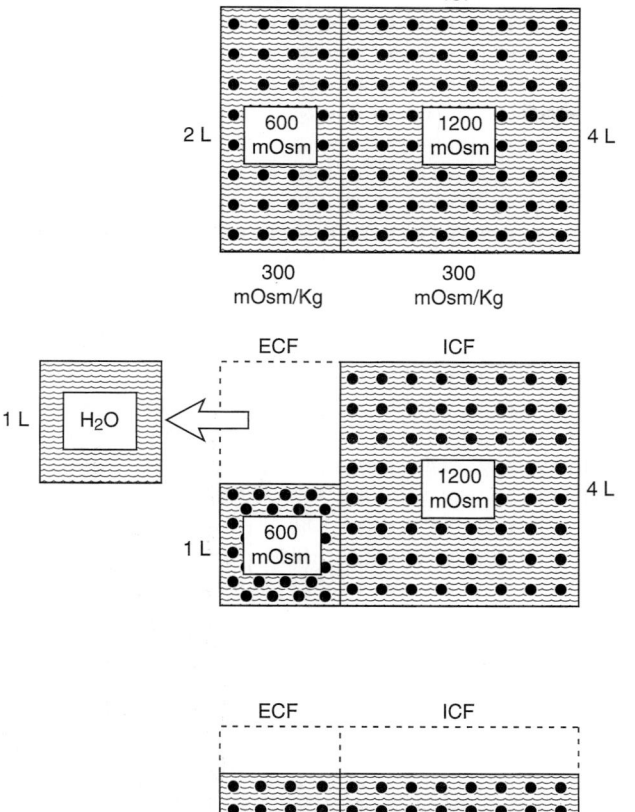

FIGURE 3-7. Effect of loss of 1 L of water on volume and tonicity of extracellular fluid (ECF) and intracellular fluid (ICF). (Drawing by Tim Vojt.)

Animals with CDI have severe polydipsia and polyuria. Their urine is typically hyposthenuric (urine osmolality 60–200 mOsm/kg), but urine osmolality may approach 400 to 500 mOsm/kg in the presence of dehydration. Variability in urine specific gravity and urine osmolality values at the time of presentation in dogs and cats with diabetes insipidus is presumably related to hydration status and severity of vasopressin deficiency. In one study, dogs were classified as having complete or partial CDI on the basis of the magnitude of increase in their urine specific gravity (USG) and urine osmolality after induction of 5% dehydration (Harb et al. 1996). Dogs with complete CDI had USG values of 1.001 to 1.007 that did not change substantially after induction of 5% dehydration, whereas dogs with partial CDI has USG values of 1.002 to 1.016 that increased to 1.010 to 1.018 after induction of 5% dehydration. In both groups, there was a substantial (>50%) increase in USG 2 h after administration of 1 to 5 U of aqueous arginine vasopressin. Affected dogs responded well to administration of desmopressin acetate (1 to 2 drops in both eyes every 12 to 24 h), but the prognosis was dependent on the underlying cause of CDI. Many older dogs with CDI had tumors in the region of the pituitary gland and developed neurologic signs.

Increased plasma osmolality and hypernatremia may occur in dogs and cats with CDI. These results suggest that some affected dogs and cats do not obtain enough water to maintain water balance and are presented in a hypertonic state. Severe hypernatremia and neurologic dysfunction may occur if the animal cannot maintain adequate water intake (Edwards et al. 1983; Reidarson et al. 1990). In contrast, with psychogenic polydipsia, plasma osmolality and serum sodium concentration may be lower than normal at presentation (Lage 1977a). Administration of vasopressin leads to an increase in urine osmolality or specific gravity in dogs and cats with CDI, but the initial response may be less than expected because of renal medullary washout of solute. In one study, USG values increased to 1.018 to 1.022 after vasopressin administration in dogs with complete CDI and to 1.018 to 1.036 in dogs with partial CDI (Harb et al. 1996).

Treatment with vasopressin restores medullary hypertonicity and normal urinary concentrating ability. Historically, vasopressin tannate in oil (Pitressin tannate) has been used to treat CDI in small animal practice. The dosage is 3 to 5 U for dogs or 1 to 2 U for cats given intramuscularly or subcutaneously every 24 to 72 h as needed to control polyuria and polydipsia. To avoid the possibility of water intoxication, it is recommended that the treatment interval be determined by recurrence of polyuria. This product is no longer commercially available.

Desmopressin is a structural analog of vasopressin (see Fig. 3-3) that has a more potent antidiuretic effect than vasopressin but minimal vasopressive effect and is relatively resistant to metabolic degradation. Desmopressin (DDAVP) is available as a nasal spray (0.1 mg/mL), injectable solution (4 μg/mL), or tablet for oral administration (0.1 and 0.2 mg). The injectable solution is much more expensive than the nasal spray, and the nasal spray has been used subcutaneously in dogs (Kraus et al. 1989) and in a cat with CDI at a dosage of 1 μg/kg (Kraus 1987) without adverse effects. Polyuria and polydipsia in a cat with CDI were controlled with 1 μg/kg administered subcutaneously q12h or 1.5 μg/kg administered conjunctivally q8h. One drop of the nasal spray contains 1.5 to 4 μg of desmopressin, and the duration of effect varies from 8 to 24 h (Feldman and Nelson 1996a).

Chlorpropamide is a sulfonylurea hypoglycemic agent that potentiates the renal tubular effects of small amounts of vasopressin and may be useful in management of animals with partial CDI. Hypoglycemia is a potential side effect of this drug. Its recommended dosage is 10 to 40 mg/kg/day orally. It has been useful in the management of CDI (up to 50% reduction in urine output) in some reports (Rogers et al. 1977) but not in others (Kraus 1987), possibly because some animals have partial and some have complete CDI.

In the broadest sense, the term nephrogenic diabetes insipidus (NDI) may be used to describe a diverse group of disorders in which structural or functional abnormalities interfere with the ability of the kidneys to concentrate

TABLE 3-5. **Causes of Nephrogenic Diabetes Insipidus**

Congenital (primary)
Acquired (secondary)
    Functional
        Drugs
            Glucocorticoids
            Lithium
            Demeclocycline
            Methoxyflurane
            Escherichia coli endotoxin (e.g., pyelonephritis, pyometra)
            Diuretics
        Electrolyte disturbances
            Hypokalemia
            Hypercalcemia
        Altered medullary hypertonicity
            Hypoadrenocorticism
        Multifactorial or unknown mechanism
            Hepatic insufficiency
            Hyperthyroidism
            Hyperadrenocorticism
        Postobstructive diuresis
        Acromegaly
    Structural
        Medullary interstitial amyloidosis (e.g., in cats, Shar Pei dog)
        Polycystic kidney disease
        Chronic pyelonephritis
        Chronic interstitial nephritis

urine (Table 3-5) (Lage 1973; Breitschwerdt et al. 1981). Congenital NDI is a rare disorder in small animal medicine (Lage 1973; Joles and Gruys 1979; Breitschwerdt et al. 1981). Affected animals are presented at a very young age for severe polyuria and polydipsia. In reported cases, urine osmolality and specific gravity have been in the hyposthenuric range. Affected animals show no response to water deprivation testing, exogenous vasopressin administration, or hypertonic saline infusion. In one case report, the plasma vasopressin concentration was markedly increased (Joles and Gruys 1979).

Thiazide diuretics (chlorothiazide 20–40 mg/kg q12h or hydrochlorothiazide 2.5–5.0 mg/kg b.i.d.) have been used to treat animals with CDI and NDI. Diuretic administration results in mild dehydration, enhanced proximal renal tubular reabsorption of sodium, decreased delivery of tubular fluid to the distal nephron, and reduced urine output. Thiazides have been reported to result in a 20 to 50% reduction in urine output in dogs with NDI (Lage 1973; Breitschwerdt et al. 1981) and in cats with CDI (Burnie and Dunn 1979; Kraus 1987). In other reports, thiazides were reported to be ineffective in reducing urine output in a dog (Henry and Sieber 1965) and a cat (Green and Farrow 1974) with CDI. Restriction of dietary sodium and protein reduces the amount of solute that must be excreted in the urine each day and thus further reduces obligatory water loss and polyuria.

Hypotonic Fluid Loss

When hypotonic fluid is lost from the extracellular compartment, the osmotic stimulus for water to move from the intracellular to the extracellular compartment is less than the stimulus for water movement created by pure water loss. Thus, hypotonic losses cause a greater reduction in the ECF volume and the animal is more likely to show clinical signs of volume depletion (e.g., changes in skin turgor, weak pulses, tachycardia). As the tonicity of the fluid lost increases toward the normal tonicity of ECF, the volume deficit of the extracellular compartment becomes progressively more severe (Fig. 3-8). In the case of isotonic losses, there is no osmotic stimulus for water movement, and the entire loss is borne by the extracellular compartment, with the result that hypovolemic shock occurs if the loss has been of sufficient magnitude (e.g., severe hemorrhage).

Consider what would occur in our previous example if our 10-kg dog suffered a loss from the extracellular compartment of 1 L of fluid with an osmolality of 150 mOsm/kg. Such a loss would leave 450 mOsm of solute and 1 L of water in the extracellular compartment. Once again, water moves from the intracellular to the extracellular compartment until the osmolality has been equalized. Thus,

$$\text{New ECF osmolality} = \text{new ICF osmolality}$$
$$450 \text{ mOsm}/(1 + x) \text{ L} = 1200 \text{ mOsm}/(4 - x) \text{ L}$$

where x is the volume of water moving between compartments:

$$450(4 - x) = 1200(1 + x)$$
$$x = 0.36 \text{ L}$$

The new volumes and osmolalities are

ECF: 450 mOsm/1.36 L = 330 mOsm/kg
ICF: 1200 mOsm/3.64 L = 330 mOsm/kg

Note that the extracellular volume deficit is more severe than in the previous example of pure water loss (0.64 L versus 0.33 L). These changes are depicted in Figure 3-9. The more closely the fluid lost approximates ECF in tonicity, the greater the volume loss from the ECF compartment.

For simplicity, these examples are based on many

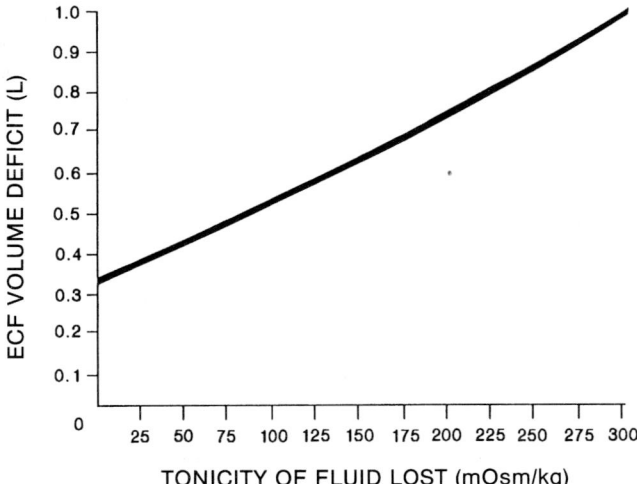

FIGURE 3-8. Magnitude of extracellular fluid (ECF) volume deficit caused by loss of 1 L of fluid of varying tonicity.

DISORDERS OF SODIUM AND WATER 57

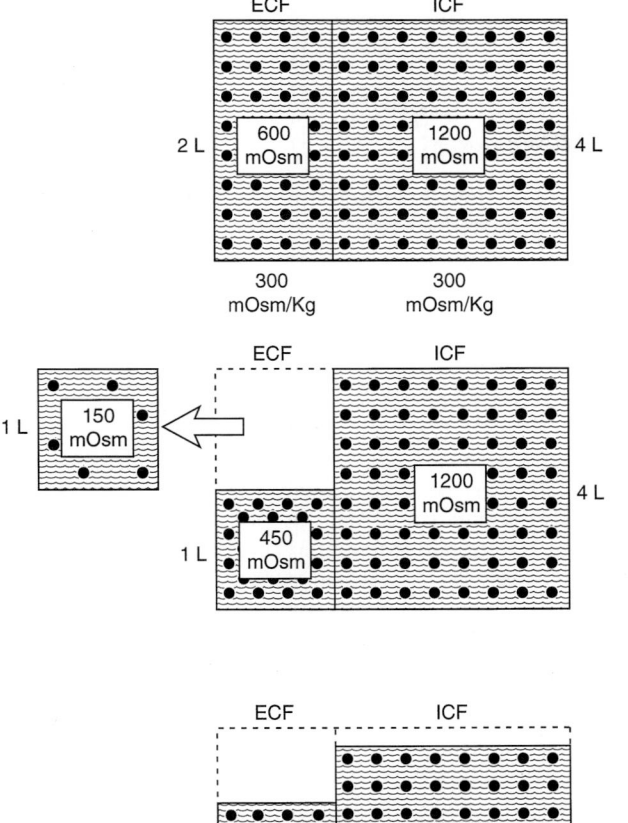

FIGURE 3-9. Effect of loss of 1 L of hypotonic fluid (150 mOsm/kg) on volume and tonicity of extracellular fluid (ECF) and intracellular fluid (ICF). (Drawing by Tim Vojt.)

assumptions that in reality may not be true. For example, total body water is not 60% of body weight in all individuals, the number of osmoles in the ECF may have been altered by electrolyte losses not detected clinically, the effects of hydrostatic forces resulting from extracellular volume depletion have not been considered, some solutes may not be strictly impermeant, and compensatory physiologic responses have not been considered. Nonetheless, such calculations are helpful in understanding the pathophysiology of hypertonic states and they provide useful clinical approximations.

Hypotonic fluid losses are the most common type encountered in small animal medicine. They may be classified as extrarenal (e.g., gastrointestinal, third-space loss, and cutaneous) or renal. Causes of gastrointestinal losses include vomiting, diarrhea, and small intestinal obstruction; causes of third-space losses include pancreatitis and peritonitis. Cutaneous losses are usually not clinically important in dogs and cats. Eccrine sweat glands are limited to the foot pads and serve no thermoregulatory function, and burns are encountered uncommonly in small animal practice. Renal losses may result from osmotically (e.g., diabetes mellitus, mannitol) or chemically (e.g., furosemide, corticosteroids) induced diuresis or from defective urinary concentrating ability related to intrinsic renal disease (e.g., chronic renal failure, nonoliguric acute renal failure, postobstructive diuresis).

Gain of Impermeant Solute

Gain of impermeant solute is uncommon in small animal medicine. The addition of a sodium salt to ECF causes hypernatremia, whereas gain of an impermeant solute that does not contain sodium (e.g., glucose, mannitol) initially causes hyponatremia because water is drawn into ECF. Hypernatremia occurs, however, as osmotic diuresis develops because urine osmolality approaches plasma osmolality and the sodium-free solute replaces sodium in urine. The sodium displaced from the urine remains in the ECF and contributes to hypernatremia.

The development of hypertonicity as a result of excessive salt ingestion is unlikely if the animal in question has an intact thirst mechanism and access to water. The addition of impermeant solute without water expands the extracellular compartment at the expense of the intracellular compartment as water moves from ICF to ECF to equalize osmolality. This volume overload may lead to pulmonary edema if the patient has underlying cardiac disease.

Consider again our example of the 10-kg dog. The addition of 200 mOsm of solute to the ECF without any water would be equivalent to ingestion of 5.85 g of sodium chloride (5.85 g NaCl = 100 mmol Na and 100 mmol Cl). The addition of this impermeant solute to ECF causes movement of water from the intracellular to extracellular compartments until osmolality has been equalized. Thus,

New ECF osmolality = new ICF osmolality
800 mOsm/$(2 + x)$ L = 1200 mOsm/$(4 - x)$ L

where x is the volume of water moving between compartments:

$$800(4 - x) = 1200(2 + x)$$
$$x = 0.4 \text{ L}$$

The new volumes and osmolalities are

ECF: 800 mOsm/2.4 L = 333 mOsm/kg
ICF: 1200 mOsm/3.6 L = 333 mOsm/kg

Note that ECF volume has been expanded by 0.4 L and that this volume has been derived from ICF. In the normal animal, this expansion of the extracellular compartment leads to natriuresis, and the volume deficit is repaired by ingestion of water in response to plasma hyperosmolality. These changes are depicted in Figure 3-10.

In one report of salt poisoning in dogs, a defective water softener resulted in delivery of drinking water containing 10% sodium chloride as compared with normal tap water containing less than 0.1% (Hughes and Sokolowski 1978). The affected dogs developed progressive ataxia, seizures, prostration, and death. Their serum so-

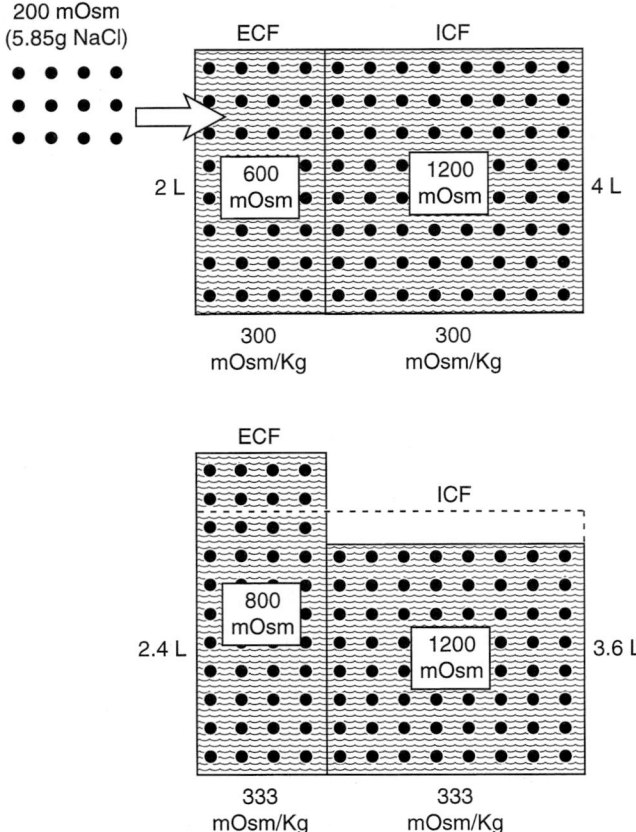

FIGURE 3-10. Effect of addition of 200 mOsm solute (5.85 g NaCl) on volume and tonicity of extracellular fluid (ECF) and intracellular fluid (ICF). (Drawing by Tim Vojt.)

dium concentrations ranged from 185 to 190 mEq/L. Histopathology showed focal areas of perivascular hemorrhage and edema in the midbrain. In another case report, presumptive salt poisoning resulted from ingestion of seawater and subsequent restriction of fresh drinking water (Chew 1969). Another dog developed fatal hypernatremia after it ingested a large amount of a salt-flour mix (Khanna et al. 1997). After ingestion of a salt-flour figurine, the dog began vomiting and developed polyuria and polydipsia. The owner removed the dog's water source and it ingested more of the salt-flour mix. Seizures, pyrexia, and sinus tachycardia developed, and the serum sodium concentration reached 211 mEq/L.

Therapeutic administration of hyperosmolar solutions containing large amounts of sodium during cardiac resuscitation can cause hypernatremia and hypertonicity (e.g., hypertonic saline, sodium bicarbonate). Sodium phosphate enemas may also result in mild hypernatremia (Atkins et al. 1985). Primary hyperaldosteronism is rare in dogs and cats, but idiopathic hyperplasia of the adrenal zona glomerulosa was associated with hypernatremia and increased plasma aldosterone concentration in one dog (Breitschwerdt et al. 1985), and hyperaldosteronism and severe hypokalemia have been reported in three dogs with adrenal adenoma or adenocarcinoma (Feldman and Nelson 1996b). An adrenocortical carcinoma was reported to cause primary hyperaldosteronism in a cat, but the cat had a normal serum sodium concentration (Eger et al. 1983). Mild hypernatremia also may occur in dogs with hyperadrenocorticism (Ling et al. 1979; Peterson 1984).

▶ Clinical Signs of Hypernatremia

The clinical signs of hypernatremia are primarily neurologic and related to osmotic movement of water out of brain cells. A rapid decrease in brain volume may cause rupture of cerebral vessels and focal hemorrhage. The severity of clinical signs is related more to the rapidity of onset of hypernatremia than to the magnitude of hypernatremia. In dogs and cats, clinical signs of hypernatremia are observed when the serum sodium concentration exceeds 170 mEq/L (Hughes and Sokolowski 1978; Hardy 1989; Reidarson et al. 1990; Khanna et al. 1997). If hypernatremia develops slowly, the brain has time to adapt to the hypertonic state by production of intracellular solutes (e.g., inositol, amino acids) called *osmolytes* or *idiogenic osmoles*. These substances prevent dehyration of the brain and allow patients with chronic hypernatremia to be relatively asymptomatic (see earlier).

Where described in dogs and cats, clinical signs of hypernatremia and hypertonicity have included anorexia, lethargy, vomiting, muscular weakness, behavioral change, disorientation, ataxia, seizures, coma, and death (Chew 1969; Hughes and Sokolowski 1978; Crawford et al. 1984; Dow et al. 1987; Reidarson et al. 1990; Van Heerden et al. 1992; Bagley et al. 1993; DiBartola et al. 1994; Khanna et al. 1997). If hypotonic losses are the cause of hypernatremia, clinical signs of volume depletion (e.g., decreased skin turgor, tachycardia, weak pulses) may be observed on physical examination. If hypernatremia has developed as a result of gain of sodium, signs of volume overload (e.g., pulmonary edema) may be observed, especially in patients with underlying cardiac disease. Patients with CDI or NDI are typically presented for evaluation of severe polydipsia and polyuria.

▶ Treatment of Hypernatremia

The main goals in treating patients with hypernatremia are to replace the water and electrolytes that have been lost and, if necessary, to facilitate renal excretion of excess sodium. The first priority in treatment should be to restore the ECF volume to normal. The next priority is to diagnose and treat the underlying disease responsible for the water and electrolyte deficits.

Pure Water Loss

Total body solute (TBS) is the product of total body water (TBW) and plasma osmolality (P_{osm}). If a patient's fluid loss has been limited to pure water, the following relationship is true:

$$\text{TBS (present)} = \text{TBS (previous)}$$
$$\text{TBW (present)} \times P_{osm}\text{ (present)} = \text{TBW (previous)} \times P_{osm}\text{ (previous)}$$

If we assume that body water (TBW) is 60% of body weight measured in kilograms (Wt) and that $2.1 \times P_{Na}$ is an estimate of P_{osm}:

$$2.1 \times P_{Na} \text{ (present)} \times 0.6 \times \text{Wt (present)}$$
$$= 2.1 \times P_{Na} \text{ (previous)} \times 0.6 \text{ Wt (previous)}$$

This equation reduces to

$$P_{Na} \text{ (present)} \times \text{Wt (present)} =$$
$$P_{Na} \text{ (previous)} \times \text{Wt (previous)}$$

$$\text{Wt (previous)} = \frac{P_{Na} \text{ (present)} \times \text{Wt (present)}}{P_{Na} \text{ (previous)}}$$

The water deficit is the difference between the previous and present body weights:

$$\text{Wt (previous)} - \text{Wt (present)} =$$
$$\frac{P_{Na} \text{ (present)} \times \text{Wt (present)}}{P_{Na} \text{ (previous)}} - \text{Wt (present)}$$

or

$$\text{Wt (present)} \times \left(\frac{P_{Na} \text{ (present)}}{P_{Na} \text{ (previous)}} - 1 \right)$$

Consider a previously normal dog that has been deprived of water for several days. The dog weighs 10 kg at presentation, and its serum sodium concentration is 170 mEq/L. Assuming a previously normal serum sodium concentration of 150 mEq/L, the dog's water deficit can be calculated:

$$\text{Water deficit} = \text{Wt (present)} \times \left(\frac{P_{Na} \text{ (present)}}{P_{Na} \text{ (previous)}} - 1 \right)$$

$$\text{Water deficit} = 10 \left[\left(\frac{170}{150} - 1 \right) \right] = 1.33 \text{ L}$$

The original estimates of total body water and serum sodium concentration may be modified on the basis of information available to the clinician at presentation. For example, if the dog's normal serum sodium concentration is known from a previous admission, this value can be substituted in place of 150 mEq/L. If the dog's previous normal body weight is known, the water deficit may simply be estimated as the difference between the previous and present body weights. The assumption inherent in the latter calculation is that the patient has not gained or lost tissue mass. Over a short time period, this is a reasonable assumption because loss of 1 kg of tissue mass requires an expenditure of approximately 1600 kcal. This caloric expenditure would require fasting for 2 to 3 days in a normal 10-kg dog with a basal energy requirement of approximately 700 kcal.

A pure water deficit can be replaced by giving 5% dextrose in water intravenously. This solution technically is only slightly hypotonic to plasma (278 mOsm/kg), but the glucose ultimately enters cells and is metabolized so that administration of 5% dextrose is equivalent to administration of water. The water deficit must be replaced and hypernatremia corrected slowly over 48 h. The brain adapts to hypertonicity by the production of osmolytes or idiogenic osmoles that prevent cellular dehydration (see earlier). Excessively rapid lowering of the serum sodium concentration may result in movement of water into brain cells and development of cerebral edema. In human patients, correction of the serum sodium concentration at a rate of less than 0.5 mEq/L/h minimizes the risk of neurologic complications related to water intoxication (Sterns et al. 1996). The animal's serum sodium concentration should be monitored serially during replacement of the water deficit.

Hypotonic Loss

As described earlier, hypotonic losses cause more severe extracellular volume contraction than do losses of pure water. As the tonicity of the fluid lost approaches the tonicity of ECF, the extracellular volume deficit becomes greater (see Fig. 3–8). As a result, signs of volume depletion are more likely with hypotonic losses, and the original replacement fluid should be isotonic so that extracellular volume repletion proceeds rapidly.

In the presence of hemorrhagic shock, whole blood, plasma, or a colloid solution is the ideal fluid to administer. The hemoglobin in whole blood improves oxygen-carrying capacity. The plasma proteins in whole blood and plasma or the dextrans in a colloid solution increase and maintain intravascular volume by increasing oncotic pressure. In many animals that have experienced severe hypotonic losses over an extended period of time, replacement of the ECF volume with an isotonic crystalloid solution (e.g., 0.9% NaCl, lactated Ringer's solution) is adequate. A volume up to four times the suspected intravascular deficit may be required because the isotonic crystalloid solution distributes rapidly throughout the ECF compartment (ECF volume is four times intravascular volume). After the extracellular volume has been expanded, hypotonic fluids (e.g., 0.45% NaCl, half-strength lactated Ringer's solution) can be administered to provide fluids for maintenance needs and ongoing losses (see Chapter 13).

Gain of Impermeant Solute

The patient with an excess of sodium-containing impermeant solute in the ECF can be treated by administration of 5% dextrose intravenously. The main disadvantage of this approach is that it causes further expansion of the extracellular compartment in a patient already suffering from ECF volume expansion. In an animal with normal cardiac and renal function, this volume expansion leads to diuresis and natriuresis and ECF volume returns to normal. In an animal with underlying cardiac disease or oliguria related to primary renal disease, this approach may lead to development of pulmonary edema. Administration of a loop diuretic (e.g., furosemide, ethacrynic acid) promotes excretion of the existing sodium load and hastens return of ECF volume to normal. As in the case of pure water deficit, it is essential that fluid administration proceed slowly and that serum sodium concentration be lowered gradually over 48 h to avoid neurologic complications.

▶ Clinical Approach to the Patient with Hyponatremia

The presence of hyponatremia usually, but not always, implies hypoosmolality. Thus, the first step in the approach to the patient with hyponatremia is to determine

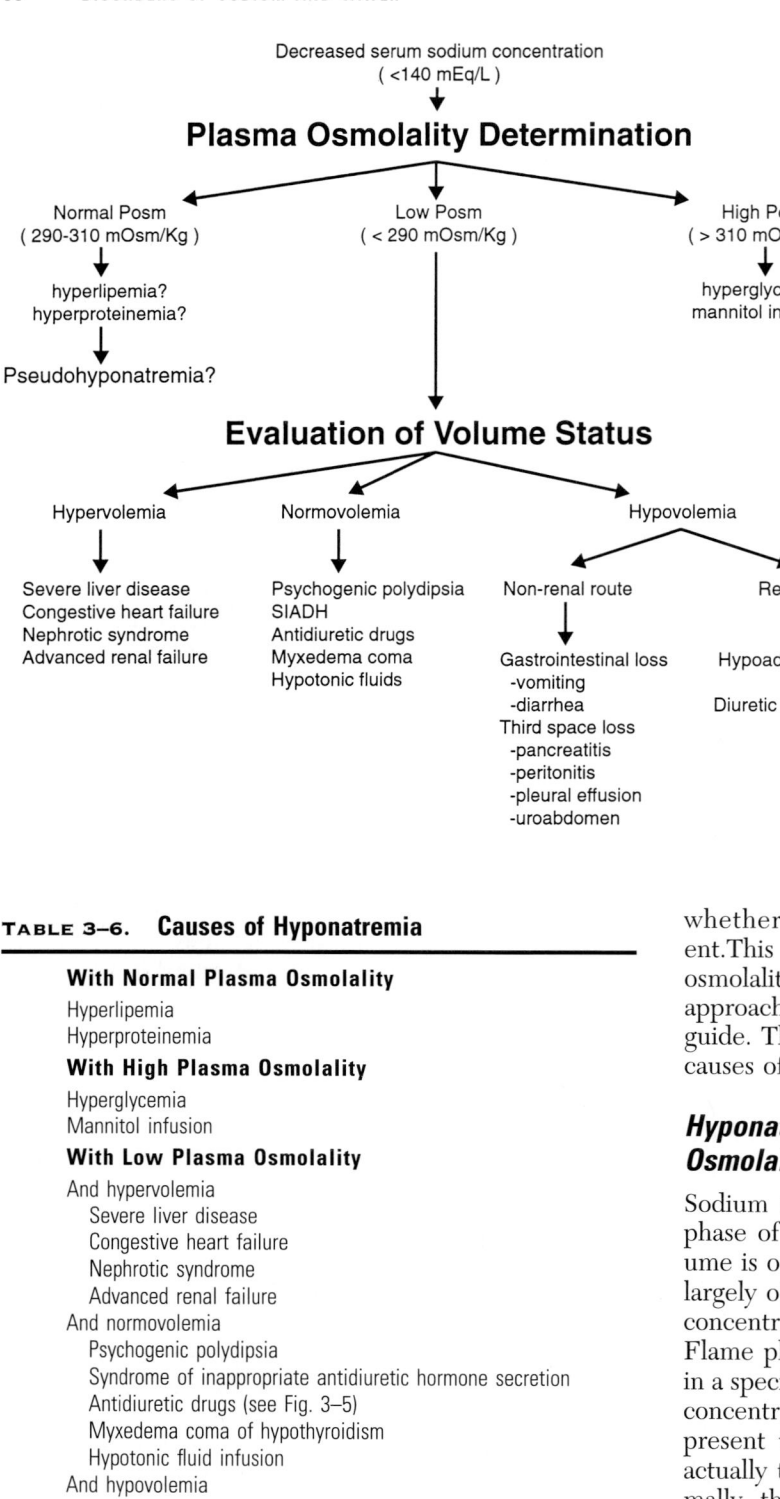

FIGURE 3–11. Clinical approach to the patient with hyponatremia. P_{osm} = plasma osmolality; SIADH = syndrome of inappropriate antidiuretic hormone. (From DiBartola SP: Hyponatremia. *Vet Clin North Am Small Anim Pract* 28:515–532, 1998.)

TABLE 3–6. Causes of Hyponatremia

With Normal Plasma Osmolality
Hyperlipemia
Hyperproteinemia

With High Plasma Osmolality
Hyperglycemia
Mannitol infusion

With Low Plasma Osmolality
And hypervolemia
  Severe liver disease
  Congestive heart failure
  Nephrotic syndrome
  Advanced renal failure
And normovolemia
  Psychogenic polydipsia
  Syndrome of inappropriate antidiuretic hormone secretion
  Antidiuretic drugs (see Fig. 3–5)
  Myxedema coma of hypothyroidism
  Hypotonic fluid infusion
And hypovolemia
  Gastrointestinal loss
    Vomiting
    Diarrhea
  Third-space loss
    Pancreatitis
    Peritonitis
    Uroabdomen
    Pleural effusion (e.g., chylothorax)
    Peritoneal effusion
  Cutaneous loss
    Burns
  Hypoadrenocorticism
  Diuretic administration

whether hypoosmolality of the ECF is actually present. This can be determined by measurement of plasma osmolality. The evaluation of hyponatremia may then be approached using the patient's plasma osmolality as a guide. This approach is outlined in Figure 3–11, and the causes of hyponatremia are listed in Table 3–6.

Hyponatremia with Normal Plasma Osmolality

Sodium is present as charged particles in the aqueous phase of body fluids. Approximately 93% of plasma volume is occupied by water and the remaining 7% consists largely of proteins and lipids. Historically, serum sodium concentration has been measured by flame photometry. Flame photometry measures the number of sodium ions in a specific volume of plasma or serum. Thus, the sodium concentration is measured as if the sodium ions were present throughout the entire sample volume, whereas actually they are active only in the aqueous phase. Normally, this error is small. In plasma or serum samples containing a large amount of lipid or protein, however, the error may be larger and the decrease in measured serum sodium concentration could be misleading to the clinician (Figure 3–12). When serum sodium concentration is measured by direct potentiometry using ion-selective electrodes, large amounts of lipid or protein in the sample should not affect the measured serum sodium concentration. If, however, the serum sample is diluted before measurement, large amounts of lipid or protein may still affect the measured serum sodium concentration (Ladenson et al. 1981) The clinician must therefore be familiar with the laboratory method employed so as to

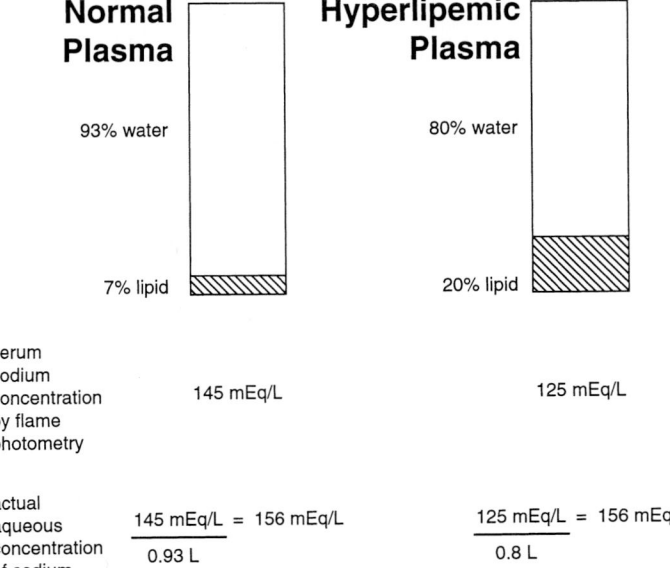

FIGURE 3-12. Effect of increased plasma lipids on serum sodium concentration (pseudohyponatremia or factitious hyponatremia). (From DiBartola SP: Hyponatremia. *Vet Clin North Am Small Anim Pract* 28:515–532, 1998.)

interpret serum sodium concentrations properly. The occurrence of a decreased serum sodium concentration as a result of laboratory methodology in the presence of normal plasma osmolality is called *pseudohyponatremia* or *factitious hyponatremia*. Pseudohyponatremia occurs in conditions associated with hyperlipidemia or severe hyperproteinemia.

Plasma osmolality in patients with pseudohyponatremia is normal because lipids and proteins are very large molecules that contribute very little to plasma osmolality. If pseudohyponatremia is present, the calculated plasma osmolality is low because of a spuriously low serum sodium concentration, whereas the measured osmolality is normal. Thus, when an abnormal osmolal gap is present and the measured osmolality is normal, pseudohyponatremia should be suspected. The diagnosis of pseudohyponatremia can be made by visual inspection of plasma for lipemia and by measurement of the total plasma protein concentration. Hyperlipemia severe enough to cause pseudohyponatremia is visible to the naked eye as lactescent plasma. Each milligram per deciliter of lipid in serum reduces the sodium concentration by 0.002 mEq/L (e.g., a serum triglyceride concentration of 1000 mg/dL would be expected to reduce the serum sodium concentration by 2 mEq/L) (Narins et al. 1982). In the case of hyperproteinemia, each gram per deciliter of protein above a concentration of 8 g/dL reduces the serum sodium concentration by approximately 0.25 mEq/L (e.g., the serum sodium concentration of a patient with a serum protein concentration of 12 g/dL would be expected to be reduced by 1 mEq/L) (Sterns et al. 1994). At such protein concentrations the plasma may be viscous, and this is likely to occur mainly in patients with plasma cell dyscrasias. Thus, whereas pseudohyponatremia may be intellectually interesting, it is unlikely to be of clinical relevance in most instances. Furthermore, pseudohyponatremia itself has no consequences for the health of the patient. Its importance lies in the ability of the clinician to recognize it and refrain from treating the patient for hyponatremia. Treatment should be directed at the underlying disorder causing hyperproteinemia or hyperlipidemia.

Hyponatremia with Increased Plasma Osmolality

If an impermeant solute is added to ECF, water moves from ICF to ECF, and the osmolality of both compartments increases (Feig and McCurdy 1977) (see Fig. 3-10). If the added solute is something other than sodium, the serum sodium concentration is reduced by the translocation of water, but the plasma osmolality is higher than normal.

Hyponatremia with hyperosmolality is usually due to hyperglycemia in diabetes mellitus, wherein each 100 mg/dL increase in glucose decreases serum sodium by 1.6 mEq/L (Katz 1973). Thus, in the diabetic patient, hyperlipidemia and hyperglycemia may both contribute to decreased serum sodium concentration. Administration of the osmotic diuretic mannitol can also cause hyponatremia with plasma hyperosmolality. The calculated osmolality is normal, the measured osmolality high, and the osmolal gap increased in the presence of mannitol, which is an unmeasured osmole. Hyperglycemia does not affect the osmolal gap because the plasma glucose concentration is part of the equation used to calculate plasma osmolality (i.e., it is a measured osmole).

Initially, total body water content is not altered in the setting of hyponatremia with hyperosmolality. Rather, there is an altered distribution of water between intracellular and extracellular compartments. A reduction in total body water content develops, however, to the extent that these substances cause an osmotic diuresis.

Hyponatremia with Decreased Plasma Osmolality

The total body sodium content and ECF volume of patients with hyponatremia and hypoosmolality may be normal, decreased, or increased. The second step in the evaluation of the patient with hyponatremia is therefore to estimate total body sodium content and ECF volume status. This is best done by clinical assessment of the patient on the basis of history, physical examination, and a few ancillary tests. A good history often indicates a source of fluid loss (e.g., vomiting, diarrhea, diuretic administration) and the physical examination provides important clues to the patient's volume status. The following physical findings should be assessed: skin turgor, moistness of the mucous membranes, capillary refill time, pulse rate and character, appearance of the jugular veins (distended or flat), and presence or absence of ascites or edema. Measurements of hematocrit and total plasma protein concentration, as well as systemic blood pressure and central venous pressure determinations, if available, further clarify the patient's ECF volume status.

HYPONATREMIA WITH VOLUME DEPLETION

For a patient with volume depletion (hypovolemia) to develop hyponatremia, the total body deficit of sodium must exceed that of water. Hyponatremic patients with volume depletion have lost fluid by renal or nonrenal routes. Gastrointestinal losses (e.g., vomiting, diarrhea) and third-space losses (e.g., pleural effusion) (Willard et al. 1991), peritoneal effusion caused by peritonitis, pancreatitis, or uroabdomen (Burrows and Bovee 1974)) are the most important nonrenal losses of fluid and NaCl. Gastrointestinal losses are often hypotonic in nature. The question thus arises, If the losses are hypotonic, how does the patient become hyponatremic? The answer follows from three physiologic events and reflects the body's tendency to preserve volume at the expense of tonicity. First, volume depletion decreases GFR, enhances isosmotic reabsorption of sodium and water in the proximal tubules, and decreases delivery of tubular fluid to distal diluting sites. These effects impair excretion of water. Second, volume depletion is a strong nonosmotic stimulus for vasopressin release, and the increased plasma vasopressin concentration further impairs water excretion. Third, the patient is thirsty because of volume depletion and continues to drink water if it is available. All of these factors have a dilutional effect on the remaining body fluids.

Recall the previous example of the loss of 1 L of fluid with an osmolality of 150 mOsm/kg and consider what would happen if the animal in question drinks 1 L of pure water after sustaining the hypotonic loss. The added water increases the ECF volume from 1.36 to 2.36 L, and the resulting hypotonicity rapidly drives water into cells to equalize osmolality:

$$\text{New ECF osmolality} = \text{new ICF osmolality}$$

$$\frac{450 \text{ mOsm}}{(2.36 - x)} = \frac{1200 \text{ mOsm}}{(3.64 + x)}$$

where x is the volume of water moving between compartments:

$$450(3.64 + x) = 1200(2.36 - x)$$
$$x = 0.72 \text{ L}$$

The new volumes and osmolalities are

$$\text{ECF:} \quad \frac{450 \text{ mOsm}}{1.64 \text{ L}} = 275 \text{ mOsm/kg}$$

$$\text{ICF:} \quad \frac{1200 \text{ mOsm}}{4.36 \text{ L}} = 275 \text{ mOsm/kg}$$

Note that in this example the intracellular compartment is expanded (4.36 L). The volume of the extracellular compartment (1.64 L) is greater than it was when the same hypotonic loss was not replaced (1.36 L) but still less than the previous normal value (2 L). Thus, hypotonic (or isotonic) losses replaced by pure water lead to expansion of the ICF space. These changes are depicted in Figure 3–13.

Renal fluid and NaCl losses resulting in hyponatremia are usually due to hypoadrenocorticism or diuretic administration. In one study, 81% of 225 dogs with hypoadrenocorticism were hyponatremic at presentation (Peterson et al. 1996). Mineralocorticoid deficiency in hypoadrenocorticism results in urinary loss of NaCl and depletion of ECF volume. Volume depletion is a strong nonosmotic stimulus for vasopressin release and impairs water excretion. Hyperkalemia typically accompanies hyponatremia in hypoadrenocorticism (Willard et al. 1982; Schaer and Chen 1983; Rakich and Lorenz 1984; Peterson et al. 1996). Some dogs with hypoadrenocorticism, however, have only glucocorticoid deficiency at the time of presentation and thus have normal serum potassium concentrations (Rogers et al. 1981). Glucocorticoids are necessary for complete suppression of vasopressin release, and in their absence impaired water excretion and hyponatremia can occur (Crow and Stockham 1985). Occasionally, dogs

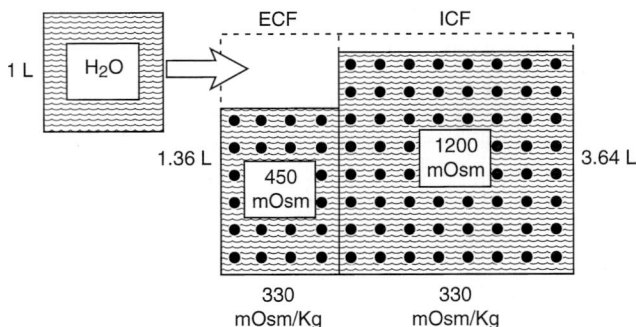

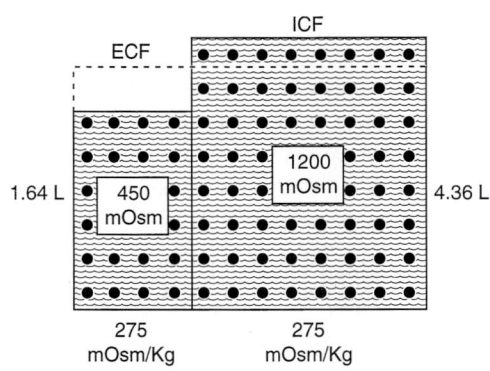

FIGURE 3–13. Effect of drinking 1 L of water after a loss of 1 L of hypotonic fluid (150 mOsm/kg) on volume and tonicity of extracellular fluid (ECF) and intracellular fluid (ICF). (Drawing by Tim Vojt.)

with gastrointestinal fluid losses develop electrolyte disturbances that mimic hypoadrenocorticism (DiBartola et al. 1985; Malik et al. 1990). Hyponatremia associated with third-space loss of fluid has been reported with pleural effusion related to chylothorax (Willard et al. 1991), lung lobe torsion (Zenger 1992), and neoplasia (Lamb and Muir 1994). In these reports, hyponatremia was attributed at least in part to removal of sodium-rich fluid by thoracocentesis. Many of these animals, however, had evidence of volume depletion, and it is likely that nonosmotic vasopressin secretion also played a role in the development of hyponatremia. Affected dogs also had mild hyperkalemia attributed to decreased renal excretion of potassium caused by volume depletion and decreased distal renal tubular flow. Similar findings haven been observed in a cat with peritoneal effusion associated with carcinomatosis (see Appendix). The pathogenesis of hyponatremia and mild hyperkalemia in dogs with gastrointestinal losses is probably similar to that described for dogs with pleural and peritoneal effusions. When the cause of hyponatremia and hyperkalemia is unclear, an ACTH stimulation test should be performed to rule out hypoadrenocorticism.

Diuretics contribute to impaired water excretion and dilution of sodium in the ECF by decreased distal delivery of tubular fluid and nonosmotic stimulation of vasopressin release, which occur in response to volume depletion. Furthermore, potassium depletion caused by diuretics can contribute to hyponatremia because shifting of intracellular potassium into the extracellular compartment in exchange for sodium may occur. Hyponatremia has been associated with chronic blood loss in dogs (Tyler et al. 1987). Defective urinary concentrating ability in these dogs was thought to be caused by impaired vasopressin release in response to plasma hypoosmolality and loss of NaCl from the renal medullary interstitium. Some of these dogs had hypoadrenocorticism and gastrointestinal fluid losses that may have contributed to their hyponatremia. Normal concentrating ability returned after resolution of hyponatremia.

HYPONATREMIA WITH VOLUME EXCESS

Hyponatremia may occur despite the presence of increased total body sodium and expansion of the ECF compartment in patients with ascites or edema. Some of the pathophysiologic events in these patients impair the excretion of ingested water and exert a dilutional effect on the serum sodium concentration. Hyponatremia with volume excess (hypervolemia) is observed in three clinical conditions: congestive heart failure, severe liver disease, and nephrotic syndrome. In these disorders, there is a perception of volume depletion by the body, and the regulatory mechanisms invoked result in volume expansion. This perceived volume deficit has been referred to as *decreased effective circulating volume* or *decreased effective arterial blood volume*.

Three major pathophysiologic mechanisms are operative in the pathogenesis of sodium retention and impaired water excretion in these clinical conditions. The renin-angiotensin system is activated by reduced renal perfusion and causes increased sodium retention by the kidneys. Decreased renal perfusion, decreased GFR, and increased proximal tubular reabsorption of sodium and water result in decreased delivery of tubular fluid to distal diluting sites and impairment of free water excretion. A decrease in effective arterial blood volume results in nonosmotic stimulation of vasopressin release and further impairment of water excretion. Impaired free water excretion causes dilution of retained sodium and results in hyponatremia despite the presence of increased total body sodium content and expansion of the ECF compartment. In addition, a primary intrarenal mechanism for sodium retention is thought to be operative in patients with the nephrotic syndrome.

In cirrhosis and the nephrotic syndrome, intravascular volume may be reduced as a result of decreased oncotic pressure caused by hypoalbuminemia. This volume depletion causes nonosmotic stimulation of vasopressin release and impaired water excretion. Reduction of cardiac output has also been observed to increase plasma concentrations of vasopressin. In congestive heart failure, decreased cardiac output is sensed by baroreceptors in the carotid and aortic sinuses, resulting in nonosmotic release of vasopressin. With chronic left atrial distention, the sensitivity of baroreceptors located in this site is presumably blunted, explaining the relative lack of vasopressin suppression that would be expected in acute left atrial distention.

The pathophysiology of sodium retention in the nephrotic syndrome appears to be complex. In some nephrotic patients with hypervolemia, the renin-angiotensin system appears to be suppressed. This conclusion is based on decreased plasma concentrations of renin and aldosterone and suggests a primary intrarenal mechanism for sodium retention (Brown et al. 1982). The site of this intrarenal mechanism of sodium retention is not clear. In one experimental study, a distal site was implicated (Ichikawa et al. 1983), whereas some investigators have suggested that alterations in filtration fraction and the glomerular ultrafiltration coefficient may be responsible (Dorhout Mees 1984).

In severe liver disease, arteriovenous shunting, splanchnic venous pooling, ascites caused by portal hypertension, and decreased oncotic pressure caused by hypoalbuminemia all may lead to decreased effective circulating volume resulting in nonosmotic stimulation of vasopressin release and activation of the renin-angiotensin system (Epstein 1985). Sodium retention and impairment of water excretion result.

Hyponatremia with hypervolemia may also be seen in advanced renal failure. Positive water balance may occur in the presence of continued polydipsia if there is an insufficient number of functional nephrons to excrete the required amount of free water. Approximately 70% of filtered water is reabsorbed isosmotically in the proximal tubules. If GFR is very low, the amount of water that can be excreted even with complete suppression of vasopressin release may be insufficient to prevent positive water balance in the presence of continued water intake. For example, consider a 10-kg dog with advanced renal failure and a GFR of 2 mL/min (approximately 5% of normal). The daily filtered load of water would be 2.88 L, and if 2.02 L (70%) is reabsorbed in the proximal tubules, the maximum volume of water that could be excreted is 860 mL. In the presence of polydipsia, it is conceivable that water intake would exceed this volume and dilutional hyponatremia would develop.

HYPONATREMIA WITH NORMAL VOLUME

Hyponatremia with normal volume (normovolemia) may occur as a result of psychogenic polydipsia, clinical conditions characterized by inappropriate secretion of vasopressin, administration of hypotonic fluids or drugs with antidiuretic effects, and myxedema coma of severe hypothyroidism. Approximately 67% of total body water is located within cells. Therefore, only 33% of the water retained in these disorders is distributed to the extracellular compartment and only 8% is located in the plasma compartment. This mild volume expansion does, however, increase GFR and decrease proximal tubular reabsorption of sodium and water, thus leading to natriuresis. If excessive water intake or inappropriate vasopressin release continues, a new steady state is achieved with a slightly expanded ECF volume and plasma hypoosmolality. Overt signs of hypervolemia are usually not present because the majority of retained water is distributed to the intracellular compartment.

Psychogenic polydipsia usually occurs in large-breed dogs. The owner may report that the dog has a nervous disposition or that polydipsia seemed to begin after some stressful event. Some hyperactive dogs placed in an exercise-restricted environment have developed psychogenic polydipsia, and some dogs with this disorder may have developed it as a learned behavior to gain attention from the owner (Feldman and Nelson 1996c). Some dogs with psychogenic polydipsia lower their water intake dramatically as a result of the stress of hospitalization, and this is sometimes a useful diagnostic observation. In one study, dogs with psychogenic polydipsia had daily water consumption of 150 to 250 mL/kg, USG of 1.001 to 1.003, urine osmolality of 102 to 112 mOsm/kg, plasma osmolality of 285 to 295 mOsm/kg, and serum sodium concentration of 131 to 140 mEq/L (Lage 1977a). Hyponatremia with plasma hypoosmolality was thus documented in this study. Approximately 67% of affected dogs had a normal response to water deprivation, whereas others had some degree of medullary washout but responded to gradual water deprivation. Psychogenic polydipsia has not yet been reported in cats.

The syndrome of inappropriate antidiuretic hormone secretion (SIADH) refers to vasopressin release in the absence of normal osmotic or nonosmotic stimuli. This syndrome occurs in human patients and may be drug induced or associated with various types of malignancies, pulmonary diseases, and central nervous system disorders (Zerbe et al. 1980). Several patterns of vasopressin secretion have been observed in human patients with SIADH: erratic changes in secretion unrelated to plasma osmolality, a normal increase in vasopressin secretion in response to changes in plasma osmolality but occurring at a lower threshold ("reset osmostat"), normal vasopressin secretion when plasma osmolality is normal or increased but inability to reduce vasopressin secretion appropriately after a water load ("vasopressin leak"), and low basal vasopressin concentration that fails to increase as plasma osmolality increases, suggesting increased renal sensitivity to vasopressin or presence of another antidiuretic substance.

SIADH is rare in dogs. In one dog it was suspected in association with dirofilariasis (Breitschwerdt and Root 1979), in one it occurred with an undifferentiated carcinoma (Giger and Gorman 1984), and in another it was reported in association with a tumor in the region of the hypothalamus (Houston et al. 1989). Inappropriate vasopressin secretion may have played a role in the pathogenesis of hyponatremia in a dog with glucocorticoid deficiency (Crow and Stockham 1985). Idiopathic SIADH has been characterized in two dogs (Rijnberk et al. 1988). Both dogs had hyponatremia, hypoosmolality, and inappropriately high vasopressin concentrations (7–30 pmol/L). Urine osmolality was inappropriately high (213–535 mOsm/kg) in one dog in the presence of plasma hypoosmolality. The threshold and sensitivity of vasopressin secretion were studied by infusion of hypertonic saline. One dog demonstrated a pattern of reset osmostat and the other a pattern consistent with vasopressin leak.

The diagnosis of SIADH must be made by excluding other causes of hyponatremia. The following criteria should be met before establishing a diagnosis of SIADH:

1. Hyponatremia with plasma hypoosmolality.
2. Inappropriately high urine osmolality in the presence of plasma hypoosmolality. (Urine osmolality is often >300 mOsm/kg in human patients with SIADH. A urine osmolality >100 mOsm/kg should be considered abnormal in a patient with hyponatremia and plasma hypoosmolality. A urine osmolality <100 mOsm/kg would normally be expected as a result of complete suppression of vasopressin release. Urine osmolality is important in distinguishing psychogenic polydipsia and SIADH. Urine is maximally dilute in psychogenic polydipsia but not in SIADH.)
3. Normal renal and adrenal function.
4. Presence of natriuresis despite hyponatremia and plasma hypoosmolality as a result of mild volume expansion (urine sodium concentration usually >20 mEq/L in human patients).
5. No evidence of hypovolemia, which could result in nonosmotic stimulation of vasopressin release.
6. No evidence of ascites or edema, which could result in hyponatremia with hypervolemia (i.e., no evidence of severe liver disease, congestive heart failure, or nephrotic syndrome).
7. Correction of hyponatremia by fluid restriction.

Drugs that stimulate the release of vasopressin or potentiate its renal effects may lead to hyponatremia with normovolemia. Nitrous oxide, barbiturates, isoproterenol, and narcotics are drugs used during anesthesia and surgery that stimulate vasopressin release from the neurohypophysis and may contribute to impaired water excretion in the postoperative period. Chlorpropamide potentiates the action of vasopressin by inhibiting vasopressin-stimulated production of prostaglandin E_2 by medullary interstitial cells. Nonsteroidal antiinflammatory drugs have a similar effect. The antineoplastic drugs vincristine and cyclophosphamide also impair water excretion. Figure 3–5 shows the effects of various drugs on the release and action of vasopressin.

Severe hypothyroidism with myxedema in humans can result in hyponatremia, possibly because of decreased distal delivery of tubular fluid and nonosmotic stimulation of vasopressin release. Hyponatremia in this setting is corrected by thyroid hormone replacement. In four reported cases of myxedema coma in dogs, hyponatremia was found in two of three dogs in which the serum sodium concentration was measured (Chastain et al. 1982; Kelly and Hill 1984).

▶ Clinical Signs of Hyponatremia

The clinical signs of hyponatremia are related more to the rapidity of onset than to the severity of the associated plasma hypoosmolality. In human patients, deaths and severe complications of hyponatremia were most common when the serum sodium concentration acutely decreased to less than 120 mEq/L or at rate greater than 0.5 mEq/L/h (Cluitmans and Meinders 1990). Cerebral edema and water intoxication occur if hyponatremia develops faster than the brain's defense mechanisms can be called into play. Reduction in plasma osmolality and influx of water into the central nervous system cause the clinical signs observed in acute hyponatremia. Clinical signs are often absent in chronic disorders characterized by slower decreases in serum sodium concentration and plasma osmolality. During hyponatremia of chronic onset, brain volume is adjusted toward normal by loss of potassium and organic osmolytes from cells (see earlier).

Acute water intoxication is likely only if the patient has some underlying cause of impaired water excretion at the time a water load occurs. For example, water-loaded dogs given repositol vasopressin developed signs of acute water intoxication (Hardy and Osborne 1982b). Early signs were mild lethargy, nausea, and slight weight gain; more severe signs included vomiting, coma, and a marked increase in body weight. One dog in this study died from pulmonary and cerebral edema. Weakness, incoordination, and seizures may also result from acute water intoxication.

▶ Treatment of Hyponatremia

The two main goals of treatment in hyponatremia are to diagnose and manage the underlying disease and, *if necessary*, increase serum sodium concentration and plasma osmolality. Severe, symptomatic hyponatremia of acute onset (<24–48 h duration) may result in seizures, cerebral edema, or death and requires prompt treatment. In human patients with acute hyponatremia, correction of serum sodium concentration may be required at rates up to 12 mEq/L/day (Sterns et al. 1994). Severe, symptomatic hyponatremia of rapid onset, however, is rare in small animal practice. Because of inexperience with the management of acute hyponatremia in dogs and cats and the known risks of overly rapid correction of hyponatremia (see later), only use of conventional crystalloid solutions (e.g., lactated Ringer's solution, 0.9% saline) is recommended. Use of 3% NaCl is not recommended.

Patients with chronic hyponatremia often have few or no clinical signs directly attributable to their hypoosmolality. This is probably due to the fact that the brain has had sufficient time to adapt to plasma hypotonicity. In fact, treatment of chronic hyponatremia can be more dangerous than the disorder itself. In human patients, complications of treatment may occur when chronic (>48 h duration) hyponatremia is corrected too rapidly (i.e., when the serum sodium concentration is increased by >12 mEq/L/24 h or >18 mEq/L/48 h) (Sterns et al. 1994).

When hyponatremia and hypoosmolality are corrected, potassium and organic osmolytes lost during adaptation must be restored to the cells of the brain. If replacement of these solutes does not keep pace with the increase in serum sodium concentration that occurs as a result of treatment, brain dehydration and injury—called osmotic demyelination syndrome—may result. Experimental studies have confirmed that this syndrome is a result of a rapid and large increase in serum sodium concentration and is not a consequence of hyponatremia and hypoosmolality. Human patients with hyponatremia of more than 72 h duration are more susceptible than those with hyponatremia of less than 24 h duration (Sterns et al. 1994). The neuroanatomic lesions of osmotic demyelination syndrome develop several days after correction of hyponatremia and are associated with areas of myelin loss in the pons and other sites in the brain (so-called central pontine myelinolysis).

Similar lesions have been reported in experimental dogs with hyponatremia with correction rates of 15 mEq/L/day even without overcorrection to hypernatremia (Laureno 1983). Myelinolysis was reported in two dogs after correction of hyponatremia associated with trichuriasis (O'Brien et al. 1994). In one dog, a serum sodium concentration of 101 mEq/L had been corrected to 136 mEq/L in less than 38 h (correction rate >22 mEq/L/day), and in the other, a serum sodium concentration of 108 mEq/L had been corrected to 134 mEq/L in less than 38 h (correction rate >16 mEq/L/day). Clinical signs developed 3 to 4 days after correction of hyponatremia and consisted of lethargy, weakness, and ataxia progressing to hypermetria and quadriparesis. Lesions were detected by magnetic resonance imaging and were located in the thalamus as compared with the typical pontine location in affected human patients. From this experience, it was recommended that dogs with asymptomatic chronic hyponatremia be treated by mild water restriction and monitoring of serum sodium concentration. Symptomatic dogs with chronic hyponatremia should be treated conservatively at correction rates less than 10 to 12 mEq/L/day (0.5 mEq/L/h). Serial monitoring of serum sodium concentration is necessary because the actual rate of correction may not correspond to the calculated rate of correction. Correction should be carried out with conventional crystalloid solutions (e.g., lactated Ringer's solution, 0.9% NaCl) in a volume calculated specifically to replace the patient's volume deficit. The clinician must remember that volume repletion in hypovolemic patients abolishes the nonosmotic stimulus for vasopressin release and allows the animal to excrete solute-free water via the kidneys. This in itself tends to correct the hyponatremia.

TABLE 3-7. Causes of Polyuria and Polydipsia in Small Animal Practice

Disease	Mechanism of Polyuria and Polydipsia	Confirmatory Tests
Chronic renal disease* (S)	Osmotic diuresis in remnant nephrons Disruption of medullary architecture by structural disease	ECC CBC Profile Urinalysis Radiography Ultrasonography
Hyperadrenocorticism* (W)	Defective ADH release and action Psychogenic	LDDST, HDDST Plasma ACTH Ultrasonography
Diabetes mellitus* (S)	Osmotic diuresis caused by glucosuria	Blood glucose Urinalysis
Hyperthyroidism* (W)	Increased medullary blood flow and MSW Psychogenic Hypercalciuria	T_4 Technetium scan
Pyometra (W)	*Escherichia coli* endotoxin Immune complex glomerulonephritis	History Physical CBC Abdominal radiographs
Postobstructive diuresis (S)	Elimination of retained solutes Defective response to ADH Defective sodium reabsorption	History Physical examination Urinalysis
Hypercalcemia (W)	Defective ADH action Increased medullary blood flow Impaired NaCl transport in loop of Henle Hypercalcemic nephropathy Direct stimulation of thirst center	Serum calcium
Liver disease (W)	Decreased urea synthesis with loss of medullary solute Decreased metabolism of endogenous hormones (e.g., cortisol, aldosterone) Psychogenic (hepatic encephalopathy) Hypokalemia	Liver enzymes Serum bile acids Blood ammonia Liver biopsy
Pyelonephritis (W)	*E. coli* endotoxin Increased renal blood flow MSW Renal parenchymal damage	Urinalysis Urine culture CBC Excretory urography Abdominal ultrasonography
Hypoadrenocorticism (W)	Renal sodium loss with MSW	Serum sodium and potassium ACTH stimulation
Hypokalemia (W)	Defective ADH action Increased medullary blood flow and loss of medullary solute	Serum potassium
Diuretic phase of oliguric ARF (S)	Elimination of retained solutes Defective sodium reabsorption	History CBC Profile Urinalysis Abdominal ultrasonography Renal biopsy
Partial urinary tract obstruction (S)	Redistribution of renal blood flow Defective sodium reabsorption Renal parenchymal damage	History Physical examination
Drugs (W)	Various mechanisms depending on drug	History
Salt administration (S)	Osmotic diuresis caused by excess sodium administered	History
Excessive parenteral fluid administration (W) (polyuria only)	Water diuresis caused by excess water administered	History
Central diabetes insipidus (CDI) (W)	Congenital lack of ADH (rare) Acquired lack of ADH (idiopathic, tumor, trauma)	Water deprivation test Exogenous ADH test ADH assay
Nephrogenic diabetes insipidus (NDI) (W)	Congenital lack of renal response to ADH (very rare) Acquired lack of renal response to ADH (see Table 3–5)	Water deprivation test Exogenous ADH test ADH assay ECC
Psychogenic polydipsia (PP) (W)	Neurobehavioral disorder (anxiety?) Increased renal blood flow MSW	Water deprivation test Exogenous ADH test Behavioral history
Renal glucosuria (S)	Solute diuresis caused by gluosuria	Blood glucose Urinalysis
Primary hypoparathyroidism (W)	Unknown (psychogenic?)	Serum calcium Serum phosphorus Serum PTH
Acromegaly (W, S)	Insulin antagonism Glucose intolerance Diabetes mellitus in affected cats	Neuroradiography Growth hormone assay
Polycythemia (W)	Unknown (increased blood viscosity?)	CBC
Multiple myeloma (W)	Unknown (increased blood viscosity?)	Serum protein electrophoresis
Renal MSW (W)	Depletion of medullary interstitial solute (urea, sodium, potassium)	Gradual water deprivation (3–5 days) Hickey-Hare test

Source: Adapted from Bruyette DS and Nelson RW: How to approach the problems of polyuria and polydipsia. *Vet Med* 81:112, 1986.
*Most common causes of polyuria and polydipsia.
Abbreviations: (W), water diuresis; (S), solute diuresis; ACTH, adrenocorticotropic hormone; ADH, antidiuretic hormone; ARF, acute renal failure; CBC, complete blood count; PTH, parathyroid hormone; ECC, endogenous creatinine clearance; MSW, medullary washout of solute; LDDST, low-dose dexamethasone suppression test; HDDST, high-dose dexamethasone suppression test.

Thus, caution should be exercised even when using conventional crystalloid fluid therapy.

Water intake should be carefully restricted to a volume less than urine output in normovolemic patients with hyponatremia (e.g., psychogenic polydipsia), or drugs causing an antidiuretic effect should be discontinued if possible. Demeclocycline and lithium inhibit vasopressin release and have been used to treat SIADH in humans (Forrest et al. 1978), but water restriction is probably the safest approach.

In edematous patients, dietary sodium restriction and diuretic therapy should be considered. A 0.9% NaCl solution can be administered concurrently with loop diuretics (e.g., furosemide) to effect more rapid correction of hyponatremia in overhydrated symptomatic patients. The occurrence of chronic hyponatremia in patients with congestive heart failure is often a sign of advanced disease and responds poorly to treatment. Administration of furosemide and an angiotensin-converting enzyme inhibitor (e.g., enalapril) may improve stroke volume and cardiac output by reducing preload and afterload and may decrease vasopressin secretion and enhance water excretion, which in turn may facilitate resolution of hyponatremia.

▶ Clinical Approach to Polyuria and Polydipsia

Normal daily water intake and urine output in dogs and cats are influenced by the nutrient, mineral, and water content of the diet. Normal water intake should not exceed 90 ml/kg/day in dogs and 45 ml/kg/day in cats. Normal urine output ranges from 20 to 45 ml/kg/day in dogs and cats. Dogs with disorders such as psychogenic polydipsia, CDI, and NDI may have water consumption as much as five times normal.

Dogs and cats with polyuria and polydipsia are encountered frequently in small animal practice. The causes of polyuria and polydipsia, their pathophysiologic mechanisms, and the necessary confirmatory laboratory tests are presented in the Table 3–7. The most common causes are chronic renal failure in dogs and cats, diabetes mellitus in dogs and cats, hyperadrenocorticism in dogs, and hyperthyroidism in cats. These common causes must always be ruled out before beginning an exhaustive diagnostic evaluation of the animal.

Determination of the specific gravity of a random urine sample from the animal is a logical starting point for evaluation of polyuria and polydipsia. If a random USG is greater than 1.030 to 1.035, the clinician should obtain additional history to rule out other disorders that may have been confused with polyuria (e.g., urinary incontinence, dysuria). If a random USG is less than 1.025 to 1.030, an initial diagnostic evaluation is warranted.

Many causes of polyuria and polydipsia can be ruled out by an initial database consisting of a complete history and physical examination, complete blood count, biochemical profile (including electrolytes), urinalysis, urine culture, and abdominal radiographs. If the animal is otherwise healthy, it is helpful to instruct the owner to quantitate and record the animal's daily water consumption at home over a 3- to 5-day period. Determination of water intake at home prevents potential reduction in water intake precipitated by the stress of hospitalization.

With some exceptions (e.g., psychogenic polydipsia), polydipsia usually occurs as a consequence of polyuria. If polydipsia occurs without polyuria, the clinician must consider causes such as high ambient temperature (i.e., increased insensible water losses), regular prolonged exercise, water consumption to replace a previous hydration deficit, and third-space distribution of consumed water. Excessive administration of parenteral fluids causes polyuria without polydipsia. The diagnostic approach to polyuria and polydipsia is summarized in Table 3–7 and Figure 3–14.

▶ Laboratory Evaluation of Polyuria and Polydipsia

Endogenous Creatinine Clearance

In chronic progressive renal disease, urinary concentrating ability is impaired after two-thirds of the nephron population has become nonfunctional, whereas azotemia does not develop until three-quarters of the nephrons have become nonfunctional. Thus, the main indication for determination of endogenous creatinine clearance is the clinical suspicion of renal disease in a patient with polyuria and polydipsia but normal BUN and serum creatinine concentrations. The only requirements for determination of endogenous creatinine clearance are an accurately timed collection of urine (usually 24 h), determination of the patient's body weight, and measurement of serum and urine creatinine concentrations. Failure to collect all urine produced results in an erroneously reduced calculated clearance value. Use of creatinine clearance as an estimate of GFR is discussed further in Chapter 2.

Water Deprivation Test

The water deprivation test is indicated in evaluation of animals with confirmed polydipsia and polyuria, the cause of which remains undetermined after the initial diagnostic evaluation. It is usually performed in animals with hyposthenuria (USG <1.007) that are suspected to have CDI, NDI, or psychogenic polydipsia. An animal that is dehydrated but has dilute urine has already failed the test and should not be subjected to water deprivation. In such an animal, failure to concentrate urine is probably due to structural or functional renal dysfunction or administration of drugs that interfere with urinary concentrating ability. The water deprivation test is also contraindicated in animals that are azotemic. The test should be performed with extreme caution in animals with severe polyuria, because such patients may rapidly become dehydrated during water deprivation if they have defective urinary concentrating ability.

At the beginning of the water deprivation test, the bladder must be emptied and baseline data collected (body weight, hematocrit, total plasma proteins, skin turgor, serum osmolality, urine osmolality, and USG). Water is then withheld and these parameters are monitored every 2 to 4 h. Urine and serum osmolalities are the best

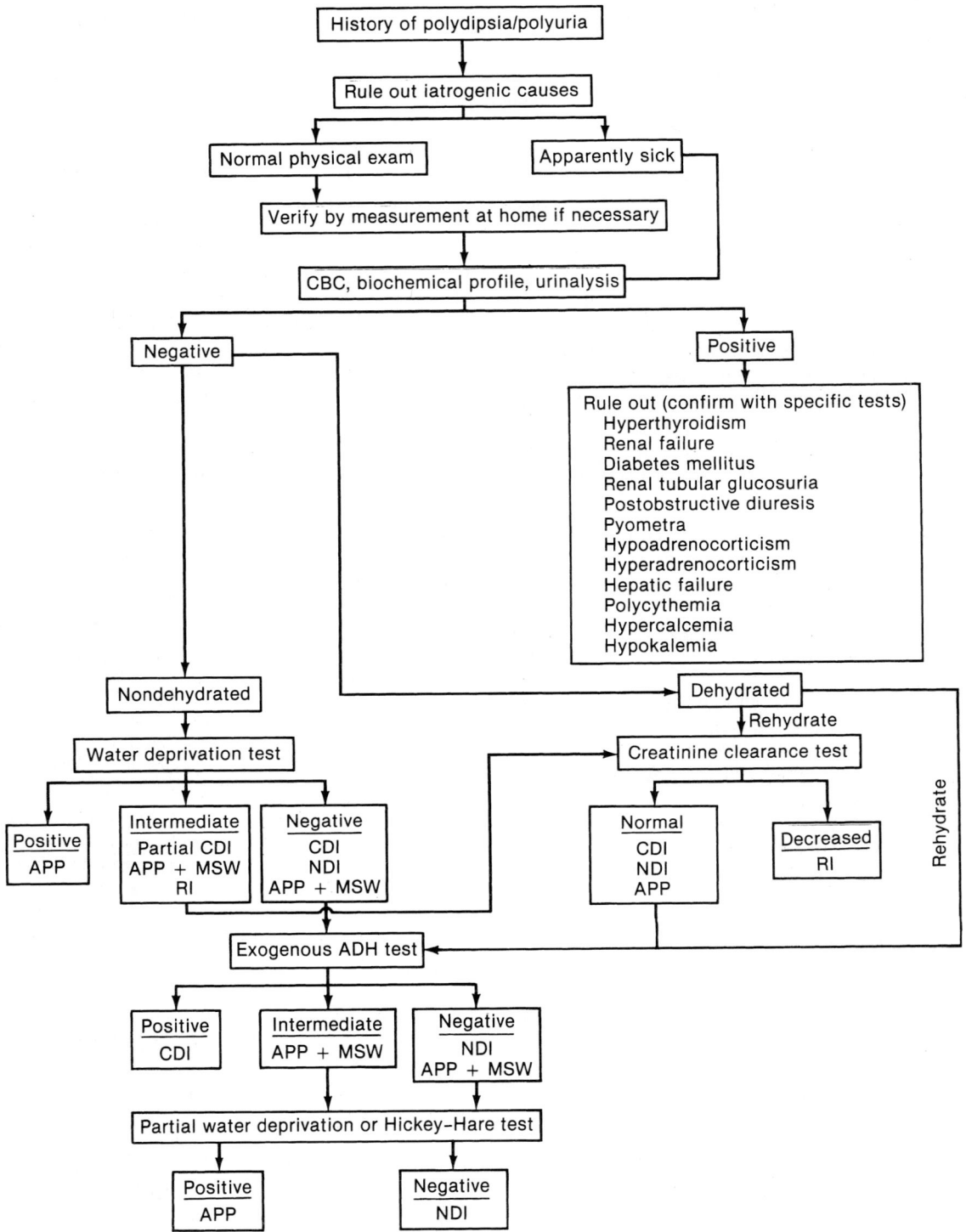

FIGURE 3-14. Clinical approach to the patient with polydipsia and polyuria. APP = apparent psychogenic polydipsia; CBC = complete blood count; CDI = central diabetes insipidus; MSW = medullary solute washout; NDI = nephrogenic diabetes insipidus; RI = renal insufficiency with solute diuresis. (From Fenner WR: *Quick Reference to Veterinary Medicine,* 2nd ed. Philadelphia, JB Lippincott, p. 110, 1991.)

parameters to follow, but osmolality results are often not immediately available to the clinician. Thus, USG and body weight assume great importance for decision making during performance of the test. An increase in total plasma protein concentration is a relatively reliable indicator of progressive dehydration, but increases in hematocrit and and changes in skin turgor are less reliable (Hardy and Osborne 1979). Serum creatinine and BUN concentrations should not increase during a properly conducted water deprivation test.

The bladder should be emptied at the time of each urine collection. Maximal stimulation of ADH release is present after loss of 5% of body weight. The test is concluded when the patient either demonstrates adequate concentrating ability or becomes dehydrated as evidenced by loss of 5% or more of its original body weight. It is important when weighing the animal to use the same scale each time and to empty the bladder at each evaluation.

In normal dogs, dehydration becomes evident after a mean of 42 h but occasionally may not occur until after 96 h (Hardy and Osborne 1979). The time required for dehydration to develop during water deprivation testing in dogs with disorders characterized by polyuria and polydipsia may be as short as a few hours or up to 12 h. By the time dehydration is evident, normal dogs develop a USG of 1.050 to 1.076, urine osmolality of 1787 to 2791 mOsm/kg, and a urine/plasma osmolality ratio of 5.7 to 8.9 (Hardy and Osborne 1979). Normal cats developed USG values of 1.047 to 1.087 and urine osmolalities of 1581 to 2984 mOsm/kg after water deprivation of sufficient duration (approximately 40 h) to induce 5% loss of body weight (Ross and Finco 1981). Failure to achieve maximal urinary solute concentration does not localize the level of the malfunction, but a structural or functional defect may be present anywhere along the hypothalamic-pituitary-renal axis. Furthermore, animals with renal medullary solute washout may have impaired concentrating capacity regardless of the underlying cause of polyuria and polydipsia.

If there has been less than 5% increase in urine osmolality or less than 10% change in USG for three consecutive determinations or if the animal has lost 5% or more of its original weight, 0.25 to 0.5 U/kg aqueous vasopressin (Pitressin) (up to a total dose of 5 U) or 5 μg of desmopressin (DDAVP) may be given subcutaneously and parameters of urinary concentrating ability monitored at 30, 60, and 120 min after ADH injection. Normal dogs and those with psychogenic polydipsia should show no additional response to ADH administration in this setting.

Modified Water Deprivation Test

A modified water deprivation test has been described for the diagnosis of polyuric disorders in dogs. Water is removed from the animal's cage and the urinary bladder emptied, after which urine osmolality or specific gravity is measured and the bladder emptied on an hourly basis. Maximal urine solute concentration is defined as occurring whenever less than 5% increase in urine osmolality occurs on sequential determinations. This maximal concentration occurred at a mean urine osmolality of 1414 mOsm/kg in normal dogs after 24 h of water deprivation (Mulnix et al. 1976). At this time, 2 to 3 U of aqueous vasopressin was administered subcutaneously and the urine osmolality determined at 1 and 2 h after injection. Further increase in urine osmolality after administration of vasopressin should not exceed 10% in normal dogs. In this study, dogs with CDI showed an average 292% increase in urine osmolality after aqueous ADH, dogs with partial CDI an average 28% increase, and dogs with hyperadrenocorticism an average 20% increase. The time required to develop dehydration ranged from 3 to 11.5 h in dogs with psychogenic polydipsia, complete or partial CDI, and hyperadrenocorticism.

Gradual Water Deprivation

Gradual water deprivation can be performed to eliminate diagnostic confusion caused by renal medullary solute washout. The owner can be instructed to restrict water consumption to 120 mL/kg/day 72 h before, to 90 mL/kg/day 48 h before, and to 60 mL/kg/day 24 h before the scheduled water deprivation test. In dogs with psychogenic polydipsia, this promotes release of endogenous vasopressin, increased permeability of the inner medullary collecting ducts to urea, and restoration of the normal gradient of medullary hypertonicity. An alternative approach is to instruct the owner to reduce water consumption by approximately 10% per day over a 3- to 5-day period (but not to less than 60 mL/kg/day). This approach should be used only in animals that are otherwise healthy on initial clinical evaluation, and the owner should provide dry food ad libitum and weigh the dog daily to monitor for loss of body weight.

Hickey-Hare Test

In the Hickey-Hare test (Lage 1977b), water (20 mL/kg) is administered by stomach tube, an indwelling urinary catheter is placed, and urine flow (mL/min) is determined. Hypertonic saline (2.5%) is administered intravenously at a rate of 0.25 mL/min/kg for 45 min. Urine volume is recorded every 15 min during the infusion and for 45 min afterward. The normal response to this procedure is a decrease in the rate of urine production caused by stimulation of ADH release by plasma hyperosmolality. It is useful in the differentiation of psychogenic polydipsia with renal medullary solute washout from NDI after negative water deprivation and exogenous ADH test results. In NDI, there should be no change or an actual increase in urine flow, whereas in psychogenic polydipsia with renal medullary solute washout, repletion of solute (e.g., NaCl) should have occurred, and the response to hypertonic saline should be normal (decreased urine volume). This test is cumbersome, is contraindicated for patients with congestive heart failure, and may lead to signs of hypernatremia in patients that cannot excrete a sodium load. It has largely been replaced by gradual water deprivation as just described.

TABLE 3–8. **Mean Maximal Values for Parameters of Total Urine Solute Concentration***

	WDT	RVPT	AVPT
U_{osm} (mOsm/kg)	2199	1518	933
Urine specific gravity	1.063	1.042	1.021
U_{osm}/P_{osm}	7.2	5.6	3.3

Sources: Hardy and Osborne 1979, 1982a, 1982b.
*Normal dogs undergoing routine water deprivation testing (WDT), repositol vasopressin testing (RVPT), and aqueous vasopressin testing (AVPT).

Exogenous Antidiuretic Hormone Testing

The exogenous vasopressin test may be used for debilitated patients in which water deprivation is considered hazardous or to further characterize a concentrating defect detected by the routine water deprivation test. In the *aqueous vasopressin test,* an intravenous infusion of aqueous vasopressin (Pitressin) at 10 mU/kg is given over 60 min. The bladder is emptied at the start of the study, and parameters of urinary concentrating ability are measured before and at 30-min intervals for 3 h after beginning the infusion. The bladder is emptied at each measurement. In one report, maximal reponse to aqueous vasopressin in water-loaded dogs usually occurred at 60 min (range, 30–90 min) and consisted of USG values of 1.012 to 1.033, urine osmolalities of 429 to 1437 mOsm/kg, and urine/plasma osmolality ratios of 1.5 to 5.1 (Hardy and Osborne 1982a). Water should be provided ad libitum during testing, but water loading should not be performed in clinical patients.

In the *repositol vasopressin test,* 3 to 5 U of vasopressin tannate in oil (Pitressin tannate) is given intramuscularly and the bladder is emptied 3 to 6 h after injection. Parameters of urinary concentrating ability are measured before and at 6, 9, 12, and 24 h after injection. Oral water loading must be avoided because of the danger of potentially lethal water intoxication (Hardy and Osborne 1982b). Maximal response to repositol vasopressin occurred 8 to 12 h after injection and consisted of USG values of 1.028 to 1.057, urine osmolalities of 1052 to 1850 mOsm/kg, and urine/plasma osmolality ratios of 3.9 to 6.7 (Hardy and Osborne 1982b).

The standard or modified water deprivation test is the preferred initial test of urinary concentrating ability, because mean maximal values are usually higher with this test and results are easier to interpret (Table 3–8). Why higher values for parameters of urinary concentrating ability are achieved with this test as compared with the exogenous vasopressin tests is unknown. Possible explanations include the actions of antidiuretic substances other than ADH that may be present in hydropenic individuals, the effect of slower renal medullary blood flow in dehydrated patients, and intensification of the medullary interstitial gradient in dehydrated individuals.

REFERENCES

Abramov M, Beauwens R, and Cogan E: Cellular events in vasopressin action. *Kidney Int* 32(suppl 21):S56, 1987.
Atkins CE, Tyler R, and Greenlee P: Clinical, biochemical, acid-base, and electrolyte abnormalities in cats after hypertonic sodium phosphate enema administration. *Am J Vet Res* 46:980, 1985.
Authement JM, Boudrieau RJ, and Kaplan PM: Transient traumatically induced central diabetes insipidus in a dog. *J Am Vet Med Assoc* 194:683, 1989.
Bagley RS, de Lahunta A, Randolph JF, et al.: Hypernatremia, adipsia, and diabetes insipidus in a dog with hypothalamic dysplasia. *J Am Anim Hosp Assoc* 29:267, 1993.
Breitschwerdt EB and Root CR: Inappropriate secretion of antidiuretic hormone in a dog. *J Am Vet Med Assoc* 175:181, 1979.
Breitschwerdt EB, Verlander JW, and Bribernik TN: Nephrogenic diabetes insipidus in three dogs. *J Am Vet Med Assoc* 179:235, 1981.
Breitschwerdt EB, Meuten DJ, Greenfield CL, et al.: Idiopathic hyperaldosteronism in a dog. *J Am Ved Med Assoc* 187:841, 1985.
Brown E, Markandu ND, Roulston JE, et al.: Is the renin-angiotensin-aldosterone system involved in the sodium retention of the nephrotic syndrome? *Nephron* 32:102, 1982.
Bruyette DS and Nelson RW: How to approach the problems of polyuria and polydipsia. *Vet Med* 81:112, 1986.
Bulger RE: Composition of renal medullary tissue. *Kidney Int* 31:557, 1987.
Burnie AG and Dunn JK: A case of central diabetes insipidus in the cat: Diagnosis and treatment. *J Small Anim Pract* 23:237, 1979.
Burrows CF and Bovee KC: Metabolic changes due to experimentally induced rupture of the canine urinary bladder. *Am J Vet Res* 35:1083, 1974.
Chastain CB, Graham CL, and Riley MG: Myxedema coma in two dogs. *Canine Pract* 9:20, 1982.
Chew DJ, Leonard M, and Muir WW: Effect of sodium bicarbonate infusion on serum osmolality, electrolyte concentrations, and blood gas tensions in cats. *Am J Vet Res* 52:12, 1991.
Chew M: Salt poisoning in a boxer bitch. *Vet Rec* 85:685, 1969.
Cluitmans FH and Meinders AE: Management of severe hyponatremia: Rapid or slow correction? *Am J Med* 88:161, 1990.
Crawford MA, Kittleson MD, and Fink GD: Hypernatremia and adipsia in a dog. *J Am Vet Med Assoc* 184:818, 1984.
Crow SE and Stockham SL: Profound hyponatremia associated with glucocorticoid deficiency in a dog. *J Am Anim Hosp Assoc* 21:393, 1985.
Davenport DJ, Chew DJ, and Johnson GC: Diabetes insipidus associated with metastatic pancreatic carcinoma in a dog. *J Am Vet Med Assoc* 189:204, 1986.
DiBartola SP, Johnson SE, Davenport DJ, et al.: Clinicopathologic findings resembling hypoadrenocorticism in dogs with primary gastrointestinal disease. *J Am Vet Med Assoc* 187:60, 1985.
DiBartola SP, Johnson SE, Johnson GC, et al.: Hypodipsic hypernatremia in a dog with defective osmoregulation of antidiuretic hormone. *J Am Vet Med Assoc* 204:922, 1994.
Dorhout Mees EJ: Edema formation in the nephrotic syndrome. *Contrib Nephrol* 43:64, 1984.
Dow SW, Fettman MJ, LeCouteur RA, et al.: Hypodipsic hypernatremia and associated myopathy in a hydrocephalic cat with transient hypopituitarism. *J Am Vet Med Assoc* 191:212, 1987.
Edwards DF, Richardson DC, and Russell RG: Hypernatremic, hypertonic dehydration in a dog with diabetes insipidus and gastric dilatation-volvulus. *J Am Vet Med Assoc* 182:973, 1983.
Eger CE, Robinson WF, and Huxtable CRR: Primary aldosteronism (Conn's syndrome) in a cat: A case report and review of comparative aspects. *J Small Anim Pract* 24:293, 1983.
Ellison DH and Velazquez H: Thiazide-sensitive sodium chloride cotransport in early distal tubule. *Am J Physiol* 253:F546, 1987.
Epstein M: Derangements of renal water handling in liver disease. *Gastroenterology* 89:1415, 1985.
Feig PU and McCurdy DK: The hypertonic state. *N Engl J Med* 297:1444, 1977.

Feldman BF and Rosenberg DP: Clinical use of anion and osmolal gaps in veterinary medicine. *J Am Vet Med Assoc* 178:396, 1981.

Feldman EC and Nelson RW: Water metabolism and diabetes insipidus. In Feldman EC and Nelson RW (eds): *Canine and Feline Endocrinology and Reproduction.* Philadelphia, WB Saunders Co., p. 33, 1996a.

Feldman EC and Nelson RW: Hyperadrenocorticism (Cushing's syndrome). In Feldman EC and Nelson RW (eds): *Canine and Feline Endocrinology and Reproduction.* Philadelphia, WB Saunders Co., p. 262, 1996b.

Feldman EC and Nelson RW: Water metabolism and diabetes insipidus. In Feldman EC and Nelson RW (eds): *Canine and Feline Endocrinology and Reproduction.* Philadelphia, WB Saunders Co., p. 15, 1996c.

Ferguson DC and Biery DN: Diabetes insipidus and hyperadrenocorticism associated with high plasma adrenocorticotropin concentration and a hypothalamic/pituitary mass in a dog. *J Am Vet Med Assoc* 193:835, 1988.

Forrest JN, Cox M, Hong C, et al.: Superiority of demeclocycline over lithium in the treatment of chronic syndrome of inappropriate secretion of antidiuretic hormone. *N Engl J Med* 298:173, 1978.

Gennari FJ: Serum osmolality: Uses and limitations. *N Engl J Med* 310:102, 1984.

Gennari FJ and Kassirer JP: Osmotic diuresis. *N Engl J Med* 291:714, 1974.

Giger U and Gorman NT: Oncologic emergencies in small animals. Part II. Metabolic and endocrine emergencies. *Compend Contin Educ Pract Vet* 6:805, 1984.

Grauer GF and Grauer RM: Veterinary clinical osmometry. *Compend Contin Educ Pract Vet* 5:539, 1983.

Green RA and Farrow CS: Diabetes insipidus in a cat. *J Am Vet Med Assoc* 164:524, 1974.

Greene CE, Wong PL, and Finco DR: Diagnosis and treatment of diabetes insipidus in two dogs using two synthetic analogs of antidiuretic hormone. *J Am Anim Hosp Assoc* 15:371, 1979.

Gross PA, Ketteler M, Hausmann C, et al.: The charted and uncharted waters of hyponatremia. *Kidney Int* 32(Suppl 21):S67, 1987.

Hall EF: Hypernatremia and adipsia in a dog (letter). *J Am Vet Med Assoc* 185:4, 1984.

Harb MF, Nelson RW, Feldman EC, et al.: Central diabetes insipidus in dogs: 20 cases (1986–1995). *J Am Vet Med Assoc* 209:1884, 1996.

Hardy RM: Hypernatremia. *Vet Clin North Am. Small Anim Pract* 19:231, 1989.

Hardy RM and Osborne CA: Water deprivation test in the dog: Maximal normal values. *J Am Vet Med Assoc* 174:479, 1979.

Hardy RM and Osborne CA: Aqueous vasopressin response test in clinically normal dogs undergoing water diuresis: Technique and results. *Am J Vet Res* 43:1987, 1982a.

Hardy RM and Osborne CA: Repositol vasopressin response test in clincally normal dogs undergoing water diuresis: Technique and results. *Am J Vet Res* 43:1991, 1982b.

Hawks D, Giger U, Miselis R, et al.: Essential hypernatremia in a young dog. *J Small Anim Pract* 32:420, 1991.

Hendriks HJ, de Bruijne JJ, and Van den Brom WE: The clinical refractometer: A useful tool for the determination of specific gravity and osmolality of canine urine. *Tijdschr Diergeneeskd* 103:1065, 1978.

Henry WB and Sieber SE: Traumatic diabetes insipidus in a dog. *J Am Vet Med Assoc* 146:1317, 1965.

Hoskins JD and Rothschmitt J: Hypernatremic thirst deficiency in a dog. *Vet Med* 79:489, 1984.

Houston DM, Allen DG, Kruth SA, et al.: Syndrome of inappropriate antidiuretic hormone secretion in a dog. *Can Vet J* 30:423, 1989.

Hughes DE and Sokolowski JH: Sodium chloride poisoning in the dog. *Canine Pract* 5:28, 1978.

Ichikawa I, Rennke HG, Hoyer JR, et al.: Role for intrarenal mechanism in the impaired salt excretion of experimental nephrotic syndrome. *J Clin Invest* 71:91, 1983.

Joles JA and Gruys E: Nephrogenic diabetes insipidus in a dog with renal medullary lesions. *J Am Vet Med Assoc* 174:830, 1979.

Katz MA: Hyperglycemia-induced hyponatremia. *N Engl J Med* 289:843, 1973.

Kelly MJ and Hill JR: Canine myxedema stupor and coma. *Compend Contin Educ Pract Vet* 6:1049, 1984.

Khanna C, Boermans HJ, and Wilcock B: Fatal hypernatremia in a dog from salt ingestion. *J Am Anim Hosp Assoc* 33:113, 1997.

Kraus KH: The use of desmopressin in diagnosis and treatment of diabetes insipidus in cats. *Compend Contin Educ Pract Vet* 9:752, 1987.

Kraus KH, Turrentine MA, Jergens AE, et al.: Effect of desmopressin acetate on bleeding times and plasma von Willebrand factor in Doberman pinscher dogs with von Willebrand's disease. *Vet Surg* 18:103, 1989.

Ladenson JH, Apple FS, and Koch DD: Misleading hyponatremia due to hyperlipemia: A method-dependent error. *Ann Intern Med* 95:707, 1981.

Lage AL: Nephrogenic diabetes insipidus in a dog. *J Am Vet Med Assoc* 163:251, 1973.

Lage AL: Apparent psychogenic polydipsia. In Kirk RW (ed): *Current Veterinary Therapy VI.* Philadelphia, WB Saunders Co., p. 1098, 1977a.

Lage AL: Nephrogenic diabetes insipidus. In Kirk RW (ed): *Current Veterinary Therapy VI.* Philadelphia, WB Saunders Co, p. 1102, 1977b.

Lamb WA and Muir P: Lymphangiosarcoma associated with hyponatremia and hyperkalemia in a dog. *J Small Anim Pract* 35:374, 1994.

Laureno R: Central pontine myelinolysis following rapid correction of hyponatremia. *Ann Neurol* 13:232, 1983.

Levitin H, Goodman A, Pigeon G, et al.: Composition of the renal medulla during water diuresis. *J Clin Invest* 41:1145, 1962.

Lieberman LL, Kircher CH, and Lein DH: Polyuria and polydipsia associated with pituitary visceral larval migrans in a dog. *J Am Anim Hosp Assoc* 15:237, 1979.

Ling GV, Stabenfeldt GH, Comer KM, et al.: Canine hyperadrenocorticism: Pretreatment clinical and laboratory evaluation of 117 cases. *J Am Vet Med Assoc* 174:1211, 1979.

Lubberink AA: Therapy for spontaneous hyperadrenocorticism. In Kirk RW (ed): *Current Veterinary Therapy VII.* Philadelphia, WB Saunders Co., p. 979, 1980.

Madewell BR, Osborne CA, Norrdin RA, et al.: Clinicopathologic aspects of diabetes insipidus in the dog. *J Am Anim Hosp Assoc* 11:497, 1975.

Malik R, Hunt GB, Hinchliffe JM, et al.: Severe whipworm infection in the dog. *J Small Anim Pract* 31:185, 1990.

Mann JFE, Johnson AK, Ganten D, et al.: Thirst and the renin angiotensin system. *Kidney Int* 32(suppl 21):S27, 1987.

Mulnix JA, Rijnberk A, and Hendriks HJ: Evaluation of a modified water-deprivation test for diagnosis of polyuric disorders in dogs. *J Am Vet Med Assoc* 169:1327, 1976.

Narins RG, Jones ER, Stom MC, et al.: Diagnostic strategies in disorders of fluid, electrolyte and acid base homeostasis. *Am J Med* 72:496, 1982.

Neer TM and Reavis DU: Craniopharyngioma and associated central diabetes insipidus and hypothyroidism in a dog. *J Am Vet Med Assoc* 182:519, 1983.

O'Brien DP, Kroll RA, Johnson GC, et al.: Myelinolysis after correction of hyponatremia in two dogs. *J. Vet Intern Med* 8:40, 1994.

O'Grady SM, Palfrey HC, and Field M: Characteristics and function of Na-K-2Cl cotransport in epithelial tissues. *Am J Physiol* 253:C177, 1987.

Palmer LG and Frindt G: Amiloride sensitive Na$^+$ channels from the apical membrane of rat cortical collecting tubule. *Proc Natl Acad Sci USA* 83:2767, 1986.

Peterson M: Hyperadrenocorticism. *Vet Clin North Am Small Anim Pract* 14:731, 1984.

Peterson ME, Kintzer PP, and Kass PH: Pretreatment clinical and laboratory findings in dogs with hypoadrenocorticism—225 cases (1979–1993). *J Am Vet Med Assoc* 208:85, 1996.

Pittari JM: Central diabetes insipidus in a cat. *Feline Pract* 24:18, 1996.

Post K, McNeill JRJ, Clark EG, et al.: Congenital central diabetes insipidus in two sibling Afghan hound pups. *J Am Vet Med Assoc* 194:1086, 1989.

Rakich PM and Lorenz MD: Clinical signs and laboratory abnormalities in 23 dogs with spontaneous hypoadrenocorticism. *J Am Anim Hosp Assoc* 20:647, 1984.

Reidarson TH, Weis DJ, and Hardy RM: Extreme hypernatremia in a dog with central diabetes insipidus: A case report. *J Am Anim Hosp Assoc* 26:89, 1990.

Rijnberk A, Biewenga WJ, and Mol JA: Inappropriate vasopressin secretion in two dogs. *Acta Endocrinol* 117:59, 1988.

Robertson GL: Thirst and vasopressin function in normal and disordered states of water balance. *J Lab Clin Med* 101:351, 1983.

Rogers W, Straus J, and Chew D: A typical hypoadrenocorticism in three dogs. *J Am Vet Med Assoc* 179:155, 1981.

Rogers WA, Valdez H, Anderson BC, et al.: Partial deficiency of antidiuretic hormone in a cat. *J Am Vet Med Assoc* 170:545, 1977.

Ross LA and Finco DR: Relationship of selected clinical renal function tests to glomerular filtration rate and renal blood flow in cats. *Am J Vet Res* 42:1704, 1981.

Schaer M and Chen CL: A clinical survey of 48 dogs with adrenocortical hypofunction. *J Am Anim Hosp Assoc* 19:443, 1983.

Schuster VL and Stokes JB: Chloride transport by the cortical and outer medullary collecting duct. *Am J Physiol* 253:F203, 1987.

Shull RM: The value of anion gap and osmolal gap determinations in veterinary medicine. *Vet Clin Pathol* 7:12, 1978.

Sterns RH, Ocdol H, Schrier RW, et al.: Hyponatremia: Pathophysiology, diagnosis and therapy. In Narins RG (ed): *Maxwell and Kleeman's Clinical Disorders of Fluid and Electrolyte Metabolism.* New York, McGraw-Hill Book Co., p. 583, 1994.

Sterns RH, Spital A, and Clark EC: Disorders of water balance. In Kokko JP and Tannen RL (eds): *Fluids and Electrolytes.* Philadelphia, WB Saunders Co., p. 63, 1996.

Tyler RD, Qualls CW, Heald RD, et al.: Renal concentrating ability in dehydrated hyponatremic dogs. *J Am Vet Med Assoc* 191:1095, 1987.

Van Heerden J, Geel J, and Moore DJ: Hypodipsic hypernatremia in a miniature Schnauzer. *J S Afr Vet Assoc* 63:39, 1992.

Willard MD, Schall WD, McCaw DE, et al.: Canine hypoadrenocorticism: Report of 37 cases and review of 39 previously reported cases. *J Am Vet Med Assoc* 180:59, 1982.

Willard MD, Fossum TW, Torrance A, et al.: Hyponatremia and hyperkalemia associated with idiopathic or experimentally induced chylothorax in four dogs. *J Am Vet Med Assoc* 199:353, 1991.

Winterbotham J and Mason K: Congenital diabetes insipidus in a kitten. *J Small Anim Pract* 24:569, 1983.

Zenger E: Persistent hyperkalemia associated with nonchylous pleural effusion in a dog. *J Am Anim Hosp Assoc* 28:411, 1992.

Zerbe R, Stropes L, and Robertson G: Vasopressin function in the syndrome of inappropriate antidiuresis. *Annu Rev Med* 31:315, 1980.

CHAPTER 4

Disorders of Chloride
HYPERCHLOREMIA AND HYPOCHLOREMIA

HELIO AUTRAN DE MORAIS

> *Whereas for a long time it was assumed that chloride ions were reabsorbed entirely passively with sodium—the "mendicant" role of chloride—more recent studies suggest that several distinctive reabsorptive transport mechanisms operate in parallel.*
>
> Schild et al. 1988

Chloride constitutes approximately two-thirds of the anions in plasma and the remainder of extracellular fluid (ECF). It is also the major anion filtered by the glomeruli and reabsorbed in the renal tubules. Chloride is important not only for maintaining osmolality but also in acid-base regulation.

Chloride is present in plasma at a mean concentration of 110 mEq/L in dogs and 120 mEq/L in cats (de Morais 1992a). Chloride concentration in venous samples is 3 to 4 mEq/L lower than in arterial samples when cells are separated from plasma anaerobically (Tietz et al. 1986). The intracellular concentration of chloride is much lower than its plasma concentration and is dependent on the resting membrane potential of the cell. Muscle cells, for example, have a resting membrane potential of approximately -68 mV and an average chloride ion concentration (Cl^-) of 2 to 4 mEq/L, whereas red blood cells have a resting membrane potential of approximately -15 mV and an average Cl^- of 60 mEq/L, although an intracellular Cl^- as high as 90 mEq/L has been reported (Jones 1987). This higher intracellular concentration of chloride ions in erythrocytes allows chloride to move in and out of the red blood cell effectively, as dictated by electrical charges on either side of the cell membrane. This is an important difference from other cells and is the basis of the so-called chloride shift in the red cell membrane (Jones 1987). The chloride ion distribution in various body fluids is summarized in Table 4–1.

▶ Chloride Metabolism

Under normal conditions, human beings produce 1 to 2 L of gastric juice daily. The Na^+ and Cl^- concentrations of gastric juice are quite variable, ranging from 20 to 100 mEq/L and 120 to 160 mEq/L, respectively (Phillips 1987). In the jejunum, sodium is absorbed actively against small electrochemical gradients and also through relatively large mucosal "pores" in the proximal bowel. Chloride absorption in the jejunum generally follows sodium to maintain electroneutrality. It is believed that chloride reabsorption in the jejunum occurs via the paracellular

TABLE 4–1. Chloride Ion in Various Body Fluids

Extracellular (ECF) and Intracellular Fluid (ICF)
Most prevalent anion in ECF
Polyvalent anions (e.g., DNA, RNA, proteins, organic phosphates) replace chloride ion in ICF
Chloride ion concentration in the ICF is dependent on the cell resting membrane potential
Intracellular chloride ion concentration:
  Muscle cells: 2–4 mEqL
  Epithelial cells: 20 mEqL
  Red blood cells: 60 mEqL

Stomach
Most prevalent anion in gastric juice
Chloride ion concentration is higher than sodium and potassium concentrations whenever gastric juice pH is below 4.0

Intestine
Most prevalent anion in small and large intestinal fluids
Higher chloride ion concentration is found in the ileum, whereas colonic fluids have the lowest chloride ion concentration

Kidneys
Most prevalent anion in glomerular ultrafiltrate
80% of filtered sodium is reabsorbed accompanied by chloride
Chloride transport in cortical collecting tubules is associated with regulation of acid-base balance

Source: de Morais HSA: Chloride ion in small animal practice: The forgotten ion. *J Vet Emerg Crit Care* 2:11–24, 1992.

route, in response to the transepithelial potential generated by active sodium transport (Dobbins 1985). The ileum is less permeable to ions than is the jejunum. Absorption of chloride and secretion of bicarbonate in the ileum are coupled by processes that may involve active transport of one or both ions. Highly efficient absorption of sodium and chloride occurs in the colon, where 90% of the sodium and chloride entering is reabsorbed. There appears to be no direct or indirect coupling between sodium and chloride or bicarbonate reabsorption in the distal colon. Active chloride reabsorption and bicarbonate secretion occur in the distal colon. Chloride can also be secreted in the jejunum, ileum, and colon (Phillips 1987; Dobbins 1985). Pancreatic juice is usually not rich in chloride ions. There is, however, a reciprocal relationship between chloride and bicarbonate concentrations in pancreatic fluid that is dependent on flow rate, with chloride being the major anion at lower rates of secretion (Dobbins 1985).

The kidneys play an important role in the regulation of plasma chloride concentration. After sodium, chloride is the most prevalent ion in the glomerular ultrafiltrate. Most of the chloride filtered is reabsorbed in the renal tubules. The traditional view of epithelial transport in the kidney represents the chloride ion as an obedient passive partner that follows the actively transported sodium ion. This view does not apply to many epithelia, including specific nephron segments. Chloride transport is intimately related to sodium and fluid transport and to cellular acid-base metabolism (Schild et al. 1988).

Chloride reabsorption in the proximal tubule is actively and passively linked to active sodium reabsorption. A formate-chloride exchange mechanism exists in the luminal membrane of proximal tubular cells and is responsible for active chloride reabsorption (Rose 1989). Reabsorbed chloride returns to the systemic circulation at the basolateral membrane primarily by a potassium chloride (KCl) cotransporter. Of filtered chloride, approximately 50 to 60% is reabsorbed by the proximal convoluted and straight tubules. Chloride reabsorption occurs transcellularly in the thick ascending limb of Henle's loop, leading to the generation of a lumen-positive transepithelial voltage. Sodium is reabsorbed transcellularly or paracellularly, and the latter process is driven by the transepithelial voltage. Chloride ion delivery is the rate-limiting step in this process and net sodium chloride (NaCl) transport increases directly with fluid Cl^- concentration. Loop diuretics such as furosemide and bumetanide act in the loop of Henle by competing for the chloride site on the Na^+-K^+-$2Cl^-$ carrier (Schild et al. 1988; Dobbins 1985; Greger 1988; Rose 1989). Parathyroid hormone inhibits reabsorption of bicarbonate and chloride in the proximal tubule, whereas angiotensin II appears to enhance chloride ion reabsorption in the proximal tubule at physiological concentrations (de Rouffignac and Elalouf 1988; Harris and Navar 1985). Glucagon, calcitonin, and antidiuretic hormone stimulate NaCl transport in the medullary thick ascending limb of Henle's loop (de Rouffignac and Elalouf 1988).

Sodium chloride transport in the distal tubule cannot be explained by a comprehensive model. This is due in part to the cellular heterogeneity of this nephron segment and differences between species and the fact that a portion of this nephron segment is not accessible to micropuncture techniques in rats, the most extensively studied species. Thiazide diuretics act by inhibiting the Na^+-Cl^- carrier in the early distal tubule, apparently at the chloride site (Greger 1988). Loop diuretics, on the other hand, do not block NaCl reabsorption at this site. Chloride ion transport in the collecting tubule is closely related to bicarbonate transport (Rose 1989).

Little is known about chloride transport in the medullary collecting tubules. In the cortical collecting tubules, however, the paracellular pathway, which is highly conductive for chloride ions, is an important route for reabsorption of chloride by diffusion down an electrochemical gradient. An increase in the lumen-positive transepithelial potential difference (TPD) decreases net chloride reabsorption, whereas a decrease in TPD increases chloride reabsorption. Hormones that change TPD in the cortical collecting tubule, therefore, can affect chloride reabsorption. Also, it has been postulated that the intercalated cells are sensitive to the acid-base status of the organism and can secrete bicarbonate ion via an HCO_3^--Cl^- exchanger that is insensitive to sodium ion transport or TPD but dependent on the presence of chloride ion in luminal fluid (de Rouffignac and Elalouf 1988).

Experimentally, administration of deoxycorticosterone acetate (DOCA) twice daily to sodium-supplemented dogs caused a significant increase in plasma sodium and bicarbonate ion concentration with no change in plasma Cl^- (Madias et al. 1984). When $NaHCO_3$ instead of NaCl was added to the diet, Na^+ and HCO_3^- increased significantly, whereas Cl^- decreased. Increased urinary loss of chloride is believed to be associated with hyperadrenocorticism. In a study of 117 dogs with hyperadrenocorticism, only 12 had Cl^- concentrations below 105 mEq/L (Ling et al. 1979). However, 25 of these dogs had hypernatremia, and the Cl^- could have been low relative to the Na^+. The mean Na^+ was 149.9 mEq/L and mean Cl^- was 108 mEq/L (mean Cl^- after correcting for changes in free water was 105 mEq/L). The cortical collecting duct is the main site of action for mineralocorticoids and glucocorticoids (de Rouffignac and Elalouf 1988). Administration of DOCA increases TPD in rats and rabbits, increasing sodium reabsorption in the cortical collecting tubules. Such an effect could explain the observed changes in chloride and sodium concentrations in dogs with hyperadrenocorticism.

▶ Chloride and Acid-Base Balance

Metabolic Acidosis

Metabolic acidoses are traditionally divided into hyperchloremic and normochloremic on the basis of the anion gap (AG). The AG is the difference between measured cations (sodium and potassium) and measured anions (chloride and bicarbonate) (see Chapters 9 and 10). Physiologically, there is no AG because electroneutrality must be maintained, and the AG is actually the difference between the unmeasured anions (UA^-) and unmeasured cations (UC^+). The AG is a simplification that is helpful clinically. It can be misleading, however, because the observed increase in HCO_3^- in cases of hyperchloremic acidosis is secondary to the decrease in Cl^-. According to one theory of acid-base regulation (Stewart 1981), addition of strong anions to the plasma causes a decrease in the strong ion difference (SID) and a secondary decrease in HCO_3^-. Strong ions are substances that are completely dissociated at body pH. If the strong anion added is chloride, the sum of the measured anions (Cl^- + HCO_3^-) remains the same and the AG does not change (so-called hyperchloremic or normal AG acidosis). If the strong anion added is an unmeasured anion (e.g., lactate), the Cl^- concentration remains normal whereas the HCO_3^- concentration decreases. The sum of the measured anions decreases, thus increasing the AG (so-called normochloremic or high-AG acidosis) (Stewart 1981).

The acid-base status of plasma is regulated by changing P_{CO_2} in the lungs and the strong ion difference (SID) in the kidneys, the latter being accomplished mainly by differential reabsorption of sodium and chloride ions in the renal tubules. Chloride is the most prevalent strong anion in the ECF. At a constant Na^+ concentration, a decrease in Cl^- concentration increases SID, causing hypochloremic alkalosis, whereas an increase in Cl^- concentration decreases SID, causing hyperchloremic acidosis.

Chloride in Metabolic Alkalosis

The role of chloride in the genesis, maintenance, and correction of metabolic alkalosis is still controversial. Decreases in Cl^-, however, increase SID, causing metabolic alkalosis. The inverse relationship between chloride and bicarbonate in metabolic alkalosis (Bia and Thier 1981), the fact that chloride depletion is accompanied by increased plasma HCO_3^- (Penman et al. 1972), and the fact that chronic metabolic alkalosis cannot be produced experimentally if chloride is available in the diet (Lemieux and Gervais 1964) have long been recognized. Compensatory increases in HCO_3^- that occur during recovery from chronic hypercapnia do not return to normal if dietary chloride is restricted (Schwartz et al. 1961).

Chloride was first linked to metabolic alkalosis in dogs when MacCallum and associates observed hypochloremia and an increase in "alkali reserve" in dogs with loss of gastric fluid caused by pyloric obstruction (MacCallum et al. 1920). The classical hypothesis associated the genesis and maintenance of metabolic alkalosis primarily with volume contraction. According to this hypothesis, volume depletion accompanying alkalosis augments fluid reabsorption in the proximal tubules. Alkalosis is maintained because bicarbonate ions are preferentially reabsorbed in this segment (Galla and Luke 1988). Volume expansion suppresses fluid and bicarbonate reabsorption, and more bicarbonate and chloride ions are delivered to distal nephron segments that have a greater capacity to reabsorb chloride than bicarbonate. Chloride is then retained, bicarbonate excreted, and alkalosis corrected (Galla and Luke 1988). Both volume expansion and provision of chloride were features of studies used to substantiate this hypothesis. The classical hypothesis can be viewed from a different perspective in which changes in chloride are the cause of the alkalosis (Galla et al. 1991). In rats, chloride ion depletion alone may play a role in the maintenance of metabolic alkalosis in a manner dissociated from its role as a marker of ECF volume (Galla et al. 1983, 1984a, 1984b; Luke and Galla, 1983). Chloride has a role more specific than merely accompanying sodium for electroneutrality in the extracellular space (Jacobson and Seldin 1983). In rats with chronic hypochloremic alkalosis, chloride repletion can be achieved without administration of sodium, without volume expansion, and without an increase in glomerular filtration rate (GFR) (Wall et al. 1987). The correction phase is associated with a decrease in plasma renin activity but with no change in plasma aldosterone concentration. It has also been shown that maintenance and correction of hypochloremic alkalosis are primarily dependent on total body chloride and its influence on renal function and not on the demands of sodium and fluid homeostasis (Galla et al. 1987). Ultimately, the correction of alkalosis is dependent on the kidney and does not occur in nephrectomized rats after infusion of chloride (Galla and Luke, 1988). The principal mechanisms by which the kidneys correct metabolic alkalosis probably operate in the collecting ducts, especially in the cortical segment, where HCO_3^- can be either secreted or reabsorbed (Galla et al. 1991).

Changes in ECF volume occur with hypochloremic alkalosis even when external losses of water and Na^+ are prevented (Garella et al. 1991). The decrease in ECF volume is an inherent feature of the hypochloremic alkalosis and is caused by internal shifts of fluid out of the ECF compartment (Garella et al. 1991). The resulting changes in GFR appear to play a minor role in the maintenance of alkalosis (Galla et al. 1991). Expanding the ECF without providing chloride does not correct hypochloremic alkalosis. Furosemide-induced hypochloremic alkalosis in humans eating an NaCl-free diet supplemented with 60 mEq of potassium per day can be corrected with orally administered KCl without changes in weight or ECF volume (Rosen et al. 1988). In this study, five NaCl-depleted control subjects were given furosemide and a combination of KCl and NaCl intravenously to maintain their sodium deficit while correcting their chloride deficit. Subjects who were selectively sodium depleted did not became alkalotic, and administration of the same amount of KCl used to treat metabolic alkalosis in the alkalotic group had no effect on plasma total carbon dioxide (CO_2) or urinary net acid excretion (Rosen et al. 1988). It has also been shown that a 25% increase in ECF volume (created by intravenous infusion of 6% bovine albumin in 5% dextrose) has no effect on hypochloremic alkalosis in a rat model of hypochloremic alkalosis (Galla et al. 1987).

These studies demonstrate that ECF volume, GFR, effective circulating volume, and sodium balance are not independent variables in the generation and maintenance of nonrespiratory alkalosis (Norris and Kurtzman 1988). It could still be concluded, however, that chloride induces potassium conservation that in turn inhibits bicarbonate reabsorption, because potassium balance was corrected even in studies in which choline-Cl instead of KCl was used to correct the alkalosis. However, when NaCl was supplied without potassium, alkalosis was corrected despite a persisting potassium deficit (Atkins and Schwartz 1962; Needle et al. 1964). Administration of potassium without chloride did not correct the alkalosis in an early study (Kassirer et al. 1965). It has been speculated that hypokalemia in rats and humans may cause hypochloremia by impairing recycling of potassium at the luminal membrane in the thick ascending limb of Henle's loop. This, in turn, impairs the effectiveness of the Na^+-K^+-$2Cl^-$ carrier, decreasing net chloride reabsorption (Galla and Luke 1988). Contrary to what occurs in rats and humans, isolated potassium deficiency in dogs causes a mild metabolic acidosis (Burnell and Dawbron 1970; Burnell et al. 1974).

Studies in rats with experimentally induced normovolemic and hypovolemic hypochloremic alkalosis showed no difference in the renal handling of chloride and bicarbonate between alkalotic and normal animals in the proximal convoluted tubule, loop of Henle, or distal convoluted tubule (Galla and Luke 1988). Key adjustments in anion excretion during the maintenance and correction of hypochloremic alkalosis were suspected to occur in the collecting tubule, especially in the cortical segment (Galla et al. 1991). Sodium-independent chloride and bicarbonate transport and secretion or reabsorption of HCO_3^- occur at this site (Galla and Luke 1988; Galla et al. 1991). Alterations in the delivery of HCO_3^- and Cl^- to the collecting tubules may also be important (Galla et al. 1991).

The chloride depletion hypothesis for the genesis and maintenance of metabolic alkalosis was proposed as an extension of the classical hypothesis (Galla and Luke 1988; Galla et al. 1991). It states that chloride alone is essential for correction of the hypochloremic alkalosis and that it does so by a renal mechanism. Volume depletion is a common but not essential feature of the maintenance phase of alkalosis, and its persistence does not preclude correction of alkalosis. If adequate chloride is provided, restoration of depleted volume may hasten correction of alkalosis by increasing GFR and decreasing proximal tubular reabsorption of fluid and bicarbonate (Galla and Luke 1988; Galla et al. 1991). The manner by which exogenous Cl^- repletion is detected and the kidney signaled to excrete HCO_3^- and the cellular mechanisms by which these events occur in the various nephron segments remain to be determined (Galla et al. 1991).

Role of Chloride in Adaptation for Acid-Base Disturbances

Chloride excretion is an important mechanism in the kidney's adaptation to metabolic acidosis and chronic respiratory acid-base disturbances. In metabolic acidosis, the kidneys increase net acid excretion (primarily by enhanced NH_4Cl excretion) beginning on day 1 and reaching a maximum after 5 to 6 days (Rose 1989). This response is due to the associated increase in intracellular hydrogen ion concentration, but glucocorticoids may also play a contributory role. The increase in chloride ion excretion without an associated increase in sodium ion excretion increases plasma SID and returns HCO_3^- and H^+ toward normal.

The increase in P_{CO_2} in chronic respiratory acidosis causes intracellular H^+ to increase in the renal tubular cells, resulting in stimulation of net acid excretion (primarily as NH_4Cl) (Rose 1989). Chloruresis, negative chloride balance, enhanced fractional and absolute bicarbonate reabsorption, and enhanced net acid excretion are typically associated with the renal response to chronic respiratory acidosis (Galla and Luke 1988). The loss of chloride ions in the urine decreases urinary SID because the Cl^- is accompanied by NH_4^+ rather than Na^+. Plasma SID and consequently HCO_3^- are thus increased. Hypochloremia is a common finding in human patients with chronic respiratory acidosis (Narins and Emmett 1980) and in dogs with experimentally induced chronic hypercapnia (Madias et al. 1985; Polak et al. 1961; Schwartz et al. 1965; van Ypersele de Strihou et al. 1962). On the other hand, in chronic hypocapnia renal H^+ excretion is decreased. This effect is probably mediated by a decrease in intracellular H^+. In this setting, there are a decrease in NH_4Cl excretion in the urine and an increase in renal reabsorption of Cl^-. The increase in Cl^- reabsorption decreases plasma SID and consequently HCO_3^- and is responsible for the hyperchloremia observed in human patients with chronic respiratory alkalosis (Narins and Emmett 1980) and in dogs with experimentally induced chronic hypocapnia (Gennari et al. 1972).

▶ Clinical Approach to Chloride Disorders

Corrected Chloride

Chloride concentration changes primarily or secondarily as a result of changes in water balance. When chloride changes because of water balance alterations, sodium concentration changes in proportion to the change in chloride. Evaluation of chloride concentration must, therefore, be done in conjunction with evaluation of changes in sodium concentration to account for changes in water balance (de Morais 1992b). A patient's chloride concentration is therefore "corrected" for changes in sodium concentration. The formula used by Fencl for humans (Leith 1990) has been adapted for use in dogs and cats (de Morais 1992b).

$$Cl^- \text{ (corrected)} = Cl^- \text{ (measured)} \times \frac{Na^+ \text{ (normal)}}{Na^+ \text{ (measured)}}$$

where Cl^- (measured) and Na^+ (measured) are the patient's chloride and sodium concentrations, respectively, and Na^+ (normal) is the mean normal sodium concentration. Assuming mean values for Na^+ of 146 mEq/L in dogs and 156 mEq/L in cats and for Cl^- of 110 mEq/L in dogs and 120 mEq/L in cats (DiBartola and de Morais 1992), the Cl^- (corrected) can be estimated (de Morais 1992b) in dogs as

$$Cl^- \text{ (corrected)} = Cl^- \times 146/Na^+$$

and in cats as

$$Cl^- \text{ (corrected)} = Cl^- \times 156/Na^+$$

Normal Cl^- (corrected) is approximately 107 to 113 mEq/L in dogs and approximately 117 to 123 mEq/L in cats

TABLE 4–2. **Classification of Chloride Disorders**

Disorder	Cl⁻	Cl⁻ Corrected	Associated Acid-base Disorder
Artifactual hyperchloremia	⇑	N	Contraction alkalosis
Artifactual hypochloremia	⇓	N	Dilutional acidosis
Corrected hyperchloremia	⇓, N, ⇑	⇑	Hyperchloremic acidosis
Corrected hypochloremia	⇓, N, ⇑	⇓	Hypochloremic alkalosis

Source: de Morais HSA: Chloride ion in small animal practice: The forgotten ion. *J Vet Emerg Crit Care* 2:11–24, 1992.
Cl⁻, chloride concentration; Cl⁻ corrected, corrected chloride concentration; ⇑, increased concentration; N, normal concentration; ⇓, decreased concentration.

(de Morais 1992b). These values may vary for different laboratories and different analyzers. With newer analyzers, higher chloride values are reported unless the chloride calibration is deliberately changed (Winter et al. 1990). Using the Cl⁻ (corrected) permits the division of chloride disorders into artifactual and corrected chloride changes (Table 4–2). In artifactual chloride changes, changes in free water are solely responsible for the chloride changes, whereas in corrected chloride changes, chloride itself is primarily changed. An algorithm for evaluation of chloride abnormalities is presented in Figure 4–1.

▶ Clinical Disturbances

Disorders Associated with Normal Cl⁻ (Corrected)

ARTIFACTUAL HYPOCHLOREMIA AND ARTIFACTUAL HYPERCHLOREMIA

A change in the water content of plasma without an imbalance in the content of electrolytes results in dilution or concentration of anions and cations. Consequently, sodium and chloride concentrations both change in parallel. These changes are usually recognized by changes in sodium concentration (hypernatremia or hyponatremia), and this ion (and changes in osmolality) should receive primary attention (see Chapter 3).

High chloride concentration with normal Cl⁻ (corrected) (artifactual hyperchloremia) is usually associated with pure water loss (e.g., diabetes insipidus, essential hypernatremia) or hypotonic losses (e.g., osmotic diuresis). Patients with hypernatremia caused by sodium gain (e.g., hypertonic saline or NaHCO₃ administration, hyperadrenocorticism) tend to have abnormal Cl⁻ (corrected). Low chloride concentration with normal Cl⁻ (corrected) (artifactual hypochloremia) has been associated with congestive heart failure, hypoadrenocorticism, and third-space loss of sodium and chloride. It is also associated with gastrointestinal loss, although in this setting one ion is often lost in excess of the other (e.g., chloride in patients with vomiting of stomach contents, sodium in patients with diarrhea) and the Cl⁻ (corrected) may be abnormal. Patients with hypoadrenocorticism may present with corrected hyperchloremia caused by mineralocorticoid deficiency.

Patients with artifactual hypochloremia tend to have decreased SID and therefore a tendency toward acidosis (dilutional acidosis), whereas patients with artifactual hyperchloremia tend to have increased SID and a tendency toward alkalosis (concentration alkalosis) (de Morais and Muir 1995). These are the only situations in which changes in HCO₃⁻ are not reciprocal and equimolar with changes in Cl⁻. In these situations both HCO₃⁻ and Cl⁻ change in the same direction, and the change in Cl⁻ is more pronounced (de Morais 1992a).

Disorders Associated with Abnormal Cl⁻ (Corrected)

CORRECTED HYPOCHLOREMIA

Decreased Cl⁻ (corrected) is associated with a tendency toward alkalosis (hypochloremic alkalosis) because of the associated increase in SID (de Morais and Muir 1995). Pseudohypochloremia may occur whenever chloride ion concentration is measured with a technique that is not ion selective in lipemic or hyperproteinemic samples (DiBartola et al. 1994; Graber et al. 1983). Chloride concentration in lipemic samples (triglyceride concentration >600 mg/dL) is underestimated by titrimetric methods but overestimated when colorimetric methods are used (Graber et al. 1983). Clinical signs associated with pure hypochloremia in dogs and cats have not been reported but are probably related to the metabolic alkalosis that

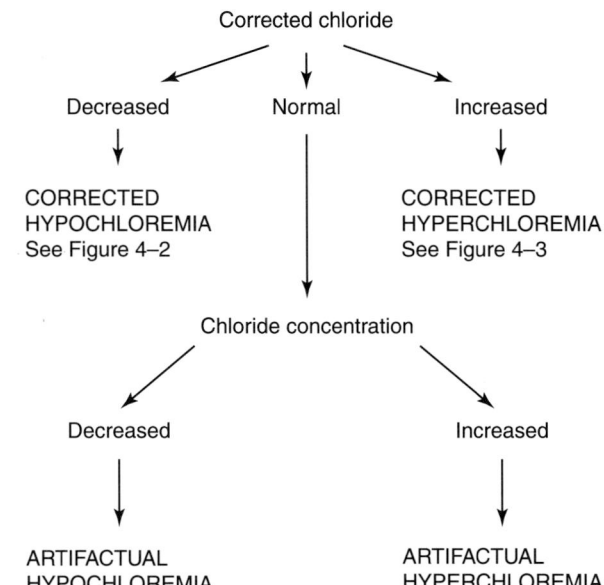

FIGURE 4–1. Algorithm for evaluation of patients with chloride abnormalities.

TABLE 4–3. Causes of Corrected Hypochloremia

Pseudohypochloremia
    Lipemic samples (titrimetric methods)
Excessive loss of chloride relative to sodium
    Vomiting of stomach contents*
    Therapy with thiazides or loop diuretics*
    Chronic respiratory acidosis
    Hyperadrenocorticism
    Exercise
Therapy with solutions containing high sodium concentration relative to chloride
Sodium bicarbonate
Sodium penicillin (extremely high doses)

Source: Adapted from de Morais HSA: Chloride ion in small animal practice: The forgotten ion. *J Vet Emerg Crit Care* 2:11–24, 1992.
*Most important causes in small animal practice.

accompanies hypochloremia (de Morais 1992b). It has been shown, however, that in euvolemic chloride depletion, the GFR decreases acutely by as much as 15 to 20%, probably as a result of changes in tubuloglomerular feedback and internal shifts of fluid out of the ECF (Garella et al. 1991; Galla and Luke 1988). The clinical importance of these experimental observations is unknown, but hypochloremia itself may potentiate the decrease in GFR associated with hypovolemia in the most common causes of corrected hypochloremia (e.g., vomiting of stomach contents, therapy with loop diuretics). Chloride ion depletion also stimulates renin secretion in rats despite concurrent volume expansion and potassium infusion (Abboud et al. 1979). Renin release caused by hypochloremia is probably mediated by the macula densa. Any resultant increase in aldosterone secretion would increase potassium excretion in the urine and contribute to hypokalemia.

Corrected hypochloremia may be caused by excessive loss of chloride relative to sodium or by administration of substances containing proportionately more sodium than chloride as compared with the normal ECF composition. The former can occur with administration of diuretics that cause chloride ion wasting (e.g., loop diuretics and thiazides) or when the fluid lost has a high Cl^- concentration, as in the case of vomiting of stomach contents or gastric conduit urinary diversions. (Fencl and Rossing 1989; de Morais and Muir 1995; McLoughlin et al. 1992). Loss of plasma during exercise in greyhounds also leads to corrected hypochloremia because of a greater loss of Cl^- than Na^+ (Toll et al. 1995). The administration of substances containing proportionately more sodium than chloride (e.g., antibiotics with Na^+ such as penicillin, $NaHCO_3$) increases Na^+ without increasing Cl^- (Fencl and Rossing 1989; Chew et al. 1991; Moon and Kramer 1995; de Morais and Muir 1995), therefore causing a decrease in Cl^-(corrected). In human patients, corrected hypochloremia rarely develops with the use of penicillin unless more than 20 g/day is administered to a hypovolemic patient (Koch and Taylor 1992). Corrected hypochloremia in dogs with hyperadrenocorticism has been discussed previously. In cats, acute tumor lysis syndrome (Calia et al. 1996), primary hypoadrenocorticism (Peterson et al. 1989), anemia (Whitehair et al. 1995), hemorragic pleural effusion (Whitehair et al. 1995), and diabetic ketoacidosis (Christopher et al. 1995) have been associated with corrected hypochloremia. Vomiting may have been a contributory factor for the corrected hypochloremia in some of these cats.

An increase in renal chloride ion excretion and decrease in plasma Cl^- have been observed in dogs with

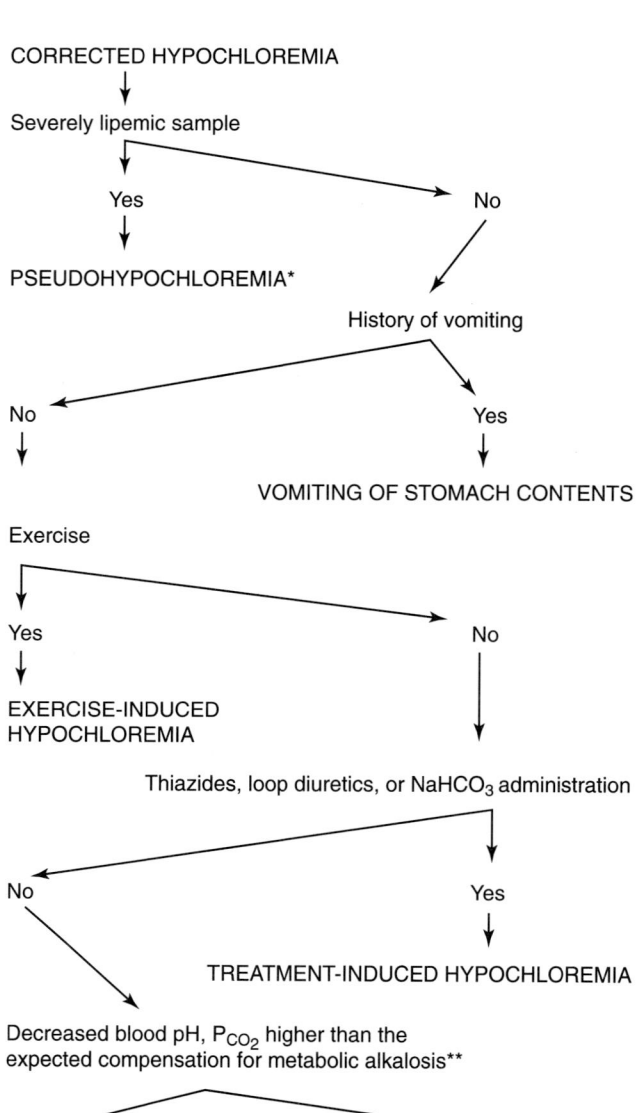

*Lipemia will underestimate chloride when chloride is measured by titrimetic methods.
**Expected compensation for metabolic alkalosis in dogs is a 0.35 mm Hg increase in P_{CO_2} for each 1 mEq/L increase in bicarbonate.

FIGURE 4–2. Algorithm for evaluation of dogs with corrected hypochloremia. (From de Morais HSA: Chloride ion in small animal practice. The forgotten ion. *J Vet Emerg Crit Care* 1:39–49, 1992.)

DISORDERS OF CHLORIDE

TABLE 4-4. Causes of Corrected Hyperchloremia

Pseudohyperchloremia
    Lipemic samples (colorimetric methods)
    Potassium bromide therapy
Excessive loss of sodium relative to chloride
    Diarrhea
Excessive gain of chloride relative to sodium
    Therapy with chloride salts (NH_4Cl, KCl)
    Total parenteral nutrition
    Fluid therapy (e.g., 0.9% NaCl, hypertonic saline, KCl-supplemented fluids)
    Salt poisoning
Renal chloride retention
    Renal failure
    Renal tubular acidosis
    Hypoadrenocorticism*
    Diabetes mellitus*
    Chronic respiratory alkalosis
    Drug-induced: acetazolamide, spironolactone

Source: Adapted from de Morais HSA: Chloride ion in small animal practice: The forgotten ion. *J Vet Emerg Crit Care* 2:11–24, 1992.
*May be associated with corrected hypochloremia in cats.

experimentally induced chronic respiratory acidosis (Madias et al. 1985; Polak et al. 1961; Schwartz et al. 1965; van Ypersele de Strihou et al. 1962). Consequently, patients with chronic hypercapnia may be presented with corrected hypochloremia. Potential causes of corrected hypochloremia are listed in Table 4–3 and an algorithm for the differential diagnosis of corrected hypochloremia is presented in Figure 4–2.

Treatment of patients with corrected hypochloremia should be directed at correction of the SID. Special attention should also be paid to the sodium concentration. Renal chloride ion conservation is enhanced in hypochloremic states, and renal chloride ion reabsorption does not return to normal until the plasma chloride concentration is restored to normal or near normal (Galla and Luke 1988). Patients with normal renal function should therefore be expected to respond to therapy if the underlying disease process is corrected and chloride is provided. In cases in which expansion of extracellular volume is desired, intravenous infusion of 0.9% NaCl is the treatment of choice (Fencl and Rossing 1989). If hypokalemia is also present, KCl should be added to the fluid administered. When volume expansion is not necessary, chloride can be administered using salts without sodium (e.g., KCl, NH_4Cl). Use of NaCl or KCl requires normal renal function to correct hypochloremia, whereas NH_4Cl requires intact hepatic and renal function (Koch and Taylor 1992).

CORRECTED HYPERCHLOREMIA

Increased Cl^- (corrected) is associated with a tendency toward acidosis (hyperchloremic acidosis) because of a decrease in SID. Pseudohyperchloremia may occur in patients receiving potassium bromide, because bromide and other halides (e.g., iodides) are measured as chloride (DiBartola et al. 1994; Emancipator and Kroll 1990). Bromide interferes with every chloride assay to some extent, although ion-selective electrodes are the most vulnerable to bromide interference (Emancipator and Kroll 1990; Driscoll and Martin 1966; Elin and Robertson 1981). If colorimetric methods are used to measure chloride concentration, other pigments such as hemoglobin and bilirubin may cause pseudohyperchloremia (DiBartola et al. 1994). Lipemia can also cause pseudohyperchloremia when colorimetric methods are used (Graber et al. 1983). Emulsified lipids in the photoelectric cell induce scattering of light resulting in overestimation of the true chloride content. This effect overcomes the decrease in chloride caused by a reduction in the plasma water fraction (Graber et al. 1983).

Specific clinical signs associated with pure hyperchloremia in dogs and cats have not been reported but are probably related to the metabolic acidosis that accompanies hyperchloremia (de Morais 1992b). Potential causes of corrected hyperchloremia are listed in Table 4–4 and an algorithm for the differential diagnosis of corrected hyperchloremia is presented in Figure 4–3.

Corrected hyperchloremia can be caused by chloride retention in renal failure (Widmer et al. 1979; Warnock 1988) or by administration of NH_4Cl to cats (Finco et al. 1986; Senior et al. 1986; Lemieux et al. 1990; Ching et al. 1989) and dogs (Halperin et al. 1985; Halperin and

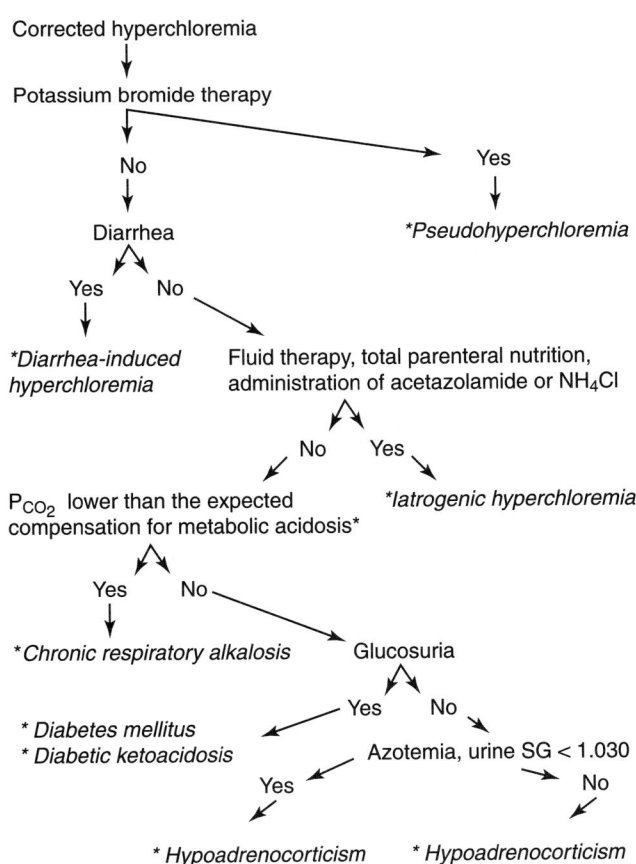

*Expected compensation for chronic respiratory alkalosis in dogs → for each 1 mm Hg decrease in P_{CO_2}, bicarbonate decreases 0.55 mEq/L

FIGURE 4-3. Algorithm for evaluation of dogs with corrected hyperchloremia. (From de Morais HSA: Chloride ion in small animal practice: The forgotten ion. *Vet Emerg Crit Care* 2:11–24, 1992.)

Bun-Chen, 1990). Type I renal tubular acidosis is also associated with hyperchloremic acidosis in dogs (DiBartola and Leonard 1982; Polzin et al. 1982) and cats (Drazner 1980; Brown et al. 1986; Watson et al. 1986). The exact mechanism whereby hyperchloremic acidosis occurs in distal renal tubular acidosis is not completely understood. There is, however, a decrease in ammonium excretion (Rose 1989), and chloride replaces bicarbonate in the plasma, causing hyperchloremia (Koch and Taylor 1992). Patients with diarrhea develop corrected hyperchloremia because of loss of a fluid with a higher sodium and a lower chloride ion concentration than those of plasma.

Patients with diabetes mellitus may have ketoacidosis with a normal AG (hyperchloremia). The ketoacids are excreted in the urine at low serum concentrations; thus, a patient with normal or near-normal extracellular volume, renal perfusion, and GFR may excrete the ketoacids as fast as they are generated. The kidneys retain chloride in place of ketones in this situation, increasing the chloride concentration while the AG remains unchanged (Gabow 1985). Patients with diabetes can also develop corrected hyperchloremia during the resolving phase of the ketoacidotic crisis (Goodkin et al. 1984; Oh et al. 1978). The hyperchloremia of the recovery phase has at least three causes. First, the administration of large volumes of isotonic saline can increase the chloride concentration more than the sodium concentration; second, KCl is often infused in large doses; and third, the ketones are lost in the urine and NaCl is reabsorbed by the kidneys (Narins and Emmett 1980; Adrogué et al. 1984). In cats, however, ketoacidosis was associated with corrected hypochloremia (Christopher et al. 1995). No information was provided about whether the cats in this report had vomited. In at least one ketoacidotic dog, corrected hypochloremia was also found (Whitehair et al. 1995).

Patients with hypoadrenocorticism and hypoaldosteronism have type IV renal tubular acidosis with chloride retention and hyperchloremic metabolic acidosis. These patients are typically presented with decreased serum chloride concentration, but because of concomitant hyponatremia caused by lack of aldosterone, Cl$^-$ (corrected) is increased (de Morais 1992b). Hyperchloremia can also be caused by drugs that cause chloride retention. Potassium-sparing diuretics such as spironolactone act by decreasing the number of open aldosterone-sensitive sodium channels in the principal cells of the cortical collecting tubules (Rose 1989). Inhibition of sodium reabsorption at this site leads to hyperkalemia and hyperchloremic acidosis. Acetazolamide inhibits carbonic anhydrase in the proximal tubule, resulting in bicarbonaturia, urinary alkalinization, and in rats, but not in dogs, reduction in renal ammoniagenesis (Fine 1986; Gougoux et al. 1987). Chloride reabsorption proceeds normally in the ascending loop of Henle, resulting in chloride retention (Kreisberg and Wood 1983), and use of acetazolamide is associated with hyperchloremia and metabolic acidosis (Rose 1989; Haskins et al. 1981; Rose and Carter 1979). Parenteral nutrition can cause hyperchloremia because some solutions have high concentrations of cationic amino acids (e.g., lysine-HCl, arginine-HCl) that release chloride and generate hydrogen ions (Heird et al. 1972).

Fluid therapy is another important cause of hyperchloremia in hospitalized patients. Administration of isotonic saline, lactated Ringer's solution, or an isotonic saline with 5% dextrose has been associated with corrected hyperchloremia in dogs and cats (Chew et al. 1991; Rose 1979). Hyperchloremia can be exacerbated by intravenous infusion of 0.9% sodium chloride (Koch and Taylor 1992). Isotonic sodium chloride solution supplemented with 20 mEq/L KCl has a final sodium concentration of 154 mEq/L and a chloride concentration of 174 mEq/L. This solution has a much higher chloride concentration than plasma and may easily cause corrected hyperchloremia, especially in patients with abnormal renal function (de Morais 1992b). Corrected hyperchloremia has also been associated with salt poisoning in dogs (DiBartola and de Morais 1992; Hughes and Sokolowski 1978) and with administration of hypertonic saline in dogs and pigs (de Morais 1992b; Moon and Kramer 1995).

Experimentally, chronic respiratory alkalosis causes renal chloride retention in dogs (Gennari et al. 1972). The observed hyperchloremia is part of the normal renal adaptation to chronic respiratory acid-base disorders. Patients with chronic hypocapnia can therefore be expected to have corrected hyperchloremia. Treatment of corrected hyperchloremia should be directed at correction of the underlying disease process. The effects of fluid therapy on chloride concentration should be anticipated, especially in patients with diabetes mellitus or abnormal renal function. Special attention should be given to plasma pH because patients with corrected hyperchloremia tend to be acidotic. Bicarbonate therapy can be instituted whenever plasma pH is below 7.2 or the bicarbonate concentration is below 12 mEq/L.

▶ Conclusions

Although it is the major anion in ECF, chloride has not received much attention in the clinical setting. It should be remembered that chloride ion is also important in the metabolic regulation of acid-base balance. The kidneys regulate acid-base balance by changing the amount of chloride that is reabsorbed with sodium (Stewart 1981). Chloride is important in determining the patient's SID, and therefore changes in chloride concentration reflect the patient's acid-base status. Corrected hypochloremia is associated with increased SID and metabolic alkalosis. Chloride is the only anion in ECF that can contribute to a substantial increase in SID. Administration of chloride is necessary for correction of hypochloremic metabolic alkalosis. Corrected hyperchloremia is associated with decreased SID and metabolic acidosis. Treatment with sodium bicarbonate should be carried out in patients with pH below 7.2.

REFERENCES

Abboud HE, Luke RG, Galla JH, and Kotchen TA: Stimulation of renin by acute selective chloride depletion in the rat. *Circ Res* 44:815–821, 1979.

Adrogué HJ, Eknoyan G, and Suki WK: Diabetic ketoacidosis: Role of the kidneys in the acid-base homeostasis re-evaluated. *Kidney Int* 25:591–598, 1984.

Atkins EL and Schwartz WB: Factors governing correction of the alkalosis associated with potassium deficiency: The critical role of chloride in the recovery process. *J Clin Invest* 41:218–229, 1962.

Bia M and Thier SO: Mixed acid-base disturbances: A clinical approach. *Med Clin North Am* 65:347–361, 1981.

Brown SA, Spyridakis LK, and Crowell WA: Distal renal tubular acidosis and hepatic lipidosis in a cat. *J Am Vet Med Assoc* 189:1350–1352, 1986.

Burnell JM and Dawbron JK: Acid base parameters in potassium depletion in the dog. *Am J Physiol* 218:1583–1589, 1970.

Burnell JM, Teubner EJ, and Simpson DP: Metabolic acidosis accompanying potassium deprivation. *Am J Physiol* 227:329–333, 1974.

Calia CM, Hohenhaus AE, Fox PR, and Meleo KA: Acute tumor lysis syndrome in a cat with lymphoma. *J Vet Intern Med* 10:409–411, 1996.

Chew DJ, Leonard M, and Muir WW III: Effect of sodium bicarbonate infusion on serum osmolality, electrolyte concentration, and blood gas tensions in cats. *Am J Vet Res* 52(1):12–17, 1991.

Ching SV, Fettman MJ, Hamar DW, et al.: The effect of chronic dietary acidification using ammonium chloride on acid-base and mineral metabolism in the adult cat. *J Nutr* 111:902–915, 1989.

Christopher MM, Broussard JD, and Peterson ME: Heinz body formation associated with ketoacidosis in cats. *J Vet Intern Med* 9:24–31, 1995.

de Morais HSA: A nontraditional approach to acid-base disorders. In DiBartola SP (ed): *Fluid Therapy in Small Animal Practice.* Philadelphia, WB Saunders Co., pp. 297–320, 1992a.

de Morais HSA: Chloride ion in small animal practice: The forgotten ion. *J Vet Emerg Crit Care* 2:11–24, 1992b.

de Morais HSA and DiBartola SP: Ventilatory and metabolic compensation in dogs with acid-base disturbances. *J Vet Emerg Crit Care* 1:39–49, 1991.

de Morais HSA and Muir WW III: Strong ions and acid-base disorders. In Bonagura JD and Kirk RW (eds): *Current Veterinary Therapy XII,* 12th ed. Philadelphia, WB Saunders Co., pp. 121–127, 1995.

de Rouffignac C and Elalouf JM: Hormonal regulation of chloride transport in the proximal and distal nephron. *Annu Rev Physiol* 50:123–140, 1988.

DiBartola SP and de Morais HSA: Case examples. In DiBartola SP (ed): *Fluid Therapy in Small Animal Practice.* Philadelphia, WB Saunders Co., pp. 599–688, 1992.

DiBartola SP and Leonard PO: Renal tubular acidosis in a dog. *J Am Vet Med Assoc* 180:70–73, 1982.

DiBartola SP, Green RA, and de Morais HSA: Electrolyte and acid-base abnormalities. In Willard MD, Tvedten H, and Turnwald GH (eds): *Small Animal Clinical Diagnosis by Laboratory Methods,* 2nd ed. Philadelphia, WB Saunders Co., pp. 97–114, 1994.

Dobbins J: Gastrointestinal disorders. In Arieff AI and DeFronzo RA (eds): *Fluid, Electrolyte, and Acid-Base Disorders.* New York, Churchill Livingstone, pp. 827–849, 1985.

Drazner FH: Distal renal tubular acidosis associated with chronic pyelonephritis in a cat. *Calif Vet* 34:15–21, 1980.

Driscoll JL and Martin HF: Detection of bromism by an automated chloride method. *Clin Chem* 12:314–318, 1966.

Elin RJ and Robertson EA: Bromide interference with determination of chloride by each of four methods (letter). *Clin Chem* 27:778–779, 1981.

Emancipator K and Kroll MH: Bromide interference: Is less really better? *Clin Chem* 8:1470–1473, 1990.

Fencl V and Rossing TH: Acid-base disorders in critical care medicine. *Annu Rev Med* 40:17–29, 1989.

Finco DR, Barsanti JA, and Brown SA: Ammonium chloride as a urinary acidifier in cats: Efficacy, safety and rationale for its use. *Mod Vet Pract* 67:537–541, 1986.

Fine A: Effects of carbonic anhydrase inhibition on renal ammoniagenesis in the dog. *Pharmacology* 33:217–220, 1986.

Gabow PA: Disorders associated with altered anion gap. *Kidney Int* 27:472–483, 1985.

Galla JH and Luke RG: Chloride transport and disorders of acid-base balance. *Annu Rev Physiol* 50:141–158, 1988.

Galla JH, Bonduris DN, and Luke RG: The correction of acute chloride-depletion alkalosis in the rat without volume expansion. *Am J Physiol* 244:F217–F221, 1983.

Galla JH, Bonduris DN, Dumbauld, SL, Luke RG: Segmental chloride and fluid handling during correction of chloride-depletion alkalosis without volume expansion in the rat. *J Clin Invest* 73:96–106, 1984a.

Galla JH, Bonduris DN, Sanders PW, Luke RG. Volume-independent reductions in glomerular filtration rate in acute chloride-depletion alkalosis in the rat. Evidence for mediation by tubuloglomerular feedback. *J Clin Invest* 74:2002–2008, 1984b.

Galla JH, Bonduris DN, Luke RG, et al.: Effects of chloride and extracellular fluid volume on bicarbonate reabsorption along the nephron in metabolic alkalosis in the rat: Reassessment of the classical hypothesis of the pathogenesis of metabolic alkalosis. *J Clin Invest* 80:41–50, 1987.

Galla JH, Gifford JD, Luke RG, et al.: Adaptations to chloride-depletion alkalosis. *Am J Physiol* 261:R771–R781, 1991.

Garella S, Cohen JJ, and Northrup TE: Chloride-depletion metabolic alkalosis induces ECF volume depletion via internal fluid shifts in nephrectomized dogs. *Eur J Clin Invest* 21:273–279, 1991.

Gennari FJ, Goldstein MB, and Schwartz W: The nature of the renal adaptation to chronic hypocapnia. *J Clin Invest* 51:1722–1730, 1972.

Goodkin DA, Krishna GG, and Narins RG: The role of the anion gap in detecting and managing mixed metabolic acid-base disorders. *Clin Endocrinol Metab* 13:333–349, 1984.

Gougoux A, Vinay P, Zizian L, et al.: Effect of acetazolamide on renal metabolism and ammoniagenesis in the dog. *Kidney Int* 31:1279–1290, 1987.

Graber ML, Quigg RJ, Slempsey WE, and Weis DO: Spurious hyperchloremia and decreased anion gap in hyperlipidemia. *Ann Intern Med* 98:607–609, 1983.

Greger R: Chloride transport in thick ascending loop, distal convolution, and collecting duct. *Annu Rev Physiol* 50:111–122, 1988.

Halperin ML and Bun-Chen C: Influence of acute hyponatremia on renal ammoniagenesis in dogs with chronic metabolic acidosis. *Am J Physiol* 258:F328–F332, 1990.

Halperin ML, Vinay P, Gougoux A, et al.: Regulation of the maximum rate of renal ammoniagenesis in the acidotic dog. *Am J Physiol* 248:F607–F615, 1985.

Harris PJ and Navar LG: Tubular transport responses to angiotensin. *Am J Physiol* 248:F621–F630, 1985.

Haskins SC, Munger RJ, Helphrey MG, et al.: Effects of acetazolamide on blood acid-base and electrolyte values in dogs. *J Am Vet Med Assoc* 179:792–796, 1981.

Heird WC, Dell B, Driscoll JM, et al.: Metabolic acidosis resulting from intravenous alimentation with synthetic amino acids. *N Engl J Med* 287:943–945, 1972.

Hughes DE and Sokolowski J: Sodium chloride poisoning in the dog. *Canine Pract* 5:28–31, 1978.

Jacobson HR and Seldin DW: On the generation, maintenance, and correction of metabolic alkalosis. *Am J Physiol* 245:F425–F432, 1983.

Jones NL: *Blood Gases and Acid Base Physiology,* 2nd ed. New York, Thieme Medical Publishers, 1987.

Kassirer JP, Berkman PM, Lawrenz DR, et al.: The critical role of chloride in the correction of hypokalemic alkalosis in man. *Am J Med* 38:172–189, 1965.

Koch SM and Taylor RW: Chloride ion in intensive care medicine. *Crit Care Med* 20:227–240, 1992.

Kreisberg RA and Wood BC: Drugs and chemical-induced metabolic acidosis. *Clin Endocrinol Metab* 12:391–411, 1983.

Leith DE: The new acid-base: Power and simplicity. *Proceedings of the 8th ACVIM Forum.* San Diego, pp. 449–455, 1990.

Lemieux G and Gervais M: Acute chloride depletion alkalosis: Effect of anions on its maintenance and correction. *Am J Physiol* 207:1279–1286, 1964.

Lemieux G, Lemieux C, Duplessis S, and Berkofsky J: Metabolic characteristics of cat kidney: Failure to adapt to metabolic acidosis. *Am J Physiol* 259:R277–R281, 1990.

Ling G, Stabenfeldt GH, Comer KM, et al.: Canine hyperadrenocorticism: Pretreatment clinical and laboratory evaluation of 117 cases. *J Am Vet Med Assoc* 174:1211–1215, 1979.

Luke RG and Galla JH: Chloride-depletion alkalosis with a normal extracellular fluid volume. *Am J Physiol* 254:F419–F424, 1983.

MacCallum WG, Lintz J, Vermilye HN, et al.: The effect of pyloric obstruction relation to gastric tetany. *Bull Johns Hopkins Hosp* 31:1–7, 1920.

Madias NE, Bossed WH, and Adrogué HJ: Ventilatory response to chronic metabolic acidosis and alkalosis in the dog. *J Appl Physiol* 56:1640–1646, 1984.

Madias NE, Wolf CJ, and Cohen JJ: Regulation of acid-base equilibrium in chronic hypercapnia. *Kidney Int* 27:538–543, 1985.

McLoughlin MA, Walshaw R, Thomas, MW, et al.: Gastric conduit urinary diversion in normal dogs. Part II. Hypochloremic metabolic alkalosis. *Vet Surg* 21:33–39, 1992.

Moon PF and Kramer GC: Hypertonic saline-dextran resuscitation from hemorragic shock induces transient mixed acidosis. *Crit Care Med* 23:323–331, 1995.

Narins RG and Emmett M: Simple and mixed acid-base disorders: A practical approach. *Medicine (Baltimore)* 59(3):161–187, 1980.

Needle MA, Kaloyanides GJ, and Schwartz WB: The effects of selective depletion of hydrochloric acid on acid-base and electrolyte equilibrium. *J Clin Invest* 43:1836–1846, 1964.

Norris SH and Kurtzman NA: Does chloride play an independent role in the pathogenesis of metabolic alkalosis? *Semin Nephrol* 7(2):101–108, 1988.

Oh MS, Carrol HJ, Goldstein DA, and Fein IA: Hyperchloremic acidosis during the recovery phase of diabetic ketosis. *Ann Intern Med* 89:925–927, 1978.

Penman RW, Luke RF, and Jarboe TM: Respiratory effects of hypochloremic alkalosis and potassium depletion in the dog. *J Appl Physiol* 33:170–174, 1972.

Peterson ME, Greco DS, and Orth DN: Primary hypoadrenocorticism in ten cats. *J Vet Intern Med* 3:55–58, 1989.

Phillips SF: Small and large intestinal disorders: Associated fluid and electrolyte complications. In Maxwell MH, Kleeman CR, and Narins RG (eds): *Clinical Disorders of Fluid and Electrolyte Metabolism.* New York, McGraw-Hill Book Co., pp. 865–877, 1987.

Polak A, Haynie GD, Hays RM, et al.: Effects of chronic hypercapnia on electrolyte and acid-base equilibrium. I. Adaptation. *J Clin Invest* 40:1223–1237, 1961.

Polzin DJ, Stevens JB, and Osborne CA: Clinical application of the anion gap in evaluation of acid-base disorders in dogs. *Compend Contin Educ Pract Vet* 4:1021–1033, 1982.

Rose BD: *Clinical Physiology of Acid-Base and Electrolyte Disorders,* 3rd ed. New York, McGraw-Hill Book Co., 1989.

Rose RJ: Some physiological and biochemical effects of the intravenous administration of five different electrolyte solutions in the dog. *J Vet Pharmacol Ther* 2:279–289, 1979.

Rose RJ and Carter J: Some physiological and biochemical effects of acetazolamide in the dog. *J Vet Pharmacol Ther* 2:215–221, 1979.

Rosen RA, Bruce JA, Dubovsky EV, et al.: On the mechanism by which chloride corrects metabolic alkalosis in man. *Am J Med* 84:449–458, 1988.

Schild L, Giebisch G, and Green R: Chloride transport in the proximal renal tubule. *Annu Rev Physiol* 50:97–110, 1988.

Schwartz WB, Hays RM, Polak A, et al.: Effects of chronic hypercapnia on electrolyte and acid-base equilibrium. II. Recovery, with special reference to the influence of chloride intake. *J Clin Invest* 40:1238–1249, 1961.

Schwartz WB, Brackelt NC, and Cohen JJ: The response of extracellular hydrogen ion concentration to graded degrees of chronic hypercapnia: The physiologic limits of defense of pH. *J Clin Invest* 44:291–301, 1965.

Senior DF, Sundslrom DA, and Wolfson BB: Testing the effects of ammonium chloride and D-methionine on the urinary pH of cats. *Vet Med* 81:88–93, 1986.

Stewart PA: *How to Understand Acid-Base.* New York, Elsevier, 1981.

Tietz NW, Pruden EL, and Sigaard-Andersen O: Electrolytes, blood gases, and acid-base balance. Section One. Electrolytes. In Tietz NW (ed): *Textbook of Clinical Chemistry.* Philadelphia, WB Saunders Co., pp. 1172–1191, 1986.

Toll PW, Gaehtgens P, Neuhaus D, et al.: Fluid, electrolyte, and packed cell volume shifts in racing greyhounds. *Am J Vet Res* 56:227–232, 1995.

van Ypersele de Strihou C, Gulyassy PF, and Schwartz WB: Effects of chronic hypercapnia on electrolyte and acid-base equilibrium. III. Characteristics of the adaptive and recovery process as evaluated by provision of alkali. *J Clin Invest* 41:2246–2253, 1962.

Wall BM, Byrum GV, Galla JH, and Luke RG: Importance of chloride for the correction of chronic metabolic alkalosis in the rat. *Am J Physiol* 253:F1031–F1039, 1987.

Warnock DG: Uremic acidosis. *Kidney Int* 34:278–287, 1988.

Watson ADJ, Culvenor JA, Middleton DJ, and Rothwell TLW: Distal renal tubular acidosis in a cat with pyelonephritis. *Vet Rec* 119:65–68, 1986.

Whitehair KJ, Haskins SC, Whitehair JG, and Pascoe PJ: Clinical applications of quantitative acid-base chemistry. *J Vet Intern Med* 9:1–12, 1995.

Widmer B, Gerhardt RE, Harrington JT, and Cohen JJ: Serum electrolyte and acid base composition: The influence of graded degrees of chronic renal failure. *Arch Intern Med* 139:1099–1102, 1979.

Winter SD, Pearson JR, Gabow PA, et al.: The fall of serum anion gap. *Arch Intern Med* 150:311–313, 1990.

CHAPTER 5

Disorders of Potassium
HYPOKALEMIA AND HYPERKALEMIA

STEPHEN P. DiBARTOLA   HELIO AUTRAN DE MORAIS

Potassium is the major intracellular cation in mammalian cells, whereas sodium is the major extracellular cation. Normally, the extracellular fluid (ECF) sodium concentration is approximately 150 mEq/L and the ECF potassium concentration is approximately 4 mEq/L. This relationship is reversed in intracellular fluid (ICF), in which the sodium concentration is approximately 10 mEq/L and the potassium concentration is approximately 150 mEq/L. In experimental studies in dogs, control values for ICF sodium and potassium concentrations in skeletal muscle were 8.4 to 13.7 and 139 to 142 mEq/L (Knochel and Schlein 1972; Bilbrey et al. 1973).

Total body potassium content in human beings is approximately 50 to 55 mEq/kg body weight, and almost all of this potassium is readily exchangeable (Alexander and Perrone 1987; Field et al. 1987). In one study of potassium depletion in dogs, the control value for total exchangeable potassium as determined by ^{42}K dilution was 47.1 mEq/kg body weight (range, 39.8–61.1 mEq/kg) (Abbrecht 1969). As much as 95% or more of total body potassium is located in cells, with muscle containing 60 to 75% of this potassium. Muscle potassium content in normal dogs and cats is approximately 400 mEq/kg (Knochel and Schlein 1972; Bilbrey et al. 1973; Patterson et al. 1983; Theisen et al. 1997). As a solute, intracellular potassium is crucial for maintenance of normal cell volume. Intracellular potassium is also important for normal cell growth because it is required for the normal function of enzymes responsible for nucleic acid, glycogen, and protein synthesis.

The remaining 5% of the body's potassium is located in the ECF. Maintaining the ECF potassium concentration within narrow limits is critical to avoid the life-threatening effects of hyperkalemia on cardiac conduction. In human beings, the serum potassium concentration is inversely correlated with the total body deficit of potassium (Fig. 5–1). Likewise, in dogs with potassium depletion induced by dietary restriction, the muscle potassium content was strongly correlated ($r = 0.87$) with the serum potassium concentration (Patterson et al. 1983). During translocation of potassium between ICF and ECF, however, the serum potassium concentration can change without any change in the total body potassium content. One of the most important functions of potassium in the body is its role in generation of the normal resting cell membrane potential.

The Resting Cell Membrane Potential

The normal relationship between ECF and ICF potassium concentrations is maintained by Na^+,K^+-adenosinetriphosphatase (Na^+,K^+-ATPase) in cell membranes. This enzyme pumps sodium ions out of and potassium ions into the cell in a 3:2 Na/K ratio so that the intracellular concentration of potassium is much higher than its extracellular concentration. As a result, K^+ ions diffuse out

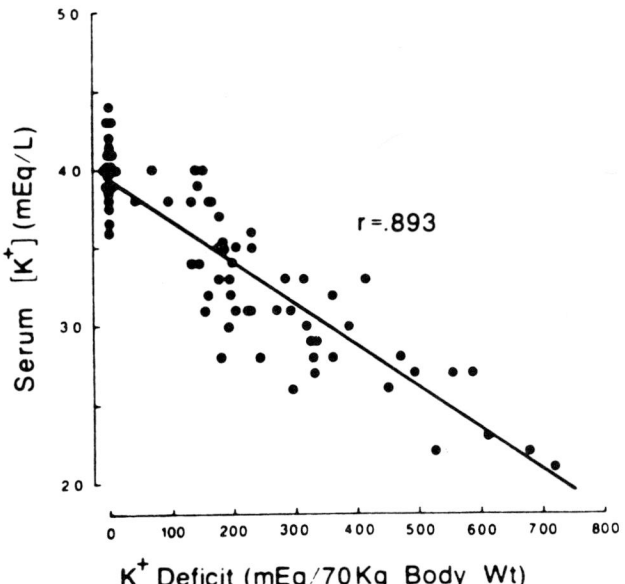

FIGURE 5–1. Relationship of serum potassium concentration to bodily potassium deficit. The data are derived from seven metabolic balance studies carried out on 24 human subjects depleted of potassium. (From Raymond KH and Kunau RT: Hypokalemic states. In Maxwell MH, Kleeman CR, and Narins RG: *Clinical Disorders of Fluid and Electrolyte Metabolism*, 4th ed. New York, McGraw-Hill Book Co, p. 519, 1987, with permission of the McGraw-Hill Companies.)

of the cell down their concentration gradient. The cell membrane, however, is impermeable to most intracellular anions (e.g., proteins, organic phosphates). A net negative charge therefore develops within the cell as K^+ ions diffuse out, and a net positive charge accumulates outside the cell. Consequently, a potential difference is generated across the cell membrane.

The principal extracellular cation is sodium, and it enters the cell relatively slowly down its concentration and electrical gradients because cell membrane permeability to potassium is 100-fold greater than that of sodium. Diffusion of K^+ ions from the cell continues until the ECF acquires sufficient positive charge to prevent further diffusion of K^+ ions out of the cell. The ratio of the intracellular to extracellular concentrations of potassium ($[K^+]_I/[K^+]_O$) is the major determinant of the *resting cell membrane potential* as described by the Nernst equation:

$$E_m = -61 \log_{10} \frac{[K^+]_I}{[K^+]_O}$$

The Goldman-Hodgkin-Katz equation is a modification of the Nernst equation that allows prediction of E_m on the basis of the ionic permeability characteristics of the cell membrane to sodium and potassium and the concentrations of these ions inside and outside the cell:

$$E_m = -61 \log_{10} \frac{rP_K[K^+]_I + P_{Na}[Na^+]_I}{rP_K[K^+]_O + P_{Na}[Na^+]_O}$$

where P_{Na} and P_K are the membrane permeabilities for sodium and potassium. The term r is included in the equation to account for the effect of the electrogenic Na^+,K^+-ATPase pump under steady-state conditions. This term is assigned the Na/K transport ratio of 3:2 so that $r = 1.5$. If the membrane permeability for potassium is assigned a value of 1.0 and the cell membrane is 100 times more permeable to potassium than sodium:

$$E_m = -61 \log_{10} \frac{1.5[K^+]_I + 0.01[Na^+]_I}{1.5[K^+]_O + 0.01[Na^+]_O}$$

For example, using the hypothetical ECF and ICF concentrations of sodium and potassium given at the beginning of this chapter:

$$E_m = -61 \log_{10} \frac{1.5[150] + 0.01[10]}{1.5[4] + 0.01[150]}$$

$$E_m = -61 \log_{10}(30) = -90 mV$$

In one study of dogs with potassium deficiency, the predicted E_m was -86.6 mV and the measured E_m in skeletal muscle of control animals was -90.1 mV (Bilbrey et al. 1973). The resting cell membrane potential plays a vital role in the normal function of skeletal and cardiac muscle, nerve, and transporting epithelia.

The Threshold Cell Membrane Potential

The *threshold cell membrane potential* is reached when sodium permeability increases to the point that sodium entry exceeds potassium exit, depolarization becomes self-perpetuating, and an action potential develops. The ability of specialized cells to develop an action potential is crucial to normal cardiac conduction, muscle contraction, and nerve impulse transmission. The excitability of a tissue is determined by the difference between the resting and threshold potentials (the smaller the difference, the greater the excitability).

Hypokalemia increases the resting potential (i.e., makes it more negative) and hyperpolarizes the cell, whereas hyperkalemia decreases the resting potential (i.e., makes it less negative) and initially makes the cell hyperexcitable (Fig. 5–2). If the resting potential decreases to less than the threshold potential, depolarization results, repolarization cannot occur, and the cell is no longer excitable. Translocation of potassium between body compartments results in a greater change in the ratio of intracellular to extracellular potassium concentrations ($[K^+]_I/[K^+]_O$) than does a change in total body potassium. In the former instance, the potassium concentrations of the two compartments change in opposite directions, whereas in the latter instance they change in the same direction.

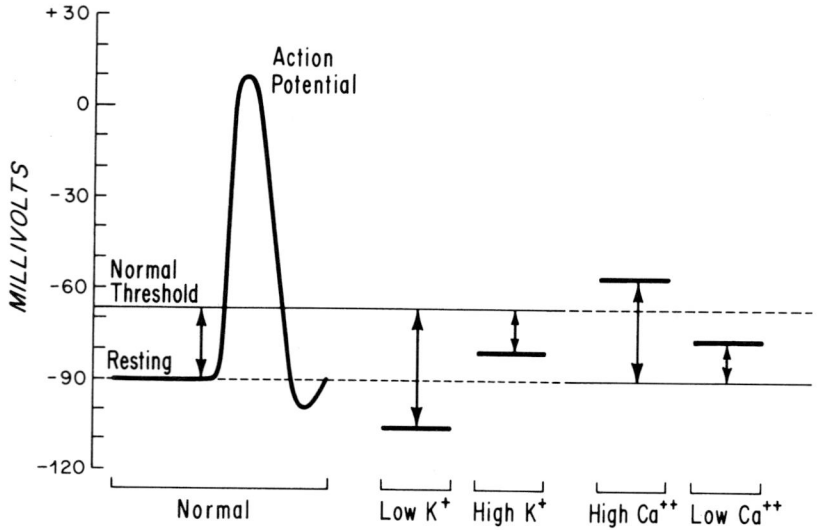

FIGURE 5–2. Effects of serum calcium and potassium on membrane potentials of excitable tissues. The concentration of potassium in extracellular fluids affects the resting potential, whereas calcium concentrations alter the threshold potential. (From Leaf A and Cotran R: *Renal Pathophysiology*. New York, Oxford University Press, p. 116, 1976.)

Membrane excitability is also affected by ionized calcium concentration and acid-base balance. Calcium affects the threshold potential rather than the resting potential. Ionized hypocalcemia increases membrane excitability by allowing self-perpetuating sodium permeability to be reached with a lesser degree of depolarization, whereas ionized hypercalcemia requires greater than normal depolarization for this threshold to be reached (see Fig. 5–2). Thus, hypercalcemia counteracts hyperkalemia by normalizing the difference between the resting and threshold potentials whereas hypocalcemia exacerbates the effect of hyperkalemia on membrane excitability. This principle is the basis for treating hyperkalemia with calcium salts (see later). Membrane excitability is increased by alkalemia and decreased by acidemia. As a result of these factors, clinical signs are not necessarily correlated with serum potassium concentrations. Electrocardiographic findings and muscle strength reflect the functional consequences of abnormalities in serum potassium concentration.

▶ Potassium Balance

External Potassium Balance

External balance for potassium is maintained by matching output (primarily in the urine) to input (from the diet). In the normal animal, potassium enters the body only through the gastrointestinal tract, and virtually all ingested potassium is absorbed in the stomach and small intestine. Transport of potassium in the small intestine is passive, whereas active transport (responsive to aldosterone) occurs in the colon. Colonic secretion of potassium may play an important role in extrarenal potassium homeostasis in some disease states (e.g., chronic renal failure) (Fig. 5–3).

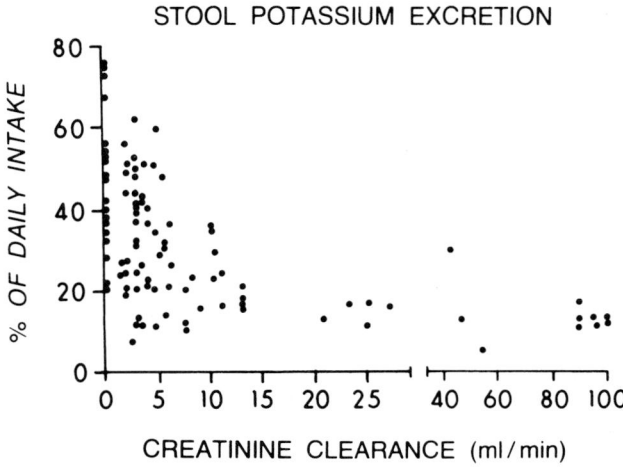

FIGURE 5–3. Relationship between the degree of renal insufficiency and fecal potassium excretion. Data points are compiled from three studies comprising 98 balance periods in 40 human patients. Variation in dietary protein or sodium intake did not produce consistent changes in fecal potassium excretion; thus data points from these balance periods were included without special designation. (From Alexander EA and Perrone RD: Regulation of extrarenal potassium metabolism. In Maxwell MH, Kleeman CR, and Narins RG: *Clinical Disorders of Fluid and Electrolyte Metabolism*, 4th ed. New York, McGraw-Hill Book Co, p. 112, 1987, with permission of the McGraw-Hill Companies.)

Potassium derived from the diet and endogenous cellular breakdown is removed from the body primarily by the kidneys and to much lesser extent by the gastrointestinal tract. During zero balance, 90 to 95% of ingested potassium is excreted in the urine and the remaining 5 to 10% is excreted in the stool. This pattern of output has been observed during control balance studies in normal dogs (Polak et al. 1961; Atkins and Schwartz 1962; Needle et al. 1964; Schwartz et al. 1965; Sapir et al. 1967). In a study of renal handling of potassium in dogs, 90 to 98% of potassium intake was eliminated from the body by the kidneys (Bourgoignie et al. 1981).

Adaptation occurs during chronic potassium loading so that the animal is protected from hyperkalemia that could occur as a result of an acute potassium load. This effect results from enhanced renal and colonic excretion of potassium as well as from enhanced uptake of potassium by liver and muscle, mediated by the effects of insulin and catecholamines. Potassium deprivation is associated with decreased aldosterone secretion, suppression of potassium secretion in the distal nephron, and increased reabsorption of potassium in the inner medullary collecting ducts (see later). Skeletal muscle potassium concentration decreases, but brain and heart potassium concentrations are minimally affected during potassium depletion (Knochel and Schlein 1972; Bilbrey et al. 1973; Schrock and Kuschinsky 1989). The colon adapts to potassium deprivation by decreasing its secretion of potassium.

Internal Potassium Balance

Internal balance for potassium is maintained by translocation of potassium between ECF and ICF. One-half to two-thirds of an acute potassium load appears in the urine within the first 4 to 6 h, and effective translocation of potassium from ECF to ICF is crucial in preventing life-threatening hyperkalemia until the kidneys have sufficient time to excrete the remainder of the potassium load. Endogenous insulin secretion and stimulation of β_2-adrenergic receptors by epinephrine promote cellular uptake of potassium in liver and muscle by increasing the activity of cell membrane Na^+,K^+-ATPase. The main effect of these hormones is to facilitate distribution of an acute potassium load and not to mediate minor adjustments in serum potassium concentration. The ECF concentration of potassium itself plays an important role in translocation, because potassium movement into cells is facilitated by the change in chemical concentration gradient resulting from addition of potassium to ECF. The fraction of an acute potassium load taken up by the body is increased during chronic potassium depletion and decreased when total body potassium is excessive. In summary, any change in serum potassium concentration must arise from a change in intake, distribution, or excretion (Fig. 5–4).

Effect of Acid-Base Balance on Potassium Distribution

The effect of acute pH changes on translocation of potassium between ICF and ECF is complex. In general, acidosis is associated with movement of potassium ions

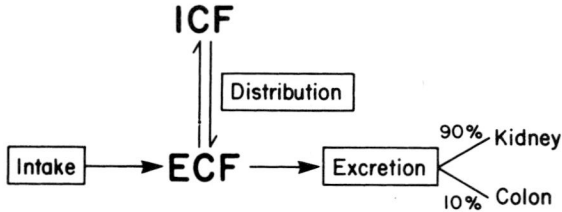

FIGURE 5-4. Components of potassium homeostasis. ECF = extracellular fluid; ICF = intracellular fluid. (From Field MJ, Berliner RW, Giebisch GH: Regulation of renal potassium metabolism. In Maxwell MH, Kleeman CR, and Narins RG: *Clinical Disorders of Fluid and Electrolyte Metabolism*, 4th ed. New York, McGraw-Hill Book Co, p. 120, 1987, with permission of the McGraw-Hill Companies.)

from ICF to ECF, and alkalosis is associated with movement of potassium ions from ECF to ICF. Early animal studies and observations in a small number of human patients (Swan and Pitts 1955; Burnell et al. 1956; Schwartz et al. 1957) led to the prediction that acute metabolic acidosis would be associated with a 0.6 mEq/L increment in serum potassium concentration for each 0.1 U decrement in pH. This rule of thumb has circulated widely among clinicians.

A critical review of experimental studies in animals and humans, however, demonstrated that changes in serum potassium concentration during acute acid-base disturbances were quite variable. (Adrogué and Madias 1981). The change in serum potassium concentration was greatest during acute mineral acidosis. In dogs, the increase in serum potassium concentration after administration of a mineral acid (e.g., HCl, NH$_4$Cl) was very variable, ranging from a 0.17 to 1.67 mEq/L increment in serum potassium concentration per 0.1 U decrement in pH (mean, 0.75 mEq/L). The increment in serum potassium concentration during acute respiratory acidosis in dogs was much lower, averaging only 0.14 mEq/L per 0.1 U decrement in pH. The decrement in serum potassium concentration during metabolic alkalosis in dogs averaged 0.18 mEq/L per 0.1 U increment in pH, whereas it averaged 0.27 mEq/L per 0.1 U increment in pH during respiratory alkalosis. In another study, respiratory alkalosis induced by hyperventilation in anesthetized dogs caused a somewhat greater decrement in serum potassium concentration (0.4 mEq/L) for each 0.1 U increment in pH (Muir et al. 1990). An increase in serum potassium concentration did not occur in acute metabolic acidosis caused by organic acids (e.g., lactic acid, ketoacids) (Tobin 1958; Oster et al. 1978, 1980; Adrogué and Madias 1981; Adrogué et al. 1985; Ilkiw et al. 1989). Acute infusion of β-hydroxybutyrate in normal dogs caused an increase in insulin in portal venous blood and hypokalemia, presumably as a result of potassium uptake by cells. Acute infusion of HCl led to hyperkalemia and increased portal vein glucagon concentration (Adrogué et al. 1985). In summary, only mineral acidosis is expected to cause any clinically relevant change in serum potassium concentration during acute acid-base disturbances.

Many factors probably contribute to the variable changes observed in serum potassium concentration during acute acid-base disturbances, including blood pH and HCO$_3^-$ concentration, nature of the acid anion (mineral versus organic), osmolality, hormonal activity (e.g., catecholamines, insulin, aldosterone), and the metabolic and excretory roles of the liver and kidney (Adrogué and Madias 1981). Hyperosmolality and lack of insulin are more likely to be responsible for hyperkalemia observed in patients with diabetic ketoacidosis than is the acidosis itself.

Hyperkalemia associated with acute metabolic acidosis induced by mineral acids is transient. In a study of acute and chronic metabolic acidosis induced in dogs by administration of HCl or NH$_4$Cl, hyperkalemia was observed after acute infusion of HCl, but hypokalemia developed after 3 to 5 days of NH$_4$Cl administration (Magner et al. 1988). The observed hypokalemia was associated with inappropriately high urinary excretion of potassium and increased plasma aldosterone concentration (Magner et al. 1988). Similar findings have been reported in rats with chronic metabolic acidosis induced by NH$_4$Cl. Despite a total body deficit of potassium, rats with chronic metabolic acidosis did not conserve potassium appropriately (Scandling and Ornt 1987). This effect may be due to a decreased filtered load of HCO$_3^-$, increased distal delivery of sodium, and increased distal tubular flow. Thus, metabolic acidosis of at least 2 to 3 days' duration is associated with increased urinary potassium excretion and mild hypokalemia rather than hyperkalemia (Gennari and Cohen 1975).

▶ Renal Handling of Potassium

The kidney is the primary regulator of potassium balance. Potassium is filtered at the glomerulus, and approximately 70% of the filtered load is reabsorbed isosmotically with water and sodium in the proximal tubule. An additional 10 to 20% of filtered potassium is reabsorbed in the ascending limb of Henle's loop. Finally, 10 to 20% of the filtered load is delivered to the distal nephron, where final adjustments in potassium reabsorption and secretion are made. Potassium experiences either net reabsorption or secretion in the connecting tubule, cortical collecting duct, and first portion of the outer medullary collecting duct, depending on the body's needs. Net movement of potassium in these segments of the nephron determines urinary excretion of potassium. Potassium once again experiences reabsorption in the last portion of the outer medullary collecting duct and inner medullary collecting duct regardless of the body's needs.

Mechanisms of Renal Tubular Transport of Potassium

The transepithelial electrical potential difference is lumen negative in the early proximal tubule, but no active transport mechanism for potassium has been discovered in this segment of the nephron. In the proximal tubule, potassium is reabsorbed along with water by solvent drag via the paracellular route. Apparently, water reabsorption increases the luminal concentration of potassium enough to overcome the unfavorable transepithelial potential difference. The transepithelial electrical potential difference becomes lumen positive in the late proximal tubule, and this facilitates reabsorption of potassium by the paracellular route. Transcellular transport of potassium in the prox-

Proximal Tubule

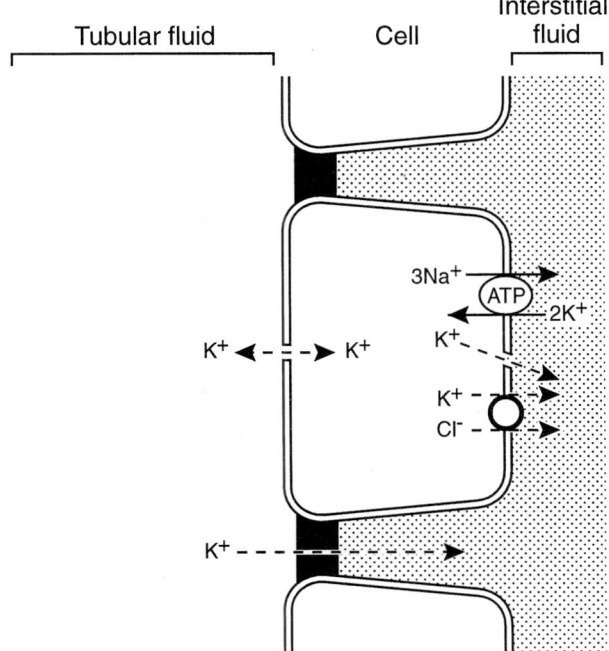

FIGURE 5-5. Renal tubular transport mechanisms for potassium in the proximal tubule. (Drawing by Tim Vojt.)

imal tubular cells occurs by means of potassium channels in both luminal and basolateral membranes and by a K^+-Cl^- cotransporter in basolateral membranes (Fig. 5-5).

In the thick ascending limb of Henle's loop, the transepithelial electrical potential difference is strongly lumen positive and most potassium reabsorption occurs by the paracellular route. Potassium channels in the luminal membranes allow potassium to exit the cell down its concentration gradient, and facilitate the electrochemical gradient for potassium reabsorption via the paracellular route. Transcellular reabsorption of potassium is facilitated by the luminal Na^+-K^+-$2Cl^-$ cotransporter and by potassium channels and a K^+-Cl^- cotransporter in the basolateral membranes (Fig. 5-6).

Principal cells are found in the connecting tubule and collecting duct and are responsible for potassium secretion. The basolateral membranes of principal cells are rich in Na^+,K^+-ATPase, which maintains a high intracellular potassium concentration. The luminal membranes of the principal cells contain an electrogenic sodium channel and sodium movement through this channel renders the tubular lumen negative (Fig. 5-7).

There are two types of intercalated cells in the distal nephron. Type A or α intercalated cells contain both H^+-ATPase and H^+,K^+-ATPase in their luminal membranes and Cl^--HCO_3^- countertransporters as well as Cl^- and K^+ channels in their basolateral membranes. They also contain carbonic anhydrase. This arrangement allows the α intercalated cell to secrete H^+ ions and reabsorb K^+ and HCO_3^- ions. Potassium is actively transported across the luminal membranes of type α intercalated cells by H^+,K^+-ATPase and then diffuses down its concentration gradient through potassium channels in the basolateral membranes (Fig. 5-8). Type α intercalated cells are found in the connecting tubule, cortical collecting duct, and outer medullary collecting duct. Type B or β intercalated cells are found only in the cortical collecting ducts and secrete HCO_3^- ions. They are able to do so because their polarity is reversed as compared with type α intercalated cells (i.e., the H^+-ATPase is in the basolateral membrane and the Cl^--HCO_3^- countertransporter is in the luminal membrane).

Potassium is reabsorbed from the last portion of the outer medullary collecting duct and throughout the inner medullary collecting duct. In these segments of the nephron, potassium is reabsorbed by the paracellular route despite a lumen-negative transepithelial potential difference because reabsorption of water increases the chemical concentration gradient sufficiently to overcome the unfavorable electrical gradient.

Determinants of Urinary Potassium Excretion

Three main factors affect potassium secretion in the distal nephron: the magnitude of the chemical concentration gradient for potassium between the tubular cells and tubular lumen, the tubular flow rate, and the transmembrane potential difference across the luminal membranes of the tubular cells. Gastrointestinal absorption of a potassium load increases the ECF concentration of potassium. This results in an increase in the number of K^+ ions available for uptake at the basolateral membranes of the distal tubular cells by Na^+, K^+-ATPase, and the resulting

Thick Ascending Limb of Henle

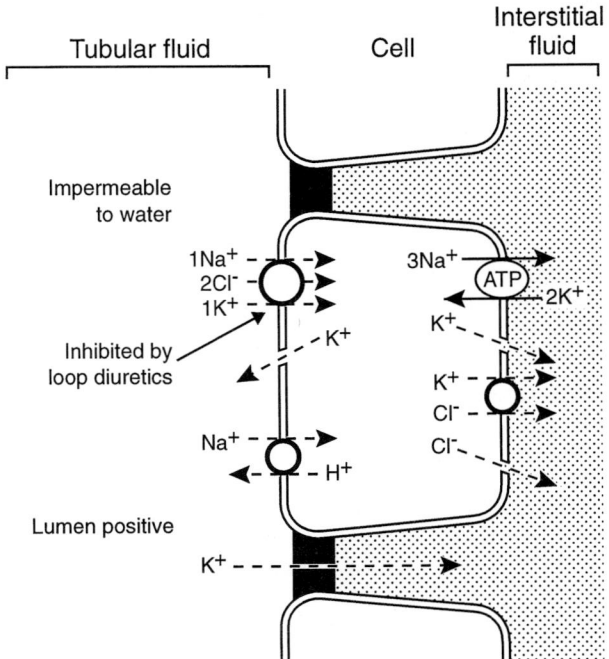

FIGURE 5-6. Renal tubular transport mechanisms for potassium in the thick ascending limb of Henle's loop. (Drawing by Tim Vojt.)

Late Distal Tubule and Collecting Duct

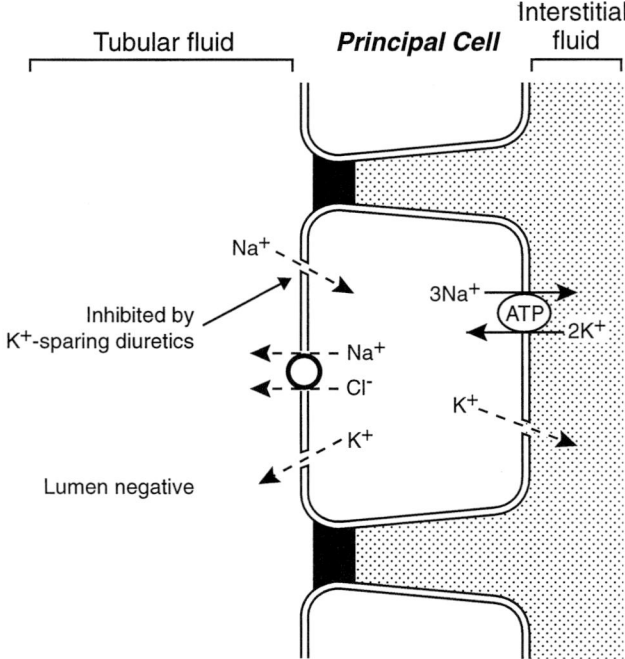

FIGURE 5–7. Renal tubular transport mechanisms for potassium in the principal cells of the late distal tubule and collecting duct. (Drawing by Tim Vojt.)

increase in intracellular potassium concentration increases the chemical concentration gradient for diffusion of K^+ ions out of the tubular cells across their luminal membranes.

Aldosterone is the most important hormone affecting urinary potassium excretion. Its secretion by the zona glomerulosa of the adrenal gland is stimulated directly by hyperkalemia and angiotensin II (produced in response to volume depletion), whereas adrenocorticotropic hormone (ACTH), hyponatremia, and decreased extracellular pH play permissive roles in promoting aldosterone secretion. Aldosterone release is inhibited by dopamine and atrial natriuretic factor, both of which are released in response to volume expansion.

Aldosterone increases reabsorption of Na^+ and secretion of K^+ and H^+ ions in the distal nephron. Its primary effect is to increase the number of open Na^+ channels in the luminal membranes of the principal cells. Sodium reabsorption via these luminal Na^+ channels is electrogenic (i.e., it generates electronegativity in the tubular lumen). This electronegativity can be dissipated either by K^+ or H^+ ion secretion or by Cl^- reabsorption in the distal nephron. Aldosterone increases the activity and number of Na^+, K^+-ATPase pumps in the basolateral membranes of the principal cells, and this effect may occur as a result of increased entry of Na^+ ions across the luminal membranes. Increased Na^+, K^+-ATPase activity in turn increases the intracellular K^+ concentration and facilitates K^+ secretion across the luminal membranes. Aldosterone also increases the number of open K^+ channels in the luminal membrane, thus facilitating K^+ exit into tubular fluid.

Aldosterone can influence H^+ secretion in two ways. It directly promotes H^+ ion secretion in H^+-secreting type α intercalated cells by stimulation of the H^+-ATPase present in their luminal membranes. Aldosterone also promotes H^+ secretion in the distal tubule by stimulating electrogenic Na^+ reabsorption in principal cells and increasing lumen electronegativity, which favors enhanced H^+ secretion.

An increase in distal tubular flow enhances potassium secretion by rapidly moving secreted K^+ ions downstream and providing new tubular fluid from upstream in the nephron. This allows maintenance of a high chemical concentration gradient for potassium secretion and provides a "sink" for movement of K^+ ions into tubular fluid. A decrease in distal tubular flow has the opposite effect and promotes dissipation of the chemical gradient for diffusion of K^+ ions from principal cells into tubular fluid.

Lumen electronegativity is generated by sodium reabsorption through Na^+ channels in the luminal membranes of principal cells. Normally, some of this electronegativity is dissipated by passive Cl^- reabsorption. If a large concentration of a relatively nonresorbable anion (e.g., SO_4^{2-}, HCO_3^-, penicillin) is present in distal tubular fluid, less dissipation of the electronegativity occurs and K^+ secretion is enhanced. This factor contributes to the pathophysiology of metabolic alkalosis. In this setting, there is less Cl^- and more HCO_3^- in the distal tubular fluid, and HCO_3^- is relatively nonresorbable in the cortical collecting duct. This is one reason metabolic alkalosis promotes urinary K^+ excretion. Amiloride is a diuretic that impairs luminal Na^+ entry into principal cells by

Late Distal Tubule and Collecting Duct

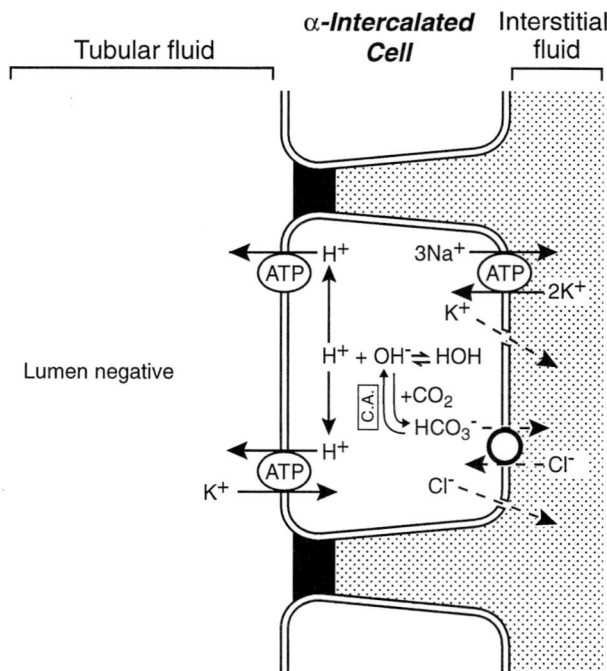

FIGURE 5–8. Renal tubular transport mechanisms for potassium in the α-intercalated cells of the late distal tubule and collecting duct. (Drawing by Tim Vojt.)

decreasing the number of open Na⁺ channels. This in turn reduces lumen electronegativity and impairs K⁺ secretion. Thus, the magnitude of distal tubular lumen electronegativity has an important effect on urinary K⁺ excretion.

The Na⁺ and Cl⁻ concentrations of distal tubular fluid usually have little effect on K⁺ secretion. When the luminal Na⁺ concentration is very low (<25–35 mEq/L), however, diffusion of Na⁺ ions into distal tubular cells may be impaired sufficiently to produce an increase in the tubular cell transmembrane potential (making the cell interior more negative) and impeding diffusion of K⁺ ions from the cell into the tubular lumen (Good et al. 1984; West et al. 1986a, 1986b). Extremely low luminal Cl⁻ concentrations (<10 mEq/L) may increase net potassium secretion, possibly because some fraction of K⁺ reabsorption or secretion may be accomplished by K⁺-Cl⁻ cotransport (Velazquez et al. 1982). Such a mechanism may also play a role in the pathophysiology of enhanced urinary K⁺ excretion during metabolic alkalosis. Antidiuretic hormone (ADH) may stimulate potassium secretion in the distal nephron. Water diuresis (which suppresses ADH release) does not stimulate potassium excretion, despite increased distal tubular flow rate. This has led to speculation that ADH may play a role in preventing disruption of potassium balance during states of water deprivation or excess (Sealey and Laragh 1974; Field et al. 1984). The factors affecting renal excretion of potassium are summarized in Figure 5–9.

Factors Influencing Renal Potassium Excretion

SODIUM INTAKE

High sodium intake is associated with increased urinary potassium excretion as a result of increased potassium secretion in the connecting tubule and cortical collecting duct. Increased delivery of sodium to the distal nephron results in more sodium crossing the luminal membranes of the distal tubular cells down its concentration gradient. This increased entry of Na⁺ ions into the tubular cells leads to increased activity of Na⁺,K⁺-ATPase in the basolateral membranes with removal of sodium to the peritubular interstitium and increased cellular uptake of potassium. This increased intracellular potassium then crosses the luminal membranes of the tubular cells and enters the tubular fluid down a favorable electrochemical gradient. Increased sodium delivery to the distal nephron also increases the distal tubular fluid flow rate, which enhances the chemical concentration gradient for potassium between the tubular cell cytoplasm and tubular fluid.

Low sodium intake is associated with decreased renal potassium excretion as a result of mechanisms opposite to those already described. Also, increased potassium reabsorption by type α intercalated cells occurs in the medullary collecting duct. One reason for this increased reabsorption may be increased recycling of potassium into the medullary interstitium, which may play a role in the urinary concentrating mechanism when sodium intake is restricted.

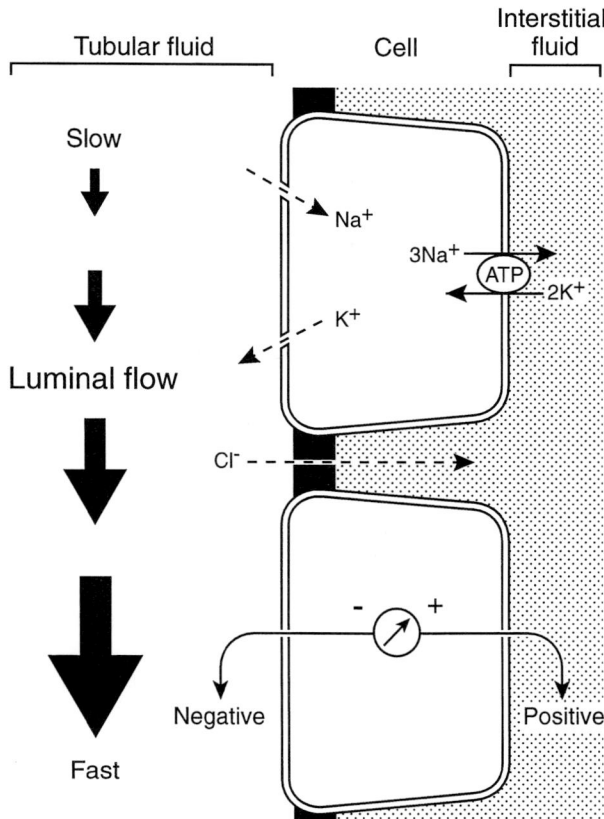

FIGURE 5–9. Factors affecting urinary excretion of potassium. (Drawing by Tim Vojt.)

POTASSIUM INTAKE

High potassium intake is associated with increased urinary potassium excretion as a result of increased tubular secretion of potassium in the connecting tubule, cortical collecting duct, and outer medullary collecting duct. This occurs because of increased numbers and activity of Na⁺,K⁺-ATPase and amplification of the basolateral membranes of principal cells, which may be due to an increased concentration of aldosterone. More potassium is therefore actively pumped into the tubular cells from the peritubular interstitium, leaves the cells down a favorable electrochemical gradient, and enters the tubular fluid.

Low potassium intake results in decreased urinary excretion of potassium. In the presence of low potassium intake there is decreased to absent tubular secretion by principal cells in the connecting tubule, cortical collecting duct, and outer medullary collecting duct and increased reabsorption by type α intercalated cells in the inner medullary collecting duct. The decrease in tubular secretion results from less potassium being available for peritubular uptake into the tubular cells by the Na⁺,K⁺-ATPase pump and a less favorable concentration gradient for potassium to leave the tubular cells and enter tubular fluid.

MINERALOCORTICOIDS

An increased concentration of aldosterone results in increased urinary excretion of potassium as a result of increased secretion of potassium by tubular cells mainly in the cortical collecting duct. The actions of aldosterone on the principal cells (see earlier) result in increased uptake of potassium from the peritubular interstitium and increased movement of potassium into tubular fluid across the luminal membranes of the principal cells. A decreased transmembrane potential difference across the luminal membrane (as Na^+ ions enter from tubular fluid) allows potassium to exit more easily into the tubular fluid (i.e., the interior of the cell is now less negative in comparison with the tubular fluid). A decreased concentration of aldosterone results in decreased urinary excretion of potassium.

HYDROGEN ION BALANCE

Acute mineral metabolic acidosis decreases urinary excretion of potassium. Chronic metabolic acidosis may actually increase urinary excretion of potassium. If distal tubular flow remains constant, acute (<8 h) mineral metabolic acidosis results in decreased urinary excretion of potassium because, during metabolic acidosis caused by administration of a mineral acid, H^+ ions enter cells to be buffered by intracellular proteins in exchange for K^+ ions that leave cells and enter the ECF (Swan and Pitts 1955; Schwartz et al. 1957). When this ion exchange occurs across the basolateral membranes of the cells of the connecting tubule and cortical collecting ducts, the resulting decreased intracellular concentration of potassium is associated with less tubular secretion of potassium because of a less favorable chemical concentration gradient.

A critical factor determining whether acute metabolic acidosis causes this exchange of H^+ and K^+ ions across the cell membranes is the permeability of the anion associated with the acid. Chloride ions are relatively impermeable and cannot follow the H^+ ions into the cell, whereas lactate and ketoacid anions are more permeable and can follow H^+ ions into the cell so that K^+ ions do not need to be exchanged with H^+ ions for electroneutrality. As a result, acute mineral metabolic acidosis may be associated with H^+-K^+ exchange across cell membranes but acute organic metabolic acidosis is not. Chronic (>3 days) metabolic acidosis caused by administration of a mineral acid leads to mild hypokalemia, possibly caused by stimulation of aldosterone secretion by the acidosis (Gennari and Cohen 1975; Scandling and Ornt 1987; Magner et al. 1988). Even in acute acidosis, a decreased filtered load of bicarbonate can reduce sodium reabsorption in the proximal tubules and increase delivery of sodium and water to the distal nephron. This increases the distal tubular flow rate and enhances urinary potassium excretion.

During alkalosis, H^+ ions leave cells to titrate bicarbonate in the ECF in exchange for K^+ ions that enter the cells. The increased concentration of potassium in the distal tubular cells results in increased secretion of potassium because of a more favorable chemical concentration gradient. Alkalosis also appears to directly stimulate the basolateral Na^+, K^+-ATPase in the principal cells of the cortical collecting duct.

DIURETICS

Many clinically important diuretics (furosemide, ethacrynic acid, thiazides, mannitol) cause increased urinary excretion of potassium and may result in depletion of body potassium stores. These diuretics increase the distal tubular delivery of sodium and the distal tubular fluid flow rate and, as a result of these effects, cause increased urinary potassium excretion for the same reason as described earlier in the discussion of the effects of high sodium intake on potassium excretion.

▶ Normal Serum Concentrations

Ion-selective potentiometry and flame photometry are methods used by clinical laboratories to measure sodium and potassium concentrations in body fluids. Electrolytes in plasma are excluded from the fraction of plasma (normally about 7%) that is occupied by solids (e.g., lipids, proteins) and are confined to the aqueous phase of plasma (about 93% of total plasma volume). Both flame photometry and indirect potentiometry are affected by the exclusion of electrolytes from the fraction of plasma that is occupied by solids, whereas direct potentiometry is not (Tietz 1986). The resulting error is usually small, but for serum sodium concentration it may be clinically relevant in patients with hyperlipemia (see Chapter 3). Potassium is present in ECF at a much lower concentration than sodium, and the effect of hyperlipemia on the measured serum potassium concentration is much less apparent.

Normal values for serum potassium concentration in dogs and cats vary slightly among laboratories but are expected to be 3.5 to 5.5 mEq/L with an average value of approximately 4.5 mEq/L. Serum potassium concentrations exceed plasma concentrations because potassium is released from platelets during the clotting process. There is a positive correlation between platelet count and serum potassium concentration in dogs (Degen 1986; Reimann et al. 1989). The difference between serum and plasma potassium concentrations is most pronounced in animals with thrombocytosis (Mandell et al. 1988; Degen et al. 1989; Reimann et al. 1989). In one study, serum potassium concentration was greater than plasma potassium concentration by a mean of 0.63 mEq/L in dogs with normal platelet counts and by a mean of 1.55 mEq/L in dogs with thrombocytosis (Reimann et al. 1989).

The potassium content of erythrocytes varies in mammalian species, and hemolysis can result in hyperkalemia in species that have high red cell potassium concentrations (Table 5–1). Normal adult canine and feline red cells usually contain potassium in concentrations similar to those of plasma (Coulter and Small 1972; Ellory and Tucker 1983; Degen 1987; Price et al. 1988; Harvey 1989) and hemolysis is not associated with hyperkalemia. In one study, storage of canine red cells in citrate-phosphate-dextrose-adenine for 40 days resulted in an increase in plasma potassium concentration from 5 to almost 9 mEq/L despite the fact that the original intracellular potassium concentration in the red cells was only 3.8 mEq/L (Price et al. 1988). Regardless of the underlying mechanism, this magnitude of increase in plasma potassium concentration would be unlikely to result in detectable hyperkalemia in

TABLE 5-1. **Sodium and Potassium Concentrations of Mammalian Erythrocytes**

Species	Sodium (mEq/L)	Potassium (mEq/L)
Human	10–21	104–155
Dog LK*	93–150	4–11
Dog HK* (Maede 1983)	54	124
Cat	104–142	6–8
Horse	4–16	80–140
Cow LK*	72–102	7–37
Cow HK*	15	70
Sheep LK*	74–121	8–39
Sheep HK*	10–43	60–88
Swine	11–19	100–124

*Sheep, cattle, and dogs demonstrate polymorphism with respect to their intracellular cation concentrations, depending on the level of Na$^+$,K$^+$-ATPase activity in the mature red cell membranes. HK, high potassium; LK, low potassium.

a recipient dog transfused with blood stored in this manner.

The potassium concentrations of red cells from neonatal dogs are higher than those of red cells from adult dogs (Coulter and Small 1972; Miles and Lee 1972; Parker 1973). Red cell concentrations of potassium decrease during the first weeks of life and reach normal adult concentrations by approximately 8 to 13 weeks of age. In one study, mean red cell potassium concentrations in puppies were 19.0 mEq/L at 1 day of age, 15.1 mEq/L at 5 weeks of age, and 8.7 mEq/L at 13 weeks of age (Coulter and Small 1972). Reticulocytes from adult dogs also contain higher potassium concentrations than do mature red cells (Maede and Inaba 1985). In adult Akitas, red cell potassium concentrations may exceed 70 mEq/L and hemolysis results in a progressive increase in plasma potassium concentration (up to 24 mEq/L) during storage of blood (Rich et al. 1986; Degen 1987).

Dogs may be divided genetically into two groups on the basis of the presence or absence of Na$^+$,K$^+$-ATPase activity in the membranes of their mature red cells (Maede et al. 1983; Inaba and Maede 1984). Dogs with red cell membrane Na$^+$,K$^+$-ATPase activity maintain high intracellular potassium contentrations, whereas those without red cell Na$^+$,K$^+$-ATPase activity maintain red cell potassium concentrations similar to those of plasma. Reticulocytes from low-potassium (LK) dogs possess Na$^+$,K$^+$-ATPase, but it is rapidly and completely degraded by a proteolytic process during cell maturation (Maede and Inaba 1985; Inaba and Maede 1986). Reticulocytes from high-potassium (HK) dogs have twice as much Na$^+$,K$^+$-ATPase activity as reticulocytes from low-potassium dogs, but in the high-potassium dogs degradation of the enzyme ceases early in maturation and sufficient activity remains in the mature red cell to account for the observed high intracellular concentration of potassium (Maede and Inaba 1985).

Red cells of English springer spaniel dogs with phosphofructokinase deficiency had potassium concentrations of 19.2 to 28 mEq/L as compared with 5.1 to 7.7 mEq/L in control dogs, and hemolytic crises in affected dogs were associated with hyperkalemia (Giger and Harvey 1987). The higher potassium concentration in the red cells of affected dogs was attributed in part to the large number of circulating reticulocytes (7–26%).

Hemolysis in Akitas (and presumably in other HK dogs) and thrombocytosis cause what has been called *pseudohyperkalemia* because these effects occur in vitro. Pseudohyperkalemia has also been reported in a dog with acute lymphoblastic leukemia before chemotherapy (Henry et al. 1996). Leakage of potassium from the leukemic cells in vitro was thought to be responsible for pseudohyperkalemia in this case. Use of plasma from small blood samples collected in an excessive volume of tripotassium ethylenediaminetetraacetic acid may also result in measured hyperkalemia.

▶ Hypokalemia
Clinical and Laboratory Features

Many dogs and cats with hypokalemia have no clinical signs. Muscular weakness, polyuria, polydipsia, and impaired urinary concentrating capacity are the clinical signs most likely to be recognized in dogs and cats with symptomatic hypokalemia. The pathophysiology of these clinical signs is discussed here.

The clinician should verify the abnormal serum potassium concentration with the laboratory, but measurement of potassium by flame photometry and ion-selective potentiometry is reliable and errors are uncommon. The clinical history often provides information about the likely source of potassium loss (e.g., chronic vomiting, diuretic administration) or the possibility of translocation (e.g., insulin administration, alkalosis).

Determination of the fractional excretion of potassium (FE_K) may help differentiate renal and nonrenal sources of potassium loss. Fractional potassium excretion can be calculated and expressed as a percentage using

$$\frac{(U_K/S_K)}{(U_{Cr}/S_{Cr})} \times 100$$

where U_K is the urine concentration of K (mEq/L), S_K is the serum concentration of K (mEq/L), U_{Cr} is the urine concentration of creatinine (mg/dL), and S_{Cr} is the serum concentration of creatinine (mg/dL).

It has been stated that FE_K should be less than 4% for nonrenal sources of loss and that, in the presence of hypokalemia, values above 4% may indicate inappropriate renal loss (Dow 1989). In one study, however, FE_K values for normal cats were 10.6 ± 2.1% (Adams et al. 1991). In another study of normal cats receiving a potassium-deficient diet, FE_K values decreased from 10 to 12% to 3 to 6% (Dow et al. 1990). Thus, FE_K values up to 6% should probably be considered normal in potassium-depleted animals with normal renal function. The clinical utility of FE_K calculations, however, is limited by the fact that FE_K does not correlate well with 24-h urinary excretion of potassium (Adams et al. 1991; Finco et al. 1997) The occurrence of hypokalemia in patients with metabolic alkalosis suggests vomiting of stomach contents or diuretic administration as likely causes of potassium loss. In patients with hypokalemia and metabolic acidosis, diarrhea caused by small intestinal disease, chronic renal failure, and distal renal tubular acidosis are more likely causes of potassium loss (Fig. 5–10).

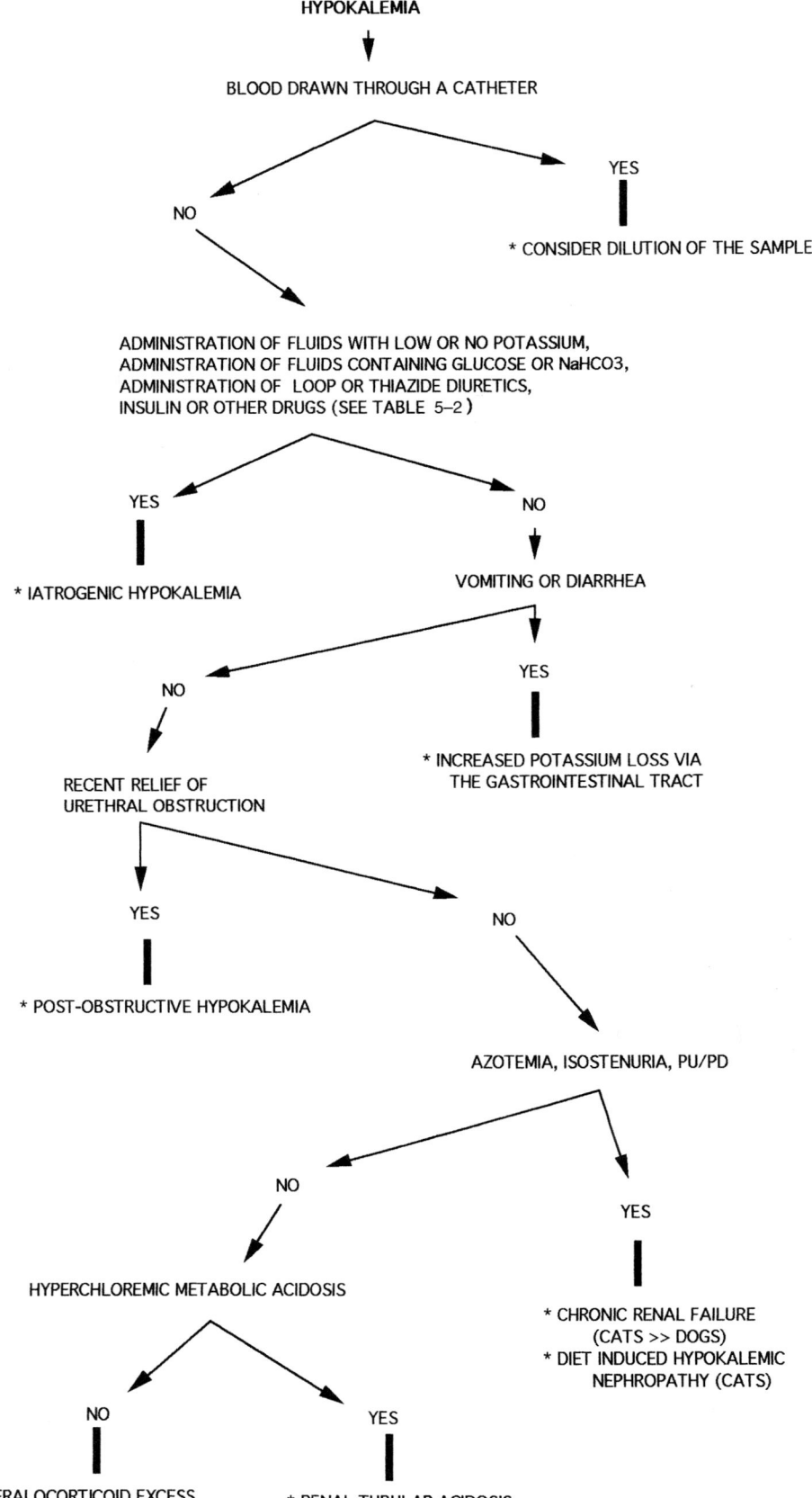

FIGURE 5-10. Algorithm for the clinical approach to hypokalemia.

The effect of aldosterone on serum potassium excretion can also be evaluated by comparing urine and serum potassium concentrations after correcting the urine potassium concentration for reabsorption of solute-free water by the kidneys. This index has been called the transtubular potassium gradient (TTKG) (West et al. 1986a, 1986b; Magner et al. 1988). A value of 5.0 or higher has been said to indicate the presence of an aldosterone effect, whereas a value of 3.0 or less is expected in the absence of mineralocorticoid activity (West et al. 1986b). Use of the TTKG is valid only when the urine osmolality is greater than 300 mOsm/kg and the urine sodium concentration is greater than 25 mEq/L. The renal TTKG may be estimated according to the equation

$$TTKG = [U_K/(U_{Osm}/S_{Osm})]/S_K$$

where U_K is the urine potassium concentration (mEq/L), S_K is the serum potassium concentration (mEq/L), U_{Osm} is the urine osmolality (mOsm/kg), and S_{Osm} is the serum osmolality (mOsm/kg) (West et al. 1986a, 1986b). Values for TTKG were estimated as 3.7 ± 0.9 in normal cats (DiBartola et al. 1993) and 4.2 ± 1.3 in normal dogs (DiBartola et al. 1980). The usefulness of the TTKG in assessment of dogs and cats with disorders of potassium balance remains to be determined. The causes of hypokalemia are listed in Table 5–2 and the diagnostic approach to hypokalemia is presented in Figure 5–10.

EFFECTS OF POTASSIUM DEPLETION ON ACID-BASE BALANCE

Hypokalemia is often said to be associated with metabolic alkalosis, but early studies employed diuretics or mineralocorticoids to induce potassium depletion. These methods probably caused disproportionate urinary loss of chloride relative to the chloride concentration of ECF, and chloride depletion was presumably the major factor responsible for development of metabolic alkalosis (see Chapter 10).

Pure potassium depletion apparently does cause metabolic alkalosis in rats, but in dogs it leads to metabolic acidosis (Bilbrey et al. 1973; Burnell et al. 1974; Garella et al. 1979). When potassium depletion was produced over a period of 2 to 4 weeks in dogs and care was taken to avoid chloride depletion, metabolic acidosis developed (Burnell et al. 1974; Garella et al. 1979). When potassium was restored to the diet, metabolic acidosis resolved within 5 days. The observed reduction in net acid excretion and metabolic acidosis that accompany dietary potassium depletion in the dog appear to be due to a distal renal tubular acidification defect, which is promptly reversed by potassium repletion (Garella et al. 1979). This acidification defect is at least partially related to decreased aldosterone secretion (Hulter et al. 1980).

Chronic potassium depletion also appears to lead to metabolic acidosis in cats. Adult cats were fed a potassium-restricted (0.2% potassium), 32% protein diet with or without 0.8% NH_4Cl (Dow et al. 1990). Serum potassium concentrations decreased from 4.3 to 4.5 mEq/L to 3.1 to 3.5 mEq/L in the NH_4Cl-treated cats and to 3.6 to 3.8 mEq/L in the cats not receiving NH_4Cl. Urinary FE_K was appropriately reduced to 3 to 6% in both groups of cats. Potassium balance was decreased in both groups but became negative only in the NH_4Cl-treated cats. Metabolic acidosis developed in both groups but was more severe in cats treated with NH_4Cl. Metabolic acidosis resolved in both groups during potassium repletion.

EFFECTS ON MUSCLE

Muscle weakness develops when serum potassium concentration falls below 3.0 mEq/L, increased creatine kinase concentrations may be observed below 2.5 mEq/L, and frank rhabdomyolysis may occur at concentrations less than 2.0 mEq/L (Knochel 1982). Rear limb weakness may be observed in dogs and cats with hypokalemia. In cats, weakness of the neck muscles with ventroflexion of the head is commonly observed (Schunk 1984; Dow et al. 1987b). Forelimb hypermetria and a broad-based hindlimb stance may also be observed in hypokalemic cats. Respiratory muscle paralysis required ventilatory support in two cats with potassium depletion (Dow et al. 1987b) and was thought to be the cause of death in an experimental study of potassium depletion in dogs (Patterson et al. 1983). Acute onset of hypokalemia and muscular weakness have also been reported in hyperthyroid cats (Nemzek et al. 1994). Three of the four cats in this study received fluid therapy with lactated Ringer's solution and were treated by surgical thyroidectomy, but one cat developed hypokalemia before treatment.

The effects of progressive potassium depletion on skeletal muscle were studied in dogs and rats (Bilbrey et al. 1973). In both species, a progressive increase in ICF sodium concentration and progressive decrease in ICF potassium concentration were observed during potassium deficiency. In rats, hyperpolarization of the cell mem-

TABLE 5–2. Causes of Hypokalemia

Decreased intake
   Alone unlikely to cause hypokalemia unless diet is aberrant
   Administration of potassium-free fluids (e.g., 0.9% NaCl, 5% dextrose in water)
Translocation (ECF → ICF)
   Alkalemia
   Insulin/glucose-containing fluids
   Catecholamines
   Hypothermia?
   Hypokalemic periodic paralysis (Burmese cats)
Increased loss
   Gastrointestinal (FE_K < 4–6%)
     Vomiting of stomach contents
     Diarrhea
   Urinary (FE_K > 4–6%)
     Chronic renal failure in cats
     Diet-induced hypokalemic nephropathy in cats
     Distal (type I) renal tubular acidosis (RTA)
     Proximal (type II) RTA after $NaHCO_3$ treatment
     Postobstructive diuresis
     Dialysis
     Mineralocorticoid excess
       Hyperadrenocorticism
       Primary hyperaldosteronism (adenoma, hyperplasia)
     Drugs
       Loop diuretics (e.g., furosemide, ethacrynic acid)
       Thiazide diuretics (e.g., chlorothiazide, hydrochlorothiazide)
       Amphotericin B
       Penicillins
       Albuterol overdosage

brane (as predicted by the Goldman-Hodgkin-Katz equation) was detected by direct measurement at all stages of potassium depletion. In dogs, there was an initial hyperpolarization of the cell membrane (mean measured E_m, -92.4 mV) during moderate potassium deficiency because $[K^+]_o$ fell proportionately more than $[K^+]_i$. There was a dramatic decrease in E_m (mean measured value, -54.8 mV) at the onset of muscle weakness and paralysis in dogs with severe potassium deficiency (serum potassium concentration 1.6 mEq/L). In rats with potassium deficiency, predicted and measured E_m values were similar during both moderate and severe potassium deficiency and paralysis was not observed. The inability to predict resting E_m in dogs with severe potassium depletion could be explained by an increase in the sodium permeability of the muscle cell membrane. This study also demonstrated the development of metabolic acidosis in dogs (pH 7.29, HCO_3^- 17.0 mEq/L) and metabolic alkalosis (pH 7.54, HCO_3^- 37.0 mEq/L) in rats with severe potassium deficiency (see earlier).

Potassium is released from muscle cells during exercise, causing vasodilatation and increased blood flow (Knochel 1982). This release of cellular potassium is impaired in states of potassium depletion, resulting in muscle ischemia. Muscle blood flow and potassium release increased markedly during exercise in normal but not in potassium-depleted dogs (serum potassium concentration 2.3 mEq/L), and exercise caused rhabdomyolysis characterized by focal necrosis and inflammatory cell infiltration in potassium-depleted dogs (Knochel and Schlein 1972). Increased creatine kinase concentrations and electromyographic abnormalities have been observed in cats with hypokalemic polymyopathy, but histopathologic lesions are usually mild or absent (Schunk 1984; Dow et al. 1987b). In dogs with experimentally induced potassium depletion, electromyographic changes were not observed, and increased serum creatine kinase concentration and muscle histopathology were observed only in dogs that had experienced extremely rapid potassium depletion induced by administration of desoxycorticosterone acetate in addition to a potassium-deficient diet (Patterson et al. 1983). Intestinal ileus has been described in human patients with potassium depletion but is usually not recognized clinically in dogs and cats.

EFFECTS ON THE CARDIOVASCULAR SYSTEM

Electrocardiographic changes and cardiac arrhythmias may develop because hypokalemia delays ventricular repolarization, increases the duration of the action potential, and increases automaticity. The electrocardiographic changes associated with hypokalemia in human patients (e.g., decreased amplitude T waves, ST segment depression, U waves) are not consistently observed in dogs and cats, but supraventricular and ventricular arrhythmias may occur. Prolongation of the QT interval and U waves have been reported in a dog with severe hypokalemia (2.0 mEq/L) caused by chronic vomiting (Grauer and Kunze 1979) and in dogs with experimentally induced potassium depletion (serum potassium concentration 2.2 mEq/L) (Bahler and Rakita 1971). In another study, development of hypokalemia in dogs over 5 days was associated with ST segment deviations, decreased amplitude T waves, and the appearance of U waves (Felkai 1985). The appearance of T waves in normal dogs is variable (e.g., positive, negative, biphasic) and interpretation of the effects of hypokalemia on ventricular repolarization is difficult unless a baseline electrocardiogram has been obtained previously. Hypokalemia potentiates the toxic effects of digitalis on cardiac conduction and may potentiate premature contractions. Hypokalemia also renders the myocardium refractory to the effects of class I antiarrhythmic agents (e.g., lidocaine, quinidine, procainamide). Therefore, serum potassium concentration should be measured and hypokalemia corrected in dogs with ventricular arrhythmias unresponsive to antiarrhythmic therapy.

EFFECTS ON THE KIDNEY

Potassium depletion produces functional and morphologic abnormalities in the kidneys, referred to as hypokalemic nephropathy. Renal vasoconstriction leads to decreases in renal blood flow and glomerular filtration rate (GFR). Polyuria and polydipsia are observed in potassium depletion and result from primary polydipsia caused by the effect of increased angiotensin II concentration on the thirst centers of the brain and by impaired responsiveness of the kidneys to ADH. Defective collecting duct responsiveness to ADH is related to decreased medullary tonicity, increased medullary blood flow, and impaired cyclic AMP generation in response to ADH.

In one study, potassium depletion in dogs for an average of 51 days led to a decrease in total exchangeable potassium from 47.1 to 35.3 mEq/kg and a decrease in serum potassium concentration from above 4.0 mEq/L to approximately 2.5 mEq/L (Abbrecht 1969). These dogs experienced decreases in GFR, renal blood flow, and urinary concentrating capacity (U_{osm} after 20 h of water deprivation) of approximately 25%. In another study, potassium depletion (serum potassium concentration 2.1 mEq/L) in dogs had little effect on GFR but caused a 45% reduction in maximal U_{osm} (1902 to 1055 mOsm/kg) (Bennett 1970). In a clinical report, a dog with chronic vomiting and hypokalemia (2.0 mEq/L) developed polyuria, polydipsia, and a urinary concentrating defect that persisted after correction of hypokalemia (Grauer and Kunze 1979). These abnormalities were attributed to medullary washout of solute and were corrected by partial water restriction and dietary supplementation with NaCl and KCl. In yet another study, dogs subjected to potassium depletion (serum potassium concentration 2.9 mEq/L) experienced a doubling of urine volume (596 to 1202 mL per 24 h) and a 40% reduction in maximal urine osmolality (2006 to 1187 mOsm/kg) (Rutecki et al. 1982).

Potassium depletion increases renal ammoniagenesis and urinary net acid excretion, whereas potassium loading tends to have the opposite effect (Tannen 1977). In the rat, increased ammoniagenesis during potassium depletion occurs primarily via enhanced phosphate-dependent glutaminase activity and increased mitochondrial ammoniagenesis in the proximal tubular cells of the renal cortex. The decrease in ammoniagenesis during potassium loading may occur in renal tubular cells from the outer medullary region. Many experimental studies on potassium depletion and renal regulation of acid-base balance have been performed in rats. The renal response of the dog to acute acidosis is known to differ somewhat from that of the rat (Tannen and Sastrasinh 1984) and care must be taken in extrapolating data about the renal response to potassium depletion in the rat to dogs.

Proximal renal tubular sodium reabsorption is increased during potassium depletion, possibly as a result of an increase in the activity of the proximal Na^+-H^+ antiporter. Distal sodium reabsorption, however, is decreased during potassium depletion. This presumably occurs as a result of decreased aldosterone secretion and is a direct effect of decreased ECF potassium concentration on the zona glomerulosa of the adrenal glands. Decreased distal sodium reabsorption decreases K^+ and H^+ ion secretion by decreasing luminal electronegativity. This reduces potassium loss in the urine but also tends to impair renal acid excretion. Thus, increased renal ammoniagenesis during potassium depletion may represent a mechanism for enhancing urinary excretion of fixed acid (as NH_4^+) at a time when distal H^+ ion secretion is impaired. Consequently, derangements in acid-base balance are minimized.

The cytoplasmic and mitochondrial enzyme activity profile of renal tubular cells during potassium depletion is strikingly similar to that observed during chronic metabolic acidosis (Tannen 1977). This similarity suggests the possibility of a common effector mechanism for stimulation of renal ammoniagenesis. Intracellular pH would be a logical candidate for such an effector. As K^+ ions leave cells to maintain ECF potassium concentration during potassium depletion, H^+ ions enter cells and presumably lower intracellular pH. Reduced intracellular pH may in turn be the signal for increased renal ammoniagenesis from glutamine. Some studies have demonstrated reduced intracellular pH in renal tubular cells during potassium depletion (Adam et al. 1986), whereas others have found no change (Schoolwerth and Culpepper 1990).

Increased ammonia concentrations may activate the third component of complement (C3) and contribute to development of chronic tubulointerstitial disease by recruitment of immune cells (Nath et al. 1985; Tolins et al. 1987). Vacuolization of proximal tubular cells is observed in human patients, whereas similar lesions are observed in the distal nephron, mainly in the medullary collecting ducts, in potassium-depleted rats. Vacuolization of proximal tubular epithelial cells has also been reported in potassium-depleted dogs (Abbrecht 1969).

Specific Causes of Hypokalemia in Dogs and Cats

Hypokalemia arises from decreased intake, translocation of potassium from ECF to ICF, and excessive loss of potassium by either the gastrointestinal or urinary route. Decreased intake of potassium alone is unlikely to cause hypokalemia, but it may be a contributing factor. In chronically ill animals, for example, prolonged anorexia, loss of muscle mass, and ongoing urinary potassium losses probably combine to cause hypokalemia. Often, a specific cause for mild hypokalemia in hospitalized dogs and cats cannot be identified. Such hypokalemia may resolve with successful treatment of the primary disease process. Also, iatrogenic hypokalemia may develop when potassium-deficient fluids are administered to anorexic patients in a hospital setting. For example, lactated Ringer's solution (potassium concentration, 4 mEq/L) is a replacement solution and does not provide sufficient potassium for maintenance needs in most animals. Solutions used for maintenance fluid therapy should contain 15 to 30 mEq/L potassium (see Chapter 13).

Translocation of potassium into cells may occur with alkalemia, insulin release, and catecholamine release. Alkalemia contributes to hypokalemia as K^+ ions enter cells in exchange for H^+ ions (see earlier). Insulin promotes uptake of glucose and potassium by hepatic and skeletal muscle cells and may contribute to hypokalemia when glucose-containing fluids are administered. The stress of illness and the associated epinephrine release may also contribute to hypokalemia. Severe hypokalemia (1.9 mEq/L) was reported in a dog that had ingested the β_2-adrenergic agonist albuterol (Vite and Gfeller 1994). The mechanism of hypokalemia was presumably rapid uptake of extracellular potassium by liver and muscle cells. Hypokalemia has been associated with hypothermia, possibly as a result of potassium entry into cells (Ross and Goldstein 1981). Mild hypokalemia was reported in 78% of dogs suffering from rattlesnake envenomation (Brown et al. 1994). Affected dogs also had transient echinocytosis that was not consistently associated with the observed hypokalemia.

A syndrome characterized by recurrent episodes of limb muscle weakness, neck ventroflexion, increased creatine kinase concentrations, and hypokalemia has been reported in related Burmese cats 4 to 12 months of age (Blaxter et al. 1986; Jones et al. 1988; Mason 1988a, 1988b; Lieveley and Gruffydd-Jones 1989). This syndrome may represent an animal model of hypokalemic periodic paralysis in humans, a familial disorder characterized by episodes of sudden translocation of potassium from ECF to ICF.

Gastrointestinal loss of potassium (e.g., vomiting of stomach contents) is an important cause of hypokalemia in small animals. Chloride depletion and sodium avidity related to volume depletion contribute to perpetuation of potassium depletion and metabolic alkalosis in this setting by enhancing urinary losses of K^+ and H^+ ions. The effects of metabolic alkalosis on potassium balance are discussed further in Chapter 10.

Urinary loss of potassium is another important cause of hypokalemia, and hypokalemia is common in cats with chronic renal failure. Approximately 20 to 30% of cats with chronic renal failure have hypokalemia at presentation (DiBartola et al. 1987; Lulich et al. 1992) and, in one study, chronic renal disease was the most common associated disorder observed in a survey of cats with hypokalemia (Dow et al. 1989). Most dogs with chronic renal failure have normal serum potassium concentrations. For example, less than 10% of dogs with chronic renal failure caused by renal amyloidosis had hypokalemia at presentation (DiBartola et al. 1989).

Renal tubular acidosis may be associated with hypokalemia (see Chapter 10). In distal (type I) renal tubular acidosis, hypokalemia is usually present before treatment, and urinary potassium losses may result in part from increased aldosterone secretion. Hypokalemia has been reported in distal renal tubular acidosis in cats (Drazner 1980; Watson et al. 1986). In proximal (type II) renal tubular acidosis, correction of acidosis requires large doses of NaHCO$_3$, and hypokalemia usually appears during therapy. This is a result of the increased delivery of Na$^+$ and HCO$_3^-$ ions to the distal nephron. These factors enhance urinary potassium excretion by increasing distal tubular flow and lumen electronegativity (HCO$_3^-$ is a relatively nonresorbable anion in the cortical collecting duct).

Finally, hypokalemic nephropathy characterized by chronic tubulointerstitial nephritis may develop in cats fed diets low in potassium and containing urinary acidifiers (Dow et al. 1987a; Dow 1989; Buffington et al. 1991; DiBartola et al. 1993). Stimulation of aldosterone secretion by chronic metabolic acidosis (Scandling and Ornt 1987) and decreased gastrointestinal absorption of potassium (Dow et al. 1990) may contribute to potassium depletion in this syndrome.

Hypokalemia commonly occurs during the postobstructive diuresis that follows relief of urethral obstruction in cats with idiopathic lower urinary tract disease. Bartter's syndrome is a rare cause of hypokalemia and metabolic alkalosis in human patients characterized by hyperreninemia, hyperaldosteronism, and hyperplasia of the juxtaglomerular apparatus with normal blood pressure. It has not yet been recognized in veterinary medicine.

Mineralocorticoid excess is an uncommon cause of urinary potassium loss and hypokalemia in dogs and cats. Primary hyperaldosteronism has been reported in a cat with an adrenocortical tumor (Eger et al. 1983), in a dog with hyperplasia of the adrenal zona glomerulosa (Breitschwerdt et al. 1985), and rarely in dogs with adrenocortical tumors (Willard et al. 1987; Feldman and Nelson 1996b). Dogs with adrenocortical tumors and hypokalemia (serum potassium concentration <3.0 mEq/L) had extremely increased plasma aldosterone concentrations and presumably had primary hyperaldosteronism (Feldman and Nelson 1996b). Hypokalemia may be observed in dogs with hyperadrenocorticism (Ling et al. 1979) because of the mineralocorticoid effects of endogenous steroids such as corticosterone and deoxycorticosterone and it is more common in dogs with adrenal-dependent disease than in those with pituitary-dependent disease (Meijer 1980). See Chapter 10 for further discussion of states of mineralocorticoid excess.

Administration of loop or thiazide diuretics may cause hypokalemia as a result of increased flow rate in the distal tubules and increased secretion of aldosterone secondary to volume depletion. In one study, dogs with heart failure receiving furosemide had significantly lower mean serum potassium concentrations (mean serum potassium concentration, 3.9 mEq/L) than did normal dogs (mean serum potassium concentration, 4.4 mEq/L) or untreated dogs with arrhythmias (mean serum potassium concentration, 4.3 mEq/L) (Cobb and Michell 1992). Of the dogs treated with furosemide, 17% had serum potassium concentrations less than 3.0 mEq/L. In another study, 10 dogs with congestive heart failure treated with captopril, furosemide, and a sodium-restricted diet did not develop significant changes in serum electrolyte concentrations (Roudebush et al. 1994). Penicillin derivatives may cause hypokalemia by acting as nonresorbable anions in the distal tubule and increasing secretion of potassium into tubular fluid. Amphotericin B may cause increased loss of potassium by binding to sterols in cell membranes and increasing permeability. Peritoneal dialysis can be complicated by hypokalemia if potassium-free dialysate is used over an extended period of time (Crisp et al. 1989).

Treatment

Preparations available for parenteral use include KCl (2 mEq K$^+$ per mL) and a potassium phosphate solution containing K$_2$HPO$_4$ and KH$_2$PO$_4$ (4.36 mEq K$^+$ per mL). Potassium chloride is the additive of choice for parenteral therapy because chloride repletion is essential if vomiting or diuretic administration is the underlying cause of hypokalemia. Replacement of chloride is also essential for resolution of the metabolic alkalosis often present in such settings (see Chapter 10). When administered intravenously, KCl should generally not be infused at rates greater than 0.5 mEq/kg/h to avoid potential adverse cardiac effects. A scale such as that shown in Table 5–3 may be used to estimate the amount of KCl to add to parenteral fluids based on serum potassium concentration (Greene 1975). Infusion rates above 0.5 mEq/kg/h are required to normalize serum potassium concentration in hypokalemic patients with diabetic ketoacidosis treated with insulin (see later). In hypokalemic human patients, potassium infusion rates up to 0.9 mEq/kg/h were used safely in one study (Hamill et al. 1991). Careful mixing of potassium choride after addition to flexible bags of fluids is extremely important to prevent the patient from receiving a high concentration of potassium that could be life threatening. In one study, inadequate mixing of potassium chloride added to flexible bags of fluid was demonstrated to result in up to a fourfold increase in the concentration of potassium in the fluids (Dhein and Wardrop 1995). For determination of serum potassium concentration, when submitting blood samples that have been drawn from intravenous catheters in patients receiving potassium-supplemented fluids, the initial volume of blood withdrawn should be discarded and a second sam-

TABLE 5–3. **Guidelines for Routine Intravenous Supplementation of Potassium in Dogs and Cats**

Serum Potassium Concentration (mEq/L)	mEq KCl to Add to 250 mL Fluid	mEq KCl to Add to 1 L Fluid	Maximal Fluid Infusion Rate* (mL/kg/h)
<2.0	20	80	6
2.1–2.5	15	60	8
2.6–3.0	10	40	12
3.1–3.5	7	28	18
3.6–5.0	5	20	25

Source: Greene RW and Scott RC: Lower urinary tract disease. In Ettinger SJ (ed): *Textbook of Veterinary Internal Medicine*. Philadelphia, WB Saunders Co., p. 1572, 1975.

*So as not to exceed 0.5 mEq/kg/h.

ple submitted to the laboratory to avoid results that may be spuriously high.

Infusion of potassium-containing fluids may initially be associated with a decrease in serum potassium concentration as a result of dilution, increased distal renal tubular flow, and cellular uptake of potassium, especially if the infused fluid also contains glucose (Dow 1989). This effect may be minimized by using a fluid that does not contain glucose, administering fluids at an appropriate rate, and beginning oral potassium supplementation as soon as possible. The concentration of potassium in the infused fluid generally should not exceed 60 mEq/L because higher concentrations of potassium may cause pain and sclerosis of peripheral veins (Rose 1994). Parenteral fluids containing up to 35 mEq/L have been used safely by the subcutaneous route (Finco 1977).

Careful potassium supplementation is important when using insulin to treat diabetic ketoacidosis. Chronic potassium depletion is usually present in affected patients as a result of loss of muscle mass, anorexia, vomiting, and polyuria. Serum potassium concentrations, however, are sometimes normal or even increased because of the effects of insulin deficiency and hyperosmolality on serum potassium concentration. As blood glucose concentration falls with insulin treatment, marked hypokalemia may develop if supplementation is not adequate.

Potassium gluconate (e.g., Kaon, Tumil-K) is recommended for oral supplementation. In one study, orally administered KCl and $KHCO_3$ were not palatable to cats (Dow et al. 1987b). Dogs may require 2 to 44 mEq potassium per day, depending on body size (Harrison et al. 1960). In cats with hypokalemic nephropathy, the initial oral dosage of potassium gluconate is 5 to 8 mEq/day divided b.i.d. or t.i.d., whereas the maintenance dosage can usually be reduced to 2 to 4 mEq/day (Dow 1989). It is difficult to estimate the amount of potassium required to reestablish normal balance from the serum potassium concentration in a given patient because potassium is an intracellular solute. Thus, the amount of potassium required for treatment must be determined by judicious supplementation and serial measurement of serum potassium concentration during treatment and recovery. Selected preparations available for oral potassium supplementation are listed in Table 5–4.

▶ Hyperkalemia

Hyperkalemia is uncommon if renal function is normal. Soon after ingestion of a potassium load, cellular uptake of potassium is mediated by insulin, epinephrine, and the resulting increase in ECF potassium concentration itself. Renal excretion of the potassium load then follows. Sustained, chronic hyperkalemia is almost always associated with some impairment in urinary excretion of potassium.

Clinical and Laboratory Features

The clinical manifestations of hyperkalemia reflect changes in cell membrane excitability and reflect the magnitude as well as the rapidity of onset of hyperkalemia. Muscle weakness develops with hyperkalemia, usually when serum potassium concentration exceeds 8.0 mEq/L. The electrocardiographic findings caused by hyperkalemia are often characteristic and the electrocardiogram may be helpful in establishing a suspicion of hyperkalemia while awaiting results for serum potassium concentration (Fig. 5–11).

The effects of hyperkalemia on the electrocardiogram have been studied in dogs and cats (Surawicz 1967a, 1967b; Cohen et al. 1971; Coulter et al. 1975). Increased amplitude and narrowing or "tenting" of the T waves may occur with mild increases in serum potassium concentration, but these changes are inconsistent in dogs and cats. Shortening of the QT interval may also be observed. These changes reflect abnormally rapid repolarization. Moderate hyperkalemia may result in prolongation of the PR interval and widening of the QRS complex because of slowing of conduction through the atrioventricular system. With progression of hyperkalemia, conduction through the atrial muscle is impaired and a decrease in the amplitude and widening of the P wave are observed. In severe hyperkalemia, atrial conduction ceases, the P waves disappear, and pronounced bradycardia with a sinoventricular rhythm may be observed. In extreme hyperkalemia, the QRS complex may merge with the T wave, creating a sine wave appearance, followed by ventricular fibrillation or ventricular asystole. During progressive hyperkalemia, atrial inexcitability, depressed conduction through the specialized tissues and ventricular muscle, and the potential for reentry lead to axis deviations, widening of the QRS complex, and ventricular asystole or ventricular fibrillation. Ventricular fibrillation in hyperkalemia is most likely due to both slow intraventricular conduction and decreased duration of the refractory period. These electrocardiographic changes have also been described in cats with hyperkalemia secondary to urethral obstruction (Parks 1975) and they represent the most life-threatening functional consequences of hyperkalemia. The causes of hyperkalemia are listed in Table 5–5 and the clinical approach to hyperkalemia is presented in Figure 5–12.

Specific Causes of Hyperkalemia in Dogs and Cats

Increased intake of potassium is unlikely to cause sustained hyperkalemia unless impaired renal excretion of potassium is present. Exceptions include iatrogenic hyperkalemia resulting from calculation errors during continuous infusion of potassium-containing fluids or administration of drugs known to predispose to hyperkalemia with concurrent potassium supplementation. Examples of the latter situation include concurrent use of nonspecific beta blockers (e.g., propranolol) or angiotensin-converting enzyme inhibitors (e.g., captopril, enalapril) with potassium supplementation (KCl used as a salt substitute contains 13.4 mEq potassium per gram) during treatment of heart failure (see Chapter 18).

Translocation of potassium from ICF to ECF can cause hyperkalemia. Acute metabolic acidosis caused by mineral acids (e.g., NH_4Cl, HCl) but not organic acids (e.g., lactic acid, ketoacids) causes potassium to shift out of cells in exchange for H^+ ions that enter cells to be buffered (see earlier). The effect of acute inorganic meta-

TABLE 5-4. **Selected Preparations Available for Oral Potassium Supplementation**

Chemical Name	Proprietary Name	Formulation	Unit	Total mg	mEq K
Potassium chloride*	Kay Ciel 10%†	Elixir	15 mL (1 T)	1500	20
	Kay Ciel†	Powder	1 packet	1500	20
	Kaon-Cl 20%‡	Elixir	15 mL (1 T)	3000	40
	Kaon-Cl‡	Sustained action tablets	1 tablet	750	10
	Kaon-Cl‡	Controlled release capsules	1 capsule	600	8
	Kaochlor 10%‡	Elixir	15 mL (1 T)	1500	20
	K-Tab SA§	Sustained action tablets	1 tablet	750	10
	Slow-K‖	Tablets	1 tablet	600	8
	Various	Tablets	1 tablet	99	1.33
		Tablets	1 tablet	600	8
		Tablets	1 tablet	750	10
		Tablets	1 tablet	1500	20
		Tablets	1 tablet	1875	40
	Micro-K Extencaps¶	Controlled release capsules	1 capsule	600	8
	Micro-K Extencaps¶	Controlled release capsules	1 capsule	750	10
Potassium gluconate	Kaon Elixir‡	Liquid	15 mL (1 T)	4680	20
	Kaon‡	Tablets	1 tablet	1170	5
	Tumil-K#	Protein-based powder	0.65 g (¼ t)	468	2
	Tumil-K#	Tablets	1 tablet	468	2
	Tumil-K#	Gel	2.34 g (½ t)	468	2
Potassium citrate	Urocit-K**	Controlled release tablets	1 tablet	540	5
	Urocit-K**	Controlled release tablets	1 tablet	1080	10
Potassium bicarbonate/potassium citrate	K-Lyte††	Effervescent tablet	1 tablet		25
	K-Lyte DS††	Double strength effervescent tablet	1 tablet		50
Potassium bicarbonate/potassium chloride	K-Lyte/Cl††	Effervescent tablet	1 tablet	1875	25
	K-Lyte/Cl††	Effervescent tablet	1 tablet	3750	50

Chemical Name	Chemical Structure	Molecular Weight	mEq K+/g
Potassium chloride	KCl	74.6	13.4
Potassium bicarbonate	KHCO$_3$	100.1	10.0
Potassium citrate	K$_3$C$_6$H$_5$O$_7$·H$_2$O	324.3	9.25
Potassium gluconate	KC$_6$H$_{11}$O$_7$	234.1	4.3

*KCl is made for injection by various manufacturers; most preparations contain 2 mEq K$^+$ per mL. A potassium phosphate preparation containing 4.36 mEq K$^+$ per mL is also available (see Chapter 7).
†Forest Pharmaceuticals, St Louis, MO 63045.
‡Savage Laboratories, Melville, NY 11747.
§Abbott Labs, Abbott Park, IL 60064.
‖Novartis, Summit, NJ 07901.
¶Wyeth-Ayerst Laboratories, Philadelphia, PA 19101.
#Daniels Pharmaceuticals, St Petersburg, FL 33713.
**Mission Pharmacal, San Antonio, TX 78296.
††Bristol-Myers Squibb, Princeton, NJ 08543.
Abbreviations: T, tablespoon; t, teaspoon.

bolic acidosis on serum potassium concentration in dogs is variable and was characterized by a 0.16 to 1.67 mEq/L increment in serum potassium concentration per 0.1 U decrement in pH in a review of previously published studies (Adrogué and Madias 1981).

Insulin deficiency and hyperosmolality contribute to hyperkalemia in diabetic patients. Hyperosmolality may increase serum potassium concentration as water moves from ICF to ECF and potassium follows because of solvent drag and as a result of the increased ICF potassium concentration resulting from cellular water loss. Most diabetic patients have total body depletion of potassium caused by urinary losses, muscle mass loss, anorexia, and vomiting. A normal or low serum potassium concentration in a patient with untreated diabetic ketoacidosis indicates serious total body depletion of potassium and the need for diligent potassium supplementation. Hypokalemia at presentation is more common than hyperkalemia in diabetic dogs and cats. In one study, 43% of dogs and 83% of cats with diabetes mellitus were hypokalemic at presentation as compared with 10% of affected dogs and 8% of affected cats that were hyperkalemic (Feldman and Nelson 1996a). Other studies of cats with diabetes mellitus have confirmed that hyperkalemia is

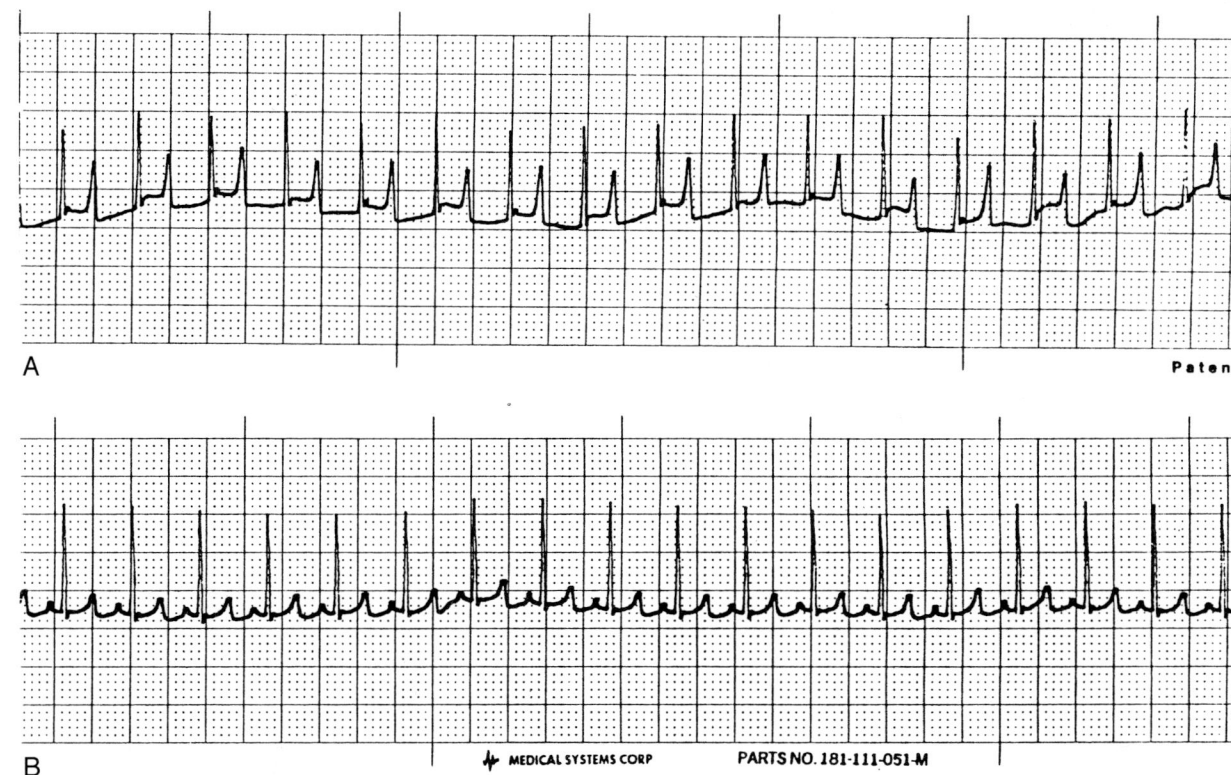
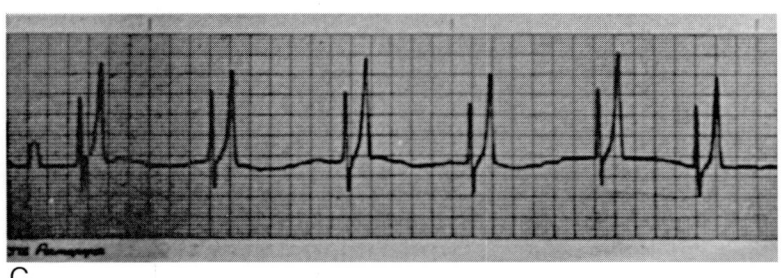
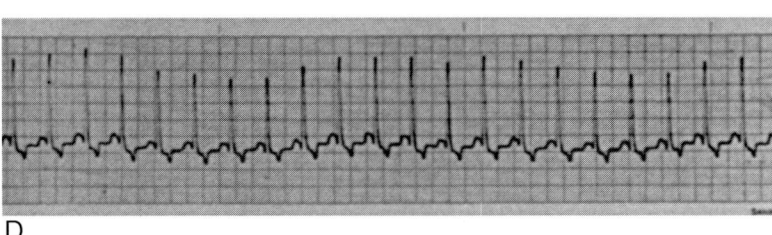

FIGURE 5-11. Electrocardiograms of a cat and dog with hyperkalemia. *(A)* Electrocardiogram from an 8-year-old female domestic shorthaired cat with oliguric acute renal failure and serum K+ concentration of 7.8 mEq/L. *(B)* Electrocardiogram of same cat after 2 mEq/kg NaHCO$_3$ administered intravenously over 30 min. *(C)* Electrocardiogram of a dog with serum K+ concentration of 9.6 mEq/L before treatment. Note tall tented T waves and absence of P waves. *(D)* Electrocardiogram of same dog 15 min after infusion of NaHCO$_3$. (Parts *C* and *D* from Chew DJ and DiBartola SP: *Manual of Small Animal Nephrology and Urology*. New York, Churchill Livingstone, p. 132, 1986.)

uncommon and that 44 to 70% of affected cats had hypokalemia at presentation (Schaer 1977; Moise and Reimers 1983; Crenshaw and Peterson 1996; Bruskiewicz et al. 1997). Hypokalemia may also develop after treatment with insulin despite potassium supplementation of fluids (Macintire 1993). Consequently, the clinician must pay close attention to potassium supplementation of patients with diabetic ketoacidosis.

Massive tissue breakdown may lead to transient hyperkalemia until released potassium is excreted by the kidneys. Severe exercise may cause release of potassium from cells and transient hyperkalemia in human beings, and this effect is less pronounced in conditioned subjects. In untrained dogs, exercise to the point of exhaustion resulted in an increase in mean serum potassium concentration from 4.4 to 6.0 mEq/L (Knochel et al. 1985). Exhaustive exercise was not associated with a significant increase in serum potassium concentration after the same dogs had been trained for 6 weeks. In racing greyhounds, no change in serum potassium concentration was observed immediately after racing, despite development of marked lactic acidosis (Ilkiw et al. 1989). Acute tumor lysis syndrome complicated by renal failure and hyperkalemia has been reported in dogs with lymphoma treated by radiation (Laing et al. 1989) and chemotherapy (Laing and Carter 1988). There is one case report of a young pit bull dog with episodic hindlimb and neck weakness. Exercise or potassium challenge resulted in mild hyperka-

TABLE 5–5. Causes of Hyperkalemia

Pseudohyperkalemia
Thrombocytosis
Hemolysis

Increased Intake
Unlikely to cause hyperkalemia in presence of normal renal function unless iatrogenic (e.g., continuous infusion of potassium-containing fluids at an excessively rapid rate)

Translocation (ICF → ECF)
Acute mineral acidosis (e.g., HCl, NH$_4$Cl)
Insulin deficiency (e.g., diabetic ketoacidosis)
Acute tumor lysis syndrome
Reperfusion of extremities after aortic thromboembolism in cats with cardiomyopathy
Hyperkalemic periodic paralysis (one case report in a pit bull)
Drugs
    Nonspecific beta blockers (e.g., propranolol)*

Decreased Urinary Excretion
Urethral obstruction
Ruptured bladder
Anuric or oliguric renal failure
Hypoadrenocorticism
Selected gastrointestinal disease (e.g., trichuriasis, salmonellosis, perforated duodenal ulcer)
Chylothorax with repeated pleural fluid drainage
Hyporeninemic hypoaldosteronism†
Drugs
    Angiotensin-converting enzyme inhibitors (e.g., captopril, enalapril)*
    Potassium-sparing diuretics (e.g., spironolactone, amiloride, triamterene)*
    Prostaglandin inhibitors (e.g., indomethacin)*
    Heparin*

*Likely to cause hyperkalemia only in conjunction with other contributing factors (e.g., decreased renal function, concurrent administration of potassium supplements).
†Not well documented in veterinary medicine.

---

lemia (Jezyk 1982). This may represent an example of hyperkalemic periodic paralysis.

Decreased urinary excretion is the most important cause of hyperkalemia in small animal practice. The most common associated disorders are urethral obstruction, ruptured bladder, anuric or oliguric renal failure, and hypoadrenocorticism. The time required for development of hyperkalemia in cats after urethral obstruction is variable, but it may occur within 48 h (Finco 1976; Finco and Cornelius 1977). After relief of obstruction, hyperkalemia resolves within 24 h whereas azotemia and hyperphosphatemia require 48 to 72 h to resolve (Finco and Cornelius 1977). After experimental bladder rupture in dogs, azotemia, hyperphosphatemia, and mild hyponatremia developed within 24 h whereas hyperkalemia did not develop until after 48 h (Burrows and Bovee 1974).

In chronic renal failure, normal potassium balance is maintained, so hyperkalemia is uncommon and develops only if oliguria occurs. This renal adaptation is accomplished by increased fractional excretion of potassium in remnant nephrons (Fig. 5–13) (Schultze et al. 1971; Bourgoignie et al. 1981, 1985). Fecal excretion of potassium also increases during chronic progressive renal disease and represents an extrarenal adaptation to maintain potassium balance (see Fig. 5–3). Patients with chronic renal disease, however, have reduced ability to tolerate an acute potassium load and may require 1 to 3 days to reestablish external potassium balance when intake of potassium is abruptly increased. Dogs with experimentally induced renal disease demonstrate a reduced ability to excrete a potassium load. In the first 5 h after a potassium load, dogs with experimentally induced renal disease excreted 30 to 37% of administered potassium whereas control dogs excreted 56 to 67%. (Bourgoignie et al. 1981, 1985). Kaliuresis was blunted in the dogs with remnant kidneys despite exaggerated hyperkalemia and increased secretion of aldosterone, and approximately 24 h was required for complete excretion of the potassium load.

Oliguria or anuria with hyperkalemia is more likely to occur in acute renal failure (e.g., ethylene glycol ingestion), but these findings may be observed terminally in chronic renal failure. Acute renal failure with oliguria or anuria is associated with hyperkalemia for several reasons. First, there has been insufficient time for renal adaptation to nephron loss, as occurs with chronic renal failure. Severe reductions in GFR and urine output result in inadequate distal tubular flow for effective urinary excretion of potassium. Finally, increased release of potassium from tissues during this catabolic state and acute metabolic acidosis may contribute to translocation of potassium from ICF to ECF.

Hyperkalemia, hyponatremia, and Na/K ratios less than 27:1 are usually (Willard et al. 1982; Schaer and Chen 1983; Rakich and Lorenz 1984; Peterson et al. 1989, 1996) but not always (Rogers et al. 1981; Lifton et al. 1996; Sadek and Schaer 1996) found in dogs and cats with hypoadrenocorticism. In dogs with hypoadrenocorticism, hyperkalemia has been reported in 74 to 96%, hyponatremia in 56 to 100%, and Na/K ratios less than 27:1 in 85 to 100% of cases. Hyperkalemia was found in 9 of 10 cats with hypoadrenocorticism, whereas hyponatremia and Na/K ratios less than 27:1 were found in all 10 affected cats (Peterson et al. 1989). Treatment is begun immediately after a presumptive diagnosis of hypoadrenocorticism is made, but conclusive diagnosis requires results of an ACTH stimulation test.

Electrolyte abnormalities similar to those found in dogs with hypoadrenocorticism (i.e., hyponatremia, hyperkalemia) can occur in dogs with gastrointestinal disease related to trichuriasis, salmonellosis, or perforated duodenal ulcer (DiBartola et al. 1985; Malik et al. 1990) and in dogs with chylothorax subjected to repeated pleural fluid drainage (Willard et al. 1991). Hyperkalemia and hyponatremia have also been reported in a dog with lung lobe torsion (Zenger 1992) and in a dog with neoplasia and pleural effusion (Lamb and Muir 1994). The hyperkalemia observed in these cases may be attributed to decreased renal excretion of potassium because of volume depletion and decreased distal renal tubular flow.

If sodium intake is sufficient to maintain normal ECF volume and distal tubular flow rate, an animal with hypoadrenocorticism may be able to maintain potassium balance. Also, treatment of dogs with hypoadrenocorticism with fluids alone often decreases serum potassium concentration into the normal range. Usually, however, these animals are presented with anorexia and vomiting that contribute to decreased ECF volume and urine output,

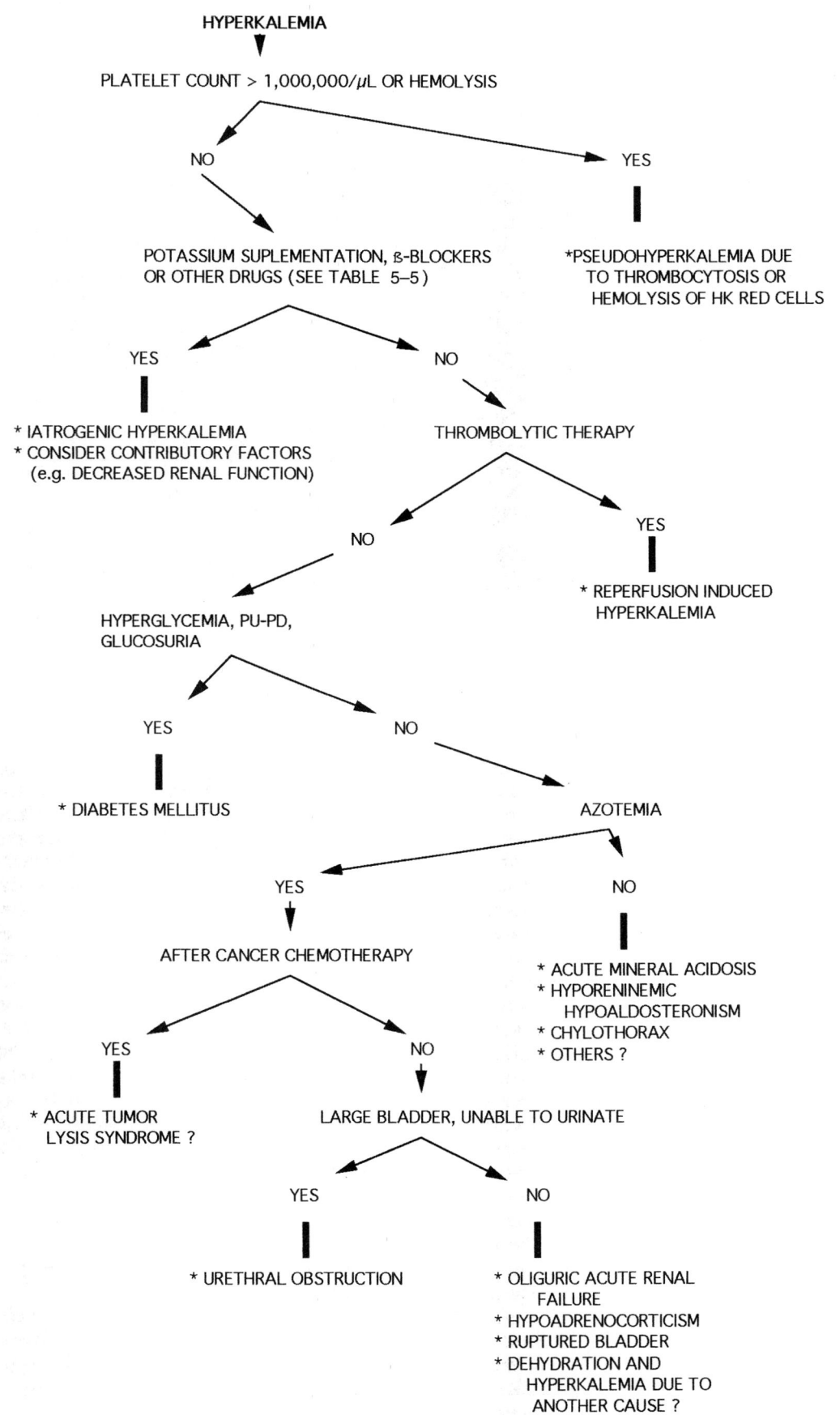

FIGURE 5-12. Algorithm for the clinical approach to hyperkalemia.

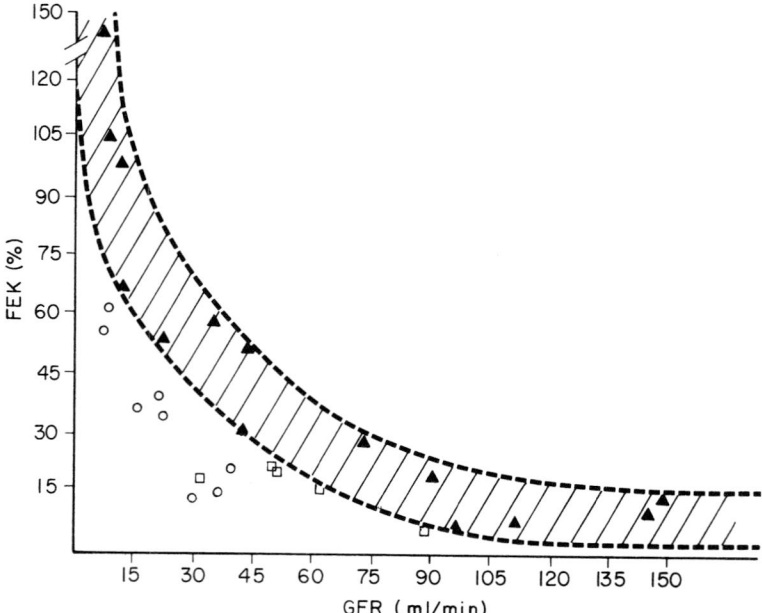

FIGURE 5-13. Nomogram relating fractional potassium excretion (FE_K) to glomerular filtration rate (GFR). Values for patients with an intact hormonal and renal tubular secretory mechanism for potassium (closed triangles) are used to delineate the hatched area. The open squares and circles indicate patients with selective aldosterone deficiency and renal tubular secretory defects, respectively. (From Batlle DC, Arruda JA, Kurtzman NA. Hyperkalemic distal renal tubular acidosis associated with obstructive uropathy. N Engl J Med 304:373–380, 1981. Reprinted by permission of The New England Journal of Medicine.)

and without adequate endogenous mineralocorticoids they are unable to excrete sufficient potassium to prevent frank hyperkalemia.

Hyporeninemic hypoaldosteronism is an important cause of unexplained asymptomatic hyperkalemia in human patients (DeFronzo 1980), but this disorder has rarely been recognized in veterinary medicine. Many affected human patients have mild to moderate renal insufficiency caused by diabetic glomerulosclerosis or interstitial renal disease. Most of them have low plasma renin and aldosterone concentrations. Even in patients with normal plasma aldosterone concentrations, the concentration of this hormone must be considered abnormal in light of the hyperkalemia. Resting plasma cortisol concentrations and response to ACTH are normal. Hyperchloremic metabolic acidosis and hypertension may be observed. It is unclear whether low aldosterone concentrations are a consequence of diminished renin secretion and lack of trophic effect of angiotensin II on the zona glomerulosa of the adrenal cortex or whether there is a primary adrenal defect in aldosterone secretion. To document this syndrome in veterinary patients would require demonstration of subnormal plasma renin and aldosterone concentrations or a subnormal increase in aldosterone after volume contraction or ACTH administration. Normally, aldosterone concentrations increase in response to ACTH in the dog (Willard et al. 1987). In this study, one dog with diabetes mellitus was suspected to have hyporeninemic hypoaldosteronism on the basis of a subnormal aldosterone response to ACTH.

Several drugs may contribute to hyperkalemia. Nonspecific beta blockers (e.g., propranolol) interfere with catecholamine-mediated uptake of potassium by liver and muscle and may cause hyperkalemia in the presence of a potassium load or decreased renal function. Similarly, angiotensin-converting enzyme inhibitors (e.g., captopril, enalapril) may cause hyperkalemia by interfering with angiotensin II–mediated aldosterone secretion if used in conjunction with potassium supplementation or in patients with decreased renal function (see Chapter 18). Prostaglandins stimulate renin release, and use of prostaglandin inhibitors (e.g., indomethacin) may contribute to development of hyperkalemia. Heparin therapy reduces aldosterone secretion and may contribute to hyperkalemia in the presence of other predisposing factors. Potassium-sparing diuretics (e.g., spironolactone, amiloride, triamterene) reduce urinary excretion of potassium and can cause hyperkalemia. Spironolactone competitively antagonizes the effect of aldosterone on the principal cells of the collecting duct and amiloride directly blocks luminal sodium channels in these cells. Triamterene may block sodium channels in the luminal membranes of principal cells in the collecting duct (Busch et al. 1996). In many hospitalized animals, the cause of mild hyperkalemia cannot be determined. In these instances, hyperkalemia often resolves with treatment of the primary disease.

Treatment

Appropriate treatment is dependent on the magnitude and rapidity of onset of the hyperkalemia as well as the underlying cause. Abnormalities of serum ionized calcium concentration and acid-base balance may aggravate the functional consequences of hyperkalemia as reflected by muscular weakness and electrocardiographic changes. Thus, if compatible electrocardiographic changes are observed, hyperkalemia should be treated regardless of its magnitude. An acute increase in serum potassium concentration to more than 6.5 mEq/L should be treated promptly. Asymptomatic animals with normal urine output and chronic hyperkalemia in the range of 5.5 to 6.5 mEq/L may not require immediate treatment, but a search for the underlying cause should be initiated.

Underlying diseases should be treated promptly (e.g., relief of urethral obstruction, establishment of urine output in patients with oliguria or anuria, 0.9% NaCl and mineralocorticoids in patients with hypoadrenocorticism). Fluid therapy with lactated Ringer's solution (potassium concentration, 4 mEq/L) ameliorates hyperkalemia by improving renal perfusion and enhancing urinary excretion of potassium. Use of a potassium-free solution (e.g., 0.9% NaCl, 0.45% NaCl), however, has a greater dilutional effect on the ECF potassium concentration.

Hyperkalemia may be treated by antagonizing the effects of potassium on cell membranes using calcium gluconate, by driving potassium from ECF to ICF with sodium bicarbonate or glucose (with or without concurrent insulin administration), or by removing potassium from the body with a cation exchange resin or dialysis. First, any source of intake must be discontinued (e.g., potassium-containing fluids, potassium penicillin). Also, the clinician should review the history to verify that the patient is not currently being treated with any drug known to contribute to hyperkalemia (e.g., prostaglandin inhibitors, beta blockers, angiotensin-converting enzyme inhibitors, potassium-sparing diuretics).

Hyperkalemia decreases the resting potential of cells. By administering calcium gluconate, the ECF concentration of calcium is increased and the threshold potential is decreased, thus normalizing the difference between the resting and threshold potential and restoring normal membrane excitability (see Fig. 5–2). Administered calcium begins to work within minutes, but its effect lasts less than an hour. The dosage of calcium gluconate is 2 to 10 mL of a 10% solution to be administered slowly with electrocardiographic monitoring.

Glucose works by increasing endogenous insulin release and moving potassium into cells. Its effects begin within an hour and last a few hours. Glucose-containing fluids (5 or 10% dextrose) or 50% dextrose (1–2 mL/kg) can be used for this purpose. The combination of insulin with glucose may result in greater reduction in serum potassium concentration (Allon et al. 1993) but there is a risk of hypoglycemia. Insulin (0.55–1.1 U/kg regular insulin added to parenteral fluids) and dextrose (2 g dextrose per unit of insulin added) have been recommended to treat hyperkalemia in cats with urethral obstruction (Schaer 1975).

Sodium bicarbonate also works by moving K^+ ions into cells as H^+ ions leave cells to titrate administered HCO_3^- in the ECF. Bicarbonate begins to work within an hour and its effects last a few hours. The usual dosage is 1 to 2 mEq/kg intravenously and it can be repeated if necessary. In normal cats, 4 mEq/kg sodium bicarbonate given intravenously caused hypokalemia, hypernatremia, hyperosmolality, and decreased ionized calcium concentrations (Chew et al. 1989, 1991). If a slow sinoventricular rhythm is present and due to hyperkalemia, atropine (0.02–0.04 mg/kg) may increase the firing rate of the sinus node. An experimental study in dogs demonstrated no beneficial effect of alkalinization in treating hyperkalemia in anesthetized dogs. In this study, the effects of sodium bicarbonate were similar to those of hypertonic saline (Kaplan et al. 1997). Sodium may have effects on cardiac muscle that account for reversal of hyperkalemic electrophysiologic changes (Ballantyne et al. 1975).

The cation exchange resin polystyrene sulfonate (Kayexalate) can be used to bind potassium and release sodium in the gastrointestinal tract. Each gram binds 1 mEq of potassium and releases 1 to 3 mEq of sodium. It can be mixed with sorbitol (to prevent constipation) and given orally or diluted in tap water and given per rectum as a retention enema using a large Foley catheter. Kayexalate must be used carefully in patients with impaired ability to excrete a sodium load (e.g., those with congestive heart failure or oliguric renal failure). This approach takes a few hours to work and lasts several hours.

Loop or thiazide diuretics increase the distal tubular flow rate and potassium secretion and may have adjunctive value in the treatment of hyperkalemia. If all of these measures fail, the clinician must consider peritoneal dialysis (see Chapter 25) (Crisp et al. 1989). Hemodialysis (see Chapter 26) is more efficient at removing potassium but is available only at selected referral institutions. The treatment of hyperkalemia is outlined in Table 5–6.

TABLE 5–6. Therapeutic Considerations in Management of Hyperkalemia*

Establish venous access and administer potassium-deficient (lactated Ringer's) or potassium-free (0.9% NaCl, 0.45% NaCl) fluids.
Discontinue potassium intake (e.g., potassium-supplemented fluids, potassium-containing salt substitutes, potassium penicillin).
If possible, discontinue drugs that promote hyperkalemia (e.g., beta blockers, angiotensin-converting enzyme inhibitors, potassium-sparing diuretics, prostaglandin inhibitors).
Administer 1–2 mEq/kg $NaHCO_3$ intravenously.†
  Or
Administer calcium gluconate 2–10 mL of a 10% solution slowly intravenously.
  Or
Administer 5–10% dextrose or 1–2 mL/kg 50% dextrose intravenously. Consider 0.55–1.1 U/kg regular insulin in parenteral fluids with 2 g dextrose per unit of insulin administered.
Consider administration of sodium polystyrene sulfonate (Kayexalate) orally (20 g with 100 mL 20% sorbitol) or by retention enema (50 g in 100–200 mL tap water).‡
Consider administration of loop (furosemide, 2–4 mg/kg) or thiazide (chlorothiazide, 10–40 mg/kg; hydrochlorothiazide, 2–4 mg/kg) diuretics.
If all other measures fail, institute peritoneal dialysis.

*The therapeutic measures to be used will vary with the clinical situation (see text for discussion).
†This is the treatment most commonly used at the Ohio State University Veterinary Teaching Hospital.
‡Oral administration of Kayexalate may cause nausea or vomiting. Sorbitol is added to the oral preparation to prevent constipation. Sorbitol should not be used when administering Kayexalate as a retention enema because of the possible risk of colonic necrosis (Lillemole et al. 1987).

REFERENCES

Abbrecht PH: Effects of potassium deficiency on renal function in the dog. *J Clin Invest* 48:432, 1969.

Adam WR, Koretsky AP, and Weiner MW: ^{32}P-NMR in vivo measurement of renal intracellular pH: Effects of acidosis and K^+ depletion in rats. *Am J Physiol* 251:F904, 1986.

Adams LG, Polzin DG, Osborne CA, et al.: Comparison of fractional excretion and 24-hour urinary excretion of sodium and potassium in clinically normal cats and cats with induced chronic renal failure. *Am J Vet Res* 52:718, 1991.

Adrogué HJ and Madias NE: Changes in plasma potassium concentration during acute acid base disturbances. *J Clin Invest* 71:456, 1981.

Adrogué HJ, Chap Z, Ishida T, et al.: Role of the endocrine pancreas in the kalemic response to acute metabolic acidosis in conscious dogs. *J Clin Invest* 75:798, 1985.

Alexander EA and Perrone RD: Regulation of extrarenal potassium metabolism. In Maxwell MH, Kleeman CR, and Narins RG (eds): *Clinical Disorders of Fluid and Electrolyte Metabolism.* New York, McGraw-Hill Book Co., pp. 105–117, 1987.

Allon M, Takeshian A, and Shanklin N: Effect of insulin-plus-glucose infusion with or without epinephrine on fasting hyperkalemia. *Kidney Int* 43:212, 1993.

Atkins EL and Schwartz WB: Factors governing correction of the alkalosis associated with potassium deficiency: The critical role of chloride in the recovery process. *J Clin Invest* 41:218, 1962.

Bahler RC and Rakita L: Cardiovascular function in potassium-depleted dogs. *Am Heart J* 81:650, 1971.

Ballantyne F, Davis LD, and Reynolds EW: Cellular basis for reversal of hyperkalemic electrocardiographic changes by sodium. *Am J Physiol* 229:935, 1975.

Bennett CM: Urine concentration and dilution in hypokalemic and hypercalcemic dogs. *J Clin Invest* 49:1447, 1970.

Bilbrey GL, Herbin L, and Carter NW: Skeletal muscle resting membrane potential in potassium deficiency. *J Clin Invest* 52:3011, 1973.

Blaxter AC, Livesley P, Gruffydd-Jones T, et al.: Periodic muscle weakness in Burmese kittens. *Vet Rec* 118:619, 1986.

Bourgoignie JJ, Kaplan M, Pincus J, et al.: Renal handling of potassium in dogs with chronic renal insufficiency. *Kidney Int* 20:482, 1981.

Bourgoignie JJ, Gavellas G, van Putten V, et al.: Potassium-aldosterone response in dogs with chronic renal insufficiency. *Miner Electrolyte Metab* 11:150, 1985.

Breitschwerdt EB, Meuten DJ, Greenfield CL, et al.: Idiopathic hyperaldosteronism in a dog. *J Am Vet Med Assoc* 187:841, 1985.

Brown DE, Meyer DJ, Wingfield WE, et al.: Echinocytosis associated with rattlesnake envenomation in dogs. *Vet Pathol* 31:654, 1994.

Bruskiewicz KA, Nelson RW, Feldman EC, et al.: Diabetic ketosis and ketoacidosis in cats: 42 cases (1980–1995). *J Am Vet Med Assoc* 211:188, 1997.

Buffington CA, DiBartola SP, Chew DJ, et al.: Effect of low potassium commercial nonpurified diet on renal function in adult cats. *J Nutr* 121:S91, 1991.

Burnell JM, Villamil MF, Uyeno BT, et al.: The effect in humans of extracellular pH change on the relationship between serum potassium concentration and intracellular potassium. *J Clin Invest* 35:935, 1956.

Burnell JM, Teubner EJ, and Simpson DP: Metabolic acidosis accompanying potassium deprivation. *Am J Physiol* 227:329, 1974.

Burrows CF and Bovee KC: Metabolic changes due to experimentally induced rupture of the canine urinary bladder. *Am J Vet Res* 35:1083, 1974.

Busch AE, Suessbrich H, Kunzelmann K, et al.: Blockade of epithelial Na^+ channels by triamterenes—Underlying mechanisms and molecular basis. *Eur J Physiol* 432:760, 1996.

Chew DJ, Leonard M, and Muir WW: Effect of sodium bicarbonate infusions on ionized calcium and total calcium concentrations in serum of clinically normal cats. *Am J Vet Res* 50:145, 1989.

Chew DJ, Leonard M, and Muir WW: Effect of sodium bicarbonate infusion on serum osmolality, electrolyte concentrations, and blood gas tensions in cats. *Am J Vet Res* 52:12, 1991.

Cobb M and Michell AR: Plasma electrolyte concentrations in dogs receiving diuretic therapy for cardiac failure. *J Small Anim Pract* 33:526, 1992.

Cohen HC, Gozo EG, and Pick A: The nature and type of arrhythmias in acute experimental hyperkalemia in the intact dog. *Am Heart J* 82:777, 1971.

Coulter DB and Small LL: Sodium and potassium concentrations of erythrocytes from perinatal, immature, and adult dogs. *Cornell Vet* 63:462, 1972.

Coulter DB, Duncan RJ, and Sander PD: Effects of asphyxia and potassium on canine and feline electrocardiograms. *Can J Comp Med* 39:442, 1975.

Crenshaw KL and Peterson ME: Pretreatment clinical and laboratory evaluation of cats with diabetes mellitus: 104 cases (1992–1994). *J Am Vet Med Assoc* 209:943, 1996.

Crisp MS, Chew DJ, DiBartola SP, et al.: Peritoneal dialysis: 27 cases (1976–1987). *J Am Vet Med Assoc* 195:1262, 1989.

DeFronzo RA: Hyperkalemia and hyporeninemic hypoaldosteronism. *Kidney Int* 17:118, 1980.

Degen M: Pseudohyperkalemia in Akitas. *J Am Vet Med Assoc* 190:541, 1987.

Degen MA: Correlation of spurious potassium elevation and platelet count in dogs. *Vet Clin Pathol* 15:20, 1986.

Degen MA, Feldman BF, Turrel JM, et al.: Thrombocytosis associated with a myeloproliferative disorder in a dog. *J Am Vet Med Assoc* 194:1457, 1989.

Dhein CR and Wardrop KJ: Hyperkalemia associated with potassium chloride administration in a cat. *J Am Vet Med Assoc* 206:1565, 1995.

DiBartola SP, Chew DJ, and Jacobs G: Quantitative urinalysis including 24-hour protein excretion in the dog. *J Am Anim Hosp Assoc* 16:537, 1980.

DiBartola SP, Johnson SE, Davenport DJ, et al.: Clinicopathologic findings resembling hypoadrenocorticism in dogs with primary gastrointestinal disease. *J Am Vet Med Assoc* 187:60, 1985.

DiBartola SP, Rutgers HC, Zack PM, et al.: Clinicopathologic findings associated with chronic renal disease in cats: 74 cases (1973–1984). *J Am Vet Med Assoc* 190:1196, 1987.

DiBartola SP, Tarr MJ, Parker AT, et al.: Clinicopathologic findings in dogs with renal amyloidosis: 59 cases (1976–1986). *J Am Vet Med Assoc* 195:358, 1989.

DiBartola SP, Buffington CA, Chew DJ, et al.: Development of chronic renal disease in cats fed a commercial diet. *J Am Vet Med Assoc* 202:744, 1993.

Dow SW: Studies on potassium depletion in cats. *Proceedings of the 12th Annual Kal Kan Symposium for the Treatment of Small Animal Diseases,* p. 61, 1989.

Dow SW, Fettman MJ, LeCouteur RS, et al.: Potassium depletion in cats: Renal and dietary influences. *J Am Vet Med Assoc* 191:1569, 1987a.

Dow SW, LeCouteur RA, Fettman MJ, et al.: Potassium depletion in cats: Hypokalemic polymyopathy. *J Am Vet Med Assoc* 191:1563, 1987b.

Dow SW, Fettman MJ, Curtis CR, et al.: Hypokalemia in cats: 186 cases (1984–1987). *J Am Vet Med Assoc* 194:1604, 1989.

Dow SW, Fettman MJ, Smith KR, et al.: Effects of dietary acidification and potassium depletion on acid-base balance, mineral metabolism and renal function in adult cats. *J Nutr* 120:569, 1990.

Drazner FH: Distal renal tubular acidosis associated with chronic pyelonephritis in a cat. *Calif Vet* 34:15, 1980.

Eger CE, Robinson WF, and Huxtable CRR: Primary aldosteronism (Conn's syndrome) in a cat: A case report and review of comparative aspects. *J Small Anim Pract* 24:293, 1983.

Ellory JC and Tucker EM: Cation transport in red blood cells. In Agar NS and Board PG (eds): *Red Blood Cells of Domestic Mammals.* Amsterdam: Elsevier Scientific Publishing Co., pp. 291–314, 1983.

Feldman EC and Nelson RW: Diabetes mellitus. In Feldman EC and Nelson RW (eds): *Canine and Feline Endocrinology.* Philadelphia, WB Saunders Co., p. 401, 1996a.

Feldman EC and Nelson RW: Hyperadrenocorticism (Cushing's syndrome). In Feldman EC and Nelson RW (eds): *Canine and Feline Endocrinology.* Philadelphia, WB Saunders Co., p. 262, 1996b.

Felkai F: Electrocardiographic signs in ventricular repolarization of

experimentally induced hypokalemia and appearance of the U wave in dogs. *Acta Vet Hung* 33:221, 1985.
Field MJ, Stanton BA, and Giebisch G: Influence of ADH on renal potassium handling: A micropuncture and microperfusion study. *Kidney Int* 25:502, 1984.
Field MJ, Berliner RW, and Giebisch GH: Regulation of renal potassium metabolism. In Maxwell MH, Kleeman GR, and Narins RG (eds): *Clinical Disorders of Fluid and Electrolyte Metabolism.* New York, McGraw-Hill Book Co., pp. 119–146, 1987.
Finco DR: Induced feline urethral obstruction: Response of hyperkalemia to relief of obstruction and administration of parenteral fluids. *J Am Anim Hosp Assoc* 12:198, 1976.
Finco DR: Fluid therapy. In Kirk RW (ed): *Current Veterinary Therapy VI.* Philadelphia, WB Saunders Co., p. 8, 1977.
Finco DR and Cornelius LM: Characterization and treatment of water, electrolyte, and acid-base imbalances of induced urethral obstruction in the cat. *Am J Vet Res* 38:823, 1977.
Finco DR, Brown SA, Barsanti JA, et al.: Reliability of using random urine samples for spot determination of fractional excretion of electrolytes in cats. *Am J Vet Res* 58:1184, 1997.
Garella S, Chang B, and Kahn SI: Alterations of hydrogen ion homeostasis in pure potassium depletion: Studies in rats and dogs during the recovery phase. *J Lab Clin Med* 93:321, 1979.
Gennari FJ and Cohen JJ: Role of the kidney in potassium homeostasis: Lessons from acid-base disturbances. *Kidney Int* 8:1, 1975.
Giger U and Harvey JW: Hemolysis caused by phosphofructokinase deficiency in English springer spaniels: Seven cases (1983–1986). *J Am Vet Med Assoc* 191:453, 1987.
Good DW, Velazquez H, and Wright FS: Luminal influences on potassium secretion: Low sodium concentration. *Am J Physiol* 246:F609, 1984.
Grauer GF and Kunze RS: Potassium depletion nephropathy and renal medullary washout: A case report. *Calif Vet* 33:8, 1979.
Greene RW and Scott RC: Lower urinary tract disease. In Ettinger SJ (ed): *Textbook of Veterinary Internal Medicine.* Philadelphia, WB Saunders Co., p. 1572, 1975.
Hamill RJ, Robinson LM, Wexler HR, et al.: Efficacy and safety of potassium infusion therapy in hypokalemic critically ill patients. *Crit Care Med* 19:694, 1991.
Harrison JB, Sussman HH, and Pickering DE: Fluid and electrolyte therapy in small animals. *J Am Vet Med Assoc* 137:637, 1960.
Harvey JW: Erythrocyte metabolism. In Kaneko JJ (ed): *Clinical Biochemistry of Domestic Animals.* New York, Academic Press, p. 196, 1989.
Henry CJ, Lanevschi A, Marks SL, et al.: Acute lymphoblastic leukemia, hypercalcemia, and pseudohyperkalemia in a dog. *J Am Vet Med Assoc* 208:237, 1996.
Hulter HN, Sebastian A, Sigala JF, et al.: Pathogenesis of renal hyperchloremic acidosis resulting from dietary potassium restriction in the dog: Role of aldosterone. *Am J Physiol* 238:F79, 1980.
Ilkiw JE, Davis PE, and Church DB: Hematologic, biochemical, blood gas, and acid base values in greyhounds before and after exercise. *Am J Vet Res* 50:583, 1989.
Inaba M and Maede Y: Increase of Na$^+$ gradient–dependent L-glutamate and L-aspartate transport in high K$^+$ dog erythrocytes associated with high activity of (Na$^+$,K$^+$)-ATPase. *J Biol Chem* 259:312, 1984.
Inaba M and Maede Y: Na,K-ATPase in dog red cells: Immunological identification and maturation-associated degradation by the proteolytic system. *J Biol Chem* 261:16099, 1986.
Jezyk PF: Hyperkalemic periodic paralysis in a dog. *J Am Anim Hosp Assoc* 18:977, 1982.
Jones BR, Swinney GW, and Alley MR: Hypokalemic myopathy in Burmese kittens. *N Z Vet J* 36:150, 1988.
Kaplan JL, Braitman LE, Dalsey WC, et al.: Alkalinization is ineffective for severe hyperkalemia in nonnephrectomized dogs. *Acad Emerg Med* 4:93, 1997.
Knochel JP: Neuromuscular manifestations of electrolyte disorders. *Am J Med* 72:521, 1982.
Knochel JP and Schlein EM: On the mechanism of rhabdomyolysis in potassium depletion. *J Clin Invest* 51:1750, 1972.
Knochel JP, Blanchley JD, Johnson JH, et al.: Muscle cell electrical hyperpolarization and reduced exercise hyperkalemia in physically conditioned dogs. *J Clin Invest* 75:740, 1985.
Laing EJ and Carter RF: Acute tumor lysis syndrome following treatment of canine lymphoma. *J Am Anim Hosp Assoc* 24:691, 1988.
Laing EJ, Fitzpatrick PJ, Binnington AG, et al.: Half-body radiotherapy in the treatment of canine lymphoma. *J Vet Intern Med* 3:102, 1989.
Lamb WA and Muir P: Lymphangiosarcoma associated with hyponatremia and hyperkalemia in a dog. *J Small Anim Pract* 35:374, 1994.
Lieveley P and Gruffydd-Jones TJ: Episodic collapse and weakness in cats. *Vet Annu* 29:261, 1989.
Lifton SJ, King LG, and Zerbe CA: Glucocorticoid deficient hypoadrenocorticism in dogs: 18 cases (1986–1995). *J Am Vet Med Assoc* 209:2076, 1996.
Lillemole KD, Romolo JL, Hamilton SR, et al.: Intestinal necrosis due to sodium polystyrene (Kayexalate) in sorbitol enemas: Clinical and experimental support for the hypothesis. *Surgery* 101:267–272, 1987.
Ling GV, Stabenfeldt GH, Comer KM, et al.: Canine hyperadrenocorticism: Pretreatment clinical and laboratory evaluation of 117 cases. *J Am Vet Med Assoc* 174:1211, 1979.
Lulich JP, Osborne CA, O'Brien TD, et al.: Feline renal failure: Questions, answers, questions. *Compend Contin Educ Pract Vet* 14:127, 1992.
Macintire DK: Treatment of diabetic ketoacidosis in dogs by continuous low-dose intravenous infusion of insulin. *J Am Vet Med Assoc* 202:1266, 1993.
Maede Y and Inaba M: (Na$^+$,K$^+$)-ATPase and ouabain binding in reticulocytes from dogs with high K and low K erythrocytes and their changes during maturation. *J Biol Chem* 260:3337, 1985.
Maede Y, Inaba M, and Taniguchi N: Increase of Na-K ATPase activity, glutamate, and aspartate update in dog erythrocytes associated with hereditary high accumulation of GSH, glutamate, glutamine, and aspartate. *Blood* 61:493, 1983.
Magner PO, Robinson L, Halperin RM, et al.: The plasma potassium concentration in metabolic acidosis: A re-evaluation. *Am J Kidney Dis* 11:220, 1988.
Malik R, Hunt GB, Hinchliffe JM, et al.: Severe whipworm infection in the dog. *J Small Anim Pract* 31:185, 1990.
Mandell CP, Goding B, Degen MA, et al.: Spurious elevation of serum potassium in two cases of thrombocythemia. *Vet Clin Pathol* 17:32, 1988.
Mason KV: A hereditary disease in Burmese cats manifested as an episodic weakness with head nodding and neck ventroflexion. *J Am Anim Hosp Assoc* 24:147, 1988a.
Mason KV: Hereditary potassium depletion in Burmese cats? *J Am Anim Hosp Assoc* 24:481, 1988b.
Meijer JC: Canine hyperadrenocorticism. In Kirk RW (ed): *Current Veterinary Therapy VII.* Philadelphia, WB Saunders Co., p. 975, 1980.
Miles PR and Lee P: Sodium and potassium content and membrane transport properties in red blood cells from newborn puppies. *J Cell Physiol* 79:367, 1972.
Moise NS and Reimers TJ: Insulin therapy in cats with diabetes mellitus. *J Am Vet Med Assoc* 182:158, 1983.
Muir WW, Wagner AE, and Buchanan C: Effects of acute hyperventilation on serum potassium in the dog. *Vet Surg* 19:83, 1990.
Nath KA, Hostetter MK, and Hostetter TH: Pathophysiology of chronic tubulointerstitial disease in rats: Interactions of dietary acid load, ammonia, and complement component C3. *J Clin Invest* 76:667, 1985.

Needle MA, Kaloyanides GJ, and Schwartz WB: The effects of selective depletion of hydrochloric acid on acid base and electrolyte equilibrium. *J Clin Invest* 43:1836, 1964.

Nemzek JA, Kruger JM, Walshaw R, et al.: Acute onset of hypokalemia and muscular weakness in four hyperthyroid cats. *J Am Vet Med Assoc* 205:65, 1994.

Oster JR, Perez GO, and Vaamonde CA: Relationship between blood pH and potassium and phosphorus during acute metabolic acidosis. *Am J Physiol* 235:F345, 1978.

Oster JR, Perez GO, Castro A, et al: Plasma potassium response to acute metabolic acidosis induced by mineral and nonmineral acids. *Miner Electrolyte Metab* 4:28, 1980.

Parker JC: Dog red blood cells—Adjustment in density in vivo. *J Gen Physiol* 61:146, 1973.

Parks J: Electrocardiographic abnormalities from serum electrolyte imbalance due to feline urethral obstruction. *J Am Anim Hosp Assoc* 11:102, 1975.

Patterson RE, Haut MJ, Montgomery CA, et al.: Natural history of potassium-deficiency myopathy in the dog: Role of adrenocorticosteroid in rhabdomyolysis. *J Lab Clin Med* 102:565, 1983.

Peterson ME, Greco DS, and Orth DN: Primary hypoadrenocorticism in ten cats. *J Vet Intern Med* 3:55, 1989.

Peterson ME, Kintzer PP, and Kass PH: Pretreatment clinical and laboratory findings in dogs with hypoadrenocorticism—225 cases (1979–1993). *J Am Vet Med Assoc* 208:85, 1996.

Polak A, Haynie GD, Hays RM, et al.: Effects of chronic hypercapnia on electrolyte and acid base equilibrium. *J Clin Invest* 40:1223, 1961.

Price GS, Armstrong PJ, McLeod DA, et al.: Evaluation of citrate-phosphate-dextrose-adenine as a storage medium for packed canine erythrocytes. *J Vet Intern Med* 2:126, 1988.

Rakich PM and Lorenz MD: Clinical signs and laboratory abnormalities in 23 dogs with spontaneous hypoadrenocorticism. *J Am Anim Hosp Assoc* 20:647, 1984.

Reimann KA, Knowlen GG, and Tvedten HW: Factitious hyperkalemia in dogs with thrombocytosis: The effect of platelets on serum potassium concentration. *J Vet Intern Med* 3:47, 1989.

Rich LJ, Berneuter DC, and Cowell RL: Elevated serum potassium associated with delayed separation of serum from clotted blood in dogs of the Akita breed. *Vet Clin Pathol* 15:12, 1986.

Rogers W, Straus J, and Chew D: Atypical hypoadrenocorticism in three dogs. *J Am Vet Med Assoc* 179:155, 1981.

Rose BD: Hypokalemia. In Rose BD (ed): *Clinical Physiology of Acid-Base and Electrolyte Disorders.* New York, McGraw-Hill Co., p. 811, 1994.

Ross LA and Goldstein M: Biochemical abnormalities associated with accidental hypothermia in a dog and cat. St. Louis, American College of Veterinary Internal Medicine, p. 66, 1981.

Roudebush P, Allen TA, Kuehn NF, et al.: The effect of combined therapy with captopril, furosemide, and a sodium-restricted diet on serum electrolyte concentrations and renal function in normal dogs and dogs with congestive heart failure. *J Vet Intern Med* 8:337, 1994.

Rutecki GW, Cox JW, Robertson GW, et al.: Urinary concentrating ability and antidiuretic hormone responsiveness in the potassium-depleted dog. *J Lab Clin Med* 100:53, 1982.

Sadek D and Schaer M: Atypical Addison's disease in the dog: A retrospective survey of 14 cases. *J Am Anim Hosp Assoc* 32:159, 1996.

Sapir DG, Levine DZ, and Schwartz WB: The effects of chronic hypoxemia on electrolyte and acid base equilibrium: An examination of normocapneic hypoxemia and of the influence of hypoxemia on the adaptation to chronic hypercapnia. *J Clin Invest* 46:369, 1967.

Scandling JD and Ornt DB: Mechanism of potassium depletion during chronic metabolic acidosis in the rat. *Am J Physiol* 252:F122, 1987.

Schaer M: The use of regular insulin in the treatment of hyperkalemia in cats with urethral obstruction. *J Am Anim Hosp Assoc* 11:106, 1975.

Schaer M: A clinical survey of thirty cats with diabetes mellitus. *J Am Anim Hosp Assoc* 13:23, 1977.

Schaer M and Chen CL: A clinical survey of 48 dogs with adrenocortical hypofunction. *J Am Anim Hosp Assoc* 19:443, 1983.

Schoolwerth AC and Culpepper RM: Measurement of intracellular pH in suspensions of renal tubules from potassium-depleted rats. *Miner Electrolyte Metab* 16:191, 1990.

Schrock H and Kuschinsky W: Consequences of chronic potassium depletion for the ionic composition of brain, heart, skeletal muscle, and cerebrospinal fluid. *Miner Electrolyte Metab* 15:171, 1989.

Schultze RG, Taggart DD, Shapiro H, et al.: On the adaptation in potassium excretion associated with nephron reduction in the dog. *J Clin Invest* 50:1061, 1971.

Schunk KL: Feline polymyopathy. *Proceedings of the American College of Veterinary Internal Medicine,* Washington DC, p. 197, 1984.

Schwartz WB, Orning KJ, and Porter R: The internal distribution of hydrogen ions with varying degrees of metabolic acidosis. *J Clin Invest* 36:373, 1957.

Schwartz WB, Brackett NC, and Cohen JJ: The response of extracellular hydrogen ion concentration to graded degrees of chronic hypercapnia: The physiologic limits of the defense of pH. *J Clin Invest* 44:291, 1965.

Sealey JE and Laragh JH: A proposed cybernetic system for sodium and potassium homeostasis: Coordination of aldosterone and intrarenal physical factors. *Kidney Int* 6:281, 1974.

Surawicz B: Arrhythmias and electrolyte disturbances. *Bull N Y Acad Med* 43:1160, 1967a.

Surawicz B: Relationship between electrocardiogram and electrolytes. *Am Heart J* 73:814, 1967b.

Swan RC and Pitts RF: Neutralization of infused acid by nephrectomized dogs. *J Clin Invest* 34:205, 1955.

Tannen RL: Relationship of renal ammonia production and potassium homeostasis. *Kidney Int* 11:453, 1977.

Tannen RL and Sastrasinh S: Response of ammonia metabolism to acute acidosis. *Kidney Int* 11:453, 1984.

Theisen SK, DiBartola SP, Radin MJ, et al.: Muscle potassium content and potassium gluconate supplementation in normokalemic cats with naturally occurring chronic renal failure. *J Vet Intern Med* 11:212, 1997.

Tietz NW, Pruden EL, and Siggaard-Andersen O: Electrolytes, blood gases, and acid-base balance. In Tietz NW (ed): *Textbook of Clinical Chemistry.* Philadelphia, WB Saunders Co., p. 1181, 1986.

Tobin RB: Varying role of extracellular electrolytes in metabolic acidosis and alkalosis. *Am J Physiol* 195:687, 1958.

Tolins JP, Hostetter MK, and Hostetter TH: Hypokalemic nephropathy in the rat: Role of ammonia in chronic tubular injury. *J Clin Invest* 79:1447, 1987.

Velazquez H, Wright FS, Good DW, et al.: Luminal influences on potassium secretion: Chloride replacement with sulfate. *Am J Physiol* 242:F46, 1982.

Vite CH and Gfeller RW: Suspected albuterol intoxication in a dog. *J Vet Emerg Crit Care* 4:7, 1994.

Watson ADJ, Culvenor JA, Middleton DJ, et al.: Distal renal tubular acidosis in a cat with pyelonephritis. *Vet Rec* 119:65, 1986.

West ML, Bendz O, Chen CB, et al.: Development of a test to evaluate the transtubular potassium concentration gradient in the cortical collecting duct in vivo. *Miner Electrolyte Metab* 12:226, 1986a.

West ML, Marsden PA, Richardson RMA, et al.: New clinical approach to evaluate disorders of potassium excretion. *Miner Electrolyte Metab* 12:234, 1986b.

Willard MD, Schall WD, McCaw DE, et al.: Canine hypoadrenocorticism: Report of 37 cases and review of 39 previously reported cases. *J Am Vet Med Assoc* 180:59, 1982.

Willard MD, Refsal K, and Thacker E: Evaluation of plasma aldosterone concentrations before and after ACTH administration in clinically normal dogs and in dogs with various diseases. *Am J Vet Res* 48:1713, 1987.

Willard MD, Fossum TW, Torrance A, et al.: Hyponatremia and hyperkalemia associated with idiopathic or experimentally induced chylothorax in four dogs. *J Am Vet Med Assoc* 199:353, 1991.

Zenger E: Persistent hyperkalemia associated with nonchylous pleural effusion in a dog. *J Am Anim Hosp Assoc* 28:411, 1992.

CHAPTER 6

Disorders of Calcium
HYPERCALCEMIA AND HYPOCALCEMIA

THOMAS J. ROSOL   DENNIS J. CHEW   LARRY A. NAGODE   PATRICIA SCHENCK

Calcium is required in the body for many vital intracellular and extracellular functions, as well as for skeletal support. Calcium ions (Ca^{2+}) are required for enzymatic reactions, membrane transport and stability, blood coagulation, nerve conduction, neuromuscular transmission, muscle contraction, vascular smooth muscle tone, hormone secretion, bone formation and resorption, control of hepatic glycogen metabolism, and cell growth and division (Rosol et al. 1995). Intracellular calcium ion is one of the primary regulators of the cellular response to many agonists and serves as "an almost universal ionic messenger, conveying signals received at the cell surface to the inside of the cell" (Rasmussen 1989). In addition to serving as an intracellular messenger, the Ca^{2+} concentration in the extracellular fluid (ECF) regulates cell function in many organs, including the parathyroid gland, kidney, and thyroid C cells by binding to a newly identified cell membrane–bound calcium-sensing receptor (Brown et al. 1995). This is the first example of a cell membrane receptor that regulates cell function in direct response to an extracellular ion.

This chapter discusses disorders that are characterized by hypercalcemia and hypocalcemia in the dog and cat. Normal homeostatic control mechanisms usually maintain the serum calcium concentration within a narrow range and guarantee an adequate supply of calcium for intracellular function. These mechanisms must be disrupted for hypercalcemia or hypocalcemia to develop. The routine use of automated serum biochemistry methods in veterinary medicine has resulted in increased detection of abnormal serum calcium concentrations (Chew and Carothers 1989). Abnormal serum calcium concentrations may be of diagnostic value and may contribute to the development of lesions and clinical signs of disease. Technologic advances in the measurement of the serum ionized calcium concentration, immunoreactive parathyroid hormone (PTH) and parathyroid hormone–related protein (PTHrP), and vitamin D metabolites have provided veterinarians with tools that allow greater diagnostic accuracy in the investigation of calcium disorders. This chapter also contains new information on the role of PTHrP in calcium balance and cancer-associated hypercalcemia, identification of the PTH-PTHrP cell membrane receptor, and development of potent bisphosphonates for therapy of hypercalcemia.

Practicing veterinarians must frequently interpret abnormal serum calcium concentrations. Large deviations of serum calcium concentration from normal occur infrequently but capture the clinician's attention and initiate urgent corrective efforts. Small deviations in serum calcium concentration may be equally important because they also provide diagnostic clues to an underlying disease. The magnitude of altered serum calcium concentration often does not suggest a specific diagnosis or the extent of disease. Hypocalcemia is more common than hypercalcemia in both dogs and cats. Furthermore, a normal serum calcium concentration does not eliminate a disorder of calcium homeostasis.

▶ Normal Physiology

Overview of Calcium Homeostasis

Regulation of serum calcium concentration is complex and requires the integrated actions of PTH, vitamin D metabolites, and calcitonin (Fig. 6–1). Parathyroid hormone and calcitriol (1,25-dihydroxyvitamin D_3) are the main regulators of calcium homeostasis and have major regulatory effects on each other (Rosol and Capen 1997). Parathyroid hormone is largely responsible for the minute-to-minute control of serum ionized calcium concentration, whereas calcitriol maintains day-to-day control. In the fetus, the parathyroid glands and placenta produce PTHrP, which binds to PTH receptors and regulates calcium balance (Tucci et al. 1996). After birth, the parathyroid glands modify their pattern of hormone secretion and produce predominantly PTH. Other hormones including adrenal corticosteroids, estrogens, thyroxine, growth hormone, glucagon, and prolactin have less influence on calcium homeostasis but may play important roles during growth, lactation, or certain disease states.

The intestine, kidney, and bone are the major target organs affected by calcium regulatory hormones. These interactions allow conservation of calcium in the ECF by

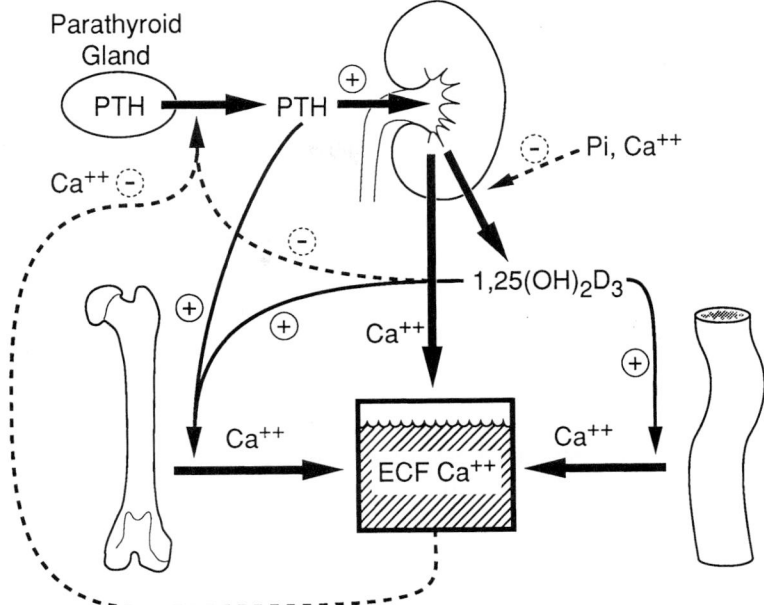

FIGURE 6–1. Regulation of extracellular fluid (ECF) calcium concentration by the effects of parathyroid hormone (PTH) and calcitriol (1,25-dihydroxyvitamin D_3) on gut, kidney, bone, and parathyroid gland. The principal effect of PTH is to increase the ECF calcium concentration by mobilizing calcium from bone, increasing tubular calcium reabsorption, and, indirectly on the gut, by increasing calcitriol synthesis. The principal effect of calcitriol is to increase intestinal absorption of calcium, but it also exerts negative regulatory control of PTH synthesis and further calcitriol synthesis. (Modified from Habner JF, Rosenblatt M, and Pott JT: Parathyroid hormone: Biochemical aspects of biosynthesis, secretion, action, and metabolism. *Physiol Rev* 64:1000, 1984.)

renal tubular reabsorption, increased intestinal transport of calcium from the diet, and internal redistribution of calcium from bone (Fig. 6–2). The intestine and kidneys are the major regulators of calcium balance in health (Favus 1992). Normally, dietary calcium intake equals the amount of calcium lost in urine and feces. The enteric absorption of calcium depends on the physiologic status of the intestines (e.g., acidity, presence of other dietary components, integrity of the villi or presence of small intestinal disease, and degree of enterocyte stimulation by calcitriol). Non–protein-bound calcium is filtered by the glomerulus and undergoes extensive renal reabsorption. This process results in reclamation of more than 98% of the filtered calcium in health (DiBartola et al. 1980; Rosol and Capen 1996).

The skeleton provides a major supply of calcium and phosphorus when intestinal absorption and renal reabsorption are inadequate to maintain normal serum calcium concentrations. Bone calcium mobilization is important in the acute regulation of blood calcium (Parfitt 1987). Calcium and phosphorus can be mobilized from readily available calcium phosphate in the bone ECF compartment, but these stores are rapidly depleted. The osteoblast is critical in limiting the distribution of calcium and phosphate between bone and ECF, and exchangeable bone water is separated from ECF water by the combined membranes of osteoblasts lining bone surfaces. For greater or prolonged release of calcium from bone, osteoclastic bone resorption must be activated. Osteoclasts secrete acid and proteases that result in dissolution of the

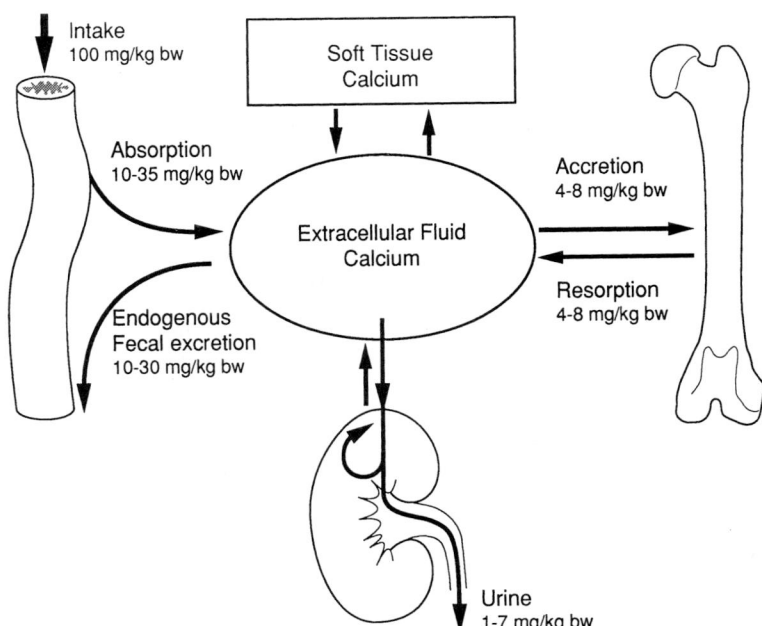

FIGURE 6–2. Normal calcium balance showing the major organs that supply or remove calcium from extracellular fluid: bone, gut, and kidney. Total calcium input into extracellular fluid equals total calcium leaving the extracellular space. (Modified from Hazewinkel HAW: Dietary influences on calcium homeostasis and the skeleton. In *Purina International Nutrition Symposium*, p. 52. Orlando, FL, Ralston Purina Company, Marriott World Center, January 15, 1991.)

mineralized matrix of bone and mobilize calcium and phosphorus. In normal states, osteoclast and osteoblast actions are "coupled" as osteoclasts initially resorb bone followed by replacement of bone by the actions of osteoblasts.

The extracellular ionized calcium concentration is the fraction of total calcium that is actively regulated (Brown 1991; Chew and Meuten 1982). When blood calcium concentration falls, PTH secretion is stimulated. Parathyroid hormone exerts direct effects on bone and kidney and indirect effects on the intestine through calcitriol. It increases synthesis of calcitriol by activating renal mitochondrial 1α-hydroxylation of 25-hydroxycholecalciferol derived from the circulation. Calcitriol, in turn, increases calcium absorption from the intestine. Calcitriol participates with PTH to stimulate osteoclastic bone resorption (Capen and Rosol 1993). Calcitriol is necessary for differentiation of osteoclasts from precursor mononuclear cells. At high pharmacologic doses, calcitriol can stimulate bone resorption (without PTH) by inducing the secretion of factors from osteoblasts that activate osteoclastic bone resorption (Stern 1990). Parathyroid hormone increases osteoclast number and stimulates osteoclast function to increase bone resorption and the release of calcium from bone to blood. Calcitriol also induces renal transport mechanisms activated by PTH that increase tubular reabsorption of calcium from the glomerular filtrate, thus preventing calcium loss in urine (Nagode and Chew 1991).

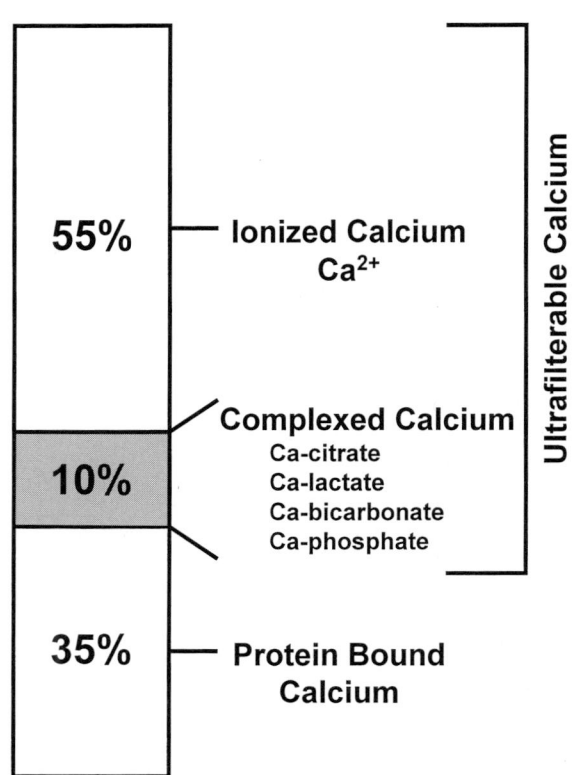

FIGURE 6-3. Serum total calcium concentration consists of ionized (free), complexed, and protein-bound fractions.

Calcium Distribution Within the Body

Approximately 99% of body calcium resides in the skeleton and is stored along with phosphate in crystalline form as hydroxyapatite, $Ca_{10}(PO_4)_6(OH)_2$. Most skeletal calcium is poorly exchangeable, and less than 1% is considered readily available. The small amount of rapidly exchangeable bone calcium arises from the ECF in bone that is present between osteoblasts and osteocytes and the bone matrix. Almost all of the nonskeletal calcium resides in the extracellular space, although small and biologically important quantities are found intracellularly (Rosol et al. 1995).

EXTRACELLULAR CALCIUM

Calcium in plasma or serum exists in three forms or fractions: ionized (free calcium), complexed or chelated (bound to phosphate, bicarbonate, sulfate, citrate, and lactate), and protein bound (Fig. 6-3). In general, between 50 and 60% of total serum calcium is ionized in normal animals. In clinically normal dogs, protein-bound, complexed, and ionized calcium account for approximately 34%, 10%, and 56% of the total serum calcium concentration, respectively (Schenck et al. 1996). Ultrafilterable (diffusible) calcium includes both ionized and complexed calcium, and the term refers to the ability of these two fractions to pass through a membrane filter. Total, ionized, and ultrafilterable calcium concentrations can be directly measured, and these values can then be used to calculate the complexed and protein-bound calcium fractions. Ionized calcium is the most important biologically active fraction in serum, although an active biologic role for complexed calcium has been suggested (Toffaletti 1983). Currently, no biologic role for protein-bound calcium has been identified other than as a storage pool or buffering system for ionized calcium.

INTRACELLULAR CALCIUM

Intracellular ionized calcium (Ca^{2+}) is an important secondary messenger in the response to biochemical signals (such as hormones) transduced through the cell membrane (Rosol et al. 1995; Rasmussen et al. 1990). Therefore, intracellular Ca^{2+} concentrations are maintained at a very low level (approximately 100 nM), 10,000-fold less than the serum concentration. This permits rapid diffusion into the cytoplasm from the ECF or endoplasmic reticulum. Intracellular calcium is rapidly buffered by cytosolic proteins and is transported into organelles or to the outside of the cell after a rise in intracellular Ca^{2+}. If intracellular Ca^{2+} is not maintained at a low concentration, it leads to toxicity and eventual cell death. Intracellular Ca^{2+} can be measured with an ionized calcium–sensitive microelectrode, microinjection of chemical indicators, or luminescent dyes that irreversibly cross the cell membrane and chelate calcium (Borle 1990; Carafoli 1987). Specialized expertise is required for these measurements, restricting them to the research environment. Fluorescence methods are most frequently employed today.

Intracellular Ca^{2+} concentrations are low because of

extrusion of calcium by membrane-bound pumps ($Ca^{2+}/2H^+$-adenosine triphosphatase [$Ca^{2+}/2H^+$-ATPase] and a $3Na^+/Ca^{2+}$ exchanger) and because plasma membrane permeability to calcium is inherently low (Rasmussen et al. 1990). It is important for cells to maintain a much lower concentration of Ca^{2+} than is observed in ECF. If they do not, cell function would be disrupted by binding of excess Ca^{2+} to intracellular phosphates and excessive stimulation of the calcium-dependent enzyme systems (Boden and Kaplan 1990). Minor changes in permeability of the plasma membrane result in major changes in cytosolic Ca^{2+} concentration (Carafoli 1987).

Although calcium-dependent systems respond to free cytosolic Ca^{2+}, most intracellular calcium is sequestered in organelles, bound to cellular membranes, or bound to cellular proteins (Irvine 1986). Total intracellular calcium can exceed 1 mM, but less than 0.1% of this calcium is ionized (free). Sequestration of Ca^{2+} in mitochondria serves to blunt rises in cytosolic Ca^{2+}, whereas endoplasmic reticulum serves as a reservoir to increase cytosolic Ca^{2+} when necessary. Cytosolic Ca^{2+} concentrations can increase 10- to 100-fold during cell activation (stimulation), largely by release from calcium stores in endoplasmic reticulum (Brown 1991). Binding of calcium to specific cytosolic or membrane proteins appears to be an efficient way for the cell to regulate its intracellular Ca^{2+} concentration. Protein binding not only provides a form of intracellular Ca^{2+} buffering but also may act as a messenger system when protein configuration and activity are altered. Calbindin, calmodulin, and troponin C are the most important intracellular calcium-binding proteins (Boden and Kaplan 1990).

▶ Parathyroid Hormone

Structure

Parathyroid hormone is an 84-amino-acid single-chain polypeptide that is synthesized and secreted by chief cells of the parathyroid gland (Rosol and Capen 1997). The amino acid sequence of PTH is known for the dog, cow, pig, rat, chicken, and human (Kronenberg et al. 1994; Rosol et al. 1996), and immunologic reactivities suggest that most mammals appear to have very similar amino-terminal portions of the molecule (Nagode and Chew 1991). Whereas the conserved amino end of PTH is vital for binding to cell membrane receptors, the role of the carboxyl terminus is to serve as a guide for PTH through the cellular secretory pathway (Lim et al. 1992). Although it is still debated, the carboxyl terminus probably has no significant role in calcium metabolism after secretion of PTH from the parathyroid gland (Orloff and Stewart 1995; Inomata et al. 1995).

Synthesis and Secretion

Synthesis, secretion, and degradation of PTH by chief cells are closely related. Little PTH is stored within the parathyroid glands compared with peptide hormones in other endocrine tissues (Capen 1983), and synthesis of new PTH is required to maintain secretion. After secretion, PTH has a short half-life (3–5 min) in serum; therefore, a steady rate of secretion is necessary to maintain serum PTH concentrations.

Chief cells initially synthesize pre-pro-PTH, a 115-amino-acid precursor of PTH. Pre-pro-PTH undergoes intracellular cleavages to form mature PTH with 84 amino acids (Rosol and Capen 1997; Kronenberg et al. 1994). The amount of PTH available for secretion is a function of the balance of synthesis and degradation within chief cells (Fig. 6–4). Calcitriol and extracellular Ca^{2+} concentration regulate these processes. In general, the parathyroid gland has evolved most of its regulatory strategies to protect against hypocalcemia with sensitive control of PTH synthesis and secretion being the dominant sites for regulation (Brown 1994; Silver and Kronenberg 1996). However, high serum Ca^{2+} concentrations increase the rate of degradation of PTH within the gland in order to protect against hypercalcemia (Kronenberg et al. 1994).

Except for minor diurnal variation, PTH secretion is relatively constant in humans. Secretion may have a mild pulsatile pattern in response to minor fluctuations in the concentration of serum Ca^{2+} (Brown 1991). Secretion of PTH is accomplished by exocytosis of secretory granules. When demand for hormone is great, PTH is secreted directly from the chief cell without packaging into secretory granules. During normal homeostasis, a relatively low rate of PTH secretion is needed to maintain serum Ca^{2+} concentration. The basal secretory rate of PTH is approximately 25% of the maximal rate in the normal parathyroid gland, and PTH is constantly secreted during normocalcemia. Complete inhibition of PTH secretion is not achieved even in the presence of severe hypercalcemia (Kronenberg et al. 1994).

Hypocalcemia is the principal stimulus for PTH secretion, but epinephrine, isoproterenol, dopamine, secretin, prostaglandin E_2, and stimulation of nerve endings within the parathyroid gland may have minor effects on PTH secretion (Habener et al. 1984). The parathyroid gland chief cells sense extracellular Ca^{2+} concentrations with a cell membrane calcium receptor that regulates intracellular Ca^{2+} concentrations. As extracellular Ca^{2+} decreases, intracellular Ca^{2+} also decreases, which results in stimulation of PTH secretion. High concentrations of serum and intracellular Ca^{2+} inhibit PTH secretion and its messenger RNA (mRNA) synthesis. The promoter of the PTH gene has a calcium response element (CaRE) that may be responsible for the inhibitory actions of Ca^{2+} on PTH mRNA synthesis (Okazaki et al. 1991).

Calcitriol also plays an important role in the regulation of PTH synthesis and secretion. Calcitriol inhibits PTH synthesis (Silver and Naveh-Many 1997) and stimulates synthesis of the cell membrane calcium receptor (Brown et al. 1996). These relationships explain the requirement for adequate blood concentrations of calcitriol to maintain the ability of the parathyroid gland to respond to changes in extracellular calcium concentrations. In addition, increased intracellular Ca^{2+} may cooperate with calcitriol to reduce PTH synthesis in chief cells by inhibiting the expression of calreticulin (a blocker of vitamin D receptor action) (Waser et al. 1997). Animals with uremia and reduced serum calcitriol concentrations have poorly regulated chief cell function that results in excess secretion of PTH (renal secondary hyperparathyroidism) because of

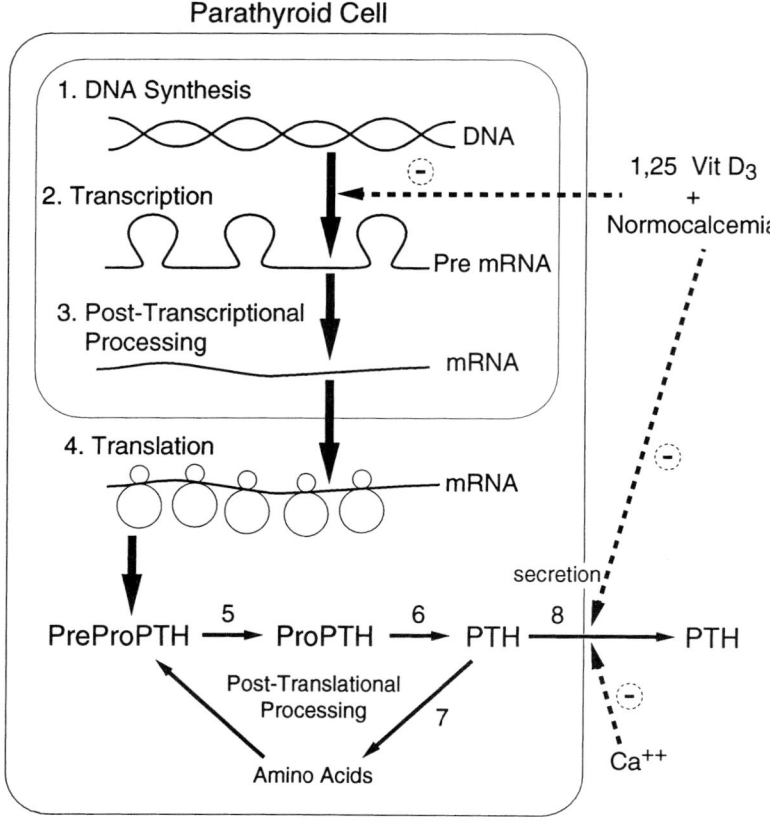

FIGURE 6–4. Synthesis and secretion of parathyroid hormone. Note sites of regulation of PTH biosynthesis by extracellular ionized calcium or calcitriol (1,25-[OH]$_2$-vitamin D$_3$) interaction. (Modified from Habner JF, Rosenblatt M, and Potts JT: Parathyroid hormone: Biochemical aspects of biosynthesis, secretion, action, and metabolism. *Physiol Rev* 64:1004, 1984.)

increased PTH synthesis and decreased responsiveness of chief cells to serum Ca^{2+} (Nagode et al. 1996).

Serum magnesium concentration has little role in the control of PTH secretion under normal conditions, but PTH secretion can be inhibited by very high concentrations of serum magnesium (Rosol and Capen 1997). Paradoxically, hypomagnesemia or magnesium depletion also results in inability to secrete PTH, but the cellular mechanism of this effect is unclear. This effect may be partially due to reduced sensitivity of cell membrane receptors to Ca^{2+} in the presence of low serum magnesium concentrations (Habener et al. 1984; Miki et al. 1997).

Serum phosphorus concentrations regulate PTH secretion principally by indirect means. Renal calcitriol synthesis is reduced early in uremia by modest hyperphosphatemia, and the plasma Ca^{2+} concentration may decrease because of reduced effects of calcitriol on the intestine, bone, and kidney. Markedly increased serum phosphorus concentrations (as seen in renal failure) can lower the serum ionized calcium concentration (mass law effect), resulting in an increase in PTH secretion. Investigations have demonstrated a direct action of phosphate on PTH synthesis by stabilization of PTH mRNA, however, the significance of this effect in vivo is unknown (Sela et al. 1997).

SET-POINT FOR PTH SECRETION

Exocytosis in most secretory cells is stimulated as intracellular Ca^{2+} increases. The opposite is true for the parathyroid gland, and PTH secretion is inhibited when intracellular Ca^{2+} concentration increases. The intracellular Ca^{2+} concentration is regulated by the cell membrane calcium receptor that monitors the extracellular Ca^{2+} concentration. It is useful for understanding the regulation of PTH secretion to define the *set-point* for PTH secretion as the ECF Ca^{2+} concentration that occurs at the serum PTH concentration that is midway between maximal and minimal values (Brown 1991). The set-point must be determined experimentally by measuring PTH concentrations during the induction of hypocalcemia (citrate or ethylenediaminetetraacetic acid [EDTA] infusion) and hypercalcemia (calcium infusion). Normal serum Ca^{2+} concentration is maintained slightly higher than the set-point, so PTH release normally is less than half-maximal (Fig. 6–5).

The rate of PTH secretion is inversely proportional to the concentration of extracellular calcium, but this proportional secretion of PTH occurs only over a narrow range corresponding to a total serum calcium concentration of 7.5 to 11.0 mg/dL (Habener et al. 1984). An inverse sigmoidal curve with a steep slope results when the relationship between serum ionized calcium concentration and PTH secretion is plotted over a larger range of calcium concentrations (Brown 1991) (see Fig. 6–5). This ensures large changes in PTH secretion for relatively small changes in ionized calcium concentration in the physiologic range and consequently more precise control of serum Ca^{2+} concentration. An approximately 10% decrease in serum Ca^{2+} concentration elicits a nearly maximal PTH secretory response. The rate of decrease of serum Ca^{2+} concentration is also important, and rapid decreases in serum Ca^{2+} result in larger increases in PTH secretion. A 2 to 3% decrease in Ca^{2+} concentration, if rapid in onset, may result in a 400% increase in PTH secretion (Brown 1991).

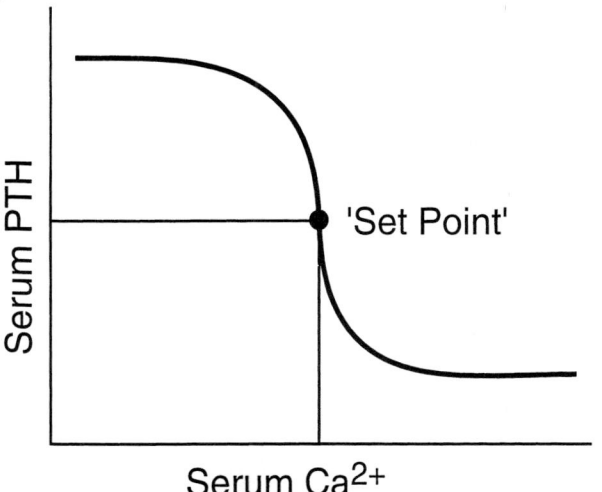

FIGURE 6–5. Relationship between secretion rate of parathyroid hormone and plasma calcium concentration. Small changes in plasma calcium concentration cause large changes in parathyroid hormone secretion, but secretion is not completely suppressed by high plasma calcium concentrations.

The cell membrane calcium receptor is responsible for establishing the relationship of the set-point for PTH secretion and extracellular Ca^{2+} concentration. The calcium receptor regulates PTH secretion indirectly by controlling the intracellular Ca^{2+} concentration by means of (1) release of Ca^{2+} from intracellular stores and (2) cell membrane calcium channels. Calcium channels span the parathyroid chief cell membrane and are important in allowing extracellular Ca^{2+} access to the interior of the cell (Fitzpatrick et al. 1986). The calcium channels are controlled by intracellular Ca^{2+} concentration (Brown 1994) and membrane regulatory G-proteins, which interact with the cell membrane calcium receptor (Schultz et al. 1990).

Calcitriol plays an important role in controlling the parathyroid gland set-point by regulating (1) synthesis of the cell membrane calcium receptor (Brown et al. 1996), (2) synthesis of cell membrane G-proteins, and (3) function of cell membrane calcium channels (Nagode and Chew 1991). Therefore, adequate calcitriol is necessary to maintain the set-point for PTH secretion (Brossard et al. 1997). Paradoxically, the parathyroid gland set-point may not be altered during chronic renal failure (calcitriol deficiency) or calcitriol therapy, but changes may be seen in the maximal secretory capacity (dependent mostly on parathyroid cell numbers) or the slope and/or position of the PTH secretion curve (Messa et al. 1994; Dunlay et al. 1989; Heidbreder et al. 1997). It is likely that increased PTH secretion in patients with uremia (renal secondary hyperparathyroidism) is due primarily to parathyroid gland hyperplasia. One important role of calcitriol in these patients is to prevent or reverse the hyperplasia (Chew and Nagode 1992; Nagode and Chew 1992).

INHIBITION OF PTH SYNTHESIS AND SECRETION

This topic has become important with understanding of the toxicity of PTH in animals and humans with chronic renal failure (CRF) and the accompanying secondary hyperparathyroidism (Nagode et al. 1996; Massry 1989).

PTH secretion is inhibited by increased serum Ca^{2+} concentration and interaction of calcitriol with its receptor in parathyroid chief cells (Silver and Naveh-Many 1997). The initial effect of increased serum Ca^{2+} concentration on decreasing PTH secretion is rapid (occurring within 2 to 3 mins), but the mechanisms involved remain unclear (Cohen et al. 1997). Slower effects are due to inhibition of synthesis of PTH mRNA and its translation to hormone (Silver and Kronenberg 1996). Increased intracellular calcium concentration inhibits adenylate cyclase and the production of cyclic AMP (cAMP) in chief cells. The cAMP facilitates PTH synthesis after phosphorylation of a nuclear transcription factor by protein kinase A. The phosphorylated transcription factor is translocated to the nucleus, where it binds to the cAMP response element of the PTH gene to enhance gene transcription (Fig. 6–6).

Calcitriol is an important inhibitor of PTH synthesis, and it completes a negative feedback loop from the kidney because PTH stimulates renal calcitriol synthesis. The calcitriol receptor (vitamin D receptor, VDR) is expressed in parathyroid chief cells at concentrations equal to those in intestinal epithelial cells that regulate calcium absorption in the gastrointestinal tract (Silver and Kronenberg 1996). This observation attests to the functional importance of calcitriol in the parathyroid gland because the concentration of the intracellular VDR is important to the response of target cells to calcitriol (Silver and Naveh-Many 1997). The VDR is induced by its own ligand, calcitriol. The VDR was found to be depleted in the parathyroid glands of dogs and humans with uremia because of lack of renal production of calcitriol (Brown et al. 1989). After the VDR binds calcitriol, the VDR-calcitriol complex acts in the nucleus of the parathyroid chief cells by binding to specific regions of the PTH gene called vitamin D response elements (VDREs) and inhibiting transcription of the PTH gene (Nagode et al. 1996; Kronenberg et al. 1994) (see Fig. 6–6). For calcitriol to suppress synthesis of PTH, a normal concentration of calcium must be present because it would be inappropriate to suppress PTH synthesis in a hypocalcemic patient. This action may be regulated by the CaRE associated with the PTH gene (Nagode et al. 1997; Okazaki et al. 1992) (see Fig. 6–6).

Short and long negative feedback loops complement each other and effectively control normal secretion of PTH (Kronenberg et al. 1994). The long negative feedback loop is completed when an increased serum Ca^{2+} concentration results from PTH stimulation of renal calcitriol production and subsequent enhanced gastrointestinal absorption of calcium. This effect takes hours to develop because calcium-binding proteins associated with calcium absorption must be induced in enterocytes (Wasserman 1997). The short negative feedback loop is mediated by the binding of calcitriol to vitamin D receptors in parathyroid cells, with inhibition of transcription of the PTH gene (Silver and Naveh-Many 1997).

Clearance and Metabolism of Parathyroid Hormone

The intact PTH molecule (84 amino acids) circulates in the bloodstream with a half-life of 2 to 5 min and is

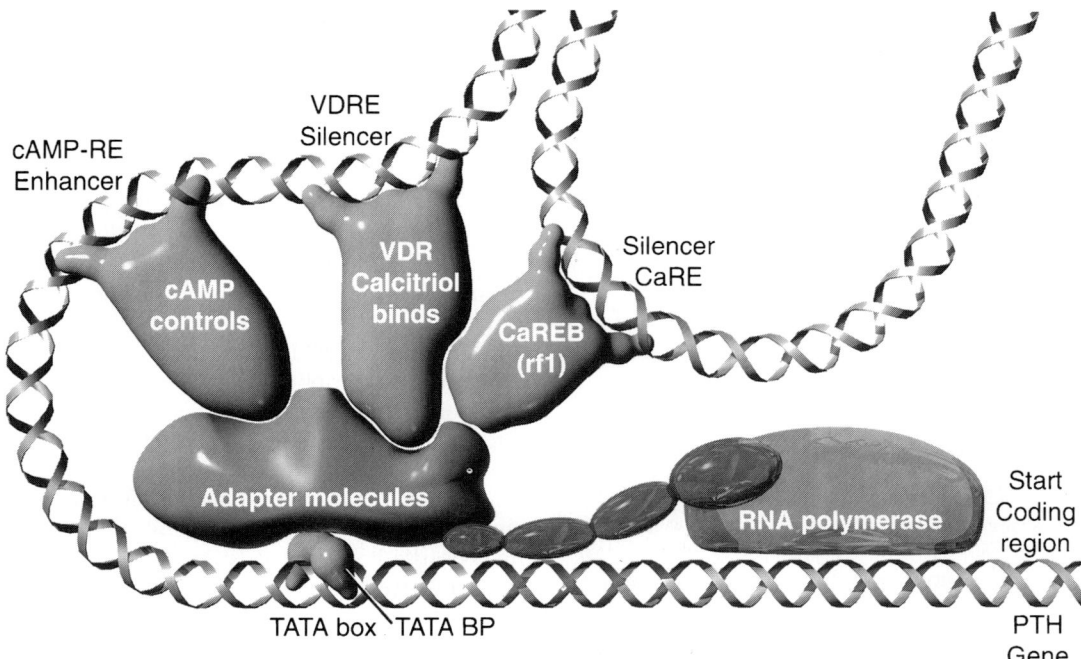

FIGURE 6–6. Simplified depiction of events regulating transcription of the parathyroid hormone (PTH) gene by RNA polymerase. Only the three transcription factors best understood to interact in this regulation are shown. Cyclic AMP stimulates phosphorylation of a transcription factor that binds to a cAMP response element (cAMP-RE) on the gene and enhances transcription. In contrast, the vitamin D receptor (VDR)–calcitriol complex and calcium response element–binding protein (CaREB, rf1) bind to their respective vitamin D (VDRE) and calcium (CaRE) response elements of the PTH gene, which function as "silencers" or negative regulators of gene transcription. Note that for calcium to exert its negative effect by means of the CaREB transcription factor, calcitriol and the vitamin D receptor must also be present. The adapter molecules (shown as a single structure) diagrammatically represent about 30 proteins termed accessory transcription factors. The TATA box is part of the gene promoter to which the TATA box binding proteins (BPs) bind. (From Nagode LA, Chew DJ, and Podell M: Benefits of calcitriol therapy and serum phosphorus control in dogs and cats with chronic renal failure. *Vet Clin North Am Small Anim Pract* 26:1293–1330, 1996.)

removed by fixed macrophages (primarily Kupffer cells in liver) (Rosol and Capen 1997; Kronenberg et al. 1994). Macrophages cleave the molecule between amino acids 33 through 43, which results in liberation of a variety of carboxyl-terminal fragments. The amino-terminal portion is completely degraded within the phagocytes. Kidney and bone also participate in degradation of intact PTH. Degradation of PTH in bone and kidney occurs by a process of receptor-mediated endocytosis. This mechanism is probably important only in conditions associated with high serum concentrations of PTH.

Intact PTH and its fragments are also filtered by the glomeruli. This mechanism of excretion is most important for the excretion of the carboxyl-terminal PTH fragments because carboxyl-terminal PTH (released from either the parathyroid gland or Kupffer cells) is cleared only by glomerular filtration (Fig. 6–7). The carboxyl-terminal fragments of PTH are not important for calcium metabolism. The circulating half-life of carboxyl-terminal PTH is much longer than that of intact PTH, and serum concentrations of carboxyl-terminal PTH can be very high during primary or secondary hyperparathyroidism or can be nonspecifically increased during renal failure. This was historically important in the interpretation of serum PTH concentrations determined by carboxyl-terminal radioimmunoassays (RIAs) but is less relevant today with the use of two-site immunoassays for intact PTH.

Actions of Parathyroid Hormone

Parathyroid hormone is the principal hormone involved in the minute-to-minute fine regulation of blood calcium concentration. It exerts its biologic actions directly by influencing the function of target cells primarily in bone and kidney and indirectly in the intestine to maintain plasma calcium at a concentration sufficient to ensure the optimal functioning of a wide variety of body cells.

In general, the most important biologic effects of PTH on calcium are to (1) increase the blood calcium concentration; (2) increase tubular reabsorption of calcium, resulting in diminished calcium loss in the urine; (3) increase bone resorption and the numbers of osteoclasts on bone surfaces; and (4) accelerate the formation of the principal active vitamin D metabolite (1,25-dihydroxyvitamin D, or calcitriol) by the kidney through a trophic effect on 1α-hydroxylase in mitochondria of renal epithelial cells in the proximal convoluted tubules.

An important action of PTH on bone is to mobilize calcium from skeletal reserves into ECF (Canalis et al. 1994). The increase in blood calcium concentration results from an interaction of PTH with receptors on osteoblasts that stimulate increased calcium release from bone and direct an increase in osteoclastic bone resorption (High et al. 1981). The mechanisms by which osteoblasts mediate increased osteoclastic bone resorption are poorly understood.

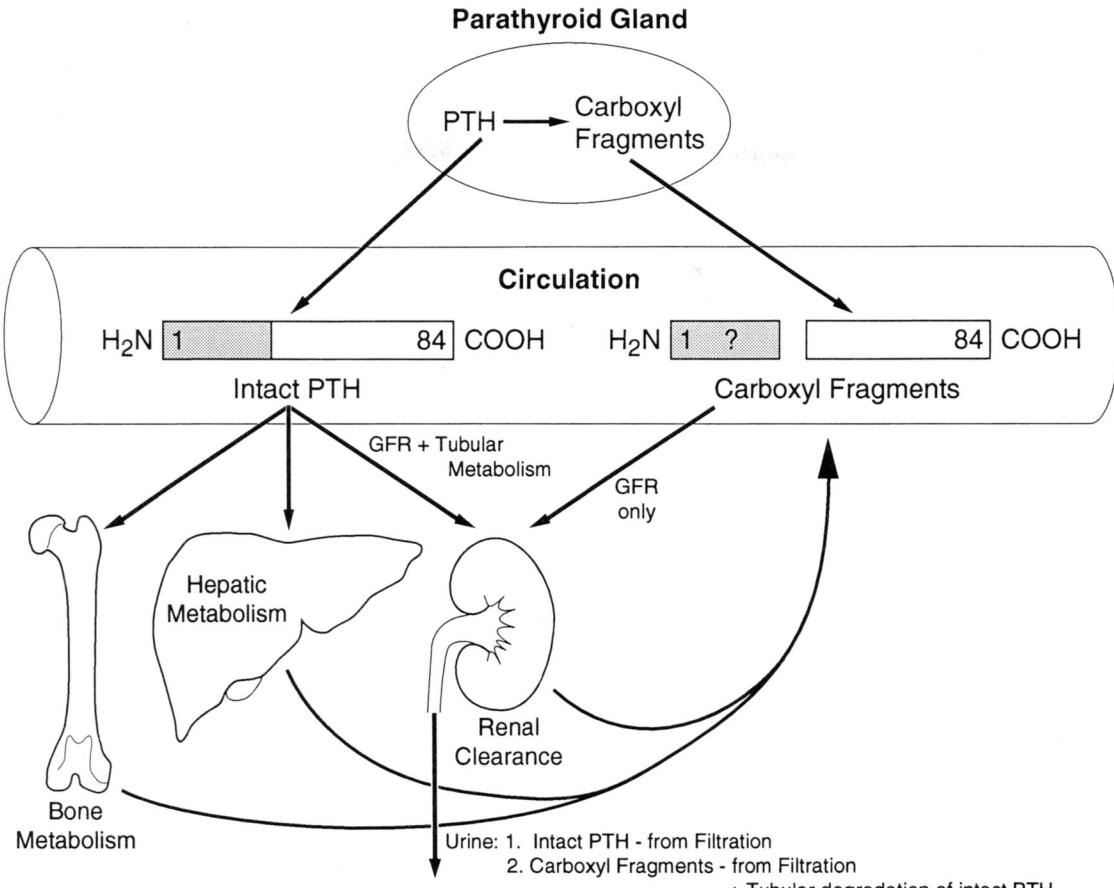

FIGURE 6-7. Degradation and clearance of parathyroid hormone (PTH). PTH (1–84) is secreted intact from the parathyroid gland into the circulation. Biologically inactive carboxy-terminal (COOH) fragments of PTH are also secreted by the parathyroid gland, but amino-terminal PTH is not secreted and does not circulate in biologically relevant concentrations. Peripheral metabolism of intact PTH to carboxy-terminal PTH fragments occurs mostly in the liver but may also occur in the kidney and bone. Both intact PTH and carboxy-terminal PTH are cleared by glomerular filtration, but only intact PTH is metabolized in the liver, kidney, and bone. The half-life of intact PTH in vivo is short compared with that of the biologically inactive carboxy-terminal fragments of PTH. (Modified from Endres DB, Villaneuva R, Sharp CF, and Singer FR: Measurement of parathyroid hormone. *Endocrinol Metab Clin North Am* 18:614, 1989.)

The response of bone to PTH is biphasic. The immediate effects are the result of increasing the activity of existing bone cells. This rapid effect of PTH depends on the continuous presence of hormone and results in an increased flow of calcium from deep in bone to bone surfaces through the action of an osteocyte-osteoblast "pump" to make fine adjustments in the blood calcium concentration (Parfitt 1997). The later effects of PTH on bone are potentially of greater magnitude and are not dependent on the continuous presence of hormone. Osteoclasts are primarily responsible for the long-term action of PTH on increasing bone resorption and overall bone remodeling (Canalis et al. 1994). This is interesting in light of findings that have failed to demonstrate receptors for PTH on osteoclasts, but receptors were present on osteoblasts (Segre 1994). Osteoblasts elaborate undefined chemical mediators to stimulate osteoclasts directly (McSheehy and Chambers 1986).

Parathyroid hormone also has the potential to serve as an anabolic agent in bone and stimulate osteoblastic bone formation (Canalis et al. 1994). The physiologic role of the anabolic action of PTH in vivo is uncertain, but intermittent administration of exogenous PTH has been reported to increase bone mass in humans and animals.

The ability of PTH to enhance the renal reabsorption of calcium is of considerable importance in the maintenance of calcium homeostasis. This effect of PTH on tubular reabsorption of calcium is due, in part, to a direct action on the distal convoluted tubule (Yanagawa and Lee 1992). PTH may also increase calcium reabsorption in the ascending thick limb of Henle's loop indirectly by increasing the net positive charge in the nephron lumen and creating a stimulus for diffusion out of the lumen. The other important effect of PTH on the kidney is regulation of the conversion of 25-hydroxycholecalciferol to calcitriol and other metabolites of vitamin D. The role of PTH as a trophic hormone in the metabolic activation of vitamin D is discussed further in the subsequent section on vitamin D.

Parathyroid hormone has been shown to promote the absorption of calcium from the gastrointestinal tract in animals under a variety of experimental conditions (Favus 1992; Nemere and Norman 1986). The effect is not as rapid as the action on the kidney and is not observed in vitamin D–deficient animals. The increased intestinal calcium transport is due principally to an indirect effect of PTH by stimulating the renal synthesis of the biologically active metabolite of vitamin D (calcitriol).

PARATHYROID HORMONE RECEPTOR

The receptor for N-terminal PTH (amino acids 1–34), the region important in calcium regulation, has been cloned and sequenced (Segre 1994; Abou-Samra et al. 1992). It is a seven-transmembrane-domain receptor that is expressed in renal epithelial cells, osteoblasts, and some other cells. The N-terminal regions of PTH and PTHrP bind this receptor with equal affinity. Binding of PTH or PTHrP to the receptor results in increased concentrations of both cytoplasmic cAMP and Ca^{2+} by stimulation of adenylate cyclase and the phosphatidylinositol pathways (Abou-Samra et al. 1992; Coleman et al. 1994). The PTH receptor is also located on many cell types, such as dermal fibroblasts, that are not associated with the action of PTH. It is assumed that the receptor functions as the binding protein for PTHrP in these tissues. Therefore, this receptor may be best termed the PTH-PTHrP receptor.

PARATHYROID HORMONE: MECHANISM OF ACTION

The calcium-mobilizing activities of PTH are mediated through the intracellular accumulation of cAMP or Ca^{2+} in target cells (Coleman et al. 1994). Binding of PTH to PTH-PTHrP receptors on target cells results in activation of the receptor, binding of the receptor to stimulatory or inhibitory G-proteins, and stimulation of adenylyl cyclase or phosphatidylinositol hydrolysis in the plasma membrane. Stimulation of adenylyl cyclase stimulates the conversion of ATP to cAMP in target cells. The accumulation of cAMP in target cells functions as an intracellular mediator or second messenger of PTH action to increase permeability for calcium ion. The cytosolic Ca^{2+} concentration may also be increased by the actions of inositol triphosphate to release Ca^{2+} from intracytoplasmic stores or by stimulation of Ca^{2+} transport through transmembrane calcium channels. The resultant increase in cytosol calcium content in combination with cAMP accumulation initiates biochemical reactions in bone cells and renal epithelial cells to conduct the intracellular functions of PTH.

▶ Parathyroid Hormone–Related Protein

PTHrP is not strictly a calcium-regulating hormone, but it was identified in 1982 as an important PTH-like factor that plays a central role in the pathogenesis of humoral hypercalcemia of malignancy (HHM) (Rosol and Capen 1992). Since its discovery, it has become known that PTHrP is produced widely in the body and has numerous actions in the normal fetus and adult animal independent of its role in cancer-associated hypercalcemia (Philbrick et al. 1996). This is in contrast to PTH, which is produced by the parathyroid glands and functions principally in regulation of calcium balance.

Some of the actions of PTHrP involve normal regulation of calcium metabolism (Rosol et al. 1995). For example, PTHrP functions as a calcium-regulating hormone in the fetus and is produced by the fetal parathyroid gland and placenta (MacIsaac et al. 1991b). In the adult, PTHrP circulates in the blood in low concentrations (<1 pM) but is produced by many different tissues and functions principally as a paracrine cellular regulator. PTHrP may play a role in the transport of calcium into milk during lactation. PTHrP acts as an abnormal systemic calcium-regulating hormone and mimics the actions of PTH in patients with HHM (see section on hypercalcemia). PTHrP not only plays a major role in most forms of HHM but also has been demonstrated in many normal tissues including epithelial cells of the skin and other organs; endocrine glands; smooth, skeletal, and cardiac muscle; lactating mammary gland; placenta; fetal parathyroid glands; bone; brain; and lymphocytes (Rosol and Capen 1997; Philbrick et al. 1996). Therefore, PTHrP functions as (1) a hormone in an endocrine manner in the fetus, (2) a paracrine factor in many fetal and adult tissues, and (3) an abnormal hormone in an endocrine manner in adults with HHM (Fig. 6–8).

PTHrP is a 139- to 173-amino-acid peptide originally isolated from human and animal tumors associated with HHM (Rosol and Capen 1992). PTHrP shares 70% sequence homology with PTH in its first 13 amino acids. The N-terminal region of PTHrP (amino acids 1–34) binds and stimulates PTH receptors in bone and kidney cells with affinity equal to that of PTH, so that PTHrP functions similarly to PTH in patients with HHM (Orloff et al. 1994). It is not known whether there is a specific receptor for PTHrP in tissues other than bone and kidney; however, the middle and C-terminal regions of PTHrP have functions that are independent of its PTH-like effects. Therefore, PTHrP is a polyhormone with multiple biologically active regions the functions of which depend on enzymatic processing of PTHrP in the serum or tissue of origin (Mallette 1994). The midregion of PTHrP is responsible for stimulating Ca^{2+} uptake by the fetal placenta (MacIsaac et al. 1991b) and the C-terminal region can inhibit osteoclastic bone resorption (Fenton et al. 1991).

The complementary DNA for canine PTHrP has been cloned and sequenced (Rosol et al. 1995). The sequence of the canine PTHrP cDNA indicated that the dog PTHrP gene is more closely related to the human PTHrP

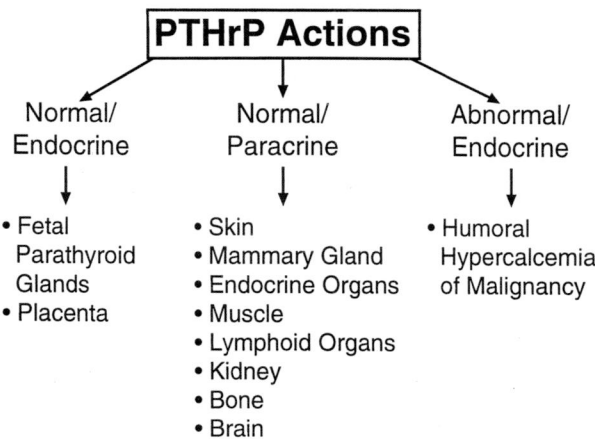

FIGURE 6–8. Actions of parathyroid hormone–related protein (PTHrP).

gene than are the PTHrP genes in rats, mice, and chickens. The coding region of canine PTHrP predicts a 177-amino-acid protein with four regions: signal peptide, N-terminal or PTH-like region, midregion, and C-terminal region (Orloff et al. 1994; Burtis 1992). The deduced amino acid sequence of the N-terminal region of the mature protein (amino acids 1–36) is identical in four mammalian species (dog, human, rat, and mouse) and there is a high degree of homology of the midregion of PTHrP in these species (Rosol et al. 1995; Suva et al. 1987; Yasuda et al. 1989; Mangin et al. 1990). The high degree of interspecies homology indicates the importance of the N-terminus and midregion in the function of PTHrP.

There is less homology of the C-terminal region of canine PTHrP with that from other species. The function of the C-terminal region is unknown. It has been reported that PTHrP (107–111) and PTHrP (107–139) inhibit osteoclastic bone resorption (Fenton et al. 1991). Increased urine concentrations of C-terminal PTHrP have been demonstrated in humans and mice with cancer-associated hypercalcemia (Imamura et al. 1991; Kasahara et al. 1992). The circulating concentrations of the C-terminal peptide are increased in patients with renal failure (Burtis et al. 1990). This mimics the finding of increased C-terminal PTH in the serum of patients with renal failure and indicates that the kidney is an important site of excretion of C-terminal PTHrP and that C-terminal PTHrP may have a longer serum half-life than N-terminal or midregion PTHrP.

Parathyroid Hormone–Related Protein in the Fetus

Fetuses maintain higher concentrations of serum Ca^{2+} than their dams. Fetal parathyroid glands produce low levels of PTH, and the mechanism for maintaining increased serum Ca^{2+} concentrations in fetuses was unknown until recently (Care 1991). Investigations have demonstrated that PTHrP functions to maintain Ca^{2+} balance in the fetus (MacIsaac et al. 1991a, 1991b). It is the major hormone secreted by fetal parathyroid chief cells, and its production by the placenta stimulates Ca^{2+} uptake by the fetus. Thyroparathyroidectomy of sheep fetuses resulted in a reduction in fetal serum Ca^{2+} concentration and reduced placental transport of Ca^{2+} (MacIsaac et al. 1991b). The midregion of PTHrP is the most active portion that stimulates Ca^{2+} and Mg^{2+} transport by the placenta.

▶ Vitamin D

Vitamin D (calciferol) is classified as a secosteroid hormone (Horst and Reinhardt 1997). The cholecalciferol (parent vitamin D_3 of animal origin) metabolites 25-hydroxyvitamin D_3 (calcidiol), 1,25-dihydroxyvitamin D_3 (calcitriol), and 24,25-dihydroxyvitamin D_3 are the most important of at least 30 metabolites. In domestic mammals, the same three metabolites derived from vitamin D_2 (ergocalciferol of plant origin) are equally bioactive, so generic use of the terms 1,25-dihydroxyvitamin D and calcitriol is assumed to include metabolites of vitamin D_3 or D_2 derived from animal or plant origin, respectively. The 25-hydroxyvitamin D that is produced in liver is the major circulating form of vitamin D (Gascon-Barré 1997) and serves as a pool for further activation by 1α-hydroxylation or catabolism by 24-hydroxylation (Henry 1997; Omdahl and May 1997). Only 25-hydroxylation and 1α-hydroxylation are important in the function of vitamin D (DeLuca et al. 1990).

Synthesis

The requirement for vitamin D can be met by consumption of vitamin D_2 or D_3 or by synthesis of vitamin D_3 (cholecalciferol) in the skin. Cholecalciferol is synthesized in the skin from 7-dehydrocholesterol after exposure to ultraviolet light. 7-Dehydrocholesterol forms previtamin D_3 in the presence of ultraviolet B light at 288 nm, followed by further thermal conversion from previtamin D_3 to vitamin D_3 (Holick 1997). Dogs and cats inefficiently photosynthesize vitamin D in their skin and consequently are dependent on vitamin D in their diet (How et al. 1994). Vitamin D ingested in the diet is absorbed intact from the intestine.

Vitamin D–binding protein is an α_2-globulin and transports vitamin D to the liver and other target sites (Cooke and Haddad 1997) (Fig. 6–9). Hydroxylation of vitamin D occurs in the liver to produce 25-hydroxyvitamin D (calcidiol). This hydroxylation reaction is not tightly regulated, and the 25-hydroxylase activity is not influenced by calcium or phosphorus (Gascon-Barré 1997). Calcidiol does not have any known action in normal animals (DeLuca et al. 1990), but during vitamin D intoxication high levels of calcidiol are produced by the liver and can induce hypercalcemia (see section on hypercalcemia and hypervitaminosis D).

The most important step in bioactivation of vitamin D occurs as 25-hydroxyvitamin D is further hydroxylated to calcitriol in the proximal tubule of the kidney (Henry 1997). This reaction is tightly regulated by ionic and hormonal control mechanisms that modulate the activity of the hydroxylase enzyme systems (Fig. 6–10). The two principal enzyme systems involved are 25-hydroxyvitamin D-1α-hydroxylase (resulting in active calcitriol formation) and 25-hydroxyvitamin D–24R-hydroxylase (the first step of catabolism to inactive vitamin D metabolites). The activities of these enzymes are reciprocally regulated (Henry 1997; Omdahl and May 1997).

The 1α-hydroxylase enzyme activity is localized within mitochondria of the convoluted and portions of the straight proximal tubule of the kidney. Little extrarenal 1α-hydroxylation of 25-hydroxyvitamin D occurs in other tissues except in human and rat placenta and skin and in some lymphoproliferative disorders (Dusso et al. 1990; Adams 1997). The 24-hydroxylation can also metabolize calcitriol, generating 1,24,25-trihydroxyvitamin D as the first step in the major catabolic pathway of calcitriol to biologically inactive calcitroic acid (Horst and Reinhardt 1997). Several inactive vitamin D catabolites are excreted through the bile into feces; less than 4% is excreted into urine (DeLuca et al. 1990).

DISORDERS OF CALCIUM

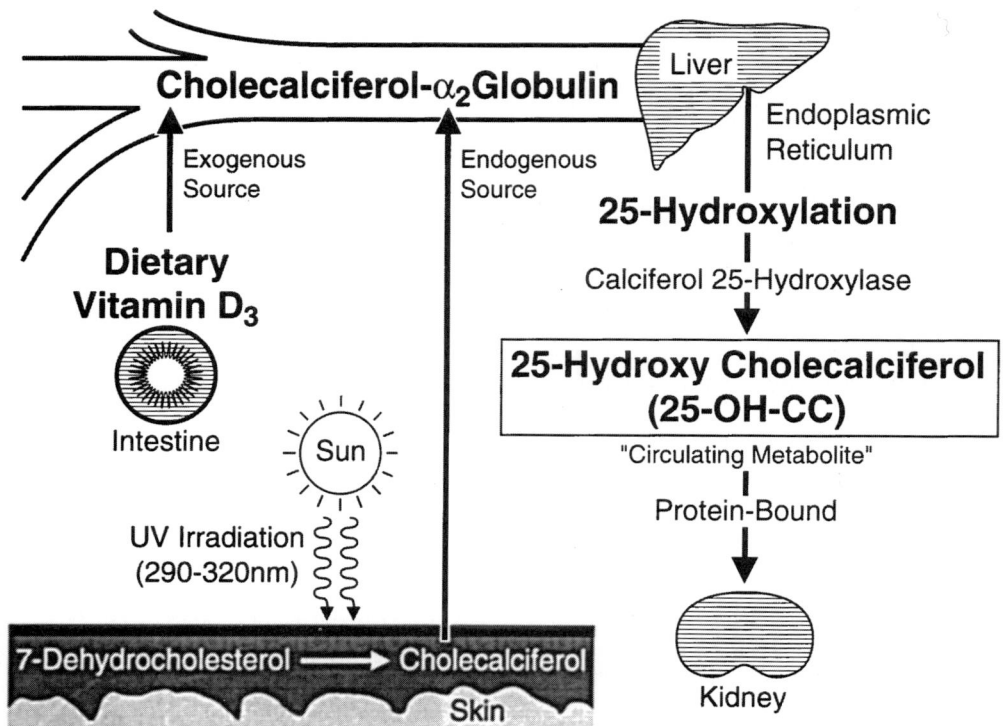

FIGURE 6-9. Metabolism of vitamin D. The initial step of metabolic activation of vitamin D_3 from endogenous (photoactivation) and dietary sources is in the liver to form 25-hydroxycholecalciferol (25-hydroxyvitamin D_3).

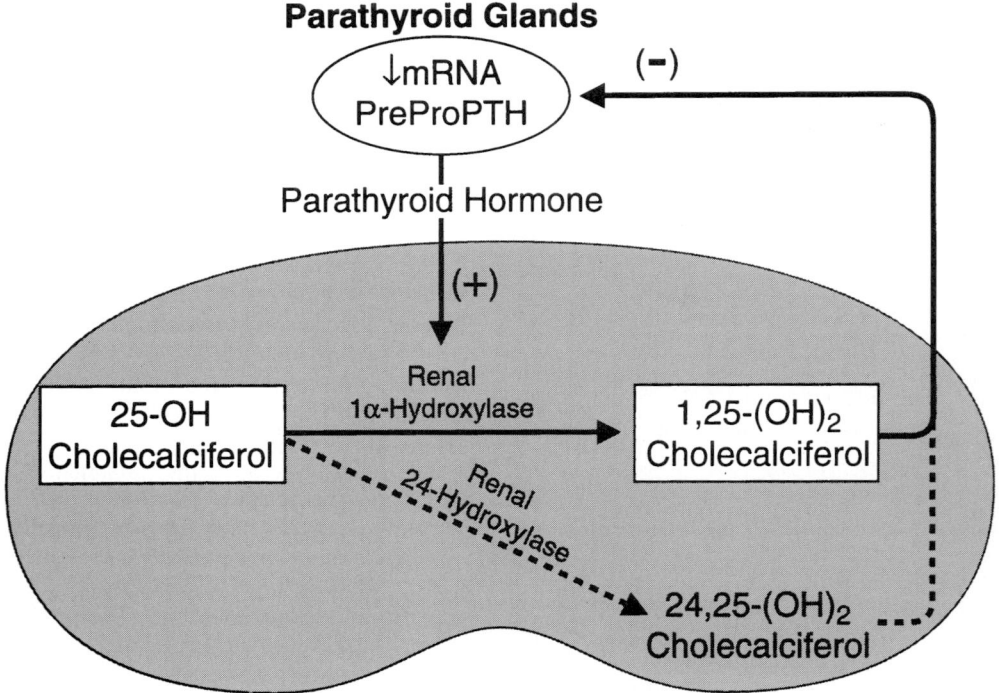

FIGURE 6-10. Parathyroid hormone increases renal synthesis of 1,25-dihydroxycholecalciferol (calcitriol) by stimulating the 1α-hydroxylase activity in renal epithelial cells that converts 25-hydroxycholecalciferol to 1,25-dihydroxycholecalciferol. Negative feedback is exerted by 1,25-dihydroxycholecalciferol (calcitriol) on parathyroid chief cells to decrease the rate of PTH synthesis and secretion, which in turn diminishes the rate of formation of 1,25-dihydroxycholecalciferol. Calcitriol also directly suppresses synthesis of the renal 1α-hydroxylase enzyme.

STIMULATION OF CALCITRIOL SYNTHESIS

Serum PTH, calcitriol, phosphorus, and calcium concentrations are the principal regulators for renal calcitriol synthesis (Henry 1997). Chronic changes in serum calcium concentration regulate the synthesis of calcitriol, and some studies suggests that these changes can override signals from serum phosphorus and PTH concentrations (Hulter et al. 1985).

Deficiencies of phosphorus, calcium, and calcitriol lead to increased calcitriol formation (Nagode et al. 1992). Low calcium or calcitriol concentrations lead to increased serum PTH concentrations. In the kidney, PTH mediates dephosphorylation of renal ferredoxin (renoredoxin) and results in increased synthesis of calcitriol (Siegel et al. 1996). Renoredoxin is the regulatory constituent of the 1α-hydroxylase enzyme system and is inhibited by phosphorylation in the presence of high concentrations of phosphorus or calcium in the renal tubule (Henry 1997; Nagode et al. 1992).

Several drugs and hormones have effects on vitamin D metabolism, some of which are stimulatory (Bowman and Epstein 1997). Hypocalcemia and calcitonin directly stimulate 1α-hydroxylation independent of PTH (Breslan 1998). Estrogens increase calcitriol synthesis after up-regulation of PTH receptors in the kidney (Breslau 1998), and testosterone may also increase calcitriol synthesis (Zelikovic and Chesney 1989). Reduced dietary calcium intake can lead to stimulation of renal 1α-hydroxylase in the absence of detectable hypocalcemia (Zelikovic and Chesney 1989).

INHIBITION OF CALCITRIOL SYNTHESIS

Calcitriol synthesis is inhibited by calcitriol, hypercalcemia, and phosphate loading (Henry 1997; Breslau 1988). Calcium directly and indirectly inhibits calcitriol synthesis (Favus and Langman 1986). The indirect action is due to inhibition of PTH synthesis and secretion. The inhibitory effects of high concentrations of phosphorus on calcitriol synthesis are particularly powerful and important (Nagode et al. 1996). The inhibitory effects of chronic hypercalcemia can override the stimulatory effects of increased PTH concentrations in calcitriol production, as may occur in hypercalcemic disorders (e.g., primary hyperparathyroidism) (Hulter et al. 1989).

Actions of Calcitriol

Calcitriol (1,25-dihydroxyvitamin D) is the only natural form of vitamin D with significant biologic activity (Reichel et al. 1989). It is approximately 1000 times as effective as parent vitamin D and 500 times as effective as its precursor calcidiol (25-hydroxyvitamin D) in binding to the natural calcitriol receptor (VDR) in target cells. Calcitriol binds with great avidity to its receptor, in part because it has three reactive hydroxyl groups, as compared with the single hydroxyl group of cholecalciferol and the two hydroxyl groups of 25-hydroxyvitamin D (Nagode and Chew 1991). Calcitriol increases serum calcium and phosphorus concentrations. Its major target organ for these effects is the intestine (Wasserman 1997). However, there is also an important contribution from bone (Suda and Takahashi 1997), and calcitriol stimulates the kidney to reabsorb both calcium and phosphorus from the glomerular filtrate. Calcitriol has multiple indirect effects on calcium balance, including up-regulation of calcitriol receptors in patients with uremia, regulation of PTH synthesis and secretion by the parathyroid gland, and prevention or reversal of parathyroid gland hyperplasia in the uremic patient (Waser et al. 1997; Nagode et al. 1992; Fukagawa et al. 1997).

In addition to its role in calcium metabolism, calcitriol has effects in many other tissues, where it functions as a regulator of cell differentiation (Walters 1997). The VDR is present in many tissues in addition to bone, kidney, intestine, and parathyroid gland (Haussler et al. 1997). Vitamin D receptors are present in pancreatic islet cells, mammary gland, keratinocytes, fibroblasts of the skin, ovary, epithelial cells, and Sertoli cells. The importance of calcitriol in a tissue is proportional to the abundance of the VDR in the cells. Intestinal epithelial cells and parathyroid gland chief cells have high concentrations of VDR, which are regulated by dietary calcium and phosphorus (Krishnan and Feldman 1997).

The VDR proteins have a molecular mass of 50,000 to 60,000 daltons, have a high affinity for calcitriol, and are stereospecific for calcitriol (Pike 1997). Investigations have identified genetic variants of the VDR that have caused controversy about the role of vitamin D in the pathogenesis of osteoporosis or the risk of prostate cancer in humans (Morrison 1997; Taylor et al. 1996; Feldman 1997).

Calcitriol initially dissociates from its serum binding protein, diffuses across the cell and nuclear membranes, and binds in the nucleus with its receptor. The calcitriol-receptor complex interacts heterodimerically with the retinoid X receptor (RXR) and then binds with nuclear DNA to regulate gene transcription (Haussler et al. 1998). In a few instances, such as in the parathyroid gland, calcitriol functions as a genetic repressor rather than gene activator, and no RXR receptor heterodimerization occurs (Mackey et al. 1996).

EFFECTS OF CALCITRIOL ON THE INTESTINE

Calcitriol enhances the transport of calcium and phosphate from the intestinal lumen to plasma across the enterocyte (Wasserman 1997). Energy in the form of ATP is required to transport calcium from the enterocytes into the blood and to absorb phosphate from the intestinal lumen. Calcitriol induces synthesis of the plasma membrane calcium pump (ATPase) that removes calcium from the enterocytes (Pannabecker et al. 1995) and the Na^+-phosphate cotransport protein that transports phosphorus into the enterocyte. Na^+-phosphate cotransport requires an Na^+ gradient established by the Na^+,K^+-ATPase that serves as the energy source for phosphorus absorption (Wasserman 1997). In addition, calcitriol increases the brush border permeability to calcium and induces the synthesis of calbindin-D (28k and 9k), which ferries calcium from the submicrovillar terminal web to the basolateral membrane of enterocytes for extrusion by both the calcium ATPase and the Na^+-Ca^{2+} exchanger (Christakos et al. 1997; Thomasset 1997). Calbindins serve as buffers to protect enterocytes from toxic concentrations of calcium ion while ferrying calcium across the cell (Wasserman 1997). Evidence suggests that calbindin-D (28k) may, like calmodulin, serve as an allosteric activator of the plasma membrane calcium ATPase, which amplifies the effect of calcitriol on transport of calcium in intestine (Wasserman 1997). Calcitriol also directly stimulates rapid calcium transport (transcaltachia) across the enterocyte (Norman 1997). Normal dogs have a progressive decrease in the number of calcitriol receptors and calbindin concentrations that regulate the efficiency of calcium absorption in enterocytes from the duodenum to the ileum (Korkor et al. 1985). Longer transit times in certain portions of the intestinal tract (e.g., ileum) can still lead to significant calcium absorption in spite of low transport efficiency (Wasserman 1997).

EFFECTS OF CALCITRIOL ON BONE

Calcitriol is necessary for bone formation and mineralization because it ensures an adequate source of calcium and phosphorus from the intestinal tract. Deficiencies in vitamin D lead to impaired bone growth, such as rickets in growing animals and osteomalacia in adults (Rosol and Capen 1997). Calcitriol is necessary for normal bone development and growth because it regulates the production of multiple bone proteins produced by osteoblasts, including alkaline phosphatase, collagen type I, osteocalcin, and osteopontin (St. Arnaud and Glorieux 1997; Aubin and Heersche 1997). The action of calcitriol in osteoblasts is dependent on the stage of osteoblast differentiation. Calcitriol is also necessary for normal bone resorption because it promotes differentiation of monocytic hematopoietic precursors in the bone marrow into osteoclasts (Suda and Takahashi 1997). This relationship between calcitriol and osteoclasts explains the dependence of PTH on calcitriol for optimal bone resorption (Nagode et al. 1992). In pharmacologic doses, calcitriol can directly stimulate bone resorption and hypercalcemia by inducing osteoblasts to secrete factors that activate osteoclasts. This can be a potential side effect of calcitriol therapy. Osteoblasts, but not osteoclasts, contain the vitamin D receptor. Other vitamin D metabolites, such as 24,25-dihydroxyvitamin D, have been studied with respect to bone, but their direct effects in bone remain controversial (Tanaka and Seino 1997).

EFFECTS OF CALCITRIOL ON THE KIDNEY

An important effect of calcitriol in the kidney is direct inhibition of 25-hydroxyvitamin D–1α-hydroxylase in the renal tubule, preventing overproduction of calcitriol (Reichel et al. 1989). In addition, calcitriol facilitates calcium and phosphorus reabsorption from the glomerular filtrate (Kumar 1997). Calcitriol induces the synthesis of calbindins in renal tubular cells that activate the plasma membrane calcium pump. Therefore, calcitriol works together with PTH to conserve urinary calcium. The type 2 Na^+-phosphate cotransport proteins in the brush border of renal epithelial cells are also induced by calcitriol, but this effect is antagonized by PTH (Hruska et al. 1997).

EFFECTS OF CALCITRIOL ON THE PARATHYROID GLAND

Calcitriol and PTH participate in an endocrine feedback loop that is important for calcium homeostasis. Calcitriol inhibits the production of PTH in the parathyroid gland by direct and indirect means (Silver and Naveh-Many 1997; Sherwood et al. 1987). Binding of calcitriol to its receptor in parathyroid chief cells directly inhibits PTH synthesis, thereby providing a short loop for negative feedback. Second, calcitriol stimulates intestinal calcium absorption, which indirectly reduces PTH secretion by increasing serum Ca^{2+} concentration and provides a long loop for negative feedback. Calcitriol suppression of PTH synthesis is dose dependent and occurs before serum Ca^{2+} concentration is increased by the delayed effects of calcitriol on intestinal calcium transport (Slatopolsky et al. 1990). Calcitriol may be considered the primary controlling factor for transcription of the PTH gene and subsequent synthesis of PTH because suppression of PTH synthesis cannot occur in the absence of calcitriol even in the presence of hypercalcemia (Silver and Naveh-Many 1997; Nagode et al. 1992) (see Fig. 6–6). Secretion of PTH decreases 12 to 24 h after exposure to calcitriol. Whereas calcitriol is a negative regulator of PTH, PTH stimulates renal calcitriol synthesis.

Long-standing calcitriol deficiency results in chief cell hypertrophy and hyperplasia, demonstrating that calcitriol is important in limiting cellular proliferation in the parathyroid gland (Silver and Naveh-Many 1997). Calcitriol treatment of uremia in dogs and humans has resulted in regression of parathyroid gland hyperplasia (Nagode and Chew 1991; Fukagawa et al. 1997).

▶ Calcitonin

Calcitonin is a 32-amino-acid polypeptide hormone that is synthesized by C cells in the thyroid gland (Rosol and Capen 1997; Mol et al. 1991). An important role of calcitonin is to limit the degree of postprandial hypercalcemia. This effect, in concert with PTH, acts to maintain serum Ca^{2+} concentration within a narrow range. Calcitonin is secreted in response to hypercalcemia and also to a calcium-rich meal. Calcitonin secretion increases during hypercalcemia, but the effects of calcitonin on normal calcium homeostasis are considered to be minor. The major target site for calcitonin is bone, where it inhibits osteoclastic bone resorption. The effects of calcitonin in bone are transitory, which has limited the usefulness of calcitonin as a treatment for hypercalcemia. At high doses, calcitonin may promote urinary calcium excretion (Brown 1991).

▶ Normal Homeostatic Response to Hypocalcemia

Hypocalcemia elicits corrective responses that are mediated by PTH and calcitriol (Rosol and Capen 1997). Acute effects occur in seconds to minutes, subacute effects occur over several hours, and chronic effects occur over days to weeks. A marked increase in PTH secretion occurs in response to mild hypocalcemia (see earlier discussion of set-point), and this response occurs in seconds. Acute secretion of preformed PTH can maintain PTH concentrations for 1 to 1.5 h during hypocalcemia. Hypocalcemia decreases the proportion of PTH that is degraded in the parathyroid chief cells, making more hormone available for secretion. This effect is relatively rapid (approximately at 40 min). During increased PTH secretion, renal calcium reabsorption and phosphorus excretion are increased within minutes, whereas bone mobilization of calcium and phosphate occurs within 1 to 2 h.

After several hours (or more) of hypocalcemia, increased PTH secretion stimulates the synthesis and secretion of calcitriol. Increased intestinal transport of calcium and phosphorus into blood follows, providing an external source of calcium in addition to the internal mobilization from bone. Hypocalcemia increases transcription of the PTH gene and synthesis of PTH mRNA, enhancing the ability of the chief cells to produce PTH. This effect also occurs within hours of hypocalcemia. Over days or weeks of hypocalcemia, further increases in PTH secretion are achieved largely by hypertrophy and hyperplasia of chief cells in the parathyroid gland (Roth and Capen 1974). In addition, the proportion of chief cells actively synthesizing PTH is increased.

▶ Normal Homeostatic Response to Hypercalcemia

Most of the effects that occur during hypercalcemia are the opposite of those described earlier for hypocalcemia (Rosol and Capen 1997). Hypercalcemia results in decreased PTH secretion, increased intracellular degradation of PTH in chief cells, and decreased PTH synthesis. Increased calcitonin secretion is stimulated in an attempt to minimize the magnitude of hypercalcemia. In addition, hyperplasia of C cells in the thyroid gland results if the hypercalcemic stimulus is sustained, but this mechanism is ineffective for controlling hypercalcemia because of the transitory effect of calcitonin on osteoclastic bone resorption (Rosol and Capen 1989; Okada et al. 1994). Calcitriol synthesis is decreased both through direct inhibition by Ca^{2+} and as a result of decreased stimulation because of decreased PTH concentration.

▶ Diagnostics

Table 6–1 lists normal values for serum total calcium (Chew and Meuten 1982), ionized calcium (Chew et al. 1989), PTH (Nagode and Chew 1991; Torrance and Nachreiner 1989), PTHrP (Rosol et al. 1992), and vitamin D metabolites that are useful in the diagnostic work-up of patients with calcium disorders (Rosol and Capen 1997).

Total Calcium

Despite the fact that only the ionized calcium fraction is physiologically active, the calcium status of animals is usually based on evaluation of the total serum calcium concentration. Reliable methods for directly measuring ionized calcium concentration are available in most clinical pathology diagnostic laboratories. Proper sample handling is necessary for accurate measurement of Ca^{2+} (see later). The total serum calcium concentration has been assumed to be directly proportional to ionized calcium. In many clinical conditions this is a valid assumption, but it may lead to erroneous interpretation of laboratory data in some instances.

TABLE 6–1. Normal Serum Concentrations

	Dog	Cat
Total calcium		
(mg/dL)	9.0–11.5	8.0–10.5
(mmol/L)	2.2–3.8	2.0–2.6
Ionized calcium		
(mg/dL)	5.0–6.0	4.5–5.5
(mmol/L)	1.2–1.5	1.1–1.4
Parathyroid hormone		
Intact (pmol/L)	2–13*	0–4*
N-terminal (pg/mL)	15–55	8–28
Parathyroid hormone–related protein (PTHrP) (pmol/L) (intact or N-terminal)	<2	<2
25-Hydroxyvitamin D (calcidiol) (nmol/L)	82–285*	
1,25-Dihydroxyvitamin D (calcitriol) (pg/mL)		
Adults	20–50	20–40
10–12 wk old	60–120	20–80

*Data from Endocrine Diagnostic Section, Animal Health Diagnostic Laboratory, Lansing, MI.

ANALYTICAL METHODS

Fasting serum or heparinized plasma samples should be submitted for analysis. Oxalate, citrate, and EDTA anticoagulants should not be used, because calcium is bound to these chemicals and becomes unavailable for analysis (Woo and Cannon 1984).

Total serum calcium concentrations vary with the method employed. Isotope dilution with subsequent mass spectrometry constitutes the definitive method for calcium measurement but is not readily available (Fraser et al. 1986). Atomic absorption spectrophotometry is another reference method that requires special equipment and technical skills (Fraser et al. 1987) and is provided by some commercial laboratories.

For the clinical determination of total serum calcium concentration, simple colorimetric reactions and spectrophotometry are usually employed using automated or manual methods. *Ortho*-cresophthalein complexone is a metal dye that is commonly used to form a color complex with calcium. This method is considered accurate and reproducible (Fraser et al. 1987). Hemolysis can result in formation of an interfering hemoglobin-chromagen complex that falsely increases measured calcium concentration, and some methods include corrective procedures to account for this error (128). High concentrations of bilirubin falsely decrease calcium concentrations, and acetaminophen and hydralazine falsely increase serum total calcium concentration. Lipemia can result in spuriously high calcium concentrations (Meuten 1984), with values exceeding 20 mg/dL in some instances of severe lipemia.

Potentiometry using ion-specific calcium electrodes can also be used to measure total serum calcium concentration after liberation of protein-bound and complexed calcium by sample acidification. Ion-specific electrodes are discussed further in the discussion of ionized calcium measurement. Potentiometric methods are not affected by lipemia. There is a strong positive correlation between total serum calcium concentrations measured by colorimetry and those measured by potentiometry (Chew and Carothers 1989). Concentrations obtained by potentiometry are often slightly lower than those obtained by colorimetry by as much as 1 mg/dL.

NORMAL VALUES

The range for total serum calcium concentration in normal dogs and cats is wide and varies among laboratories (see Table 6–1). Each laboratory should establish normal values. Variability may result from differences in age, diet, duration of fasting before sampling, and time of sampling, in addition to differences in analytical method. Repeated calcium concentrations vary much less than concentrations in samples obtained from different individuals.

Normal total serum calcium concentrations in mature dogs and cats are approximately 10.0 and 9.0 mg/dL, respectively. No difference in total serum calcium concentration has been ascribed to breed or sex in normal dogs and cats, but an effect of aging has been observed in the dog (Chew and Meuten 1982; Hazewinkel 1991). Dogs younger than 3 months of age have slightly higher mean serum calcium concentrations (approximately 11.0 mg/dL) than those for dogs older than 1 year (approximately 10.0 mg/dL), probably because of normal bone growth. In a small percentage of normal young dogs, total serum calcium concentrations may be greater than 12.0 mg/dL and as high as 15.0 mg/dL (Ralston-Purina, 1975). Dietary calcium, phosphorus, and vitamin D supplementation should be evaluated in dogs with serum calcium concentrations greater than 12.0 mg/dL.

ADJUSTED TOTAL CALCIUM

It has been reported that total serum calcium concentrations should be "corrected" or "adjusted" relative to the total serum protein or albumin concentration in order to improve diagnostic interpretation (Meuten et al. 1982; Finco 1983). Such correction seems logical because binding of serum calcium to protein is substantial and 80 to 90% of the calcium bound to proteins is bound to albumin. The correlation between total serum calcium and serum albumin or total protein concentrations was moderate, and adjustment formulas were developed for use in dogs older than 1 year. Total serum calcium concentration in dogs is partially dependent on serum albumin or total protein content but can be standardized using one of the following formulas (Meuten et al. 1982):

$$\text{Adjusted Ca (mg/dL)} = \text{Ca (mg/dL)} - \text{albumin (g/dL)} + 3.5$$

or

$$\text{Adjusted Ca (mg/dL)} = \text{Ca (mg/dL)} - 0.4[\text{total serum protein (g/dL)}] + 3.3$$

The formula based on albumin is preferred because of the stronger relationship between serum albumin and total calcium concentrations. The formulas are not appropriate for use in young dogs (6 to 24 weeks old) because high values may be obtained (Meuten et al. 1982). Also, the formulas should not be used for cats because there is no linear relationship between serum total calcium and serum albumin and total protein concentrations in this species (Flanders et al. 1989).

Application of the correction formula is most helpful for patients with hypoproteinemia or hypoalbuminemia. In the absence of direct ionized calcium measurements, an advantage of the adjusted calcium concentration is identification of physiologic hypercalcemia or hypocalcemia, previously unrecognized because of the masking effect of serum proteins. It has been assumed that total serum calcium concentrations that correct into the normal range are associated with normal serum ionized calcium concentration. Likewise, samples with values that fail to correct into the normal range are presumed to have abnormal serum ionized calcium concentrations. These formulas, however, were developed without verification by serum ionized calcium measurements. Correction of total serum calcium concentration for albumin did not improve the correlation between serum total and ionized calcium concentrations (Mischke et al. 1996). Despite this, use of the correction formulas with data for dogs has been clinically helpful in deciding whether a primary disorder of calcium metabolism exists or an abnormal total serum calcium concentration can be attributed to altered serum albumin or total protein concentrations.

Ionized Calcium

Ionized calcium is the biologically active form of calcium and its homeostasis is important for many physiologic functions (Rosol and Capen 1997). Calcium ion regulates its own homeostasis directly by binding to cell membrane receptors specific for Ca^{2+} (Brown and Hebert 1997). The cell membrane calcium receptors are present in parathyroid chief cells and C cells of the thyroid gland, in which Ca^{2+} regulates PTH and calcitonin secretion, respectively. In addition, calcium receptors are present on renal tubular cells, and Ca^{2+} directly regulates its own tubular reabsorption rate. Therefore, serum Ca^{2+} concentration is controlled by many interacting feedback loops that involve Ca^{2+}, phosphate, PTH, calcitriol, and calcitonin. These mechanisms help maintain serum Ca^{2+} concentration in a narrow range for normal function of the body.

Measurement of total calcium concentration is more readily available than ionized calcium measurement, but it may not always reflect the ionized calcium concentration of the patient. In many clinical conditions, however, the total calcium concentration can be used as an indirect measure of the ionized calcium concentration. In dogs with lymphoma and hypercalcemia, serum ionized and total calcium concentrations correlated well, and serum ionized calcium measurement was not an advantage over total calcium measurement (Teachout et al. 1997). In contrast, some dogs with lymphoma and ionized hypercalcemia may have normal serum total calcium concentrations. Mild hypercalcemia can be overlooked in these patients without measurement of serum ionized calcium concentration. In cats, serum ionized calcium concentrations were only moderately correlated with total serum calcium concentrations (Deniz and Mischke 1997). It is ideal to measure serum ionized calcium concentration directly, and these measurements may be superior to total calcium measurements in hyperparathyroidism, renal disease, hypo- and hyperproteinemia, acid-base disturbances, and critical illnesses (Gosling 1986; Zaloga et al. 1987). In humans with disorders of calcium balance, measurement of total serum calcium concentrations failed to predict serum ionized calcium concentrations in 31% of all patients (Thode et al. 1989) and in 26% of patients with renal disease (Burritt et al. 1980). Changes in the magnitude of serum protein concentration, individual protein binding capacity and affinity, serum pH, and complexed calcium all interact to determine the ionized calcium concentration, independent of the total calcium concentration. Effects of circadian rhythm, gender, and dietary calcium have not been critically evaluated in veterinary medicine. Consequently, fasting serum samples collected at the same time in the morning are advised.

ANALYTICAL METHODS

Evaluation of calcium homeostasis in animals has been limited largely to determination of total serum calcium concentration. Improved instrumentation has permitted serum ionized calcium concentration to be measured more routinely. Use of automated equipment with a calcium ion-selective electrode allows easy and accurate measurement of ionized calcium in blood, plasma, or serum (Bowers et al. 1986). New electrodes have been developed that minimize interference by other ions (e.g., magnesium, lithium, potassium), protein, or hemolysis (Gouget et al. 1988). Nevertheless, differences among analyzers exist, and it is recommended that reference ranges be established for each analyzer (Hristova et al. 1995).

SAMPLE HANDLING TECHNIQUES

The accurate determination of ionized calcium concentration requires that samples be collected and processed anaerobically to ensure that no increase in pH occurs because of loss of CO_2. The pH of blood or serum has a significant effect on serum ionized calcium concentration. Acidic pH favors dissociation of calcium from protein and increases the amount of ionized calcium in the sample. Alkaline pH occurs with loss of CO_2 and favors calcium binding to protein, thus decreasing the amount of ionized calcium. Samples must be collected and handled anaerobically because mixing serum and air results in increased pH and decreased ionized calcium, because of loss of CO_2 from the sample (Schenck et al. 1995). Ionized calcium concentration can be determined in whole blood, serum, or plasma. Heparinized canine blood provided stable ionized calcium measurements when stored up to 9 h at 4°C, but pH was significantly increased after 3 h (Szenci et al. 1991). In practice, it may be impossible to analyze the sample within this time period, especially if the sample must be sent to a reference laboratory. The amount and type of heparin used for whole blood or plasma samples may also affect the measurement of ionized calcium, usually by displacing calcium from protein (Lyon et al. 1995).

Ionized calcium and pH are more stable in serum than in whole or heparinized blood. The analysis of serum eliminates the potential interference of heparin and allows longer storage period before analysis. Serum may be stored for subsequent ionized calcium analysis as long as it has been handled anaerobically. Silicone separator tubes should not be used; the ionized calcium concentration was increased in serum separated by use of silicone separator tubes because of release of calcium from the silicone gel (Larsson and Ohman 1985). Measured ionized calcium in canine and equine serum was stable after storage for 72 h at 23 or 4°C and for 7 days at 4°C (Schenck et al. 1995, 1996). Use of serum collected anaerobically and stored at 4°C allows sufficient time for shipment to a reference laboratory for measurement of ionized calcium.

NORMAL VALUES

The range for serum ionized calcium concentration in normal dogs and cats varies among laboratories but is approximately 5.1 to 5.8 mg/dL in adult dogs (Schenck et al. 1996) and 4.6 to 5.4 mg/dL in adult cats (Deniz and Mischke 1995). An effect of aging has been observed in both the dog and cat. Young dogs and cats (up to 2 years of age) have serum ionized calcium concentrations that are 0.1 to 0.4 mg/dL higher than those reported in older animals (Mischke et al. 1996; Deniz and Mischke 1995). Normal values should be established for each laboratory on the basis of age of animal, type of sample, and analyzer used.

CORRECTION OR STANDARDIZATION OF IONIZED CALCIUM TO pH

Some instruments mathematically manipulate the ionized calcium concentration and actual pH value of the sample and yield an adjusted value for ionized calcium concentration that theoretically would occur at a pH of 7.4. These correction formulas were developed for use in humans and are based on the assumption that pH and ionized calcium concentration change in a predictable inverse logarithmic manner. Corrected ionized calcium concentrations have not been advocated for use in humans because insight into the pathophysiology of the patient is gained by evaluation of the in vivo ionized calcium concentration and pH (Fraser et al. 1986). This is especially true for patients with renal disease (Rudnicki et al. 1992). Mathematical formulas have also been developed to correct the ionized calcium concentration in samples exposed to air (i.e., with increased pH) to the actual pH of the patient (Lincoln and Lane 1990; Nachreiner and Refsal 1990). These formulas have not been validated for use in small animals. In horses, it was reported that the percentage of ionized calcium in serum did not correlate well with pH (Kohn and Brooks 1990). Therefore, when it is important to evaluate the calcium status of a patient, direct measurement of ionized calcium concentration in a sample handled anaerobically is best.

FRACTIONATION OF SERUM CALCIUM

In addition to measuring the ionized concentration in serum, the protein-bound and complexed fractions of calcium can be quantified using fractionation techniques. Ionized calcium and complexed calcium are diffusible and together are referred to as ultrafilterable calcium. To separate protein-bound from ultrafilterable serum calcium, a micropartition system based on the filtration method has been used (Schenck et al. 1996; Farese et al. 1970). This method was originally developed to estimate the concentration of ionized calcium in serum before the availability of ion-selective electrodes. The micropartition system contains a filter through which ultrafilterable calcium (complexed and ionized) passes. By determining the total serum calcium concentration and subtracting the total calcium concentration of the ultrafilterable fraction, the amount of protein-bound calcium in serum can be calculated. The serum ionized calcium concentration may be measured accurately using an ion-selective electrode, and this amount can be subtracted from the total calcium concentration of the ultrafiltrate to determine the complexed fraction of serum calcium. It is important that serum be collected anaerobically before ultrafiltration to allow accurate measurement of the calcium fractions and to prevent changes in serum pH.

In normal dogs, protein-bound, ionized, and complexed calcium fractions in serum were 34, 56, and 10%, respectively (Schenck et al. 1996). Ultrafilterable calcium (ionized and complexed fractions) in dogs and horses accounted for 66% and 63% of total serum calcium, respectively (Schenck et al. 1996; Holley and Evans 1977). In humans, ultrafilterable calcium accounted for 50% of total serum calcium (Farese et al. 1970). In normal dogs, the ionized calcium fraction has the smallest variation, with larger variations occurring in the protein-bound and complexed fractions. This observation supports the concept that the ionized calcium fraction is tightly regulated and represents the biologically active fraction of serum calcium.

The ultrafiltration method provides a rapid means for fractionating serum calcium and with ionized calcium measurements allows an accurate assessment of the protein-bound and complexed calcium fractions. Biologic roles of these calcium fractions have been suggested, but they have not been assessed in metabolic disorders associated with abnormal calcium concentrations. Measurement of the protein-bound and complexed calcium fractions in addition to the ionized calcium fraction may facilitate detection of disease processes that affect calcium metabolism.

Parathyroid Hormone

Parathyroid hormone circulates predominantly as intact PTH (1–84) and carboxyl-terminal fragments. Only intact PTH is biologically active, and it is best to measure this form in serum or plasma. Samples should be stored and shipped frozen to prevent degradation of intact PTH. Stability is best in plasma collected with EDTA, but serum is adequate if stored frozen after separation from blood. Because of sequence homology of human and animal PTH, commercial assays developed for humans have been used successfully for some veterinary species (Chew et al. 1995). An amino-terminal–specific RIA was used for over 50 mammalian species but is no longer commercially available (Nagode et al. 1992). Newer two-site immunoassays utilize antibodies to amino- and carboxyl-terminal regions of PTH and are very sensitive. The two-site assays have proved useful for some species, including dogs, cats, and horses. A two-site immunoradiometric (IRMA) assay for intact human PTH has been validated in the dog and cat (Torrance and Nachreiner 1989; Barber et al. 1993). In the cat, the assay works best in detection of primary hyperparathyroidism, because sample dilution may be required to avoid the effects of high concentrations of carboxyl-terminal fragments in cats with uremia (Barber et al. 1994). Normal values for serum PTH concentration are 2 to 13, 0 to 4, and 0 to 2 pmol/L in the dog, cat, and horse, respectively (Endocrine Diagnostic Section, Animal Health Diagnostic Laboratory, Lansing, MI). The two-site assays have not proved useful for measurement of PTH in reptiles, such as iguanas or turtles. For the rat and mouse, PTH can be detected by an IRMA that uses two antigenic determinants located on the amino terminus of PTH (Rucinski et al. 1995; Meyer et al. 1994). The commercial IRMA kit previously available for the rat (Nichols Institute Diagnostic, San Juan Capistrano, CA) has worked well for measurement of mouse PTH, but changes in the antibodies have been made and cross-reactivity with mouse PTH must be confirmed. Two-site immunochemiluminometric assays for intact PTH in humans use antibodies similar to those in the intact PTH IRMA assays and have the same range of applicability to animal sera (Michelangeli et al. 1997).

CLINICAL UTILITY OF PTH ASSAYS

Serum PTH concentrations should always be evaluated in relation to simultaneous measurement of serum total or ionized calcium concentration. If the parathyroid glands are normal, hypercalcemia should be associated with a low PTH concentration, whereas a high PTH concentration should occur during hypocalcemia. Serum PTH concentration is increased in most patients with primary hyperparathyroidism related to an adenoma of the chief cells in the parathyroid gland (Rosol et al. 1992). In some animals with primary hyperparathyroidism, serum PTH concentration may be in the high-normal range, and serum ionized calcium concentration may be mildly increased early in the course of disease. This finding represents inappropriate response of PTH to high serum calcium concentration and is suggestive of hyperparathyroidism. Animals with end-stage renal failure and secondary hyperparathyroidism have increased serum PTH concentrations (Nagode and Chew 1991). Humoral hypercalcemia of malignancy may be associated with a low or low-normal PTH concentration (Rosol et al. 1992).

The kidney plays an important role in the degradation and excretion of PTH and normally serves as the major source for clearance of carboxyl-terminal fragments of PTH by glomerular filtration (Kronenberg et al. 1994). Consequently, renal disease creates special problems in the interpretation of serum PTH concentrations. Renal failure markedly impedes the clearance of intact PTH and fragments of PTH by glomerular filtration and decreases the metabolic degradation of intact PTH. Of these two mechanisms, failure to eliminate PTH carboxyl-terminal fragments by glomerular filtration is more important. High concentrations of inactive carboxyl-terminal PTH fragments accumulate in serum to a much greater extent than do intact PTH or amino-terminal fragments (Nagode and Chew 1991). High concentrations of carboxyl-terminal PTH fragments, which occur in cats with CRF, can interfere with intact PTH immunoassays (Barber et al. 1994).

Parathyroid Hormone–Related Protein

Two-site IRMA and N-terminal RIA are available for the measurement of human PTHrP (Bilezikian 1992; Kremer and Goltzman 1994). These assays are useful for measuring biologically active PTHrP in the dog (see later section on cancer-associated hypercalcemia) (Rosol et al. 1992; Chew et al. 1995) because of the high degree of sequence homology of PTHrP between species, especially in the N-terminal 111 amino acids (Burtis 1992). An N-terminal RIA for human PTHrP did not prove useful for measuring circulating PTHrP in a small number of horses (Rosol et al. 1994). PTHrP is susceptible to degradation by serum proteases, and PTHrP concentrations must be measured in fresh or frozen plasma using EDTA as an anticoagulant. The EDTA complexes with plasma calcium, which is required for function of many proteases. The addition of protease inhibitors such as aprotinin and leupeptin may provide further inhibition of proteolysis in plasma (Pandian et al. 1992). Serum is not recommended for measurement of PTHrP; PTHrP concentrations measured in serum are inaccurate because of proteolysis during clotting and sample handling.

The circulating forms of PTHrP are not completely understood because PTHrP rapidly undergoes proteolysis intracellularly and extracellularly after secretion into blood (Pandian et al. 1992). The natural proteolytic cleavage sites of PTHrP (1–141) have not been identified (Orloff et al. 1994; Burtis 1992; Bowden et al. 1993). The forms of PTHrP that are present in vivo include intact PTHrP, an N-terminal peptide, a combined N-terminal and midregion peptide, a midregion peptide, and a C-terminal peptide (Yang et al. 1994; Burtis et al. 1994).

Proteolysis of PTHrP makes proper sample collection and storage important for accurate measurement of circulating PTHrP. The fragments that would be expected to have PTH-like biologic activity in vivo include N-terminal PTHrP (1–36), PTHrP (1–86), and intact PTHrP (1–141). The two-site immunologic assays measure intact PTHrP (1–141) and PTHrP (1–86) because antibodies bind to the N terminus and midregion. The N-terminal RIAs measure intact PTHrP (1–141), PTHrP (1–86), and N-terminal PTHrP (1–36). The C-terminal PTHrP accumulates in the serum of human patients with renal failure, which suggests that C-terminal PTHrP peptides are excreted by the kidney, as occurs with PTH (Burtis et al. 1990).

Vitamin D Metabolites

Measurement of vitamin D metabolites, although not common in veterinary medicine, is occasionally helpful in the diagnosis of disorders of calcium homeostasis (see Table 6-1). 25-Hydroxyvitamin D (calcidiol) and 1,25-dihydroxyvitamin D (calcitriol) are the metabolites of greatest clinical interest for detection of hypovitaminosis D, hypervitaminosis D, and abnormalities of the renal hydroxylase system (e.g., renal failure). The metabolites are stable during refrigeration and freezing, but samples should not be exposed to light for long periods.

The metabolites of vitamin D are chemically identical in all species. Consequently, receptor-binding assays or RIAs developed for use in humans are satisfactory for the measurement of the same metabolites in animals (Horst et al. 1990; Hollis et al. 1996). Assays for calcidiol are more frequently available from commercial laboratories than are assays for calcitriol. Young growing dogs have higher calcitriol concentrations than those in mature dogs, and most mammals appear to share this attribute during rapid growth (Meller et al. 1984). Calcidiol concentrations are a good indicator of vitamin D ingestion or production in vivo and can be use to diagnose hypo- or hypervitaminosis D (vitamin D intoxication) (Carothers et al. 1994). Calcitriol assays can be used to detect genetic errors of vitamin D metabolism, low concentrations of calcitriol in patients with renal failure, or high concentrations of calcitriol in some patients with cancer-associated hypercalcemia (Rosol and Capen 1997).

Bone Biopsy and Bone Marrow Aspiration

Bone biopsy is occasionally useful in the evaluation of disorders of calcium homeostasis. Bone marrow aspiration or core biopsy is frequently part of the diagnostic evaluation of animals without an obvious cause of hypercalcemia. Its greatest utility is in the discovery of lymphoma, myeloproliferative disease, or multiple myeloma. Biopsy of the iliac crest is recommended to standardize the evaluation of a generalized bone process, particularly when histomorphometric analysis is available for the quantitative evaluation of bone formation and bone resorption. A procedure for iliac crest bone biopsy utilizing a trephine has been described for use in the lightly anesthetized dog (Rosol et al. 1992) and in the cat (Ching and Norrdin 1990). Directly biopsy of focal bone lesions may be diagnostic, particularly when such lesions are due to lymphoma, multiple myeloma, or a metastatic bone tumor.

▶ Hypercalcemia

Hypercalcemia is an uncommon but important electrolyte disturbance of dogs and cats. It is much more common in dogs than in cats. Hypercalcemia can serve as a marker of disease or can create disease. Increases in biologically active ionized serum calcium concentration above normal often have adverse pathophysiologic consequences. Hypercalcemia represents a clinically relevant increase above an individual animal's own normal serum calcium concentration, usually defined as a fasting serum total calcium concentration above 12.0 mg/dL in dogs or above 11.0 mg/dL in cats. Ionized calcium measurements can provide greater sensitivity and specificity for the diagnosis of some hypercalcemic disorders. An ionized serum calcium concentration above 6.0 mg/dL in dogs and above 5.5 mg/dL in cats constitutes ionized hypercalcemia.

Mechanisms and Differential Diagnosis of Hypercalcemia

Increased entry of calcium into ECF, decreased egress of calcium from ECF, reduced plasma volume, or a combination of these factors must occur for hypercalcemia to develop (Fig. 6–11). Increased calcium input can arise from increased intestinal absorption, increased bone resorption, or increased renal tubular reabsorption of calcium. Decreased glomerular filtration and decreased bone accretion result in decreased egress of calcium from ECF. Volume contraction is common in the presence of hypercalcemia because of the effects of anorexia, vomiting, and obligatory polyuria. The mechanisms of hypercalcemia vary with the specific causes, but much attention has been focused on the importance of increased bone resorption.

Table 6–2 provides a list of possibilities in the differential diagnosis for hypercalcemia by category. Characterization of the hypercalcemia as transient or persistent, pathologic or nonpathologic, mild or severe, progressive or static, and acute or chronic is helpful in determining its cause. Persistent, pathologic hypercalcemia occurs most often in association with malignancy. Most studies in dogs attribute hypercalcemia to malignancy in over 50% of the cases (Bienzle et al. 1993; Uehlinger et al. 1998; Elliott et al. 1991), although in one series malignancy accounted for only one-third of the cases (Kruger et al. 1996). Hypoadrenocorticism, renal failure, primary hyperparathyroidism, hypervitaminosis D, and inflammatory disorders sporadically account for hypercalcemia in dogs. It is often difficult to determine the cause of hypercalcemia in animals with mild or transient hypercalcemia. No definitive diagnosis could be made for 2 to 9% of hypercalcemic dogs in two reports (Uehlinger et al. 1998; Elliott et al. 1991).

Nonpathologic Hypercalcemia

Serum calcium concentrations in animals may be mildly increased after feeding; consequently, a 12-h fast is recommended before blood sampling. Laboratory error or detergent contamination of the serum or sample tube may result in artifactual hypercalcemia (Meuten 1984). Lipemia frequently causes erroneously high serum calcium concentrations because of colorimetric interference. Normal young growing dogs may have mildly higher serum calcium concentrations than older dogs (Mischke et al. 1996).

TRANSIENT OR INCONSEQUENTIAL HYPERCALCEMIA

Inconsequential hypercalcemia refers to a condition in which hypercalcemia does not cause injury, resolves rapidly, or is only mild. Dehydration can result in mild hypercalcemia, which is usually attributed to hemoconcentration with an increase in all calcium fractions. Furthermore, dehydration and volume contraction stimulate increased sodium and calcium reabsorption in the kidney. An increased serum concentration of protein, especially albumin, can result in an increased total serum calcium concentration as more calcium binds to protein. Dehydration in dogs is occasionally associated with total serum calcium concentrations of 12.0 to 13.5 mg/dL that rapidly return to normal after dehydration is corrected. Increased serum total calcium and decreased ionized calcium concentrations can occur transiently after plasma transfusion because of excess citrate–calcium ion complexes (Mischke et al. 1996).

HYPOADRENOCORTICISM

Hypoadrenocorticism is probably the second most common cause of hypercalcemia in dogs (after malignancy), accounting for 11 to 45% of cases in five studies (Chew and Meuten 1982; Uehlinger et al. 1998; Elliott et al. 1991; Kruger et al. 1996; Willard et al. 1982), but no cases were reported in one study (Bienzle et al. 1993). Hypercalcemia was reported in 28 to 31% of dogs with

TABLE 6–2. Conditions Associated with Hypercalcemia

Nonpathologic
Nonfasting (minimal increase)
Physiologic growth of young
Laboratory error
Spurious
  Lipemia
  Detergent contamination of sample or tube

Transient or Inconsequential
Hemoconcentration
Hyperproteinemia
Hypoadrenocorticism
Severe environmental hypothermia

Pathologic or Consequential—Persistent
Malignancy-associated
  Humoral hypercalcemia of malignancy
    Lymphoma (common)
    Anal sac apocrine gland adenocarcinoma (common)
    Carcinoma (sporadic): lung, pancreas, skin, nasal cavity, thyroid, mammary gland, adrenal medulla
    Thymoma (rare)
  Hematologic malignancies (bone marrow osteolysis)
    Lymphoma
    Multiple myeloma
    Myeloproliferative disease (rare)
    Leukemia (rare)
  Metastatic or primary bone neoplasia (very uncommon)
Chronic renal failure
Hypervitaminosis D
  Iatrogenic
  Plants (calcitriol glycosides)
  Rodenticide
Granulomatous disease
  Blastomycosis
  Dermatitis
Primary hyperparathyroidism
  Adenoma (common)
  Adenocarcinoma (rare)
  Hyperplasia (uncommon)
Acute renal failure
Skeletal lesions (nonmalignant) (uncommon)
  Osteomyelitis (bacterial or mycotic)
  Hypertrophic osteodystrophy
  Disuse osteoporosis (immobilization)
Excessive calcium-containing intestinal phosphate binders
Excessive calcium supplementation (calcium carbonate)
Hypervitaminosis A
Hypercalcemic conditions in human medicine
  Milk-alkali syndrome (rare in dogs)
  Thiazide diuretics
  Acromegaly
  Thyrotoxicosis
  Postrenal transplantation
  Aluminum exposure (dogs?)

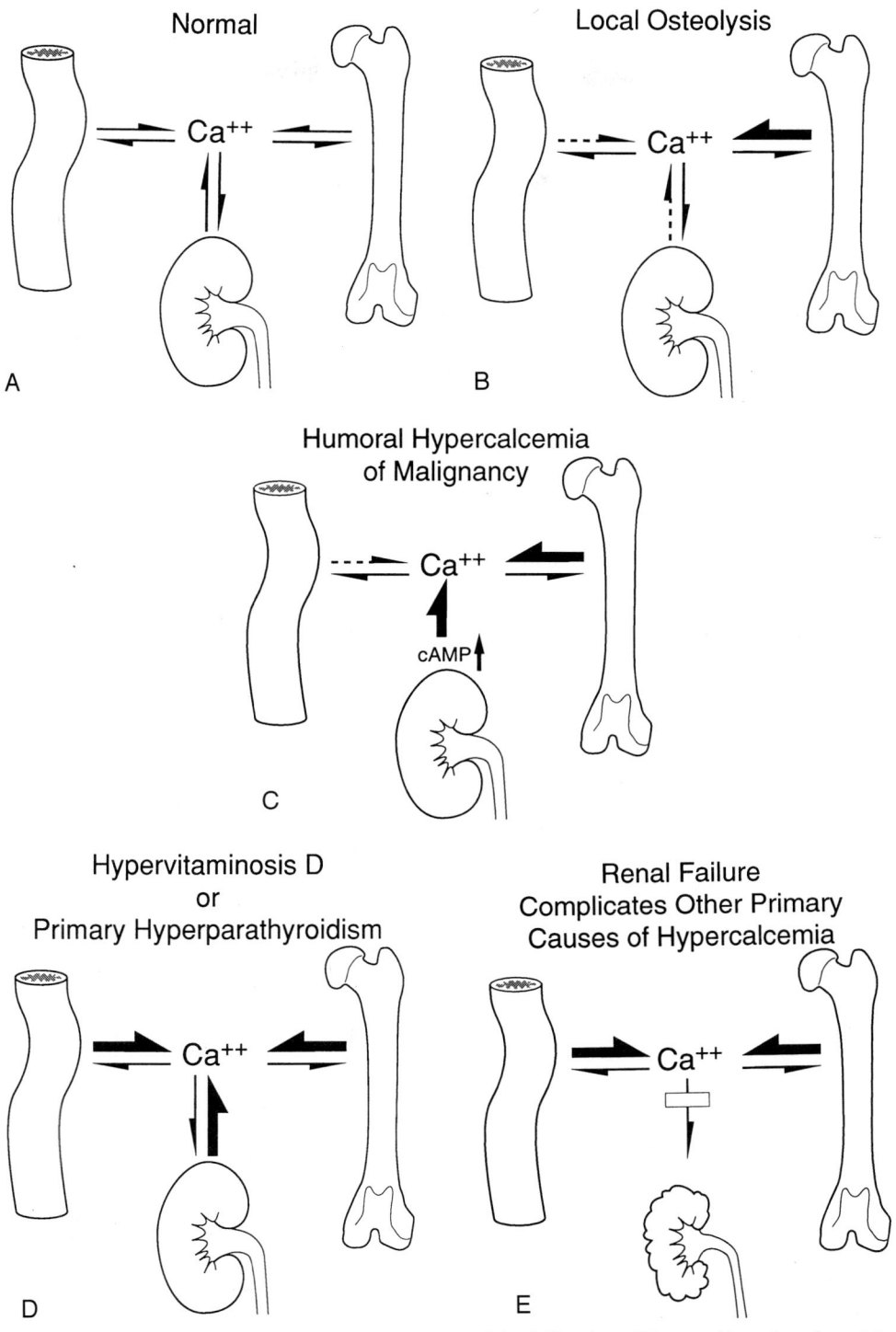

FIGURE 6–11. Patterns of calcium transport between extracellular fluid and gut, kidney, and bone in various states of hypercalcemia. *(A)* Normal; *(B)* osteolysis; *(C)* humoral hypercalcemia of malignancy; *(D)* hypervitaminosis D or primary hyperparathyroidism; *(E)* hypercalcemia complicated by renal failure. Size of arrows is proportional to the degree of calcium influx or efflux. Dashed arrows indicate possible response of decreased PTH secretion to hypercalcemia of nonparathyroid origin. (Modified from Mundy GR: Malignancy and hypercalcemia—humoral hypercalcemia of malignancy, hypercalcemia associated with osteolytic metastases. In Mundy GR [ed]: *Calcium Homeostasis: Hypercalcemia and Hypocalcemia.* London, Martin Dunitz, p. 65, 1989.)

glucocorticoid- and mineralocorticoid-deficient hypoadrenocorticism (Peterson and Feinman 1982; Peterson et al. 1996) and in 1 of 10 cats (Peterson et al. 1989). Mean serum total calcium concentration in dogs with hypoadrenocorticism and hypercalcemia is often approximately 13.0 mg/dL but may be as high as 16.0 mg/dL. The magnitude of hypercalcemia was greatest in the most severely affected dogs, but the mechanism was not readily apparent. Hypercalcemia was also present in some dogs with glucocorticoid-deficient hypoadrenocorticism (Lifton et al. 1996). A correlation between the degree of hyperkalemia and hypercalcemia was detected when the serum potassium concentration was greater than 6.0 to 6.5 mEq/L, and serum calcium concentration was often 11.4 to 13.5 mg/dL in these instances (Feldman and Nelson 1996).

This form of hypercalcemia is not considered to be dangerous to the animal. In experimental hypoadrenocorticism in dogs, ionized hypercalcemia did not develop despite increased total serum calcium concentration (Walser et al. 1963). Increased total serum calcium concentration rapidly returns to normal after 1 to 2 days of corticosteroid replacement therapy in dogs (Peterson and Feinman 1982), and intravenous volume expansion with 0.9% NaCl alone can return serum calcium concentration to normal within a few hours. Hypercalcemia in untreated dogs with hypoadrenocorticism can persist for days to weeks. Moderate to severe azotemia and hyperphosphatemia are also present at the time of diagnosis in most dogs with hypoadrenocorticism (Peterson et al. 1996). Hypoadrenocorticism should always be included in the differential diagnosis of hypercalcemia, especially because the signs of hypoadrenocorticism are similar to those attributed to hypercalcemia. Hyponatremia and hyperkalemia usually alert the clinician to the possibility of hypoadrenocorticism, and definitive diagnosis is established by finding a blunted or absent response of plasma cortisol concentration to adrenocorticotropic hormone stimulation.

CHRONIC RENAL FAILURE

The finding of hypercalcemia and primary renal azotemia poses a special diagnostic problem because hypercalcemia can cause renal failure or develop as a consequence of CRF. Serum PTH concentration is often increased in patients with hypercalcemia related to renal failure, and these animals must be differentiated from those with primary hyperparathyroidism. Serum ionized calcium concentration is increased in primary hyperparathyroidism but is usually normal or low in patients with CRF (Kruger et al. 1996; Chew and Nagode 1990). Deleterious effects of hypercalcemia occur in patients with renal failure only if it is associated with increases in serum ionized calcium concentration; consequently, clinical signs of hypercalcemia are uncommon in CRF patients. Hypercalcemia can be attributed to underlying renal disease in patients with a history of long-standing azotemia that initially have normal serum total calcium concentrations and subsequently develop increased serum total calcium concentrations. Therefore, renal failure–associated hypercalcemia is usually characterized by increased total serum calcium concentration, normal or low ionized serum calcium concentration, and increased PTH concentrations. Approximately 6% of dogs with CRF have increased serum ionized calcium concentrations (Chew and Nagode 1990).

Most dogs and cats with CRF have normal total serum calcium concentrations (Meuten 1984; Finco and Rowland 1978; DiBartola et al. 1987). Hypercalcemia based on measurement of total serum calcium concentration occurs sporadically in dogs and cats with CRF and is usually listed as second or third in frequency of causes of hypercalcemia in dogs. A mild degree of hypercalcemia (maximal serum total calcium concentration of 12.7 mg/dL) was reported in 11.5% of cats with chronic renal failure (DiBartola et al. 1987). Ten of 300 uremic dogs had hypercalcemia ≥12.5 mg/dL (mean, 13 mg/dL) (Nagode et al. 1988) and 14% of dogs with CRF had serum total calcium concentrations ≥12.0 mg/dL (Chew and Nagode 1990). In another series, seven dogs with CRF and hypercalcemia had a mean serum total calcium concentration of 12.8 mg/dL with a range of 12.1 to 13.6 mg/dL (Kruger et al. 1996). Finally, the maximal serum total calcium concentration was 15.2 mg/dL in four young dogs with CRF and hypercalcemia (Finco and Rowland 1978). Hypercalcemia was not correlated with serum phosphorus concentration in dogs with experimental renal failure (Norrdin et al. 1980; Tuma and Mallette 1983).

Some cases of hypercalcemia and CRF may be associated with the use of calcium carbonate intestinal phosphate binders (both total and ionized calcium concentrations are increased). In these cases, serum calcium concentration rapidly returns to normal after discontinuation of treatment. Hypercalcemia (both total and ionized) occurs in patients with CRF that receive excessive doses of calcitriol used to treat renal secondary hyperparathyroidism and replace decreased renal production of calcitriol. Hypercalcemia is very uncommon in animals treated with the lower dosages of calcitriol (2.5 to 4.0 ng/kg daily) that are commonly used. If hypercalcemia is caused by excessive calcitriol, the serum calcium concentration declines during the week after its discontinuation. Most CRF patients that develop hypercalcemia during low-dose calcitriol treatment have normal or low serum ionized calcium concentrations. Serum calcium concentration may not decline when calcitriol is discontinued if the increased total serum calcium concentration is due to increased complexed calcium.

The mechanisms of increased total serum calcium concentration in CRF have not been well characterized but include several possibilities (Rosol and Capen 1997; Kruger et al. 1996; Finco and Rowland 1978; Tuma and Mallette 1983). Reduced glomerular filtration rate (GFR) caused by loss of renal mass could cause increased serum calcium concentration as the filtered load of calcium declines. Increased PTH-mediated bone resorption as a consequence of CRF could increase total serum calcium concentration. Increased concentrations of organic anions capable of complexing with calcium could increase total serum calcium concentration but not ionized serum calcium concentration. Such anions include citrates, phosphates, lactates, and bicarbonates. In addition, PTH can stimulate hypercitricemia. Results of preliminary studies of serum calcium concentrations in dogs with primary renal failure have shown increased protein-bound and complexed calcium fractions. Autonomous secretion of PTH from the parathyroid gland is unlikely, but the setpoint for PTH secretion may be altered in CRF such that higher concentrations of calcium are necessary to inhibit PTH secretion (Goodman et al. 1998). Decreased serum calcitriol concentrations, decreased numbers of calcitriol receptors in the parathyroid gland, and decreased calcitriol–vitamin D receptor interactions with chief cell DNA caused by uremic toxins may contribute to this increase in set-point (Brown et al. 1989; Hsu and Patel 1995; Patel et al. 1995). Finally, hyperplasia of parathyroid gland chief cells could account for increased PTH secretion and serum calcium concentration independent of changes in set-point, because chief cells secrete small amounts of PTH that are nonsuppressible regardless of serum ionized calcium concentration (Goodman et al. 1995). Ionized calcium concentration should be increased with all of these mechanisms except when excess anions in serum form complexes with calcium.

The role of increased PTH in the pathogenesis of hypercalcemia is apparent in both experimental and naturally occurring CRF in dogs. The parathyroid glands must be present for hypercalcemia to develop in nephrectomized dogs (Tuma and Mallette 1983), and partial parathyroidectomy ameliorated hypercalcemia in some dogs with CRF (Finco and Rowland 1978). Treatment of dogs with CRF and hypercalcemia with low-dose calcitriol to reduce PTH synthesis and secretion can result in decreased serum calcium concentration. Low-dose calcitriol therapy does not appreciably increase intestinal calcium absorption (Nagode et al. 1992, 1996). In patients with CRF, increased serum PTH concentration (renal secondary hyperparathyroidism) contributes to the progression of renal disease (Nagode et al. 1992). Oral administration of low doses of calcitriol reduces toxic concentrations of PTH, improves quality of life, reduces progression of renal disease, and leads to prolongation of life (Nagode and Chew 1992; Schwarz et al. 1998).

Tertiary hyperparathyroidism refers to the condition of a subset of patients with CRF that develop ionized hypercalcemia and excessive PTH secretion that is not inhibited by high serum calcium concentration. It is likely that such patients had high PTH concentrations in association with normal or low serum ionized calcium concentration (typical of renal secondary hyperparathyroidism) earlier in the clinical course of CRF. Ten dogs with naturally occurring renal failure and increased total serum calcium concentration were compared with those with normal total serum calcium concentration after being matched for age and serum creatinine and phosphorus concentrations (Fig. 6–12). Serum amino-terminal PTH concentration was markedly increased in both groups of uremic dogs, but those with hypercalcemia had higher PTH concentrations. Calcitriol concentration was decreased to a similar extent in both groups. It was proposed that the hypercalcemic and more markedly hyperparathyroid uremic dogs may have had greater calcitriol receptor (VDR) deficits in their parathyroid cells, which would lead to poorly controlled PTH synthesis and chief cell hyperplasia (Nagode et al. 1988).

A role for aluminum accumulation in the development of hypercalcemia in dogs or cats with renal disease during treatment with aluminum-containing intestinal phosphate binders has not been investigated despite the fact that such treatment is common. Experimental dogs exposed to aluminum developed mild hypercalcemia within minutes of a single intravenous injection. In these dogs, mean total serum calcium concentration increased by 1.7 mg/dL. The increase in calcium concentration could have been due to acute mobilization of calcium from the skeleton or caused by an acute blockade of normal calcium entry into bone. During chronic daily exposure to aluminum over a period of weeks, serum calcium concentration progressively increased and azotemia developed. Total serum calcium concentration increased by a mean of 1.1 mg/dL, but severe increases (total serum calcium concentrations of 15 to 20 mg/dL) occurred in three dogs and were associated with abrupt development of azotemia. The mechanisms responsible for these findings were not clear (Henry et al. 1984). Ionized calcium concentration was decreased at the time of increased total serum calcium concentration in a study of rats given aluminum acutely. Increased binding of calcium to constituents in plasma was suspected as the underlying mechanism (Rodriguez et al. 1987).

Pathologic or Consequential Hypercalcemia

CANCER-ASSOCIATED HYPERCALCEMIA

The most common cause of hypercalcemia in dogs and cats is cancer-associated hypercalcemia. There are three mechanisms (Fig. 6–13) of increased serum calcium concentration induced by neoplasms: (1) HHM, (2) hypercalcemia induced by metastases of solid tumors to bone, and (3) hematologic malignancies growing in the bone marrow (Rosol and Capen 1992).

HUMORAL HYPERCALCEMIA OF MALIGNANCY

Humoral hypercalcemia of malignancy is a syndrome associated with many tumors in people and animals (Rosol and Capen 1992). Characteristic clinical findings in patients with HHM include hypercalcemia, hypophosphatemia, hypercalciuria (often with decreased fractional calcium excretion), increased fractional excretion of phosphorus, increased nephrogenous cAMP, and increased osteoclastic bone resorption. Hypercalcemia is induced by humoral effects on bone, kidney, and possibly the intestine (Fig. 6–14) (Rosol and Capen 1988). Increased osteoclastic bone resorption is a consistent finding in HHM and increases calcium release from bone. The kidney plays a critical role in the pathogenesis of hypercalcemia, because calcium reabsorption is stimulated by PTHrP, which binds and activates renal PTH-PTHrP receptors. The level of renal function in the patient may also contribute to development of hypercalcemia. Animals with dehydration or impaired renal function are more susceptible to developing hypercalcemia or may have more severe hypercalcemia because of decreased renal excretion of calcium. In some forms of HHM, increased serum 1,25-dihydroxyvitamin D concentrations may increase calcium absorption from the intestine (Rosol et al. 1992).

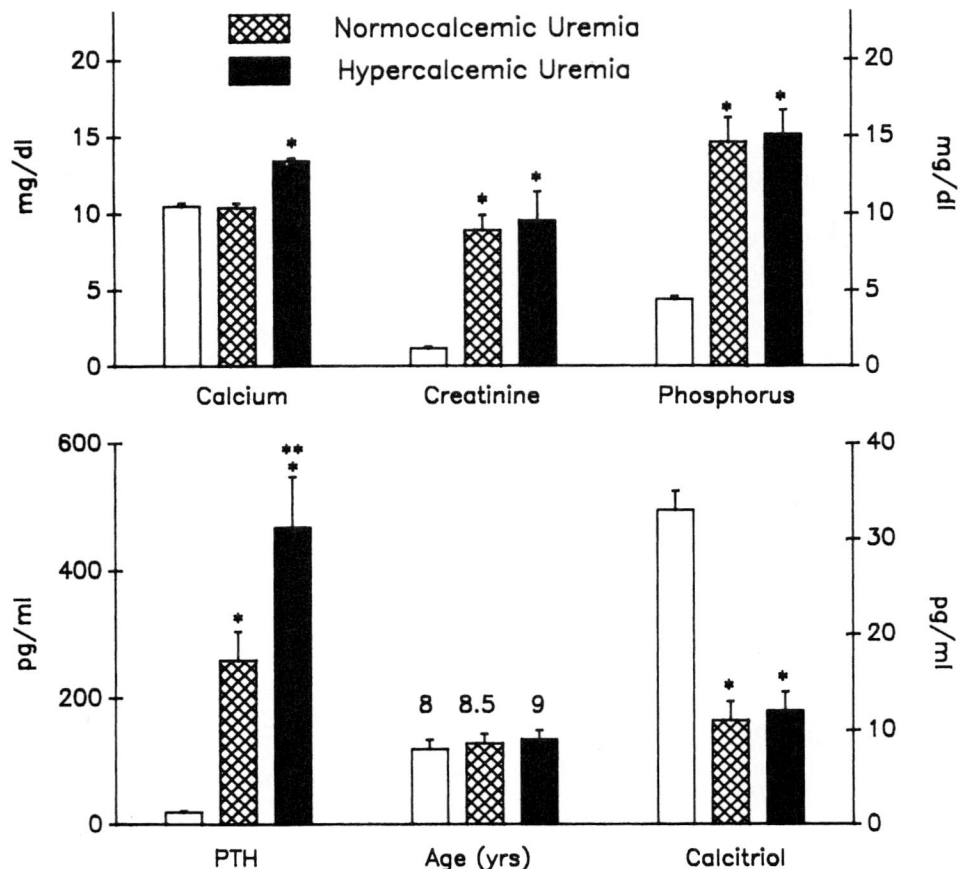

FIGURE 6–12. Comparison of biochemical data for dogs with renal failure and hypercalcemia or normocalcemia. Dogs with renal failure were normalized for age and had similar concentrations of serum creatinine, phosphorus, and calcitriol. Serum concentrations of PTH were greater in the hypercalcemic dogs than in the normocalcemic dogs. Data are means ± SEM. For normal and hypercalcemic uremic dogs, $n = 10$; for normocalcemic uremic dogs, $n = 20$. Significant differences were *$p < .0001$ (from normal) and **$p < .02$ (from normocalcemic uremia PTH) by Student's t-test. (From Nagode LA, Steinmeyer CL, Chew DJ, et al.: Hyper- and normo-calcemic dogs with chronic renal failure: Relations of serum PTH and calcitriol to parathyroid gland Ca^{++} set-point. In Norman AW, Schaefer K, Grigoleit HG, and Herrath DV [eds]: *Vitamin D 1988. Chemical, Biochemical and Clinical Endocrinology.* Berlin, Walter de Gruyter & Co., pp. 799–800, 1988.)

Malignancies that are commonly associated with HHM in dogs include T-cell lymphoma (approximately 30% of all dogs with lymphoma have HHM) and adenocarcinomas derived from the apocrine glands of the anal sac (approximately 70% of affected dogs have HHM) (Rosol and Capen 1992; Weir et al. 1988). Lymphoma is an uncommon cause of mild HHM in cats (Engelman et al. 1985) and ferrets (Kawasaki 1991). In addition, sporadic cases of HHM occur in dogs and cats with thymoma or carcinomas originating in the lungs, pancreas, thyroid gland, skin, mammary gland, nasal cavity, and adrenal medulla (Rosol and Capen 1988, 1992). Excessive secretion of biologically active PTHrP plays a central role in the pathogenesis of hypercalcemia in most forms of HHM, but cytokines such as interleukin-1, tumor necrosis factor-α, and transforming growth factor-α and -β or calcitriol may have synergistic or cooperative actions with PTHrP (see Fig. 6–14). Before PTHrP was identified, it was recognized that tumors associated with HHM induced a syndrome that mimicked primary hyperparathyroidism with secretion of a PTH-like factor that was antigenically unrelated to PTH. Purification of the PTH-like activity from human and animal tumors associated with HHM resulted in the characterization of PTHrP (Moseley et al. 1987; Weir et al. 1988).

PTHrP binds to the N-terminal PTH-PTHrP receptor in bone and kidney but does not cross-react immunologically with native PTH (Fig. 6–15). PTHrP stimulates adenyl cyclase and increases intracellular calcium in bone and kidney cells by binding to and activating the cell membrane PTH-PTHrP receptors. This results in stimulation of osteoclastic bone resorption, increased renal tubular calcium reabsorption, and decreased renal tubular phosphate reabsorption. Interleukin-1 stimulates bone resorption in vivo and in vitro and is synergistic with PTHrP (Rosol and Capen 1992; McCauley et al. 1991). Transforming growth factors-α and -β can stimulate bone resorption in vitro and have been identified in tumors associated with HHM, including adenocarcinomas derived from apocrine glands of the anal sac in dogs (Merryman et al. 1989).

LYMPHOMA

Hypercalcemia is found in 20 to 40% of dogs with lymphoma (Fig. 6–16A and B). Most dogs with lymphoma

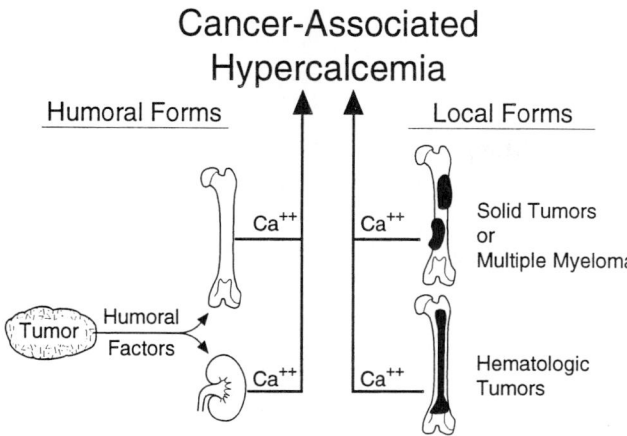

FIGURE 6-13. Pathogenesis of cancer-associated hypercalcemia. Humoral and local forms of cancer-associated hypercalcemia increase circulating concentrations of calcium by stimulation of osteoclastic bone resorption and increased renal tubular reabsorption of calcium.

and hypercalcemia have HHM, because increased osteoclastic resorption is present in bones without evidence of tumor metastasis. Lymphomas associated with HHM are usually of the T-cell type (Weir et al. 1988). The pathogenesis of hypercalcemia in dogs with lymphoma and HHM resembles that occurring in humans with lymphoma or leukemia induced by human T-cell lymphotropic virus type I (HTLV-I). Neoplastic cells from humans with HTLV-I–induced lymphoma have increased PTHrP production because of stimulation of PTHrP transcription by the virally encoded Tax transcription factor (Prager et al. 1994).

Most dogs with lymphoma and HHM have increased circulating PTHrP concentrations, but concentrations are lower (2–15 pM) than in dogs with carcinomas and HHM, and PTHrP concentrations are not correlated with serum calcium concentration (Fig. 6–17) (Rosol et al. 1992).

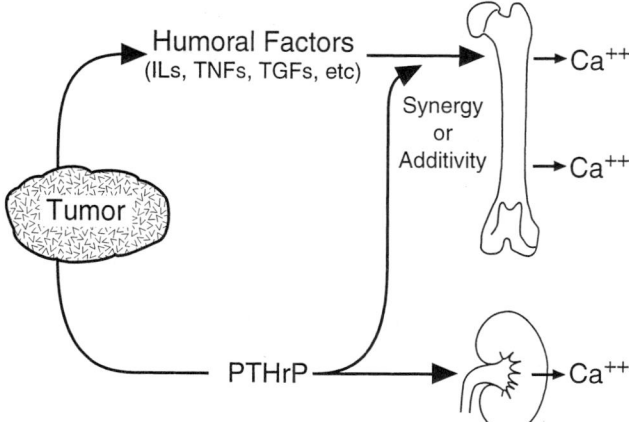

FIGURE 6-14. Humoral factors such as parathyroid hormone–related protein (PTHrP), interleukin-1 (IL-1), tumor necrosis factors (TNFs), or transforming growth factors (TGFs) produced by tumors induce humoral hypercalcemia of malignancy (HHM) by acting as systemic hormones and stimulating osteoclastic bone resorption or increasing tubular reabsorption of calcium.

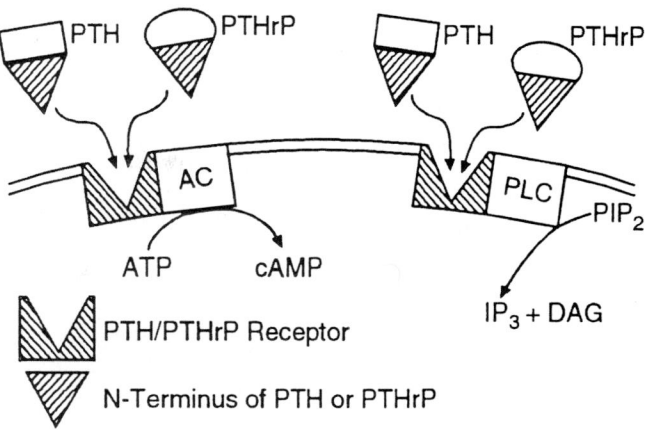

FIGURE 6-15. Parathyroid hormone–related protein (PTHrP) induces many of the effects of parathyroid hormone (PTH) by interacting with the PTH receptor in bone and kidney and activating adenylate cyclase (AC) to form cyclic AMP (cAMP) and phospholipase C (PLC) to form inositol triphosphate (IP_3) and diacylglycerol (DAG) from phosphatidylinositol (PIP_2). Stimulation of the PTH receptor results in increased osteoclastic bone resorption and renal tubular reabsorption of calcium, inhibition of renal tubular reabsorption of phosphorus, and stimulation of renal production of 1,25-dihydroxyvitamin D_3 (calcitriol).

These findings indicate that PTHrP is an important marker of HHM in dogs with lymphoma but is not the sole humoral factor responsible for stimulation of osteoclasts and development of hypercalcemia. It is likely that cytokines such as interleukin-1 or tumor necrosis factor function synergistically with PTHrP to induce HHM in dogs with lymphoma (see Fig. 6–14) (Rosol and Capen 1992).

Some dogs and human patients with lymphoma and hypercalcemia have increased serum calcitriol concentrations, which may be responsible for or contribute to the induction of hypercalcemia (Rosol et al. 1992; Seymour and Gagel 1993). Some lymphocytes contain the 1α-hydroxylase (similar that found in renal tubules) that converts 25-hydroxyvitamin D to the active metabolite, 1,25-dihydroxyvitamin D (calcitriol). Therefore, lymphomas that retain this capability may synthesize excessive calcitriol, which could increase calcium absorption from the intestinal tract and facilitate development of hypercalcemia.

CANINE ADENOCARCINOMA DERIVED FROM APOCRINE GLANDS OF THE ANAL SAC

The adenocarcinoma derived from apocrine glands of the anal sac of dogs consistently fulfills the criteria for HHM (Meuten et al. 1981, 1983). This unique tumor appears primarily in middle-aged (mean, 10 years) female dogs and rarely metastasizes to bone. German shepherd dogs (Meuten et al. 1981; Ross et al. 1991) and longhaired German pointers may be overrepresented (Rijnberk et al. 1978). Clinical signs are referable to hypercalcemia (polyuria, polydipsia, anorexia, weakness) or a mass in the perineum (tenesmus, ribbonlike stools, increased odor, protruding mass). Apocrine adenocarcinomas may require rectal palpation to confirm their presence because their size ranges from 7 mm to 6 × 8 cm (Fig. 6–18). Dogs with this tumor and HHM have hypercalcemia (12 to 24

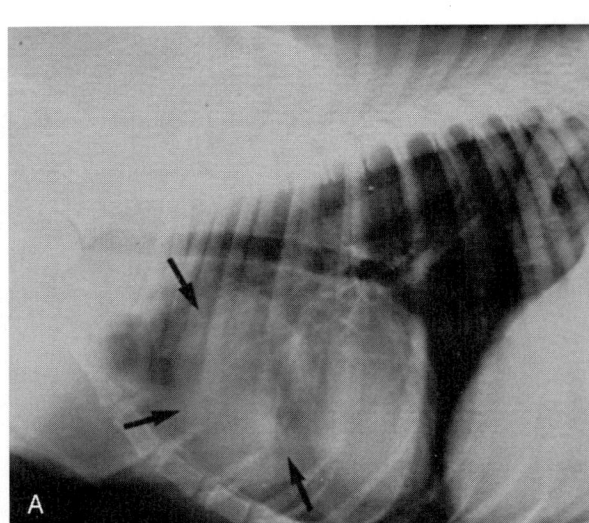
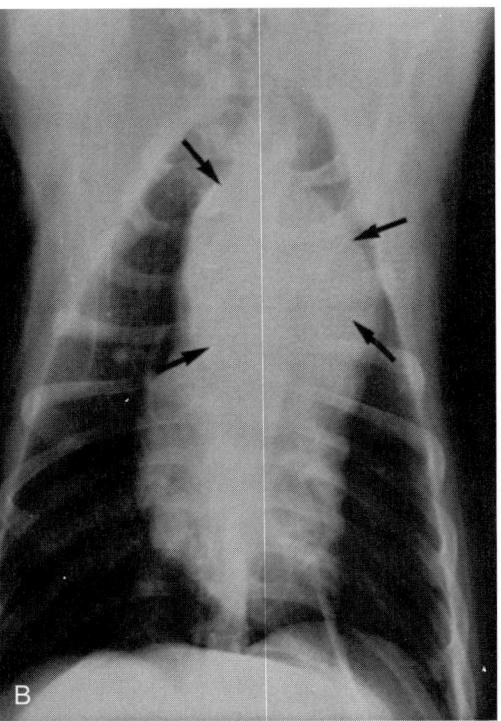

FIGURE 6-16. Lateral (A) and ventrodorsal (B) thoracic radiographs of a 5-year-old boxer dog with hypercalcemia of malignancy caused by mediastinal lymphoma (arrows). Severe hypercalcemia (serum total calcium concentration, 20.6 mg/dL) was detected on initial presentation. (From Chew DJ and Carothers M: Hypercalcemia. Vet Clin North Am 19(2): 272, 1989.)

mg/dL); hypophosphatemia; decreased immunoreactive PTH concentration; increased urinary excretion of calcium, phosphorus, and cAMP; and increased osteoclastic bone resorption (Meuten et al. 1983). This tumor should not be confused with the common perianal adenomas or the uncommon perianal adenocarcinomas that arise from the circumanal glands and have entirely different biologic behavior. Perianal adenomas and adenocarcinomas affect primarily male dogs and are not associated with hypercalcemia (Vail et al. 1990).

Hypercalcemia was present at the time of diagnosis in 80 to 100% of affected dogs in early studies (Meuten et al. 1983; Rijnberk et al. 1978). The incidence of hypercalcemia is lower (33%) in dogs with earlier detection (Ross et al. 1991). In some instances, the finding of hypercalcemia during routine serum biochemistry testing prompts rectal palpation and subsequent discovery of an apocrine gland adenocarcinoma. Surgical removal or radiation therapy of the adenocarcinoma results in rapid return to normal of serum calcium and phosphorus concentrations, increased serum PTH concentration, and decreased calcitriol concentration (Rosol et al. 1992). Post-surgical survival of dogs with apocrine gland adenocarcinoma and hypercalcemia ranged from 2 to 21 months, with a mean of 8.8 months. Sublumbar metastases occur in a high percentage (94%) of affected dogs and are associated with recrudescence of the biochemical alterations in serum and urine.

Most dogs with HHM have increased concentrations of circulating PTHrP (see Fig. 6–17). Plasma concentrations of PTHrP are highest (10–100 pM) in dogs with apocrine adenocarcinomas of the anal sac and sporadic carcinomas associated with HHM (Rosol et al. 1992). Serum calcium concentrations in affected dogs correlate well with circulating PTHrP concentrations, which is consistent with the concept that PTHrP plays a primary role in the pathogenesis of HHM in these dogs. Dogs with apocrine adenocarcinomas and normocalcemia may have increased plasma PTHrP concentrations (2–15 pM), but the concentrations are lower than in dogs with hypercalcemia.

Some dogs with apocrine adenocarcinomas have inappropriate concentrations (normal or increased) of calcitriol for the degree of hypercalcemia (Rosol et al. 1992). This finding suggests that the humoral factors produced by the neoplastic cells are capable of stimulating renal 1α-hydroxylase and increasing the formation of calcitriol even in the presence of increased serum calcium concentration. Plasma immunoreactive PTH concentrations were not increased in hypercalcemic dogs and were significantly lower than those observed in dogs with primary hyperparathyroidism. Parathyroid glands from dogs with apocrine adenocarcinoma were atrophic or inactive and there was nodular hyperplasia of C cells in the thyroid glands because of prolonged hypercalcemia (Menten et al. 1983).

HEMATOLOGIC MALIGNANCIES

Some types of hematologic malignancies present in the bone marrow produce hypercalcemia by inducing bone resorption locally (Rosol and Capen 1992). This effect occurs most commonly in multiple myeloma and lymphoma. Hypercalcemia has been reported in 17% of dogs

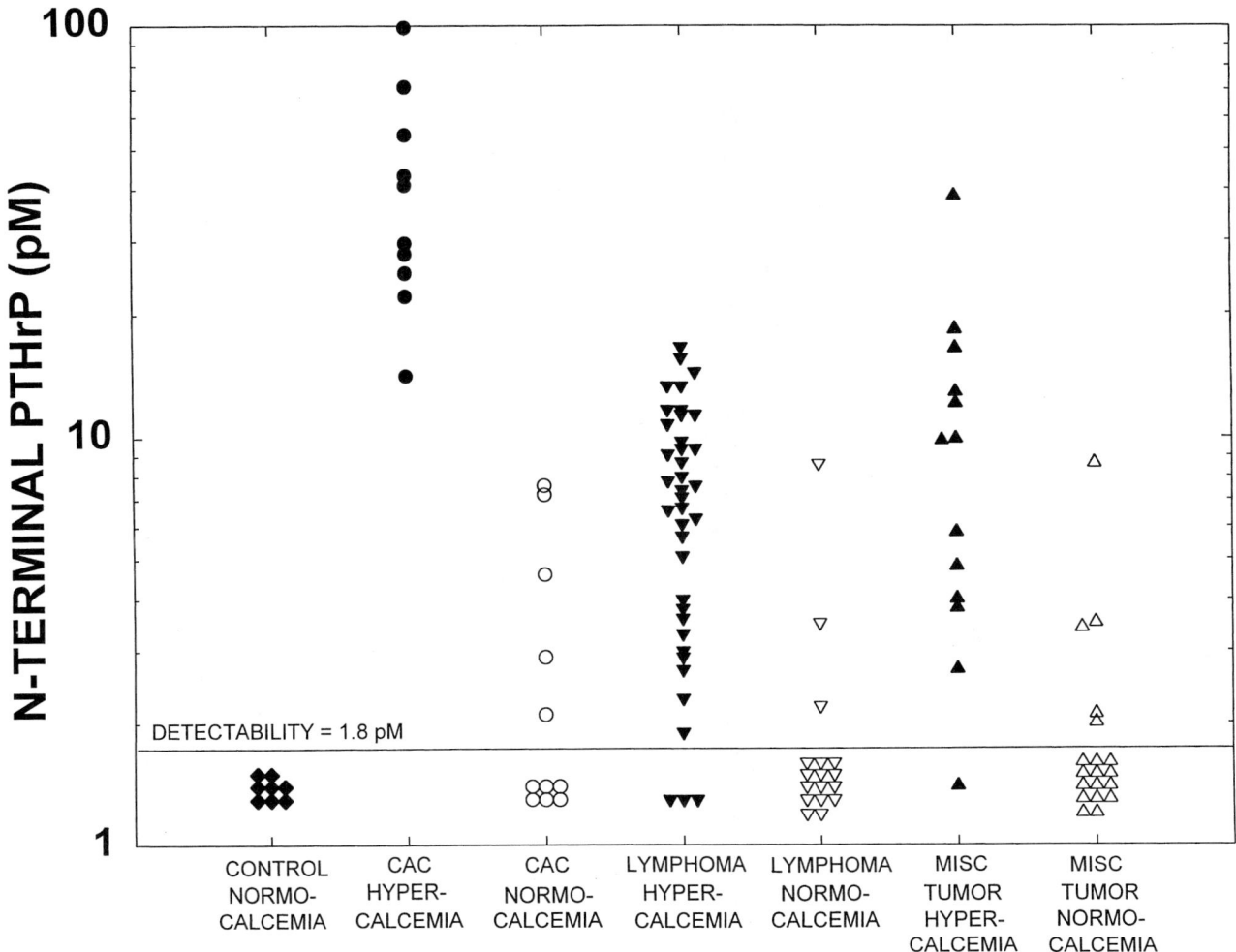

FIGURE 6-17. Circulating N-terminal parathyroid hormone–related protein (PTHrP) concentrations in normal dogs (CONTROL); dogs with hypercalcemia (>12 mg/dL) and anal sac adenocarcinomas (CAC), lymphoma, or miscellaneous tumors (MISC TUMOR); and dogs with normocalcemia (<12 mg/dL) and anal sac adenocarcinomas, lymphoma, or miscellaneous tumors. (From Rosol TJ, Nagode LA, Couto CG, et al.: Parathyroid hormone–related protein, parathyroid hormone, and 1,25-dihydroxyvitamin D in dogs with cancer-associated hypercalcemia. *Endocrinology* 131:1157, 1992. © The Endocrine Society.)

with multiple myeloma (Matus et al. 1986). A number of paracrine factors or cytokines may be responsible for the stimulation of bone resorption in this setting. The cytokines most often implicated in the pathogenesis of local bone resorption are interleukin-1, tumor necrosis factor-α, and tumor necrosis factor-β (lymphotoxin) (Martin and Grill 1992). Other cytokines or factors that may play a role include interleukin-6, transforming growth factor-α and -β, and PTHrP (Black and Mundy 1994). Production of small amounts of PTHrP by a tumor in bone may stimulate local bone resorption without inducing a systemic response. Prostaglandins (especially prostaglandin E_2) may also be responsible for local stimulation of bone resorption.

Some dogs with lymphoma and hypercalcemia have localized bone resorption associated with metastases to medullary cavities without evidence of increased bone resorption at sites distant from the tumor metastases (Meuten et al. 1983). Hypercalcemic dogs with lymphoma and bone metastases had decreased serum PTH and calcitriol concentrations; increased excretion of calcium, phosphorus, and hydroxyproline; and increased serum concentrations of the prostaglandin E_2 metabolite 13,14-dihydro-15-ketoprostaglandin E_2. The mediator of local bone resorption has not been conclusively identified, but prostaglandin E_2 may be an important primary or secondary local mediator of bone resorption in these dogs. Other potential mediators include interleukin-1 and tumor necrosis factors.

TUMORS METASTATIC TO BONE

Solid tumors that metastasize widely to bone can produce hypercalcemia by the induction of local bone resorption associated with tumor growth. This effect is not common in animals but is an important cause of cancer-associated hypercalcemia in human beings (Rosol and Capen 1992). Tumors that often metastasize to bone and induce hypercalcemia in human patients include breast and lung carcinomas. Carcinomas of the mammary gland, prostate, liver, and lung were most frequently reported to metastasize to bone in dogs, and the humerus, femur, and vertebrae were the most common sites of metastasis (Meuten 1984).

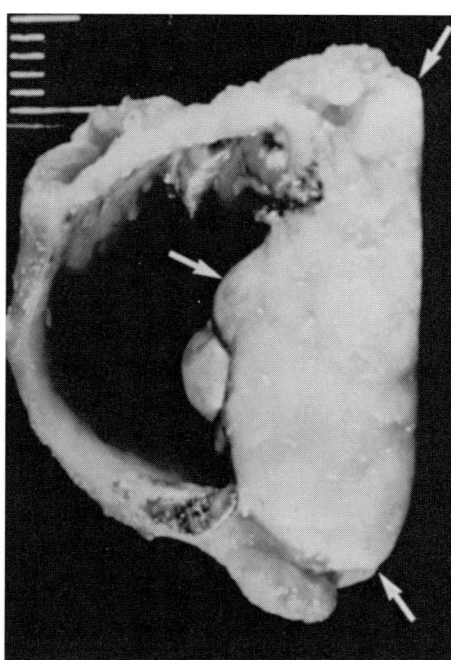

FIGURE 6-18. Hypercalcemia of malignancy associated with apocrine gland adenocarcinoma of the anal sac in an elderly female dog. Transverse section of the anal sac and associated malignancy (arrows). (From Chew DJ and Meuten DJ: Disorders of calcium and phosphorus metabolism. *Vet Clin North Am* 12[3]:417, 1982.)

Primary bone tumors are not often associated with hypercalcemia in dogs or cats.

The pathogenesis of enhanced bone resorption in this setting is not well understood, but two primary mechanisms are secretion of cytokines or factors that stimulate local bone resorption and indirect stimulation of bone resorption by tumor-induced cytokine secretion from local immune or bone cells (Garrett 1993). Cytokines or factors that may be secreted by tumor cells and stimulate local bone resorption include PTHrP (Powell et al. 1991), transforming growth factor-α and -β, and prostaglandins (especially prostaglandin E_2). In some cases, bone resorbing activity can be inhibited by indomethacin, which suggests that prostaglandins are either directly or indirectly associated with stimulation of bone resorption. The cytokines most often implicated in indirect stimulation of bone resorption by local immune cells include interleukin-1 and tumor necrosis factors.

Malignant neoplasms with osseous metastases may cause moderate to severe hypercalcemia and hypercalciuria, but serum alkaline phosphatase activity and phosphorus concentrations are usually normal or only moderately increased. These changes are believed to be due to release of calcium and phosphorus into the blood from areas of bone destruction at rates greater than can be cleared by the kidney and intestine. Bone involvement can be multifocal but is usually sharply demarcated and localized to the area of metastasis.

PRIMARY HYPERPARATHYROIDISM

Primary hyperparathyroidism is an important and treatable, but uncommon, cause of hypercalcemia in dogs (Berger and Feldman 1987; Bruyette and Feldman 1988). It is even less common in cats (Kallet et al. 1991; den Hertog et al. 1997). Excessive and inappropriate secretion of PTH by the parathyroid glands relative to the serum calcium concentration characterizes this condition. Primary hyperparathyroidism was caused by a solitary parathyroid gland adenoma in approximately 90% of dogs, whereas parathyroid gland carcinoma and parathyroid gland hyperplasia each accounted for 5% of cases in one large series (Feldman and Nelson 1996). Adenomas occurred with nearly equal frequency in the external and internal parathyroid glands in one study (Berger and Feldman 1987), but external gland adenomas predominated in another report in dogs (Wisner et al. 1997). Idiopathic parathyroid gland hyperplasia may affect one or more glands and has been reported in six older dogs (DeVries et al. 1993). Although remnant parathyroid tissue may be found in the cranial mediastinum near the base of the heart, neoplastic transformation has not been reported at this site in dogs or cats. An ectopic parathyroid gland adenoma cranial to the thoracic inlet has been described in one dog (Wisner and Nyland 1998).

Primary parathyroid gland hyperplasia has been reported in two German shepherd puppies (Thompson et al. 1984). Diffuse hyperplasia was present in all four parathyroid glands. In retrospect, this family of German shepherd dogs probably had an inactivating mutation in the gene for the calcium-sensing receptor. The calcium receptor plays an important role in the regulation of extracellular calcium homeostasis and is present on parathyroid chief cells, C-cells, and renal epithelial cells. It is responsible for sensing serum ionized calcium concentration and modifying PTH secretion (Chattopadhyay et al. 1996). Mutations in one or both of the calcium-sensing receptor genes in humans result in familial hypocalciuric hypercalcemia or neonatal severe hypercalcemia, respectively, because of inadequate ability to sense extracellular calcium concentration and coordinate the appropriate cellular response (Pollak et al. 1993). Familial hypocalciuric hypercalcemia is a benign condition characterized by mild hypercalcemia, decreased urinary excretion of calcium, and inappropriately normal PTH concentrations. In contrast, neonatal severe hypercalcemia is lethal unless total parathyroidectomy is performed early in life to markedly reduce increased PTH concentrations. The affected German shepherd puppies had a disease syndrome that mimicked neonatal severe hypercalcemia in humans.

Dogs with primary hyperparathyroidism are older, with a mean age of 10.5 years (range, 5–15 years) in one series (Feldman and Nelson 1996). The mean age in affected cats was 12.9 years (range, 8–15 years) (Kallet et al. 1991). No sex predisposition has been noted, but Keeshonds constituted 36% of affected dogs, and five of eight cats were Siamese (Kallet et al. 1991). Parathyroid gland masses usually cannot be palpated in dogs, but 50% of cats with primary hyperparathyroidism had a palpable cervical mass (Kallet et al. 1991; den Hertog et al. 1997). Clinical signs related to hypercalcemia are either mild (e.g., lethargy, polydipsia, polyuria, weakness) or absent in many affected dogs (Feldman and Nelson 1996; Berger and Feldman 1987). In one study, most owners of affected dogs were not convinced that their dogs had a serious illness (Berger and Feldman 1987), but some owners retrospectively recognized subtle signs after hypercalcemia resolved (Feldman and Nelson 1996). More prominent clinical signs and serious consequences can occur when hyperparathyroidism and severe hypercalcemia are long-standing and associated with renal failure (Chew and Meuten, 1982, 1983). Clinical signs referable to the lower urinary tract have been reported to occur in 27% of dogs as a result of urolithiasis or bacterial urinary tract infection (Feldman and Nelson 1996). Calcium-containing uroliths (calcium phosphate, calcium oxalate, or mixtures) occurred in approximately 30% of dogs and in a cat with primary hyperparathyroidism (Feldman and Nelson 1996; Klausner et al. 1986; Marquez et al. 1995). Urolithiasis is attributed to hypercalcemia and subsequent hypercalciuria. Interestingly, hypercalcemia arising from other causes has not been associated with urolithiasis.

The diagnostic work-up to confirm primary hyperparathyroidism often begins with the fortuitous finding of increased serum calcium concentration on routine clinical chemistry testing for some nonspecific or unrelated condition (Feldman and Nelson 1996). The diagnosis of primary hyperparathyroidism is easy in dogs and cats that have increased serum total calcium concentration, normal renal function, and increased concentration of immunoreactive PTH. The appropriateness of the PTH concentration must be interpreted in relation to the serum calcium concentration, preferably the ionized calcium concentration. Additional support for the diagnosis of primary hyperparathyroidism is provided by the finding of increased serum ionized calcium concentration, increased serum alkaline phosphatase, low serum phosphorus concentration, increased or normal calcitriol concentration, undetectable PTHrP, and calcium-containing uroliths. The most consistent laboratory abnormality in dogs with primary hyperparathyroidism is increased total serum calcium concentration. Mean serum calcium concentration was 15.6 mg/dL, with a range of 12.1 to 23.0 mg/dL, in one reported series of dogs (Feldman and Nelson 1996).

Hypercalcemia results from a combination of effects following PTH binding to receptors in kidney and bone. PTH also acts indirectly to increase serum calcium concentration by enhancing renal conversion of 25-hydroxyvitamin D to calcitriol. Hypophosphatemia secondary to PTH-enhanced urinary excretion of phosphorus was observed in 5 of 21 dogs (Berger and Feldman 1987). Serum phosphorus concentration is typically low to low-normal and was less than 4.0 mg/dL in most dogs (Feldman and Nelson 1996). Calcitriol concentrations were mildly increased or in the high-normal range in three of four dogs with primary hyperparathyroidism (Rosol et al. 1992).

The diagnosis of primary hyperparathyroidism is more challenging when concentrations of PTH are still within the reference range. Such concentrations should be considered abnormally high when they occur in combination with hypercalcemia. Confirmed primary hyperparathyroidism has been noted in some dogs and cats with hypercalcemia and PTH concentrations within the reference range when measured using intact molecule assays (Feldman and Nelson 1996; Kallet et al. 1991). In a cat with persistent hypercalcemia related to primary hyperparathyroidism, PTH concentration was increased on two occasions but within the reference range on five other occasions (den Hertog et al. 1997). PTH concentrations measured in blood collected from either the left or right jugular vein did not differ, and sampling from a specific side was not valuable for localizing the site of an enlarged parathyroid gland (Feldman et al. 1997). Circulating PTHrP concentrations were undetectable in six dogs with primary hyperparathyroidism (Rosol et al. 1992).

Ultrasonography of the neck is helpful in the diagnosis of primary hyperparathyroidism, but it requires an ultrasound unit with a high-frequency (7.5- to 10-MHz) transducer to achieve the necessary level of resolution rather than the widely available 5- or 7.5-MHz units used for abdominal studies (Feldman and Nelson 1996; Wisner and Nyland 1998). The anatomy of the cervical region is complex and the experience of the ultrasonographer influences the ability to detect enlarged parathyroid glands. The parathyroid glands of normal dogs and cats are not usually seen during ultrasonography (Wisner and Nyland 1998). Parathyroid gland masses greater than 5 mm can usually be identified and some masses as small as 2 mm may be detected. Enlarged parathyroid glands are expected to be hypoechoic or anechoic, well margined, and easily contrasted with thyroid tissue. False-positive results are rare but false-negative findings may occur. A solitary parathyroid gland that measured 4 mm or more in its greatest dimension was associated with parathyroid gland adenoma ($n = 15$) or adenocarcinoma ($n = 5$) (Wisner et al. 1997). Most of the enlarged parathyroid glands were found in either the cranial or caudal pole of the thyroid lobe and occasionally in the middle of the thyroid lobe. The right cranial thyroid lobe had parathyroid gland enlargement in the majority of dogs with either parathyroid gland adenoma or adenocarcinoma. One or more parathyroid glands smaller than 4 mm were associated with either primary or secondary hyperplasia of the parathyroid gland (Wisner et al. 1997). Parathyroid glands could not be seen in two of three dogs with renal secondary hyperparathyroidism or in three of four dogs with nonparathyroid malignancy-associated hypercalcemia. An ectopic parathyroid gland adenoma was located cranial to the thoracic inlet of one dog. Consequently, it is important to conduct a complete ultrasound study of the ventral cervical region in patients with hypercalcemia when there are negative results during routine examination of the thyroid region (Wisner and Nyland 1998). Ultrasonography correctly identified the presence and location of a solitary parathyroid gland mass in 10 of 11 dogs in a prospective study in which the mass was confirmed at surgery and serum total calcium concentration remained normal after removal of the mass (Feldman et al. 1997). Sonography of the cervical region identifies the location of the parathyroid gland tumor and allows presurgical planning.

Double-phase scintigraphy of the parathyroid glands using ^{99m}Tc sestamibi was useful in the diagnosis of parathyroid gland adenoma in two dogs (Matwichuk et al. 1996; Wright et al. 1995). Differential washout from a parathyroid adenoma compared with normal parathyroid tissue forms the basis for this test. This method may be particularly useful when results of routine diagnostic studies for other causes of hypercalcemia are negative and serum PTH concentration is within the normal range.

Surgical exploration of the cervical region in patients with parathyroid gland adenoma or carcinoma usually reveals enlargement of one parathyroid gland, and the remaining three are small or impossible to identify because hypercalcemia results in atrophy of normal parathyroid tissue. Primary parathyroid gland hyperplasia may affect more than one gland, and clinical signs can recur if only the largest gland is removed surgically. Parathyroid gland tumors may be difficult to identify if the tumor is embedded in fat or if it arises from the internal parathyroid gland. Failure to visualize a parathyroid gland tumor is rarely attributed to the occurrence of a tumor in ectopic parathyroid tissue. Methylene blue infusion to enhance visualization of parathyroid glands should be reserved for patients in which a tumor is strongly suspected but not readily identified during surgery, because clinically relevant side effects of methylene blue administration include hemolytic anemia and acute renal failure (Fingeroth and Smeak 1988).

HYPERVITAMINOSIS D

Hypervitaminosis D refers to toxicity resulting from excess cholecalciferol (vitamin D_3) or ergocalciferol (vitamin D_2) in the body, because these are the two common forms of naturally occurring vitamin D. Metabolites of vitamin D can also exert toxicity and the term hypervitaminosis D has been extended clinically to include toxicity from 25-hydroxyvitamin D, dihydrotachysterol, and 1,25-dihydroxyvitamin D (calcitriol), as well as newer analogues of calcitriol. Vitamin D toxicity is better referred to as 25-hydroxyvitamin D toxicity, because vitamin D is rapidly transformed into this metabolite in vivo (Fraser et al. 1986). Vitamin D and its immediate metabolite, 25-hydroxyvitamin D, have little biologic activity at physiologic concentrations because they have low binding affinity for the vitamin D receptor. Pharmacologic concentrations of 25-hydroxyvitamin D that occur during hypervitaminosis D, however, exert hypercalcemic effects because 25-hydroxyvitamin D completes with calcitriol for binding to the vitamin D receptor in target tissues (Nagode and Chew 1991; Dzanis and Kallfelz 1988). Hypercalcemia results primarily from increased intestinal absorption of calcium, but increased osteoclastic bone resorption and calcium reabsorption from renal distal tubules may also contribute.

Vitamin D intoxication and hypercalcemia may result from excessive dietary supplementation by an owner or a breeder or may be caused iatrogenically during the treatment of hypoparathyroidism. Accurate dosing with cholecalciferol and ergocalciferol is difficult because they have a slow onset and prolonged duration of action (Berger and Feldman 1987; Sherding et al. 1980). Hypercalcemia developed in 7 of 16 hypoparathyroid dogs during treatment with vitamin D and calcium salt supplementation (Berger and Feldman 1987). Ingestion of toxic plants that contain glycosides of calcitriol (e.g., *Cestrum diurnum, Solanum malacoxylon, Trisetum flavescens*) is a potential cause of hypercalcemia in small animals. Vitamin D toxicity associated with ingestion of *C. diurnum* has been reported in a cat (Drazner 1981). *C. diurnum*, day-blooming jessamine, has achieved increasing popularity as a house plant and should not be confused with jasmine, which is an indoor climbing plant without active vitamin D metabolites (Brownie 1987).

Hypervitaminosis D and hypercalcemia in dogs and cats became a more frequent diagnosis with the introduction of cholecalciferol-containing rodenticides in 1985, but it appears that this source of intoxication is less common today. Cholecalciferol bait is delivered as pellets that are apparently palatable to some animals and are very toxic when ingested. One manufacturer claimed a low hazard to dogs (oral median lethal dose, 88 mg/kg) but toxicity at a lower dosage (10 mg/kg) was demonstrated (Dzaner and Kallfelz 1988; Gunther et al. 1988). High-risk groups include dogs weighing 12 kg or less and those younger than 9 months. Toxicity in cats has also been reported. Clinical signs are usually vague and include anorexia, lethargy, vomiting, tremors, constipation, and polyuria. These signs are usually attributed to the effects of hypercalcemia. Hypercalcemia is reversible with early and aggressive therapy by providing enough time for 25-hydroxyvitamin D to be eliminated from the body (Dzaner and Kallfelz 1988; Carothers et al. 1994; Dougherty et al. 1990). Death occurred in approximately 45% of dogs after developing hypercalcemia from hypervitaminosis D in early reports (Dzaner and Kallfelz 1988; Gunther et al. 1988; MacKenzie et al. 1987; Garlock et al. 1991), but the survival rate was higher in dogs of a later series (Carothers et al. 1994).

Laboratory abnormalities usually include hypercalcemia that develops within 24 h after ingestion (Gunther et al. 1988). At presentation, hypercalcemia is often severe (15–20 mg/dL) unless serum samples were obtained within 24 h of ingestion. Mild hyperphosphatemia (7–8 mg/dL) is often found simultaneously. Azotemia is initially absent but can develop subsequently. Usually, serum creatinine concentration is <3 mg/dL unless treatment has been delayed, in which case azotemia may be marked. It may take as long as 72 h for azotemia to develop as a result of renal lesions caused by hypercalcemia. Measurement of serum 25-hydroxyvitamin D concentration can provide conclusive evidence for hypervitaminosis D after exposure to cholecalciferol or ergocalciferol. Measurement of serum 25-hydroxyvitamin D is now available commercially at modest cost. Serum concentrations of 25-hydroxyvitamin D were increased to at least twice the upper limit of normal, with a mean concentration approximately 10 times normal in dogs with hypervitaminosis D (Carothers et al. 1994). Serum 25-hydroxyvitamin D concentrations were increased for weeks to months in some instances (Dougherty et al. 1990). Serum calcitriol concentrations were also increased early in the syndrome in some dogs, but suppression of calcitriol synthesis is expected later in the syndrome.

Hypercalcemia attributed to the effects of increased calcitriol occasionally occurs during calcitriol treatment in dogs with hypoparathyroidism and rarely during treatment of renal secondary hyperparathyroidism. High serum concentrations of calcitriol have been observed in some dogs with lymphoma and hypercalcemia (Rosol et al. 1992), but it is not clear whether the excess calcitriol was synthesized by the tumor or by the kidneys under stimulation of PTHrP.

GRANULOMATOUS DISEASE

Hypercalcemia can result from calcitriol synthesis by activated macrophages during granulomatous inflammation. Normal macrophages express 1α-hydroxylase activity (which converts 25-hydroxyvitamin D to calcitriol) when stimulated by interferon or lipopolysaccharide. Macrophages in granulomatous inflammation express such activity without stimulation (Dusso et al. 1990). The activity of 1α-hydroxylase and subsequent synthesis of calcitriol by macrophages are not under regulatory control by calcitriol, PTH, or calcium concentration (Holick 1995). Granulomatous diseases such as systemic mycosis, sarcoidosis, tuberculosis, leprosy, and silicone-induced granulomas occasionally induce hypercalcemia in humans. Blastomycosis is a granulomatous disease in dogs that is occasionally (6–14% of cases) associated with hypercalcemia. Hypercalcemia is usually mild (11.5 to 13 mg/dL), but can be severe (>17 mg/dL) (Dow et al. 1986; Arceneaux et al. 1998). Increased production of calcitriol by granulomatous tissue results in hypercalcemia, but metabolites of vitamin D have not been measured. Reports of other granulomatous diseases associated with hypercalcemia include two of eight cats with disseminated histoplasmosis (Hodges et al. 1994) and dogs with coccidioidomycosis or schistosomiasis (Feldman and Nelson 1996; Troy et al. 1987). We have observed hypercalcemia in a cat with tuberculosis and severe hypercalcemia in association with noninfectious granulomatous dermatitis in two dogs in which excess synthesis of calcitriol was suspected (Barrett et al. 1998). PTH, PTHrP, and 25-hydroxyvitamin D concentrations were not increased, but calcitriol concentrations were not determined. Hypercalcemia resolved as the inflammation subsided. Nodular panniculitis with hypercalcemia has been reported in dogs, and calcitriol concentrations were two to three times normal in one instance (Elliott et al. 1981; Petrie 1996). Topical ointments containing potent vitamin D analogues designed for treatment of psoriasis in people have been approved for use in the United States and can result in hypercalcemia if excessively absorbed or ingested. One dog developed hypercalcemia and hyperphosphatemia after ingestion of Dovonex, which contains calcipotriene or calcipotriol as the vitamin D analogue (Refsal et al. 1998). Telephone calls to animal poison control centers indicate that exposure to this ointment has been increasing in dogs (Martin 1998).

IDIOPATHIC HYPERCALCEMIA OF CATS

Hypercalcemia is less common in cats than in dogs, but an important new hypercalcemic syndrome in cats has emerged since 1992 (Refsal et al. 1998). Directors of national and regional veterinary biochemistry and endocrinology laboratories have noted an increased frequency of hypercalcemia in cats without obvious explanation. We have observed several young to middle-aged cats with mild to moderate hypercalcemia that have no identifiable cause after standard diagnostic testing. Serum total calcium concentration has been increased in some cats for months to more than 1 year, often without obvious clinical signs. Serum ionized calcium concentration is increased, sometimes out of proportion to the increase in total serum calcium concentration. Nephrocalcinosis may be observed on radiographs or renal ultrasonography, but renal function, based on blood urea nitrogen and serum creatinine concentration, is usually normal initially. CRF eventually develops in most affected cats, followed by death or euthanasia. Urinary calculi have developed in some of the affected cats. Affected cats have no evidence of malignancy on thoracic and skeletal radiography, abdominal sonography, bone marrow evaluation, and (in some instances) full necropsy. Results of serology testing for feline leukemia virus and feline immunodeficiency virus have been negative and serum thyroxine concentrations have been normal. Serum PTH concentrations have been normal or low, PTHrP has not been detectable, and 25-hydroxyvitamin D concentrations have been within normal limits. Serum calcitriol concentrations have also been normal in the few cats in which they were measured. Chronic acidosis may explain chronic ionized hypercalcemia (Ching et al. 1989), but venous blood gas analysis has not revealed significant acid-base disturbances. Exploration of the cervical region has not identified primary hyperparathyroidism, and subtotal parathyroidectomy has not resolved hypercalcemia in cats in which this procedure was performed. A change to a high-fiber diet was recommended for most affected cats in the hope that dietary calcium would be less available for intestinal absorption, but this dietary modification did not change serum calcium concentration in any affected cat. Treatment with prednisone has resulted in long-term decreases in serum ionized and total serum calcium concentrations in several cats.

Approximately 33% of cats with calcium oxalate urolithiasis from the records of the University of Minnesota Urolithiasis Center have had hypercalcemia. Some of these hypercalcemic cats experienced decreases in their serum calcium concentrations after changes to diets with increased fiber. Idiopathic hypercalcemia in some calcium oxalate stone–forming cats has also been reported from the University of Georgia (McClain and Barsanti 1999). The occurrence of ureterolithiasis in cats was very uncommon before 1993. Eleven cases of calcium oxalate ureterolithiasis were recently described in cats, 3 of which had mild hypercalcemia and 1 of which had moderate hypercalcemia (Kyles et al. 1998). Analysis of calcitropic hormones was not reported in this study.

It is not clear whether the pathophysiology of idiopathic hypercalcemia in oxalate stone–forming cats is the same as in cats that do not form stones. It is possible that these different clinical presentations represent different phases of the same disease process. Additional studies that include measurements of calcium regulatory hormones and serum ionized calcium concentrations are needed to characterize this syndrome further. The role of diet in the hypercalcemic syndrome also requires further investigation. It is likely that studies of calcium balance that include dietary intake, intestinal absorption, fecal excretion, bone resorption, and urinary excretion will be needed to discover the mechanism of hypercalcemia. Urinary markers of increased bone turnover may prove useful in determining whether bone resorption contributes to this form of hypercalcemia. Measurement of vitamin A metabolites and aluminum would also be valuable to evaluate some of the unusual possibilities for the development of hypercalcemia. Alkali treatment can be used as a challenge to assess the role of chronic dietary acidification in the pathogenesis of this syndrome and to determine whether hypercalcemia resolves with alkali therapy. Bisphosphonate treatment could also be used to determine whether bone resorption contributes to the observed hypercalcemia.

UNCOMMON CAUSES OF HYPERCALCEMIA

Acute intrinsic renal failure in dogs is occasionally associated with mild hypercalcemia. Hypercalcemia may occur more commonly after conversion of oliguria to polyuria, possibly as calcium salts that were deposited during oliguria are mobilized from soft tissues. Sudden improvement in renal function also may result in rapid lowering of serum phosphorus concentration, changing mass law interactions between phosphorus and calcium and resulting in transient hypercalcemia. We have observed mild hypercalcemia (11.5–12.5 mg/dL) uncommonly in some dogs with severe oliguria and decreased GFR during intrinsic renal failure, but it is usually transient and the mechanisms were not studied. Animals with severe hyperphosphatemia during acute intrinsic renal failure usually have normal or low serum calcium concentrations.

Nonmalignant skeletal lesions are occasionally associated with hypercalcemia in dogs. Bacterial and fungal osteomyelitis can potentially result in hypercalcemia if the rate of osteolysis is sufficient (Chew and Capen 1980). The relative contribution to hypercalcemia from lysis of bone in contact with fungal infection as opposed to that resulting from calcitriol synthesis in macrophages of granulomatous inflammation (see earlier) is not known. Neonatal septicemia has been associated with hypercalcemia on rare occasion in puppies after septic embolization of bone and subsequent osteolysis (Chew and Capen 1980). We have observed mild hypercalcemia in some dogs with hypertrophic osteodystrophy, and results of experimental studies of hypertrophic osteodystrophy suggest that hypercalcemia may be aggravated by ascorbic acid supplementation (Teare et al. 1979). Disuse osteoporosis after prolonged immobilization can rarely contribute to the development of mild hypercalcemia, because weight bearing is necessary to maintain the balance between new bone formation and resorption of old bone.

Toxicity of Hypercalcemia and Clinical Signs

Ionized calcium is the serum calcium fraction that is important for pathophysiologic effects as well as for normal physiology (Rosol and Capen 1996). Excessive numbers of calcium ions are toxic to cells (Rasmussen et al. 1990). Increased serum ionized calcium concentration decreases cellular function by causing alterations in cell membrane permeability and cell membrane calcium pump activity. Increased intracellular calcium content can ultimately result in cell death caused by deranged cellular function and reduced energy production. Although all tissues may be subject to the dangerous effects of hypercalcemia, effects on the central nervous system, gastrointestinal tract, heart, and kidneys are of most importance clinically.

Polydipsia, polyuria, anorexia, lethargy, and weakness are the most common clinical signs in animals with hypercalcemia (Chew and Carothers 1989; Feldman and Nelson 1996), but individual animals often display remarkable differences in clinical signs despite similar magnitudes of hypercalcemia. The severity of clinical signs and development of lesions of hypercalcemia depends not only on the magnitude of hypercalcemia but also on its rate of development and duration. Simultaneous disturbances in other electrolyte concentrations and in acid-base balance, as well as organ dysfunction secondary to hypercalcemia, all contribute to clinical signs, laboratory abnormalities, and lesions. Table 6–3 lists the signs and conditions associated with hypercalcemia.

Clinical signs are most severe when hypercalcemia develops rapidly, as can occur with vitamin D intoxication or during rapid infusion of calcium-containing fluids. Dogs with similar magnitudes of hypercalcemia may display minimal clinical signs when hypercalcemia has developed gradually. Regardless of the rate of increase in serum calcium concentration, clinical signs become more severe as the magnitude of hypercalcemia increases. Serum total calcium concentrations of 12.0 to 14.0 mg/dL may not be associated with severe clinical signs, but most animals with concentrations >15.0 mg/dL show systemic signs. Dogs with serum calcium concentrations >18 mg/dL are often severely ill, and concentrations >20 mg/dL may constitute a life-threatening crisis. Exceptions do occur, however, and some dogs are severely affected by mild hypercalcemia whereas others are relatively unaffected by severe hypercalcemia. Clinical signs and histopathologic changes are more likely to develop the longer hypercalcemia has been present, regardless of its magnitude. Progressive hypercalcemia may also contribute to the severity of clinical signs, as occurs in animals with malignant neoplasia or hypervitaminosis D related to rat bait ingestion.

Changes in serum sodium and potassium concentrations can magnify the clinical signs of hypercalcemia by their effects on cell membrane excitability, particularly in nerve and muscle (see Chapter 5). Acidosis increases the proportion of serum calcium that is ionized, worsening clinical signs, whereas alkalosis lessens toxicity and clinical signs by decreasing the proportion of calcium that is ionized.

TABLE 6–3. Clinical Signs and Conditions Associated with Hypercalcemia

Common	Uncommon
Polydipsia and polyuria	Constipation
Anorexia	Cardiac arrhythmia
Dehydration	Seizures or twitching
Lethargy	Death
Weakness	Acute intrinsic renal failure
Vomiting	Calcium urolithiasis
Prerenal azotemia	
Chronic renal failure	

Mineralization of soft tissues (especially the heart and kidneys) is an important complication of hypercalcemia. The serum phosphorus concentration at the time hypercalcemia develops is important in determining the extent of soft tissue mineralization. Soft tissue mineralization is most severe when the calcium (mg/dL) times phosphorus (mg/dL) product is greater than 60 (Chew and Meuten 1982). Soft tissue mineralization occurs regardless of the serum phosphorus concentration in severe hypercalcemia.

RENAL EFFECTS OF HYPERCALCEMIA

Abnormal renal function frequently accompanies hypercalcemia and is due to functional and structural changes, and rapid deterioration in renal function occasionally occurs. The functional effects of hypercalcemia on the kidneys are readily reversible, but the structural changes may not be reversible if the renal lesions are advanced. Azotemia occurred commonly in 34 dogs with hypercalcemia related to malignancy, hypoadrenocorticism, CRF, and hypervitaminosis D (Kruger et al. 1996). The frequency of azotemia was higher in dogs with malignancy (71%) than in those with hypercalcemia related to primary hyperparathyroidism (11%). Azotemia caused by hypercalcemia can result from any combination of the following: prerenal reduction in ECF volume (anorexia, hypodipsia, vomiting, and polyuria); renal vasoconstriction from ionized hypercalcemia; decreased permeability coefficient of the glomerulus (K_f); acute tubular necrosis from the ischemic and toxic effects of hypercalcemia; and CRF caused by nephron loss, nephrocalcinosis, tubulointerstitial inflammation, and interstitial fibrosis.

Decreased urinary concentrating ability and polyuria are early functional effects of hypercalcemia. The concentrating defect is often out of proportion to the observed reduction in GFR and increase in serum creatinine or blood urea nitrogen concentration. Urine specific gravity is consistently <1.030 and was <1.020 in over 90% of hypercalcemic dogs in one study (Kruger et al. 1996). Defective urinary concentrating ability results from a combination of reduced tubular reabsorption of sodium and impaired action of antidiuretic hormone on tubular cells of the collecting duct. This results in a form of nephrogenic diabetes insipidus characterized by hyposthenuria if the diluting segment of the nephron (medullary thick ascending limb of Henle's loop) is unaffected. These effects are due to intrinsic responses of the kidney to hypercalcemia and are mediated by calcium-sensing receptors on the renal epithelial cells (Brown and Hebert 1997). Additional direct effects of hypercalcemia on the kidney include reduced tubular calcium reabsorption and antagonism of the actions of PTH. These responses by the kidney facilitate calcium excretion and help to ameliorate the clinical effects of hypercalcemia. Renal medullary blood flow is increased in dogs with experimental hypercalcemia (Brunette et al. 1974) and can result in medullary washout as another mechanism contributing to hyposthenuria. Isosthenuria develops if the diluting segments have been structurally altered by long-standing hypercalcemia. Polydipsia occurs as compensation for obligatory polyuria, but there is evidence that polydipsia can be due to direct stimulation of the thirst center by hypercalcemia (Chew and Meuten 1982). Mineralization of renal tubules, basement membranes, or the interstitium; tubular degeneration; and interstitial fibrosis are structural changes that may occur in the kidney secondary to hypercalcemia and can contribute to impaired urinary concentrating ability. A review of calcium nephropathy is available for more detailed information (Kruger et al. 1996).

Dehydration is common owing to increased fluid losses from vomiting and polyuria. Substantial contraction of the ECF volume results in reduced GFR that may be severe enough to increase blood urea nitrogen and serum creatinine concentrations and cause prerenal azotemia. The clinical axiom that dilute urine in association with azotemia is usually caused by intrinsic renal lesions may not be true in animals with hypercalcemia, because the urinary concentrating defect can occur without structural renal lesions. This condition is commonly misdiagnosed as primary renal failure when it is actually prerenal failure caused by dehydration and a renal concentrating defect early in the course of hypercalcemia.

Intrarenal causes of azotemia during hypercalcemia can be functional or structural. Hypercalcemia can induce renal vasoconstriction resulting in decreased renal blood flow (RBF) and GFR (Chew and Capen 1980). In an acute model of hypercalcemia, reduced RBF and GFR were observed consistently in conscious dogs when serum calcium concentration exceeded 20 mg/dL, but only half of the dogs had significant reductions in GFR and RBF when serum calcium concentration was 15 to 20 mg/dL. Little effect on RBF and GFR was observed when serum calcium concentration was <15 mg/dL. These findings are in contrast to those in studies of anesthetized dogs, which demonstrated much more severe functional changes during hypercalcemia (Lins 1979). The effects of chronic hypercalcemia on GFR and RBF have not been studied. Impaired renal autoregulation related to the effects of hypercalcemia may result in azotemia at early stages of dehydration, because GFR would otherwise be maintained by afferent arteriolar vasodilatation.

Acute intrinsic renal failure occasionally develops as a consequence of hypercalcemia, but chronic intrinsic renal failure is more common. Sustained renal vasoconstriction related to hypercalcemia may result in ischemic tubular injury, promoting development of both acute and chronic intrinsic renal failure and potentiating the direct toxic effects of calcium on tubular cells. Tubular cells are exposed to toxic calcium concentrations as increased amounts of ionized and complexed calcium traverse the glomerulus into tubular fluid and come in contact with luminal tubular surfaces. Basolateral tubular membranes are exposed to a high concentration of calcium by postglomerular blood flow. Both of these mechanisms result in increased concentrations of calcium within tubular cells and mitochondria, leading to disrupted cell function and lethal cell injury. The toxic effects of ionized hypercalcemia are enhanced by high concentrations of PTH in animals with CRF, as excess PTH increases calcium entry into cells (Nagode and Chew 1992). The ascending limb of Henle's loop and distal convoluted tubule show the earliest structural lesions, but lesions in the collecting system are ultimately the most pronounced. Thickening and mineralization of tubular basement membranes are most apparent in the proximal tubule. Tubular atrophy, mononuclear cell infiltration, and interstitial fibrosis occur in the chronic stages. Degenerative and necrotic tubules also are observed. Granular and tubular cell casts contribute to intrarenal obstruction and azotemia (Kruger et al. 1996; Chew and Capen 1980).

Calcium-oxalate urolithiasis occasionally occurs in animals with long-standing hypercalcemia and can be detected by radiography or ultrasonography. This complication has been described in dogs and cats with primary hyperparathyroidism. Nephrocalcinosis and linear mineralization along the renal diverticula are nonspecific findings discovered by radiography or ultrasonography in some dogs with long-standing hypercalcemia. Increased renal echogenicity and the medullary rim sign have been described during renal ultrasonography in dogs with hypercalcemia (Biller et al. 1992; Barr et al. 1989). These changes can occur in other normocalcemic conditions as well as in forms of dystrophic mineralization.

EFFECTS OF HYPERCALCEMIA ON OTHER ORGANS
Anorexia, vomiting, and constipation can result from hypercalcemia by reduction of the excitability of gastrointestinal smooth muscle as well as from direct effects on the central nervous system. Gastric hyperacidity and subsequent gastric ulceration caused by increased secretion of gastrin and direct stimulation of hydrogen ion secretion from parietal cells by hypercalcemia may account for some of the vomiting. Pancreatitis secondary to hypercalcemia occurs in experimental animals, but its importance in dogs and cats with clinical hypercalcemia is not clear (Frick et al. 1995; Mithöfer et al. 1995). Decreased excitability of skeletal muscle contributes to generalized weakness. Lethargy is commonly observed in severe hypercalcemia because of direct effects on the central nervous system and rarely can progress to stupor and coma. Seizures and muscle twitching are unusual neuromuscular manifestations of hypercalcemia (Ihle et al. 1988).

Clinically important cardiac effects of hypercalcemia are not commonly detected in dogs and cats, but PR interval prolongation and QT interval shortening can be observed on the electrocardiogram. Serious arrhythmias (including ventricular fibrillation) can be due to the direct effects of severe hypercalcemia or may be a consequence of mineralization of cardiac tissue. Hypertension has been convincingly demonstrated in human beings and rats during both acute and chronic hypercalcemia. The rise in blood pressure is proportional to the rise in serum calcium concentration in acute studies (Campese 1989). Whether hypertension is a clinically relevant complication in dogs and cats with hypercalcemia is unknown.

Treatment of Hypercalcemia

PHILOSOPHY OF TREATMENT
There is no absolute serum calcium concentration that can be used as a guideline for the decision to treat hypercalcemia aggressively (Chew and Carothers 1989; Finco 1983). The magnitude of hypercalcemia, its rate of development, whether the serum calcium concentration is stable or progressively increasing, and the modifying effects of other electrolyte and acid-base disturbances must all be considered when deciding on a treatment plan. The clinical condition of the animal ultimately dictates how aggressive treatment should be, but a serum calcium concentration ≥16 mg/dL has been recommended as a basis for aggressive therapy (Finco 1983). Animals with serum calcium concentrations approaching 20 mg/dL should be considered candidates for crisis management. Animals with serum calcium concentrations below 16 mg/dL may also require aggressive treatment, depending on the degree of neurologic, cardiac, and renal dysfunction induced by the hypercalcemia and concurrent deleterious factors. Acidosis can magnify the effects of hypercalcemia at all serum calcium concentrations by shifting more calcium to the ionized fraction. The serum phosphorus concentration at the time of hypercalcemia is also an important modulating factor in clinical decision making because soft tissue mineralization is potentiated by hyperphosphatemia. Animals with rapid and progressive development of hypercalcemia usually display serious clinical signs that require aggressive therapy.

DEFINITIVE THERAPY
Removal of the underlying cause is the definitive treatment for hypercalcemia, but this is not always immediately possible. Most animals with pathologic hypercalcemia have an associated malignancy that is quickly diagnosed but often not readily treated. Complete excision of isolated neoplasms (e.g., apocrine gland adenocarcinoma of the anal sac, parathyroid gland adenoma) abolishes hypercalcemia. In animals with disseminated metastases, multicentric neoplasia, or nonresectable primary malignancy, the tumor burden and hypercalcemia may be decreased by appropriate chemotherapy, radiation therapy, and immunotherapy. Chemotherapy may disrupt neoplastic cellular metabolism to such an extent that the tumor may no longer be able to synthesize enough humoral factors to sustain hypercalcemia. Decreased serum calcium concentrations can occur despite lack of obvious reduction in tumor size in these instances.

TABLE 6–4. General Treatment of Hypercalcemia

Definitive
    Remove underlying cause
Supportive
    Initial considerations
        Fluids (0.9% sodium chloride)
        Furosemide
        Sodium bicarbonate
        Glucocorticosteroids
    Secondary considerations
        Bisphosphonates
        Calcitonin
    Tertiary considerations
        Mithramycin
        Ethylene diamine tetraacetic acid (EDTA)
        Peritoneal dialysis
    Future considerations
        Calcium channel blockers
        Somatostatin congeners
        Calcium receptor agonists
        Nonhypercalcemic calcitriol analogues

Antifungal treatment with amphotericin B, ketoconazole, or itraconazole effectively lowers increased serum calcium concentrations in dogs with systemic mycoses as the infectious agent is eradicated and inflammation resolves. For animals with hypercalcemia associated with hypoadrenocorticism, replacement therapy with mineralocorticoids and glucocorticoids after fluid volume replacement definitively manages the condition. Discontinuing all vitamin D supplementation in animals with hypervitaminosis D and hypercalcemia removes the external cause of intoxication, but excessive body stores of vitamin D may continue to contribute to hypercalcemia for several weeks.

SUPPORTIVE THERAPY

Supportive therapy is often necessary to decrease serum calcium concentration to a less toxic level while waiting for a definitive diagnosis to be established, for definitive treatment to reduce serum calcium concentration permanently, or for chronic management of hypercalcemia when the underlying cause cannot be removed. Tables 6–4 and 6–5 list general and specific treatments for the management of hypercalcemia. Unfortunately, no single treatment protocol is consistently effective for all causes of hypercalcemia. Consequently, regimens must be tailored for the individual patient. Supportive treatments reduce the magnitude of hypercalcemia by increasing

TABLE 6–5. **Specific Treatment of Hypercalcemia**

Treatment	Dose	Indications	Comments
Volume Expansion			
SQ saline (0.9%)*	75–100 mL/kg/day	Mild hypercalcemia	Contraindicated if peripheral edema is present.
IV saline (0.9%)*	100–125 mL/kg/day	Moderate to severe hypercalcemia	Contraindicated in congestive heart failure and hypertension.
Diuretics			
Furosemide	2–4 mg/kg b.i.d. to t.i.d. IV, SQ, PO	Moderate to severe hypercalcemia	Volume expansion is necessary before use of this drug.
Alkalinizing Agent			
Sodium bicarbonate	1 mEq/kg IV slow bolus; may continue at 0.3 × base deficit × wt in kg/day	Severe hypercalcemia	Requires close monitoring.
Glucocorticoids			
Prednisone	1–2.2 mg/kg b.i.d. PO, SQ, IV	Moderate to severe hypercalcemia	Use of these drugs before identification of etiology may make definitive diagnosis difficult!
Dexamethasone	0.1–0.22 mg/kg b.i.d. IV, SQ		
Bone Resorption Inhibitors			
Calcitonin	4–6 IU/kg SQ b.i.d. to t.i.d.	Hypervitaminosis D	Response may be short-lived. Vomiting may occur.
Bisphosphonates			
EHDP-Didronel	15 mg/kg q24h to b.i.d.	Moderate to severe hypercalcemia	All are expensive and use in dogs is limited.
Clodronate	20–25 mg/kg in a 4-h IV infusion		Clodronate is approved for use in humans in Europe; availability in United States may be limited.
Pamidronate	1.3 mg/kg in 150 mL 0.9% saline in a 2-h IV infusion, can repeat in 1 wk		
Mithramycin	25 µg/kg IV in 5% dextrose over 2–4 h q2–4 wk	Severe hypercalcemia, refractory HHM	Limited use in dogs and cats. Nephrotoxicity, hepatotoxicity, thrombocytopenia.
Miscellaneous			
Sodium EDTA	25–75 mg/kg/h	Severe hypercalcemia	Nephrotoxicity
Peritoneal dialysis	Low calcium dialysate	Severe hypercalcemia	Short duration of response. Use in hypercalcemia not reported.

*Potassium supplementation is necessary. Add 5–40 mEq KCl/L depending on serum potassium concentration.
Abbreviation: HHM, Humoral hypercalcemia of malignancy.

renal calcium excretion, inhibiting bone resorption, promoting soft tissue deposition of calcium, causing a shift of intravascular calcium to other body compartments, promoting extrarenal calcium loss, reducing calcium transport across the gut, or some combination of these effects (Chew and Carothers 1989; Martin 1998; Kruger et al. 1986).

INITIAL CONSIDERATIONS FOR TREATMENT

Parenteral fluids, furosemide, sodium bicarbonate, glucocorticoids, or combinations of these treatments effectively reduce serum calcium concentrations in most animals with hypercalcemia. It is wise to confirm that hypercalcemia is a repeatable finding before prescribing aggressive treatments. It is not always necessary or possible to reduce serum calcium concentration to within normal limits, but substantial resolution of serious clinical signs may still be accomplished when serum calcium concentration declines by as little as 1 to 3 mg/dL in some animals with very high serum calcium concentrations.

FLUID THERAPY

Parenteral fluid therapy is an important first treatment for all animals that have systemic signs from hypercalcemia. The first goal of fluid therapy is to correct dehydration, because hemoconcentration contributes to increased serum calcium concentration. In addition, the kidney responds during ECF volume contraction with more avid reabsorption of sodium and calcium from the glomerular ultrafiltrate. Correction of dehydration abrogates this effect and allows calciuresis and natriuresis to occur.

Dehydration should be corrected with intravenous fluids within 4 to 6 h of presentation in animals with severe clinical signs attributable to hypercalcemia. Additional expansion of ECF volume with parenteral fluids is then indicated, but sufficient fluid for rehydration and volume expansion is often provided simultaneously. Fluid therapy alone may be sufficient in some animals to reduce the magnitude of hypercalcemia adequately when the initial serum calcium concentration is below 14 mg/dL, but often other treatments must be added. Normocalcemia may be restored by fluid therapy alone if hypercalcemia was initially mild (12–13 mg/dL), in which case persistent pathologic hypercalcemia is probably not present.

Physiologic saline (0.9% NaCl) is the solution of choice for correction of the intravascular volume deficit and for further slight volume expansion. Slight volume expansion with 0.9% NaCl promotes calcium loss in urine secondary to increased GFR and increased filtered load of calcium, and competition from the additional sodium ions results in reduced renal tubular calcium reabsorption and enhanced calciuresis.

Extracellular fluid volume expansion with lactated Ringer's solution (6 mg/dL calcium) in dogs resulted in decreased total protein, total calcium, and ionized calcium concentrations. Decreases in total calcium concentration, however, were greater (12.4%) than those observed for ionized calcium concentration (3.5%) (Renoe et al. 1979). Thus, volume expansion with solutions that contain some calcium can be beneficial, because the dilutional effect supersedes the effect of the additional calcium that is administered. Physiologic saline (0.9% NaCl) is preferred, however, because it is devoid of additional calcium and contains more sodium than that in lactated Ringer's solution (154 versus 130 mEq/L). Consequently, 0.9% NaCl results in a more rapid reduction in serum calcium concentration. An initial fluid volume of two to three times maintenance needs (120–180 mL/kg/day) usually corrects dehydration, provides maintenance needs, and results in mild volume expansion.

Other parenteral fluid regimens have been used in the treatment of hypercalcemia in humans, including infusions of sodium sulfate or sodium phosphate. Veterinary experience with either one of these solutions is lacking. Sodium sulfate provides a nonresorbable anion that promotes calciuresis, whereas phosphates promote soft tissue mineralization. The use of sodium phosphate is not recommended because of the potential detrimental effects of soft tissue mineralization (Finco 1983).

DIURETICS (CALCIURETICS)

Administration of furosemide (Lasix) follows rehydration and fluid volume expansion as second in importance for treatment of persistent hypercalcemia. The diuretic action of furosemide promotes enhanced urinary calcium loss, but calciuresis does not follow the use of all diuretics. In particular, thiazides should not be used because they may result in hypocalciuria and potentially may aggravate hypercalcemia. Furosemide (5 mg/kg IV followed by 5 mg/kg/h as an infusion) can be helpful in acutely decreasing serum calcium concentration by a maximum of approximately 3 mg/dL in experimental animals (Ong et al. 1974). If the hourly regimen is selected, it is important to match the increased volume of urine lost after administration of the diuretic with an increased volume of parenteral fluids to prevent dehydration and to gain maximal calciuresis. Less aggressive regimens of furosemide administration may be effective in combination with other treatments or for chronic management of hypercalcemia, but this approach has not been adequately studied in animals. Adequate hydration before and during furosemide administration is essential; otherwise diuresis may actually increase serum calcium concentration through hemoconcentration.

SODIUM BICARBONATE

Infusion of sodium bicarbonate has been advocated for acute or crisis management of hypercalcemia, but most often it is mentioned for use in the presence of metabolic acidosis (Chew and Carothers 1989; Kruger et al. 1996; Martin 1998). Serum ionized calcium concentration is reduced as acidosis is corrected or mild alkalosis created, because more calcium becomes bound to serum proteins. Not all of the decrease in ionized calcium concentration can be explained by increased protein binding, and some of the decrease may result from increased binding of calcium to bicarbonate (Renoe et al. 1979). Decreases in ionized and total calcium concentrations after bicarbonate infusions have been observed in dogs (Meuten 1984) and cats (Chew et al. 1989). These studies suggest that additional mechanisms (beyond shifting of calcium among its serum fractions) cause both ionized and total serum calcium concentrations to decrease simultaneously. This observation could be the result of an expanded volume of distribution for calcium. A dosage of 1 to 4 mEq/kg sodium bicarbonate has been recommended to obtain the desired reduction in calcium concentration (Chew et al. 1989; Kruger et al. 1996), but it may not be necessary to provide continuous bicarbonate infusion because the effect can last for as long as 3 h after a single dose of bicarbonate in normal cats (Chew et al. 1989). The magnitude of reduction in serum calcium concentration is slight after administration of sodium bicarbonate alone, but the effect increases with larger doses. Consequently, sodium bicarbonate infusion is most likely to be helpful in combination with other treatments.

STEROIDS

Glucocorticosteroids can contribute to a significant reduction in serum calcium concentration in hypercalcemic animals with lymphoma, multiple myeloma, thymoma, hypoadrenocorticism, hypervitaminosis D, hypervitaminosis A, or granulomatous disease, but they have little effect on serum calcium concentration in animals with other causes of hypercalcemia (Table 6–6). Some cats with idiopathic hypercalcemia also have a substantial decrease in serum calcium concentration after glucocorticoid treatment. Steroids exert their effect mainly by reducing bone resorption, decreasing intestinal calcium absorption, and increasing renal calcium excretion (Chew and Capen 1980; Mahgoub et al. 1997).

Cytotoxicity against neoplastic lymphocytes after glucocorticoids can result in a dramatic and rapid reduction in serum calcium concentration in dogs with lymphoma. Whenever possible, however, glucocorticoids should be withheld from animals for which a diagnosis has not yet been established, because lymphocytolysis can make a definitive histopathologic diagnosis of lymphoma much more difficult or impossible. Evaluation of the magnitude of change in hypercalcemia after treatment with glucocorticoids (glucocorticoid challenge or response test) can suggest a group of steroid-responsive disorders, but this is strongly discouraged until efforts to establish a definitive diagnosis have been exhausted (Feldman and Nelson 1996). An alternative challenge test for the diagnosis of occult lymphoma has been proposed using L-asparaginase at 20,000 IU/m^2 IV in an effort to disturb tumor cell metabolism but not cause cytolysis. Calcium concentrations are measured at baseline and then every 12 to 24 for 72 h. A complete return of serum calcium concentration to normal suggests occult lymphoma (Feldman and Nelson 1996). Once a diagnosis of lymphoma has been made, prednisone is usually administered at 1 to 2 mg/kg twice daily concomitant with chemotherapy. Oral prednisone at 1 mg/kg/day resulted in decreased serum total calcium and increased serum phosphorus concentrations in three dogs with apocrine gland adenocarcinoma of the anal sac but did not return the calcium concentration to normal (Rijnberk et al. 1978).

Decreased bone resorption after administration of glucocorticoids may be the result of impaired osteoclast maturation and decreased numbers of calcitriol receptors in bone (Stern 1990). Cortisol antagonizes the effects of vitamin D on the intestine in rats (Harrison and Harrison 1960). In dogs, chronic oral administration of prednisone (1.2 to 1.5 mg/kg/day) resulted in decreased serum calcitriol concentrations but caused no change in the number of calcitriol receptors or calcium-binding proteins in enterocytes (Korkor et al. 1985). Granulomatous diseases associated with increased calcitriol synthesis and hypercalcemia are often sensitive to the effects of glucocorticoids in reducing the serum calcium concentration (Reichel et al. 1989; Sharma 1996). Caution is advised, however, because the underlying disease (e.g., systemic mycosis) may be worsened. Hypercalcemia associated with hypervitaminosis A can also be steroid responsive (Bergman et al. 1988).

CALCITONIN

Calcitonin is an adjunctive treatment that may be useful in the management of animals with severe hypercalcemia or in those in which IV fluids and furosemide have not sufficiently reduced serum calcium concentration. Calcitonin should also be considered instead of prednisone for treatment of animals without a definitive diagnosis. Calcitonin rapidly decreases the magnitude of hypercalcemia primarily by reducing the activity and formation of osteoclasts. A maximal decrement in serum calcium concentration of approximately 3 mg/dL can be expected (Chew and Meuten 1982). The only known adverse effects of calcitonin are anorexia and vomiting, but relatively few treated dogs and cats have been evaluated. Calcitonin treatment is expensive, the magnitude of its effect is unpredictable, its effects may be short-lived (hours), and resistance often develops in a few days. Receptor down-regulation is thought to be responsible for development of resistance, a phenomenon that may be delayed by concurrent glucocorticoid treatment. The effectiveness of calcitonin may be restored after discontinuing treatment for 24 to 48 h (Martin 1998). Despite these limitations, calcitonin in combination with pamidronate is considered the best therapy for severe hypercalcemia associated with malignancy in humans after hydration with 0.9% NaCl (Chisholm et al. 1996; Sekine and Takami 1998).

The dosage of calcitonin in animals has been extrapolated from that used in humans (4 IU/kg IV followed by 4–8 IU/kg SQ once or twice daily) (Kruger et al. 1986). Calcitonin is listed as an antidote on packages of cholecalciferol-containing (vitamin D) rat poison, and treatment with calcitonin has been reported in dogs with hypercalcemia resulting from cholecalciferol toxicity. The dosage of calcitonin used in these dogs was 8 IU/kg SQ q24h (Fooshee and Forrester 1990), 5 IU/kg SQ q6h (Garlock et al. 1991), and 4 to 7 IU/kg SQ q6h to q8h (Dougherty et al. 1990). Calcitonin treatments were discontinued in two dogs because of anorexia and vomiting, and mild intermittent vomiting was reported in the third dog. The usefulness of calcitonin for treatment of a cat with hyper-

TABLE 6–6. Steroid-Sensitive Causes of Hypercalcemia

Lymphoma or leukemia	Vitamin A toxicity
Multiple myeloma	Granulomatous disease
Thymoma	Hypoadrenocorticism
Vitamin D toxicity	Idiopathic hypercalcemia in cats

calcemia caused by hypervitaminosis D was not clear because the cat died from complications of hypercalcemia shortly after treatment (Peterson et al. 1991).

BISPHOSPHONATES

Bisphosphonates (formerly misnamed diphosphonates) are a relatively new class of drugs (pyrophosphate analogues) that have been developed to inhibit bone resorption (Rodan and Batena 1993; Body et al. 1996). The hypocalcemic effects of bisphosphonates during malignancy are accounted for by their actions in bone as there is no effect on tumor mass. Bisphosphonates decrease osteoclast activity and function, despite increased numbers of osteoclasts present as a result of local or humoral mechanisms of osteolysis. Inhibition of resorption requires 1 to 2 days and supports the concept that bisphosphonates must first enter the osteoclast after it comes in contact bisphosphonate-containing bone mineral. Several important synthetic and metabolic functions required for osteoclastic bone resorption are impaired. Long-term bisphosphonate administration can lead to decreased osteoclast numbers through lethal injury of osteoclasts and decreased recruitment of new osteoclasts. Etidronate was the first bisphosphonate to be used clinically and the activity of newer bisphosphonates is often compared with that of etidronate. Clodronate, pamidronate, alendronate, and residronate have potencies 10, 100, 1000, and 5000 times as great as that of etidronate, respectively (Fleisch 1991).

Oral bisphosphonate therapy is generally designed for maintenance treatment after a course of IV bisphosphonates has been effective in the control of hypercalcemia. Less than 5% of bisphosphonates are absorbed from the gastrointestinal tract (Fleisch 1997), which limits the usefulness of oral forms of etidronate, clodronate, and alendronate (Green 1997). Etidronate is generally administered orally to dogs at 10 to 40 mg/kg/day in divided doses, and it has had some effectiveness in reduction of hypercalcemia associated with lymphoma, myeloma, primary hyperparathyroidism, and hypervitaminosis D in dogs treated at our hospital. A puppy with hypercalcemia and primary hyperparathyroidism was also successfully treated using etidronate (Thompson et al. 1984). Etidronate is available for IV administration at a lower dosage, but we have no clinical experience with etidronate administered by this route. Inhibition of bone resorption by pamidronate occurs earlier and is maintained longer than that induced by etidronate. Pamidronate is the main agent for treatment of severe hypercalcemia associated with malignancy in humans (Chisholm et al. 1996; Coukell and Markham 1998). Dogs with experimental cholecalciferol intoxication were treated with an infusion of pamidronate at a dosage of 1.3 mg/kg in 150 mL of 0.9% saline given over 2 h on days 1 and 8. Pamidronate treatment resulted in less weight loss, lower ionized and total serum calcium concentrations, lower serum phosphorus concentration, and better renal function than in control dogs (Rumbeiha et al. 1997). Clodronate is a second-generation bisphosphonate that was used to treat hypercalcemia of malignancy in one dog and hypervitaminosis D in another dog. Serum ionized and total calcium concentrations were normal when measured at 36 and 48 h after a 4-h infusion of clodronate at 20 to 25 mg/kg but long-term results were not reported (Petrie 1996).

Bisphosphonate treatment occasionally has been associated with the development of renal impairment in humans and acute intrinsic renal failure in experimental animals (Machado and Flombaum 1996). Therefore, dehydration should be corrected with 0.9% saline before bisphosphonates are administered. Depending on the bisphosphonate used, several hours of 0.9% saline infusion may be required to attenuate potential adverse effects. Pamidronate infusion in humans with hypercalcemia and underlying renal failure was shown to be safe (Machado and Flombaum 1996).

OTHER MISCELLANEOUS TREATMENTS

Mithramycin is a cytotoxic antibiotic developed for its antineoplastic properties, but it is also a potent inhibitor of osteoclastic bone resorption (Rosol et al. 1992; Rosol and Capen 1987). Significant toxicity, including thrombocytopenia, hepatic necrosis, renal necrosis, and hypocalcemia, unfortunately has been reported with the use of this drug (Chew and Meuten 1982; Finco 1983; Kruger et al. 1996). Mithramycin was safe when two doses of 0.1 mg/kg were administered IV 1 week apart to eight normal beagle dogs. Mithramycin decreased serum ionized calcium concentration in these normal dogs without adverse side effects such as hepatotoxicity, nephrotoxicity, or bone marrow hypoplasia, but some shivering occurred during the infusion. Osteoclastic bone resorption was significantly reduced (Rosol et al. 1992). Mithramycin was used to treat cancer-associated hypercalcemia in client-owned dogs in another study (Rosol et al. 1994). A single infusion of 0.1 mg/kg to two dogs resulted in normal serum total calcium concentration within 24 h, but severe hepatocellular necrosis associated with marked vomiting, diarrhea, and fever resulted in death shortly thereafter. Hypercalcemia may have increased the toxicity of mithramycin compared with that in normal dogs. To decrease additional episodes of toxicity, the dosage of mithramycin was decreased to 25 µg/kg for the remaining dogs in this study. Serum calcium concentration returned to the normal range in six of nine dogs within 24 to 48 h of treatment. Toxicity at this dosage was minimal but the calcium-lowering effect lasted only 24 to 72 h in three dogs. PTHrP concentrations and tumor size remained unchanged after treatment, and the lowering of serum calcium concentration was attributed to decreased osteoclastic bone resorption. Mithramycin is seldom prescribed because of its toxicity in hypercalcemic dogs at higher dosages and the short-lived effect at lower dosages.

During a hypercalcemic crisis, EDTA can be infused at a dosage of 25 to 75 mg/kg/h. Administered EDTA combines with circulating calcium to form a soluble complex that then is excreted by the kidneys (Chew and Meuten 1982). This treatment is considered a rescue method designed to allow other modalities time to take effect. Use of EDTA should be reserved for crisis situations because EDTA is nephrotoxic at higher dosages. A 2-h infusion of EDTA in normal dogs at 25 mg/kg/h did not have detrimental effects on the kidneys (Torrance and Nachreiner 1989).

Hemodialysis or peritoneal dialysis with calcium-free

dialysate may be used to lower serum calcium concentration when other methods fail (Camus et al. 1996; Koo et al. 1996). Dialysis may be particularly helpful in animals with severe intrinsic renal failure caused by hypercalcemia. Clinical experience with this method of treatment in animals is limited.

FUTURE CONSIDERATIONS

The calcium channel blocker diltiazem has been shown to reduce the magnitude of hypercalcemia and soft tissue mineralization in a model of vitamin D toxicosis in chicks (Dzanis and Kallfelz 1988) and may be effective in hypercalcemia of other causes. The toxic effects of hypercalcemia on the cardiovascular system of dogs can be blunted by verapamil (Basoglu et al. 1997; Zaloga et al. 1987; Zawada et al. 1990) and this drug may prove useful for stabilizing dogs and cats with severe hypercalcemia until other measures to decrease serum calcium concentration become effective.

Most treatments for HHM have focused on counteracting the effects of excess PTHrP rather than inhibiting PTHrP secretion. Somatostatin congeners inhibit secretion of certain hormones and one congener, lanreotide, successfully reduced serum calcium and PTHrP concentrations in a human patient with HHM (Anthony et al. 1995). Similar results were observed in other tumors in humans treated with octreotide (Mosdell and Visconti 1994; Pezzilli et al. 1997; Tweedy and Rees 1992; Miller and Edmonds 1991).

Nonhypercalcemic analogues of calcitriol have been reported to inhibit cell proliferation and PTHrP production by neoplastic tissue in vitro (Yu et al. 1995; McElwain et al. 1997). These new modalities for treating hypercalcemia in conditions associated with increased PTHrP are attractive for use in clinical patients because they appear to be safe, are easy to use, and are effective (Kruger et al. 1996). There are no reports yet of their use for control of PTHrP-associated hypercalcemia in veterinary patients.

Gallium nitrate is an antineoplastic, radioprotectant drug that has hypocalcemic properties related to its ability to reduce the solubility of hydroxyapatite in bone and inhibit osteoclast function. Gallium nitrate has been considered for treatment of refractory hypercalcemia, but it requires constant infusion (Okada et al. 1994; Kruger et al. 1986; Warrell et al. 1991; Bilezikian et al. 1994). The cytoprotectant amifostine (investigational drug WR-2721) inhibits PTH secretion and may have effectiveness in animals with hyperparathyroidism (Weaver et al. 1989). Use of amifostine has been limited to humans, and its adverse effects include nausea, vomiting, somnolence, and hypotension (Bilezekian et al. 1994). New calcium receptor agonists currently in development bind to and stimulate the cell membrane calcium receptor on parathyroid chief cells and other cells in the body. These compounds will be tested for their ability to inhibit PTH secretion and may be useful in patients with primary or renal secondary hyperparathyroidism.

ADDITIONAL SPECIFIC TREATMENTS FOR HYPERVITAMINOSIS D

In hypervitaminosis D associated with cholecalciferol intoxication, treatment may be necessary for several weeks because of the long half-lives of cholecalciferol and vitamin D metabolites. Consequently, aggressive fluid therapy for a week or more may be required to correct the severe hypercalcemia that is often encountered. Prednisone and furosemide therapy should be continued as maintenance therapy for 1 month. In addition, a low-calcium diet is important to reduce intestinal absorption of calcium. The diet provided can be a commercially available veterinary food or a homemade diet consisting mostly of macaroni and lean ground beef. Dairy products should be strictly avoided. Non–calcium-containing intestinal phosphorus binders may also be beneficial to counteract the effects of hyperphosphatemia. This treatment may be particularly important because the magnitude of soft tissue mineralization is most severe in animals with hypercalcemia induced by vitamin D toxicosis. Aluminum hydroxide at 30 to 90 mg/kg/day in divided doses is recommended during the first 2 weeks, with dosage and duration of treatment adjusted on the basis of serial measurements of serum phosphorus concentration. Decreased exposure to sunlight to lessen the conversion of 7-dehydrocholesterol to vitamin D in the skin has been advocated, but dogs do not efficiently photobioactivate cholecalciferol precursors (How et al. 1994), precluding the benefit of such therapy. Other unproven methods for treatment include anticonvulsants to increase hepatic metabolism of cholecalciferol, intestinal calcium binders to reduce intestinal calcium absorption, and calcium channel blockers to decrease the toxic intracellular effects of persistent hypercalcemia (Dzamis and Kallfelz 1988).

When hypervitaminosis D is due to excess calcitriol in patients with granulomatous disease, chloroquine, hydroxychloroquine, and ketoconazole may be used as supplemental therapeutic agents or as substitutes for glucocorticoids, because they impair conversion of 25-hydroxyvitamin D to 1,25-dihydroxyvitamin D by macrophages (Reichel et al. 1989; Sharma 1996).

▶ Hypocalcemia

Introduction

Hypocalcemia is a relatively common laboratory abnormality and was observed in 13.5% of serum biochemical profiles of dogs in one clinical study (Chew and Meuten 1982). On the basis of total serum calcium concentration, *hypocalcemia* is usually defined as a concentration lower than 8.0 mg/dL in dogs and lower than 7.0 mg/dL in cats. When serum ionized calcium concentration is used, hypocalcemia is generally defined as a concentration lower than 5.0 mg/dL in dogs and lower than 4.5 mg/dL in cats. In human patients, much larger and unexplained differences between ionized and total calcium concentrations have been found in hypocalcemic conditions as compared with hypercalcemic disorders (Ladenson et al. 1979).

Consequences of Hypocalcemia and Clinical Signs

Clinical signs related to hypocalcemia are identical regardless of the underlying cause (Table 6–7). Most of our

TABLE 6–7. **Clinical Signs Associated with Hypocalcemia**

Common
- None
- Muscle tremors or fasciculations
- Facial rubbing (paresthesia?)
- Muscle cramping
- Stiff gait
- Behavioral change
    - Restlessness or excitation
    - Aggression
    - Hypersensitivity to stimuli
    - Disorientation

Occasional
- Panting
- Pyrexia
- Lethargy
- Anorexia
- Prolapse of third eyelid (cats)
- Posterior lenticular cataracts
- Tachycardia or electrocardiographic alterations (prolonged QT interval)

Uncommon
- Polyuria or polydipsia
- Hypotension
- Respiratory arrest or death

---

knowledge about the clinical signs of hypocalcemia has been derived from animals with hypoparathyroidism. Low serum ionized calcium increases excitability of neuromuscular tissue, which accounts for many of the clinical signs of hypocalcemia. Animals with mild decreases in ionized calcium concentration may display no obvious clinical signs. The duration and magnitude of ionized hypocalcemia and the rate of decline in ionized calcium concentration interact to determine the severity of clinical signs. Clinical signs in dogs often are not obvious until serum total calcium concentration is below 6.5 mg/dL and some dogs show surprisingly few signs despite severe hypocalcemia (total serum calcium concentration <5.0 mg/dL), especially if the underlying disease has been chronic and there has been sufficient time for physiologic adaptation. Acute development of hypocalcemia is usually associated with severe clinical signs. In its most severe forms, hypocalcemia can cause death as a result of circulatory effects (e.g., hypotension, decreased myocardial contractility) and respiratory arrest from paralysis of respiratory muscles. Serum total calcium concentration below 4.0 mg/dL can cause left-sided myocardial failure (Drop 1985) and death (Feldman and Nelson 1996), especially if the decline in serum calcium concentration was rapid.

Other electrolyte and acid-base abnormalities can either magnify or diminish the signs of hypocalcemia. Correction of hypokalemia in cats with concurrent hypocalcemia may precipitate the onset of clinical signs of hypocalcemia (Nemzek et al. 1994; Dhupa and Proulx 1998). Patients with chronic hypocalcemia often display intermittent clinical signs despite seemingly stable total serum calcium concentrations. Although unpredictable, clinical signs often follow periods of exercise or excitement that may be associated with respiratory alkalosis and subsequent decreases in ionized calcium concentration. Rapid infusion of alkali to correct metabolic acidosis can cause seizures in animals with marginal or previously compensated hypocalcemia through further reduction in ionized calcium concentration. We have observed this phenomenon during treatment of primary renal failure in dogs and cats.

Clinical signs in dogs with chronic hypocalcemia (primary hypoparathyroidism) include seizures, muscle tremors or fasciculations, muscle cramping, stiff gait, and behavioral changes (e.g. restlessness, excitation, aggression, hypersensitivity to stimuli, disorientation) (Chew and Meuten 1982; Bruyette and Feldman 1988; Sherding et al. 1980; Dhupa and Proulx 1998). Tetany following hypocalcemia is initiated by central mechanisms, because experimental dogs with transected spinal cords and hypocalcemia exhibit tetany only above the level of the transection (Feldman and Nelson 1996). Seizures often begin as focal muscle tremors that become more widespread. Most dogs in one series had a seizure during the initial 24 to 48 h of hospitalization, a much higher frequency than encountered with idiopathic epilepsy (Feldman and Nelson 1996). Seizure activity associated with hypocalcemia may not be similar to that in idiopathic epilepsy because affected dogs may remain partially conscious and retain urinary continence during the seizure (Feldman and Nelson 1996; Peterson 1986). Seizures are often preceded by apprehension or nervousness. The seizures may be as short as 60 s or as long as 30 min in some dogs. Most seizures resolve without treatment but often recur despite treatment with anticonvulsants. Growling attributable to pain or behavior change occurred in approximately 40% of dogs, and intense rubbing of the face with the paws or on the ground was observed in more than 50% of dogs. These signs were attributed to either paresthesias or pain from facial muscle spasms (Bruyette and Feldman 1988; Feldman and Nelson 1996).

Pyrexia may be due to increased muscular activity with or without seizures. Lethargy and weakness are seen in approximately 33% of cases. Polyuria and polydipsia occur in approximately 25% of cases, possibly as a result of psychogenic mechanisms or renal injury (nephrocalcinosis) from hypercalciuria associated with PTH deficiency in animals with hypoparathyroidism (Sherding et al. 1980; Lees 1983; Russo and Lees 1986). Anterior and posterior lenticular cataracts occurred in over 33% of affected dogs (Bruyette and Feldman 1988; Kornegay 1982) and also in cats (Feldman and Nelson 1996; Peterson et al. 1991). Tachycardia and electrocardiographic abnormalities (increased QT interval) may also be encountered. Both hypertension and hypotension have been reported during hypocalcemia in humans (Campese 1989; Drop 1985). Whether blood pressure changes occur in dogs and cats with hypocalcemia is not known.

Neuromuscular signs in cats with chronic hypocalcemia associated with primary hypoparathyroidism are similar to those in dogs (e.g., muscle tremors, weakness, generalized seizures) (Peterson et al. 1991). Anorexia and lethargy appear to be more common in cats than in dogs with primary hypoparathyroidism, but seizures have not been reported to be induced by excitement, as occurs in dogs. Prolapse of the third eyelid is occasionally observed in cats with acute hypocalcemia but is not a prominent finding during chronic hypocalcemia.

Clinical signs associated with acute postoperative hypocalcemia are similar in dogs and cats and are related to neuromuscular excitability. Focal twitching of facial muscles and vibrissae may be noticed before more generalized muscle tremors or seizures develop. Tetany or facial twitching has not been observed in cats after thyroidectomy until serum total calcium concentration is lower than 6.9 mg/dL (Feldman and Nelson 1996; Peterson 1986; Peterson et al. 1991). Severe hypocalcemia (<6.5 mg/dL) is often associated with muscular twitching, tetany, or seizures. Anorexia and lethargy are not often considered primary signs of hypocalcemia, but both signs diminish in cats during calcium infusion after thyroidectomy, suggesting a relationship between hypocalcemia and these signs.

Differential Diagnosis and Mechanisms of Hypocalcemia

The conditions associated with hypocalcemia in dogs and cats are listed in Table 6–8 according to their relative frequency regardless of clinical signs or severity of de-

TABLE 6–8. Conditions Associated with Hypocalcemia

Common
- Hypoalbuminemia
- Chronic renal failure
- Puerperal tetany (eclampsia)
- Acute renal failure
- Acute pancreatitis
- Undefined cause (mild hypocalcemia)

Occasional
- Soft tissue trauma or rhabdomyolysis
- Hypoparathyroidism
    - Primary
        - Idiopathic or spontaneous
        - Postoperative bilateral thyroidectomy
    - After sudden reversal of chronic hypercalcemia
- Ethylene glycol intoxication
- Phosphate enema
- After NaHCO$_3$ administration

Uncommon
- Laboratory error
- Improper sample anticoagulant (EDTA)
- Infarction of parathyroid gland adenoma
- Rapid intravenous infusion of phosphates
- Acute calcium-free intravenous infusion (dilutional)
- Intestinal malabsorption or severe starvation
- Hypovitaminosis D
- Blood transfusion (citrated anticoagulant)
- Hypomagnesemia
- Nutritional secondary hyperparathyroidism
- Tumor lysis syndrome

Human
- Pseudohypoparathyroidism
- Drug-induced
- Hypercalcitonism
- Osteoblastic bone neoplasia (prostate cancer)

creased serum calcium concentration. Hypoalbuminemia is the most common associated condition but perhaps the least important for clinical consequences, and it occurred in nearly half of the dogs with hypocalcemia in one clinical study (Chew and Meuten 1982). Hypocalcemia associated with hypoalbuminemia is usually mild (total serum calcium concentration 7.5–9.0 mg/dL in dogs), and no signs referable to the functional effects of low serum calcium concentration are observed. Application of calcium correction formulas to serum total calcium concentrations in dogs or cats with hypoproteinemia or hypoalbuminemia usually results in values that are within normal limits. The correction to normal limits implies that serum ionized calcium concentration is normal and that total serum calcium concentration is low as a result of reduction of the protein-bound fraction of serum calcium. Unfortunately, ionized calcium concentrations may still be low despite "correction" to normal values. A correction formula has been widely used for both dogs and cats, but it was originally designed for use based only on data for dogs (Meuten et al. 1982). In addition, this formula was derived using serum albumin concentrations obtained by a different analytic method from that employed by autoanalyzers today, and the normal range for serum albumin concentration was considerably lower in the original report. Although there was a positive correlation, only 33% of the variability in serum total calcium concentration could be attributed to serum albumin concentration and 17% of the variability could be attributed to serum total proteins in a study of dogs (Meuten et al. 1982). In cats, there was no relationship between serum total protein and serum calcium concentrations and only 18% of the variability of serum total calcium concentration could be attributed to serum albumin concentrations (Flanders et al. 1989). Seventeen percent of the variability in total serum calcium concentration in dogs and 29% of the variability in cats could be attributed to serum albumin concentration in another study (Bienzle et al. 1993). The routine use of correction formulas is not advocated because the association between total serum calcium concentration and serum protein or albumin concentration is weak.

Renal failure was the second most common disorder associated with hypocalcemia in dogs (Chew and Meuten 1982). Total serum calcium concentration was 8.0 mg/dL or lower in 10% of dogs with CRF, and when the diagnosis was based on serum ionized calcium concentrations of 5.0 mg/dL or lower, hypocalcemia was detected in 40% of affected dogs (Chew and Nagode 1990). Approximately 15% of cats with CRF were hypocalcemic, and 6.7 mg/dL was the lowest total serum calcium concentration observed (DiBartola et al. 1987). Decreased calcitriol synthesis by the diseased kidneys and to a lesser extent mass law interactions of calcium with markedly increased serum phosphorus concentration are probable causes of the hypocalcemia observed in dogs and cats with CRF. In order to decrease ionized calcium concentration by 0.1 mg/dL, serum phosphorus concentration must increase by 3.7 mg/dL (Adler et al. 1985). Calcitriol deficits are more important because hypocalcemia results from reduced intestinal calcium absorption and increased skeletal resistance to PTH (Nagode and Chew 1991). Animals with CRF and decreased total serum calcium concentration are most often asymptomatic, possibly because of an increase in ionized calcium concentration that accompanies metabolic acidosis. Acute intrinsic renal failure and postrenal failure can result in hypocalcemia that is more likely to be symptomatic, because the degree of hyperphosphatemia is often greater than that observed in CRF. Dogs with acute intrinsic renal failure had a mean serum total calcium concentration of 9.8 ± 1.7 mg/dL, but ionized calcium was not reported (Vaden et al. 1997). Twenty-six percent of male cats with urethral obstruction were hypocalcemic at initial presentation on the basis of measurement of total serum calcium concentration, whereas 75% were hypocalcemic on the basis of evaluation of ionized calcium concentrations. Ionized hypocalcemia was considered severe in 12.5%, moderate in 25%, and mild in 37.5% of affected cats (Drobatz and Hughes 1997).

Puerperal tetany (eclampsia) typically occurs between 1 and 3 weeks post partum in small bitches and is attributed to loss of calcium into milk during lactation, although parathyroid gland dysfunction has not been conclusively excluded (Feldman and Nelson 1996; Austad and Bjerkas 1976). Hypophosphatemia may accompany the hypocalcemia of eclampsia (Capen and Martin 1977). Puerperal tetany is rare in cats (Waters and Scott-Moncrieff 1992).

HYPOPARATHYROIDISM

Hypoparathyroidism is a state of absolute or relative deficiency of PTH secretion that can be permanent or transient. Hypocalcemia and clinical signs referable to low ionized calcium concentration are the hallmarks of advanced hypoparathyroidism. Hypoparathyroidism in dogs is most commonly idiopathic, whereas surgical removal of or injury to the parathyroid gland during thyroidectomy to correct hyperthyroidism is the most common cause in cats.

Inappropriately low concentrations of PTH result in hypocalcemia, hyperphosphatemia, and decreased concentrations of 1,25-dihydroxyvitamin D (calcitriol). Hypocalcemia results from increased urinary loss of calcium (hypercalciuria), reduced bone resorption, and decreased intestinal absorption of calcium (secondary to the calcitriol deficit). Hyperphosphatemia results from decreased urinary loss of phosphorus (hypophosphaturia) that overrides the effects of decreased bone resorption and decreased intestinal absorption of phosphorus (secondary to calcitriol deficit) on serum phosphorus concentration. PTH is a potent stimulator, and phosphorus a potent inhibitor, of the 25-hydroxyvitamin D–1α-hydroxylase enzyme system in renal tubules. Consequently the absence of PTH and the presence of hyperphosphatemia act together to decrease renal synthesis of calcitriol. Decreased concentrations of calcitriol contribute to hypocalcemia largely through decreased intestinal calcium absorption. Hypocalcemia unrelated to low PTH concentrations may arise from increased uptake of calcium by bone after rapid correction of long-standing hyperparathyroidism or hyperthyroidism, both of which are associated with loss of bone calcium before treatment ("hungry bone" syndrome) (Feldman and Nelson 1996; Reber and Heath 1995; Tohme and Bilezikian 1993).

Diagnosis of hypoparathyroidism requires evaluation of inclusionary and exclusionary criteria related to the causes of hypocalcemia (see Table 6–8). Hypoparathyroidism is the only possibility in the differential diagnosis with the combination of low serum calcium concentration, high serum phosphorus concentration, normal renal function, and low PTH concentration. Low serum calcium and high serum phosphorus concentrations can be encountered during nutritional and renal secondary hyperparathyroidism, after phosphate-containing enema, and during tumor lysis syndrome, but PTH is increased in all of these conditions. A presumptive diagnosis of hypoparathyroidism can be made on the basis of low serum calcium concentration, high serum phosphorus concentration, normal renal function, and the absence of obvious alternative diagnoses.

PTH should be measured in patients with chronic hypocalcemia of undetermined etiology. Primary hypoparathyroidism requires lifelong treatment, and confirmation of the diagnosis with PTH measurement is recommended. It is not necessary to measure PTH routinely in patients with postsurgical hypocalcemia probably caused by hypoparathyroidism because this effect is usually transient and the cause obvious. PTH concentrations should be determined for patients in which hypocalcemia does not resolve. The definitive diagnosis of hypoparathyroidism requires finding an inappropriately low serum PTH concentration during hypocalcemia, because hypocalcemia normally provides a strong stimulus to the parathyroid gland to secrete PTH. Absolute hypoparathyroidism is present if a PTH concentration below the reference range is detected simultaneously with hypocalcemia. Relative hypoparathyroidism is present if PTH concentration is inappropriately low but remains within the normal reference range. Increased serum phosphorus and decreased calcitriol concentrations provide further support for a diagnosis of hypoparathyroidism (Halabe et al. 1994).

The causes of hypoparathyroidism can be divided into three categories: (1) suppressed secretion of PTH without parathyroid gland destruction (Chew and Meuten 1982; Dhupa and Proulx 1998), (2) sudden correction of chronic hypercalcemia, and (3) absence or destruction of the parathyroid glands. The most common category of hypoparathyroidism in dogs and cats is absence or destruction of the parathyroid glands.

Postoperative hypocalcemia develops 1 to 3 days after thyroidectomy in approximately 20 to 30% of cats (Birchard et al. 1984; Flanders et al. 1987; Welches et al. 1989; Flanders 1994; Graves 1995). Some cats developed hypocalcemia as late as 1 to 2 weeks after surgery. The surgical technique employed for thyroidectomy influences the chances that hypocalcemia will develop, and hypocalcemia occurred in over 80% of cats when original extracapsular technique was used (Flanders et al. 1987). Bilateral thyroidectomy results in loss of the two internal parathyroid glands. Hypoparathyroidism is permanent in patients in which the external parathyroid glands are completely removed during bilateral thyroidectomy. Hypocalcemia and hypoparathyroidism do not develop if the two external parathyroid glands are not excised or damaged during thyroidectomy. Normocalcemia can be maintained with one completely functional parathyroid gland.

Hypoparathyroidism is usually transient when the external parathyroid glands are retained but have their blood supply disrupted (parathyroid gland ischemia after physical trauma, vessel stretching, suture, cautery, or transection) during surgery. Permanent hypoparathyroidism is rare but it may take as long as 3 months to be certain whether remaining parathyroid tissue can recover by hyperplasia (Peterson 1986; Russo and Lees 1986; Birchard et al. 1984). Similar injury to parathyroid glands can occur during any extensive surgery of the neck in dogs (Henderson et al. 1991; Klein et al. 1995) or cats or after exploration of the neck for unilateral parathyroid gland removal. Restored vascular supply to damaged parathyroid tissue seems unlikely as the mechanism for recovery from hypocalcemia. It is more likely that hyperplasia and hypertrophy of parathyroid gland remnants left behind during surgery or ectopic parathyroid tissue achieve sufficient mass to synthesize adequate amounts of PTH. Experimental cats subjected to parathyroidectomy predictably developed hypocalcemia and low serum PTH concentration, but, interestingly, the hypocalcemia resolved although the PTH concentrations remained low (Flanders et al. 1991). Reimplantation of parathyroid gland tissue into muscle near the surgical site may prevent hypocalcemia in humans when the external parathyroid glands are inadvertently removed during thyroidectomy, and cryopreservation of parathyroid tissue can also be performed for later use if the initial transplant fails (Walker et al. 1994). Autotransplantation of parathyroid tissue after bilateral thyroparathyroidectomy was associated with reduced morbidity and rapid return of serum calcium concentrations to normal in experimental cats (Padgett et al. 1998).

Radiation treatment for hyperthyroidism with radioactive iodine is a rare cause of hypocalcemia in humans, in whom parathyroid as well as thyroid tissue is destroyed by this therapy (Reber and Heath 1995). This phenomenon has not been reported yet in hyperthyroid cats treated with ^{131}I.

Long-standing ionized hypercalcemia causes normal parathyroid tissue to atrophy. If the hypercalcemia is nonparathyroid in origin, PTH concentrations will already be low. Rapid correction of the cause of hypercalcemia results in hypocalcemia because the atrophic parathyroid glands cannot respond immediately to the need for increased PTH secretion. Surgical removal of a single parathyroid gland tumor (usually an adenoma) commonly causes postoperative hypocalcemia in this manner. PTH concentrations rapidly decrease after removal of a parathyroid gland adenoma, achieving the greatest decrease in the first 8 h postoperatively in humans (Reber and Heath 1995). Hypocalcemia severe enough to require treatment is likely to develop within 24 to 48 h. Nearly 50% of dogs with primary hyperparathyroidism can be expected to develop clinical signs of hypocalcemia 3 to 6 days after surgical removal of a parathyroid gland tumor. Total serum calcium concentration may range from 5.4 to 8.4 mg/dL in those that develop hypocalcemia (Berger and Feldman 1987; Feldman and Nelson 1996; Peterson 1986). Hypocalcemia is more likely to develop in dogs with the highest presurgical serum calcium concentrations. Over half of hyperparathyroid dogs have rapidly decreased serum calcium concentrations that enter the normal range within 24 h of surgery. Serum calcium concentrations in the remaining dogs usually enter the normal range by 2 or 3 days after surgery, but some require as long as 5 days. Hypoparathyroidism resolves for most affected dogs in 8 to 12 weeks. Cats develop hypocalcemia less frequently than dogs after surgery for correction of primary hyperparathyroidism and have not been reported to be symptomatic if they develop hypocalcemia (Kallet et al. 1991; den Hertog et al. 1997). As in dogs, the cats that develop hypocalcemia are those with the highest presurgical serum calcium concentrations. Spontaneous infarction of a parathyroid gland tumor previously causing hypercalcemia is a rare condition that can result in acute hypocalcemia in dogs (Rosol et al. 1988). Rapid correction of cancer-associated hypercalcemia (e.g., with tumor excision, chemotherapy) can be associated with hypocalcemia, but it is usually minor and transient.

Serum calcium concentrations are often suppressed to a mild degree as a nonspecific and transient response to surgery and anesthesia after thyroidectomy or parathyroidectomy for parathyroid gland adenoma (Peterson 1986). The mechanisms of this form of hypocalcemia have not been studied, but it may be due to a transient decrease in parathyroid gland responsiveness or minor reduction in parathyroid gland mass.

Suppressed secretion of PTH without destruction of the parathyroid glands occurs in humans after exposure to aluminum, asparaginase, doxorubicin, cytosine arabinoside, and intravenously (but not orally administered) H_2 receptor blockers. Acute hypermagnesemia and severe magnesium depletion also may suppress PTH secretion (Reber and Heath 1995; Tohme and Bilezikian 1993; Bourke and Delaney 1993). As with hypocalcemia, mild acute hypomagnesemia stimulates PTH secretion, but severe magnesium depletion decreases PTH secretion, increases end-organ resistance to PTH, and may impair calcitriol synthesis. The end-organ resistance to PTH that develops during magnesium depletion may persist for days after magnesium repletion and resumption of normal PTH concentrations in humans. Hypomagnesemia has been reported rarely in dogs and cats with hypoparathyroidism, but the actual frequency of hypomagnesemia in veterinary medicine remains unknown because measurement of magnesium is not common. Critical illness in human medicine can be associated with hypocalcemia involving decreased PTH secretion, hypercalcitonism, and altered calcium binding to proteins (Reber and Heath 1995). These relationships have not been investigated in veterinary medicine.

Magnesium depletion can cause functional hypoparathyroidism, and measurement of serum magnesium concentration is recommended to exclude or identify this form of hypoparathyroidism. Serum magnesium concentrations in dogs and cats with primary hypoparathyroidism usually have been normal when measured (Bruyette and Feldman 1988; Peterson et al. 1991). The potential role of magnesium depletion in development of postthyroidectomy hypocalcemia in cats has not been explored. Magnesium depletion could play a role in the development of postoperative hypocalcemia in cats with hyperthyroidism, because hyperthyroidism can be associated with magnesium depletion (Feldman and Nelson 1996).

Idiopathic chronic inflammation of parathyroid tissue occurs sporadically in both dogs and cats, but more commonly in dogs. It is presumed that the parathyroiditis has an immune-mediated mechanism. Histopathologic study of affected parathyroid glands reveals inflammatory cell infiltration (lymphocytes, plasma cells, neutrophils), fibrosis, and loss of secretory cells (Bruyette and Feldman 1988; Sherding et al. 1980; Feldman and Nelson 1996; Peterson 1986; Peterson et al. 1991). Clinical signs occurred 1 to 26 weeks (mean, 7 weeks) before diagnosis of primary hypoparathyroidism in cats (Peterson et al. 1991) and 1 day to 25 weeks (mean, 3 weeks) before diagnosis in dogs (Bruyette and Feldman 1988). Primary hypoparathyroidism and parathyroiditis occur in dogs and cats of any age but more frequently in female dogs and male cats. Toy poodles, miniature schnauzers, Labrador retrievers, German shepherds, and terriers are overrepresented dog breeds.

Serum total calcium concentration is usually below 6.5 mg/dL (often 4.0 to 4.9 mg/dL) in dogs with primary hypoparathyroidism. Dogs that have episodes of tetany or seizures often have serum total calcium concentration <6.0 mg/dL. Serum phosphorus concentration is greater than serum calcium concentration in nearly all affected dogs, and most dogs have hyperphosphatemia. Most reference laboratories do not provide separate reference ranges for serum phosphorus concentrations in young and mature animals. Dogs older than 6 months usually have serum phosphorus concentrations lower than 5.5 mg/dL, whereas puppies often have serum phosphorus concentrations as high as 8 or 9 mg/dL. Severe hypocalcemia (total serum calcium concentration 2.8 to 4.2 mg/dL) associated with hyperphosphatemia is also characteristic of primary hypoparathyroidism in cats, and serum phosphorus concentration is usually greater than serum calcium concentration as observed in dogs. Parathyroid gland biopsy may confirm the diagnosis of lymphocytic parathyroiditis as the cause of primary hypoparathyroidism, but the parathyroid glands can be difficult or impossible to locate during surgical exploration because of atrophy and fibrosis. It is usually necessary to remove one thyroid gland to be sure that the internal parathyroid gland is harvested. Parathyroid gland biopsy is neither essential nor recommended to confirm hypoparathyroidism since the advent of validated PTH assays for use in the dog and cat.

MISCELLANEOUS CAUSES OF HYPOCALCEMIA

Pancreatitis, ethylene glycol poisoning, maldigestion or intestinal malabsorption, transfusion with citrate anticoagulated blood, and precipitation of calcium salts in injured soft tissues are occasional causes of hypocalcemia (Chew and Meuten 1982). Acute pancreatitis and hypocalcemia occur together occasionally. Deposition of calcium salts in tissues surrounding the inflamed pancreas (i.e., saponification of adipose tissue) is often cited as the cause of the observed hypocalcemia, but this represents only one part of a poorly understood process (Dhupa and Proulx 1998; Bhattacharya et al. 1985; Izquierdo et al. 1985; Ryzen and Rude 1990). Severely traumatized or necrotic tissue can rapidly take up calcium in some instances, resulting in mild hypocalcemia. Metabolites of ethylene glycol can chelate calcium and become deposited in soft tissues, resulting in hypocalcemia with or without tetany (Thrall et al. 1984). Administration of phosphate enemas can result in hypocalcemia after rapid absorption of phosphate, hyperphosphatemia, and subsequent mass law interaction with serum calcium. This is particularly a problem in cats and small dogs (Schaer et al. 1977; Atkins et al. 1985; Jorgensen et al. 1985). Sodium bicarbonate infusion has been associated with development of hypocalcemia in a cat with salicylate intoxication (Abrams 1987) and in experimental cats (Chew et al. 1989).

Tumor lysis syndrome occurs after acute release of intracellular contents during chemotherapy for highly sensitive neoplasms (usually lymphoid or bone marrow tumors) (Persons et al. 1998). Multiple metabolic abnormalities occur in acute tumor lysis syndrome and include decreased serum calcium concentration related to mass law interactions of calcium with markedly increased serum phosphorus concentration (Page 1986; Calia et al. 1996; Piek and Teske 1996). Tumor lysis syndrome with clinical signs is rare in dogs and cats receiving chemotherapy. Hypocalcemia occurs in 15 to 40% of human patients with critical illness and probably occurs in critical care veterinary patients as well (Dhupa and Proulx 1998). The mechanism of hypocalcemia in this setting (sepsis or systemic inflammatory response syndrome) appear to be multifactorial and are not completely understood (Dhupa and Proulx 1998; Zaloga and Chernow 1987; Lind et al. 1995).

Vitamin D deficiency and nutritional secondary hyperparathyroidism associated with low calcium and high phosphorus concentrations in the diet result in low serum ionized calcium and phosphorus concentrations, and PTH secretion is increased. Increased PTH secretion tends to return serum calcium concentration to normal but further lowers serum phosphorus concentration (Woo and Cannon 1984). Dietary deficiency of calcium alone rarely causes hypocalcemia.

Acute decreases in ionized calcium concentrations are most commonly caused by acute respiratory alkalosis in humans (Reber and Heath 1995). It is likely that this phenomenon also occurs in dogs and cats subjected to the stresses of hypocalcemia and a visit to a veterinary clinic. This could explain the phenomenon of mild stress-induced seizures or tetany in dogs that have hypocalcemia, as the alkalosis shifts some calcium to the protein-bound state, causing more severe ionized hypocalcemia. Caution should be exercised in the interpretation of ionized calcium measured with portable analyzers because results for dogs and cats are lower than those obtained with standard methodology (Grosenbaugh et al. 1998). The use of dry heparin syringes for sample collection may negate this difference.

Treatment of Hypocalcemia

Puerperal tetany is the condition in general practice most likely to require specific correction of hypocalcemia acutely, but chronic treatment is not needed. Hypoparathyroidism is the only condition requiring acute and chronic treatment to alleviate clinical signs associated with hypocalcemia. Other conditions associated with hypocalcemia are transient or result in minimal decreases in serum calcium concentration, do not cause obvious clinical signs, and only occasionally necessitate calcium replacement therapy. No treatment is indicated for animals with hypocalcemia that is attributable entirely to hypoalbuminemia or hypoproteinemia, assuming that the ionized calcium fraction is normal.

Treatment is individualized on the basis of the severity of clinical signs, the magnitude of hypocalcemia, the rapidity of decline in serum calcium concentration, and trend of serial serum calcium measurements (i.e., further decrease or stability). More aggressive treatment is prescribed for patients with severe clinical signs of hypocalcemia, patients with severe ionized hypocalcemia with or without signs, and patients in which serum calcium concentration is steadily or rapidly declining. Acute, subacute, and chronic rescue treatment regimens are available using supplementation with calcium salts and vitamin D metabolites. The goal of therapy is to increase serum calcium concentration predictably and smoothly to a level that alleviates the signs of hypocalcemia, minimizes the likelihood of the development of hypercalcemia, and reduces the magnitude of hypercalciuria (especially in patients with hypoparathyroidism). It is usually not necessary or desirable to return serum calcium concentration completely to normal, as many clinical signs improve dramatically with slight increases in serum calcium concentration, and the consequences of overcorrection can be serious. For suspected temporary postsurgical hypoparathyroidism, it is desirable to keep the serum calcium concentration relatively low to maximize compensatory hypertrophy of remaining parathyroid glands.

In patients with hypoparathyroidism, no treatment regimen completely compensates for the full range of physiologic actions of the absent PTH. Vitamin D metabolite treatment corrects the low intestinal absorption of calcium but does not completely protect the kidneys from hypercalciuria as would occur in the presence of PTH. Similarly, vitamin D metabolites do not exert as powerful an effect on bone in the absence of PTH. Replacement therapy with once-daily subcutaneous injections of human PTH (1–34) in human subjects was highly effective in providing good 24-h control of serum calcium concentration in one study (Winer et al. 1996). Better control of serum phosphorus concentration and less hypercalciuria were additional benefits of PTH (1–34) treatment compared with calcitriol treatment. Use of synthetic human amino-terminal PTH for treatment of veterinary patients is possible because the amino-terminal portions of PTH are highly conserved, function in vivo in animals, and would be unlikely to elicit an immune response.

Hypocalcemia severe enough to cause clinical signs should be anticipated in dogs undergoing parathyroidectomy as treatment for hypercalcemia related to a parathyroid gland adenoma. Animals with very high concentrations of serum calcium, PTH, and serum alkaline phosphatase may be at greater risk of developing postoperative hypocalcemia. Postoperative hypocalcemia in this instance is the consequence of acute hypoparathyroidism resulting from chronic suppression of remaining parathyroid glands as well as calcium uptake into "hungry" bones. Hypocalcemia should be anticipated in cats that undergo bilateral thyroidectomy, because up to 30% of cats can be expected to have transiently lowered serum calcium concentrations.

We do not agree with previous recommendations to wait for signs of tetany before instituting therapy to increase serum calcium concentration. Preemptive therapy to increase serum calcium concentration may be a good choice for animals with marked hypocalcemia despite absence of clinical signs or for those in which serum calcium concentration is steadily or rapidly declining. Prophylactic therapy to prevent hypocalcemia in dogs undergoing surgery for hyperparathyroidism should be considered, especially in dogs with more severe hypercalcemia. Active vitamin D metabolites should be started before surgery in these instances because there is a lag time until maximal effect is achieved. Vitamin D metabolites given at the time of surgery or just after surgery fail to prevent development of hypocalcemia.

ACUTE MANAGEMENT OF HYPOCALCEMIA CAUSING TETANY OR SEIZURES

Tetany or seizures caused by hypocalcemia require treatment with intravenously administered calcium salts. Calcium is administered to effect at a dosage of 5 to 15 mg/kg of elemental calcium (0.5 to 1.5 mL/kg of 10% calcium gluconate) over a 10- to 20-min period (Chew and Meuten 1982; Feldman and Nelson 1996; Peterson 1982, 1986). The calcium content of different calcium salts varies considerably (Table 6–9). There is no difference in effectiveness of calcium salts administered IV to correct hypocalcemia when the dose is based on elemental calcium content. Calcium gluconate is often the calcium salt of choice because it is nonirritating if the solution is inadvertently injected perivascularly. In contrast, calcium chloride is extremely irritating to tissues but provides more elemental calcium in each milliliter of solution (see Table 6–9).

The heart rate and electrocardiogram should be monitored during acute infusions of calcium salts. Bradycardia may signal the onset of cardiotoxicity arising from excessively rapid infusion of calcium. Sudden elevation of the ST segment or shortening of the QT interval also may indicate cardiotoxicity resulting from the calcium infusion. Not all clinical signs abate immediately after acute correction of hypocalcemia. Some clinical signs may persist for 30 to 60 min. Nervousness, panting, and behavioral changes may persist despite return of normocalcemia during this period, perhaps reflecting a lag in equilibration between cerebrospinal fluid and ECF calcium concentrations (Feldman and Nelson 1996; Russo and Lees 1986; Kirk et al. 1974). Hyperthermia that resulted from increased muscle activity or seizures may also take time to dissipate.

SUBACUTE MANAGEMENT OF HYPOCALCEMIA

The initial bolus injection of elemental calcium can be expected to decrease signs of hypocalcemia for as little as 1 h to as long as 12 h if the underlying cause of hypocalcemia has not been corrected. Vitamin D metabolites should be administered as soon as possible, because some of them require a few days before intestinal calcium

TABLE 6–9. Treatment of Hypocalcemia

Drug	Preparation	Available Calcium	Dose	Comment(s)	
Parenteral Calcium*					
Calcium gluconate	10% solution	9.3 mg Ca/mL	(a) Slow IV to effect (0.5–1.5 mL/kg IV) (b) 5–15 mg/kg/h IV (c) 1–2 mL/kg diluted 1:1 with saline SQ t.i.d.	Stop if bradycardia or shortened QT interval occurs Infusion to maintain normal Ca	
Calcium chloride	10% solution	27.2 mg Ca/mL	5–15 mg/kg/h IV	Given only IV as extremely caustic perivascularly	
Oral Calcium†					
Calcium carbonate	Many sizes	40% tablet	25–50 mg/kg/day	Most common calcium supplement	
Calcium lactate	325, 650 mg tablets	13% tablet	25–50 mg/kg/day		
Calcium chloride	Powder	27.2%	25–50 mg/kg/day	May cause gastric irritation	
Calcium gluconate	Many sizes	10%	25–50 mg/kg/day		
Vitamin D					
				Time for maximal effect to occur:	*Time for toxicity effect to resolve:*
Vitamin D_2 (ergocalciferol)			Initial: 4000–6000 U/kg/day Maintenance: 1000–2000 U/kg once daily to once weekly	5–21 days	1–18 wk
Dihydrotachysterol			Initial: 20–30 ng/kg/day Maintenance: 10–20 ng/kg q 24–48 h	1–7 days	1–3 wk
1,25-Dihydroxyvitamin D_3 (calcitriol)			Initial: 20–30 ng/kg/day for 3–4 days Maintenance: 5–15 ng/kg/day	1–4 days	2–14 days

*Do not mix calcium solutions with bicarbonate-containing fluids as precipitation may occur.
†Calculate dose on the basis of elemental calcium content.

transport is maximized. Calcitriol exerts initial effects on the intestine within 3 to 4 h (Wasserman 1997). Additional parenteral calcium salt administration is necessary until therapy with vitamin D metabolites is effective at maintaining serum calcium concentration at an acceptable level.

Multiple intermittent IV injections of calcium salts can be administered to control clinical signs, but this method is not recommended because wide fluctuations in serum calcium concentration are likely to be encountered. The remaining two options are continuous infusion or intermittent SQ injection of calcium salts.

Continuous IV infusion of calcium is recommended at 60 to 90 mg/kg/day elemental calcium (2.5 to 3.75 mg/kg/h) until oral medications provide control of serum calcium concentration (Bruyette and Feldman 1988; Feldman and Nelson 1996; Peterson 1982, 1986). Initial doses in the higher range are administered to patients with more severe hypocalcemia, and the dose decreases according to the serum calcium concentration achieved. The IV dose of calcium is further reduced as oral calcium salts and vitamin D metabolites become more effective.

Ten milliliters of 10% calcium gluconate provides 93 mg of elemental calcium. A convenient method for infusing calcium is available when IV fluids are given at a maintenance volume of 60 mL/kg/day (2.5 mL/kg/h). Approximately 1, 2, or 3 mg/kg/h elemental calcium is provided by adding 10, 20, or 30 mL of 10% calcium gluconate, respectively, to each 250-mL bag of fluids. Calcium salts should not be added to fluids that contain lactate, acetate, bicarbonate, or phosphates, as calcium salt precipitates can occur. Alkalinizing fluids containing sodium bicarbonate should be avoided because they can decrease ionized calcium and may unmask clinical signs of hypocalcemia in animals with borderline hypocalcemia. Alternatively, fluids containing calcium can be administered SQ. Calcium gluconate should be diluted at least 1:1 before SQ injection, and calcium chloride should not be used because it is highly irritating to tissues. The dose of calcium initially needed to control tetany can be given q6h or q8h, or a dosage of 60 to 90 mg/kg/day can be divided in SQ fluids given several times a day. Doses of calcium administered SQ should be tapered as described for continuous infusion of calcium.

SUBACUTE AND CHRONIC MAINTENANCE

Supplemental elemental calcium is administered orally (see Table 6–9) to guarantee adequate calcium for intestinal absorption after treatment with vitamin D metabolites. Oral calcium administered by pill or slurry is most important during initial treatment, especially if the animal is not eating. Active intestinal transport of calcium is under the control of calcitriol when calcium intake is low, but vitamin D–independent (passive) intestinal absorption of calcium occurs when calcium intake is high. The passive mechanisms for intestinal calcium transport can be utilized therapeutically before the actions of vitamin D take effect in the intestine. In most patients, normal dietary intake of calcium is sufficient to maintain adequate serum calcium concentrations in the presence of vitamin D metabolite treatment. Consequently, oral calcium salt supplementation can be tapered and discontinued in many instances as vitamin D compounds reach maximal effect.

Calcium carbonate is the most widely used oral preparation of the calcium salts because it contains the greatest percentage of elemental calcium. This approach allows fewer pills to be administered. The degree of calcium ionization from its salt and its bioavailability for absorption vary for each calcium salt and with conditions in the intestine. Consequently, it is not a simple matter to determine the bioavailable elemental calcium content of a specific oral calcium salt. Oral calcium is usually administered at 25 to 50 mg/kg/day elemental calcium in divided doses. Oral calcium carbonate serves as an intestinal phosphate binder in addition to providing calcium for intestinal absorption. It is advisable to continue oral calcium carbonate therapy for its intestinal phosphate-binding effects if serum phosphorus concentration remains increased. Lower serum phosphorus concentrations may allow increased endogenous synthesis of calcitriol, because phosphate inhibits renal synthesis of calcitriol.

Vitamin D preparations (see Table 6–9) include ergocalciferol, cholecalciferol, dihydrotachysterol (DHT), 25-hydroxycholecalciferol (calcidiol), 1α-hydroxycholecalciferol, and 1,25-dihydroxycholecalciferol (calcitriol). Ergocalciferol, DHT, and calcitriol are the preparations most commonly used in veterinary medicine. Lifelong treatment with some form of vitamin D metabolite is necessary for patients with primary hypoparathyroidism or postoperative hypocalcemia that fails to resolve spontaneously.

Ergocalciferol is favored by some because of its low cost (Reber and Heath 1995), but it has several features that make it the least attractive agent for treatment of hypocalcemia. Ergocalciferol and its immediate metabolite, 25-hydroxyergocalciferol, have low vitamin D receptor avidity and consequently high doses are necessary. Ergocalciferol is highly lipid soluble, and several weeks are required to saturate body stores and achieve a maximal effect. It also has a long half-life. Consequently, prolonged periods of hypercalcemia occur after overdose with ergocalciferol. In addition, there is extreme individual variation in the dose of ergocalciferol required to achieve a target serum calcium concentration. Use of loading doses reduces the time required to achieve a maximal effect on serum calcium concentration (see Table 6–9).

DHT is a synthetic vitamin D analogue with onset of maximal effect and biologic half-life between those of ergocalciferol and calcitriol. DHT possesses both 1α- and 25-hydroxyl groups after 25-hydroxylation in the liver but lacks a 3β-hydroxyl group, which dramatically reduces its efficiency of binding to the vitamin D receptor. The polarity and lower dose requirements of DHT limit its storage in fat compared with ergocalciferol. Toxicity resulting from hypercalcemia still can be prolonged (up to 30 days), and there is wide variation in the dose required to achieve a target serum calcium concentration. Use of loading doses reduces the time to maximal effect (as observed with ergocalciferol).

Calcitriol is the vitamin D metabolite of choice to provide calcemic actions because it has the most rapid onset of maximal action and the shortest biologic half-life. Calcitriol is approximately 1000 times as effective as parent vitamin D and 500 times as effective as its precursor, calcidiol (25-hydroxyvitamin D), in binding to the vitamin D receptor. The dose of calcitriol can be adjusted frequently because of its short half-life and rapid effects on serum calcium concentration. If hypercalcemia occurs, it abates quickly after dose reduction. The half-life of calcitriol in blood is 4 to 6 h, whereas its biologic half-life is 2 to 4 days. Loading protocols for use of calcitriol in animals have not been reported, but it is logical to employ a loading protocol when more rapid correction of serum calcium concentration is desirable. A calcitriol dosage of 30 to 60 ng/kg/day has been recommended (Bruyette and Feldman 1988; Feldman and Nelson 1996). This dosage may be satisfactory as a loading dose, but in our experience it is too high for chronic maintenance therapy. Calcitriol dosages for chronic maintenance therapy in humans range from 10 to 40 ng/kg/day, and doses are divided and given twice daily (Reber and Heath 1995; Halabe et al. 1994; Winer et al. 1996). We have employed loading dosages of 20 to 30 ng/kg/day for 3 to 4 days and maintenance dosages of 10 to 20 ng/kg/day in most patients. The dose of calcitriol is divided and given twice daily to ensure sustained priming effects on intestinal epithelium for calcium transport. Calcitriol is commercially available in 0.25- and 0.50-μg capsules (250 and 500 ng per capsule, respectively; Rocaltrol, Hoffman-LaRoche). It is likely that reformulation of calcitriol in doses suitable for a variety of animal sizes will be necessary. It may be useful to prescribe calcitriol in liquid formulation so that small adjustments in dosage can be made accurately. A number of specialty pharmacies reformulate human drugs for veterinary use and can create any calcitriol dose needed.

Thiazide diuretics are sometimes used to treat humans with primary hypoparathyroidism to reduce hypercalciuria. This approach is especially useful for humans in whom hypercalciuria continues despite normalization of serum calcium concentration (Tohme and Bilezikian 1993; Halabe et al. 1994). It is likely that a reduction of the vitamin D metabolite dose would be necessary after treatment with thiazides, because serum calcium concentrations would be higher as a result of greater reabsorption of calcium by the kidney. The effects of thiazide diuretics on urinary calcium excretion in dogs or cats are not well understood.

▶ Clinical Follow-up and Potential Complications

Periods of hypocalcemia and hypercalcemia occur sporadically in patients during initial efforts to manage serum calcium concentration. Daily measurement of serum total calcium concentration during stabilization is necessary. Weekly serum calcium measurements should suffice during maintenance therapy until the target serum calcium concentration has been achieved and maintained. Measurement of serum total calcium concentration is recommended every 3 months thereafter in animals with permanent hypoparathyroidism. Serum calcium concentration should be adjusted to just below the reference range. This not only lessens the likelihood that hypercalcemia will develop but also reduces the magnitude of hypercalciuria that occurs in patients with PTH deficiency. Maintaining a mildly decreased serum calcium concentration also ensures a continued stimulus for hypertrophy of the remaining parathyroid tissue in patients with postoperative hypoparathyroidism.

It is important to change the dose of vitamin D metabolite gradually after evaluation of serum calcium concentrations and to be certain that enough time has passed to see the maximal effect before the dose is changed again. The time lag for this effect varies with the different vitamin D metabolites (see Table 6–9). Dosage increases of 10 to 25% are recommended when serum calcium concentration is still below the target level (Peterson 1982, 1986). Vitamin D metabolite and calcium salt supplementation should be discontinued temporarily in patients that develop hypercalcemia.

Hypercalcemia is a serious adverse effect that can result in death of the animal or renal damage severe enough to cause acute or CRF (Chew and Meuten 1982; Kruger et al. 1996; Chew and Capen 1980). The early signs of hypercalcemia should be explained to the owners, who should be instructed to seek veterinary attention for measurement of serum calcium concentration if clinical signs suggest hypercalcemia. Clinical signs of hypercalcemia that clients are likely to recognize include polydipsia, polyuria, anorexia, vomiting, and lethargy. Animals with severe hypercalcemia require hospitalization and appropriate therapy. Fluids, furosemide, corticosteroids, bisphosphonates, calcitonin, or some combination may be required. All patients with symptomatic, vitamin D metabolite–induced hypercalcemia should be given a calcium-restricted diet because hypervitaminosis D is a form of hypercalcemia in which increased intestinal absorption of calcium contributes substantially to the development of hypercalcemia.

Patients that maintain serum calcium concentrations in the target zone are often managed successfully for years. Twenty-four of 25 dogs with primary hypoparathyroidism were managed successfully for over 5 years (Feldman and Nelson 1996), and long-term management was successful in a small number of cats (Peterson et al. 1991). Patients that develop episodic or prolonged hypercalcemia during treatment have a poor prognosis. Management with calcitriol is easier and more successful in inducing and maintaining serum calcium concentrations in the target zone than are older therapeutic approaches.

Hypercalciuria, nephrocalcinosis, urolithiasis, and reduced renal function have occurred in humans treated for chronic hypoparathyroidism (Tohme and Bilezikian 1993; Halabe et al. 1994; Winer et al. 1996). As many as 80% of human patients treated for 2 years or longer have decreased creatinine clearance (Winer et al. 1996). These abnormalities can be attributed to episodes of hypercalcemia and hyperphosphatemia and to hypercalciuria that occurs in the absence of the actions of PTH on the renal tubules. In the absence of PTH, hypercalciuria occurs more readily at all serum calcium concentrations and is especially severe as calcium concentrations approach the normal range, which increases the filtered load of calcium. Nephrocalcinosis, reduced renal function, and CRF have also been suspected in veterinary patients receiving long-term treatment for hypoparathyroidism, but the risk for these disorders has not been critically evaluated (Peterson 1986).

Care is taken to adjust the dosage of vitamin D metabolites in humans to both the serum calcium concentration and degree of hypercalciuria achieved during treatment. Maintaining a mildly decreased serum calcium concentration does not guarantee that hypercalciuria will not occur. Hypercalciuria is monitored by measuring 24-h urinary calcium excretion or by determining the ratio of urinary calcium to creatinine (Halabe et al. 1994). Guidelines for assessing the magnitude of hypercalciuria in veterinary patients have not yet been developed.

Vitamin D metabolite treatment is gradually tapered and then discontinued in patients with postsurgical hypoparathyroidism, because hypocalcemia is usually transient. Most cats are able to maintain normal serum calcium concentrations 2 weeks after thyroidectomy, although some may take as long as 3 months. Dogs with hypocalcemia usually require 6 to 12 weeks of treatment after removal of a parathyroid gland adenoma. We usually begin to reduce the dose of vitamin D metabolites 1 month after initiation of therapy. If serum calcium concentration declines substantially, the previous dose is resumed and reduction is attempted again 1 or 2 months later. Permanent hypoparathyroidism is likely if failure to maintain acceptable serum calcium concentration occurs after reduction of the vitamin D metabolite dose at 3 months.

REFERENCES

Abou-Samra A-B, Jüppner H, Force T, et al.: Expression cloning of a common receptor for parathyroid hormone and parathyroid hormone–related peptide from rat osteoblast-like cells: A single receptor stimulates intracellular accumulation of both cAMP and inositol triphosphates and increases intracellular calcium. *Proc Natl Acad Sci U S A* 89:2732–2736, 1992.

Abrams KL: Hypocalcemia associated with administration of sodium bicarbonate for salicylate intoxication in a cat. *J Am Vet Med Assoc* 191:235–236, 1987.

Adams JS: Extrarenal production and action of active vitamin D metabolites in human lymphoproliferative diseases. In Feldman D (ed): *Vitamin D*. New York, Academic Press, pp. 903–921, 1997.

Adler AJ, Ferran N, and Berlyne GM: Effect of inorganic phosphate on serum ionized calcium concentration in vitro: A reassessment of the "trade-off hypothesis." *Kidney Int* 28:932–935, 1985.

Anthony LB, May ME, and Oates JA: Case report: Lanreotide in the management of hypercalcemia of malignancy. *Am J Med Sci* 309:312–314, 1995.

Arceneaux KA, Taboada J, and Hosgood G: Blastomycosis in dogs: 115 cases (1980–1995). *J Am Vet Med Assoc* 213:658–664, 1998.

Atkins CE, Tyler R, and Greenlee P: Clinical, biochemical, acid-base, and electrolyte abnormalities in cats after hypertonic sodium phosphate enema administration. *Am J Vet Res* 46:980–988, 1985.

Aubin JE and Heersche JN: Vitamin D and osteoblasts. In Feldman D (ed): *Vitamin D*. New York, Academic Press, pp. 313–328, 1997.

Austad R and Bjerkas E: Eclampsia in the bitch. *J Small Anim Pract* 17:793–798, 1976.

Barber PJ, Elliott J, and Torrance AG: Measurement of feline intact parathyroid hormone: Assay validation and sample handling studies. *J Small Anim Pract* 34:614–620, 1993.

Barber PJ, Torrance AG, and Elliott J: Carboxyl fragment interference in assay of feline parathyroid hormone. *J Vet Intern Med* 8:168, 1994.

Barr FJ, Patterson MW, Lucke VM, et al.: Hypercalcemic nephropathy in three dogs: Sonographic appearance. *Vet Radiol* 30:169–173, 1989.

Barrett S, Sheafor S, Hillier A, et al.: Challenging cases in internal medicine "What's your diagnosis?" *Vet Med* 93:35–44, 1998.

Basoglu A, Sevinc M, Sen I, et al.: The blocking effect of verapamil in hypercalcemic dogs. *Turkish J Vet Anim Sci* 21:331–333, 1997.

Berger B and Feldman EC: Primary hyperparathyroidism in dogs: 21 cases (1976–1986). *J Am Vet Med Assoc* 191:350–356, 1987.

Bergman SM, O'Mailia J, Krane NK, et al.: Vitamin-A–induced hypercalcemia: Response to corticosteroids. *Nephron* 50:362–364, 1988.

Bhattacharya SK, Luther RW, Pate JW, et al.: Soft tissue calcium and magnesium content in acute pancreatitis in the dog: Calcium accumulation, a mechanism for hypocalcemia in acute pancreatitis. *J Lab Clin Med* 105:422–427, 1985.

Bièmle D, Jacobs RM, and Lumsden JH: Relationship of serum total calcium to serum albumin in dogs, cats, horses, and cattle. *Can Vet J* 34:360–364, 1993.

Bilezikian JP: Clinical utility of assays for parathyroid hormone–related protein. *Clin Chem* 38:179–181, 1992.

Bilezikian JP and Singer FR: Acute management of hypercalcemia due to parathyroid hormone and parathyroid hormone-related protein. In Bilezikian JP, Levine MA, and Marcus R (eds): *The Parathyroids*. New York, Raven Press, pp. 359–372, 1994.

Biller DS, Bradley GA, and Partington BP: Renal medullary rim sign: Ultrasonographic evidence of renal disease. *Vet Radiol Ultrasound* 33:286–290, 1992.

Birchard SJ, Peterson ME, and Jacobson A: Surgical treatment of feline hyperthyroidism: Results of 85 cases. *J Am Anim Hosp Assoc* 20:705–709, 1984.

Black KS and Mundy GR: Other causes of hypercalcemia: Local and ectopic secretion syndromes. In Bilezikian JP, Marcus R, and Levine MA (eds): *The Parathyroids*. New York, Raven Press, pp. 341–358, 1994.

Boden SD and Kaplan FS: Calcium homeostasis. *Orthop Clin North Am* 21:31–42, 1990.

Body JJ, Coleman RE, and Piccart M: Use of bisphosphonates in cancer patients. *Cancer Treat Rev* 22:265–287, 1996.

Borle AB: An overview of techniques for the measurement of calcium distribution, calcium fluxes, and cytosolic free calcium in mammalian cells. *Environ Health Perspect* 84:45–56, 1990.

Bourke E and Delaney V: Assessment of hypocalcemia and hypercalcemia. *Clin Lab Med* 13:157–181, 1993.

Bowden SJ, Hughes SV, and Ratcliffe WA: Molecular forms of parathyroid hormone–related protein in tumours and biological fluids. *Clin Endocrinol* 38:287–294, 1993.

Bowers GN Jr, Brassard C, and Sena SF: Measurement of ionized calcium in serum with ion-selective electrodes: A mature technology that can meet the daily service needs. *Clin Chem* 32:1437–1447, 1986.

Bowman AR and Epstein S: Drug and hormone effects on vitamin D metabolism. In Feldman D (ed): *Vitamin D*. New York, Academic Press, pp. 797–829, 1997.

Breslau NA: Normal and abnormal regulation of 1,25-$(OH)_2$D synthesis. *Am J Med Sci* 296:417–425, 1988.

Brossard JH, Roy L, Lepage R, et al.: Intravenous 1,25-$(OH)_2$D therapy increases the intact parathyroid hormone secretion set point in hemodialyzed patients. *Miner Electrolyte Metab* 23:25–32, 1997.

Brown EM: Extracellular Ca^{2+} sensing, regulation of parathyroid cell function, and role of Ca^{2+} and other ions as extracellular (first) messengers. *Physiol Rev* 71:371–411, 1991.

Brown EM: Homeostatic mechanisms regulating extracellular and intracellular calcium metabolism. In Bilezikian JP, Marcus R, and Levine MA (eds): *The Parathyroids*. New York, Raven Press, pp. 15–54, 1994.

Brown EM and Hebert SC: Calcium-receptor-regulated parathyroid and renal function. *Bone* 20:303–309, 1997.

Brown AJ, Dusso A, Lopez-Hilker S, et al.: 1,25-$(OH)_2$D receptors are decreased in parathyroid glands from chronically uremic dogs. *Kidney Int* 35:19–23, 1989.

Brown EM, Pollak M, Seidman CE, et al.: Calcium-ion-sensing cell-surface receptors. *N Engl J Med* 333:234–240, 1995.

Brown AJ, Zhong M, Finch J, et al.: Rat calcium-sensing receptor is regulated by vitamin D but not by calcium. *Am J Physiol* 39:F454–F460, 1996.

Brownie CF: Confusion over jasmine and jessamine (letter). *J Am Vet Med Assoc* 191:613–614, 1987.

Brunette MG, Vary J, and Carriere S: Hyposthenuria in hypercalcemia. A possible role of intrarenal blood-flow (IRBF) redistribution. *Pflügers Arch* 350:9–23, 1974.

Bruyette DS and Feldman EC: Primary hypoparathyroidism in the dog. Report of 15 cases and review of 13 previously reported cases. *J Vet Intern Med* 2:7–14, 1988.

Burchard KW, Simms HH, Robinson A, et al.: Hypocalcemia during sepsis. Relationship to resuscitation and hemodynamics. *Arch Surg* 127:265–272, 1992.

Burritt MF, Pierides AM, and Offord KP: Comparative studies of total and ionized calcium values in normal subjects and patients with renal disorders. *Mayo Clin Proc* 55:606–613, 1980.

Burtis WJ: Parathyroid hormone–related protein: Structure, function, and measurement. *Clin Chem* 38:2171–2183, 1992.

Burtis WJ, Brady TG, Orloff JJ, et al.: Immunochemical characterization of circulating parathyroid hormone–related protein in patients with humoral hypercalcemia of malignancy. *N Engl J Med* 322:1106–1112, 1990.

Burtis WJ, Dann P, Gaich GA, et al.: A high abundance midregion species of parathyroid hormone-related protein: Immunological and chromatographic characterization in plasma. *J Clin Endocrinol Metab* 78:317–322, 1994.

Calia CM, Hohenhaus AE, Fox PR, et al.: Acute tumor lysis syndrome in a cat with lymphoma. *J Vet Intern Med* 10:409–411, 1996.

Campese VM: Calcium, parathyroid hormone, and blood pressure. *Am J Hypertens* 2:34S–44S, 1989.

Camus C, Charasse C, Jouannic-Montier I, et al.: Calcium free hemodialysis: Experience in the treatment of 33 patients with severe hypercalcemia. *Intensive Care Med* 22:116–121, 1996.

Canalis E, Hock JM, and Raisz LG: Anabolic and catabolic effects of parathyroid hormone on bone and interactions with growth factors. In Bilezikian JP, Marcus R, and Levine MA (eds): *The Parathyroids*. Raven Press, New York, pp. 65–82, 1994.

Capen CC: Structural and biochemical aspects of parathyroid gland function in animals. In Jones TC, Mohr U, and Hunt RD (eds): *Monograph on Pathology of Laboratory Animals:* Vol. 1, *Endocrine System*. International Life Sciences Institute Series. New York, Springer-Verlag, pp. 217–247, 1983.

Capen CC and Martin SL: Calcium metabolism and disorders of parathyroid glands. *Vet Clin North Am* 7:513–555, 1977.

Capen CC and Rosol TJ: Hormonal control of mineral metabolism.

In Bojrab MJ (ed): *Disease Mechanisms in Small Animal Surgery.* Philadelphia, Lea & Febiger, pp. 841–857, 1993.

Carafoli E: Intracellular calcium homeostasis. *Annu Rev Biochem* 56:395–433, 1987.

Care AD: Placental transfer of calcium. *J Dev Physiol* 15:253–257, 1991.

Carothers MA, Chew DJ, and Nagode LA: 25-OH-cholecalciferol intoxication in dogs. *Proc Am Coll Vet Intern Med Forum* 12:822–825, 1994.

Chattopadhyay N, Mithal A, and Brown EM: The calcium-sensing receptor: A window into the physiology and pathophysiology of mineral ion metabolism. *Endocr Rev* 17:289–307, 1996.

Chew DJ and Capen CC: Hypercalcemic nephropathy and associated disorders. In Kirk RW (ed): *Current Veterinary Therapy VII.* Philadelphia, WB Saunders Co., pp. 1067–1072, 1980.

Chew DJ and Carothers MA: Hypercalcemia. *Vet Clin North Am Small Anim Pract* 19:265–288, 1989.

Chew DJ and Meuten DJ: Disorders of calcium and phosphorus metabolism. *Vet Clin North Am Small Anim Pract* 12:411–438, 1982.

Chew DJ and Meuten DJ: Primary hyperparathyroidism. In Kirk RW (ed): *Current Veterinary Therapy VIII.* Philadelphia, WB Saunders Co., pp. 880–884, 1983.

Chew DJ and Nagode LA: Renal secondary hyperparathyroidism. *Proc Soc Comp Endocrinol* 17–26, 1990.

Chew DJ and Nagode LA: Calcitriol in the treatment of chronic renal failure. In Kirk RW and Bonagura J (eds): *Current Veterinary Therapy XI: Small Animal Practice.* Philadelphia, WB Saunders Co., pp. 857–860, 1992.

Chew DJ, Leonard M, and Muir W III: Effect of sodium bicarbonate infusions on ionized calcium and total calcium concentrations in serum of clinically normal cats. *Am J Vet Res* 50:145–150, 1989.

Chew DJ, Nagode LA, Rosol TJ, et al: Utility of diagnostic assays in the evaluation of hypercalcemia and hypocalcemia: Parathyroid hormone, vitamin D metabolites, parathyroid hormone–related protein, and ionized calcium. In Bonagura JD (ed): *Kirk's Current Veterinary Therapy XII: Small Animal Practice.* Philadelphia, WB Saunders Co., pp. 378–383, 1995.

Ching SV and Norrdin RW: Histomorphometric comparison of measurements of trabecular bone remodeling in iliac crest biopsy sites and lumbar vertebrae in cats. *Am J Vet Res* 51:447–450, 1990.

Ching SV, Fettman MJ, Hamar DW, et al.: The effect of chronic dietary acidification using ammonium chloride on acid-base and mineral metabolism in the adult cat. *J Nutr* 119:902–915, 1989.

Chisholm MA, Mulloy AL, and Taylor AT: Acute management of cancer-related hypercalcemia. *Ann Pharmacother* 30:507–513, 1996.

Christakos S, Beck JD, and Hyliner SJ: Calbindin-D 28K. In Feldman D (ed): *Vitamin D.* New York, Academic Press, pp. 209–221, 1997.

Cohen Y, Rahamimov R, Navehmany T, et al.: Where is the "inverting factor" in hormone secretion from parathyroid cells? *Am J Physiol* 36:E630–E637, 1997.

Coleman DT, Fitzpatrick LA, and Bilezikian JP: Biochemical mechanisms of parathyroid hormone action. In Bilezikian JP, Marcus R, and Levine MA (eds): *The Parathyroids.* New York, Raven Press, pp. 239–258, 1994.

Cooke NE and Haddad JG: Vitamin D binding protein. In Feldman D (ed): *Vitamin D.* New York, Academic Press, pp. 87–101, 1997.

Coukell AJ and Markham A: Pamidronate. A review of its use in the management of osteolytic bone metastases, tumour-induced hypercalcaemia and Paget's disease of bone. *Drugs Aging* 12:149–168, 1998.

DeLuca HF, Krisinger J, and Darwish H: The vitamin D system: 1990. *Kidney Int* 38(suppl 29):S2–S8, 1990.

den Hertog E, Goossens MM, van der Linde-Sipman JS, et al.: Primary hyperparathyroidism in two cats. *Vet Q* 19:81–84, 1997.

Deniz A and Mischke R: Ionized calcium and total calcium in the cat. *Berl Münch Teirarztl Wochenschr* 108:105–108, 1995.

DeVries SE, Feldman EC, Nelson RW, et al.: Primary parathyroid hyperplasia in dogs: Six cases (1982–1991). *J Am Vet Med Assoc* 202:1132–1136, 1993.

Dhupa N and Proulx J: Hypocalcemia and hypomagnesemia. *Vet Clin North Am Small Anim Pract* 28:587–608, 1998.

DiBartola SP, Chew DJ, and Jacobs G: Quantitative urinalysis including 24-hour protein excretion in the dog. *J Am Anim Hosp Assoc* 16:537–546, 1980.

DiBartola SP, Rutgers HC, Zack PM, et al.: Clinicopathologic findings associated with chronic renal disease in cats: 74 cases (1973–1984). *J Am Vet Med Assoc* 190:1196–1202, 1987.

Dougherty SA, Center SA, and Dzanis DA: Salmon calcitonin as adjunct treatment for vitamin D toxicosis in a dog. *J Am Vet Med Assoc* 196:1269–1272, 1990.

Dow SW, Legendre AM, Stiff M, et al.: Hypercalcemia associated with blastomycosis in dogs. *J Am Vet Med Assoc* 188:706–709, 1986.

Drazner FH: Hypercalcemia in the dog and cat. *J Am Vet Med Assoc* 178:1252–1256, 1981.

Drobatz KJ and Hughes D: Concentration of ionized calcium in plasma from cats with urethral obstruction. *J Am Vet Med Assoc* 211:1392–1395, 1997.

Drop LJ: Ionized calcium, the heart, and hemodynamic function. *Anesth Analg* 64:432–451, 1985.

Dunlay R, Rodriguez M, Felsenfeld AJ, et al.: Direct inhibitory effect of calcitriol on parathyroid function (sigmoidal curve) in dialysis. *Kidney Int* 36:1093–1098, 1989.

Dusso AS, Finch JL, Delmez JA, et al.: Extrarenal production of calcitriol. *Kidney Int* 38:S36–S40, 1990.

Dzanis DA and Kallfelz FA: Recent knowledge of vitamin D toxicity in dogs. *Proc Am Coll Vet Intern Med Forum* 6:289–292, 1998.

Elliott J, Dobson J, Dunn J, et al.: Hypercalcaemia in the dog: A study of 40 cases. *J Small Anim Pract* 32:564–571, 1991.

Engelman RW, Tyler RD, Good RA, et al.: Hypercalcemia in cats with feline-leukemia-virus–associated leukemia-lymphoma. *Cancer* 56:777–781, 1985.

Farese G, Mager M, and Blatt WF: A membrane ultrafiltration procedure for determining diffusable calcium in serum. *Clin Chem* 16:226–228, 1970.

Favus MJ: Intestinal absorption of calcium, magnesium, and phosphorus. In Coe FL and Favus MJ (eds): *Disorders of Bone and Mineral Metabolism.* New York, Raven Press, pp. 57–81, 1992.

Favus MJ and Langman CB: Evidence for calcium-dependent control of 1,25-dihydroxyvitamin D_3 production by rat kidney proximal tubules. *J Biol Chem* 261:11224–11229, 1986.

Feldman D: Androgen and vitamin D receptor gene polymorphisms: The long and short of prostate cancer risk. *J Natl Cancer Inst* 89:109–111, 1997.

Feldman EC and Nelson RW: Hypercalcemia and primary hyperparathyroidism. In Feldman EC (ed): *Canine and Feline Endocrinology and Reproduction.* Philadelphia, WB Saunders Co., pp. 455–496, 1996.

Feldman EC and Nelson RW: Hypocalcemia and primary hypoparathyroidism. In Feldman EC (ed): *Canine and Feline Endocrinology and Reproduction.* Philadelphia, WB Saunders Co., pp. 497–524, 1996.

Feldman EC, Wisner ER, Nelson RW, et al.: Comparison of results of hormonal analysis of samples obtained from selected venous sites versus cervical ultrasonography for localizing parathyroid masses in dogs. *J Am Vet Med Assoc* 211:54–56, 1997.

Fenton AJ, Kemp BE, Hammonds RG Jr, et al.: A potent inhibitor of osteoclastic bone resorption within a highly conserved pepta-peptide region of parathyroid hormone–related protein: PTHrP[107–111]. *Endocrinology* 129:3424–3426, 1991.

Fenton AJ, Kemp BE, Kent GN, et al.: A carboxy-terminal peptide from the parathyroid hormone–related protein inhibits bone resorption by osteoclasts. *Endocrinology* 129:1762–1768, 1991.

Finco DR: Interpretations of serum calcium concentration in the dog. *Comp Contin Educ* 5:778–787, 1983.

Finco DR and Rowland GN: Hypercalcemia secondary to chronic renal failure in the dog: A report of four cases. *J Am Vet Med Assoc* 173:990–994, 1978.

Fingeroth JM and Smeak DD: Intravenous methylene blue infusion for intraoperative identification of parathyroid gland tumors in dogs. Part III: Clinical trials and results in three dogs. *J Am Anim Hosp Assoc* 24:673–678, 1988.

Fitzpatrick LA, Brandi ML, and Aurbach GD: Control of PTH secretion is mediated through calcium channels and is blocked by pertussis toxin treatment of parathyroid cells. *Biochem Biophys Res Commun* 138:960–965, 1986.

Flanders JA: Surgical therapy of the thyroid. *Vet Clin North Am Small Anim Pract* 24:607–621, 1994.

Flanders JA, Harvey HJ, and Erb HN: Feline thyroidectomy. A comparison of postoperative hypocalcemia associated with three different surgical techniques. *Vet Surg* 16:362–366, 1987.

Flanders JA, Scarlett JM, Blue JT, et al.: Adjustment of total serum calcium concentration for binding to albumin and protein in cats: 291 cases (1986–1987). *J Am Vet Med Assoc* 194:1609–1611, 1989.

Flanders JA, Neth S, Erb HN, et al.: Functional analysis of ectopic parathyroid activity in cats. *Am J Vet Res* 52:1336–1340, 1991.

Fleisch H: Bisphosphonates. Pharmacology and use in the treatment of tumour-induced hypercalcaemic and metastatic bone disease. *Drugs* 42:919–944, 1991.

Fleisch H: Mechanisms of action of the bisphosphonates. *Medicina (Buenos Aires)* 57:65–75, 1997.

Fooshee SK and Forrester SD: Hypercalcemia secondary to cholecalciferol rodenticide toxicosis in two dogs. *J Am Vet Med Assoc* 196:1265–1268, 1990.

Fraser D, Jones G, Kooh SW, et al.: Calcium and phosphate metabolism. Philadelphia, WB Saunders Co., pp. 1317–1372, 1986.

Fraser D, Jones G, Kooh SW, et al.: Calcium and phosphate metabolism. In Tietz NW (ed): *Fundamentals of Clinical Chemistry.* Philadelphia, WB Saunders Co., pp. 705–728, 1987.

Frick TW, Mithöfer K, Fernandez-del Castillo C, et al.: Hypercalcemia causes acute pancreatitis by pancreatic secretory block, intracellular zymogen accumulation, and acinar cell injury. *Am J Surg* 169:167–172, 1995.

Fukagawa M, Kitaoka M, and Kurokawa K: Renal failure and hyperparathyroidism. In Feldman D (ed): *Vitamin D.* New York, Academic Press, pp. 1227–1239, 1997.

Garlock SM, Matz ME, and Shell LG: Vitamin D_3 rodenticide toxicity in a dog. *J Am Anim Hosp Assoc* 27:356–360, 1991.

Garrett IR: Bone destruction in cancer. *Semin Oncol* 20:4–9, 1993.

Gascon-Barré M: The vitamin D 25-hydroxylase. In Feldman D (ed): *Vitamin D.* New York, Academic Press, pp. 41–56, 1997.

Goodman WG, Belin T, Gales B, et al.: Calcium-regulated parathyroid hormone release in patients with mild or advanced secondary hyperparathyroidism. *Kidney Int* 48:1553–1558, 1995.

Goodman WG, Veldhuis JD, Belin TR, et al.: Calcium-sensing by parathyroid glands in secondary hyperparathyroidism. *J Clin Endocrinol Metab* 83:2765–2772, 1998.

Gosling P: Analytical reviews in clinical biochemistry: Calcium measurement. *Ann Clin Biochem* 23:146–156, 1986.

Gouget B, Gourmelin Y, Blanchet F, et al.: Ca^{2+} measurement with ion selective electrode. The French coordinated evaluation of seven analyzers for a better clinical relevance and acceptance. *Ann Biol Chem* 46:419–434, 1988.

Graves TK: Complications of treatment and concurrent illness associated with hyperthyroidism in cats. In Bonagura JD (ed): *Kirk's Current Veterinary Therapy XII: Small Animal Practice.* Philadelphia, WB Saunders Co., pp. 369–372, 1995.

Green MD: Oral bisphosphonates and malignancy. *Med J Aust* 167:211–212, 1997.

Grosenbaugh DA, Gadawski JE, and Muir WW: Evaluation of a portable clinical analyzer in a veterinary hospital setting. *J Am Vet Med Assoc* 213:691–694, 1998.

Gunther R, Felice LJ, Nelson RK, et al.: Toxicity of vitamin D_3 rodenticide to dogs. *J Am Vet Med Assoc* 193:211–214, 1988.

Habener JF, Rosenblatt M, and Potts JT: Parathyroid hormone: Biochemical aspects of biosynthesis, secretion, action, and metabolism. *Physiol Rev* 64:985, 1984.

Halabe A, Arie R, Mimran D, et al.: Hypoparathyroidism—A long-term follow-up experience with 1-α-vitamin D_3 therapy. *Clin Endocrinol* 40:303–307, 1994.

Harrison HE and Harrison HC: Transfer of [45]Ca across intestinal wall in vitro in relation to action of vitamin D and cortisol. *Am J Physiol* 199:265–271, 1960.

Haussler MR, Jurutka PW, Hsieh JC, et al.: Nuclear vitamin D receptor: Structure-function, phosphorylation, and control of gene transcription. In Feldman D (ed): *Vitamin D.* New York, Academic Press, pp. 149–177, 1997.

Haussler MR, Whitfield GK, Haussler CA, et al.: The nuclear vitamin D receptor: Biological and molecular regulatory properties revealed. *J Bone Miner Res* 13:325–349, 1998.

Hazewinkel HAW: Dietary influences on calcium homeostasis and the skeleton. *Proc 1st Purina Int Nutr Symp*, pp. 51–59, 1991.

Heidbreder E, Naujoks H, Brosa U, et al.: The calcium–parathyroid hormone regulation in chronic renal failure. Investigation of its dynamic secretion pattern. *Horm Metab Res* 29:70–75, 1997.

Henderson RA, Powers RD, and Perry L: Development of hypoparathyroidism after excision of laryngeal rhabdomyosarcoma in a dog. *J Am Vet Med Assoc* 198:639–643, 1991.

Henry DA, Goodman WG, Nudelman RK, et al.: Parenteral aluminum administration in the dog: I. Plasma kinetics, tissue levels, calcium metabolism, and parathyroid hormone. *Kidney Int* 25:362–369, 1984.

Henry H: The 25-hydroxyvitamin D 1-α-hydroxylase. In Feldman D (ed): *Vitamin D.* New York, Academic Press, pp. 57–68, 1997.

High WB, Black HE, and Capen CC: Histomorphometric evaluation of the effects of low dose parathyroid hormone administration on cortical bone remodeling in adult dogs. *Lab Invest* 44:449–454, 1981.

Hodges RD, Legendre AM, Adams LG, et al.: Itraconazole for the treatment of histoplasmosis in cats. *J Vet Intern Med* 8:409–413, 1994.

Holick MF: Defects in the synthesis and metabolism of vitamin D. *Exp Clin Endocrinol Diabetes* 103:219–227, 1995.

Holick MF: Photobiology of vitamin D. In Feldman D (ed): *Vitamin D.* New York, Academic Press, pp. 33–40, 1997.

Holley DC and Evans JW: Determination of total and ultrafilterable calcium and magnesium in normal equine serum. *Am J Vet Res* 38:259–262, 1977.

Hollis BW, Kamerud JQ, Kurkowski A, et al.: Quantification of circulating 1,25-dihydroxyvitamin D by radioimmunoassay with an ^{125}I-labeled tracer. *Clin Chem* 42:586–592, 1996.

Horst RL, Reinhardt TA, and Hollis BW: Improved methodology for the analysis of plasma vitamin D metabolites. *Kidney Int* 38:S28–S35, 1990.

Horst RL and Reinhardt TA: Vitamin D metabolism. In Feldman D (ed): *Vitamin D.* New York, Academic Press, pp. 13–31, 1997.

How KL, Hazewinkel HA, and Mol JA: Dietary vitamin D dependence of cat and dog due to inadequate cutaneous synthesis of vitamin D. *Gen Comp Endocrinol* 96:12–18, 1994.

Hristova EN, Cecco S, Niemela JE, et al.: Analyzer-dependent differences in results for ionized calcium, ionized magnesium, sodium, and pH. *Clin Chem* 41:1649–1653, 1995.

Hruska K, Gupta A, Bonjour JP, et al.: Regulation of phosphate transport. In Feldman D (ed): *Vitamin D.* New York, Academic Press, pp. 499–519, 1997.

Hsu CH and Patel SR: Altered vitamin D metabolism and receptor interaction with the target genes in renal failure: Calcitriol receptor interaction with its target gene in renal failure. *Curr Opin Nephrol Hypertens* 4:302–306, 1995.

Hulter HN, Halloran BP, Toto RD, et al.: Long-term control of plasma calcitriol concentration in dogs and humans. Dominant role of plasma calcium concentration in experimental hyperparathyroidism. *J Clin Invest* 76:695–702, 1985.

Ihle SL, Nelson RW, and Cook JR: Seizures as a manifestation of primary hyperparathyroidism in a dog. *J Am Vet Med Assoc* 192:71–72, 1988.

Imamura H, Sato K, Shizume K, et al.: Urinary excretion of parathyroid hormone–related protein fragments in patients with humoral hypercalcemia of malignancy and hypercalcemia tumor-bearing nude mice. *J Bone Min Res* 6:77–84, 1991.

Inomata N, Akiyama M, Kubota N, et al.: Characterization of a novel parathyroid hormone (PTH) receptor with specificity for the carboxyl-terminal region of PTH-(1–84). *Endocrinology* 136:4732–4740, 1995.

Irvine RF: Calcium transients: Mobilization of intracellular Ca^{2+}. *Br Med Bull* 42:369–374, 1986.

Izquierdo R, Bermes EJ, Sandberg L, et al.: Serum calcium metabolism in acute experimental pancreatitis. *Surgery* 98:1031–1037, 1985.

Jorgensen LS, Center SA, Randolph JF, et al.: Electrolyte abnormalities induced by hypertonic phosphate enemas in two cats. *J Am Vet Med Assoc* 187:1367–1368, 1985.

Kallet AJ, Richter KP, Feldman EC, et al.: Primary hyperparathyroidism in cats: Seven cases (1984–1989). *J Am Vet Med Assoc* 199:1767–1771, 1991.

Kasahara H, Tsuchiya M, Adachi R, et al.: Development of a C-terminal-region-specific radioimmunoassay of parathyroid hormone–related protein. *Biomed Res* 13:155–161, 1992.

Kawasaki T: Creatinine unreliable indicator of renal failure in ferrets. *J Small Anim Exotic Med* 1:28–29, 1991.

Kirk GR, Breazile JE, and Kenny AD: Pathogenesis of hypocalcemic tetany in the thyroparathyroidectomized dog. *Am J Vet Res* 35:407–408, 1974.

Klausner JS, Fernandez FR, O'Leary TP, et al.: Canine primary hyperparathyroidism and its association with urolithiasis. *Vet Clin North Am Small Anim Pract* 16:227–239, 1986.

Klein MK, Powers BE, Withrow SJ, et al.: Treatment of thyroid carcinoma in dogs by surgical resection alone: 20 cases (1981–1989). *J Am Vet Med Assoc* 206:1007–1009, 1995.

Kohn CW and Brooks CL: Failure of pH to predict ionized calcium percentage in healthy horses. *Am J Vet Res* 51:1206–1210, 1990.

Koo WS, Jeon DS, Ahn SJ, et al.: Calcium-free hemodialysis for the management of hypercalcemia. *Nephron* 72:424–428, 1996.

Korkor AB, Kuchibotla J, Arrieh M, et al.: The effects of chronic prednisone administration on intestinal receptors for 1,25-dihydroxyvitamin D_3 in the dog. *Endocrinology* 117:2267–2273, 1985.

Kornegay JN: Hypocalcemia in dogs. *Compend Contin Educ* 4:1785–1792, 1982.

Kremer R and Goltzman D: Assays for parathyroid hormone–related protein. In Bilezikian JP, Marcus R, and Levine MA (eds): *The Parathyroids*. New York, Raven Press, pp. 321–340, 1994.

Krishnan AV and Feldman D: Regulation of vitamin D receptor abundance. In Feldman D (ed): *Vitamin D*. New York, Academic Press, pp. 179–200, 1997.

Kronenberg HM, Bringhurst FR, Segre GV, et al.: Parathyroid hormone biosynthesis and metabolism. In Bilezikian JP, Marcus R, and Levine MA (eds): *The Parathyroids*. New York, Raven Press, pp. 125–138, 1994.

Kruger JM, Osborne CA, and Polzin DJ: Treatment of hypercalcemia. In Kirk RW (ed): *Current Veterinary Therapy IX*. Philadelphia, WB Saunders Co., pp. 75–90, 1986.

Kruger JM, Osborne CA, Nachreiner RF, et al.: Hypercalcemia and renal failure: Etiology, pathophysiology, diagnosis, and treatment. *Vet Clin North Am Small Anim Pract* 26:1417–1445, 1996.

Kumar R: Vitamin D and the kidney. In Feldman D (ed): *Vitamin D*. New York, Academic Press, pp. 275–292, 1997.

Kyles AE, Stone EA, Gookin J, et al.: Diagnosis and surgical management of obstructive ureteral calculi in cats: 11 cases (1993–1996). *J Am Vet Med Assoc* 213:1150–1156, 1998.

Ladenson JH, Lewis JW, McDonald JM, et al.: Relationship of free and total calcium in hypercalcemic conditions. *J Clin Endocrinol Metab* 48:393–397, 1979.

Larsson L and Ohman S: Effect of silicone-separator tubes and storage time on ionized calcium in serum. *Clin Chem* 31:169–170, 1985.

Lees GE: *Hypoparathyroidism*. Philadelphia, WB Saunders Co, pp. 876–879, 1983.

Lifton SJ, King LG, and Zerbe CA: Glucocorticoid deficient hypoadrenocorticism in dogs: 18 cases (1986–1995). *J Am Vet Med Assoc* 209:2076–2081, 1996.

Lim SK, Gardella TJ, Baba H, et al.: The carboxy-terminus of parathyroid hormone is essential for hormone processing and secretion. *Endocrinology* 131:2325–2330, 1992.

Lincoln SD and Lane VM: Serum ionized calcium concentration in clinically normal dairy cattle, and changes associated with calcium abnormalities. *J Am Vet Med Assoc* 197:1471–1474, 1990.

Lind L, Bucht E, and Ljunghall S: Pronounced elevation in circulating calcitonin in critical care patients is related to the severity of illness and survival. *Intensive Care Med* 21:63–66, 1995.

Lins BE: Renal function in hypercalcemic dogs during hydropenia and during saline infusion. *Acta Physiol Scand* 106:177–186, 1979.

Lyon ME, Guajardo M, Laha T, et al.: Zinc heparin introduces a preanalytical error in the measurement of ionized calcium concentration. *Scand J Clin Lab Invest* 55:61–65, 1995.

Machado CE and Flombaum CD: Safety of pamidronate in patients with renal failure and hypercalcemia. *Clin Nephrol* 45:175–179, 1996.

MacIsaac RJ, Caple IW, Danks JA, et al.: Ontogeny of parathyroid hormone–related protein in the ovine parathyroid gland. *Endocrinology* 129:757–764, 1991a.

MacIsaac RJ, Heath JA, Rodda CP, et al.: Role of the fetal parathyroid glands and parathyroid hormone–related protein in the regulation of placental transport of calcium, magnesium, and inorganic phosphate. *Reprod Fertil Dev* 3:447–457, 1991b.

MacKenzie CP, Burnie AG, and Head KW: Poisoning in four dogs by a compound containing warfarin and calciferol. *J Small Anim Pract* 28:433–445, 1987.

Mackey SL, Heymont JL, Kronenberg HM, et al.: Vitamin D receptor binding to the negative human parathyroid hormone vitamin D response element does not require the retinoid X receptor. *Mol Endocrinol* 10:298–305, 1996.

Mahgoub AM, Hirsch PF, and Munson PL: Calcium-lowering action of glucocorticoids in adrenalectomized-parathyroidectomized rats. Specificity and relative potency of natural and synthetic glucocorticoids. *Endocrine* 6:279–283, 1997.

Mallette LE: Parathyroid hormone and parathyroid hormone-related protein as polyhormones. In Bilezikian JP, Marcus R, and Levine MA (eds): *The Parathyroids*. New York, Raven Press, pp. 171–184, 1994.

Mangin M, Ikeda K, and Broadus AE: Structure of the mouse gene encoding parathyroid hormone–related protein. *Gene* 95:195–202, 1990.

Marquez GA, Klausner JS, and Osborne CA: Calcium oxalate urolithiasis in a cat with a functional parathyroid adenocarcinoma. *J Am Vet Med Assoc* 206:817–819, 1995.

Martin LG: Hypercalcemia and hypermagnesemia. *Vet Clin North Am Small Anim Pract* 28:565–585, 1998.

Martin TJ and Grill V: Hypercalcemia and cancer. *J Steroid Biochem Mol Biol* 43:123–129, 1992.

Massry SG: Pathogenesis of uremic toxicity. In Massry SG and Glassock RJ (eds): *Textbook of Nephrology.* Baltimore, Williams & Wilkins, 1989, pp. 1126–1144, 1989.

Matus RE, Leifer CE, MacEwen EG, et al.: Prognostic factors for multiple myeloma in the dog. *J Am Vet Med Assoc* 188:1288–1292, 1986.

Matwichuk CL, Taylor SM, Wilkinson AA, et al.: Use of technetium Tc 99m sestamibi for detection of a parathyroid adenoma in a dog with primary hyperparathyroidism. *J Am Vet Med Assoc* 209:1733–1736, 1996.

McCauley LK, Rosol TJ, Stromberg PC, et al.: In vivo and in vitro effects of interleukin-1α and cyclosporin A on bone and lymphoid tissues in mice. *Toxicol Pathol* 19:1–10, 1991.

McClain HM, Barsanti JA, and Bartges JW: Hypercalcemia and calcium oxalate urolithiasis in cats: A report of five cases. *J Am Anim Hosp Assoc* 35(4):297–301, 1999.

McElwain MC, Modzelewski RA, Yu WD, et al.: Vitamin D: An antiproliferative agent with potential for therapy of squamous cell carcinoma. *Am J Otolaryngol* 18:293–298, 1997.

McSheehy PM and Chambers TJ: Osteoblastic cells mediate osteoclastic responsiveness to parathyroid hormone. *Endocrinology* 118:824–828, 1986.

Meller Y, Kestenbaum RS, Yagil R, et al.: The influence of age and sex on blood levels of calcium-regulating hormones in dogs. *Clin Orthop* 187:296–309, 1984.

Merryman JI, Rosol TJ, Brooks CL, et al.: Separation of parathyroid hormone-like activity from transforming growth factor-α and -β in the canine adenocarcinoma (CAC-8) model of humoral hypercalcemia of malignancy. *Endocrinology* 124:2456–2563, 1989.

Messa P, Vallone C, Mioni G, et al.: Direct in vivo assessment of parathyroid hormone–calcium relationship curve in renal patients. *Kidney Int* 46:1713–1720, 1994.

Meuten DJ: Hypercalcemia. *Vet Clin North Am Small Anim Pract* 14:891–910, 1984.

Meuten DJ, Cooper BJ, Capen CC, et al.: Hypercalcemia associated with an adenocarcinoma derived from the apocrine glands of the anal sac. *Vet Pathol* 18:454–471, 1981.

Meuten DJ, Chew DJ, Capen CC, et al.: Relationship of serum total calcium to albumin and total protein in dogs. *J Am Vet Med Assoc* 18:63–67, 1982.

Meuten DJ, Kociba GJ, Capen CC, et al.: Hypercalcemia in dogs with lymphosarcoma: Biochemical, ultrastructural, and histomorphometric investigations. *Lab Invest* 49:553–562, 1983.

Meuten DJ, Segre GV, Capen CC, et al.: Hypercalcemia in dogs with adenocarcinoma derived from apocrine glands of the anal sac: Biochemical and histomorphometric investigations. *Lab Invest* 48:428–435, 1983.

Meyer RA, Morgan PL, and Meyer MH: Measurement of parathyroid hormone in the mouse: Secondary hyperparathyroidism in the X-linked hypophosphatemic (Gyro, Gy) mouse. *Endocrine* 2:1127–1132, 1994.

Michelangeli VP, Heyma P, Colman PG, et al.: Evaluation of a new, rapid and automated immunochemiluminometric assay for the measurement of serum intact parathyroid hormone. *Ann Clin Biochem* 34:97–103, 1997.

Miki H, Maercklein PB, and Fitzpatrick LA: Effect of magnesium on parathyroid cells: Evidence for two sensing receptors or two intracellular pathways? *Am J Physiol* 35:E1–E6, 1997.

Miller D and Edmonds MW: Hypercalcemia due to hyperparathyroidism treated with a somatostatin analogue. *Can Med Assoc J* 145:227–228, 1991.

Mischke R, Hanies R, Lange K, et al.: The effect of the albumin concentration on the relation between the concentration of ionized calcium and total calcium in the blood of dogs. *Dtsch Tierarztl Wochenschr* 103:199–204, 1996.

Mithöfer K, Castillo CF-D, Frick TW, et al.: Acute hypercalcemia causes acute pancreatitis and ectopic trypsinogen activation in the rat. *Gastroenterology* 109:239–246, 1995.

Mol JA, Kwant MM, Arnold ICJ, et al.: Elucidation of the sequence of canine (pro)-calcitonin. A molecular biological and protein chemical approach. *Regul Peptides* 35:189–195, 1991.

Morrison N: Vitamin D receptor gene variants and osteoporosis: A contributor to the polygenic control of bone density. In Feldman D (ed): *Vitamin D.* New York, Academic Press, pp. 713–731, 1997.

Mosdell KW and Visconti JA: Emerging indications for octreotide therapy, Part 1. *Am J Hosp Pharm* 51:1184–1192, 1994.

Moseley JM, Kubota M, Diefenbach-Jagger H, et al.: Parathyroid hormone–related protein purified from a human lung cancer cell line. *Proc Natl Acad Sci U S A* 84:5048–5052, 1987.

Nachreiner RF and Refsal KR: The use of parathormone, ionized calcium and 25-hydroxyvitamin D assays to diagnose calcium disorders in dogs. *Proc Am Coll Vet Intern Med Forum* 8:251–254, 1990.

Nagode LA and Chew DJ: The use of calcitriol in treatment of renal disease of the dog and cat. *Proc 1st Purina Int Nutr Symp,* pp. 39–49, 1991.

Nagode LA and Chew DJ: Nephrocalcinosis caused by hyperparathyroidism in progression of renal failure: Treatment with calcitriol. *Semin Vet Med Surg Small Anim* 7:202–220, 1992.

Nagode LA, Steinmeyer CL, Chew DJ, et al.: Hyper- and normocalcemic dogs with chronic renal failure: Relations of serum PTH and calcitriol to PTG Ca^{++} set-point. In Norman AW, Schaefer K, Grigoleit HG, and Herrath DV (eds): *Vitamin D. Molecular, Cellular and Clinical Endocrinology.* Berlin, Walter de Gruyter, pp. 799–800, 1988.

Nagode LA, Chew DJ, and Steinmeyer CL: The use of low doses of calcitriol in the treatment of renal secondary hyperparathyroidism. *15th Waltham Symposium (Endocrinology),* pp. 49–63, 1992.

Nagode LA, Chew DJ, and Podell M: Benefits of calcitriol therapy and serum phosphorus control in dogs and cats with chronic renal failure. *Vet Clin North Am Small Anim Pract* 26:1293–1330, 1996.

Nagode LA, Chew DJ, Podell M, et al.: Clinical benefits of calcitriol therapy in dogs and cats with naturally occurring chronic renal failure. In Norman AW, Bouillon R, and Thomasset M (eds): *Vitamin D: Chemistry, Biology and Clinical Applications of the Steroid Hormone.* Riverside, University of California, pp. 865–866, 1997.

Nemere I and Norman AW: Parathyroid hormone stimulates calcium transport in perfused duodena from normal chicks: Comparison with the rapid (transcaltachic) effect of 1,25-dihydroxyvitamin D_3. *Endocrinology* 119:1406–1408, 1986.

Nemzek JA, Kruger JM, Walshaw R, et al.: Acute onset of hypokalemia and muscular weakness in four hyperthyroid cats. *J Am Vet Med Assoc* 205:65–68, 1994.

Norrdin RW, Miller CW, LoPresti CA, et al.: Observations on calcium metabolism, ^{47}Ca absorption, and duodenal calcium-binding activity in chronic renal failure: Studies in beagles with radiation-induced nephropathy. *Am J Vet Res* 41:510–515, 1980.

Norman AW: Rapid biological responses mediated by 1,25-dihydroxyvitamin D_3: A case study of transcaltachia (rapid hormonal stimulation of intestinal calcium transport). In Feldman D (ed): *Vitamin D.* New York, Academic Press, pp. 233–256, 1997.

Okada H, Merryman JI, Rosol TJ, et al.: Effects of humoral hypercalcemia of malignancy and gallium nitrate on thyroid C-cells in nude mice: Immunohistochemical and ultrastructural investigations. *Vet Pathol* 31:349–357, 1994.

Okazaki T, Zajac JD, Igarashi T, et al.: Negative regulatory elements in the human parathyroid hormone gene. *J Biol Chem* 266:21903–21910, 1991.

Okazaki T, Ando K, Igarashi T, et al.: Conserved mechanism of negative gene regulation by extracellular calcium–parathyroid hormone gene versus atrial natriuretic polypeptide gene. *J Clin Invest* 89:1268–1273, 1992.

Omdahl J and May B: The 25-hydroxyvitamin D 24-hydroxylase. In Feldman D (ed): *Vitamin D*. New York, Academic Press, pp. 69–86, 1997.

Ong SC, Shalhoub RJ, Gallagher P, et al.: Effect of furosemide on experimental hypercalcemia in dogs. *Proc Soc Exp Biol Med* 145:227–233, 1974.

Orloff JJ and Stewart AF: The carboxy-terminus of parathyroid hormone—Inert or invaluable? *Endocrinology* 136:4729–4731, 1995.

Orloff JJ, Reddy D, dePapp AE, et al.: Parathyroid hormone–related protein as a prohormone: Posttranslational processing and receptor interactions. *Endocr Rev* 15:40–60, 1994.

Padgett SL, Tobias KM, Leathers CW, et al.: Efficacy of parathyroid gland autotransplantation in maintaining serum calcium concentrations after bilateral thyroparathyroidectomy in cats. *J Am Anim Hosp Assoc* 34:219–224, 1998.

Page RL: Acute tumor lysis syndrome. *Semin Vet Med Surg Small Anim* 1:58–60, 1986.

Pandian MR, Morgan CH, Carlton E, et al.: Modified immunoradiometric assay of parathyroid hormone–related protein: Clinical application in the differential diagnosis of hypercalcemia. *Clin Chem* 38:282–288, 1992.

Pannabecker TL, Chandler JS, and Wasserman RH: Vitamin-D–dependent transcriptional regulation of the intestinal plasma membrane calcium pump. *Biochem Biophys Res Commun* 213:499–505, 1995.

Parfitt AM: The cellular basis of bone turnover and bone loss. *Clin Orthop* 127:236–247, 1977.

Parfitt AM: Bone and plasma calcium homeostasis. *Bone* 8(suppl 1):S1–S8, 1987.

Patel SR, Ke HQ, Vanholder R, et al.: Inhibition of calcitriol receptor binding to vitamin D response elements by uremic toxins. *J Clin Invest* 96:50–59, 1995.

Persons DA, Garst J, Vollmer R, et al.: Tumor lysis syndrome and acute renal failure after treatment of non–small cell lung carcinoma with combination irinotecan and cisplatin. *Am J Clin Oncol* 21:426–429, 1998.

Peterson ME: Treatment of canine and feline hypoparathyroidism. *J Am Vet Med Assoc* 181:1434–1436, 1982.

Peterson ME: Hypoparathyroidism. In Kirk RW (ed): *Current Veterinary Therapy IX: Small Animal Practice*. Philadelphia, WB Saunders Co., pp. 1039–1045, 1986.

Peterson ME and Feinman JM: Hypercalcemia associated with hypoadrenocorticism in sixteen dogs. *J Am Vet Med Assoc* 181:802–804, 1982.

Peterson ME, Greco DS, and Orth DN: Primary hypoadrenocorticism in ten cats. *J Vet Intern Med* 3:55–58, 1989.

Peterson ME, James KM, Wallace M, et al.: Idiopathic hypoparathyroidism in five cats. *J Vet Intern Med* 5:47–51, 1991.

Peterson EN, Kirby R, Sommer M, et al.: Cholecalciferol rodenticide intoxication in a cat. *J Am Vet Med Assoc* 199:904–906, 1991.

Peterson ME, Kintzer PP, and Kass PH: Pretreatment clinical and laboratory findings in dogs with hypoadrenocorticism: 225 cases (1979–1993). *J Am Vet Med Assoc* 208:85–91, 1996.

Petrie G: Management of hypercalcemia using dichloromethylene bisphosphonate (clodronate). *Proc Cong Eur Soc Vet Intern Med* 6:80, 1996.

Pezzilli R, Billi P, Barakat B, et al.: Octreotide for the treatment of hypercalcemia related to B cell lymphoma (letter). *Oncology* 54:517–518, 1997.

Philbrick WM, Wysolmerski JJ, Galbrath S, et al.: Defining the roles of parathyroid hormone–related protein in normal physiology. *Physiol Rev* 76:127–173, 1996.

Piek CJ and Teske E: Tumor lysis syndrome in a dog. *Tijdschr Diergeneeskd* 121:64–66, 1996.

Pike JW: The vitamin D receptor and its gene. In Feldman D (ed): *Vitamin D*. New York, Academic Press, pp. 105–125, 1997.

Pollak MR, Brown EM, Chou Y-HW, et al.: Mutations in the human Ca^{2+}-sensing receptor gene cause familial hypocalciuric hypercalcemia and neonatal severe hypercalcemia. *Cell* 75:1297–1303, 1993.

Powell GJ, Southby J, Danks JA, et al.: Localization of parathyroid hormone–related protein in breast cancer metastases: Increased incidence in bone compared to other sites. *Cancer Res* 51:3059–3061, 1991.

Prager D, Rosenblatt JD, and Ejima E: Hypercalcemia, parathyroid hormone–related protein expression and human T-cell leukemia virus infection. *Leuk Lymphoma* 14:395–400, 1994.

Ralston-Purina Co.: *Normal Blood Values for Cats and Normal Blood Values for Dogs*. St. Louis, 1975.

Rasmussen H: The cycling of calcium as an intracellular messenger. *Sci Am* 261:66–73, 1989.

Rasmussen H, Barrett P, Smallwood J, et al.: Calcium ion as an intracellular messenger and cellular toxin. *Environ Health Perspect* 84:17–25, 1990.

Reber PM and Heath H: Hypocalcemic emergencies. *Med Clin North Am* 79:93–106, 1995.

Refsal KR, Nachreiner RF, and Graham PA: Laboratory assessment of hypercalcemia. *Proc Am Coll Vet Intern Med Forum* 16:646–647, 1998.

Reichel H, Koeffler HP, and Norman AW: The role of the vitamin D endocrine system in health and disease. *N Engl J Med* 320:980–991, 1989.

Renoe BW, McDonald JM, and Ladenson JH: Influence of posture on free calcium and related variables. *Clin Chem* 25:1766–1769, 1979.

Rijnberk A, Elsinghorst AM, Koeman JP, et al.: Pseudohyperparathyroidism associated with perirectal adenocarcinomas in elderly female dogs. *Tijdschr Diergeneeskd* 103:1069–1075, 1978.

Rodriguez M, Felsenfeld AJ, and Llach F: The role of aluminum in the development of hypercalcemia in the rat. *Kidney Int* 31:766–771, 1987.

Rodan GA and Balena R: Bisphosphonates in the treatment of metabolic bone diseases. *Ann Med* 25:373–378, 1993.

Rosol TJ and Capen CC: The effect of low calcium diet, mithramycin, and dichlorodimethylene bisphosphonate on humoral hypercalcemia of malignancy in nude mice transplanted with the canine adenocarcinoma tumor line (CAC-8). *J Bone Mine Res* 2:395–405, 1987.

Rosol TJ and Capen CC: Pathogenesis of humoral hypercalcemia of malignancy. *Domest Anim Endocrinol* 5:1–21, 1988.

Rosol TJ and Capen CC: Tumors of the parathyroid gland and circulating parathyroid hormone–related protein associated with persistent hypercalcemia. *Toxicol Pathol* 17:346–356, 1989.

Rosol TJ and Capen CC: Biology of disease: Mechanisms of cancer-induced hypercalcemia. *Lab Invest* 67:680–702, 1992.

Rosol TJ and Capen CC: Pathophysiology of calcium, phosphorus, and magnesium metabolism in animals. *Vet Clin North Am Small Anim Pract* 26:1155–1184, 1996.

Rosol TJ and Capen CC: Calcium-regulating hormones and diseases of abnormal mineral (calcium, phosphorus, magnesium) metabolism. In Kaneko JJ, Harvey JW, and Bruss ML (eds): *Clinical Biochemistry of Domestic Animals*. San Diego, Academic Press, pp. 619–702, 1997.

Rosol TJ, Chew DJ, Capen CC, et al.: Acute hypocalcemia associated with infarction of parathyroid gland adenomas in two dogs. *J Am Vet Med Assoc* 192:212–214, 1988.

Rosol TJ, Chew DJ, Couto GC, et al.: Effects of mithyramycin on calcium metabolism and bone in dogs. *Vet Pathol* 29:223–229, 1992.

Rosol TJ, Nagode LA, Couto CG, et al.: Parathyroid hormone (PTH)–related protein, PTH, and 1,25-dihydroxyvitamin D in

Rosol TJ, Chew DJ, Capen CC, et al.: dogs with cancer-associated hypercalcemia. *Endocrinology* 131:1157–1164, 1992.

Rosol TJ, Chew DJ, Hammer AS, et al.: Effect of mithramycin on hypercalcemia in dogs. *J Am Anim Hosp Assoc* 30:244–250, 1994.

Rosol TJ, Nagode LA, Robertson JT, et al.: Humoral hypercalcemia of malignancy associated with ameloblastoma in a horse. *J Am Vet Med Assoc* 204:1930–1933, 1994.

Rosol TJ, Chew DJ, Nagode LA, et al.: Pathophysiology of calcium metabolism. *Vet Clin Pathol* 24:49–63, 1995.

Rosol TJ, Steinmeyer CL, McCauley LK, et al.: Sequences of the cDNAs encoding canine parathyroid hormone–related protein and parathyroid hormone. *Gene* 160:241–243, 1995.

Rosol TJ, McCauley LK, Steinmeyer CL, et al.: Nucleotide sequence of canine preproparathyroid hormone. In Dacke C, Danks J, Caple I, and Flik G (eds): *The Comparative Endocrinology of Calcium Regulation*. Bristol, Journal of Endocrinology Ltd., pp. 201–203, 1996.

Ross JT, Scavelli TD, Matthiesen DT, et al.: Adenocarcinoma of the apocrine glands of the anal sac in dogs: A review of 32 cases. *J Am Anim Hosp Assoc* 27:349–355, 1991.

Roth SI and Capen CC: Ultrastructural and functional correlations of the parathyroid glands. *Int Rev Exp Pathol* 13:162–221, 1974.

Rucinski B, Mann GN and Epstein S: A new rapid and reproducible homologous immunoradiometric assay for amino-terminal parathyroid hormone in the rat. *Calcif Tissue Int* 56:83–87, 1995.

Rudnicki M, Frolich A, Haaber A, et al.: Actual ionized calcium (at actual pH) vs. adjusted ionized calcium (at pH 7.4) in hemodialyzed patients (letter). *Clin Chem* 38:1384–1384, 1992.

Rumbeiha WK, Kruger J, Fitzgerald S, et al.: The use of pamidronate disodium for treatment of vitamin D_3 toxicosis in dogs. *Proc Am Assoc Vet Lab Diagnost* 40:71, 1997.

Russo EA and Lees GE: Treatment of hypocalcemia. In Kirk RW (ed): *Current Veterinary Therapy IX: Small Animal Practice*. Philadelphia, WB Saunders Co., pp. 91–94, 1986.

Ryzen E and Rude RK: Low intracellular magnesium in patients with acute pancreatitis and hypocalcemia. *West J Med* 152:145–148, 1990.

Schaer M, Cavanaugh P, Hause W, et al.: Iatrogenic hyperphosphatemia, hypocalcemia, and hypernatremia in a cat. *J Am Anim Hosp Assoc* 13:39, 1977.

Schenck PA, Chew DJ, and Brooks CL: Effects of storage on normal canine serum ionized calcium and pH. *Am J Vet Res* 56:304–307, 1995.

Schenck PA, Chew DJ, Brooks CL, et al: Effects of storage on serum ionized calcium and pH from horses with normal and abnormal ionized calcium concentrations. *Vet Clin Pathol* 25:118–120, 1996.

Schenck PA, Chew DJ, and Brooks CL: Fractionation of canine serum calcium, using a micropartition system. *Am J Vet Res* 57:268–271, 1996.

Schultz G, Rosenthal W, Hescheler J, et al.: Role of G-proteins in calcium channel modulation. *Annu Rev Biochem* 52:275–292, 1990.

Schwarz U, Amann K, Orth SR, et al.: Effect of $1,25(OH)_2$ vitamin D_3 on glomerulosclerosis in subtotally nephrectomized rats. *Kidney Int* 53:1696–1705, 1998.

Segre GV: Receptors for parathyroid hormone and parathyroid hormone–related protein. In Bilezikian JP, Marcus R, and Levine MA (eds): *The Parathyroids*. New York, Raven Press, pp. 213–230, 1994.

Sekine M and Takami H: Combination of calcitonin and pamidronate for emergency treatment of malignant hypercalcemia. *Oncol Rep* 5:197–199, 1998.

Sela A, Kilav R, Naveh-Many T, et al.: Regulation of parathyroid hormone gene expression and parathyroid cell proliferation by vitamin D, calcium and phosphate. In Norman AW, Bouillon R, and Thomasset M (eds): *Vitamin D: Chemistry, Biology and Clinical Applications of the Steroid Hormone*. Riverside, University of California, pp. 260–267, 1997.

Seymour JF and Gagel RF: Calcitriol: The major humoral mediator of hypercalcemia in Hodgkin's and non-Hodgkin's lymphomas. *Blood* 82:1383–1394, 1993.

Sharma OP: Vitamin D, calcium, and sarcoidosis. *Chest* 109:535–539, 1996.

Sherding RG, Meuten DJ, Chew DJ, et al.: Primary hypoparathyroidism in the dog. *J Am Vet Med Assoc* 176:439–444, 1980.

Sherwood LM, Cantley L, and Russell J: Effects of calcium and $1,25\text{-}(OH)_2D_3$ on the synthesis and secretion of parathyroid hormone. In Cohn DV, Martin TJ, and Meunier PJ (eds): *Calcium Regulation and Bone Metabolism: Basic and Clinical Aspects*. Amsterdam, Elsevier Science Publishers, pp. 778–781, 1987.

Siegel N, Wongsurawat N, and Ambrecht HJ: Parathyroid hormone stimulates dephosphorylation of the renoredoxin component of the 25-hydroxyvitamin D_3-1 alpha hydroxylase from rat renal cortex. *J Biol Chem* 261:16998–17003, 1986.

Silver J and Kronenberg HM: Parathyroid hormone—Molecular biology and regulation. In Bilezikian JP, Raisz LG, and Rodan GA (eds): *Principles of Bone Biology*. San Diego, Academic Press, pp. 325–337, 1996.

Silver J and Naveh-Many T: Vitamin D and the parathyroid glands. In Feldman D (ed): *Vitamin D*. San Diego, Academic Press, pp. 353–367, 1997.

Slatopolsky E, Lopez-Hilker S, Delmez J, et al.: The parathyroid-calcitriol axis in health and chronic renal failure. *Kidney Int* 38:S41–S47, 1990.

Sperber SJ, Blevins DD, and Francis JB: Hypercalcitoninemia, hypocalcemia, and toxic shock syndrome. *Rev Infect Dis* 12:736–739, 1990.

St. Arnaud R and Glorieux FH: Vitamin D and bone development. In Feldman D (ed): *Vitamin D*. San Diego, Academic Press, pp. 293–303, 1997.

Stern PH: Vitamin D and bone. *Kidney Int* 38:S17–S21, 1990.

Suda T and Takahashi N: Vitamin D and osteoclastogenesis. In Feldman D (ed): *Vitamin D*. San Diego, Academic Press, pp. 329–340, 1997.

Suva LJ, Winslow GA, Wettenhall REH, et al.: A parathyroid hormone–related protein implicated in malignant hypercalcemia: Cloning and expression. *Science* 237:893–896, 1987.

Szenci O, Brydl E, and Bajcsy CA: Effect of storage on measurement of ionized calcium and acid-base variables in equine, bovine, ovine, and canine venous blood. *J Am Vet Med Assoc* 199:1167–1169, 1991.

Tanaka H and Seino Y: Vitamin D metabolites and bone. In Feldman D (ed): *Vitamin D*. New York, Academic Press, pp. 305–311, 1997.

Taylor JA, Hirvonen A, Watson M, et al.: Association of prostate cancer with vitamin D receptor gene polymorphism. *Cancer Res* 56:4108–4110, 1996.

Teachout DJ, Taylor SM, and Archer PJ: A comparison of serum ionized calcium concentrations and serum total calcium concentrations in dogs with lymphoma. *Zentralbl Veterinarmed A* 44:195–200, 1997.

Teare JA, Krook L, Kallfelz FA, et al.: Ascorbic acid deficiency and hypertrophic osteodystrophy in the dog: A rebuttal. *Cornell Vet* 69:384–401, 1979.

Thode J, Juul-Jorgensen B, Bhatia HM, et al.: Comparison of serum total calcium, albumin-corrected total calcium, and ionized calcium in 1213 patients with suspected calcium disorders. *Scand J Clin Lab Invest* 49:217–223, 1989.

Thomasset M: Calbindin-D 9K. In Feldman D (ed): *Vitamin D*. New York, Academic Press, pp. 223–232, 1997.

Thompson KG, Jones LP, Smylie WA, et al.: Primary hyperparathyroidism in German shepherd dogs: A disorder of probable genetic origin. *Vet Pathol* 21:370–376, 1984.

Thrall MA, Grauer GF, and Mero KN: Clinicopathologic findings in dogs and cats with ethylene glycol intoxication. *J Am Vet Med Assoc* 184:37–41, 1984.

Toffaletti J: Ionized calcium measurement: Analytical and clinical aspects. *Lab Manage* 20:31–35, 1983.

Tohme JF and Bilezikian JP: Hypocalcemic emergencies. *Endocrinol Metab Clin North Am* 22:363–375, 1993.

Torrance AG and Nachreiner R: Human-parathormone assay for use in dogs: Validation, sample handling techniques, and parathyroid function testing. *Am J Vet Res* 50:1123–1127, 1989.

Torrance AG and Nachreiner R: Intact parathyroid hormone assay and total calcium concentration in the diagnosis of disorders of calcium metabolism in dogs. *J Vet Intern Med* 3:86–89, 1989.

Troy GC, Forrester D, Cockburn C, et al.: *Heterobilharzia americana* infection and hypercalcemia in a dog: A case report. *J Am Anim Hosp Assoc* 23:35–40, 1987.

Tucci J, Hammond V, Senior PV, et al.: The role of fetal parathyroid hormone–related protein in transplacental calcium transport. *J Mol Endocrinol* 17:159–164, 1996.

Tuma SN and Mallette LE: Hypercalcemia after nephrectomy in the dog: Role of the kidneys and parathyroid glands. *J Lab Clin Med* 102:213–219, 1983.

Tweedy CR and Rees GM: Octreotide acetate in the treatment of hypercalcemia accompanying small cell carcinoma (letter; comment). *South Med J* 85:561–561, 1992.

Uehlinger P, Glaus T, Hauser B, et al.: Differential diagnosis of hypercalcemia—A retrospective study of 46 dogs. *Schweiz Arch Tierheilkd* 140:188–197, 1998.

Vaden SL, Levine J, and Breitschwerdt EB: A retrospective case-control study of acute renal failure in 99 dogs. *J Vet Intern Med* 11:58–64, 1997.

Vail DM, Withrow SJ, Schwarz PD, et al.: Perianal adenocarcinoma in the canine male: A retrospective study of 41 cases. *J Am Anim Hosp Assoc* 26:329–334, 1990.

Walker RP, Paloyan E, Kelley TF, et al.: Parathyroid autotransplantation in patients undergoing a total thyroidectomy: A review of 261 patients. *Otolaryngol Head Neck Surg* 111:258–264, 1994.

Walser M, Robinson BH, and Duckett JW Jr: The hypercalcemia of adrenal insufficiency. *J Clin Invest* 42:456–465, 1963.

Walters MR: Other vitamin D target tissues: Vitamin D actions in cardiovascular tissue and muscle, endocrine and reproductive tissues, and liver and lung. In Feldman D (ed): *Vitamin D*. New York, Academic Press, pp. 463–482, 1997.

Warrell RP, Murphy WK, Schulman P, et al.: A randomized double-blind study of gallium nitrate compared with etidronate for acute control of cancer-related hypercalcemia. *J Clin Oncol* 9:1467–1475, 1991.

Waser M, Mesaeli N, Spencer C, et al.: Regulation of calreticulin gene expression by calcium. *J Cell Biol* 138:547–557, 1997.

Wasserman RH: Vitamin D and the intestinal absorption of calcium and phosphorus. In Feldman D (ed): *Vitamin D*. New York, Academic Press, pp. 259–273, 1997.

Waters CB and Scott-Moncrieff JC: Hypocalcemia in cats. *Compend Contin Educ* 14:497–506, 1992.

Weaver ME, Morrissey J, McConkey CJ, et al.: WR-2721 inhibits parathyroid adenylate cyclase. *Am J Physiol* 252:E197–E201, 1987.

Weir EC, Burtis WJ, Morris CA, et al.: Isolation of 16,000-dalton parathyroid hormone–like proteins from two animal tumors causing humoral hypercalcemia of malignancy. *Endocrinology* 123:2744–2751, 1988.

Weir EC, Norrdin RW, Matus RE, et al.: Humoral hypercalcemia of malignancy in canine lymphosarcoma. *Endocrinology* 122:602–608, 1988.

Welches CD, Scavelli TD, Matthiesen DT, et al.: Occurrence of problems after three techniques of bilateral thyroidectomy in cats. *Vet Surg* 18:392–396, 1989.

Willard MD, Schall WD, McCaw DE, et al.: Canine hypoadrenocorticism: Report of 37 cases and review of 39 previously reported cases. *J Am Vet Med Assoc* 180:59–62, 1982.

Winer KK, Yanovski JA, Cutler GB Jr: Synthetic human parathyroid hormone 1–34 vs calcitriol and calcium in the treatment of hypoparathyroidism. *JAMA* 636, 1996.

Wisner ER and Nyland TG: Ultrasonography of the thyroid and parathyroid glands. *Vet Clin North Am Small Anim Pract* 28:973–991, 1998.

Wisner ER, Penninck D, Biller DS, et al.: High-resolution parathyroid sonography. *Vet Radiol Ultrasound* 38:462–466, 1997.

Woo J and Cannon DC: *Metabolic Intermediates and Inorganic ions*. 17th ed. Philadelphia, WB Saunders Co., pp. 133–179, 1984.

Wright KN, Breitschwerdt EB, Feldman JM, et al.: Diagnostic and therapeutic considerations in a hypercalcemic dog with multiple endocrine neoplasia. *J Am Anim Hosp Assoc* 31:156–162, 1995.

Yanagawa N and Lee DBN: Renal handling of calcium and phosphorus. In Coe FL and Favus MJ (eds): *Disorders of Bone and Mineral Metabolism*. New York, Raven Press, pp. 3–40, 1992.

Yang KH, dePapp AE, Soifer NE, et al.: Parathyroid hormone–related protein: Evidence for isoform- and tissue-specific post-translational processing. *Biochemistry* 33:7460–7469, 1994.

Yasuda T, Banville D, Rabbani S, et al.: Rat parathyroid hormone–like peptide: Comparison with the human homologue and expression in malignant and normal tissue. *Mol Endocrinol* 3:518–525, 1989.

Yu J, Papavasiliou V, Rhim J, et al.: Vitamin D analogs: New therapeutic agents for the treatment of squamous cancer and its associated hypercalcemia. *Anticancer Drugs* 6:101–108, 1995.

Zaloga GP and Chernow B: The multifactorial basis for hypocalcemia during sepsis. *Ann Intern Med* 107:36–41, 1987.

Zaloga GP, Malcolm D, Holaday J, et al.: Verapamil reverses calcium cardiotoxicity. *Ann Emerg Med* 16:637–639, 1987.

Zaloga GP, Willey S, Tomasic P, et al.: Free fatty acids alter calcium binding: A cause for misinterpretation of serum calcium values and hypocalcemia in critical illness. *J Clin Endocrinol Metab* 64:1010–1014, 1987.

Zawada Jr ET, Saelens DA, and Lembke JM: Influence of calcium infusion on plasma atrial natriuretic peptide in conscious dogs: Intervention with calcium antagonist, verapamil. *Miner Electrolyte Metab* 16:369–377, 1990.

Zelikovic I and Chesney RW: Vitamin D and mineral metabolism: The role of the kidney in health and disease. *World Rev Nutr Diet* 59:156–216, 1989.

CHAPTER 7

Disorders of Phosphorus
HYPOPHOSPHATEMIA AND HYPERPHOSPHATEMIA

M. D. WILLARD   STEPHEN P. DiBARTOLA

Phosphorus plays an essential role in cellular structure and function (Kreisberg 1977). A constituent of structural phospholipids in cell membranes and of hydroxyapatite in bone, phosphorus is also an integral component of nucleic acids and of phosphoproteins involved in mitochondrial oxidative phosphorylation. Energy for essential metabolic processes (e.g., muscle contraction, neuronal impulse conduction, epithelial transport) is stored in high-energy phosphate bonds of adenosine triphosphate (ATP). The compound 2,3-diphosphoglycerate (2,3-DPG) decreases the affinity of hemoglobin for oxygen and facilitates the delivery of oxygen to tissues. Cyclic adenosine monophosphate (cAMP) is an intracellular second messenger for many polypeptide hormones. Phosphate is also an important urinary buffer, and urinary phosphate constitutes the majority of titratable acidity (see Chapter 9).

Phosphorus is important in the intermediary metabolism of protein, fat, and carbohydrate and as a component of glycogen. It stimulates glycolytic enzymes (e.g., hexokinase, phosphofructokinase) and participates in the phosphorylation of many glycolytic intermediates. Nicotinamide adenine dinucleotide phosphate ($NADP^+$) is a coenzyme for important biochemical reactions. Phosphate regulates the activity of enzymes such as the glutaminase essential for ammoniagenesis (stimulated by increased phosphate concentrations) and the 1α-hydroxylase required for vitamin D activation (stimulated by decreased phosphate concentrations).

▶ Physical Chemistry

Phosphorus exists in organic (phospholipids and phosphate esters) and inorganic (orthophosphoric and pyrophosphoric acids) forms in the body. Almost all serum phosphorus is in the form of orthophosphate. Orthophosphoric acid is governed by the following set of equilibria:

$$H_3PO_4 \rightleftharpoons H_2PO_4^{1-} + H^+ \rightleftharpoons HPO_4^{2-} + H^+ \rightleftharpoons PO_4^{3-} + H^+$$
$$\text{pKa 2.0} \qquad \text{pKa 6.8} \qquad \text{pKa 12.4}$$

The pKa for the reaction between $H_2PO_4^{1-}$ and HPO_4^{2-} is 6.8 at the ionic strength and temperature of extracellular fluid, and these are the two prevailing ionic species at the normal extracellular fluid pH of 7.4. At this pH, H_3PO_4 and PO_4^{3-} are present in negligible amounts; thus, plasma inorganic phosphorus principally consists of $H_2PO_4^{1-}$ and HPO_4^{2-}. At pH 7.4, the $HPO_4^{2-}:H_2PO_4^{1-}$ ratio is 4.0, and the average valence of phosphate in serum reflects this ratio. There is four times as much HPO_4^{2-} as $H_2PO_4^{1-}$ at pH 7.4; therefore, the average valence of phosphate at this pH is $(4/5)(-2) + (1/5)(-1) = -1.8$. Because the valence and number of milliequivalents (mEq) of phosphate in extracellular fluid are influenced by pH, it is easier to measure phosphate in millimoles (mmol) or milligrams (mg) of elemental phosphorus. Serum phosphorus concentrations are typically reported as elemental phosphorus and expressed as milligrams of elemental phosphorus per deciliter of serum. One mmol of phosphate contains 31 mg of elemental phosphorus. To convert mg/dL to mmol/L, divide mg/dL by 3.1. At pH 7.4, 1 mmol of phosphate equals 1.8 mEq and conversion from mmol/L to mEq/L requires multiplication by 1.8.

Even though phosphorus circulates in organic and inorganic forms, clinical laboratories typically measure inorganic phosphate. Approximately 10 to 20% of the inorganic phosphate in serum is protein bound and the remainder circulates as free anion or is complexed to sodium, magnesium, or calcium. The free and complexed fractions are available for ultrafiltration by the renal glomeruli.

▶ Body Stores and Distribution

Phosphate is the body's major intracellular anion, and translocation in and out of the intracellular compartment can rapidly change serum phosphorus concentration. Gradual changes in total body phosphate can be accommodated without noticeable changes in serum phosphorus concentration, resembling the situation with potassium (the major intracellular cation). Approximately 80 to 85% of total body phosphate is inorganic hydroxyapatite in bone, whereas 15% is in soft tissues such as muscle (Knochel 1977; Fitzgerald 1978). Most soft tissue phosphorus is organic and can be readily converted to the inorganic form as needed. The extracellular fluid compartment contains less than 1% of total body phosphorus stores.

▶ Normal Serum Concentrations

Normal serum phosphorus concentrations in adult dogs range from 2.5 to 6.0 mg/dL (Bloom 1960), but they are usually higher in dogs younger than 1 year. Serum phosphorus concentrations up to 8.7 mg/dL occur in normal giant breed dogs younger than 1 year (Fletch and Smart 1973). Sex-related changes are not reported (Ralston Purina 1975). The effect of age is less pronounced in cats, although immature cats have a tendency for higher serum concentrations (Chew and Meuten 1982). Growth hormone increases the renal tubular reabsorption of phosphorus and presumably contributes to this age effect. Feeding affects serum phosphorus concentration; carbohydrates decrease serum phosphorus concentration because phosphate shifts into intracellular fluid as a result of stimulation of glycolysis and formation of phosphorylated glycolytic intermediates in muscle, liver, and adipose cells. In contrast, protein intake increases serum phosphorus concentration because of the relatively high phosphorus content of protein-rich diets.

Time of sampling affects the observed serum phosphorus concentration. People have substantial variation in serum phosphorus concentrations throughout the day (Levine and Kleeman 1994). Acid-base balance influences serum phosphorus concentration. Respiratory alkalosis stimulates glycolysis (by activating phosphofructokinase) and decreases serum phosphorus concentration. Thus, a measured serum phosphorus concentration is affected by several variables and does not accurately indicate total body phosphorus stores. Measuring serum phosphorus after a 12-h fast minimizes confounding factors, but the clinician must understand that the magnitude of hypo- or hyperphosphatemia may be incorrectly assessed if only one serum or plasma sample is analyzed.

Hemolysis may affect laboratory results because phosphate is present in erythrocytes. Human erythrocytes contain 8 μmol/dL red cells, whereas canine erythrocytes contain 35 μmol/dL and feline erythrocytes 26 μmol/dL (Carlson 1989). Hyperlipidemia (Leehey et al. 1985) and hyperproteinemia (Busse et al. 1987) sometimes cause overestimation of serum phosphorus concentration, depending on the methodology used (Glick et al. 1991). Thrombocytosis (Lutomski and Bower 1994) and monoclonal gammopathy (Mavrikakis et al. 1996) may also cause spurious increases in serum phosphorus. Mannitol and other drugs may interfere with some assay systems, leading to erroneous measured values (Fraser et al. 1987; Young 1995). Icterus and hemolysis were shown to result in artifactual hypophosphatemia in dogs with immune-mediated hemolytic anemia (Harkin et al. 1998). Artifactual hypophosphatemia can occur in some automated systems but not in others. Thus, occurrence of hypophosphatemia in patients without known predisposing factors should prompt consideration of laboratory error.

▶ Dietary Intake

The average phosphorus content of commercial pet foods is approximately 1% on a dry matter basis. Dogs and cats ingest 0.5 to 3.0 g of phosphorus per day, depending on their body size and energy requirements. The source of dietary phosphorus markedly affects absorption and excretion of phosphorus in cats (Finco et al. 1989). The amount of phosphorus absorbed by the gastrointestinal tract, the amount excreted in the urine, and the extent of postprandial hyperphosphatemia were increased when monobasic and dibasic salts of phosphorus were fed but decreased when phosphorus originated from poultry, meat, and fish meal.

▶ Intestinal Absorption

Ingested organic phosphate is hydrolyzed in the gastrointestinal tract, liberating inorganic phosphate for absorption. Net intestinal phosphate absorption (i.e., the difference between dietary and fecal phosphate) is approximately 60 to 70% of the ingested load, and absorption is a linear function of phosphorus intake. In an animal in zero phosphorus balance, urinary phosphate excretion equals net intestinal phosphate absorption.

Intestinal phosphate absorption occurs via two mechanisms. Passive diffusion is the principal route and occurs primarily through the paracellular pathway. Active mucosal phosphate transport is a sodium-dependent, saturable carrier-mediated process. Calcitriol (1,25-dihydroxycholecalciferol) increases active intestinal mucosal phosphate transport, but this mechanism is probably important only during dietary phosphate deficiency. Both transport mechanisms function in the duodenum, whereas diffusion is the primary mechanism in the jejunum and ileum. Intestinal alkaline phosphatases may help by freeing inorganic phosphate for transport. Optimal phosphate transport occurs in an alkaline environment. Decreased intestinal phosphate absorption may occur with vitamin D deficiency and in malabsorptive states.

There is no evidence of a direct effect of parathyroid hormone (PTH) on intestinal phosphate absorption, and observed effects are probably mediated by PTH converting 25-hydroxycholecalciferol to calcitriol. High dietary ratios of calcium to phosphorus (>3–4) may suppress intestinal phosphate absorption, presumably through binding of phosphate by calcium and formation of poorly absorbed calcium phosphate complexes. During phosphate deprivation, the kidney dramatically reduces phosphate excretion to almost nonexistent amounts in less than 3 days. Obligatory gastrointestinal loss continues for at least 3 weeks, but there is a diminution in the amount lost (Levine and Kleeman 1994). This gastrointestinal loss may cause a cumulative negative phosphorus balance during phosphate deprivation.

▶ Renal Handling

The kidney adjusts tubular reabsorption of filtered phosphate to maintain zero balance. Normally, 80 to 90% of the filtered phosphate load is reabsorbed by the renal tubules, and renal dysfunction is the most common cause of hyperphosphatemia (Slatopolsky et al. 1977; Chew and Meuten 1982). PTH is the most important regulator of renal phosphate transport; it reduces the tubular transport maximum for phosphate reabsorption (T_{maxPi}) in the proximal tubule (i.e., where most phosphate reabsorption occurs). Phosphate reabsorption is also inhibited in the early proximal tubule by volume expansion with saline, but there is a more distal reabsorptive site (at some point beyond the last portion of the proximal tubule accessible by micropuncture) that is PTH sensitive and unaffected by saline volume expansion.

The effects of calcitriol on renal phosphate transport are difficult to separate from effects of calcitriol on PTH secretion and on phosphate transport in other organs (e.g., intestine, bone). Growth hormone increases proximal renal tubular phosphate reabsorption, which partially accounts for the increased serum phosphorus concentrations found in immature animals. Calcitonin inhibits renal tubular phosphate reabsorption, whereas thyroxine stimulates renal phosphate reabsorption. High doses of adrenocorticotropic hormone or glucocorticoids increase renal phosphate excretion and may decrease serum phosphorus concentration.

The kidney is also sensitive to dietary phosphate intake; urinary excretion increases with increased intake and decreases during deprivation. Volume expansion increases urinary phosphate excretion and natriuresis. This may be because phosphate is cotransported with sodium in the proximal tubule. Increased urinary phosphate excretion also occurs when urinary bicarbonate excretion is increased.

▶ Hypophosphatemia

Clinical Effects of Hypophosphatemia

Hypophosphatemia can have many detrimental effects. The most severe cellular damage seems to occur when there is concurrent phosphate depletion (Levine and Kleeman 1994). Hypophosphatemia decreases erythrocyte concentrations of ATP, which increases erythrocyte fragility, leading to hemolysis. Hemolysis is usually not observed until serum phosphorus concentration decreases to 1.0 mg/dL or less. Hypophosphatemia also reduces erythrocyte 2,3-DPG concentrations, which impairs oxygen delivery to tissues. Leukocytes in hypophosphatemic patients have impaired chemotaxis, phagocytosis, and bacterial killing (Craddock et al. 1974). This altered function may promote sepsis in hypophosphatemic patients receiving total parenteral nutrition. Platelet-associated abnormalities include shortened survival time, impaired clot retraction, megakaryocytosis of the bone marrow, and thrombocytopenia. In starved dogs made hypophosphatemic by infusion of amino acids, hemolytic anemia, thrombocytopenia, and impaired clot retraction resulted (Yawata et al. 1974), ostensibly because of depletion of cellular ATP stores. Clinically, hemolysis has been reported in hypophosphatemic dogs and cats with diabetic ketoacidosis, hepatic lipidosis, and various other disorders (Willard et al. 1987; Adams et al. 1993; Justin and Hohenhaus 1995). Hemolysis was reported in four other hypophosphatemic diabetic cats, but cause and effect were obscured by the possibility of Heinz body anemia (Brushkiewicz et al. 1997).

Neuromuscular effects of hypophosphatemia include weakness and pain associated with rhabdomyolysis (Knochel 1977, 1978) as well as anorexia, vomiting, and nausea secondary to intestinal ileus. Decreased phosphate may impair central nervous system glucose utilization and ATP production, leading to metabolic encephalopathy (Yawata et al. 1973), which has a wide range of manifestations in people (e.g., coma, seizure, confusion, irritability) (Levine and Kleeman 1994). Reversible impairment of cardiac contractility occurs in dogs with experimentally induced hypophosphatemia (Fuller et al. 1976, 1978) and people with spontaneous hypophosphatemia (Zazzo et al. 1995). Hypophosphatemia also causes proximal tubular bicarbonate wasting, reduction in titratable acidity, and impaired renal ammoniagenesis. Serious acid-base disturbances, however, do not arise in phosphate-deprived dogs (Schmidt 1978). Phosphate deficiency produces bone demineralization via effects of PTH and calcitriol, and release of carbonate from bone may prevent serious metabolic acidosis. Hypomagnesemia is frequently found in hypophosphatemic people, but the reasons are not clear (Clark et al. 1995).

Causes of Hypophosphatemia

Hypophosphatemia may be caused by translocation of phosphate from extracellular to intracellular fluid (maldistribution), increased loss (decreased renal reabsorption of phosphate), or decreased intake (decreased intestinal absorption of phosphate) (Ritz 1982; Levine and Kleeman 1994). Clinical conditions associated with hypophosphatemia are presented in Table 7–1.

Translocation related to administration of a carbohydrate load (e.g., 5% dextrose infusion) is a common cause of hypophosphatemia in hospitalized people (Betro and Pain 1972; Juan and Elrazak 1979). Insulin facilitates entry of glucose and phosphate into cells, where glucose is phosphorylated to glycolytic intermediates. Interestingly, infusion of a higher concentration (e.g., 10%) for a shorter time seems to be less detrimental than infusing 4% glucose constantly (Levine and Kleeman 1994). Malnour-

TABLE 7–1. Causes of Hypophosphatemia

Maldistribution (Translocation)
    Treatment of diabetic ketoacidosis
    Carbohydrate load or insulin administration
    Respiratory alkalosis or hyperventilation
    Total parenteral nutrition or nutritional recovery
    Hypothermia
Increased loss (Reduced renal reabsorption)
    Primary hyperparathyroidism
    Renal tubular disorders (e.g., Fanconi's syndrome)
    Proximally acting diuretics (e.g., carbonic anhydrase inhibitors) (?)*
    Eclampsia
    Hyperadrenocorticism (?)
Decreased intake (Reduced intestinal absorption)
    Dietary deficiency (?)
    Vomiting (?)
    Malabsorption (?)
    Phosphate binders
    Vitamin D deficiency
Laboratory error (e.g., mannitol administration)

*(?) Importance in veterinary medicine uncertain.

ished patients receiving total parenteral nutrition are particularly susceptible to hypophosphatemia because of the accelerated rate of tissue repair as phosphate is incorporated into new cells (Knochel 1977; Ritz 1982) and phosphate utilization during glycolysis. Respiratory alkalosis likewise causes translocation because it stimulates glycolysis by activating phosphofructokinase (Knochel 1977). This effect has been demonstrated in experimental dogs but was marked only when hyperventilation was combined with glucose administration (Brautbar et al. 1983). It is hypothesized that an increased intracellular pH is more important than an increased extracellular pH for causing hypophosphatemia in respiratory alkalosis, which could explain why severe hypophosphatemia may occur in people with severe respiratory failure who are mechanically ventilated (Levine and Kleeman 1994).

Diabetic patients are especially at risk for hypophosphatemia. They often have total body phosphate deficits because of loss of muscle mass, urinary phosphate losses, and impaired tissue use of phosphate related to insulin deficiency. Most diabetic cats in one study had mild hypophosphatemia at presentation (Schaer 1977), whereas 20 of 48 ketotic cats in another study were hypophosphatemic (Bruskiewicz et al. 1997). Another study found only 7 of 104 diabetic cats to be hypophosphatemic. However stratification of the cats into ketoacidotic and nonketoacidotic groups revealed that 5 of 38 ketoacidotic cats were hypophosphatemic and only 2 of 66 nonketotic cats were hypophosphatemic (Crenshaw and Peterson 1996). Interestingly, serum phosphorus concentrations are often normal to increased at presentation in diabetic people (Kebler et al. 1985), perhaps because of metabolic acidosis by organic acids (e.g., β-hydroxybutyrate) (Oster et al. 1978), insulin deficiency, osmotic effects of hyperglycemia, or renal insufficiency.

Administration of large doses of insulin makes hypophosphatemia even more likely in diabetic ketoacidotic patients. Severe hypophosphatemia has been reported in dogs and cats treated for diabetic ketoacidosis (Willard et al. 1987; Adams et al. 1993; Bruskiewicz et al. 1997). Hypophosphatemia developed or worsened after insulin administration, and clinical signs (e.g., hemolysis, seizures) thought related to hypophosphatemia developed in 11 animals. Interestingly, four of these cats developed hemolytic anemia despite intravenous supplementation of potassium phosphate, and it is not clear whether the anemia was due to inadequate phosphate supplementation or Heinz body formation (Bruskiewicz et al. 1997).

Although it is not documented in dogs and cats, hypophosphatemia may occur in people with certain rapidly growing tumors. Ostensibly, the rapidly dividing cells utilize the phosphorus, removing it from the blood (Levine and Kleeman 1994).

Increased loss of phosphorus often produces moderate hypophosphatemia in primary hyperparathyroidism, but clinical signs are caused by hypercalcemia (Wilson et al. 1974; Legendre et al. 1976; Carillo et al. 1979; Weir et al. 1986; Berger and Feldman 1987; Klausner et al. 1987). If 2.5 mg/dL is considered the lower limit of normal, serum phosphorus concentration was decreased in approximately one-third of reported cases associated with parathyroid adenoma but six of six cases associated with parathyroid hyperplasia (DeVries et al. 1993). Hypophosphatemia was seen in only two of seven cats with primary hyperparathyroidism (Kallet et al. 1991). The fractional excretion of phosphorus was increased in a few affected dogs (Weir et al. 1986). The normal fractional excretion of phosphorus (FE_{Pi}) was found to be 7.5 ± 4.6% in 10 normal dogs but 10 to 23% in a dog with primary hyperparathyroidism (Carillo et al. 1979).

Fanconi's syndrome in basenjis is associated with reduced renal fractional reabsorption of phosphate, but serum phosphorus concentrations are normal (Bovee et al. 1979). The renal tubular transport abnormality may be caused by metabolic or membrane defects affecting sodium transport, and the observed phosphaturia may be secondary to natriuresis (McNamara et al. 1989). Loop diuretics (e.g., furosemide) and distally acting diuretics (e.g., thiazides) have little effect on renal phosphate excretion, but proximally acting diuretics (e.g., carbonic anhydrase inhibitors) may increase renal excretion of phosphate secondary to their effects on proximal tubular sodium reabsorption. In one study, acetazolamide (10 mg/kg IV t.i.d.) did not cause hypophosphatemia when administered to dogs over a 7-day period (Rose and Carter 1979). Eclampsia in the bitch may be associated with hypophosphatemia and hypocalcemia (Austad and Bjerkas 1976). Presumably, increased PTH secretion in response to hypocalcemia leads to decreased renal reabsorption of phosphate.

Hypophosphatemia caused by dietary deficiency is unlikely in animals eating commercial diets with adequate protein content. A low-protein, low-phosphorus diet designed to dissolve struvite calculi (Prescription Diet S/D) did not cause significant hypophosphatemia when fed to dogs over a 6-month period (Abdullahi et al. 1984). Urinary phosphorus excretion decreased and calcium excretion increased in this study. Although vomiting and malabsorptive diseases can potentially cause phosphate loss, these disorders rarely cause hypophosphatemia in dogs or cats (Chew and Meuten 1982). Canine malabsorptive intestinal disorders are often characterized by hypocalcemia related to hypoalbuminemia, but serum phosphorus concentrations are typically normal (Breitschwerdt et al. 1980; Finco et al. 1973).

People have become hypophosphatemic after administration of magnesium and aluminum-containing antacids (Lotz et al. 1968). Whether phosphate depletion occurs during such administration depends on the patient's phosphorus intake, dosage of the phosphate binding agent, duration of administration, and preexisting phosphate balance of the patient. Vitamin D deficiency may cause hypophosphatemia because hypocalcemia increases PTH secretion, which increases renal phosphate excretion. Decreased intestinal phosphate absorption presumably also plays a role in this setting.

It has been stated that 38% of hyperadrenocortical dogs have hypophosphatemia (Peterson 1984), but actual serum phosphorus concentrations were not reported. An identifiable cause of hypophosphatemia could not be found in the majority of dogs with this serum biochemical abnormality (Chew and Meuten 1982). Hypophosphatemia, hypercalcemia, hyperglycemia, azotemia, hypokalemia, and acidosis have been reported in a dog and cat with hypothermia caused by exposure to low environmental temperature (Ross and Goldstein 1981). The mechanisms responsible for these electrolyte and acid-base disturbances are uncertain, but translocation seems likely.

Treatment of Hypophosphatemia

Prevention, when possible, is preferred to therapy. Astute clinicians anticipate potential hypophosphatemia and either administer supplemental phosphorus (e.g., patients receiving total parenteral nutrition (TPN) or insulin treatment for diabetic ketoacidosis) or carefully monitor the patient for hypophosphatemia (e.g., patients receiving phosphate binders).

If hypophosphatemia occurs, one should seek to correct the underlying condition responsible for it. Whether or not phosphorus is administered depends on the magnitude of the hypophosphatemia and whether clinical signs are present. Asymptomatic animals with low serum phosphorus concentrations but without phosphorus depletion and those with serum phosphorus concentrations above 1.8 mg/dL that are unlikely to fall any lower (e.g., primary hyperparathyroidism) often do not require phosphate administration.

Phosphate supplementation is appropriate for asymptomatic patients deemed to be at risk for developing symptomatic hypophosphatemia (e.g., diabetic ketoacidotic cat with serum phosphorus = 1.6 mg/dL) and patients with clinical signs believed to be due to hypophosphatemia. Interestingly, treatment of asymptomatic hypophosphatemia in diabetic people is controversial and is recommended only when severe (<2.0 mg/dL) (Kassirer et al. 1989); however, experience suggests that anticipatory phosphorus supplementation is reasonable in some ketoacidotic cats.

Oral phosphate administration is safe but slow and unacceptable in vomiting patients and perhaps in diarrheic patients. If the enteral route is chosen, feeding skim or low-fat milk or a buffered laxative (e.g., Phospho-Soda) is usually effective. Patients symptomatic because of hypophosphatemia generally need parenteral replacement therapy. Administering phosphate intravenously is potentially dangerous because it may cause hypocalcemia, tetany, soft tissue mineralization, renal failure, or hyperphosphatemia (Knochel 1977). Therefore, phosphorus administration has classically consisted of injecting small amounts slowly over hours to days and monitoring the patient repeatedly (e.g., 0.01–0.06 mmol/kg/h in dogs and cats with measurement of serum phosphorus concentration every 6 to 8 h) (Willard et al. 1987; Justin and Hohenhaus 1995). Although such caution is wise, it is noteworthy that more aggressive phosphorus administration has been used in people (i.e., 0.16–0.64 mmol/kg over 4 to 12 h in patients receiving total parenteral nutrition) (Clark et al. 1995). Other groups have used similarly large doses over even shorter times (e.g., 0.4–0.8 mmol/kg depending on the degree of hypophosphatemia over 30 min in patients with cardiac disease) (Zazzo et al. 1995), also without problems. Sodium phosphate and potassium phosphate are commonly used, but administration of glucose phosphate has been reported (Zazzo et al. 1995). Selection of the particular form of phosphorus to administer is based on the patient's serum electrolyte concentrations.

Currently, it seems safest to administer phosphate by constant-rate infusion at rates that have been used successfully in dogs and cats and to monitor the serum phosphorus concentration every 6 to 8 h. Theoretically, adding phosphorus to fluids containing calcium may cause precipitation of calcium phosphate, but this appears to depend on relative concentrations of calcium and phosphorus. Phosphorus is usually administered after diluting it in physiologic saline solution. The volume of distribution for administered phosphate varies tremendously among hypophosphatemic people, and redistribution of phosphate can occur rapidly. Therefore, the dose necessary to replete a patient and the patient's response to therapy cannot be predicted. In two studies of hypophosphatemic cats, total amounts of phosphorus infused intravenously ranged from 0.138 to 1.26 mmol/kg (Adams et al. 1993; Justin and Hohenhaus 1995), indicating a wide range of total body phosphate deficits.

A conservative approach is to assume that intravenously administered phosphate remains in the extracellular fluid compartment (actually, much of it enters the intracellular fluid). Development of hypophosphatemia is unlikely with this approach. Prophylactic parenteral phosphate therapy (such as may be used for patients with diabetic ketoacidosis) may be reasonably estimated by giving one-fourth to one-half of the supplemented potassium as potassium phosphate and the rest as potassium chloride. However, decreased urinary phosphate excretion that develops during hypophosphatemia may persist during treatment and predispose to hyperphosphatemia. The products available for oral and parenteral use are summarized in Tables 7–2 and 7–3.

▶ Hyperphosphatemia

Clinical Effects of Hyperphosphatemia

Increased serum phosphorus concentration may decrease serum calcium concentration so that the calcium phosphate solubility product ([Ca] × [Pi]) remains constant. Hypocalcemia (which may cause tetany) and soft tissue mineralization are the major clinical consequences of hyperphosphatemia (Thatte et al. 1995). After phosphate administration, deposition of calcium and phosphate in bone and soft tissue may contribute to hypocalcemia. The magnitude of hypocalcemia is related to the rate at which serum phosphorus concentration increases, but the exact relationship is unpredictable. The risk of soft tissue mineralization increases when the [Ca] × [Pi] solubility product exceeds 60 to 70.

Causes of Hyperphosphatemia

Hyperphosphatemia in dogs and cats is due primarily to decreased renal excretion, although increased intake and translocation may also be responsible (Table 7–4) (Thatte et al. 1995). Translocation occurring during treatment of hemolymphatic malignancies may cause tumor lysis syndrome (i.e., hyperphosphatemia, hypocalcemia, hyper-

TABLE 7-2. **Oral Preparations of Compounds Used as Phosphate Binders or for Phosphate Supplementation**

Name of Product	Chemical Name	Company	Preparations
Basaljel	Aluminum carbonate gel	Wyeth-Ayerst	Capsules, suspension, tablets
ALternaGEL	Aluminum hydroxide gel	Johnson & Johnson-Merck	Liquid
Amphojel	Aluminum hydroxide gel	Wyeth-Ayerst	Suspension, tablets
Alu-Cap	Aluminum hydroxide gel	3M Pharmaceuticals	Capsules
Alu-Tab	Aluminum hydroxide gel	3M Pharmaceuticals	Tablets
Aluminum hydroxide	Aluminum hydroxide gel	Roxane	Liquid, concentrate
Calcium carbonate	Calcium carbonate	Roxane	Suspension
Caltrate 600	Calcium carbonate	Lederle	Tablets
Os-Cal 500	Calcium carbonate	SmithKline Beecham	Tablets
Tums	Calcium carbonate	SmithKline Beecham	Tablets
Phos-Ex	Calcium acetate	Vitaline	Tablets
PhosLo	Calcium acetate	Braintree	Tablets
Citracal	Calcium citrate	Mission	Tablets
K-Phos Neutral	Dibasic sodium phosphate, monobasic potassium phosphate, monobasic sodium phosphate	Beach	Tablets
K-Phos Original	Monobasic potassium phosphate	Beach	Tablets

kalemia, hyperuricemia, and oliguric acute renal failure). Myeloblasts and lymphoblasts may contain up to four times as much phosphate as normal cells, and destruction of the cells causes release of phosphate. This syndrome is uncommon in small animal practice. In one study of dogs with multicentric lymphosarcoma, serum phosphorus concentrations were normal before therapy and did not change after treatment (Page et al. 1986). Urinary phosphorus excretion increased but probably because urine volume increased. There was no change in fractional phosphorus excretion or renal function (as assessed by endogenous creatinine clearance). Chemotherapy in these dogs consisted of prednisone, vincristine, and L-asparaginase. However, acute tumor lysis syndrome has been reported in some animals with lymphosarcoma treated with chemotherapy with or without radiation therapy (Laing and Carter 1988; Laing et al. 1989; Calia et al. 1996). Severe hyperphosphatemia (23.6 and 13.7 mg/dL) occurred in a dog and a cat (respectively), and mild hyperphosphatemia (7.4 and 7.7 mg/dL) occurred in two other affected dogs (Laing and Carter 1988; Calia et al. 1996). Thus, it may be prudent to promote diuresis by intravenous administration of fluids before beginning chemotherapy in patients with lymphosarcoma suspected of having large tumor burdens (e.g., hepatosplenomegaly).

Massive tissue injury with rhabdomyolysis may cause hyperphosphatemia. Subsequent development of acute renal failure related to myoglobinuria further contributes to hyperphosphatemia (Spangler and Muggli 1978). Hemolysis can produce hyperphosphatemia because of the phosphorus content of erythrocytes. Lactic acidosis and diabetic ketoacidosis can be associated with hyperphosphatemia because acidosis caused by organic acids apparently breaks down ATP to AMP and releases inorganic phosphate (Oster et al. 1978).

Increased intake of phosphorus may occur with intravenous administration of phosphate-containing fluids. Such therapy is uncommon in veterinary practice, except in treatment of diabetic ketoacidosis (Willard et al. 1987, Bruskiewicz et al. 1997) and total parenteral nutrition. Increased absorption of phosphorus from the alimentary tract may occur with colonic infusion of hypertonic enema solutions or oral administration of sodium phosphate (DiPalma et al. 1996). Such enemas have caused severe hyperphosphatemia in small dogs and cats (Atkins et al. 1985; Schaer et al. 1977; Jorgensen et al. 1985). Clinical signs in cats receiving phosphate enemas include lethargy, ataxia, vomiting, bloody diarrhea, mucous membrane pallor, and stupor. Laboratory abnormalities included marked hyperglycemia and hyperphosphatemia, mild

TABLE 7-3. **Injectable Preparations for Parenteral Phosphate Supplementation**

Compound	Composition (per mL)	pH	Osmolality (mOsm/kg)	Phosphate (mmol/mL)	Sodium (mEq/mL)	Potassium (mEq/mL)
Sodium phosphate	142 mg Na_2HPO_4, 276 mg $NaH_2PO_4 \cdot H_2O$	5.70	5580	3.000	4.0	0
Potassium phosphate	236 mg K_2HPO_4, 224 mg KH_2PO_4	6.60	5840	3.003	0	4.36

Source: Adapted from Lentz RD, Brown DM, and Kjellstrand CM: Treatment of severe hypophosphatemia. *Ann Intern Med* 89:941–944, 1978.

TABLE 7–4. **Causes of Hyperphosphatemia**

> Maldistribution (translocation)
>   Tumor cell lysis
>   Tissue trauma or rhabdomyolysis
>   Hemolysis
>   Metabolic acidosis
> Increased intake
>   Gastrointestinal
>   Phosphate enemas
>   Vitamin D intoxication
>   Parenteral
>   Intravenous phosphate
> Decreased loss
>   Acute or chronic renal failure
>   Uroabdomen or urethral obstruction
>   Hypoparathyroidism
>   Acromegaly (?)*
>   Hyperthyroidism
> Physiologic: young growing animal
> Laboratory error (e.g., lipemia, hyperproteinemia, depending on methodology)

*(?) Importance in veterinary medicine uncertain.

hypernatremia, and lactic acidosis (Atkins et al. 1985). Severe hyperphosphatemia, azotemia, and metabolic acidosis were reported in a cat treated with a phosphate-containing urinary acidifier (pHos-pHaid) at twice the recommended dosage (Fulton and Fruechte 1991).

Vitamin D increases intestinal absorption of calcium and phosphorus and may produce hyperphosphatemia as well as hypercalcemia. In one study, administration of vitamin D_2 to dogs for 3 weeks caused hypercalcemia and azotemia, but serum phosphorus concentrations remained normal (Spangler et al. 1979). However, intoxication with cholecalciferol-containing rodenticides causes azotemia, hypercalcemia, and hyperphosphatemia in dogs and cats (MacKenzie et al. 1987; Gunther et al. 1988; Moore et al. 1988; Fooshee and Forrester 1990; Dougherty et al. 1990).

Decreased excretion is the main cause of hyperphosphatemia, and chronic renal failure is probably the most common cause of hyperphosphatemia in adult dogs and cats (Chew and Meuten 1982). Chronic renal disease causes a progressive decrease in glomerular filtration rate (GFR), and the filtered load of phosphate (GFR × serum phosphorus concentration) decreases as GFR decreases. If phosphorus intake remains constant, phosphorus retention and transient hyperphosphatemia result. Sustained hyperphosphatemia does not usually develop in early chronic renal failure, however, because there is a compensatory increase in phosphate excretion by remnant nephrons. This increase in the fractional urinary excretion of phosphate (FE_{Pi}) is mediated by the effects of PTH on the kidney. When GFR decreases to 20% of normal or lower (i.e., late chronic renal failure), this compensatory mechanism is exhausted and hyperphosphatemia develops.

Renal secondary hyperparathyroidism is a consistent finding in progressive renal disease (Slatopolsky et al. 1971, 1977). Hyperphosphatemia inhibits renal 1α-hydroxylase, which is present in the renal tubules (this inhibition impairs conversion of 25-hydroxycholecalciferol to calcitriol and thus reduces intestinal calcium absorption) and decreases serum ionized calcium concentration by the mass law effect ([Ca] × [Pi] = constant). The resultant hypocalcemia and the decreased serum calcitriol concentration stimulate PTH secretion. This increased PTH secretion increases renal excretion of phosphate and release of calcium and phosphate from bone. It also stimulates production of calcitriol. These actions normalize serum phosphorus and ionized calcium concentrations. Thus, calcium and phosphorus balance is maintained by a progressive increase in serum PTH concentration (in early chronic renal failure). However, as renal tubular destruction progresses, there are fewer proximal renal tubules and a decrease in the amount of 1α-hydroxylase enzyme present. This reduction in 1α-hydroxylase means that it is harder for increased concentrations of PTH to increase serum calcium concentration. It also means that calcitriol is not available to inhibit PTH secretion (Nagode et al. 1996). As serum phosphate concentrations persistently remain increased, other changes also occur. Persistent hyperphosphatemia in rats increases the number and size of parathyroid cells. This is important because some percentage of each cell's secretion is autonomous, and parathyroid hyperplasia means that there is a greater amount of nonsuppressible PTH secretion. Chronically increased PTH concentration leads to bone demineralization and other toxic effects of uremia (e.g., bone marrow suppression, uremic encephalopathy). In addition, uremia decreases the number of parathyroid gland calcitriol receptors (Korkor 1987; Merke et al. 1987; Brown et al. 1989), which subsequently decreases the responsiveness of parathyroid glands to the inhibitory effect of calcitriol on PTH release (Slatopolsky et al. 1990). Thus, both decreased calcitriol production and decreased numbers of parathyroid gland calcitriol receptors promote development of renal secondary hyperparathyroidism.

Renal secondary hyperparathyroidism can be prevented or reversed in dogs with experimentally induced chronic renal disease by reducing dietary phosphorus intake in proportion to the decrease in GFR (Slatopolsky et al. 1972; Slatopolsky and Bricker 1973; Kaplan et al. 1979). Early in the course of chronic renal disease, decreased phosphorus intake stimulates renal 1α-hydroxylase activity, which increases calcitriol production. Increased calcitriol enhances intestinal calcium absorption, increases serum ionized calcium concentration, and decreases PTH secretion. Phosphorus restriction in advanced renal disease still decreases PTH secretion by unknown mechanisms independent of serum ionized calcium or calcitriol concentrations (Slatopolsky et al. 1990). These observations form the basis for restricting phosphorus in the medical management of chronic renal failure.

Phosphorus restriction may also prevent renal disease progression by minimizing renal interstitial mineralization (Alfrey 1988). In rats with experimentally induced chronic renal failure, detrimental histologic changes (e.g., interstitial mineralization, inflammation, and fibrosis) could be prevented and residual renal function maintained by dietary phosphorus restriction (Ibels et al. 1978; Karlinsky et al. 1980). In cats with experimentally induced renal disease, histologic changes were prevented by phosphorus restriction (Ross et al. 1982). In a study in rats with 80% nephrectomy, diet was carefully controlled so that only phosphorus intake differed between groups, and a beneficial effect of phosphorus restriction was clearly demonstrated with regard to mortality, proteinuria, histologic changes, creatinine clearance, and serum lipid concentrations over a period of 14 weeks (Lumlertgul et al. 1986). Similar beneficial effects were observed in dogs with 90% nephrectomy fed diets differing only in phosphorus content and followed for 12 months (Brown et al. 1987). A similar experiment utilizing 48 dogs with experimentally induced renal failure found that the amount of dietary phosphorus was more important in clinical management than the amount of dietary protein (Finco et al. 1992).

In contrast to findings in early chronic renal failure, hyperphosphatemia is typical in acute renal failure because of insufficient time for compensatory mechanisms to develop. Hyperphosphatemia also occurs in uroabdomen or urethral obstruction because of urine reabsorption from the peritoneal cavity or decreased GFR caused by increased intratubular pressure resulting from urinary tract obstruction (Burrows and Bovee 1974; Finco and Cornelius 1977).

Hypoparathyroidism in people causes mild hyperphosphatemia because renal reabsorption of phosphate is increased in the absence of PTH. Mild hyperphosphatemia also occurs in dogs with hypoparathyroidism but is overshadowed by the effects of hypocalcemia (e.g., muscle tremors, tetany, seizures, ataxia, and behavioral aberrations) (Burk and Schaubhut 1975; Meyer and Terrell 1976; Sherding et al. 1980; Bruyette and Feldman 1988). Hyperphosphatemia has also been reported in cats with hypoparathyroidism (Peterson et al. 1991).

Acromegalic people may develop hyperphosphatemia because of growth hormone's effects on renal tubular phosphate reabsorption. Mild hyperphosphatemia has been reported in some acromegalic dogs (Feldman and Nelson 1996) and cats (Peterson et al. 1986, 1990; Peterson 1988). Thyroxine increases renal tubular phosphate reabsorption, which contributes to the increased serum phosphorus concentrations observed in hyperthyroid cats (Peterson 1984; Turrel et al. 1988; Taylor et al. 1989). Hyperphosphatemia was reported in 21% of hyperthyroid cats in one study (Peterson et al. 1983).

Treatment of Hyperphosphatemia

Volume expansion with saline dilutes extracellular fluid phosphate and enhances renal phosphate excretion in dehydrated patients. Increasing GFR by volume expansion increases the filtered load of phosphate, and natriuresis impairs proximal tubular phosphate reabsorption. Administration of glucose (and insulin if necessary) may temporarily decrease serum phosphorus concentration by promoting phosphorus entry into cells, although such therapy is rarely if ever necessary. All sources of phosphorus intake should be curtailed. In the diet, phosphorus restriction is accomplished primarily by protein restriction. As a rule, low-protein diets are also low in phosphorus.

In patients with severe, chronic renal failure, low-phosphorus diets are helpful but often insufficient. Dialysis is unpredictable because phosphate is a poorly diffusible ion. Therefore, the most practical and effective way to treat hyperphosphatemia in patients with stable chronic renal failure is to decrease intestinal phosphate absorption by orally administered phosphate binders. Such administration helps prevent ingested as well as endogenously secreted phosphate from being absorbed. Phosphate binders work because the cation in the binder combines with dietary phosphate, producing insoluble, nonabsorbable phosphate compounds. Adsorption of phosphate ions on the surface of binder particles may also contribute to their effect. The rate at which a binder dissolves depends on its water solubility, the pH of the environment, and the dosage (Sheikh et al. 1989).

The most widely used oral phosphorus-binding agents contain aluminum or calcium and hydroxide, carbonate, or acetate (Slatopolsky et al. 1977; Hercz and Coburn 1987; Coburn and Salusky 1989) (see Table 7–2). The appropriate dosage must be determined empirically, but 90 to 100 mg/kg/day divided b.i.d. to t.i.d. is a reasonable starting point. Lower dosages of calcium acetate (50–60 mg/kg/day) may be sufficient, because it has a greater capacity to bind phosphate than does calcium carbonate (Mai et al. 1989). Magnesium-containing compounds are efficacious (Delmez et al. 1996) but should usually be avoided for patients with renal failure because limited ability to excrete magnesium increases the risk of hypermagnesemia. However, use of magnesium carbonate has allowed continued use of calcitriol in human patients with renal failure who became hypercalcemic when receiving oral calcium carbonate (Delmez et al. 1996).

Aluminum hydroxide and aluminum carbonate are commonly used phosphate binders. Aluminum hydroxide reduces intestinal phosphorus absorption in normal and uremic people (Clarkson et al. 1972). Aluminum is a better binding agent for phosphate than calcium or magnesium in the acidic gastric environment (Sheikh et al. 1989). This effect is less important at the higher intestinal pH. Aluminum-containing gels are better tolerated by many dogs and cats when given as tablets or capsules, but the desiccated form has a lower phosphate binding capacity than the liquid gel (Rutherford et al. 1973). Aluminum oxide gel prepared to maximize phosphate binding has been studied in dogs (Rutherford et al. 1973, 1980). Constipation is a common side effect of aluminum-containing phosphate binders.

In people undergoing hemodialysis, osteomalacia and dialysis encephalopathy have been correlated with the aluminum content of dialysis water (Parkinson et al. 1981). In one study, encephalopathy occurred in dialysis patients receiving aluminum hydroxide despite a negligible aluminum content of dialysis water (Alfrey et al. 1976). Aluminum can be absorbed from the intestinal tract in normal people (Kaehny et al. 1977) and uremic people (Berlyne et al. 1970; Clarkson et al. 1972), and aluminum-induced bone disease can occur in nondialyzed patients after oral administration of aluminum hydroxide (Andreoli et al. 1984). It is unclear whether aluminum-containing phosphate binders represent a hazard to dogs with chronic renal failure.

Calcium carbonate also decreases intestinal phosphate absorption in normal and uremic people (Clarkson et al. 1966; Lopez et al. 1984; Slatopolsky et al. 1986; Fournier et al. 1986; Andreoli et al. 1987; Malberti et al. 1988) and has been advocated as a phosphate binder. One approach is to give calcium-containing phosphate binders after the serum phosphorus concentration has been decreased into the normal range by using aluminum-containing compounds, thus reducing the risk of soft tissue mineralization. Calcium citrate has also been advocated as a phosphate binder (Cushner et al. 1988) but should not be given with aluminum-containing compounds because citrate enhances aluminum absorption (Slanina et al. 1984; Partridge et al. 1989; Froment et al. 1989; Molitoris et al. 1989). Nausea, constipation, and hypercalcemia are potential side effects of calcium-containing phosphate binders. In one study, calcium acetate bound more phosphate than either calcium citrate or calcium carbonate, and less calcium was absorbed from the intestine during its use (Sheikh et al. 1989). Calcium acetate binds phosphate better than aluminum carbonate at the neutral pH found in the small intestine, but aluminum carbonate is better at the lower gastric pH (Sheikh et al. 1989). In vivo, both were about equally effective.

Phosphate binders are most effective when given with meals. In one study, calcium acetate reduced intestinal absorption of phosphate best when ingested just before or after a meal but was much less effective if given 2 h after eating (Schiller et al. 1989). Approximately one-third as much phosphate was removed from the body when calcium acetate was given during fasting versus as when it was given with a meal. The endogenous phosphate removed probably originated from basal intestinal secretions or passive diffusion into the intestine. Ingestion of a meal also decreased the absorption of calcium from the calcium acetate. Thus, calcium-containing phosphate binders should be given with meals to reduce the risk of hypercalcemia.

Phosphate binder effectiveness is monitored by measuring fasting serum phosphorus concentration. The goal is to maintain the serum phosphorus concentration in the normal range. In normophosphatemic patients with early renal insufficiency, one may monitor fasting fractional excretion of phosphate (FE_{Pi}) to determine the efficacy of phosphate restriction. Dogs with spontaneous chronic renal failure (mean serum creatinine concentration, 2.3 mg/dL) had significantly higher FE_{Pi} values than control dogs (23% vs. 5%) respectively, and FE_{Pi} decreased in both groups after feeding of Prescription Diet K/D (Hansen et al. 1992). In one dog with chronic renal failure, FE_{Pi} was below the mean value for the chronic renal failure group despite increased serum PTH concentration. It has been suggested that FE_{Pi} values less than 30% are indicative of adequate phosphate restriction (Finco 1983). This method is limited by the wide range of normal values for FE_{Pi} (DiBartola et al. 1980; Russo et al. 1986). The response to phosphate binders may be relatively slow because the pool of accumulated phosphate is large and the persistent osteolytic effects of PTH provide a large endogenous phosphate load. Thus, the clinician should not be discouraged if the patient responds slowly to phosphate binder therapy.

REFERENCES

Abdullahi SU, Osborne CA, Leininger JR, et al.: Evaluation of a calculolytic diet in female dogs with induced struvite urolithiasis. *Am J Vet Res* 45:1508–1519, 1984.

Adams LG, Hardy RM, Weiss DJ, et al.: Hypophosphatemia and hemolytic anemia associated with diabetes mellitus and hepatic lipidosis in cats. *J Vet Intern Med* 7:266–271, 1993.

Alfrey AC: Effect of dietary phosphate restriction on renal function and deterioration. *Am J Clin Nutr* 47:153–156, 1988.

Alfrey AC, LeGendre GR, and Kaehny WD: The dialysis encephalopathy syndrome: Possible aluminum intoxication. *N Engl J Med* 294:184–188, 1976.

Andreoli SP, Bergstein JM, and Sherrard DJ: Aluminum intoxication from aluminum-containing phosphate binders in children with azotemia not undergoing dialysis. *N Engl J Med* 310:1079–1084, 1984.

Andreoli SP, Dunson J, and Bergstein JM: Calcium carbonate is an effective phosphorus binder in children with chronic renal failure. *Am J Kidney Dis* 9:206–210, 1987.

Atkins CE, Tyler R, and Greenlee P: Clinical, biochemical, acid-base, and electrolyte abnormalities in cats after hypertonic sodium phosphate enema administration. *Am J Vet Res* 46:980–988, 1985.

Austad R and Bjerkas E: Eclampsia in the bitch. *J Small Anim Pract* 17:795–798, 1976.

Berger B and Feldman EC: Primary hyperparathyroidism in dogs: 21 cases (1976–1986). *J Am Vet Med Assoc* 191:350–356, 1987.

Berlyne GM, Ben-Ari J, Pest D, et al.: Hyperaluminemia from aluminum resins in renal failure. *Lancet* 2:494–496, 1970.

Betro MG and Pain RW: Hypophosphatemia and hyperphosphatemia in a hospital population. *Lancet* 1:273–276, 1972.

Bloom F: *The Blood Chemistry of the Dog and Cat.* New York, Gamma Publications, 1960.

Bovee KC, Joyce T, Blazer-Yost B, et al.: Characterization of renal defects in dogs with a syndrome similar to Fanconi syndrome in man. *J Am Vet Med Assoc* 174:1094–1099, 1979.

Brautbar N, Leibovici H, and Massry SG: On the mechanism of hypophosphatemia during acute hyperventilation: Evidence for increased muscle glycolysis. *Miner Electrolyte Metab* 9:45–50, 1983.

Breitschwerdt EB, Halliwell WH, Foley CW, et al.: A hereditary diarrhetic syndrome in the basenji characterized by malabsorption, protein losing enteropathy, and hypergammaglobulinemia. *J Am Anim Hosp Assoc* 16:551–560, 1980.

Brown AJ, Dusso A, Lopez-Hilker S, et al.: 1,25-$(OH)_2$D receptors are decreased in parathyroid glands from chronically uremic dogs. *Kidney Int* 35:19–23, 1989.

Brown S, Finco D, Crowell WA, et al.: Beneficial effect of moderate phosphate restriction in partially nephrectomized dogs on a low protein diet (abstract). *Kidney Int* 31:380, 1987.

Bruskiewicz KA, Nelson RW, Feldman EC, et al.: Diabetic ketosis and ketoacidosis in cats: 42 cases (1980–1995). *J Am Vet Med Assoc* 211:188–192, 1997.

Bruyette DS and Feldman EC: Primary hypoparathyroidism in the dog. *J Vet Intern Med* 2:7–14, 1988.

Burk RL and Schaubhut CW: Spontaneous primary hypoparathyroidism in a dog. *J Am Anim Hosp Assoc* 11:784–785, 1975.

Burrows CF and Bovee KC: Metabolic changes due to experimentally-induced rupture of the canine urinary bladder. *Am J Vet Res* 35:1083–1088, 1974.

Busse JC, Gelbard MA, Byrnes JJ, et al.: Pseudohyperphosphatemia and dysproteinemia. *Arch Intern Med* 147:2045–2046, 1987.

Calia CM, Hohenhaus AE, Fox PR, et al.: Acute tumor lysis syndrome in a cat with lymphoma. *J Vet Intern Med* 10:409–411, 1996.

Carillo JM, Burk RL, and Bode C: Primary hyperparathyroidism in a dog. *J Am Vet Med Assoc* 174:67–71, 1979.

Carlson GP: Fluid, electrolyte, and acid base balance. In Kaneko JJ (ed): *Clinical Biochemistry of Domestic Animals*, 4th ed. New York, Academic Press, pp. 543–575, 1989.

Chew DJ and Meuten DJ: Disorders of calcium and phosphorus metabolism. *Vet Clin North Am* 12:411–438, 1982.

Clark CL, Sacks GS, Dickerson RN, et al.: Treatment of hypophosphatemia in patients receiving specialized nutrition support using a graduated dosing scheme. Results from a prospective clinical trial. *Crit Care Med* 23:1504–1511, 1995.

Clarkson EM, McDonald SJ, and deWardener HE: The effect of a high intake of calcium carbonate in normal subjects and patients with chronic renal failure. *Clin Sci* 30:425–438, 1966.

Clarkson EM, Luck VA, Hynson WV, et al.: The effect of aluminum hydroxide on calcium, phosphorus, and aluminum balances, the serum parathyroid hormone concentration and the aluminum content of bone in patients with chronic renal failure. *Clin Sci* 43:519–531, 1972.

Coburn JW and Salusky IB: Control of serum phosphorus in uremia. *N Engl J Med* 320:1140–1142, 1989.

Craddock PR, Yawata Y, VanSanten L et al.: Acquired phagocyte dysfunction. *N Engl J Med* 290:1403–1407, 1974.

Crenshaw KL and Peterson ME: Pretreatment of clinical and laboratory evaluation of cats with diabetes mellitus: 104 cases (1992–1994). *J Am Vet Med Assoc* 209:943–949, 1996.

Cushner HM, Copley JB, Lindberg JS, et al.: Calcium citrate, a non–aluminum-containing phosphate-binding agent for treatment of CRF. *Kidney Int* 33:95–99, 1988.

Delmez JA, Kelber J, Norword KY, et al.: Magnesium carbonate as a phosphorus binder: A prospective controlled crossover study. *Kidney Int* 49:163–167, 1996.

DeVries SE, Feldman EC, Nelson RW, et al.: Primary parathyroid gland hyperplasia in dogs: Six cases (1982–1991). *J Am Vet Med Assoc* 202:1132–1136, 1993.

DiBartola SP, Chew DJ, and Jacobs G: Quantitative urinalysis including 24-hour urinary protein excretion in the dog. *J Am Anim Hosp Assoc* 16:537–546, 1980.

DiPalma JA, Buckley SE, Warner BA, et al.: Biochemical effects of oral sodium phosphate. *Dig Dis Sci* 41:749–753, 1996.

Dougherty SA, Center SA, and Dzanis DA: Salmon calcitonin as adjunct treatment for vitamin D toxicosis in a dog. *J Am Vet Med Assoc* 196:1269–1272, 1990.

Feldman EC and Nelson RW: Disorders of growth hormone. In *Canine and Feline Endocrinology and Reproduction*, 2nd ed. Philadelphia, WB Saunders Co., p. 60, 1996.

Finco DR: The role of phosphorus restriction in the management of chronic renal failure in the dog and cat. *Proc 7th Kal Kan Symposium*, pp. 131–134, 1983.

Finco DR and Cornelius LM: Characterization and treatment of water, electrolyte, and acid-base imbalances of induced urethral obstruction in the cat. *Am J Vet Res* 38:823–830, 1977.

Finco DR, Duncan JR, Schall WD, et al.: Chronic enteric disease and hypoproteinemia in 9 dogs. *J Am Vet Med Assoc* 163:262–271, 1973.

Finco DR, Barsanti JA, and Brown SA: Influence of dietary source of phosphorus on fecal and urinary excretion of phosphorus and other minerals by male cats. *Am J Vet Res* 50:263–266, 1989.

Finco DR, Brown SA, Crowell WA, et al.: Effects of dietary phosphorus and protein in dogs with chronic renal failure. *Am J Vet Res* 53:2264–2271, 1992.

Fitzgerald F: Clinical hypophosphatemia. *Annu Rev Med* 29:177–189, 1978.

Fletch SM and Smart ME: Blood chemistry of the giant breeds: bone profile. *Bull Am Soc Vet Clin Pathol* 2:30–31, 1973.

Fooshee SK and Forrester SD: Hypercalcemia secondary to cholecalciferol rodenticide toxicosis in two dogs. *J Am Vet Med Assoc* 196:1265–1268, 1990.

Fournier A, Moriniere P, Sebert JL, et al.: Calcium carbonate, an aluminum-free agent for control of hyperphosphatemia, hypocalcemia, and hyperparathyroidism in uremia. *Kidney Int* 29:S114–S119, 1986.

Fraser D, Hones G, Kooh SW, et al.: Calcium and phosphate metabolism. In Tietz NW (ed): *Fundamentals of Clinical Chemistry*. Philadelphia, WB Saunders Co., pp. 705–728, 1987.

Froment DH, Molitoris BA, Buddington B, et al.: Site and mechanism of enhanced gastrointestinal absorption of aluminum by citrate. *Kidney Int* 36:978–984, 1989.

Fuller TJ, Carter NW, Barcenas C, et al.: Reversible changes of the muscle cell in experimental phosphorus deficiency. *J Clin Invest* 57:1019–1024, 1976.

Fuller TJ, Nichols WW, Brenner BJ, et al.: Reversible depression in myocardial performance in dogs with experimental phosphorus deficiency. *J Clin Invest* 62:1194–1200, 1978.

Fulton RB and Fruechte LK: Poisoning induced by administration of a phosphate-containing urinary acidifier in a cat. *J Am Vet Med Assoc* 198:883–885, 1991.

Glick MR, Ryder KW, and Glick SJ: *Interferographs*. Indianapolis, Science Enterprises Inc., 1991.

Gunther R, Felice LJ, and Nelson RK: Toxicity of a vitamin D_3 rodenticide to dogs. *J Am Vet Med Assoc* 193:211–214, 1988.

Hansen B, DiBartola SP, Chew DJ, et al.: Clinical and metabolic findings in dogs with spontaneous chronic renal failure fed two different diets. *Am J Vet Res* 53:326–334, 1992.

Harkin KR, Braselton WE, and Tvedten H: Pseudohypophosphatemia in two dogs with immune-mediated hemolytic anemia. *J Vet Intern Med* 12:178–181, 1998.

Hercz G and Coburn JW: Prevention of phosphate retention and hyperphosphatemia in uremia. *Kidney Int* 32:S215–S220, 1987.

Ibels LS, Alfrey AC, Haut L, et al.: Preservation of function in experimental renal disease by dietary restriction of phosphate. *N Engl J Med* 298:122, 1978.

Jorgensen LS, Center SA, Randolph JF, et al.: Electrolyte abnormalities induced by hypertonic phosphate enemas in two cats. *J Am Vet Med Assoc* 187:1367–1368, 1985.

Juan D and Elrazak MA: Hypophosphatemia in hospitalized patients. *J Am Med Assoc* 242:163–164, 1979.

Justin RB and Hohenhaus AE: Hypophosphatemia associated with enteral alimentation in cats. *J Vet Intern Med* 9:228–233, 1995.

Kaehny WD, Hegg AP, and Alfrey AC: Gastrointestinal absorption of aluminum from aluminum-containing antacids. *N Engl J Med* 296:1389–1390, 1977.

Kallet AJ, Richter KP, Feldman EC, et al.: Primary hyperparathyroidism in cats: Seven cases (1984–1989). *J Am Vet Med Assoc* 199:1767–1771, 1991.

Kaplan MA, Canterbury JM, Bourgoignie JJ, et al.: Reversal of hyperparathyroidism in response to dietary phosphorus restriction in the uremic dog. *Kidney Int* 15:43, 1979.

Karlinsky ML, Haut L, Buddington B, et al.: Preservation of renal function in experimental glomerulonephritis. *Kidney Int* 17:293, 1980.

Kassirer JP, Hricik DE, and Cohen JJ: Phosphate. In *Repairing Body Fluids: Principles and Practice*. Philadelphia, WB Saunders Co., pp. 110–117, 1989.

Kebler R, McDonald FD, and Cadnapaphornchai P: Dynamic changes in serum phosphorus level in diabetic ketoacidosis. *Am J Med* 79:571–576, 1985.

Klausner JS, O'Leary TP, and Osborne CA: Calcium urolithiasis in two dogs with parathyroid adenomas. *J Am Vet Med Assoc* 191:1423–1426, 1987.

Knochel JP: The pathophysiology and clinical characteristics of severe hypophosphatemia. *Arch Intern Med* 137:203–220, 1977.

Knochel JP: Skeletal muscle in hypophosphatemia and phosphorus deficiency. *Adv Exp Med Biol* 103:357–366, 1978.

Korkor AB: Reduced binding of [^{3}H]1,25-dihydroxyvitamin D_3 in the parathyroid glands of patients with renal failure. *N Engl J Med* 316:1573, 1987.

Kreisberg RA: Phosphorus deficiency and hypophosphatemia. *Hosp Pract* 12:121–128, 1977.

Laing EJ and Carter RF: Acute tumor lysis syndrome following treatment of canine lymphoma. *J Am Anim Hosp Assoc* 24:691–696, 1988.

Laing EJ, Fitzpatrick PJ, Norris AM, et al.: Half-body radiotherapy in the treatment of canine lymphoma. *J Vet Intern Med* 3:102–108, 1989.

Leehey DJ, Daugirdas JT, Ing TS et al.: Spurious hyperphosphatemia due to hyperlipidemia. *Arch Intern Med* 145:743–744, 1985.

Legendre AM, Merkley DF, Carrig CB, et al.: Primary hyperparathyroidism in a dog. *J Am Vet Med Assoc* 168:694–696, 1976.

Levine BS and Kleeman CR: Hypophosphatemia and hyperphosphatemia: Clinical and pathophysiologic aspects. In Narins RG (ed): *Clinical Disorders of Fluid and Electrolyte Metabolism*, 5th ed. New York, McGraw-Hill Book Co., pp. 1045–1090, 1994.

Lopez S, Galceran T, and Slatopolsky E: Evaluation of calcium carbonate as an effective phosphorus-binding agent in the dog. *Clin Res* 32:452A, 1984.

Lotz M, Zisman E, and Bartter FC: Evidence for a phosphorus depletion syndrome in man. *N Engl J Med* 278:409–415, 1968.

Lumlertgul D, Burke TJ, Gillum DM, et al.: Phosphate depletion arrests progression of chronic renal failure independent of protein intake. *Kidney Int* 29:658, 1986.

Lutomski DM and Bower RH: The effect of thrombocytosis on serum potassium and phosphorus concentrations. *Am J Med Sci* 307:255–258, 1994.

MacKenzie CP, Burnie AG, and Head KW: Poisoning in four dogs by a compound containing warfarin and calciferol. *J Small Anim Pract* 28:433–445, 1987.

Mai ML, Emmett ME, Sheikh MS, et al.: Calcium acetate, an effective phosphorus binder in patients with renal failure. *Kidney Int* 36:690–695, 1989.

Malberti F, Surian M, Colussi G, et al.: Calcium carbonate: A suitable alternative to aluminum hydroxide as phosphate binder. *Kidney Int* 33:S184–S185, 1988.

Mavrikakis M, Vaiopoulos G, Athanassiades P, et al.: Pseudohyperphosphatemia in multiple myeloma. *Am J Hematol* 51:178–179, 1996.

McNamara PD, Rea CT, Bovee KC, et al.: Cystinuria in dogs: Comparison of the cystinuric component of the Fanconi syndrome in basenji dogs to isolated cystinuria. *Metabolism* 38:8–15, 1989.

Merke J, Hugel U, Zlotkowski A, et al.: Diminished parathyroid 1,25-dihydroxycholecalciferol receptors in experimental uremia. *Kidney Int* 32:350–353, 1987.

Meyer DJ and Terrell TG: Idiopathic hypoparathyroidism in a dog. *J Am Vet Med Assoc* 168:858–860, 1976.

Molitoris BA, Froment DH, MacKenzie TA, et al.: Citrate: A major factor in the toxicity of orally administered aluminum compounds. *Kidney Int* 36:949–953, 1989.

Moore FM, Kudisch M, Richter K, et al.: Hypercalcemia associated with rodenticide poisoning in three cats. *J Am Vet Med Assoc* 193:1099–1100, 1988.

Nagode LA, Chew DJ, and Podell M: Benefits of calcitriol therapy and serum phosphorus control in dogs and cats with renal failure. *Vet Clin North Am* 26:1293–1330, 1996.

Oster JR, Perez GO, and Vaamonde CA: Relationship between blood pH and potassium and phosphorus during acute metabolic acidosis. *Am J Physiol* 235:F345–F351, 1978.

Page RL, Leifer CE, and Matus RE: Uric acid and phosphorus excretion in dogs with lymphosarcoma. *Am J Vet Res* 47:910–912, 1986.

Parkinson IS, Ward MK, and Kerr DNS: Dialysis encephalopathy, bone disease, and anemia: The aluminum intoxication syndrome during regular hemodialysis. *J Clin Pathol* 34:1285–1294, 1981.

Partridge NA, Regnier FE, White JL, et al.: Influence of dietary constituents on intestinal absorption of aluminum. *Kidney Int* 35:1413–1417, 1989.

Peterson ME: Hyperadrenocorticism. *Vet Clin North Am* 14:731–749, 1984.

Peterson ME: Endocrine disorders in cats: Four emerging diseases. *Comp Contin Educ Pract Vet* 10:1353–1362, 1988.

Peterson ME, Kintzer PP, Cavanagh PG, et al.: Feline hyperthyroidism: Pretreatment clinical and laboratory evaluation of 131 cases. *J Am Vet Med Assoc* 183:103–110, 1983.

Peterson ME, Taylor RS, Greco DS, et al.: Spontaneous acromegaly in the cat. *Proc Am Coll Vet Intern Med* Washington, DC, pp. 14–43, 1986.

Peterson ME, Taylor RS, Greco DS, et al.: Acromegaly in 14 cats. *J Vet Intern Med* 4:192–201, 1990.

Peterson ME, James KM, Wallace M, et al.: Idiopathic hypoparathyroidism in five cats. *J Vet Intern Med* 5:47–51, 1991.

Ralston Purina Company: *Normal Blood Values for Cats and Normal Blood Values for Dogs*. St. Louis, Ralston Purina Company, 1975.

Ritz E: Acute hypophosphatemia. *Kidney Int* 22:84–94, 1982.

Rose RJ and Carter J: Some physiological and biochemical effects of acetazolamide in the dog. *J Vet Pharmacol Ther* 2:215–221, 1979.

Ross LA and Goldstein M: Biochemical abnormalities associated with accidental hypothermia in a dog and cat. Abstract. *Proc Am Coll Vet Intern Med*, St. Louis, p. 66, 1981.

Ross LA, Finco DR, Crowell WA, et al.: Effect of dietary phosphorus restriction on the kidneys of cats with reduced renal mass. *Am J Vet Res* 43:1023, 1982.

Russo EA, Lees GE, and Hightower D: Evaluation of renal function in cats, using quantitative urinalysis. *Am J Vet Res* 47:1308–1312, 1986.

Rutherford E, Mercado A, Hruska K, et al.: An evaluation of a new and effective phosphorus binding agent. *Trans Am Soc Artif Intern Organs* 19:446–449, 1973.

Rutherford E, King S, Perry B, et al.: Use of a new phosphate binder in chronic renal insufficiency. *Kidney Int* 17:528–534, 1980.

Schaer M: A clinical survey of 30 cats with diabetes mellitus. *J Am Anim Hosp Assoc* 13:23–27, 1977.

Schaer M, Cavanagh P, Hause W, et al.: Iatrogenic hyperphosphatemia, hypocalcemia and hypernatremia in a cat. *J Am Anim Hosp Assoc* 13:39–41, 1977.

Schiller LR, Santa Ana CA, Sheikh MS, et al.: Effect of the time of administration of calcium acetate on phosphorus binding. *N Engl J Med* 320:1110–1113, 1989.

Schmidt RW: Effects of phosphate depletion on acid-base status in dogs. *Metabolism* 27:943–952, 1978.

Sheikh MS, Maguire JA, Emmett M, et al.: Reduction of dietary phosphorus absorption by phosphorus binders: A theoretical, in vitro, and in vivo study. *J Clin Invest* 83:66–73, 1989.

Sherding RF, Meuten DJ, Chew DJ, et al.: Primary hypoparathyroidism in the dog. *J Am Vet Med Assoc* 176:439–444, 1980.

Slanina P, Falkeborn Y, Frech W, et al.: Aluminum concentration in the brain and bone of rats fed citric acid, aluminum citrate or aluminum hydroxide. *Food Chem Toxicol* 27:391–397, 1984.

Slatopolsky E and Bricker NS: The role of phosphorus restriction in the prevention of secondary hyperparathyroidism in chronic renal disease. *Kidney Int* 4:141, 1973.

Slatopolsky E, Caglar S, Pennell JP, et al.: On the pathogenesis of hyperparathyroidism in chronic renal insufficiency in the dog. *J Clin Invest* 50:492, 1971.

Slatopolsky E, Caglar S, Gradowska L, et al.: On the prevention of secondary hyperparathyroidism in experimental chronic renal disease using "proportional reduction" of dietary phosphorus intake. *Kidney Int* 2:147, 1972.

Slatopolsky E, Rutherford WE, Rosenbaum R, et al.: Hyperphosphatemia. *Clin Nephrol* 7:138–146, 1977.

Slatopolsky E, Weerts C, Lopez-Hilker S, et al.: Calcium carbonate as a phosphate binder in patients with chronic renal failure undergoing dialysis. *N Engl J Med* 315:157–161, 1986.

Slatopolsky E, Lopez-Hilker S, Delmez J, et al.: The parathyroid-calcitriol axis in health and chronic renal failure. *Kidney Int* 38:S41–S47, 1990.

Spangler WL and Muggli FM: Seizure-induced rhabdomyolysis accompanied by renal failure in a dog. *J Am Vet Med Assoc* 172:1190–1194, 1978.

Spangler WL, Gribble DH, and Lee TC: Vitamin D intoxication and the pathogenesis of vitamin D nephropathy in the dog. *Am J Vet Res* 40:73–83, 1979.

Taylor JA, Jacobs RM, Lumsden JH, et al.: Perspectives on the diagnosis of feline hyperthyroidism. *Can Vet J* 30:477–481, 1989.

Thatte L, Oster JR, Singer I, et al.: Review of the literature: Severe hyperphosphatemia. *Am J Med Sci* 310:167–174, 1995.

Turrel JM, Feldman EC, Nelson RW, et al.: Thyroid carcinoma causing hyperthyroidism in cats: 14 cases (1981–1986). *J Am Vet Med Assoc* 193:359–364, 1988.

Weir EC, Morrdin RW, Barthold SW, et al.: Primary hyperparathyroidism in a dog: Biochemical, bone, histomorphometric, and pathologic findings. *J Am Vet Med Assoc* 189:1471–1474, 1986.

Willard MD, Zerbe CA, Schall WD, et al.: Severe hypophosphatemia associated with diabetes mellitus in six dogs and one cat. *J Am Vet Med Assoc* 190:1007–1010, 1987.

Wilson JW, Harris SG, Moor WD, et al.: Primary hyperparathyroidism in a dog. *J Am Vet Med Assoc* 164:942–946, 1974.

Yawata Y, Craddock P, Hebbel R, et al.: Hyperalimentation hypophosphatemia: Hematologic and neurologic dysfunction due to ATP depletion. *Clin Res* 31:729A, 1973.

Yawata Y, Hebbel RP, Silvis S, et al.: Blood cell abnormalities complicating the hypophosphatemia of hyperalimentation: Erythrocyte and platelet ATP deficiency associated with hemolytic anemia and bleeding in hyperalimented dogs. *J Lab Clin Med* 84:643–653, 1974.

Young DS: *Effects of Drugs on Clinical Laboratory Tests*. Washington, DC, AACC Press, 1995.

Zazzo JF, Troche G, Ruel P, et al.: High incidence of hypophosphatemia in surgical intensive care patients. Efficacy of phosphorus therapy on myocardial function. *Intensive Care Med* 21:826–831, 1995.

APPENDIX TO CHAPTER 7

Calculation of Amount of PO_4^{3-} and H_3PO_4 Present in Extracellular Fluid at pH 7.4

The Henderson-Hasselbalch equation is derived from the formula for the dissociation constant of an acid. For the ionic species of phosphate of interest:

$$pH = pKa + \log([PO_4^{3-}]/[HPO_4^{2-}])$$
$$7.4 = 12.4 + \log(x)$$
$$\log(x) = -5.0$$
$$x = 0.00001$$
$$[PO_4^{3-}]/[HPO_4^{2-}] = 0.00001$$
$$[HPO_4^{2-}]/[PO_4^{3-}] = 100,000$$

Thus, at pH 7.4, there are 100,000 molecules of HPO_4^{2-} for every molecule of PO_4^{3-}.

$$pH = pKa + \log([H_2PO_4^{1-}]/[H_3PO_4])$$
$$7.4 = 2.0 + \log(x)$$
$$\log(x) = 5.4$$
$$x = 251,189$$
$$[H_2PO_4^{1-}]/[H_3PO_4] = 251,189$$

Thus, at pH 7.4, there are 251,189 molecules of $H_2PO_4^{1-}$ for every molecule of H_3PO_4.

$$pH = pKa + \log([HPO_4^{2-}]/[H_2PO_4^{1-}])$$
$$7.4 = 6.8 + \log(x)$$
$$\log(x) = 0.6$$
$$x = 4.0$$
$$[HPO_4^{2-}]/[H_2PO_4^{1-}] = 4.0$$

From these calculations, it can be determined that, at pH 7.4, there will be 1,004,756 molecules of HPO_4^{2-}, 251,189 molecules of $H_2PO_4^{1-}$, and 10 molecules of PO_4^{3-} for every molecule of H_3PO_4. It can be seen, therefore, that the amounts of H_3PO_4 and PO_4^{3-} present in extracellular fluid at pH 7.4 can be safely ignored.

CHAPTER 8

Disorders of Magnesium

BERNIE HANSEN

Although magnesium has been recognized as an important nutrient throughout this century, the medical profession has become widely interested in its therapeutic uses only in the past two decades. This relatively recent interest stems from the realization that borderline dietary deficiencies are common in humans, that magnesium depletion often coexists with severe illness, and that magnesium is an effective therapeutic agent for certain disorders.

Magnesium is the eighth most abundant element on the earth's surface, where it is found in large deposits of composites such as magnesite and dolomite. It is the fourth most abundant cation in the mammalian body and is second in intracellular abundance only to potassium. It is an essential nutrient responsible for many physiologic functions. Despite recognition of the neuromuscular effects of pharmacologic doses of magnesium 140 years ago (Gordon and Iams 1995), the primary focus of biomedical research on this element for the next 100 years was description of its biologic functions and identification of signs of deficiency states.

By the second half of the 20th century, growing interest in the pharmacologic actions of magnesium prompted its use as a treatment for preeclampsia in women in 1966. Reports of its use as therapy for arrhythmias, ischemic heart disease, and asthma published in the 1980s led to wider appreciation of the therapeutic potential of magnesium when used to induce magnesium overload in patients without preexisting deficiencies. At the same time, several investigators reported that hypomagnesemia was common in human intensive care unit patients without classical symptoms of magnesium depletion. The finding that these patients had higher morbidity and mortality than patients with a normal serum magnesium concentration spurred interest in routine determination of magnesium status and treatment of patients with hypomagnesemia. The discovery of a statistical correlation between ischemic heart disease and habitation in regions with magnesium-deficient soil and water has also stimulated interest in a possible role of magnesium deficiency in human heart disease and hypertension.

Hypomagnesemia occurs in approximately 9 to 12% of human medical patients (Brautbar and Massry 1987). This observation may be related to inadequate intake in the general population. Roughly 15 to 20% of the population of western societies are estimated to have inadequate dietary intake and the potential for inadequate body stores of magnesium (Durlach 1989; Durlach et al. 1994). The mean daily intake of magnesium in some countries is approximately 4 mg/kg/day, significantly less than the routinely recommended daily allowance of 4.5 to 6 mg/kg/day (Durlach 1989; Durlach and Mareschi 1991; Wangemann et al. 1993).

The importance of adequate dietary intake of magnesium to the health of lactating dairy cattle has been recognized for decades. However, with the exception of research investigating the role of magnesium in urinary tract disease of dogs and cats, magnesium was essentially ignored in companion animal practice until the 1990s. This previous lack of interest was probably due at least in part to the rarity of clinical signs of magnesium deficiency in a pet population fed commercial diets that contain abundant magnesium. However, some epidemiologic surveys of hospitalized companion animals have identified hypomagnesemic patients in proportions similar to those found in human intensive care unit patients. Given this striking prevalence, it seems likely that magnesium depletion complicates some veterinary disease syndromes and could affect disease outcome.

▶ Magnesium Metabolism
Chemistry and Biology

Magnesium and calcium are the major divalent cations found in biologic systems. The hydrated magnesium ion is larger than hydrated calcium, and the hydrated forms of magnesium salts are more soluble than hydrated calcium salts. This difference may account for magnesium's wider participation in metabolic processes and for the vastly different roles these cations play in biologic systems.

The atomic weight of magnesium is 24.32. Therefore, 1 mEq (0.5 mmol) of Mg^{2+} is equal to 12.16 mg of magnesium. Magnesium content per unit of body mass appears to be similar among most mammals. The adult human body contains 21 to 28 g of magnesium. Newborn puppies and kittens contain roughly 0.2 g/kg, and adult cats contain 0.4 g/kg, a concentration that is reportedly

175

slightly higher than that found in adult dogs (Kienzle et al. 1991). Approximately 50 to 60% of total body magnesium is distributed in bone, and only about one-third of this magnesium is exchangeable. Most of the remaining body content of magnesium resides within cells, but only a small fraction of this reservoir is available for exchange with extracellular fluid magnesium. Less than 2% of total body magnesium is present in extracellular fluid. The intracellular and extracellular distribution of magnesium is similar to that of potassium. Unlike changes in potassium, however, marked changes in the intracellular concentration of magnesium do not produce rapid changes in extracellular magnesium concentration, and intracellular stores do not provide effective replacement for acute changes in extracellular fluid concentration. This observation is probably related to the fact that most intracellular magnesium is bound to ligands that render it relatively unavailable for exchange (Alfrey and Miller 1973). Thus, only a small fraction of intracellular magnesium is exchangeable with extracellular fluid, and the earliest biochemical change observed in experimental magnesium depletion in humans or animals is a fall in extracellular fluid magnesium concentration (Alfrey 1974a, 1974b).

The wide participation by magnesium in many intracellular biologic functions reflects its importance as a nutrient. Magnesium serves as a cofactor for many intracellular enzymes, including those concerned with the generation and storage of energy via hydrolysis of adenosine triphosphate (ATP). Its primary biologic function is to complex with ATP to form Mg^{2+}-ATP^{2-}. This compound is the actual substrate for adenosinetriphosphatases (ATPases), including the enzymes responsible for controlling intracellular electrolyte concentrations. Magnesium is also a necessary cofactor for some enzymatic processes involving DNA synthesis and transcription, nucleic acid polymerization, binding of ribosomes to RNA, phosphorylation of glucose, and is indirectly involved in mitochondrial oxidative metabolism.

Nutrition

SOURCES OF MAGNESIUM

Most magnesium intake occurs via ingestion of foodstuffs containing the nutrient, but in some areas of the country high concentrations in ground water provide an important source ("hard" water contains approximately 10 to 30 mg/L magnesium) (Marier 1982). The best dietary sources of magnesium for humans include nuts, green vegetables, soybeans, chocolate, and whole cereal grains, where it is found in high concentrations. In the average American diet, consumption of magnesium correlates with caloric intake provided that few calories are derived from sugar or alcohol. The ideal diet of humans should contain approximately 600 ppm magnesium to provide positive magnesium balance (Durlach 1989). The 1989 Food and Nutrition Board, Commission on Life Sciences of the National Research Council (NRC) recommended daily allowance (RDA) for magnesium is 4.5 mg/kg/day for adults (Subcommittee on the tenth edition of the recommended dietary allowances, 1989). The Department of Agriculture determined that only 25% of Americans had a magnesium intake at or greater than the RDA (Elin 1994).

When a balanced diet is consumed, the minimal dietary concentration of magnesium required by adult dogs is probably 80 ppm, by growing dogs more than 120 ppm, and by cats 190 ppm (Bunce et al. 1962a, 1962b; Pastoor et al. 1995). The NRC recommendation for magnesium content in the diet of growing dogs and cats is 400 ppm (0.11 g per 1000 kcal metabolizable energy). The Association of American Feed Control Officials recommendation for magnesium content for growth, reproduction, and adult maintenance for dogs and maintenance of adult cats is 400 ppm and for growth and reproduction of cats is 800 ppm. The maximum recommended magnesium content is 3000 ppm. Commercially available pet foods in the United States are fortified with magnesium and generally provide the mineral in higher concentrations than the minimum recommendation of the NRC. Thus, dietary deficiency of magnesium in the United States is less likely to occur in healthy companion animals fed commercial diets than in their human providers.

ABSORPTION

Under normal conditions, most magnesium absorption occurs in the jejunum and ileum. The fraction of magnesium absorbed is dependent on its concentration in the diet, and low dietary intake promotes increased fractional absorption. Approximately 30 to 50% of ingested magnesium is absorbed in humans consuming an average diet. In normal humans fed a low-magnesium diet, 74% of ingested magnesium is absorbed, and absorption falls to 24% when they are fed a high-magnesium diet (Graham et al. 1960). The rectum and colon are able to absorb magnesium, and development of hypermagnesemia is a potential complication of administration of enemas containing magnesium sulfate. Absorption in the small intestine occurs via both a saturable facilitated diffusion cellular transport system and an extracellular unsaturable passive transport system. The latter mechanism is driven by the electrochemical gradient across the mucosa and by the phenomenon of solvent drag.

No single hormonal mechanism appears responsible for controlling intestinal magnesium transport. Vitamin D and its active metabolites may enhance the absorption of magnesium, but the magnitude of this effect appears to be much less than it is with calcium (Brannan et al. 1976; Hodgkinson et al. 1979). Vitamin D–deficient humans maintain magnesium absorption at nearly normal rates, and repletion of vitamin D stores produces only a small increase in absorption (Hodgkinson et al. 1979).

Binding of magnesium to other ingested nutrients appears to affect absorption. Excessive intake of fatty acids, phytate, oxalate, phosphate, and fiber may bind magnesium and impair absorption. Dietary calcium concentration does not appear to influence absorption (Brannan et al. 1976; Spencer et al. 1980).

RENAL REGULATION OF MAGNESIUM

Excess body magnesium is excreted in the urine. The kidneys are responsible for maintenance of plasma magnesium concentration within a narrow range and are essential for physiologic control of magnesium balance. Renal impairment is associated with hypermagnesemia in dogs and cats (Martin et al. 1994). In normal humans fed an average diet, approximately 2400 mg of magnesium is filtered at the glomeruli each day, and only about 120 mg is excreted in the urine. Renal handling of magnesium is a function of balance between glomerular filtration and tubular reabsorption. At present, there is no evidence for active tubular secretion of magnesium. Approximately two-thirds of magnesium presented to the glomeruli passes into the glomerular filtrate. In contrast to other electrolytes, only a small fraction of filtered magnesium is reabsorbed in the proximal nephron, and over 70% travels to the loop of Henle. It is here, in the thick ascending limb, that most magnesium is reabsorbed. Magnesium reabsorption in the thick ascending limb of Henle's loop is closely linked to sodium chloride transport. The active transcellular transport of NaCl creates a positive luminal potential in the cortical thick ascending limb that provides a favorable electrical gradient for the movement of Mg^{2+} into the peritubular fluid.

MAMMARY SECRETION DURING LACTATION

Large quantities of magnesium are secreted in milk. The magnesium content of milk from lactating cats is approximately 5.7 to 6.6 mEq/L. The concentration of magnesium in colostrum is higher (9 mEq/L) (Adkins et al. 1997). The concentration of magnesium in milk from beagle dogs is slightly lower, ranging from 4.5 to 5 mEq/L. By comparison, the milk of dairy cattle has a magnesium concentration of approximately 10 mEq/L. In that species, secretion of magnesium is unchanged in the presence of inadequate dietary intake, predisposing lactating cows to reduced total milk production and magnesium depletion.

▶ Assessment of Magnesium Status

Magnesium status may be evaluated by several methods, including measurement of tissue magnesium concentrations, measurement of ionized magnesium in serum or cells, and physiologic assessment of magnesium balance and excretion.

Tissue Magnesium Concentration and Ionized Magnesium

Serum magnesium concentration is the most widely used initial screening test for disorders of magnesium balance in both humans and animals. The major limitation of this test is that plasma contains only 0.3% of total body stores of magnesium and the plasma magnesium concentration may be normal or high in the presence of intracellular magnesium depletion in some humans. Although serum magnesium concentration routinely falls during deficiency states, it is a weak predictor of the magnesium status of human patients. Nevertheless, it is the least expensive and most convenient assay, and it is the initial diagnostic test for evaluation of disorders of magnesium metabolism.

The definitive method for measurement of serum magnesium concentration is isotope dilution and mass spectrometry, and the reference method established by the National Reference System for Clinical Laboratories of the National Committee for Clinical Laboratory Standards is flame atomic absorption spectrometry (FAAS) (Elin 1994). Most commercial laboratories utilize a colorimetric assay, using primarily calmagite or methylthymol blue as a chromophore. These assays are more susceptible to interference by other compounds than is the FAAS method.

Serum magnesium exists in three distinct fractions: protein bound, anion complexed, and ionized. Some examples of published normal values for ionized and total serum magnesium concentrations in dogs and cats are listed in Table 8–1. As with calcium, the ionized fraction of magnesium is the only form available to participate in biologic functions in extracellular fluid. Consequently, there has been interest in measuring serum ionized magnesium concentrations in clinical patients (Martin et al. 1993; Mann et al. 1998). The equipment necessary to perform this measurement, however, is either expensive (e.g., ion-selective electrode detectors) or limited to research use (e.g., fluorescent probes of intracellular ionized magnesium). In addition, the value and meaning of this measurement as opposed to measurement of total serum magnesium concentration in animals are currently unknown, and it may offer little advantage over other measures. Therefore, its routine use may not be justified until the relationship of ionized magnesium concentration to magnesium balance and disease outcome has been more thoroughly characterized.

The concentration of magnesium in other tissues has been examined for use as a way to evaluate magnesium balance. Tissues that have been evaluated most extensively include bone, skeletal muscle, erythrocytes, and leukocytes. Of these tissues, only the blood components are easily accessible and practical for clinical use.

Red blood cell or whole-blood magnesium concentration has been evaluated as an alternative to serum measurement (Elin 1994). There appears to be a limited correlation between the red cell magnesium content and that of other body storage pools. Thus, red cell magnesium content may not offer improved diagnostic power over measurement of serum magnesium concentration. Reduced red cell magnesium content has been identified in humans with essential hypertension, premenstrual syndrome, and chronic fatigue syndrome, suggesting a role for this assay in people afflicted with these conditions.

TABLE 8–1. **Observed Ranges of Serum Magnesium Concentration in Normal Dogs and Cats**

Species	Total Mg (mg/dL)	pH-Normalized Ionized Mg (mg/dL)
Dog		
<16 wk (Mann et al. 1998)	1.23–1.99	0.99–1.35
>16 wk (Mann et al. 1998)	1.05–1.37	1.04–1.36
Adult (Martin et al. 1994)	1.89–2.51	
Any (Dhupa 1995)	1.7–2.4	
Cat (Kallfelz et al. 1980)	1.7–2.3	
Cat (Lewis et al. 1978)	2.7	

No similar correlation with disease syndromes has been reported in companion animals. The magnesium content of mononuclear white blood cells has been evaluated and compared with the magnesium content of muscle. To date, however, evidence for a strong correlation is lacking (Elin 1994). Thus, measurement of the magnesium content in blood components has not proved to be a reliable method for evaluating magnesium stores in humans or animals.

Physiologic Assessment

Tests to assess the physiologic balance of magnesium in the patient provide insight into overall magnesium balance. Some such studies are limited to the research laboratory (e.g., isotope studies, balance studies). However, renal excretion of magnesium into the urine may be used to evaluate magnesium balance by taking advantage of that organ's ability to conserve magnesium during periods of deficiency or excrete it during excess intake.

URINE EXCRETION

The normal fractional urinary excretion of filtered magnesium is approximately 5% in humans. In magnesium deficiency states, 24-h urinary magnesium excretion falls to less than 1 mmol, usually with no initial decrease in plasma magnesium concentration (Sutton and Domrongkitchaiporn 1993). Most veterinary studies of urine magnesium excretion in companion animals have focused on urine magnesium concentration in animals fed various dietary concentrations to evaluate the effectiveness of diet in treating or preventing urolithiasis (Barker and Povey 1973; Finco and Barsanti 1984; Lewis and Morris 1984a, 1984b; Finco et al. 1985; Tarttelin 1987a, 1987b; Buffington et al. 1990; Osborne et al. 1990). In general, dietary intake of magnesium has little effect on plasma or tissue concentration of the element unless it is present in the diet in concentrations substantially higher than those found in commercial diets. Even the relationship between ingested magnesium and urine magnesium concentration may be quite unpredictable because other factors may influence the intestinal absorption of the element (Finco et al. 1985). Other factors such as urine pH may be equally important determinants of urolith formation (Tarttelin 1987a; Buffington et al. 1990).

The primary value of measuring urine magnesium excretion is to look for evidence of a magnesium-wasting nephropathy as a cause of hypomagnesemia. In humans, renal magnesium wasting may be defined as urinary excretion greater than 1 mmol/day in the presence of hypomagnesemia. Similar guidelines have not been established for companion animals, but presumably many of the disorders associated with excessive renal losses (Table 8–2) could be evaluated by this method.

MAGNESIUM RETENTION TEST

This test consists of intravenous administration of magnesium and measurement of the total amount of magnesium excreted within a standardized time period (usually 24 h). The magnesium tolerance test has proved to be a useful method for assessing magnesium status in humans.

The principle behind this assay is that in magnesium-deficient states not caused by excessive renal losses, the kidneys attempt to retain a large portion of any administered magnesium. Patients with excessive renal losses of magnesium may not be accurately assessed. One protocol for the test in humans is as follows (Nadler and Rude, 1995):

1. Empty the bladder and collect a baseline urine sample for determination of the magnesium and creatinine

TABLE 8–2. Causes of Magnesium Depletion in Humans

Inadequate Dietary Intake
Protein-calorie malnutrition
Magnesium-free fluids and total parenteral nutrition

Gastrointestinal Disorders
Prolonged nasogastric suction
Chronic diarrhea
Malabsorption syndromes
Extensive bowel resection
Intestinal and biliary fistulas
Primary infantile hypomagnesemia

Renal Loss
Chronic parenteral fluid therapy with magnesium-free fluids
Intrinsic tubular disorders
    Chronic interstitial nephritis, pyelonephritis, glomerulonephritis
    Acute tubular necrosis (diuretic phase)
    Postobstructive diuresis
    Renal tubular acidosis
    Congenital magnesium wasting
    Drug injury
        Aminoglycosides
        Amphotericin B
        Cisplatin
        Cyclosporine
Loop diuretics
Osmotic diuretics: glucose, mannitol, urea
Hypercalcemia
Hypokalemia
Alcohol

Metabolic
Hypercalcemia
Hypophosphatemia

Endocrine
Diabetes mellitus
Hyperthyroidism
Primary hyperparathyroidism
Hyperadrenocorticism
Inappropriate secretion of antidiuretic hormone

Redistribution
Pancreatitis
Hyperadrenergic states
Massive blood transfusion
Insulin therapy, refeeding
Hypothermia
Acute respiratory alkalosis
Sepsis
Cardiopulmonary bypass

Miscellaneous
Severe burns
Excessive lactation
Excessive sweating

Sources: Brautbar and Massry 1987; Martin et al. 1993; al-Ghamdi et al. 1994.

concentrations to calculate the magnesium/creatinine ratio.
2. Infuse magnesium at 0.2 mEq/kg lean body weight in 50 mL of 5% dextrose over 4 h.
3. Collect urine for 24 h beginning at the start of the infusion. Pool the urine and determine the urine magnesium and creatinine concentrations.
4. The percentage of magnesium retained is calculated by:

$$\%Mg \text{ retained} = [1 - \{(U_{Mg} - (R \cdot U_{Cr}))/Mg_{inf}\}] \times 100$$

where U_{Mg} = postinfusion 24-h urine magnesium in mg; R = preinfusion urine magnesium-to-creatinine ratio ($[U_{Mg}]/[U_{Cr}]$); U_{Cr} = postinfusion 24-h urine creatinine in mg; and Mg_{inf} = total elemental magnesium infused in mg.
5. The criteria for magnesium deficiency include the following:
   a. >50% retention at 24 h indicates definite deficiency.
   b. >25% retention at 24 h indicates probable deficiency.

Normal humans in one study retained a mean of 14%, whereas patients thought to be at risk for magnesium deficiency retained 85% (Nadler and Rude 1995). Thus, this assay may be a sensitive method for detecting magnesium deficiency states in humans. Thus far there are no reports of evaluation of similar tests in companion animals, although a modification of the test has been recommended for evaluating the magnesium status of dogs (Martin 1994).

▶ Magnesium Depletion

Magnesium depletion may be caused by impaired intestinal absorption or by increased renal losses. Hypomagnesemia may also be a consequence of redistribution of magnesium from extracellular to intracellular fluid. Causes of magnesium deficit in humans have been reviewed (see Table 8–2), and many of the conditions known to be associated with magnesium depletion or hypomagnesemia in humans also occur in companion animals.

Clinical Findings in Humans with Magnesium Deficiency

Magnesium deficiency is associated with well-characterized signs and symptoms in humans. Most patients with hypomagnesemia are asymptomatic. Signs and symptoms may develop when serum magnesium concentration falls below 1.2 mg/dL. However, many patients with serum magnesium concentrations substantially below 1.2 mg/dL remain asymptomatic, and development of clinical signs may depend as much on the rate of decline as on the absolute serum concentration or tissue content of magnesium.

NEUROMUSCULAR AND NERVOUS SYSTEM MANIFESTATIONS

The most dramatic and easily recognized clinical signs of magnesium deficiency are related to neuromuscular dysfunction. Clinical manifestations of experimental or naturally occurring magnesium deficiency include neural and neuromuscular hyperexcitability. These create a constellation of clinical findings termed tetany syndrome. Tetany syndrome symptoms include muscle spasms, cramps, hyperarousal, hyperventilation, and asthenia. Physical signs (Chvostek's, Trousseau's, or von Bonsdorff's) and abnormalities of the electromyogram or electroencephalogram can usually be elicited. Muscle cramps, fasciculations, and tremors may occur. Clinical signs in infants are usually more dramatic than those in adults and often include generalized convulsions that respond only to magnesium therapy. Neurologic signs include vertigo, ataxia, nystagmus, and twitching and athetoid (unwanted, involuntary) movements (Brautbar and Massry 1987; Whang et al. 1994). Psychiatric abnormalities include depression and psychosis.

The pathogenesis of neuromuscular signs in magnesium deficiency is unclear. They are most likely a manifestation of the interaction between magnesium and calcium in the neuromuscular system. A decrease in the concentration of either ion lowers the depolarization threshold of excitable tissue, thereby increasing neuronal excitability and enhancing transmission at the motor end plate. Hypomagnesemia also stimulates release of acetylcholine at the motor end plate (Vallee et al. 1960). Low magnesium concentrations enhance muscular contraction, and magnesium acts as a calcium antagonist inside the myocyte (al-Ghamdi et al. 1994). Low intracellular magnesium concentrations enhance release of calcium from the sarcoplasmic reticulum, whereas increased concentrations block this process.

CARDIAC MANIFESTATIONS

Several cardiac arrhythmias responsive to treatment with magnesium have been described in people with hypomagnesemia or probable magnesium deficiency (al-Ghamdi et al. 1994; Nadler and Rude 1995). The mechanisms thought to be responsible for development of arrhythmias in magnesium depletion include inhibition of Na^+,K^+-ATPase and excessive outward movement of potassium from cells. Magnesium normally interferes with the movement of potassium out of myocardial cells by blocking the movement of potassium through specific potassium channels. If magnesium is unavailable, myocardial loss of potassium is enhanced, leading to depolarization of the cell. Magnesium deficiency also increases myocardial uptake of digoxin and augments digoxin's inhibition of Na^+,K^+-ATPase, thus enhancing digoxin toxicity.

Magnesium-responsive arrhythmias that have been identified in magnesium-deficient humans include ventricular premature depolarizations, ventricular tachycardia, ventricular fibrillation, junctional rhythm, atrial premature contractions, atrial fibrillation, supraventricular tachycardia, and torsades de pointes. Prolongation of the PR and QT intervals is also seen in magnesium deficiency.

The role of magnesium in myocardial infarction has received intense research scrutiny. Observations in animal models of coronary infarction suggest that magnesium deficiency increases the size of myocardial infarction after coronary occlusion and that administration of magnesium before restoration of blood flow inhibits reperfusion injury

(Antman 1996). The permissive effect of magnesium depletion on reperfusion injury after myocardial ischemia is at least in part due to fluxes of calcium and loss of cellular energy reserves. After coronary occlusion, myocardial energy production and contractility fall precipitously, and magnesium is lost from the myocyte in exchange for calcium. Loss of magnesium further impairs energy production, predisposing the heart to arrhythmias as sarcolemmal ion gradients deteriorate, calcium influx progresses, and mitochondrial structural abnormalities occur. These findings are consistent with the idea that magnesium depletion predisposes humans to death resulting from myocardial disease, as has been suggested by epidemiologic surveys (Rylander 1996).

DISTURBANCE OF OTHER ELECTROLYTES

CALCIUM

Hypocalcemia was observed in 40% of hypomagnesemic intensive care unit patients in one survey (Reinhart and Desbiens 1985). Hypocalcemia in patients with concurrent hypomagnesemia is often refractory to calcium therapy unless magnesium is administered first. Several factors have been implicated in this finding, including impaired release of parathyroid hormone (PTH) in response to ionized hypocalcemia as well as end-organ resistance to PTH at the skeleton. Skeletal resistance to the effects of PTH in humans with magnesium depletion may be due to impaired uptake of PTH by bone as well as decreased exchange of calcium for magnesium at the bone matrix. Low serum calcitriol concentration has been identified in affected patients but may not be a factor in the development of hypocalcemia because normocalcemia may be achieved after magnesium supplementation before any clinically relevant increase in serum calcitriol concentration is achieved.

POTASSIUM

As many as 40 to 50% of hypomagnesemic human patients in intensive care units have concurrent hypokalemia (Reinhart and Desbiens 1985; Whang et al. 1992). Hypokalemia and kaliuresis develop in normal humans subjected to experimentally induced magnesium depletion. There are several points of interaction between magnesium and potassium that may explain these findings. Magnesium deficiency has been associated with loss of cellular potassium in a number of tissues. Loss of potassium from skeletal muscle, kidney, and cardiac tissue has been identified in rats with experimentally induced magnesium deficiency, and effective restoration of potassium balance was possible only after correction of magnesium depletion (Martindale and Heaton 1964; Whang et al. 1967). Inability to restore cellular potassium stores in animals with experimental magnesium deficiency parallels the clinical observation in humans that it is difficult to restore normokalemia in patients with hypomagnesemia without concurrent correction of magnesium deficiency. Hypokalemia, alkalosis, reduced muscle potassium content, and increased muscle sodium content are common in humans with magnesium deficiency, and these alterations may respond to magnesium therapy (Khilnani 1992; al-Ghamdi et al. 1994; Hamill-Ruth and McGory 1996). This association is strong enough to warrant the general recommendation that magnesium status be investigated in any patient with hypokalemia refractory to potassium supplementation.

Most available evidence suggests that this relationship is a consequence of both increased renal losses of magnesium and direct effects of magnesium on potassium transport across cell membranes. The enzyme Na^+, K^+-ATPase has an absolute requirement for magnesium complexed with ATP. Magnesium depletion may therefore impair cell membrane regulation of those electrolytes. Magnesium also has direct effects on potassium channels and favors net inward movement of potassium. This may be an important factor in preventing excessive loss of potassium from excitable tissue during the plateau phase of the action potential (Whang et al. 1992).

Clinical Findings in Dogs and Cats with Magnesium Deficiency

Perhaps because of the ubiquity of magnesium in the diet, magnesium deficiency in otherwise healthy companion animals appears rare. Several reports describe magnesium depletion in dogs or cats with concurrent disease, but there have been no reports describing this syndrome in otherwise healthy companion animals. Magnesium depletion has been induced experimentally in dogs by feeding diets containing very low magnesium concentrations. From this work, it appears that the minimal dietary concentration of magnesium required by adult dogs is between 80 and 180 ppm and by growing dogs is at least 120 to 140 ppm (Bunce et al. 1962a, 1962b). Adult ovariectomized cats appear to be in magnesium balance when fed purified diets containing 190 ppm magnesium (Pastoor et al. 1995).

In addition to daily intake, at least two other factors influence the rate of development of magnesium deficiency. First, at any given level of dietary magnesium shortfall, the syndrome of magnesium depletion occurs more rapidly and is more severe in immature dogs than in adults. For example, a dietary concentration of 80 ppm induces severe magnesium deficiency within 8 weeks in puppies but adults may not develop signs for as long as 23 weeks (Bunce et al. 1962a). In one study, the average latency to death in puppies younger than 4 months old fed a magnesium-free diet was 60 days, whereas for 4- to 8-month-old puppies the latency was 87 days and for two dogs older than 16 months the latency was over 10 months (Wener et al. 1964).

Second, the dietary requirement for magnesium to maintain magnesium balance is also influenced by the dietary concentration of phosphorus. Weanling dogs fed a diet containing 0.4% phosphorus required approximately 140 ppm (on a dry weight basis) of elemental magnesium (Bunce et al. 1962b). An increase in the concentration of dietary phosphorus to 0.9% increased the severity of magnesium deficiency syndrome in dogs fed a magnesium-deficient diet (80 ppm). Alterations of dietary calcium and fat content did not appear to influence the onset or severity of magnesium deficiency signs in dogs (Bunce et al. 1962a).

The clinical findings in dogs with experimentally induced magnesium deficiency have been described (Orent et al. 1932; Syllm-Rapoport and Strassburger 1961; Vitale et al. 1961; Ono 1962; Syllm-Rapoport 1962; Bunce et al. 1962a, 1962b; Barnes and Mendelson 1963; Wener et al. 1964). In general, the clinical signs are more severe and develop more rapidly when the syndrome is induced in rapidly growing weanling dogs as compared with adults. Clinical signs develop in 6- to 8-week-old puppies after eating a severely magnesium-restricted diet for 2 weeks. The first change noted by one investigator was hyperemia of the nail beds (Orent et al. 1932). This finding was followed by development of hyperemia of the tongue, eyelids, and oral mucous membranes. After 4 to 6 weeks of the magnesium-deficient diet, hyperemia of the ears developed, and this observation appears to be the last change suggesting superficial vasodilatation. Hyperemia of these tissues may subsequently disappear, but it recurs in some dogs at variable intervals.

Orthopedic abnormalities develop after feeding a magnesium-deficient diet for 4 to 6 weeks. Abnormalities are most prominent in the thoracic limbs. The phalanges spread apart, and the paws distal to the proximal metacarpal bones increase in size, possibly because of tissue edema (Wener et al. 1964). The dogs then assume a plantigrade posture of the limbs, bearing their weight primarily on the metacarpus, and the nails arch out horizontally. The nails become brittle and are easily broken.

Generalized hair loss develops but is especially severe around the eyes and on the legs, tail, and abdomen. Some small circumscribed areas become completely denuded. Hairless skin becomes erythematous, desquamates, and may ulcerate. All of the skin is scaly and dry. The ears become thick, leathery, and mottled. Lacrimal secretion may be persistent, and the urine may become deeply pigmented but is free of blood. Mild hypothermia may develop, possibly as a consequence of impaired utilization of food (Syllm-Rapoport and Strassburger 1961).

NEUROMUSCULAR AND NERVOUS SYSTEM MANIFESTATIONS

After a month of the deficient diet, many but not all animals develop neurologic signs including hyperexcitability. Stimuli ignored by normal dogs (e.g., sharp noises) are capable of provoking convulsions in magnesium-deficient dogs. A sharp drop in rectal temperature precedes some, but not all, convulsions.

Convulsions appear in the puppies after feeding a magnesium-deficient diet for 5 to 7 weeks. The convulsions are strikingly uniform in appearance. Typically, the dog becomes restless and uneasy, paces, and then collapses on its side in extensor rigidity and opisthotonus. These findings rapidly progress to generalized tonic-clonic convulsions. Respirations cease during the seizure and then gradually return to normal. Respirations may stop abruptly, followed by cardiac arrest. Affected animals often die when recovery from the seizure appears imminent. In one study, 13 of 15 dogs died during apparent recovery from their first convulsion, whereas other affected dogs survived several different episodes of seizures (Orent et al. 1932).

Myocyte electrolyte disturbances in beagle dogs with magnesium depletion induced by feeding a magnesium-free diet included reductions in cell content of phosphorus and gains in cell content of calcium, sodium, and chloride (Cronin et al. 1982). Despite the development of severe hypomagnesemia in affected dogs, muscle content of magnesium remained relatively stable.

CARDIAC MANIFESTATIONS

Electrocardiographic changes in dogs with experimentally induced magnesium deficiency have been described in several reports. Abnormalities generally did not occur until the serum magnesium concentration fell below 0.8 mg/dL (Ono 1962). The changes observed most often included peaked T waves and mild ST segment depression (Vitale et al. 1961; Ono 1962; Wener et al. 1964). Peaked T waves occurred at the same time potassium depletion became evident, prompting speculation that this change was related to altered potassium status. One author hypothesized that peaking of the T waves represented a change associated with serum concentrations that were *relatively* high compared with intracellular potassium concentrations. These changes may not occur until marked signs of magnesium deficiency have been present for several weeks. Although some investigators suggested that there is predictable shortening of the PQ and QRS intervals during progressive magnesium depletion (Syllm-Rapoport 1962), others have found that this change is not consistent or specific enough to differentiate magnesium depletion from other electrolyte disturbances (Ono 1962; Wener et al. 1964).

In spite of the reported electrocardiographic changes, the magnesium-deficient dogs described in these reports did not exhibit marked problems with arrhythmias. One study (Ono 1962) observed premature beats in 3 of 18 dogs with serum magnesium concentrations less than 1 mg/dL. However, electrocardiographic surveillance in each of these studies was limited to periodic recordings for brief periods, which reduced the likelihood of observing intermittent arrhythmias.

DISTURBANCE OF OTHER ELECTROLYTES

In general, the electrolyte disturbances observed in magnesium-deficient humans also occur in other species. Experimental magnesium depletion reliably reduced serum potassium concentration by 0.2 to 1.0 mEq/L in some (Vitale et al. 1961; Ono 1962; Zawada et al. 1988) but not all (Wener et al. 1964) studies in dogs. Serum calcium concentration may fall (Zawada et al. 1988) or remain unchanged (Ono 1962).

▶ Therapy for Magnesium Depletion

Role of Magnesium Depletion in Illness in Dogs and Cats

Hypomagnesemia appears to be common in sick, hospitalized dogs and cats (Martin et al 1994; Dhupa 1994; Khanna et al. 1998). Although it has not been proved, it is likely that hypomagnesemia is a consequence of magnesium depletion in these patients. The etiology of hypomagnesemia in hospitalized veterinary patients is likely to be multifactorial. Reduced magnesium intake may be partly responsible for this finding. However, reduced intake alone is unlikely to produce magnesium deficiency in dogs, as this species can efficiently conserve magnesium during fasting. For example, healthy dogs fasted for 3 weeks lost only 6% of their body stores of magnesium (de Bruijne 1979). Therefore, other factors are probably involved in development of hypomagnesemia in sick companion animals.

One group found a high frequency of hypomagnesemia in critically ill dogs in a veterinary teaching hospital intensive care unit (26 of 48 dogs; insufficient information was provided to determine whether there was sampling bias). Abnormal conditions found in those dogs included trauma and gastrointestinal, cardiopulmonary, renal, and metabolic diseases (Martin et al. 1994). There was no statistically significant difference in the prevalence of hypomagnesemia between dogs affected with each disease syndrome. However, each of these conditions has been associated with magnesium depletion in humans and probably predisposed the dogs described in that report to hypomagnesemia.

With the exception of disturbances of other electrolytes (e.g., hyponatremia and hypokalemia), the dogs and cats afflicted with hypomagnesemia in veterinary hospital surveys did not exhibit typical clinical signs or complications associated with magnesium depletion in dogs. In spite of this, magnesium therapy for known or suspected deficiency states may be justified even in animals not showing classical signs of deficiency.

As described earlier, magnesium depletion is most often suspected after identification of hypomagnesemia as opposed to documenting reduced tissue magnesium content. At present, there is no evidence that correcting magnesium deficiency or hypomagnesemia in asymptomatic patients has any positive effect on the outcome of a concurrent illness. Hypomagnesemia was associated with higher mortality in sick animals, but it is not currently known whether the increased risk of death was due to that abnormality or whether hypomagnesemia was simply an epiphenomenon that accompanied serious underlying disease (Martin et al. 1994; Dhupa 1994). Nevertheless, correction of magnesium deficiency certainly fits the general critical care philosophy of support of homeostasis and organ system function, and there are several logical reasons to justify supplementation. Hypokalemia and other electrolyte disturbances may be difficult to correct without concurrent restoration of magnesium stores. Furthermore, there is experimental evidence that magnesium depletion increases mortality in animals with some clinically relevant experimentally induced disorders. For example, progressive magnesium deficiency was strongly associated with increased mortality in rats subjected to endotoxin challenge, and magnesium replacement therapy provided significant protection (Salem et al. 1995). Finally, it has been suggested that magnesium deficiency intensifies the neuroendocrine stress response to environmental stimuli and may reduce survival after stressful insults (Seelig 1994).

Administration of Magnesium to Treat Deficiency States

Magnesium depletion may be treated by oral or parenteral supplementation with magnesium salts. In clinical practice, magnesium depletion is most often suspected on the basis of the patient's history and identification of hypomagnesemia in sick animals. Serum magnesium concentration is most often determined as part of a diagnostic biochemical profile of animals sick enough to require hospitalization. Many of these patients are either anorectic or unable to eat enough to make oral supplementation practical. Therefore, supplementation is most often accomplished by administration of magnesium salts by injection. Intramuscular injections of magnesium salts are painful (Salem et al. 1995), and the intravenous route best accomplishes parenteral administration.

Magnesium may be administered by slow intravenous injection or by oral supplementation. Chronic primary magnesium deficiency is the most common disorder in humans and is typically managed with oral supplementation. Contraindications to magnesium supplementation include hypermagnesemia and myasthenia. Renal failure is a relative contraindication, because some patients with severely impaired renal function are hypermagnesemic or have low tolerance for supplementation.

Dogs and cats may be at higher risk for chronic magnesium depletion when afflicted with disorders known to predispose humans to this condition. Such disorders might include chronic diarrhea (particularly in diseases associated with malabsorption syndromes), diabetes mellitus, hyperparathyroidism, therapy with loop diuretics, and some causes of chronic renal failure. If definitive therapy for the underlying disease is possible (e.g., successful insulin therapy for diabetes mellitus or surgical excision of a parathyroid tumor), chronic oral therapy may be unnecessary. Definitive information about the frequency of magnesium depletion in companion animals with these disorders is lacking. Nevertheless, chronic oral supplementation may be warranted if hypomagnesemia is identified in animals afflicted with any of these disorders. The daily dosage required to achieve positive magnesium balance in these patients must be determined on an individual basis by repeated measurement of serum magnesium concentration. The typical initial daily dosage of magnesium used for humans is 300 to 600 mg of elemental magnesium (approximately twice the normal daily dietary intake) divided into three or four doses to avoid catharsis (Rude 1993).

Recommendations for the administration of magnesium to dogs are based on extrapolation of the dosage used in human beings as well as clinical experience. An initial dosage of 0.75 to 1.0 mEq/kg/day (approximately 90 to 120 mg/kg/day magnesium sulfate) administered by slow intravenous infusion has been recommended for treatment of magnesium depletion in dogs (Dhupa 1995). This may be followed by a slower rate (0.3 to 0.5 mEq/kg/day or 40 to 60 mg/kg/day of magnesium sulfate) for 3 to 5 days (Dhupa 1995).

There are no simple magnesium salts approved for veterinary use. All of the magnesium salts available for oral supplementation have comparable bioavailability, including mineral salts (e.g., chloride) and organic salts (e.g., acetate, aspartate, citrate, glutamate, lactate, methionate, and pyrrolidone carboxylate). When these products are administered at physiologic replacement dosages, tolerance is generally excellent. Magnesium sulfate (Epsom salt) is widely available as an over-the-counter agent and is inexpensive but is not often used to treat magnesium deficiency. At high dosages, Epsom salt produces catharsis. Several combination products (also containing one or more of potassium, chloride, calcium, phosphorus, dextrose, selenium, and cobalt) are marketed for use in treating hypomagnesemia and other electrolyte disturbances in ruminants. Magnesium gluconate tablets and liquid (Magonate, Fleming and Company, Fenton, MO), magnesium oxide tablets (Mag-Ox 400, Blaine Company, Erlanger, KY), magnesium oxide capsules (Uro-Mag, Blaine Company, Erlanger, KY), and magnesium carbonate (Mag-Carb, R&D Laboratories, Marina Del Ray, CA) are examples of oral magnesium supplements available as over-the-counter products for human use.

Urgent treatment of magnesium depletion is best accomplished by injection of the sulfate or chloride salt. Injectable solutions are prescription drugs. Generic magnesium sulfate is available as 10% (0.8 mEq/mL), 12.5% (1 mEq/mL), and 50% (4 mEq/mL) solutions. Magnesium chloride injection is available at a concentration of 200 mg/mL (1.98 mEq Mg^{2+}/mL). Despite the nearly universal practice of using the sulfate salt for parenteral therapy, at least one author has pointed out potential advantages of the oral administration of the chloride salt preparation, including better absorption, less urinary loss, and better cell penetration than the sulfate salt (Durlach et al. 1996).

▶ Magnesium as a Therapeutic Agent

Magnesium is also administered as a pharmacologic agent to patients that are not magnesium depleted. In this case, a state of therapeutic magnesium overload is induced to produce specific therapeutic effects. These actions may be effective components of management of some disease states. Pharmacodynamic properties include antispasmodic, curariform, and ganglioplegic effects on muscle, bradycardia, arrhythmia suppression, vasodilatation, and bronchodilatation. Magnesium loading has been used to treat a variety of disorders in humans, but with the exception of treatment of ventricular arrhythmias, little information is available concerning the administration of pharmacologic dosages of magnesium to dogs or cats.

The most common method of administration of pharmacologic doses of magnesium to adult humans is intravenous administration of 1 to 6 g of magnesium sulfate over 20 to 30 min. The clinical conditions most often treated with intravenous magnesium include premature labor, preeclampsia, eclampsia, severe asthma, and some arrhythmias. Magnesium is also used in the treatment of myocardial infarction and some forms of headache, although those uses are more controversial.

The most well-established uses of magnesium by physicians in the United States are to relax uterine contractions in women with preterm labor and to treat preeclampsia. The therapeutic use of magnesium for tocolysis is based on two possible actions: suppression of nerve transmission to uterine smooth muscle and a direct effect on myometrial cells. Magnesium overload inhibits release of acetylcholine by motor end plates within the neuromuscular junction and prevents neuronal calcium influx to block neuromuscular transmission. Furthermore, magnesium overload induces hypocalcemia in some patients, probably by suppression of PTH and by enhancing calciuria (Cruikshank et al. 1981).

Preeclampsia is defined as blood pressure exceeding 140/90 mm Hg accompanied by proteinuria or edema in a previously normotensive pregnant woman. Eclampsia is the same condition accompanied by seizures. Magnesium sulfate is frequently used to treat preeclampsia and prevent eclamptic seizures, based on studies demonstrating its safety and efficacy (Frakes and Richardson 1997). Once seizures occur, magnesium sulfate is still used therapeutically, although many prefer anticonvulsant drugs. A systematic review and meta-analysis of studies comparing magnesium sulfate with other therapies for preeclampsia and eclampsia concluded that magnesium sulfate is superior to other therapies (phenytoin or diazepam) for prevention of recurrent seizures in eclampsia and for seizure prophylaxis in preeclampsia (Chien et al. 1996).

Magnesium has been advocated as therapy for severe (McLean 1994; Schiermeyer and Finkelstein 1994; Frakes and Richardson 1997) but not chronic stable (Bernstein et al. 1995) human bronchial asthma. The mechanisms of action in acute asthma attacks are not known but are postulated to include smooth muscle relaxation secondary to inhibition of calcium uptake, impaired acetylcholine release, and increased respiratory strength. Magnesium is typically recommended for patients with severe signs not responsive to other therapies, as it has little effect on respirations in asthmatics with mild respiratory impairment (Bernstein et al. 1995; Frakes and Richardson 1997).

Magnesium has been used as a treatment for cardiac arrhythmias in humans for many years. Among the electrophysiologic actions of magnesium on the heart, effects on repolarizing potassium currents and potassium conductance are perhaps the most important (Farrow 1994). The net result of these effects is to limit the cellular loss of potassium and maintain the plateau phase of the action potential. Magnesium concentration also influences transmembrane calcium flow and calcium channel function. When administered at therapeutic dosages, magnesium inhibits both early and delayed after-depolarizations and the triggered ventricular rhythms induced by them. Rhythm disturbances that respond to magnesium loading include torsades de pointes, a discrete form of ventricular tachycardia characterized by QRS complexes that "twist" around the isoelectric baseline and have a long QT interval. One instance of using magnesium for therapy of a torsades de pointes–like arrhythmia has been reported in a dog (Baty et al. 1994). Other arrhythmias reliably treated by magnesium in humans include those associated with digoxin toxicity and magnesium deficiency–induced atrial fibrillation. Acceptable uses also include treatment of ventricular extrasystole or ventricular tachycardia associated with myocardial infarction and multifocal atrial tachycardia (Fazekas et al. 1993).

The role of magnesium as therapy for myocardial infarction is controversial, although there is growing evidence that it is effective in limiting myocardial necrosis when administered before or during thrombolytic therapy

(Antman 1996). Beneficial effects may be related to maintenance of cellular energy stores during ischemia, prevention of cellular calcium overload, stabilization of function of injured cell membranes, inhibition of free-radical injury, inhibition of intracoronary thrombosis, coronary and systemic vasodilatation, and slowing of the heart rate. Research using a dog model of myocardial ischemia has demonstrated that magnesium at moderately high dosages (100 mg/kg of magnesium sulfate intravenously) protects myocardial function when administered at the time of release of the occlusion (Mass et al. 1994). These findings might indicate a role of magnesium loading as therapy for myocardial injury and arrhythmias resulting from ischemia associated with severe shock syndrome.

In dogs with life-threatening complications including ventricular arrhythmia, an intravenous dosage of 0.15 to 0.3 mEq/kg (19 to 38 mg/kg magnesium sulfate) over 5 to 15 min has been recommended. In normal anesthetized beagle dogs, 0.1 to 0.2 mEq/kg may be infused within 2 min without producing hemodynamic effects (Nakayama et al. 1999). However, excessive administration of magnesium produces toxicity. Administration of magnesium at a rate of 0.12 mEq/kg/min produced hemodynamic alterations after infusion of 0.2 mEq/kg and death caused by arrhythmia occurred when the cumulative dosage exceeded 5.9 mEq/kg (Fig. 8–1).

▶ Hypermagnesemia

Hypermagnesemia is a relatively uncommon diagnosis in humans, most likely because of the ability of the kidneys to increase excretion of magnesium markedly in the presence of high dietary intake. It is therefore not surprising that the patients most often affected by hypermagnesemia are those with renal insufficiency or failure who ingest large quantities of magnesium. The most common sources of excessive dietary magnesium are over-the-counter magnesium-containing antacids and magnesium salt cathartics. Hypermagnesemia may be less common than hypomagnesemia in sick companion animals. In one survey of dogs admitted to a critical care unit of a veterinary teaching hospital, 6 of 48 were hypermagnesemic whereas 26 of 48 were hypomagnesemic (Martin et al. 1994). The highest serum magnesium concentrations were found in dogs with renal failure. Although the mean serum concentration in those dogs (2.4 mg/dL) was substantially lower than concentrations associated with cardiovascular toxicity in dogs with induced hypermagnesemia (>6 mg/dL) (Nakayama et al. 1999), hypermagnesemic dogs were 2.6 times more likely to die than normomagnesemic dogs. Although none of the clinical signs in those dogs were attributed to hypermagnesemia, the depression and other clinical signs associated with renal failure could mask subtle signs of hypermagnesemia.

Clinical findings in hypermagnesemic humans include depression, weakness, and hypotension. With more severe hypermagnesemia, loss of deep tendon reflexes, electrocardiographic changes, and respiratory depression develop. Electrocardiographic abnormalities include prolongation of the PR interval and QRS duration.

Therapy of hypermagnesemia includes cessation of all magnesium intake, maneuvers to increase renal excretion, and, when it is severe, administration of calcium to antagonize the effects of hypermagnesemia at the cell membrane. Renal excretion may be enhanced by administration of sufficient sodium-containing fluids to promote diuresis and administration of a loop diuretic. When using this approach, serum potassium concentrations should be monitored carefully because hypokalemia is a common complication of therapy in these patients. Intravenous administration of calcium is reserved for human patients demonstrating unresponsiveness, respiratory depression, arrhythmias, or hemodynamic instability. If used in veterinary patients, 50 to 150 mg of calcium gluconate or 15 to mg 50 of calcium chloride may be administered intravenously over 5 to 10 min.

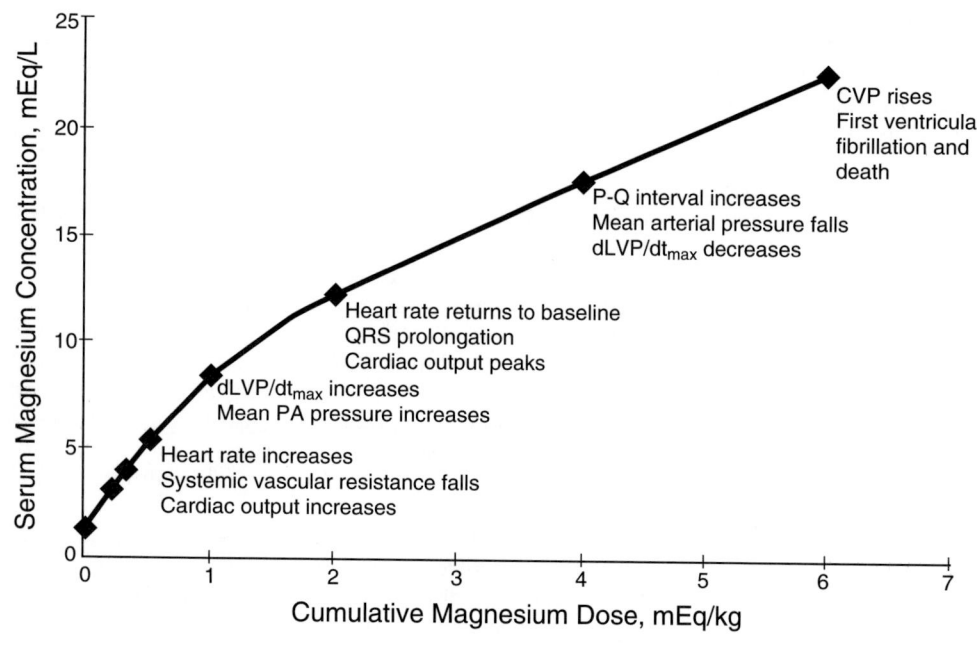

FIGURE 8–1. Sequence of events in eight beagle dogs receiving intravenous magnesium sulfate at the rate of 0.12 mEq/kg/min. The curve shows the mean serum magnesium concentration during the progressive infusion, and the text boxes describe events occurring at various points during the infusion. Note that these events occurred at specific cumulative doses of magnesium, not at specific serum magnesium concentrations. (Data from Nakayama T et al. 1999.)

REFERENCES

Adkins Y, Zicker SC, Lepine A, et al.: Changes in nutrient and protein composition of cat milk during lactation. *Am J Vet Res* 58:370–375, 1997.

Alfrey AC: Effect of age and magnesium depletion on bone magnesium pools in rats. *J Clin Invest* 54:1074–1081, 1974a.

Alfrey AC: Evaluation of body magnesium stores. *J Lab Clin Med* 84:153–162, 1974b.

Alfrey AC and Miller N: Bone magnesium pools in uremia. *J Clin Invest* 52:3019–3027, 1973.

al-Ghamdi SM, Cameron EC, and Sutton RA: Magnesium deficiency: Pathophysiologic and clinical overview. *Am J Kidney Dis* 24:737–752, 1994.

Antman EM: Magnesium in acute myocardial infarction: Overview of available evidence. *Am Heart J* 132:487–495, 1996.

Barker J and Povey RC: The feline urolithiasis syndrome: A review and an inquiry into the alleged role of dry cat foods in its aetiology. *J Small Anim Pract* 14:445–457, 1973.

Barnes BA and Mendelson J: The measurement of exchangeable magnesium in dogs. *Metabolism* 12:184–193, 1963.

Baty CJ, Sweet DC, and Keene BW: Torsades de pointes–like polymorphic ventricular tachycardia in a dog. *J Vet Intern Med* 8:439–442, 1994.

Bernstein WK, Khastgir T, Khastgir A, et al.: Lack of effectiveness of magnesium in chronic stable asthma. A prospective, randomized, double-blind, placebo-controlled, crossover trial in normal subjects and in patients with chronic stable asthma. *Arch Intern Med* 155:271–276, 1995.

Brannan P, Vergne-Marini P, Pak C, et al.: Magnesium absorption in human small intestine. Results in normal subjects, patients with chronic renal disease, and patients with absorptive hypercalciuria. *J Clin Invest* 57:1412–1418, 1976.

Brautbar N and Massry SG: Hypomagnesemia and hypermagnesemia. In Maxwell MH, Kleeman CR, and Narins RG (eds): *Clinical Disorders of Fluid and Electrolyte Metabolism*. New York, McGraw-Hill Book Co., pp. 831–849, 1987.

Buffington CA, Rogers QR, and Morris JG: Effect of diet on struvite activity product in feline urine. *Am J Vet Res* 51:2025–2030, 1990.

Bunce GE, Chiemchaisri Y, and Phillips PH: The mineral requirements of the dog. IV. Effect of certain dietary and physiologic factors upon the magnesium deficiency syndrome. *J Nutr* 76:23–29, 1962a.

Bunce GE, Jenkins KJ, and Phillips PH: The mineral requirements of the dog. III. The magnesium requirement. *J Nutr* 76:17–22, 1962b.

Chien PF, Khan KS, and Arnott N: Magnesium sulphate in the treatment of eclampsia and pre-eclampsia: An overview of the evidence from randomised trials. *Br J Obstet Gynaecol* 103:1085–1091, 1996.

Cronin RE, Ferguson ER, Shannon WA Jr, and Knochel JP: Skeletal muscle injury after magnesium depletion in the dog. *Am J Physiol* 243:F113–F120, 1982.

Cruikshank D, Pitkin R, Donnelly E, et al.: Urinary magnesium, calcium, and phosphate excretion during magnesium phosphate infusion. *Obstet Gynecol* 58:430–434, 1981.

de Bruijne JJ: Biochemical observations during total starvation in dogs. *Int J Obesity* 3:239–247, 1979.

Dhupa N: Serum magnesium abnormalities in a small animal intensive care unit population (abstract). *J Vet Intern Med* 8:157, 1994.

Dhupa N: Magnesium therapy. In Bonagura JD (ed): *Kirk's Current Veterinary Therapy*. Philadelphia, WB Saunders Co., pp. 132–133, 1995.

Durlach J: Recommended dietary amounts of magnesium: Mg RDA. *Magnes Res* 2:195–203, 1989.

Durlach J and Mareschi JP: Recommended dietary amounts for magnesium: II. Updated European Consensus and future prospects. In Lasserre B and Durlach J (eds): *Magnesium: A Relevant Ion*. London, John Libbey, pp. 39–49, 1991.

Durlach J, Durlach V, Bac P, et al: Magnesium and therapeutics. *Magnes Res* 7:313–328, 1994.

Durlach J, Bara M, and Theophanides T: A hint on pharmacological and toxicological differences between magnesium chloride and magnesium sulphate, or of scallops and men. *Magnes Res* 9:217–219, 1996.

Elin RJ: Magnesium: The fifth but forgotten electrolyte. *Clin Chem* 102:616–622, 1994.

Farrow CS: Postural radiography in dogs. *J Am Vet Med Assoc* 205:878–887, 1994.

Fazekas T, Scherlag BJ, Vos M, et al.: Magnesium and the heart: Antiarrhythmic therapy with magnesium. *Clin Cardiol* 16:768–774, 1993.

Finco DR and Barsanti JA: Diet-induced feline urethral obstruction. *Vet Clin North Am Small Anim Pract* 14:529–536, 1984.

Finco DR, Barsanti JA, and Crowell WA: Characterization of magnesium-induced urinary disease in the cat and comparison with feline urologic syndrome. *Am J Vet Res* 46:391–400, 1985.

Frakes MA and Richardson LE: Magnesium sulfate therapy in certain emergency conditions. *Am J Emerg Med* 15:182–187, 1997.

Gordon MC and Iams JD: Magnesium sulfate. *Clin Obstet Gynecol* 38:706–712, 1995.

Graham LA, Caessar JJ, and Burgen ASV: Gastrointestinal absorption of Mg28 in man. *Metabolism* 9:646–659, 1960.

Hamill-Ruth RJ and McGory R: Magnesium repletion and its effect on potassium homeostasis in critically ill adults: Results of a double-blind, randomized, controlled trial. *Crit Care Med* 24:38–45, 1996.

Hodgkinson A, Marshall DH, and Nordin BEC: Vitamin D and magnesium absorption in man. *Clin Sci* 57:121–123, 1979.

Kallfelz FA, Bressett JD, and Wallace RJ: Urethral obstruction in random source and SPF male cats induced by high levels of dietary magnesium or magnesium and phosphorus. *Feline Pract* 10:25–35, 1980.

Khanna C, Lund EM, Raffe M, et al.: Hypomagnesemia in 188 dogs: A hospital population-based prevalence study. *J Vet Intern Med* 12:304–309, 1998.

Khilnani P: Electrolyte abnormalities in critically ill children. *Crit Care Med* 20:241–250, 1992.

Kienzle E, Stratmann B, and Meyer H: Body composition of cats as a basis for factorial calculation of energy and nutrient requirements for growth. *J Nutr* 121:S122–S123, 1991.

Lewis LD and Morris MLJ: Diet as a causative factor of feline urolithiasis. *Vet Clin North Am Small Anim Pract* 14:513–527, 1984a.

Lewis LD and Morris MLJ: Treatment and prevention of feline struvite urolithiasis. *Vet Clin North Am Small Anim Pract* 14:649–660, 1984b.

Lewis LD, Chow FHC, Taton GF, et al.: Effect of various dietary mineral concentrations on the occurrence of feline urolithiasis. *J Am Vet Med Assoc* 172:559–563, 1978.

Mann FA, Boon GD, Wagner-Mann MA, et al.: Ionized and total magnesium concentrations in blood from dogs with naturally acquired parvoviral enteritis. *J Am Vet Med Assoc* 212:1398–1401, 1998.

Marier JR: Quantitative factors regarding magnesium status in the modern-day world. *Magnesium* 1:3–15, 1982.

Martin LG: Intravenous magnesium loading test as a method of evaluating magnesium status in the dog. *Proceedings of the Fourth International Veterinary Emergency Critical Care Symposium*, pp. 1–3, 1994.

Martin LG, Wingfield WE, Van Pelt DR, et al.: Magnesium in the 1990's: Implications for veterinary critical care. *J Vet Emerg Crit Care* 3:105–114, 1993.

Martin LG, Matteson VL, Wingfield WE, et al.: Abnormalities of serum magnesium in critically ill dogs: Incidence and implications. *J Vet Emerg Crit Care* 4:15–20, 1994.

Martindale L and Heaton FW: Magnesium deficiency in the adult rat. *Biochem J* 92:119, 1964.

Mass H, Santoni F, Feliciano I, et al.: Parenteral magnesium sulfate restores regional contractile function in the post-ischaemic canine myocardium. *Magnes Res* 7:255–266, 1994.

McLean RM: Magnesium and its therapeutic uses: A review. *Am J Med* 96:63–76, 1994.

Nadler JL and Rude RK: Disorders of magnesium metabolism. *Endocrinol Metab Clin North Am* 24:623–641, 1995.

Nakayama T, Nakayama H, Miyamoto M, and Hamlin RL: Hemodynamic and electrocardiographic effects of magnesium sulfate in healthy dogs. *J Vet Intern Med* 13:485–490, 1999.

Ono I: The effect of varying dietary magnesium on the electrocardiogram and blood electrolytes of dogs. *Jpn Circ J* 26:677–685, 1962.

Orent ER, Kruse HD, and McCollum EV: Studies on magnesium deficiency in animals. II. Species variation in symptomatology of magnesium deprivation. *Am J Physiol* 101:454–461, 1932.

Osborne CA, Lulich JP, Kruger JM, et al.: Medical dissolution of feline struvite urocystoliths. *J Am Vet Med Assoc* 196:1053–1063, 1990.

Pastoor FJH, Van't Klooster AT, Opitz R, Beynen AC: Effect of dietary magnesium level on urinary and faecal excretion of calcium, magnesium and phosphorus in adult, ovariectomized cats. *Br J Nutr* 74:77–84, 1995.

Reinhart RA and Desbiens NA: Hypomagnesemia in patients entering the ICU. *Crit Care Med* 13:506–507, 1985.

Rude RK: Magnesium metabolism and deficiency. *Endocrinol Metab Clin North Am* 22:377–395, 1993.

Rylander R: Environmental magnesium deficiency as a cardiovascular risk factor. *J Cardiovasc Risk* 3:4–10, 1996.

Salem M, Kasinski N, Munoz R, et al.: Progressive magnesium deficiency increases mortality from endotoxin challenge: Protective effects of acute magnesium replacement therapy. *Crit Care Med* 23:108–118, 1995.

Schiermeyer RP and Finkelstein JA: Rapid infusion of magnesium sulfate obviates need for intubation in status asthmaticus. *Am J Emerg Med* 12:164–166, 1994.

Seelig MS: Consequences of magnesium deficiency on the enhancement of stress reactions; preventive and therapeutic implications (a review). *J Am Coll Nutr* 13:429–446, 1994.

Spencer H, Lesniak K, Gatza CA, et al.: Magnesium absorption and metabolism in patients with chronic renal failure and in patients with normal renal function. *Gastroenterology* 79:26–34, 1980.

Subcommittee on the tenth edition of the recommended dietary allowances. *Recommended Dietary Allowances*. Washington, DC, National Research Council, 1989.

Sutton RA and Domrongkitchaiporn S: Abnormal renal magnesium handling. *Miner Electrolyte Metab* 19:232–240, 1993.

Syllm-Rapoport I: Electrocardiographic studies in dogs with experimental magnesium deficiency. *J Pediatr* 60:801–804, 1962.

Syllm-Rapoport I and Strassburger I: Über den experimentellen magnesium-mangel beim hund. *Acta Biol Med Ger* 7:467–475, 1961.

Tarttelin MF: Feline struvite urolithiasis: Factors affecting urine pH may be more important than magnesium levels in food. *Vet Rec* 121:227–230, 1987a.

Tarttelin MF: Feline struvite urolithiasis: Fasting reduced the effectiveness of a urinary acidifier (ammonium chloride) and increased the intake of a low magnesium diet. *Vet Rec* 121:245–248, 1987b.

Vallee BL, Wacker WEC, and Ulmer DD: The magnesium deficiency-tetany syndrome in man. *N Engl J Med* 262:155–161, 1960.

Vitale JJ, Hellerstein EE, Nakamura M, et al.: Effects of magnesium-deficient diet upon puppies. *Circ Res* 9:387–394, 1961.

Wangemann M, Selzer A, Leitzmann C, et al.: On the magnesium supply of a normal diet. *Magnes Res* 6:402–403, 1993.

Wener J, Pintar K, Simon MA, et al.: The effects of prolonged hypomagnesemia on the cardiovascular system in young dogs. *Am Heart J* 67:221–231, 1964.

Whang R, Morosi HJ, Rogers D, et al.: The influence of sustained magnesium deficiency on muscle potassium repletion. *J Lab Clin Med* 70:895–902, 1967.

Whang R, Whang DD, and Ryan MP: Refractory potassium repletion: A consequence of magnesium deficiency. *Arch Intern Med* 152:40–45, 1992.

Whang R, Hampton EM, and Whang DD: Magnesium homeostasis and clinical disorders of magnesium deficiency. *Ann Pharmacother* 28:220–226, 1994.

Zawada ET, TerWee JA, and McClung DE: Canine renal and systemic hemodynamic measurements after 4 weeks of a magnesium deficient diet. *Nephron* 50:253–257, 1988.

SECTION 3

Acid-Base Disorders

CHAPTER 9

Introduction to Acid-Base Disorders

STEPHEN P. DiBARTOLA

> To Faraday we are indebted for naming the products of dissociation, ions—and thus we came by "hydrogen ions," a term now synonymous with proton. Tiny though it is, I suppose no constituent of living matter has so much power to influence biological behavior....
>
> A. Baird Hastings, Ann N Y Acad Sci 133:16, 1966

Metabolic processes each day yield 50 to 100 mEq of H^+ ions (*fixed* or *nonvolatile acid*) from the metabolism of proteins and phospholipids and 10,000 to 15,000 mmol of CO_2 (*volatile acid*) from the metabolism of carbohydrate and fat. Carbon dioxide is potentially an acid by virtue of its ability to combine with H_2O in the presence of carbonic anhydrase to form carbonic acid (H_2CO_3). Carbon dioxide is continuously removed by alveolar ventilation so that the partial pressure of CO_2 ($P{CO_2}$) is kept constant at approximately 40 mm Hg in the normal individual.

▶ Concept of Acidity

The most commonly employed concept of acids and bases is that of Brönsted and Lowry, who stated that an *acid* is a proton donor and a *base* a proton acceptor. In the following equation, HA is an acid and A^- is a base:

$$HA \rightleftarrows H^+ + A^-$$

In aqueous solutions, protons or H^+ ions are normally bound by electrostatic interaction to H_2O, resulting in the formation of hydronium ions, designated H_3O^+. Conventionally, however, the term *hydrogen ion* and the symbol H^+ are used to refer to protons in aqueous solutions.

The acidity of a solution refers to the chemical *activity* of its constituent H^+ ions. Chemical activity is related to chemical *concentration* by the *activity coefficient*, a factor that varies directly with temperature and inversely with the ionic strength of the solution. Physiologic control of body temperature and osmolality and the dilute nature of body fluids result in this factor being near unity and the difference between activity and concentration being negligible in body fluids. Thus, concentration and activity are considered the same in body fluids and subsequently only the term concentration is used.

The concentrations of most important electrolytes in body fluids (e.g., Na^+, K^+, Cl^-, HCO_3^-) are in the range of milliequivalents per liter, whereas the concentration of H^+ is in the range of nanoequivalents per liter. That is, hydrogen ions are present at one-millionth the concentration of other electrolytes. What, then, accounts for the emphasis on hydrogen ions in biology and medicine? The answer lies in the fact that hydrogen ions are highly reactive. The proteins of the body have many dissociable groups. These may gain or lose protons as $[H^+]$ changes, resulting in alterations in charge and molecular configuration that may adversely affect protein structure and function. The $[H^+]$ of body fluids must be kept constant so that detrimental changes in enzyme function and cellular structure do not occur. The range of $[H^+]$ compatible with life is 16 to 160 nEq/L.

▶ Concept of pH

The concept of pH was introduced by Sørensen to allow easier notation for the wide range of $[H^+]$ found in chemical systems. The term pH is defined as the negative base 10 logarithm of the hydrogen ion concentration expressed in equivalents per liter or the base 10 logarithm of the reciprocal of the hydrogen ion concentration:

$$pH = -\log_{10}[H^+] = \log_{10}\left(\frac{1}{[H^+]}\right)$$

Thus, at the normal extracellular fluid $[H^+]$ of 40 nEq/L (4×10^{-8} Eq/L):

$$[H^+] = 4 \times 10^{-8} \text{ Eq/L}$$
$$pH = -\log_{10}(4 \times 10^{-8})$$
$$= -\log_{10}4 - \log_{10}10^{-8}$$
$$= -(0.602) - (-8)$$
$$= 8 - 0.602$$
$$= 7.398$$

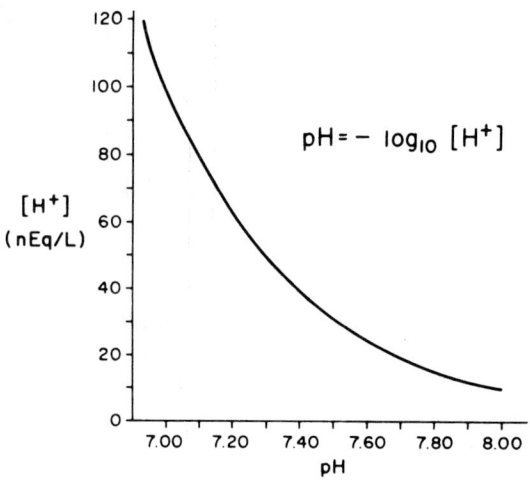

FIGURE 9-1. Exponential relationship between [H+] and pH. (From Madias NE and Cohen JJ: Acid-base chemistry and buffering. In Cohen JJ and Kassirer JP (eds): *Acid-Base*. Boston, Little, Brown & Co., p. 5, 1982.)

There is an inverse relationship between pH and [H$^+$]. The greater the [H$^+$], the lower the pH. Furthermore, pH and [H$^+$] vary not linearly with one another but exponentially as shown in Figure 9-1. The [H$^+$] for a given pH within the physiologic range is given in Table 9-1.

▶ Law of Mass Action

The *law of mass action* states that the velocity of a reaction is proportional to the product of the concentrations of the reactants. For the acid just described, there are two opposing reactions:

$$HA \rightarrow H^+ + A^-$$
$$H^+ + A^- \rightarrow HA$$

The velocity of the first reaction can be written:

$$v_1 = k_1[HA]$$

and the velocity of the second reaction:

$$v_2 = k_2[H^+][A^-]$$

At equilibrium, the rates of the two opposing reactions exactly counterbalance one another and the two velocities are equal:

$$k_1[HA] = k_2[H^+][A^-]$$

Rearranging and substituting a new constant, K_a, the ionization, or dissociation, constant for the acid HA:

$$k_1/k_2 = K_a = \frac{[H^+][A^-]}{[HA]}$$

The ionization, or dissociation, constant for an acid is an indication of the strength of that acid. A large value for K_a means that [H$^+$] and [A$^-$] are much greater than [HA]; that is, the acid is a strong one and is largely dissociated. A small value for K_a means that [H$^+$] and [A$^-$] are much smaller than [HA]; that is, the acid is a weak one and little of it is dissociated. Hydrochloric acid (HCl) and sulfuric acid (H$_2$SO$_4$) are strong acids and dissociate almost completely in aqueous solutions, whereas NH$_4^+$ is a weak acid (i.e., it is a strong base) and dissociates to a small extent.

Taking the base 10 logarithm of both sides of the dissociation equilibrium equation yields

$$\log K_a = \log \frac{[H^+][A^-]}{[HA]}$$

$$\log K_a = \log([H^+]) + \log \frac{[A^-]}{[HA]}$$

Multiplying by -1 yields:

$$-\log K_a = -\log([H^+]) - \log \frac{[A^-]}{[HA]}$$

Applying the concept of pH to both the hydrogen ion concentration and dissociation constant, K_a,

$$pK_a = pH - \log\left(\frac{[A^-]}{[HA]}\right)$$

$$pH = pK_a + \log\left(\frac{[A^-]}{[HA]}\right)$$

This is the commonly used Henderson-Hasselbalch form of the dissociation equilibrium equation. Occasionally, the term *salt* or *base* is substituted for A$^-$ and the term *acid* for HA:

$$pH = pK_a + \log \frac{[salt]}{[acid]}$$

▶ Concept of Buffering

A *buffer* is a compound that can accept or donate protons (hydrogen ions) and minimize a change in pH. A buffer solution consists of a weak acid and its conjugate salt. When a strong acid is added to a buffer solution containing a weaker acid and its salt, the dissociated protons from the strong acid are donated to the salt of the weak acid and the change in pH is minimized.

Consider an aqueous solution with equal amounts of Na$_2$HPO$_4$ and NaH$_2$PO$_4$. The pK_a for this buffer pair is 6.8:

$$pH = pK_a + \log \frac{[salt]}{[acid]}$$

$$pH = 6.8 + \log \frac{[Na_2HPO_4]}{[NaH_2PO_4]}$$

If the amounts of Na$_2$HPO$_4$ and NaH$_2$PO$_4$ are equal, their ratio is 1.0:

$$pH = 6.8 + \log(1.0)$$
$$= 6.8$$

Consider adding 1 mmol of HCl to this solution. The protons from the HCl are donated to the salt of the buffer pair (Na$_2$HPO$_4$), converting it to its conjugate acid (NaH$_2$PO$_4$). If 10 mmol of each phosphate salt was present initially, the new ratio of Na$_2$HPO$_4$/NaH$_2$PO$_4$ would be 9/11 or 0.82 and

$$pH = 6.8 + \log(0.82)$$
$$= 6.8 + (-0.086)$$
$$= 6.71$$

TABLE 9-1. **Conversions Between pH and [H⁺]**

pH Units	[H⁺]* (nEq/L)	pH Units	[H⁺] (nEq/L)	pH Units	[H⁺] (nEq/L)	pH Units	[H⁺] (nEq/L)
8.00	10	7.64	23	7.29	51	6.94	115
7.99	10	7.63	23	7.28	52	6.93	117
7.98	10	7.62	24	7.27	54	6.92	120
7.97	11	7.61	25	7.26	55	6.91	123
7.96	11	7.60	25	7.25	56	6.90	126
7.95	11	7.59	26	7.24	58	6.89	129
7.94	11	7.58	26	7.23	59	6.88	132
7.93	12	7.57	27	7.22	60	6.87	135
7.92	12	7.56	28	7.21	62	6.86	138
7.91	12	7.55	28	7.20	63	6.85	141
7.90	13	7.54	29	7.19	65	6.84	145
7.89	13	7.53	30	7.18	66	6.83	148
7.88	13	7.52	30	7.17	68	6.82	151
7.87	13	7.51	31	7.16	69	6.81	155
7.86	14	7.50	32	7.15	71	6.80	159
7.85	14	7.49	32	7.14	72	6.79	162
7.84	14	7.48	33	7.13	74	6.78	166
7.83	15	7.47	34	7.12	76	6.77	170
7.82	15	7.46	35	7.11	78	6.76	174
7.81	15	7.45	35	7.10	79	6.75	178
7.80	16	7.44	36	7.09	81	6.74	182
7.79	16	7.43	37	7.08	83	6.73	186
7.78	17	7.42	38	7.07	85	6.72	191
7.77	17	7.41	39	7.06	87	6.71	196
7.76	17	7.40	40	7.05	89	6.70	200
7.75	18	7.39	41	7.04	91	6.69	204
7.74	18	7.38	42	7.03	93	6.68	209
7.73	19	7.37	43	7.02	95	6.67	214
7.72	19	7.36	44	7.01	98	6.66	219
7.71	19	7.35	45	7.00	100	6.65	224
7.70	20	7.34	46	6.99	102	6.64	229
7.69	20	7.33	47	6.98	105	6.63	234
7.68	21	7.32	48	6.97	107	6.62	240
7.67	21	7.31	49	6.96	110	6.61	245
7.66	22	7.30	50	6.95	112	6.60	251
7.65	22						

Source: Cohen JJ and Kassirer JP: Clinical evaluation of acid-base disorders. In Cohen JJ and Kassirer JP (eds): *Acid-Base*. Boston, Little, Brown & Co., p. 409, 1982.
*Values for [H⁺] are given to the nearest nEq/L.

By contrast, an aqueous solution containing 1 mmol/L HCl (10^{-3} Eq/L) would have a pH of 3.0.

The same thing can be shown by solving the dissociation equilibrium equation for $[H^+]$:

$$[H^+] = K_a \frac{[HA]}{[A^-]}$$

For the previously described solution of sodium phosphate:

$$[H^+] = K_a \frac{[NaH_2PO_4]}{[Na_2HPO_4]}$$

The K_a for this reaction is 1.6×10^{-7} Eq/L and if there are equal amounts of the two phosphate salts present ($[NaH_2PO_4] = [Na_2HPO_4]$),

$$[H^+] = 1.6 \times 10^{-7} \text{ Eq/L}$$
$$= 160 \text{ nEq/L (pH 6.80)}$$

After addition of 1 mmol of HCl:

$$[H^+] = (1.6 \times 10^{-7})(11 \times 10^{-3})/(9 \times 10^{-3})$$
$$= 1.95 \times 10^{-7} \text{ Eq/L}$$
$$= 195 \text{ nEq/L (pH 6.71)}$$

By contrast, an aqueous solution containing 1 mmol/L HCl would have $[H^+]$ = .001 mol/L or 1 million nmol/L. Thus, 99.98% of the added hydrogen ions have been buffered by the sodium phosphate solution.

If the amount of strong acid (e.g., HCl) or base (e.g., NaOH) added to a solution of a weak acid and its salt (i.e., a buffer solution) is plotted against pH, the resulting relationship is called a *titration* or *buffer* curve (Fig. 9–2). The curve is sigmoidal, and its slope is greatest in the midregion, over which the curve is approximately linear. In the pH range associated with the midregion of the curve, the change in pH is smallest for a given amount of added acid or base and buffer capacity is greatest at

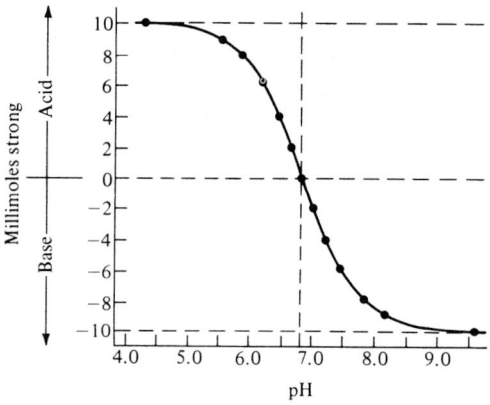

FIGURE 9-2. Titration curve for an aqueous solution containing a phosphate buffer. (From Rose BD: *Clinical Physiology of Acid-Base and Electrolyte Disorders*, 3rd ed. New York, McGraw-Hill Book Co., p. 269, 1989, with permission of the McGraw-Hill Companies.)

the midpoint of the curve. At this point, there are equal amounts of the weak acid and its conjugate salt and, as shown by the Henderson-Hasselbalch equation, pH = pK_a. The region of best buffer capacity extends approximately 1.0 pH unit on either side of the pK_a. Thus, a buffer is most effective within one pH unit of its pK_a. The pK_a values for some important biologic compounds are listed in Table 9–2.

▶ Isohydric Principle

Regardless of the number of buffers present, a solution can have only one [H$^+$] and one pH. Using the law of mass action or the Henderson-Hasselbach equation, the ratio of acid to salt forms of any buffer in the solution can be calculated. This has been called the *isohydric principle*. The implication of the isohydric principle is that the behavior of any buffer pair in a complex solution can be predicted by knowledge of the dissociation constant and concentrations of any one buffer pair. In clinical practice, the bicarbonate–carbonic acid buffer pair is the one used to monitor acid-base balance in body fluids.

The relative importance of a given buffer in the body is based on its concentration in the relevant body fluid, its pK_a, and the prevailing [H$^+$] (40 nmol/L in extracellular fluid). The bicarbonate–carbonic acid system is unique among buffers in that carbonic acid is in equilibrium with dissolved CO_2, the concentration of which normally is kept constant by alveolar ventilation.

▶ The Bicarbonate–Carbonic Acid System: Physical Chemistry

Gaseous CO_2 produced in the tissues is soluble in water and the concentration of dissolved CO_2 in body fluids is proportional to the partial pressure of CO_2 in the gas phase (P_{CO_2}):

$$[CO_{2\,diss}] = \alpha(P_{CO_2})$$

where α is a factor called the *solubility coefficient of CO_2*. The solubility coefficient of CO_2 has a value of 0.0301 mmol/L/mm in arterial plasma at 37°C. Thus,

$$[CO_{2\,diss}] = 0.0301 P_{CO_2}$$

Dissolved CO_2 combines with water to form carbonic acid:

$$CO_{2\,diss} + H_2O \rightarrow H_2CO_3$$

The uncatalyzed reaction proceeds slowly but its rate is dramatically increased by the enzyme carbonic anhydrase, which is present in abundance in the body (e.g., red cells, renal tubular cells). In the body, therefore, the hydration of CO_2 to form H_2CO_3 reaches equilibrium almost instantaneously. Normally, the equilibrium is so far to the left that there are approximately 340 molecules of dissolved CO_2 for each molecule of carbonic acid (Malnic and Giebisch 1972).

The dissociation of carbonic acid can be expressed by the law of mass action:

$$K_a = \frac{[H^+][HCO_3^-]}{[H_2CO_3]}$$

K_a for this reaction is 2.72×10^{-4} mol/L ($pK_a = 3.57$). The ratio of bicarbonate to carbonic acid at the normal [H$^+$] of body fluids can be calculated by rearranging this equation:

$$\frac{[HCO_3^-]}{[H_2CO_3]} = \frac{K_a}{[H^+]}$$
$$= 2.72 \times 10^{-4}/4 \times 10^{-8}$$
$$= 6.8 \times 10^3$$

Thus, at [H$^+$] = 40 nmol/L (pH 7.40), there are 6800 bicarbonate ions and 340 molecules of dissolved CO_2 for each molecule of carbonic acid.

TABLE 9–2. pK_a Values of Biologically Important Compounds*

Compound	pK_a
Phosphoric acid	2.0
Citric acid	2.9
Carbonic acid (pK_a)	3.6
Acetoacetic acid	3.6
Lactic acid	3.9
Citrate^{1-}	4.3
Acetic acid	4.6
3-Hydroxybutyric acid	4.7
Creatinine	5.0
Citrate^{2-}	5.6
Uric acid	5.8
Organic phosphates	6.0–7.5
Carbonic acid (pK_a')	6.1
Imidazole group of histidine	6.4–7.0
Oxygenated hemoglobin	6.7
Phosphate^{1-}	6.8
α-Amino (amino terminal)	7.4–7.9
Deoxygenated hemoglobin	7.9
Ammonium	9.2
Bicarbonate	9.8
Phosphate^{2-}	12.4

*Compounds with pK_a values in the range of 6.4–8.4 are most useful as buffers in biologic systems. The pK_a values for the imidazole group of histidine and for α-amino (amino-terminal) amino groups are for those side groups in proteins. The pK_a range for organ phosphates refers to such intracellular compounds as ATP, ADP, and 2,3-diphosphoglycerate.

The reaction of dissolved CO_2 in aqueous body fluids can be summarized as:

$$CO_{2diss} + H_2O \rightleftarrows H_2CO_3 \rightleftarrows H^+ + HCO_3^-$$

The number of carbonic acid molecules, however, is negligible in comparison with the numbers of dissolved CO_2 molecules and HCO_3^- ions. Therefore, this equation can be simplified:

$$CO_{2diss} + H_2O \rightleftarrows H^+ + HCO_3^-$$

The law of mass action for this equilibrium can be expressed as

$$K_a = \frac{[H^+][HCO_3^-]}{[CO_{2diss}][H_2O]}$$

The concentration of water in dilute body fluids remains virtually unchanged by this reaction and can be incorporated into K_a to yield another constant, K'_a:

$$K'_a = \frac{[H^+][HCO_3^-]}{[CO_{2diss}]}$$

Solving for $[H^+]$ yields:

$$[H^+] = \frac{K'_a[CO_{2diss}]}{[HCO_3^-]}$$

In body fluids at 37°C, K'_a is approximately equal to 8×10^{-7} mol/L and pK'_a equals 6.1. An approximate value of 6.1 for this pK'_a is valid at temperatures ranging from 30 to 40°C (86 to 104°F) and pH values ranging from 7.0 to 7.6 (Madias and Cohen 1982).

A formula for $[H^+]$ in nanomoles per liter or nanoequivalents per liter is obtained by expressing K'_a in nanomoles per liter or nanoequivalents per liter:

$$[H^+] = \frac{800[CO_{2diss}]}{[HCO_3^-]}$$

Using the solubility coefficient for carbon dioxide yields

$$[H^+] = \frac{800(0.0301)P_{CO_2}}{[HCO_3^-]} = \frac{24 P_{CO_2}}{[HCO_3^-]}$$

This is the Henderson equation and has been used extensively in the clinical evaluation of acid-base disturbances. It shows clearly that the $[H^+]$ (and thus pH) of body fluids is determined by the *ratio* of P_{CO_2} to HCO_3^- concentration. The Henderson-Hasselbalch equation is derived by expressing $[H^+]$ and K'_a in moles per liter or equivalents per liter and converting the equation to logarithmic form:

$$[H^+] = K'_a \frac{[CO_{2diss}]}{[HCO_3^-]}$$

$$\log[H^+] = \log K'_a + \log \frac{[CO_{2diss}]}{[HCO_3^-]}$$

Multiplying by -1, we obtain

$$-\log[H^+] = -\log K'_a - \log \frac{[CO_{2diss}]}{[HCO_3^-]}$$

$$pH = pK'_a + \log \frac{[HCO_3^-]}{[CO_{2diss}]}$$

Substituting 6.1 for the value of pK'_a and applying the solubility coefficient for CO_2, we obtain

$$pH = 6.1 + \log \frac{[HCO_3^-]}{0.03 P_{CO_2}}$$

This is the clinically relevant form of the equation and shows that in body fluids, pH is a function of the *ratio* between HCO_3^- concentration and P_{CO_2}.

▶ Body Buffers

Body buffers can be divided into *bicarbonate*, which is the primary buffer system of *extracellular* fluid, and *nonbicarbonate* buffers (e.g., proteins and inorganic and organic phosphates), which constitute the primary *intracellular* buffer system. Bone is a prominent source of buffer and can contribute calcium carbonate and, to a lesser extent, calcium phosphate during chronic metabolic acidosis. Bone may even account for up to 40% of the buffering of an acute acid load in the dog (Burnell 1971). After administration of $NaHCO_3$, carbonate can be deposited in bone.

Bicarbonate as a Buffer in Extracellular Fluid

If a buffer is most effective within 1 pH unit of its pK_a, what accounts for the importance of the bicarbonate system (pK'_a 6.1 vs. extracellular fluid pH 7.4)? One factor is the high concentration of HCO_3^- (approximately 24 mEq/L vs. 2 mEq/L for phosphate). The most important factor, however, is that the bicarbonate–carbonic acid buffer pair functions as an open system. In a *closed* system, the bicarbonate and carbonic acid or dissolved CO_2 concentrations must change in a reciprocal manner as the following reaction is driven to the left or right:

$$CO_{2diss} + H_2O \rightleftarrows H_2CO_3 \rightleftarrows H^+ + HCO_3^-$$

In the body, the system is *open* and carbonic acid, in the presence of carbonic anhydrase, forms CO_2, which is eliminated entirely from the system by alveolar ventilation. Thus, the "acid" member of the buffer pair is free to change directly with the "salt" member as compensation for metabolic acidosis occurs. If P_{CO_2} is kept constant at 40 mm Hg, the effectiveness of the bicarbonate–carbonic acid system is increased dramatically. In response to metabolic acidosis, however, the body goes even further and P_{CO_2} is reduced below the normal value of 40 mm Hg, thus increasing the effectiveness of this buffer pair even more.

Consider a closed system in which the bicarbonate–carbonic acid system is the only buffer pair. We will assume the following conditions at the start: $[H^+]$ = 40 nmol/L, $[HCO_3^-]$ = 24 mmol/L, P_{CO_2} = 40 mm Hg (dissolved CO_2 = 1.2 mmol/L), and pH = 7.40. If 5 mmol of HCl is added to this closed system, $[HCO_3^-]$ is titrated and decreases to 19 mmol/L, P_{CO_2} increases to 206 mm Hg (dissolved CO_2 = 1.2 + 5 = 6.2 mmol/L), $[H^+]$ increases to 260 nmol/L, and pH decreases to 6.58, a value incompatible with life.

Consider now what would happen if the system was

open and the P_{CO_2} kept constant at 40 mm Hg by a factor external to the system (e.g., alveolar ventilation). What would happen now if 5 mmol of HCl was added, assuming the same starting conditions? The $[HCO_3^-]$ again decreases to 19 mmol/L, but P_{CO_2} is fixed at 40 mm Hg (dissolved CO_2 = 1.2 mmol/L). The $[H^+]$ can be calculated from the Henderson equation: $[H^+]$ = 24(40)/19 = 50 nmol/L. The pH is 7.30.

Consider now what would happen if, rather than being kept constant, the P_{CO_2} actually decreased to 36.5 mm Hg. This is what would be expected in a patient with metabolic acidosis if we use the rule of thumb that P_{CO_2} decreases by 0.7 mm Hg per 1.0 mEq/L decrement in plasma HCO_3^- concentration. In this setting, $[HCO_3^-]$ still decreases to 19 mmol/L, but P_{CO_2} is 36.5 mm Hg, and dissolved CO_2 = 0.0301(36.5) = 1.1 mmol/L. Again, the $[H^+]$ can be calculated from the Henderson relationship: $[H^+]$ = 24(36.5)/19 = 46 nmol/L. The pH in this setting is 7.34, just slightly below the starting pH of 7.40. This, in essence, is what happens in the body in response to metabolic acidosis and illustrates the dramatic effect achieved because the bicarbonate–carbonic acid system is an open system with P_{CO_2} closely regulated by alveolar ventilation.

Proteins as Buffers

Plasma proteins play a limited role in extracellular buffering, whereas intracellular proteins play an important role in the total buffer response of the body. The buffer effect of proteins is due to their dissociable side groups. For most proteins, including hemoglobin, the most important of these dissociable groups is the imidazole ring of histidine residues (pK_a 6.4–7.0). Amino-terminal amino groups (pK_a 7.4–7.9) also contribute somewhat to the buffer effect of proteins. Other side groups are relatively unimportant, because their pK_a values are either too high or too low to be useful in the normal physiologic range of pH. The pK_a values for the dissociable groups of proteins are listed in Table 9–3.

Hemoglobin is responsible for over 80% of the nonbicarbonate buffering capacity of whole blood, whereas plasma proteins contribute 20%. Of the plasma proteins, albumin is much more important than are the globulins.

TABLE 9–3. pK'_a Values for Dissociable Groups Found in Proteins

Dissociable Group (Amino Acid)	pK'_a
α-Carboxyl	3.6–3.8
β-Carboxyl (aspartic acid)	≈4.0
γ-Carboxyl (glutamic acid)	≈4.0
Imidazole (histidine)	6.4–7.0
α-Amino	7.4–7.9
Sulfhydryl (cysteine)	≈9.0
ε-Amino (lysine)	9.8–10.6
Phenolic (tyrosine)	8.5–10.9
Guanidino (arginine)	11.9–13.3

Source: Madias NE and Cohen JJ: Acid-base chemistry and buffering. In Cohen JJ and Kassirer JF (eds). *Acid-Base*. Boston, Little, Brown & Co., p. 16, 1982.

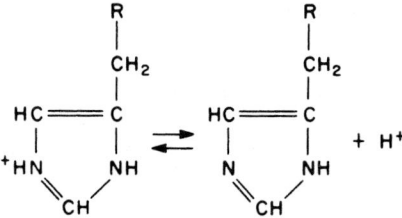

FIGURE 9–3. The imidazole group of histidine. (From Madias NE and Cohen JJ: Acid-base chemistry and buffering. In Cohen JJ and Kassirer JP [eds]: *Acid-Base*. Boston, Little, Brown & Co., p. 16, 1982.)

The buffer value of albumin is 0.12 to 0.14 mmol/g/pH unit, whereas that of globulins is 0 to 0.08 mmol/g/pH unit (van Slyke et al. 1928; van Leeuwen 1964; Madias and Cohen 1982). The difference results from a larger number of histidine (Fig. 9–3) residues in albumin.

The *isoelectric point* (pI) is the pH at which a substance has no tendency to move in an electric field and thus has no net charge. For proteins, this means that the sum of the charges on the negative side groups (e.g., R–COO$^-$) equals the sum of the charges on the positive side groups (e.g., R–NH$_3^+$). At physiologic pH (7.4), plasma proteins are polyanions because their isoelectric points range from 5.1 to 5.7. The net negative charge on plasma proteins in mEq/L can be calculated as (Madias and Cohen 1982)

$$[Pr] \times \beta \times (pH - pI)$$

where [Pr] is the concentration of plasma proteins in grams per liter, β is the buffer value of plasma proteins in millimoles per gram per pH unit, pH is the extracellular fluid pH, and pI is the isoelectric point of plasma proteins. Using this formula, it can be calculated that, at a normal plasma protein concentration of 7 g/dL, average buffer value of 0.1 mmol/g/pH unit, and pI range of 5.1 to 5.7, plasma proteins contribute 12 to 16 mEq/L of negative charge. In dogs, the mean contribution of charge by plasma proteins was estimated to be just over 16 mEq/L (Zweens et al. 1977).

Phosphates as Buffers

The most important intracellular buffers are proteins and inorganic and organic (e.g., ATP, ADP, 2,3-diphosphoglycerate, etc.) phosphates. The pK_a value for $H_2PO_4^-$ is 6.8 and pK_a values for organic phosphates range from 6.0 to 7.5. Inorganic phosphate is a more important buffer intracellularly, where its concentration is high (approximately 40 mEq/L in skeletal muscle cells), and less important in extracellular fluid, where its concentration is much lower (approximately 2 mEq/L). Inorganic phosphate is an important buffer in urine because the range of pH in tubular fluid (6.0–7.0) includes the pK_a of the Na_2HPO_4/NaH_2PO_4 system (6.8). This buffer pair functions in the excretion of *titratable acidity* in urine (see section on titratable acidity later in this chapter).

▶ Physiologic Lines of Defense in Acid-Base Disturbances

An overview of the body buffer response is provided by contrasting the body's response to a nonvolatile, or fixed, acid (e.g., HCl) and its response to the volatile acid CO_2. The hydrogen ions from a fixed acid load immediately titrate bicarbonate ions in extracellular fluid and then titrate intracellular buffers (e.g., proteins, phosphates). This physicochemical response occurs within minutes and protects extracellular fluid pH. Alveolar ventilation is stimulated and P_{CO_2} is decreased to below normal. This response, which begins immediately and is complete within hours, further minimizes the change in pH because the ratio of HCO_3^- to P_{CO_2} is normalized. Finally, the kidneys regenerate titrated HCO_3^-, pH increases, alveolar ventilation decreases, and P_{CO_2} returns to normal. The renal response begins within hours but requires 2 to 5 days to reach maximal effectiveness.

The volatile acid CO_2 cannot be buffered by HCO_3^-, and the hydrogen ions resulting from the dissociation of carbonic acid must titrate intracellular buffers, such as proteins (especially hemoglobin in red cells) and phosphates. Renal adaptation is characterized by increased HCO_3^- reabsorption and net acid excretion, mechanisms that require 2 to 5 days to achieve maximal effectiveness. The buffer response of the body to the primary acid base disorders is considered in more depth in the chapters on those disorders (Chapters 10 and 11).

▶ Terminology

The terms *acidosis* and *alkalosis* refer to the pathophysiologic processes that cause net accumulation of acid or alkali in the body. The terms *acidemia* and *alkalemia* refer specifically to the pH of extracellular fluid. In *acidemia* the extracellular fluid pH is lower than normal and the [H^+] higher than normal. In *alkalemia* the extracellular fluid pH is higher than normal and the [H^+] lower than normal. The distinction between these terms is important. For example, a patient with chronic respiratory alkalosis may have a blood pH within the normal range because of effective renal compensation in this setting. Such a patient has *alkalosis* but does not have *alkalemia*. Patients with *mixed* acid-base disturbances can have blood pH values within the normal range as a result of the presence of two counterbalancing acid-base disturbances (see following section on simple and mixed acid-base disorders).

▶ Primary Acid-Base Disturbances

Acidosis and *alkalosis* can each be of *metabolic* or *respiratory* origin and, as a result, there are four *primary* acid base disturbances: *metabolic acidosis, respiratory acidosis, metabolic alkalosis,* and *respiratory alkalosis*. The *metabolic* disturbances refer to a net excess or deficit of *nonvolatile*, or *fixed* acid, whereas the *respiratory* disturbances refer to the net excess or deficit of *volatile* acid (dissolved CO_2).

Metabolic acidosis is characterized by a decreased plasma HCO_3^- concentration and decreased pH (increased [H^+]) caused by either HCO_3^- loss or buffering of a noncarbonic (nonvolatile or fixed) acid. *Metabolic alkalosis* is characterized by an increased plasma HCO_3^-

TABLE 9-4. Characteristics of Primary Acid-Base Disturbances

Disorder	pH	[H^+]	Primary Disturbance	Compensatory Response
Metabolic acidosis	↓	↑	↓ [HCO_3^-]	↓ P_{CO_2}
Metabolic alkalosis	↑	↓	↑ [HCO_3^-]	↑ P_{CO_2}
Respiratory acidosis	↓	↑	↑ P_{CO_2}	↑ [HCO_3^-]
Respiratory alkalosis	↑	↓	↓ P_{CO_2}	↓ [HCO_3^-]

Source: Rose BD: *Clinical Physiology of Acid-Base and Electrolyte Disorders.* 3rd ed. New York, McGraw-Hill, p. 470, 1989, with permission of the McGraw-Hill Companies.

concentration and increased pH (decreased [H^+]), usually caused by a disproportionate loss of chloride ions from the body (i.e., loss of fluid with a chloride concentration greater than that of extracellular fluid) or hypoalbuminemia (because albumin is a weak acid). In the absence of volume depletion or renal dysfunction, it is extremely difficult to produce metabolic alkalosis by administration of alkali. *Respiratory acidosis* is characterized by increased P_{CO_2} (hypercapnia) caused by alveolar hypoventilation. *Respiratory alkalosis* is characterized by decreased P_{CO_2} caused by alveolar hyperventilation (hypocapnia). In one study, metabolic acidosis was the most common acid-base disturbance encountered in dogs (Cornelius and Rawlings 1981).

Each *primary* metabolic or respiratory acid-base disturbance is accompanied by a *secondary*, or *adaptive*, change in the opposing component of the system (Table 9–4). The adaptive response involves the component opposite the one disturbed and returns the pH of the system toward but not completely to normal. Overcompensation does not occur. For example, metabolic acidosis is accompanied by a secondary or adaptive respiratory alkalosis. Respiratory acidosis is accompanied by a secondary or adaptive metabolic alkalosis.

▶ Simple and Mixed Acid-Base Disorders

An acid-base disorder is said to be *simple* if it is limited to the *primary* disorder and the *expected* secondary, or adaptive, response. The magnitude of the *expected* responses is considered in detail in the chapters devoted to the *primary* acid-base disorders (Chapters 10 and 11). A *mixed* acid-base disorder is one that is characterized by the presence of at least two separate primary acid-base abnormalities occurring in the same patient. A *mixed* acid-base disorder should be suspected whenever the secondary, or adaptive, response exceeds or falls short of that expected. In dogs, for example, the expected response to metabolic acidosis is a 0.7 mm Hg decrease in P_{CO_2} for each 1.0 mEq/L decrement in plasma HCO_3^- concentration caused by metabolic acidosis (see Chapter 10 for more details).

Consider a dog with these normal blood gas values: pH 7.39, [H^+] = 41 nEq/L, [HCO_3^-] = 21 mEq/L, and P_{CO_2} = 36 mm Hg. This dog becomes ill and is observed to have the following blood gas values: pH 7.22,

$[H^+] = 60$ nEq/L, $[HCO_3^-] = 14$ mEq/L, and $P_{CO_2} = 35$ mm Hg. If the dog had a *simple* metabolic acidosis, using the rule of thumb described before, we would have expected the following results: pH 7.27, $[H^+] = 53$ nEq/L, $[HCO_3^-] = 14$ mEq/L, and $P_{CO_2} = 31$ mm Hg. Thus, the dog has a *mixed* acid-base disorder characterized by both metabolic and respiratory acidoses.

Consider a patient with the following blood gas values: pH 7.40, $[H^+] = 40$ nEq/L, $[HCO_3^-] = 31$ mEq/L, and $P_{CO_2} = 51$ mm Hg. This patient is neither *alkalemic* nor *acidemic* because blood pH is 7.40 but, on the basis of the P_{CO_2} and $[HCO_3^-]$, the patient is not normal. This patient has a *mixed* disorder characterized by metabolic alkalosis and respiratory acidosis. The two disorders have counterbalancing effects, resulting in a normal pH. Mixed acid-base disorders are considered in detail in Chapter 12.

▶ Compensatory Responses for Primary Acid-Base Disturbances

The guidelines for secondary or adaptive responses are listed in Table 9–5 for reference. Note that there are single rules of thumb for each of the *metabolic* acid-base disorders but two rules of thumb (one each for acute and chronic disorders) for the *respiratory* acid-base disorders. This is a consequence of the fact that the adaptive respiratory response to metabolic disorders begins immediately and is complete within hours. On the other hand, the response to respiratory disorders occurs in two phases. In the first phase, there is immediate titration of predominantly intracellular nonbicarbonate buffers resulting in an initial change in plasma HCO_3^- concentration. The second phase is carried out by the kidneys and is characterized by alterations in net acid excretion and bicarbonate reabsorption. This response begins within hours but takes 2 to 5 days to achieve maximal effectiveness. Thus, there are two expected compensatory responses: acute (<24 h) and chronic (>48 h). One caution about rules of thumb is that they define the *average* response and not 95% confidence intervals. Acid-base maps depict 95% confidence intervals and, although more awkward to use, allow the clinician to consider normal variation in response (Fig. 9–4). Thus, a patient should be considered to have a mixed disorder only when the blood gas value in question deviates considerably from the calculated expected value. Guidelines for establishing a diagnosis of mixed acid-base disorder are discussed in Chapter 12.

▶ Measurement of Blood Gases

Most blood gas analyzers measure pH and P_{CO_2}. The HCO_3^- concentration is calculated. *Total CO_2 content* is determined by adding a strong acid to plasma or serum and measuring the amount of CO_2 produced according to the following reaction:

$$H^+ + HCO_3^- \rightleftarrows H_2CO_3 \rightleftarrows CO_2 + H_2O$$

The term *total CO_2 content* refers to the fact that this method includes both dissolved CO_2 and HCO_3^- present in the sample. As a result, total CO_2 content is greater than HCO_3^- concentration in normal individuals by approximately 1 to 2 mEq/L:

$$\begin{aligned} CO_{2\text{diss}} + HCO_3^- &= 0.0301 P_{CO_2} + HCO_3^- \\ &= 0.0301(40) + 24 \\ &= 25.2 \text{ mEq/L} \end{aligned}$$

If a sample to be analyzed for total CO_2 content is handled aerobically, the dissolved CO_2 is released to the atmosphere and the value obtained is approximately equal to the HCO_3^- concentration.

Total CO_2 concentrations determined by automated chemistry analysis may differ substanstially from those obtained by standard blood gas analysis. In one study of normal dogs and cats, factors implicated in this discrepancy included underfilling of blood collection tubes, delays between sampling and analysis, and freshness of laboratory reagents (James et al. 1997). According to the results of this study, values for total CO_2 obtained by routine blood gas analysis may be as much as 5 mmol/L higher than those obtained by automated analysis. Another study comparing total CO_2 measurement by three different methods (radiometer blood gas analyzer, Coulter DACOS analyzer, and Kodak Ektachem DTE analyzer) found lower than expected agreement among the different methods of analysis (Kilborn et al. 1995). In this study, sample storage for 7 h resulted in a decrease of approximately 2 mmol/L in total CO_2 concentration.

CO_2 combining power is the total CO_2 content of a plasma sample that has been equilibrated in vitro at 37°C with CO_2 at a partial pressure of 40 mm Hg. This method overestimates total CO_2 content when the patient's P_{CO_2} is < 40 mm Hg and underestimates total CO_2 content when the patient's P_{CO_2} is > 40 mm Hg. It is no longer commonly used in clinical medicine.

Standard bicarbonate is the concentration of bicarbonate in the plasma of fully oxygenated whole blood

TABLE 9–5. **Expected Renal and Respiratory Compensations to Primary Acid-Base Disorders in Dogs**

Disorder	Primary Change	Compensatory Response
Metabolic acidosis	↓ $[HCO_3^-]$	0.7 mm Hg decrement in P_{CO_2} for each 1 mEq/L decrement in $[HCO_3^-]$
Metabolic alkalosis	↑ $[HCO_3^-]$	0.7 mm Hg increment in P_{CO_2} for each 1 mEq/L increment in $[HCO_3^-]$
Acute respiratory acidosis	↑ P_{CO_2}	1.5 mEq/L increment in $[HCO_3^-]$ for each 10 mm Hg increment in P_{CO_2}
Chronic respiratory acidosis	↑ P_{CO_2}	3.5 mEq/L increment in $[HCO_3^-]$ for each 10 mm Hg increment in P_{CO_2}
Acute respiratory alkalosis	↓ P_{CO_2}	2.5 mEq/L decrement in $[HCO_3^-]$ for each 10 mm Hg decrement in P_{CO_2}
Chronic respiratory alkalosis	↓ P_{CO_2}	5.5 mEq/L decrement in $[HCO_3^-]$ for each 10 mm Hg decrement in P_{CO_2}

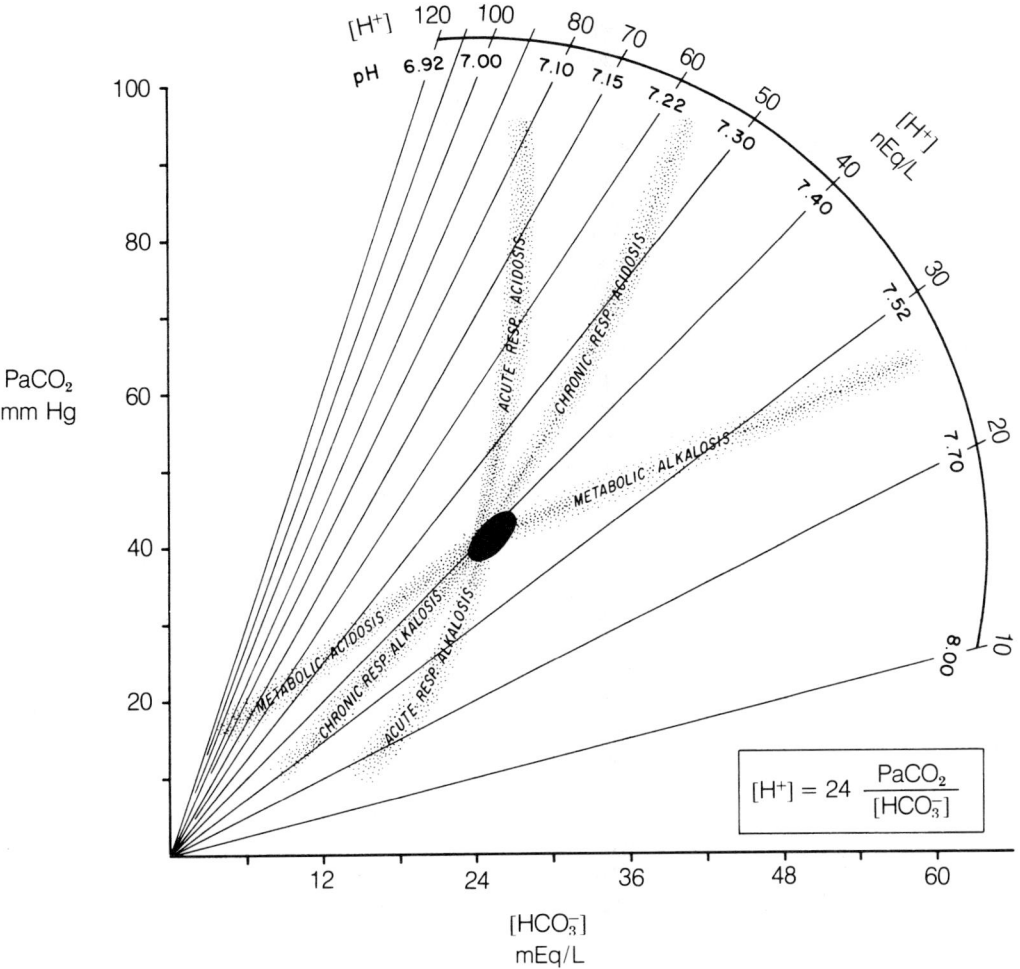

FIGURE 9–4. Acid-base map or template. The shaded areas exemplify the ranges of P_{aCO_2}-bicarbonate relationships characteristic of graded degrees of simple acid-base disorders. (From Harrington JT, Cohen JJ, and Kassirer JP: Mixed acid-base disturbances. In Cohen JJ and Kassirer JP [eds]: *Acid-Base*. Boston, Little, Brown & Co., p. 379, 1982.)

after equilibration with CO_2 at a partial pressure of 40 mm Hg at 37°C. The *base excess* (BE) is the amount of strong acid or base required to titrate 1 L of blood to pH 7.40 at 37°C while P_{CO_2} is held constant at 40 mm Hg (Astrup et al. 1960; Siggaard-Andersen et al. 1960; Astrup 1961). It is usually derived from the Siggaard-Andersen alignment nomogram using measurements of pH, P_{CO_2}, and hematocrit. *Base excess* is changed only by nonvolatile, or fixed, acids and thus is considered to reflect metabolic acid-base disturbances. In general, a negative value for *base excess* (i.e., a *base deficit*) indicates metabolic acidosis, whereas a positive value indicates metabolic alkalosis.

One problem with the concept of standard bicarbonate is the assumption that the CO_2 titration curve of a whole-blood sample is similar to that of the intact organism. This is not true, because in the isolated blood sample all of the buffering of the CO_2 equilibrated with the sample is done by the hemoglobin and other nonbicarbonate buffers in the sample, and the HCO_3^- generated can be distributed only within that sample. In vivo, however, other intracellular buffers are involved, the HCO_3^- produced has a larger volume of distribution, and the observed increase in HCO_3^- concentration would be less (Cohen et al. 1964) (Fig. 9–5). Another problem with standard bicarbonate and base excess determinations is that abnormalities of these values do not necessarily imply the presence of a primary metabolic acid-base disturbance. Rather, the change in HCO_3^- concentration may represent the normal adaptive change resulting from renal compensation for a respiratory acid-base disturbance. Debate continues about whether or not standard bicarbonate and base excess are any more useful than bicarbonate in the evaluation of acid-base disturbances (Schwartz and Relman 1963; Severinghaus 1993). Regardless of the approach used, all of the aids devised to facilitate interpretation of blood gas data are merely graphic representations of the classic Henderson-Hasselbalch equation and there is no substitute for a thorough understanding of the underlying principles of acid-base physiology (Valtin and Gennari 1987).

Whole-blood buffer base is the sum of the concentrations of all buffer anions contained in whole blood and includes HCO_3^-, hemoglobin, plasma proteins, phosphates, and any other potential buffer anions (Singer and Hastings 1948). Its normal value is 40 to 50 mEq/L and is similar to Stewart's *strong ion difference* (Stewart 1981, 1983; Whitehair et al. 1995). Changes in the P_{CO_2} of the

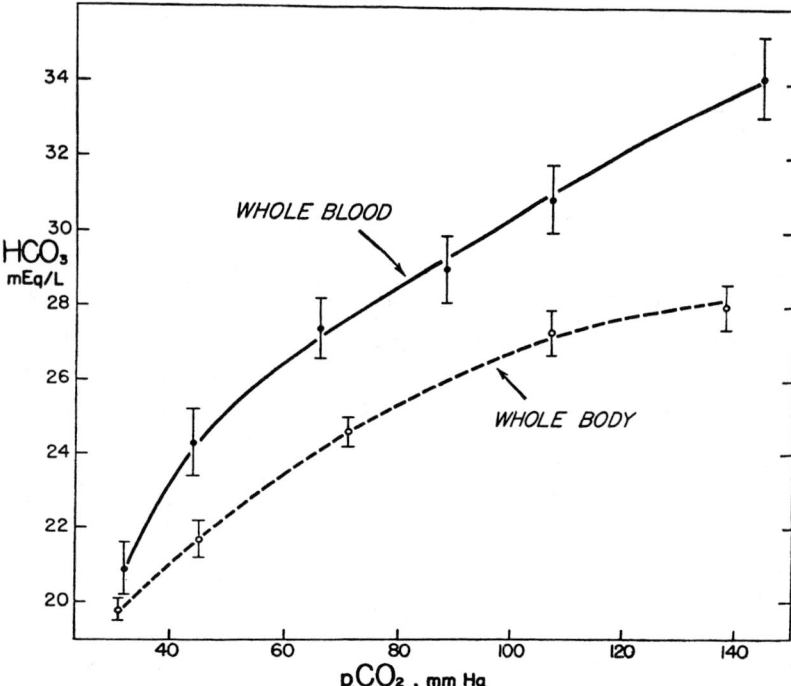

FIGURE 9–5. Comparison of the CO_2 titration curves for whole blood and whole body using data derived from the dog. (Reproduced from the *Journal of Clinical Investigation*, 1964, Vol. 43, p. 783, by copyright permission of the American Society for Clinical Investigation.)

whole-blood sample do not change the value of the *whole-blood buffer base*, because a change in the nonbicarbonate buffers results in a reciprocal change in HCO_3^- concentration. The *whole-body buffer base* decreases with metabolic acidosis and increases with metabolic alkalosis, regardless of changes in Pco_2 in the sample.

The calculations of *standard bicarbonate* and *whole-blood buffer base* were introduced before the concept of whole-body titration was developed (Harrington et al. 1982), and represented an attempt to use in vitro titration of whole-blood samples to separate the respiratory and metabolic components of acid-base disturbances. These methods do not account for other buffering effects in the body (e.g., intracellular proteins other than hemoglobin, intracellular organic phosphates, bone carbonate).

Sample Collection and Handling

Proper collection and handling of samples for blood gas analysis are as important as accurate measurement of pH and Pco_2 by the blood gas analyzer (Haskins 1977a). In small animals, arterial samples are usually taken from the femoral artery. This procedure can be performed in unanesthetized dogs with minimal discomfort and restraint but is difficult in unanesthetized cats. Samples for venous blood gas analysis are usually taken from the jugular vein. Venous stasis and muscular activity, however, can result in accumulation of acid metabolites. Thus, an attempt should be made to obtain a free-flowing venous sample by releasing digital pressure on the vein after venipuncture has been achieved.

For femoral artery samples, the hair over the medial thigh is clipped and the puncture site disinfected. A 3-mL syringe with a 25-gauge needle is coated with a small amount of heparin (1000 U/mL). Enough heparin is drawn into the syringe to coat the interior of the entire barrel and air is expelled, leaving the dead space of the syringe filled with heparin. The dead space of 1- to 5-mL syringes is 0.1 to 0.2 mL, and this volume provides more than enough heparin for anticoagulation (Pruden et al. 1996). Dilution of the sample with heparin should be avoided because it can cause erroneously low values for pH, Pco_2, and HCO_3^- (Haskins 1977b; Hutchison et al. 1983; Pruden et al. 1996).

The dog is restrained in lateral recumbency by an assistant and the rear limb closest to the table extended. The artery is located by palpating the femoral pulse and immobilized beneath the first and second fingers of the operator's free hand. The artery is punctured with the needle directed at an angle approximately perpendicular to the course of the vessel. At least 1.5 mL of blood is withdrawn and the site of puncture manually compressed for 3 to 5 min after needle withdrawal to prevent hematoma formation. If necessary, air bubbles are dislodged by flicking the barrel of the syringe with the index finger and expelling any air from the hub of the syringe. Usually, the needle is inserted into a rubber stopper to prevent exposure of the sample to room air. A tightly fitting cap placed over the hub of the syringe may be superior (Pruden et al. 1996). The syringe is rolled between the palms of the hands to mix the sample.

The Pco_2 of dry room air is extremely low, and the Pco_2 of the blood sample decreases and its pH increases if it is exposed to air (Pruden et al. 1996). The Po_2 of room air is higher than that of arterial or venous blood and the Po_2 of the sample increases if it is exposed to air. The increase is much greater for venous than arterial blood samples. Air bubbles may also cause an increase in

Po_2 and a decrease in Pco_2 if they occupy 10% or more of the sample volume.

Analysis of the sample within 15 to 30 min of collection is desirable. The Pco_2 of a blood sample increases and the pH decreases as the sample is allowed to stand before analysis. The rate of change is much greater at 25°C than at 4°C. These changes in Pco_2 and pH are accompanied by decreased glucose and increased lactate concentrations and are attributed to glycolysis by white cells, red cells, and platelets. Aerobic metabolism by white cells also decreases Po_2. These changes are minimized by cooling the blood sample. Therefore, if the sample cannot be analyzed soon after collection, the syringe should be immersed in a mixture of ice and water. Samples are stable for up to 2 h at 4°C, but Pco_2 begins to increase and pH to decrease after 20 to 30 min at 25°C (Madiedo et al. 1980).

Arterial samples are preferred to venous ones because oxygenation of blood can be evaluated and the sample is not affected by stasis of blood flow and local tissue metabolism. The most conspicuous difference between arterial and venous samples is the difference in Po_2, which reflects oxygenation of blood in the lungs and utilization in the tissues. Conversely, arterial samples may not reflect the acid-base status in peripheral tissues. This may present a problem during cardiopulmonary resuscitation (see Chapter 10). The Pco_2 is slightly higher and the pH slightly lower in venous samples because of local tissue metabolism. Free-flowing capillary blood that has been "arterialized" by warming the skin puncture site is used as an alternative to arterial samples in human medicine.

Capillary blood obtained from the caudal medial ear margin of unanesthetized dogs had blood gas values similar to those of arterial samples and did not require induction of arteriolar vasodilatation by warming ("arterialization") (Rodkey et al. 1978). In a study of cats, arterialized capillary blood was obtained from the cut claw after previously warming the paw (Solter et al. 1988). In this study, mean Po_2 and Pco_2 did not differ from those of arterial blood, but mean pH was significantly higher (7.432 vs. 7.419). Capillary blood is collected directly into a heparinized capillary tube, a small metal "flea" is added for mixing, and the ends of the tube are sealed with clay. During states of peripheral vascular collapse (e.g., hypovolemic shock), capillary blood does not provide meaningful blood gas values for comparison with those of arterial samples (Rodkey et al. 1978; van Sluijs et al. 1983).

Normal Values

Normal blood gas values for dogs and cats should be established by the laboratory performing the analysis. Extreme care must be taken in obtaining blood samples to establish a normal range because hyperventilation related to fear or pain, increased muscular activity related to struggling, and delays during sample transport and analysis may have effects on the resulting normal range. A review of previously published data provided the following guidelines for normal arterial blood gas values in dogs and cats (Haskins 1983):

	Dog	Cat
pH	7.407	7.386
	(7.351–7.463)	(7.310–7.462)
Pco_2 (mm Hg)	36.8 (30.8–42.8)	31.0 (25.2–36.8)
HCO_3^- (mEq/L)	22.2 (18.8–25.6)	18.0 (14.4–21.6)
Po_2 (mm Hg)	92.1 (80.9–103.3)	106.8 (95.4–118.2)

Studies of normal unanesthetized dogs yielded venous blood gas results as follows: pH 7.397 (7.351–7.443), Pco_2 37.4 (33.6–41.2) mm Hg, and HCO_3^- 22.5 (20.8–24.2) mEq/L (Zweens et al. 1977; Rodkey et al. 1978). In one of these studies, venous Po_2 values were reported to be 52.1 (47.9–56.3) mm Hg (Rodkey et al. 1978). Studies of normal unanesthetized cats indicated venous blood gas values as follows: pH 7.343 (7.277–7.409), Pco_2 38.7 (32.7–44.7) mm Hg, and HCO_3^- 20.6 (18.0–23.2) mEq/L (Herbert and Mitchell 1971; Middleton et al. 1981; Chew et al. 1991).

When sampling sites were compared using unanesthetized normal dogs, blood gas data from three different venous sites (jugular vein, pulmonary artery, cephalic vein) were similar, but Pco_2 was higher and pH lower when venous data were compared with results obtained for the carotid artery (Ilkiw et al. 1991). The respiratory compensation for metabolic acidosis in these dogs ranged from 1.1 to 1.3 mm Hg decrement in Pco_2 for each 1 mEq/L decrement in HCO_3^-, whereas the respiratory compensation for metabolic alkalosis ranged from 0.4 to 0.6 mm Hg increment in Pco_2 for each 1 mEq/L increment in HCO_3^- for arterial, mixed venous, and jugular venous samples. The increment was 1.3 mm Hg per 1 mEq/L increment in HCO_3^- for the cephalic samples, which had the highest Pco_2 values, presumably because they were the only samples not collected under free-flowing conditions. Data for the normal dogs in this study are reproduced in Table 9–6.

Aging in human beings has been associated with a decrease in PaO_2 and an increase in the alveolar-to-arterial Po_2 gradient, $P(A - a)O_2$. Mild or no changes in these values were observed in geriatric dogs, and no significant changes in acid-base balance were found in geriatric dogs (King et al. 1992; Aguilera-Tejero et al. 1997).

Interpretation of Blood Gas Data

Correct identification of acid-base disturbances may provide a clue to an underlying primary disease process and aids in determining appropriate therapy for the patient. A routine methodical approach to interpretation of blood gas data facilitates the clinician's approach to the patient. The clinician should try to answer the following four questions:

1. Is an acid-base disturbance present?
2. What is the primary disturbance?
3. Is the secondary, or adaptive, response as expected (i.e., is the disturbance simple or mixed)?
4. What underlying disease process(es) is (are) responsible for the acid-base disturbance(s)?

TABLE 9-6. Blood Gas and Acid-Base Measurements (Mean ± Standard Deviation) in Five Normal Unanesthetized Dogs

Value	Arterial	Mixed Venous	Jugular Venous	Cephalic Venous
pH (U)	7.395 ± 0.028	7.361 ± 0.021	7.352 ± 0.023	7.360 ± 0.022
P_{CO_2} (mm Hg)	36.8 ± 2.7	43.1 ± 3.6	42.1 ± 4.4	43.0 ± 3.2
P_{O_2} (mm Hg)	102.1 ± 6.8	53.1 ± 9.9	55.0 ± 9.6	58.4 ± 8.8
HCO_3^- (mEq/L)	21.4 ± 1.6	23.0 ± 1.6	22.1 ± 2.0	23.0 ± 1.4
T_{CO_2} (mEq/L)	22.4 ± 1.8	24.1 ± 1.7	23.2 ± 2.1	24.1 ± 1.4
BE (mEq/L)	−1.8 ± 1.6	−1.1 ± 1.4	−2.1 ± 1.7	−1.2 ± 1.1
$SHCO_3^-$ (mEq/L)	22.8 ± 1.3	23.0 ± 1.2	22.2 ± 1.3	23.2 ± 1.1

Source: Ilkiw JE, Rose RJ, and Martin ICA: A comparison of simultaneously collected arterial, mixed venous, jugular venous and cephalic venous blood samples in the assessment of blood gas and acid base status in dogs. J Vet Intern Med 5:294, 1991.
Abbreviations: BE, Base excess; $SHCO_3^-$, standard bicarbonate.

The possibility of an acid-base disturbance should be considered when the history (e.g., vomiting, diarrhea) or the pathophysiology of the patient's disease (e.g., renal failure, diabetes mellitus) is suggestive or when abnormalities in total CO_2 or electrolytes (Na^+, K^+, Cl^-) are observed in the biochemical profile. Total CO_2 may be increased as a result of metabolic alkalosis or renal adaptation to respiratory acidosis. Total CO_2 may be decreased as a result of metabolic acidosis or renal adaptation to respiratory alkalosis. Thus, the acid-base disturbance cannot be classified on the basis of the total CO_2 concentration alone. Objective physical findings suggestive of an acid-base disturbance (e.g., hyperventilation) are unreliable as indicators of acid-base disturbances and are often not present. Blood gas analysis is required to identify and classify acid-base disorders conclusively.

The clinician should first consider the patient's blood pH. Evaluation of pH often provides the answer to the question of whether or not an acid-base disturbance is present. If the pH is outside the normal range, an acid-base disturbance is present. If the pH is within the normal range, an acid-base disturbance may or may not be present. If the patient is acidemic and plasma HCO_3^- concentration is decreased, metabolic acidosis is present. If the patient is acidemic and P_{CO_2} is increased, respiratory acidosis is present. If the patient is alkalemic and plasma HCO_3^- concentration is increased, metabolic alkalosis is present. If the patient is alkalemic and P_{CO_2} is decreased, respiratory alkalosis is present. These relationships are summarized in Table 9–4. Complicating acid-base disturbances that would alter pH in the same direction as the primary disturbance, however, cannot be ruled out at this point in the evaluation.

The next step is to calculate the expected compensatory response in the opposing component of the system (e.g., respiratory alkalosis as compensation for metabolic acidosis, metabolic alkalosis as compensation for respiratory acidosis) using the rules of thumb listed in Table 9–5. If the patient's secondary or adaptive response in the compensating component of the system falls within the expected range, a simple acid-base disturbance is probably present. If the adaptive response falls outside the expected range, a mixed disorder may be present.

Considering the magnitude of change in pH can help in assessment of mixed disorders. This can be seen by consideration of the Henderson equation:

$$[H^+] = \frac{24 P_{CO_2}}{[HCO_3^-]}$$

The effect on extracellular pH of a mixed disorder is minimized if the disorders change P_{CO_2} and HCO_3^- in the same direction (e.g., respiratory acidosis and metabolic alkalosis) and is maximized if the disorders change P_{CO_2} and HCO_3^- in opposite directions (e.g., respiratory acidosis and metabolic acidosis). In the former instance, blood pH may remain within the normal range, whereas in the latter instance blood pH is markedly abnormal. Mixed acid-base disorders are discussed in detail in Chapter 12.

Once the clinician has classified the disturbance as simple or mixed and has defined the type of disturbance(s) present, an attempt should be made to determine whether the acid-base disturbance(s) is (are) compatible with the patient's history and clinical findings. Examples include metabolic acidosis in renal failure, acute diarrhea, ethylene glycol ingestion, or diabetic ketoacidosis; respiratory acidosis in advanced pulmonary disease; metabolic alkalosis in vomiting of stomach contents or loop diuretic administration; and respiratory alkalosis in pulmonary disease or sepsis. The original interpretation of the blood gas data must be questioned if the acid-base disturbance does not fit the patient's history, clinical findings, and other laboratory data. Diagnostic difficulties are most likely in mild acid-base disturbances with blood gas results still within the normal range, in mixed disturbances with counterbalancing components that result in a pH within the normal range, and in acute, rapidly changing disorders without adequate time for achievement of a compensated steady state.

▶ Anion Gap

The major cations of extracellular fluid are sodium, potassium, calcium, and magnesium; the major anions are chloride, bicarbonate, plasma proteins, organic acid anions (including lactate), phosphate, and sulfate. The approximate charge contributions of these ions in dogs and cats are listed in Table 9–7. Automated clinical chem-

TABLE 9–7. **Approximate Concentrations of Cations and Anions in Plasma in Normal Dogs and Cats (mEq/L)**

Cations	Dog	Cat	Anions	Dog	Cat
Sodium	145	155	Chloride	110	120
Potassium	4	4	Bicarbonate	21	21
Calcium	5	5	Phosphate	2	2
Magnesium	2	2	Sulfate	2	2
Trace elements	1	1	Lactate	2	2
			Other organic acids	4	4
			Protein	16	16
Total:	157	167		157	167

istry analyzers provide values for serum sodium, potassium, chloride, and total CO_2 concentrations. Thus, the sum of the concentrations of commonly measured cations exceeds the sum of the concentrations of commonly measured anions, and the difference has been called the *anion gap* (Emmett and Narins 1977; Oh and Carrol 1977):

$$(Na^+ + K^+) - (Cl^- + HCO_3^-)$$

The serum concentration of potassium varies little and its charge contribution is small compared with that of sodium. Therefore, the anion gap is often defined as

$$Na^+ - (Cl^- + HCO_3^-)$$

From several reported studies, the normal anion gap calculated as $(Na^+ + K^+) - (Cl^- + HCO_3^-)$ is approximately 12 to 24 mEq/L in dogs (Bleich et al. 1964; Madias et al. 1977, 1979a, 1984; Adrogue et al. 1978; Shull 1978; Polzin et al. 1982) and 13 to 27 mEq/L in cats (Atkins et al. 1985; Ching et al. 1989; Christopher et al. 1990; Chew et al. 1991). In one study, the anion gap was significantly increased in aged dogs compared with young dogs (16.7 ± 0.7 vs. 14.3 ± 0.8 mEq/L). The increase in anion gap was attributed to a slight decrease in serum chloride concentration that was balanced by an increase in the net negative charge associated with plasma proteins and phosphate (Aguilera-Tejero et al. 1997).

In reality, there is no anion gap because the law of electroneutrality must always be satisfied. This can be indicated by including terms for unmeasured cations (UC) and unmeasured anions (UA) as follows:

$$Na^+ + K^+ + UC = Cl^- + HCO_3^- + UA$$
$$UA - UC = (Na^+ + K^+) - (Cl^- + HCO_3^-)$$

Thus, the anion gap is the difference between unmeasured anions and unmeasured cations and may be affected by changes in the concentration of either component. The magnitude of change in the concentration of any of the unmeasured cations (e.g., calcium, magnesium) necessary to cause an appreciable change in the anion gap, however, would probably be incompatible with life (Gabow 1985). As a result, most discussions of the anion gap focus on changes in unmeasured anions.

Normally, plasma proteins contribute approximately two-thirds of unmeasured anion charge in mEq/L (Madias et al. 1979b). Albumin contributes 2.0 to 2.8 mEq/L for each g/dL and globulins 1.3 to 1.9 mEq/L for each g/dL (Gabow 1985). For each 0.1 U increment in pH, there is an approximate 0.1 mEq/L increase in negative charge on plasma proteins (van Slyke et al. 1928; van Leeuwen 1964; Madias et al. 1979b; Gabow 1985).

Increases in anion gap are much more common than decreases, and the concept of anion gap is usually used as an aid in differentiating the causes of metabolic acidosis (see Chapter 10). In organic acidoses (e.g., diabetic ketoacidosis, lactic acidosis), HCO_3^- is titrated by H^+ ions from organic acids. Theoretically, the extracellular fluid HCO_3^- concentration should fall in reciprocal fashion with the increase in concentration of organic acid anions and the serum chloride concentration should not change (so-called normochloremic metabolic acidosis). The anion gap in this setting should increase proportionately. In practice, however, the decrement in HCO_3^- concentration rarely equals the increment in anion gap for several reasons. For example, buffers other than HCO_3^- are titrated by hydrogen ions from the organic acid, the volume of distribution of the organic anion may differ from that of HCO_3^-, and the prevailing concentration of the organic anion in extracellular fluid is affected by its urinary excretion. Furthermore, the patient's HCO_3^- concentration and anion gap before illness are usually not known, and the changes in HCO_3^- concentration and anion gap must by necessity be calculated from available normal values.

The anion gap may be useful in identifying mixed acid-base disturbances. Consider, for example, a mixed disturbance characterized by metabolic alkalosis and lactic acidosis (e.g., chronic vomiting severe enough to have caused hypotension and impaired tissue perfusion). The pH in such a setting could be normal if HCl loss from the stomach was exactly counterbalanced by accumulation of lactic acid from anaerobic metabolism. A markedly increased anion gap suggests the presence of the complicating organic acidosis. The usefulness of the anion gap in this situation is hampered by the fact that alkalemia itself can cause an increase in the anion gap by several mechanisms (Madias et al. 1979b; Gabow 1985). Alkalemia results in loss of protons from plasma proteins and an increase in their net negative charge. Hemoconcentration related to volume depletion increases the concentration of plasma proteins and the concentration of their net negative charge. Finally, alkalemia increases lactic acid generation by stimulating phosphofructokinase. The net effect is an increase in the concentration of unmeasured anions (lactate and anionic plasma proteins) and an increase in anion gap. The utility of the anion gap concept in considered further in Chapter 12.

Acidosis resulting from administration of NH_4Cl causes a decrease in HCO_3^- concentration because hydrogen ions are released during ureagenesis. There is a reciprocal increase in serum chloride concentration and, as a result, there is no change in the anion gap (so-called hyperchloremic metabolic acidosis). Gastrointestinal loss of HCO_3^- has the same end result because the kidney conserves NaCl in response to volume depletion. The use of the anion gap in the classification of metabolic acidosis is considered further in Chapter 10.

A decreased anion gap may be observed in immunoglobin G (IgG) multiple myeloma because the pI of IgG paraproteins is greater than 7.4. Hypoalbuminemia or dilution of plasma proteins by crystalloid infusion can decrease the anion gap by decreasing the concentration of net negative charge associated with plasma proteins. Hypoalbuminemia may be the most common cause of a decreased anion gap, and each 1.0 g/dL decrease in albumin is associated with an approximately 2.4 to 3.0 mEq/L decrease in anion gap (Gabow 1985; McAuliffe et al. 1986).

▶ Nontraditional Approach to Acid-Base Evaluation

The traditional approach to acid-base evaluation focuses on the relationship between pH, HCO_3^-, and $P{CO_2}$ as described by the Henderson-Hasselbalch equation. In this approach, pH is shown to be a function of HCO_3^- concentration and $P{CO_2}$. The $P{CO_2}$ is viewed as the *respiratory* component and is determined by alveolar ventilation, whereas the HCO_3^- concentration is considered the *metabolic* (or nonrespiratory) component and is regulated by the kidneys. This approach may lead to the impression that $P{CO_2}$ and HCO_3^- are independent variables. In reality, only $P{CO_2}$ is independent. When a primary increase in $P{CO_2}$ occurs, the hydrogen ions that are produced by dissociation of H_2CO_3 are buffered by proteins (notably hemoglobin) and the HCO_3^- concentration increases secondarily. Furthermore, an understanding of the effects of changes in other electrolytes (e.g., Na^+, K^+, Cl^-) and plasma proteins on acid-base balance is not facilitated by the traditional approach. The nontraditional approach allows the clinician to better understand the complexity of the acid-base disturbances in some patients.

Stewart formulated a model of acid-base chemistry in biologic systems governed by three physical laws: (1) maintenance of electroneutrality; (2) satisfaction of dissociation equilibria for incompletely dissociated solutes; and (3) conservation of mass (Stewart 1981, 1983). The equations that satisfy these laws were solved simultaneously to identify variables that control $[H^+]$. Independent variables are those that may be altered from outside the system, whereas dependent variables are internal to the system and change only in response to changes in independent variables. Simultaneous solution of Stewart's equations identified three independent variables: strong ion difference (SID), the total concentration of weak acid ($HA + A^-$) or $[A_{tot}]$, and $P{CO_2}$.

The SID changes if the difference between the sum of strong cations and the sum of strong anions changes. Ions are considered strong if they are almost completely dissociated at the pH of body fluids. The strong cations consist of sodium, potassium, calcium, and magnesium. Of these, only Na^+ is present at high enough concentration in extracellular fluid that a change in its concentration is likely to have a substantial effect on SID. The strong anions consist of chloride and several other anions that are not routinely measured clinically and collectively are referred to as *unmeasured* strong anions (e.g., lactate, acetoacetate, β-hydroxybutyrate, sulfate). Chloride and some unmeasured strong anions can be sufficiently altered in certain disease states to have a substantial effect on SID. The average concentrations of all cations and anions in the plasma of normal dogs and cats are presented in Table 9–7.

The weak anions in extracellular fluid are HCO_3^-, plasma proteins, and phosphate. Of these, plasma proteins and phosphate constitute the independent variable A_{tot}, whereas HCO_3^- is a dependent variable. Hypoproteinemia has been shown to be associated with metabolic alkalosis in critically ill human patients in whom a decrease in serum albumin concentration of 1 g/dL caused an increase in standard base excess of +3.7 mEq/L (McAuliffe et al. 1986). Serum phosphorus concentration (normally approximately 2 mEq/L) cannot decrease enough to cause alkalosis, but hyperphosphatemia in patients with renal failure can make a substantial contribution to A_{tot} and metabolic acidosis.

Fencl and Leith (Fencl and Rossing 1989; Leith 1991; Fencl and Leith 1993) applied Stewart's concepts to human patients by characterizing four components of base excess: changes in free water (as indicated by changes in serum sodium concentration), abnormalities of chloride (after correcting serum chloride concentration for the effect of changes in free water), changes in serum albumin concentration, and unmeasured anions. The portion of the base excess related to unmeasured anions was calculated by subtracting the effects of the other three components from the total base excess. Phosphate was not considered separately and remained a portion of the unmeasured anion component. Consequently, hyperphosphatemic patients with renal failure have high calculated values for unmeasured anions because of the presence of phosphate. Formulas for using this approach are as follows:

$$\Delta BE \text{ (free water)} = z(\text{measured } [Na^+] - \text{normal } [Na^+])$$

where z is estimated as 0.25 for dogs and 0.22 for cats (de Morais 1992)

$$\Delta BE \text{ (chloride)} = \text{normal } [Cl^-] \text{ for species} - \text{corrected } [Cl^-]$$

where the $[Cl^-]$ is corrected for the effects of water excess or deficit by the formula $[Cl^-]$ corrected = $[Cl^-]$ measured × (normal $[Na^+]$/measured $[Na^+]$)

$$\Delta BE \text{ (albumin)} = 3.7([\text{albumin}] \text{ normal} - [\text{albumin}] \text{ measured})$$

$$\Delta BE \text{ (unmeasured anions)} = \Delta BE \text{ (total)} - \Delta BE \text{ (free water)} - \Delta BE \text{ (chloride)} - \Delta BE \text{ (albumin)}$$

This method has been successfully applied in veterinary medicine to understand the genesis of complex acid-base disorders in small and large animals (Whitehair et al. 1995). The ΔBE (unmeasured anions) estimated in human patients using these calculations has shown very good agreement with the estimate of unidentified anions obtained using Stewart's original formula (Gifix et al. 1993).

Figge and colleagues (1992) modified Stewart's approach to increase the accuracy of the unmeasured anion calculation and account separately for phosphate. The modified approach calculates an *apparent* SID using the concentrations of all strong ions that can be measured in clinical laboratories:

Apparent SID:
$$Na^+ + K^+ + Ca^{+2} + Mg^{+2} - Cl^-$$
(all concentrations in mEq/L)

Extracellular fluid, however, also contains several other strong anions that are not routinely measured (e.g., lactate, acetoacetate, β-hydroxybutyrate, sulfate). Thus, *effective* SID is defined as

Effective SID:
$$Na^+ + K^+ + Ca^{+2} + Mg^{+2} - Cl^- - XA^-$$
(all concentrations in mEq/L)

where XA^- refers to the unmeasured strong anions and

$$XA^- = SID_{apparent} - SID_{effective}$$

The *effective* SID includes HCO_3^-, proteins, and phosphate. The value for HCO_3^- is obtained from the biochemical profile or (preferably) blood gas analysis and the formulas for calculating the contributions of proteins and phosphate are (Figge et al. 1992):

$$\text{Proteins (mEq/L)} = 10 \times \text{serum albumin} \times (0.123 \times pH - 0.631)$$

$$\text{Phosphate (mEq/L)} = \text{serum phosphate (mmol/L)} \times (0.309 \times pH - 0.469)$$

The latter approach more accurately estimates the charge contribution of unmeasured strong anions but unfortunately requires data that are not typically available from a serum biochemical profile (e.g., serum magnesium concentration, pH).

In summary, the apparent SID is composed of HCO_3^-, proteins, phosphate, and unmeasured strong anions, whereas the effective SID includes HCO_3^-, proteins, and phosphate. The apparent SID is the same as the quantity buffer base originally described by Singer and Hastings (1948). The anion gap includes proteins, phosphate, and unmeasured strong anions, and its value is affected by changes in serum albumin concentration and hyperphosphatemia. The ΔBE (unmeasured anions) in the unmodified Stewart approach includes phosphate and unmeasured strong anions.

The nontraditional approach defines a primary acid-base disturbance as a change in one or more of the independent variables ([SID], P_{CO_2}, [A_{tot}]). Compensatory changes occur in response to the primary disturbance (Fencl and Rossing 1989; de Morais 1992). For example, a primary alteration in [SID] results in a secondary change in P_{CO_2} brought about by a modification of alveolar ventilation. A primary alteration in P_{CO_2} is accompanied by a secondary change in [SID] brought about by modifications in renal excretion of chloride relative to sodium. The three main ways in which [SID] may change are changes in the water content of plasma, changes in [Cl^-]$_{corrected}$, and changes in the concentration of unmeasured strong anions (Table 9–8). Changes in A_{tot} do not occur in response to primary acid-base disturbances because albumin synthesis by the liver arises primarily as a result of the need to maintain normal plasma oncotic pressure. Changes in A_{tot} can, however, affect the patient's acid-base status (e.g., hypoproteinemic alkalosis).

TABLE 9–8. Causes of Primary Acid-Base Disturbances Classified According to the Nontraditional Approach

Respiratory disturbances
  Abnormalities of P_{CO_2}
    Increased: respiratory acidosis
    Decreased: respiratory alkalosis
Nonrespiratory disturbances
  Abnormalities of [A_{tot}]
    Decreased: hypoproteinemic alkalosis
    Increased: hyperproteinemic acidosis; hyperphosphatemic acidosis
  Abnormalities of [SID]
    Free-water abnormalities
      Deficit: contraction (concentration) alkalosis
      Excess: expansion acidosis
    Isonatremic chloride abnormalities
      Decreased: hypochloremic alkalosis
      Increased: hyperchloremic acidosis
    Isonatremic organic acid abnormalities
      Increased: organic acidosis

From de Morais HSA: A non-traditional approach to acid-base disorders. In DiBartola SP (ed): *Fluid Therapy in Small Animal Practice*. Philadelphia, WB Saunders Co., 1992, p. 301.

The Stewart approach as modified by Fencl and Figge extends the traditional assessment of acid-base disturbances by allowing the clinician to evaluate the effects of alterations in plasma proteins, free water, chloride, and phosphate on the patient's acid-base status (see Table 9–8). This method is most helpful in the assessment of patients with mixed metabolic disorders. If the nontraditional approach seems cumbersome, the clinician should evaluate the anion gap and a rough estimate of the apparent SID calculated simply as [Na^+] − [Cl^-] (normally 32–40 mEq/L). If the anion gap is increased and the estimated apparent SID ([Na^+] − [Cl^-]) decreased, the concurrent presence of hyperchloremic metabolic acidosis and unmeasured strong anion acidosis (e.g., lactic acidosis, ketoacidosis) should be considered. If the anion gap is high and the estimated apparent SID ([Na^+] − [Cl^-]) is also high, the presence of metabolic alkalosis and unmeasured strong anion acidosis should be considered. If the anion gap is increased and the estimated apparent SID ([Na^+] − [Cl^-]) is normal, an unmeasured strong anion acidosis is probably present (Table 9–9).

The Stewart method for evaluation of acid-base disorders remains controversial and has been subject to criticism because of some of the assumptions required by the original model, the complex calculations required, and uncertainty about the value of clinical application (Cameron 1989; Siggaard-Andersen and Fogh-Andersen 1995; Schlichtig 1997). The nontraditional approach has been applied in veterinary medicine (de Morais 1992; de Morais and Muir 1995; Whitehair et al. 1995; Russell et al. 1996) but difficulties remain, and the method requires certain assumptions and simplifications for practical application. The limitations of the model include the error that arises if phosphate is not calculated as a separate component of base excess, variablity in protein concentra-

TABLE 9-9. Use of Anion Gap and [Na⁺] − [Cl⁻] to Assess Metabolic Acid-Base Disorders

	Normal Anion Gap	High Anion Gap
↓ [Na⁺] − [Cl⁻]	Hyperchloremic acidosis	Hyperchloremic acidosis and increased unmeasured anion acidosis
Normal [Na⁺] − [Cl⁻]	Normal	Increased unmeasured anion acidosis
↑ [Na⁺] − [Cl⁻]	Metabolic alkalosis	Metabolic alkalosis and increased unmeasured anion acidosis

Modified from de Morais HSA: A non-traditional approach to acid-base disorders. In DiBartola SP (ed): *Fluid Therapy in Small Animal Practice*. Philadelphia, WB Saunders Co., 1992, p. 285.

tion and charge in different species, lack of agreement on which cations and anions should be included in the calculation of *apparent* SID, the risk that error will be compounded when individual potentially inaccurate calculations are summed, and concern about the complexity of the original equations and calculations (Cameron 1989; Frischmeyer and Moon 1994; Constable 1997). Despite these concerns, [H⁺] can be adequately predicted in rabbits with experimentally induced metabolic acidosis using the original Stewart formula in the pH range 7.3 to 7.6. Addition of phosphate, calcium, and magnesium to the calculation allowed adequate prediction of the [H⁺] throughout the physiologic range (Waters et al. 1995). It has also been shown in running greyhounds that [H⁺] can be adequately predicted using the Stewart formula whenever SID is between 30 and 50 mEq/L (Fedde and Pieschl 1995). When SID was below 30 mEq/L, however, the variability between measured and calculated [H⁺] increased.

A more thorough understanding of the pathophysiology underlying acid-base disorders should serve to improve care of patients, but it is unclear whether insight from this type of analysis actually alters the treatment strategies and outcome. Furthermore, thorough analysis cannot be done without information (e.g., base excess, pH) previously available only by blood gas analysis. This problem may be circumvented in the future by increased use of point-of-care testing in the critical care setting (Dirks 1996). Regardless of the laboratory data available and diagnostic approach used, the clinician must determine whether the patient's history, physical findings, and working diagnosis fit the interpretation of the laboratory data.

Using Stewart's approach, the biochemical profile can provide useful information about the acid-base status of the patient (de Morais and Muir 1995). First, the total CO_2 should be used to estimate $[HCO_3^-]$. Unfortunately, the respiratory component cannot be assessed using the biochemical profile, and therefore decreases in total CO_2 related to respiratory alkalosis or increases in total CO_2 related to respiratory acidosis cannot be predicted. The second step is to look at the strong (Na^+, Cl^-) and weak (albumin, phosphate) ions that affect $[HCO_3^-]$. Total CO_2 increases (i.e., $[HCO_3^-]$ increases) with decreases in chloride (hypochloremic alkalosis), increases in sodium (contraction or concentration alkalosis), or decreases in albumin (hypoalbuminemic alkalosis) concentrations. Total CO_2 decreases (i.e., $[HCO_3^-]$ decreases) with increases in chloride (hyperchloremic acidosis), decreases in sodium (expansion or dilutional acidosis), increases in unidentified strong anion (organic acidosis), or increases in phosphate (hyperphosphatemic acidosis) concentrations. Unmeasured strong anions cannot be accurately evaluated using the biochemical profile. They can, however, be estimated from the anion gap. An increase in anion gap in the absence of hyperphosphatemia strongly suggests the presence of an organic acidosis. Chloride disorders can be identified easily whenever the sodium concentration is normal merely by evaluating the $[Na^+] - [Cl^-]$ difference. In this setting, an increase in $[Na^+] - [Cl^-]$ suggests the presence of metabolic alkalosis whereas a decrease in $[Na^+] - [Cl^-]$ suggests the presence of a hyperchloremic acidosis.

▶ Concept of External Hydrogen Ion Balance

External balance for hydrogen ions is maintained by renal excretion of a number of hydrogen ions equal to that consumed in the diet and produced each day by metabolic processes. The majority of hydrogen ions originate from metabolic processes and little fixed acid originates as such from the diet. A small amount of base is lost each day from the gastrointestinal tract (primarily as organic anions) and this is equivalent to a gain of fixed acid. These processes result in a net daily gain of 50 to 100 mEq of hydrogen ions. Bicarbonate ions that have been titrated by these hydrogen ions must be regenerated. The kidney is the only *regulated* route for H⁺ loss from the body.

Metabolic processes that convert cationic compounds to neutral products generate hydrogen ions, whereas those that convert anionic compounds to neutral products consume hydrogen ions (Halperin and Jungas 1983; Walser 1986; Cohen et al. 1997). The main sources of acid are oxidation of the sulfur-containing (e.g., cysteine, methionine) and cationic (e.g., lysine, arginine) amino acids and hydrolysis of organic phosphate diesters, such as phospholipids and nucleic acids. Oxidation of the sulfur-containing amino acids is the major source of acid produced each day:

$C_5H_{11}O_2NS$ (methionine) + $7\frac{1}{2}O_2 \rightarrow$
$\frac{1}{2}CH_4ON_2$ (urea) + $4\frac{1}{2}CO_2$ + $3\frac{1}{2}H_2O$ + SO_4^{2-} + $2H^+$
$C_3H_7O_2NS$ (cysteine) + $5\frac{1}{2}O_2 \rightarrow$
$\frac{1}{2}CH_4ON_2$ (urea) + $2\frac{1}{2}CO_2$ + $1\frac{1}{2}H_2O$ + SO_4^{2-} + $2H^+$

The main sources of base are metabolism of anionic amino acids (e.g., glutamate, aspartate) and the oxidation or utilization for gluconeogenesis of other organic anions (e.g., lactate, citrate).

▶ Whole-Body Regulation of Acid-Base Balance

Acid-base balance requires the cooperation of three major organs: liver, kidneys, and lungs. By the process of alveolar ventilation, the lungs remove the tremendous amount of volatile acid (10,000–15,000 mmol CO_2) produced each day by metabolic processes. The liver metabolizes amino acids derived from protein catabolism to glucose or triglyceride and releases NH_4^+ in the process. When urea is synthesized in the liver from NH_4^+ and CO_2, H^+ is produced and HCO_3^- is titrated. Consequently, the liver produces much of the fixed or nonvolatile acid that must be excreted each day. The kidneys excrete NH_4^+ in the urine, thus diverting it from ureagenesis and producing a net gain of HCO_3^- and net loss of H^+.

▶ Renal Regulation of Acid-Base Balance

The kidneys maintain normal extracellular fluid HCO_3^- concentration by reabsorbing virtually all filtered HCO_3^- and by regenerating HCO_3^- that has been titrated during the daily endogenous production of fixed, or nonvolatile, acid. The latter process is accomplished by excretion of *titratable acidity* (primarily phosphate salts) and *ammonium* salts. The term *net acid excretion* is defined as the sum of titratable acidity and ammonium minus HCO_3^- in the urine. Normally, there is a negligible amount of HCO_3^- in urine.

All three of the functions described are accomplished by renal tubular secretion of H^+. Hydrogen ion secretion occurs by means of a luminal Na^+-H^+ antiporter in the proximal tubules and loop of Henle and by a luminal H^+-adenosinetriphosphatase (H^+-ATPase) in all H^+-secreting tubular segments. The H^+,K^+-ATPase found in the luminal membranes of the type A intercalated cells of the collecting ducts is quantitatively less important for H^+ secretion but mediates K^+ reabsorption. These transport mechanisms depend on the presence of carbonic anhydrase in tubular cells. Of the filtered HCO_3^-, 90 to 95% is reabsorbed in the first portion of the proximal tubule and 5 to 10% is reabsorbed in the loop of Henle, distal tubule, and collecting duct (Fig. 9–6).

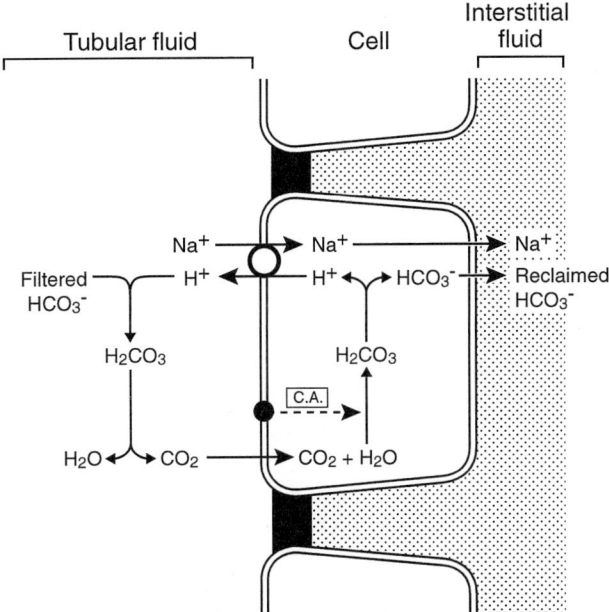

FIGURE 9–7. Reabsorption of filtered HCO_3^- by H^+ ion secretion in the proximal tubule. (Drawing by Tim Vojt.)

If secreted H^+ titrates filtered HCO_3^-, HCO_3^- is effectively reabsorbed because one HCO_3^- is added to extracellular fluid for each filtered HCO_3^- titrated by a secreted H^+ (Fig. 9–7). This process occurs primarily in the proximal tubules. Net acid excretion and generation of "new" HCO_3^- occur whenever secreted H^+ titrates phosphate in tubular fluid or whenever NH_4^+ is excreted in the urine with Cl^- or in exchange for Na^+ (Figs. 9–8 and 9–9). These processes occur primarily in the distal nephron.

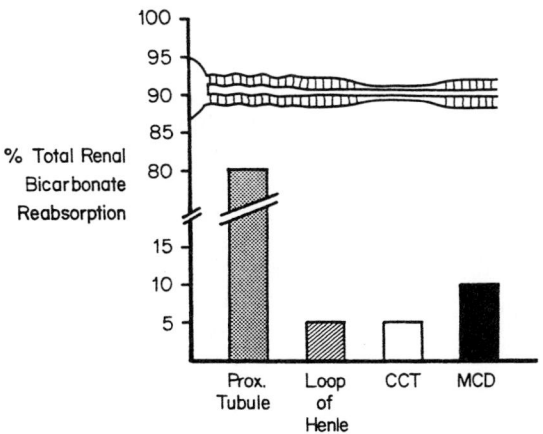

FIGURE 9–6. Segmental reabsorption of bicarbonate along the nephron. The major portion of filtered bicarbonate is reabsorbed proximally. Fine tuning of bicarbonate reabsorption occurs in distal nephron segments, including the medullary and cortical collecting ducts, as well as the thick ascending limb of Henle's loop. (From Kokko JP and Tannen RL: *Fluids and Electrolytes*, 3rd ed. Philadelphia, WB Saunders Co., p. 208, 1996.)

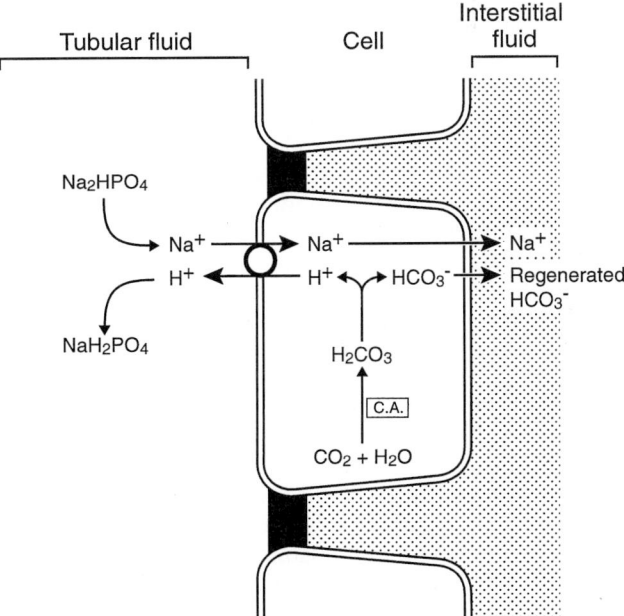

FIGURE 9–8. Regeneration of new HCO_3^- by titration of phosphate by secreted H^+ ion in renal tubule. (Drawing by Tim Vojt.)

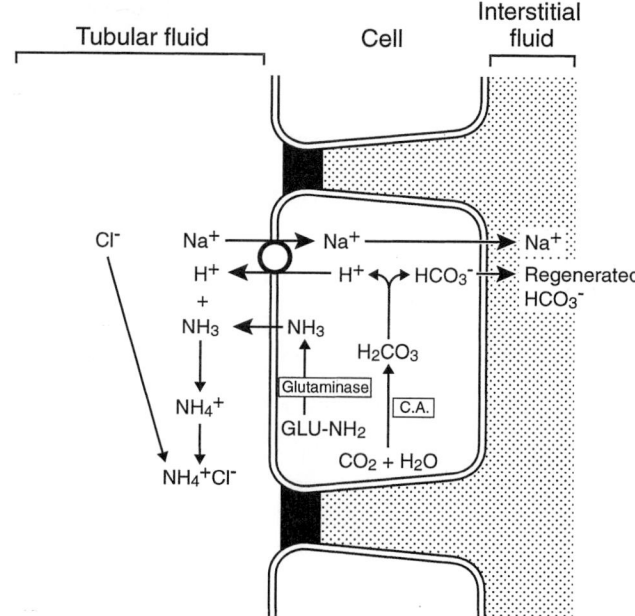

FIGURE 9-9. Regeneration of new HCO_3^- by ammonium excretion in renal tubules. (Drawing by Tim Vojt.)

Factors Affecting Renal Bicarbonate Reabsorption

If the glomerular filtration rate (GFR) and extracellular fluid volume (ECFV) are constant, the amount of HCO_3^- reabsorbed by the kidneys is equal to the filtered load. Under these conditions, HCO_3^- appears to have a tubular maximum (T_M) of approximately 3 mEq/min and a renal threshold of 25 mEq/L. Renal reabsorption of HCO_3^-, however, is closely tied to reabsorption of sodium and defense of ECFV. A primary expansion of ECFV leads to natriuresis and a transient decrease in renal HCO_3^- reabsorption. Contraction of the ECFV increases renal tubular reabsorption of sodium and HCO_3^-. When hypovolemia is induced experimentally, renal HCO_3^- reabsorption continues to increase even at extremely high plasma HCO_3^- concentrations (Slatopolsky et al. 1970; Malnic and Mellow Aires 1971). Thus, the *apparent* T_M for HCO_3^- changes depending on renal sodium avidity, being increased during volume depletion and decreased during volume expansion.

The anionic composition of glomerular ultrafiltrate determines, to a large extent, the effect that sodium avidity has on the electrolyte composition of the reabsorbed tubular fluid. If an adequate amount of chloride is present in the filtrate, the kidney reabsorbs chloride with sodium and alkalosis does not develop. If, however, there is insufficient chloride in the filtrate, sodium is reabsorbed with HCO_3^- and alkalosis develops. The prevailing acid-base status of the extracellular fluid can be viewed as a consequence of factors governing sodium and chloride reabsorption in the kidney (Schwartz and Cohen 1978). At a given rate of renal sodium reabsorption, a change in the reabsorption of either Cl^- or HCO_3^- must be accompanied by a reciprocal change in reabsorption of the other anion.

Renal HCO_3^- reabsorption is increased by an increase in arterial P_{CO_2} and decreased by a decrease in arterial P_{CO_2}. This effect may be mediated by a decrease (or increase) in pH within renal tubular cells and increased (or decreased) availability of H^+ for secretion. There is an inverse relationship between serum chloride concentration and the rate of renal HCO_3^- reabsorption that results from the requirement for electroneutrality during sodium reabsorption (see preceding paragraph). When serum chloride concentration is reduced, the filtered load of chloride decreases and the kidneys reabsorb more sodium with HCO_3^-. When serum chloride concentration is increased, the filtered load of chloride increases and the kidneys reabsorb more sodium with chloride and less with HCO_3^-. The fact that chloride and HCO_3^- are the only important resorbable anions in tubular fluid is important in understanding the pathophysiology of chloride-responsive metabolic alkalosis (see Chapters 4 and 10).

Hyperkalemia is associated with decreased renal HCO_3^- reabsorption in the distal nephron, and hypokalemia is associated with increased HCO_3^- reabsorption. During hypokalemia, transcellular shifting of potassium ions out of renal tubular cells into extracellular fluid occurs in exchange for hydrogen ions. This results in greater availability of H^+ for secretion by the tubular cells. When H^+ is secreted into tubular fluid, HCO_3^- is added to extracellular fluid. The opposite effect occurs with hyperkalemia, and there are fewer hydrogen ions in tubular cells available for secretion into tubular fluid. Aldosterone increases HCO_3^- reabsorption in the collecting ducts directly by stimulating the luminal H^+-ATPase responsible for H^+ secretion and indirectly by increasing lumen electronegativity by enhancement of sodium reabsorption.

Titratable Acidity

Titratable acidity refers to the amount of strong base needed to titrate a 24-h urine sample back to a pH of 7.40 and represents the amount of H^+ excreted in the urine in combination with weak acid anions, primarily phosphate. When urine pH is very low (e.g., 5.0–5.5), other weak acids such as creatinine ($pK_a = 5.0$) and urate ($pK_a = 5.8$) contribute to titratable acidity. Frequently, however, the term titratable acidity is considered synonymous with urinary phosphate ($pK_a = 6.8$). Of the daily 50 to 100 mEq of fixed or nonvolatile acid produced by metabolic processes, approximately 20 to 40 mEq (40%) is excreted as titratable acidity.

The pK_a of a weak acid is the pH at which one-half of the buffer is in the salt and one-half in the acid form (i.e., the ratio of salt to acid is 1.0) and buffers are most effective within 1.0 pH unit of their pK_a. Phosphate is a very effective urinary buffer because its pK_a (6.8) falls between the pH of distal tubular fluid (6.0) and that of glomerular filtrate (7.4). The amount of phosphate available for buffering tubular fluid is the product of serum phosphorus concentration and GFR (i.e., the filtered load of phosphate). The filtered load of phosphate is relatively constant in a normal individual in phosphorus balance.

Ammonium Excretion

Excretion of ammonium by the kidney is essential for eliminating the daily fixed acid load and regenerating titrated bicarbonate. Most of the ammonium to be excreted is produced from glutamine in the proximal tubule by action of the enzyme glutaminase (Good 1989; Halperin 1989):

$$\text{glutamine} \rightarrow \alpha\text{-ketoglutarate}^{2-} + 2NH_4^+$$
$$\alpha\text{-ketoglutarate}^{2-} + 2H^+ \rightarrow CO_2 + H_2O \text{ (oxidation)}$$

or

$$\alpha\text{-ketoglutarate}^{2-} + 2H^+ \rightarrow \text{glucose (gluconeogenesis)}$$
$$2NH_4^+ + CO_2 \rightarrow \text{urea} + 2H^+ \text{ (urea cycle)}$$

It can be seen from these reactions that two H^+ are consumed when the α-ketoglutarate produced from glutamine is either oxidized or converted to glucose. This results in the simultaneous generation of two new bicarbonate ions. If an equal number of ammonium ions are used by the liver for urea synthesis, two H^+ are produced, two HCO_3^- are titrated, and there is no net gain of HCO_3^-. If, however, the NH_4^+ is excreted in the urine along with Cl^- or in exchange for Na^+, a net gain of HCO_3^- occurs.

The classic theory of ammonium excretion by the kidney suggests that NH_3 diffuses passively through the luminal membrane of the tubular cell into tubular fluid. Hydrogen ions derived from the dissociation of carbonic acid could then combine with NH_3 to form NH_4^+ because the pK_a for this reaction is 9.2. In the pH range of tubular fluid (6.0–7.0), only 0.1 to 1% of this buffer pair would exist as NH_3. Thus, the associated H^+ is strongly attached to NH_3 by forming NH_4^+ and does not affect urine pH (Fig. 9–10).

The classic theory of ammonium excretion by the kidney was based on diffusion trapping of NH_3 in tubular fluid. According to this theory, the lipid-soluble, nonionized NH_3 diffuses passively into tubular fluid, where it is trapped by combination with H^+ to form less permeant NH_4^+. This theory dictates that diffusion equilibrium occurs for NH_3 and that renal tubular cells do not transport NH_4^+. These assumptions have been questioned (Good 1989).

Several renal transport mechanisms contribute to the ultimate appearance of NH_4^+ in urine. Ammonium is secreted into the lumen of the early proximal tubule, primarily by active transport. It is thought that NH_4^+ is substituted for H^+ in the proximal Na^+-H^+ antiporter. Much of the NH_4^+ secreted into the proximal tubules is reabsorbed from the loop of Henle, possibly by substitution for K^+ in the Na^+-K^+-$2Cl^-$ carrier in the thick ascending limb of Henle's loop. This results in countercurrent multiplication of interstitial NH_4^+ in the same fashion as occurs for NaCl and generates a transepithelial concentration gradient favoring secretion of NH_4^+ into the medullary collecting ducts and excretion of large amounts of NH_4^+ in the urine. Thus NH_4^+, like NaCl, undergoes medullary recycling.

The ability of the kidneys to excrete an acid load despite their inability to reduce urine pH below 5.0 (in dogs and cats) is explained by the high pK_a (9.2) of the NH_3-NH_4^+ buffer pair (Valtin and Schafer 1995) (see Fig. 9–10). In the normal animal, 30 to 60 of the 50 to 100 (60%) mEq of the fixed or nonvolatile acid produced each day is excreted in the urine as ammonium, either as the chloride salt or in exchange for sodium. The more acidic the urine, the greater the proportion of ammonium existing as NH_4^+. The kidney can also increase its production of ammonium from glutamine during acidosis. At any given urine pH, the rate of ammonium salt excretion is higher in the presence of acidosis (Valtin and Schafer 1995) (Fig. 9–11). Renal ammonium excretion can increase fivefold in response to metabolic acidosis.

▶ Potassium and Acid-Base Balance

The distribution of potassium ions between intracellular and extracellular fluids may be affected by acid-base disorders. When HCl was infused acutely into nephrectomized dogs, approximately 50% of the H^+ load was buffered intracellularly (Swan and Pitts 1955; Schwartz et al. 1957). Intracellular sodium and potassium ions entered extracellular fluid in exchange for the H^+ entering cells, and serum potassium concentration increased. These early animal studies and observations in a small number of human patients (Burnell et al. 1956) led to the predic-

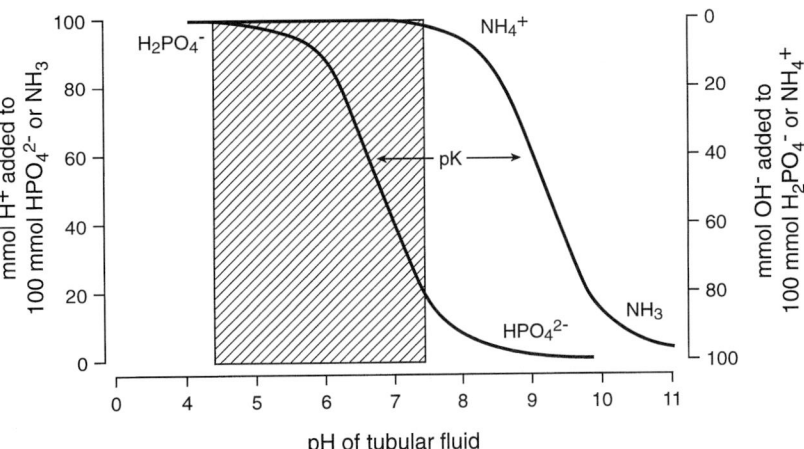

Figure 9–10. Explanation of how NH_4^+ excretion allows removal of acid without affecting urine pH (see text for details). (Drawing by Tim Vojt.)

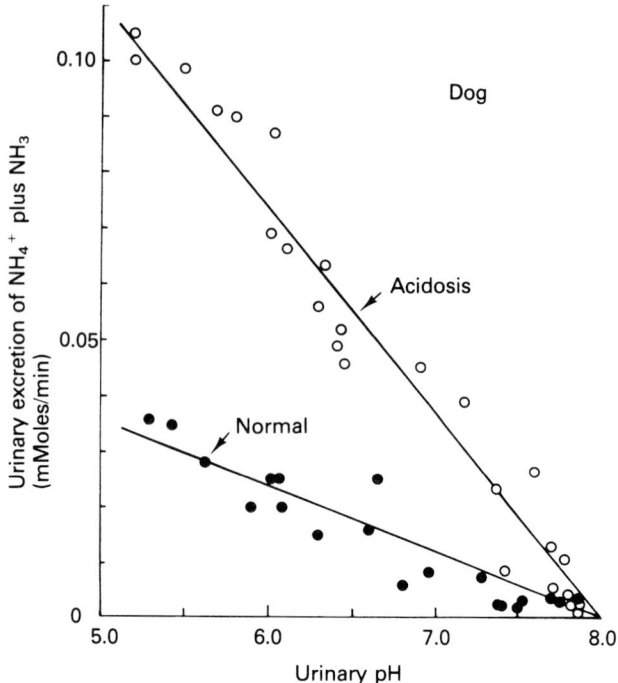

FIGURE 9-11. Effect of acidosis on urinary ammonium excretion. (From Valtin H: *Renal Function: Mechanisms Preserving Fluid and Solute Balance in Health*. Boston, Little, Brown & Co., p. 238, 1983.)

tion that metabolic acidosis would be associated with a 0.6 mEq/L increase in serum potassium concentration for each 0.1 U decrease in pH. A review of animal studies demonstrated that the change in serum potassium concentration observed during acute metabolic acidosis caused by mineral acids (e.g., HCl, NH$_4$Cl) was variable (Adrogue and Madias 1981). Furthermore, an increase in serum potassium concentration does not occur in acute metabolic acidosis caused by organic acids (e.g., lactic acid, ketoacids) (Tobin 1958; Oster et al. 1978, 1980; Adrogue and Madias 1981; Adrogue et al. 1985; Ilkiw et al. 1989). Acute infusion of β-hydroxybutyrate in normal dogs caused an increase in insulin in portal venous blood and hypokalemia, presumably as a result of potassium uptake by cells (Adrogue et al. 1985). Acute infusion of HCl led to hyperkalemia and increased portal vein glucagon concentration (Adrogue et al. 1985). These acute changes in serum potassium concentration are not due to changes in renal excretion of potassium (Oster et al. 1978; Adrogue et al. 1985).

The hyperkalemia associated with acute metabolic acidosis caused by mineral acids is transient. In a study of acute and chronic metabolic acidosis induced in dogs by administration of HCl or NH$_4$Cl, hyperkalemia was observed after acute infusion of HCl, but hypokalemia developed after 3 to 5 days of NH$_4$Cl administration (Magner et al. 1988). The observed hypokalemia was associated with inappropriately high urinary excretion of potassium and increased plasma aldosterone concentration (Magner et al. 1988). Similar findings in rats with chronic metabolic acidosis induced by NH$_4$Cl have been reported (Scandling and Ornt 1987). Acute metabolic acidosis induced by administration of mineral acid decreases renal proximal tubular reabsorption of sodium, leading to volume contraction and increased distal delivery of sodium. Increased Na$^+$-H$^+$ and Na$^+$-K$^+$ exchange then occurs in the distal nephron, mediated by increased distal tubular fluid flow and hyperaldosteronism. These findings suggest that mild hypokalemia and potassium depletion are likely to develop during chronic metabolic acidosis caused by administration of a mineral acid. The observation of hyperkalemia during chronic metabolic acidosis should prompt consideration of impaired renal potassium excretion or some other cause of hyperkalemia (see Chapter 5).

REFERENCES

Adrogue HJ and Madias NE: Changes in plasma potassium concentration during acute acid base disturbances. *J Clin Invest* 71:456, 1981.

Adrogue HJ, Brensilver J, and Madias NE: Changes in the plasma anion gap during chronic metabolic acid-base disturbances. *Am J Physiol* 235:F291, 1978.

Adrogue HJ, Chap Z, Ishida T, et al.: Role of the endocrine pancreas in the kalemic response to acute metabolic acidosis in conscious dogs. *J Clin Invest* 75:798, 1985.

Aguilera-Tejero E, Fernandez H, Estepa JC, et al.: Arterial blood gases and acid-base balance in geriatric dogs. *Res Vet Sci* 63:253, 1997.

Astrup P: New approach to acid-base metabolism. *Clin Chem* 7:1, 1961.

Astrup P, Jorgensen K, Siggaard-Andersen O, et al.: Acid-base metabolism: New approach. *Lancet* 1:1035, 1960.

Atkins CE, Tyler R, and Greenlee P: Clinical, biochemical, acid-base, and electrolyte abnormalities in cats after hypertonic sodium phosphate enema administration. *Am J Vet Res* 46:980, 1985.

Bleich HL, Berkman PM, and Schwartz WB: The response of cerebrospinal fluid composition to sustained hypercapnia. *J Clin Invest* 43:11, 1964.

Burnell JM: Changes in bone sodium and carbonate in metabolic acidosis and alkalosis in the dog. *J Clin Invest* 50:327, 1971.

Burnell JM, Villamil MF, Uyeno BT, et al.: The effect in humans of extracellular pH change on the relationship between serum potassium concentration and intracellular potassium. *J Clin Invest* 35:935, 1956.

Cameron JN: Acid-base homeostasis: Past and present perspectives. *Physiol Zool* 62:845, 1989.

Chew DJ, Leonard M, and Muir WW: Effect of sodium bicarbonate infusion on serum osmolality, electrolyte concentrations, and blood gas tensions in cats. *Am J Vet Res* 52:12, 1991.

Ching SV, Fettman MJ, Harnar DW, et al.: The effect of chronic dietary acidification using ammonium chloride on acid-base and mineral metabolism in the adult cat. *J Nutr* 119:902, 1989.

Christopher MM, Eckfeld JH, and Eaton JW: Propylene glycol ingestion causes D-lactic acidosis. *Lab Invest* 62:114, 1990.

Cohen JJ, Brackett NC, and Schwartz WB: The nature of the carbon dioxide titration curve in the normal dog. *J Clin Invest* 43:777, 1964.

Cohen RM, Feldman GM, and Fernandez PC: The balance of acid, base and charge in health and disease. *Kidney Int* 52:287, 1997.

Constable PD: A simplified strong ion model for acid-base equilibria: Application to horse plasma. *J Appl Physiol* 83:297, 1997.

Cornelius LM and Rawlings CA: Arterial blood gas and acid base values in dogs with various diseases and signs of disease. *J Am Vet Med Assoc* 178:992, 1981.

de Morais HSA: A non-traditional approach to acid-base disorders. In DiBartola SP (ed): *Fluid Therapy in Small Animal Practice*. Philadelphia, WB Saunders Co., p. 297, 1992.

de Morais HSA and Muir WW: Strong ions and acid-base disorders. In Bonagura JD (ed): *Kirks's Current Veterinary Therapy XII*. Philadelphia, WB Saunders Co., p. 121, 1995.

Dirks JL: Diagnostic blood analysis using point-of-care technology. *AACN Clin Issues* 7:249, 1996.

Emmett M and Narins RG: Clinical use of the anion gap. *Medicine (Baltimore)* 56:38, 1977.

Fedde MR and Pieschl RL: Extreme derangements of acid-base balance in exercise: Advantages and limitations of the Stewart analysis. *Can J Appl Physiol* 20:369, 1995.

Fencl V and Leith DE: Stewart's quantative acid-base chemistry: Applications in biology and medicine. *Respir Physiol* 91:1, 1993.

Fencl V and Rossing TH: Acid-base disorders in critical care medicine. *Annu Rev Med* 40:17, 1989.

Figge J, Mydosh T, and Fencl V: Serum proteins and acid-base equilibria: A follow-up. *J Lab Clin Med* 120:713, 1992.

Frischmeyer KJ and Moon PF: Evaluation of quantitative acid-base balance and determination of unidentified anions in swine. *Am J Vet Res* 55:1153, 1994.

Gabow PA: Disorders associated with an altered anion gap. *Kidney Int* 27:472, 1985.

Gifix BM, Mique M, and Magder S: A physical chemical approach to the analysis of acid base balance in the clinical setting. *J Crit Care* 8:187, 1993.

Good DW: New concepts in renal ammonium excretion. In Seldin DW and Giebisch G (eds): *The Regulation of Acid-Base Balance*. New York, Raven Press, p. 169, 1989.

Halperin ML: How much "new" bicarbonate is formed in the distal nephron in the process of net acid excretion? *Kidney Int* 35:1277, 1989.

Halperin ML and Jungas RL: Metabolic production and disposal of hydrogen ions. *Kidney Int* 24:709, 1983.

Harrington JT, Cohen JJ, and Kassirer JP: Introduction to the clinical acid-base disturbances. In Cohen JJ and Kassirer JP (eds): *Acid-Base*. Boston, Little, Brown & Co., p. 119, 1982.

Haskins SC: An overview of acid-base physiology. *J Am Vet Med Assoc* 170:423, 1977a.

Haskins SC: Sampling and storage of blood for pH and blood gas analysis. *J Am Vet Med Assoc* 170:429, 1977b.

Haskins SC: Blood gases and acid-base balance: Clinical interpretation and therapeutic implications. In Kirk RW (ed): *Current Veterinary Therapy VIII*. Philadelphia, WB Saunders Co., p. 201, 1983.

Herbert DA and Mitchell RA: Blood gas tensions and acid-base balance in awake cats. *J Appl Physiol* 30:434, 1971.

Hutchison AS, Ralston SH, Drybaugh FJ, et al.: Too much heparin: Possible source of error in blood gas analysis. *Br Med J* 287:1131, 1983.

Ilkiw JE, Davis PE, and Church DB.: Hematologic, biochemical, blood gas, and acid base values in greyhounds before and after exercise. *Am J Vet Res* 50:583, 1989.

Ilkiw JE, Rose RJ, and Martin ICA: A comparison of simultaneously collected arterial, mixed venous, jugular venous and cephalic venous blood samples in the assessment of blood gas and acid base status in dogs. *J Vet Intern Med* 5:294, 1991.

James KM, Polzin DJ, Osborne CA, et al.: Effects of sample handling on total carbon dioxide concentrations in canine and feline serum and blood. *Am J Vet Res* 58:343, 1997.

Kilborn SH, Bonnett BN, and Pook HA: Comparison of three different methods of total carbon dioxide measurement. *Vet Clin Pathol* 24:22, 1995.

King LG, Anderson JG, Rhodes WH, et al.: Arterial blood gas tensions in healthy aged dogs. *Am J Vet Res* 53:1744, 1992.

Leith DE: The new acid-base: Power and simplicity. *Proceedings of the 8th ACVIM Forum*, New Orleans, p. 611, 1991.

Madias NE and Cohen JJ: Acid-base chemistry and bufferin. In Cohen JJ and Kassirer JP (eds): *Acid-Base*. Boston, Little, Brown & Co., p. 13, 1982a.

Madias NE and Cohen JJ: Acid-base chemistry and buffering. In Cohen JJ and Kassirer JP (eds): *Acid-Base* Boston, Little, Brown & Co., p. 17, 1982b.

Madias NE, Schwartz WB, and Cohen JJ: The maladaptive renal response to secondary hypocapnia during chronic HCl acidosis in the dog. *J Clin Invest* 60:1393, 1977.

Madias NE, Adrogue JH, and Cohen JJ: Effect of natural variations in PaCO$_2$ on plasma HCO$_3^-$ in dogs: A redefinition of normal. *Am J Physiol* 236:F30, 1979a.

Madias NE, Ayus JC, and Adrogue HJ: Increased anion gap in metabolic alkalosis: The role of plasma protein equivalency. *N Engl J Med* 300:1421, 1979b.

Madias NE, Bossert WH, and Adrogue HJ: Ventilatory response to chronic metabolic acidosis and alkalosis in the dog. *J Appl Physiol* 56:1640, 1984.

Madiedo G, Sciacca R, and Hause L: Air bubbles and temperature effect on blood gas analysis. *J Comp Pathol* 33:864, 1980.

Magner PO, Robinson L, Halperin RM, et al.: The plasma potassium concentration in metabolic acidosis: A re-evaluation. *Am J Kidney Dis* 11:220, 1988.

Malnic G and Giebisch G: Mechanism of renal hydrogen ion secretion. *Kidney Int* 1:280, 1972.

Malnic G and Mellow Aires M: Kinetic study of bicarbonate reabsorption in proximal tubule of the rat. *Am J Physiol* 220:1759, 1971.

McAuliffe JJ, Lind LJ, Leith DE, et al.: Hypoproteinemic alkalosis. *Am J Med* 81:86, 1986.

Middleton DJ, Ilkiw JE, and Watson ADJ: Arterial and venous blood gas tensions in clinically healthy cats. *Am J Vet Res* 42:1609, 1981.

Oh MS and Carrol JH: The anion gap. *N Engl J Med* 297:814, 1977.

Oster JR, Perez GO, and Vaamonde CA: Relationship between blood pH and potassium and phosphorus during acute metabolic acidosis. *Am J Physiol* 235:F345, 1978.

Oster JR, Perez GO, Castro A, et al.: Plasma potassium response to acute metabolic acidosis induced by mineral and nonmineral acids. *Miner Electrolyte Metab* 4:28, 1980.

Polzin DJ, Stevens JB, and Osborne CA: Clinical evaluation of the anion gap in evaluation of acid-base disorders in dogs. *Compend Contin Educ Pract Vet* 4:102, 1982.

Pruden EL, Siggaard-Andersen O, and Tietz NW: Blood gases and pH. In Burtis CA and Ashwood ER (eds): *Tietz Fundamentals of Clinical Chemistry*. Philadelphia, WB Saunders Co., p. 506, 1996.

Rodkey WG, Hannon JP, Dramise JG, et al.: Arterialized capillary blood used to determine the acid-base and blood gas status of dogs. *Am J Vet Res* 39:459, 1978.

Russell KE, Hansen BD, and Stevens JB: Strong ion difference approach to acid-base imbalances with clinical applications to dogs and cats. *Vet Clin North Am* 26:1185, 1996.

Scandling JD and Ornt DB: Mechanism of potassium depletion during chronic metabolic acidosis in the rat. *Am J Physiol* 252:F122, 1987.

Schlichtig R: [Base excess] vs [strong ion difference]: Which is more helpful? *Adv Exp Med Biol* 411:91, 1997.

Schwartz WB and Cohen JJ: The nature of the renal response to chronic disorders of acid-base equilibrium. *Am J Med* 64:417, 1978.

Schwartz WB and Relman AS: A critique of the parameters used in the evaluation of acid-base disorders. "Whole blood buffer base" and "standard bicarbonate" compared with blood pH and plasma bicarbonate concentration. *N Engl J Med* 268:1382, 1963.

Schwartz WB, Orning KJ, and Porter R: The internal distribution of hydrogen ions with varying degrees of metabolic acidosis. *J Clin Invest* 36:373, 1957.

Severinghaus JW: Siggard-Andersen and the "Great Transatlantic acid-base debate." *Scand J Clin Lab Invest* 54(suppl 214):99, 1993.

Shull RM: The value of anion gap and osmolal gap determinations in veterinary medicine. *Vet Clin Pathol* 7:12, 1978.

Siggaard-Andersen O, Engel K, Jorgensen K, et al.: A micro method for determination of pH, carbon dioxide tension, base excess and standard bicarbonate in capillary blood. *Scand J Clin Lab Invest* 12:172, 1960.

Siggaard-Andersen O and Fogh-Andersen N: Base excess or buffer base (strong ion difference) as measure of a non-respiratory acid-base disturbance. *Acta Anaesthesiol Scand* 39:123, 1995.

Singer RB and Hastings AB: An improved clinical method for the estimation of disturbances of the acid-base balance of human blood. *Medicine (Baltimore)* 27:223, 1948.

Slatopolsky E, Hoffsten P, Purkerson M, et al.: On the influence of extracellular fluid volume expansion and of uremia on bicarbonate reabsorption in man. *J Clin Invest* 49:988, 1970.

Solter PF, Haskins SC, and Patz JD: Comparison of P_{O_2}, P_{CO_2} and pH in blood collected from the femoral artery and a cut claw of cats. *Am J Vet Res* 49:1882, 1988.

Stewart PA: *How to Understand Acid-Base*. New York, Elsevier, 1981.

Stewart PA: Modern quantitative acid-base chemistry. *Can J Physiol Pharmacol* 61:1444, 1983.

Swan RC and Pitts RF: Neutralization of infused acid by nephrectomized dogs. *J Clin Invest* 34:205, 1955.

Tobin RB: Varying role of extracellular electrolytes in metabolic acidosis and alkalosis. *Am J Physiol* 195:687, 1958.

Valtin H and Gennari FJ: *Acid-Base Disorders: Basic Concepts and Clinical Management*. Boston, Little, Brown & Co., 1987.

Valtin H and Schafer JA: *Renal Function*. Boston, Little, Brown & Co., 1995.

van Leeuwen AM: Net cation equivalency ("base binding power") of the plasma proteins: A study of ion-protein interaction in human plasma by means of in vivo ultrafiltration and equilibrium dialysis. *Acta Med Scand* 422(suppl):1, 1964.

van Sluijs FJ, de Vries HW, de Bruijne JJ, et al.: Capillary and venous blood compared with arterial blood in the measurement of acid-base and blood gas status of dogs. *Am J Vet Res* 44:459, 1983.

van Slyke DD, Hastings AB, Hiller A, et al.: Studies of gas and electrolyte equilibria in blood. XIV. The amounts of alkali bound by serum albumin and globulin. *J Biol Chem* 79:769, 1920.

Walser M: Roles of urea production, ammonium excretion, and amino acid oxidation in acid-base balance. *Am J Physiol* 250:F181, 1986.

Waters JH, Scanlon TS, Howard RS, et al.: Role of minor electrolytes when applied to Stewart's acid-base approach in an acidotic rabbit model. *Anesth Analg* 81:1043, 1995.

Whitehair KJ, Haskins SC, Whitehair JG, et al.: Clinical applications of quantitative acid-base chemistry. *J Vet Intern Med* 9:1, 1995.

Zweens J, Frankena H, van Kampen EJ, et al.: Ionic composition of arterial and mixed venous plasma in the unanesthetized dog. *Am J Physiol* 233:F412, 1977.

CHAPTER 10

Metabolic Acid-Base Disorders

STEPHEN P. DiBARTOLA

Metabolic disturbances of acid-base balance are associated with many disease states, and identification of the acid-base disturbance may facilitate diagnosis of the underlying disease process. For example, observation of hypochloremic metabolic alkalosis on a serum biochemical profile of a vomiting dog may lead to recognition of gastrointestinal obstruction as the cause. The regulation of normal acid-base balance is considered in detail in Chapter 9.

▶ Metabolic Acidosis

Metabolic acidosis is characterized by a primary decrease in plasma HCO_3^- concentration, increased $[H^+]$, decreased pH, and a secondary, or adaptive, decrease in P_{CO_2}. In one study, metabolic acidosis was the most common acid-base disturbance in dogs and cats (Cornelius and Rawlings 1981).

Metabolic acidosis can be caused by loss of HCO_3^--rich fluid from the body, addition of fixed acid to the body or its production by metabolism within the body, or failure of renal excretion of fixed acid. Loss of HCO_3^--rich fluid usually occurs via the gastrointestinal tract (e.g., small-bowel diarrhea) but may also occur via the kidneys (e.g., carbonic anhydrase inhibitors, proximal renal tubular acidosis). The HCO_3^- concentration of diarrheal fluid exceeds that of plasma, whereas its Cl^- concentration is lower. The loss of such fluid results in a hyperchloremic metabolic acidosis. Examples of the addition of fixed acid to the body include toxins (e.g., ethylene glycol, salicylate) and compounds used therapeutically (e.g., ammonium chloride, cationic amino acids). Examples of metabolic production of fixed acid within the body include lactic acidosis and diabetic ketoacidosis. Renal failure, hypoadrenocorticism, and distal renal tubular acidosis are examples of impaired urinary excretion of fixed acid. Small-bowel diarrhea, renal failure, hypoadrenocorticism, diabetic ketoacidosis, and lactic acidosis during cardiovascular collapse are the most common causes of metabolic acidosis in small animal practice.

Body Buffer Response to an Acute Acid Load

When HCl was infused acutely into nephrectominzed dogs, approximately 40% of the acid was buffered by extracellular HCO_3^-, 10% by red cell buffers (primarily hemoglobin), and 50% by intracellular buffers of soft tissues and bone (primarily proteins and phosphates) (Swan and Pitts 1955). In nonnephrectomized unanesthetized dogs infused intermittently with HCl, intracellular buffers contributed approximately 50% of the buffer response, regardless of the magnitude of the H^+ load (Schwartz et al. 1957). Within a few minutes of an acute fixed acid load, administered H^+ is buffered by HCO_3^- in plasma water. Plasma proteins and phosphates play a minor role in this acute response. Some of the administered acid enters red cells and is buffered by hemoglobin. The CO_2 produced by the combination of the H^+ with HCO_3^- ions is rapidly removed from the body by alveolar ventilation. Within 30 min, the acid load has been distributed to the interstitial fluid, where HCO_3^- again plays the dominant role in the acute buffer response. After several hours, H^+ enters intracellular water in exchange for sodium and potassium ions. These hydrogen ions are buffered within cells by proteins and phosphates. In early studies (Swan and Pitts 1955; Schwartz et al. 1957), serum potassium concentration increased, but serum sodium concentration decreased after infusion of HCl. The relative roles of these buffers are depicted in Figure 10–1.

Respiratory Response to an Acute Acid Load

A fixed acid load increases $[H^+]$ and thereby stimulates peripheral and central chemoreceptors to increase alveolar ventilation. This effect begins within hours and is complete within 12 to 24 h. In humans, there is an approximately 1.2 mm Hg reduction in P_{CO_2} for each 1 mEq/L decrement in plasma HCO_3^- concentration to a minimum P_{CO_2} of approximately 10 mm Hg (Harrington and Cohen 1982a; Rose 1994a). In dogs with uncomplicated metabolic acidosis induced by chronic feeding of HCl, the observed compensatory respiratory response is an approximately 0.7 mm Hg decrement in P_{CO_2} per 1 mEq/L decrement in plasma HCO_3^- concentration (Lowance et al. 1972; DeSousa et al. 1974; Cohen et al. 1976; Madias et al. 1977; Adrogue et al. 1983; Clark et al. 1983; Madias et al. 1985; Madias and Zelman 1986). In these studies, the smallest observed respiratory re-

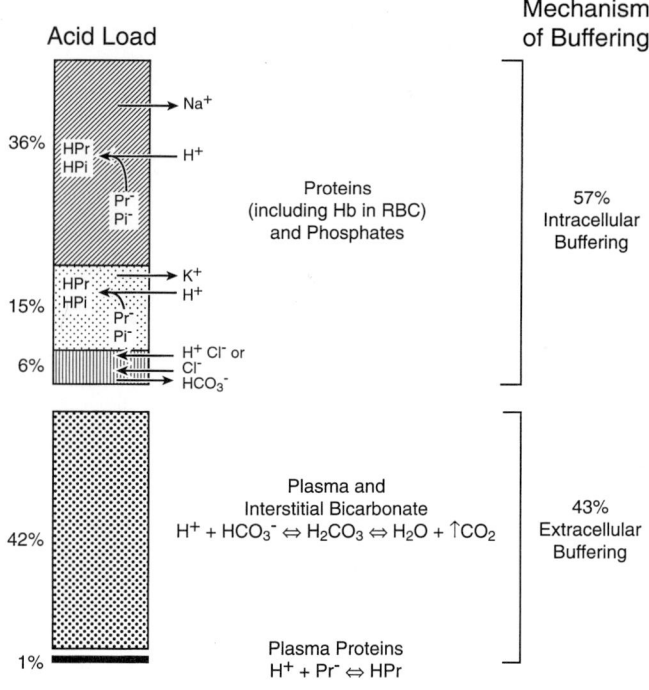

FIGURE 10-1. Distribution of buffer response to a fixed acid load. (Drawing by Tim Vojt. Adapted from Pitts RF: *Physiology of the Kidney and Body Fluids*, 2nd ed. Chicago, Year Book Medical Publishers, p. 171, 1968.)

sponse was an approximately 0.5 mm Hg decrement in P_{CO_2} per mEq/L decrement in plasma HCO_3^- concentration (Adrogue et al. 1983) and the largest response was a 1.1 mm Hg decrement in P_{CO_2} per mEq/L decrement in plasma HCO_3^- concentration (DeSousa et al. 1974). Data are limited on the respiratory response of cats to metabolic acidosis, but there is some evidence that the cat fails to develop respiratory compensation to the same extent as observed in the dog in spontaneous (Watson et al. 1986) and NH_4Cl-induced metabolic acidosis (Finco et al. 1986; Senior et al. 1986a, 1986b; Ching et al. 1989; Lemieux et al. 1990).

The classic explanation of the respiratory response to metabolic acidosis is that the increase in [H^+] (decrease in pH) stimulates ventilation, and the resultant decrease in P_{CO_2} returns the HCO_3^-/P_{CO_2} ratio and pH toward normal. This is true in acute metabolic acidosis, but the resultant secondary hypocapnia has been observed to decrease plasma HCO_3^- concentration further in chronic metabolic acidosis, presumably by reducing renal HCO_3^- reabsorption. This secondary hypocapnia contributes to 40% of the observed decrease in plasma HCO_3^- concentration during chronic HCl acidosis (Madias et al. 1977). Thus, chronic metabolic acidosis decreases plasma HCO_3^- concentration by two mechanisms: the effect of the administered HCl on body buffers and a reduction in renal HCO_3^- reabsorption that accompanies secondary hyperventilation. In this study, serum potassium concentration decreased during development of chronic HCl acidosis (contrary to what is typically described for acute metabolic acidosis caused by mineral acids), whereas serum sodium concentration was unchanged (Madias et al. 1977).

Renal Response to an Acute Acid Load

The role of the kidney is to excrete the fixed acid load imposed by the underlying disease process responsible for metabolic acidosis. The kidney accomplishes this task primarily by augmenting its excretion of NH_4^+. Titratable acidity changes little unless there is a change in the filtered load of phosphate. Chloride ions accompany the NH_4^+ into urine while HCO_3^- is regenerated and reabsorbed into extracellular fluid (ECF) to restore HCO_3^- that was titrated during the acute fixed acid load. Within 48 h of a fixed acid load, approximately 25% of the added acid has been excreted in the urine, and the remainder is excreted over the next 4 days (Valtin and Gennari 1987). The kidney can increase its NH_4^+ excretion three- to fivefold during chronic metabolic acidosis (Simpson 1971; Welbourne et al. 1972; Warnock 1988). There is some evidence that cats do not adapt to metabolic acidosis by enhanced renal ammoniagenesis (Lemieux et al. 1990). The role of the kidney in regulation of acid base balance is discussed further in the Chapter 9.

Clinical Features of Metabolic Acidosis

The clinical signs in small animals with metabolic acidosis are more likely to be due to the underlying disease responsible for metabolic acidosis than to the acidosis itself. In humans, respiratory compensation for metabolic acidosis leads to characteristic hyperventilation, recognized by a deep, rhythmic breathing pattern (i.e., Kussmaul's respirations). Such a characteristic respiratory pattern has not been described in small animal patients, and metabolic acidosis is usually suspected by observation of a low total CO_2 content on a biochemical profile and confirmed by blood gas analysis.

Severe acidosis has serious detrimental effects on cardiovascular function including decreased cardiac output, decreased arterial blood pressure, and decreased hepatic and renal blood flow (Adrogue and Madias 1998). Myocardial contractility is decreased when blood pH falls below 7.20 (Mitchell et al. 1972; Orchard and Kentish 1990). Impaired contractility may result from a decrease in myocardial intracellular pH and displacement of calcium ions from critical binding sites on contractile proteins. Acidosis may predispose the heart to ventricular arrhythmias or ventricular fibrillation. Acidosis has a direct arterial vasodilating effect that is offset by increased release of endogenous catecholamines. The inotropic response to catecholamines, however, is impaired, and this may be associated with a reduction in the number of β-adrenergic receptors (Marsh et al. 1988). Acidosis has a direct vasoconstrictive effect on the venous side of the circulation, which tends to centralize blood volume and predisposes to pulmonary congestion. Acidosis shifts the oxygen-hemoglobin dissociation curve to the right, thus enhancing O_2 release from hemoglobin, but this effect is offset by a decrease in red cell 2,3-diphosphoglycerate, which develops after 6 to 8 h of acidosis and shifts the curve back to the left (Mitchell et al. 1972).

Acidemia produces insulin resistance that impairs peripheral uptake of glucose and inhibits anaerobic glycolysis by inhibiting phosphofructokinase (Adrogue and Madias 1998). During severe acidosis, the liver may be converted from a consumer to a producer of lactate (Madias 1986). Severe acidosis also impairs the ability of the brain to regulate its volume, leading to obtundation and coma. Acute mineral acidosis causes hyperkalemia by a transcellular shifting of potassium from intracellular to extracellular fluid in exchange for hydrogen ions. This effect causes a very variable change in serum potassium concentration and is not observed with organic acidosis (Adrogue and Madias 1981). Acute reduction in blood pH causes displacement of calcium ions from negatively charged binding sites (e.g., $-COO^-$ groups) on proteins (primarily albumin) as these sites become protonated and an increase in ionized serum calcium concentration results. Chronic metabolic acidosis leads to release of buffer (mainly calcium carbonate) from bone and osteodystrophy and hypercalciuria result.

Diagnosis of Metabolic Acidosis

Metabolic acidosis is associated with several different diseases and should be considered in any severely ill patient. Often, the diagnosis is first suspected by review of the electrolyte and total CO_2 results on the patient's biochemical profile. It is confirmed by blood gas analysis. The causes of metabolic acidosis may be divided into those associated with a normal anion gap (hyperchloremic metabolic acidosis) and those associated with an increased anion gap (normochloremic metabolic acidosis) (see Table 10–1).

TABLE 10–1. Causes of Metabolic Acidosis

Increased Anion Gap (Normochloremic)
Ethylene glycol intoxication
Salicylate intoxication
Other rare intoxications (e.g., paraldehyde, methanol)
Diabetic ketoacidosis*
Uremic acidosis†
Lactic acidosis

Normal Anion Gap (Hyperchloremic)
Diarrhea
Renal tubular acidosis
Carbonic anhydrase inhibitors (e.g., acetazolamide)
Ammonium chloride
Cationic amino acids (e.g., lysine, arginine, histidine)
Posthypocapnic metabolic acidosis
Dilutional acidosis (e.g., rapid administration of 0.9% saline)
Hypoadrenocorticism‡

*Patients with diabetic ketoacidosis may have some component of hyperchloremic metabolic acidosis in conjunction with increased anion gap acidosis (Adrogue et al. 1982, 1984).
†The metabolic acidosis early in renal failure may be hyperchloremic and later convert to typical increased anion gap acidosis (Widmer et al. 1979).
‡Patients with hypoadrenocorticism typically present with hypochloremia due to impaired water excretion, absence of aldosterone, impaired renal function, and lactic acidosis. These factors prevent manifestation of hyperchloremia.

The anion gap represents the difference between the commonly measured plasma cations and the commonly measured anions. This concept is discussed in detail in Chapters 9 and 12. The normal electrolyte composition of canine plasma is compared with that in normal (hyperchloremic) and increased (normochloremic) anion gap metabolic acidosis in Figure 10–2. The anion gap concept is useful in the diagnostic approach to the patient with metabolic acidosis, but it must not be taken literally. In reality, electroneutrality is maintained and there is no actual anion gap. Normally, the anion gap is made up of the net negative charge on sulfates, phosphates, plasma proteins, and organic anions (e.g., lactate, citrate). Factors other than metabolic acidosis may also affect the value of the anion gap, and these are discussed in the Chapter 12.

When the anion gap is calculated as $[(Na^+ + K^+) - (Cl^- + HCO_3^-)]$, normal values in dogs are in the range 12 to 25 mEq/L (Adrogue et al. 1978; Shull 1978; Polzin et al. 1982). Values for anion gaps in cats are probably similar. For example, the mean anion gap for normal cats (calculated as just described) is approximately 20 mEq/L (Christopher et al. 1989; Christopher et al. 1990; Chew et al. 1991). If the observed metabolic acidosis is characterized by a high anion gap, it is assumed to have arisen from an acid that does not contain chloride as its anion. Examples include some inorganic acids (e.g., phosphates, sulfates) or organic acids (e.g., lactate, ketoacids, salicylate, metabolites of ethylene glycol). In this setting, titration of body buffers by the acid results in accumulation of an anion other than chloride. If the observed metabolic acidosis is characterized by a normal anion gap, there is a reciprocal increase in the plasma chloride concentration to balance the decrease in plasma HCO_3^- concentration. In the following discussion below, the causes of metabolic acidosis have been divided into those associated with a normal anion gap and those associated with an increased anion gap.

Disorders Associated with a Normal Anion Gap

DIARRHEA

The concentration of HCO_3^- in intestinal fluid is usually higher than that of plasma, whereas its Cl^- concentration is lower. This results from the addition of alkaline pancreatic and biliary secretions to luminal contents and from secretion of HCO_3^- in exchange for Cl^- in the ileum (Fig. 10–3 and Table 10–2). In some diseases of the small intestine, increased delivery of ileal contents to the colon may overwhelm the considerable capacity of the colon for reabsorption of fluid and electrolytes. As a result, severe acute small-bowel diarrhea may cause loss of HCO_3^- in excess of Cl^- with resultant hyperchloremic metabolic acidosis. The acidosis is not purely hyperchloremic but rather is mixed if volume depletion and impaired tissue perfusion lead to lactic acid accumulation.

In one study of 134 dogs with gastroenteritis caused by parvoviral infection, only 13% had low total CO_2 concentrations (Jacobs et al. 1980). In another study of 17 dogs with parvoviral gastroenteritis, 59% had normal pH at presentation (Heald et al. 1986). In the animals with abnormal blood gas results, alkalemia (6 of 17) was more

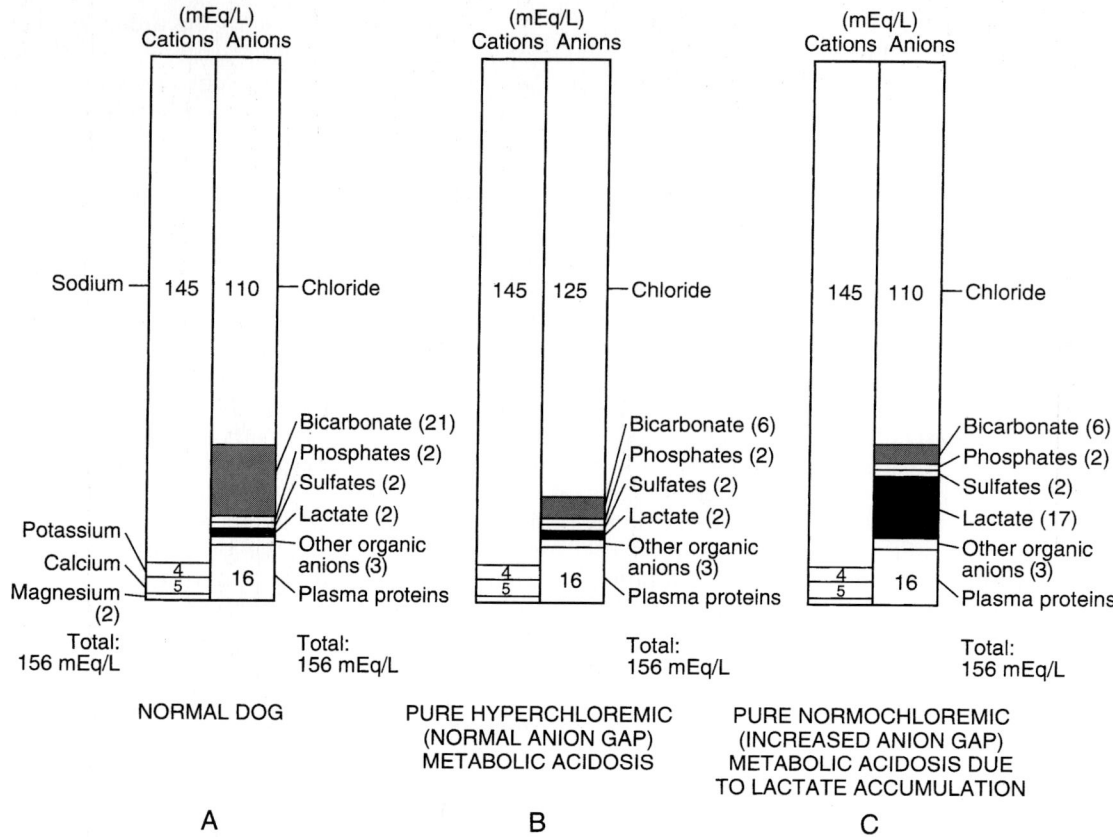

FIGURE 10-2. Theoretical examples of electrolyte distribution in (A) normal canine plasma, (B) a dog with pure hyperchloremic (normal anion gap) metabolic acidosis, and (C) a dog with normochloremic (increased anion gap) metabolic acidosis caused by lactate accumulation (i.e., lactic acidosis). (Adapted from Toto RD: Metabolic acid-base disorders. In Kokko JP and Tannen RL: *Fluids and Electrolytes*, 2nd ed. Philadelphia, WB Saunders Co., p. 324, 1990.)

common than acidemia (1 of 17). The majority (64%) of the dogs in this study were presented for both vomiting and diarrhea. Hypochloremia is much more common than hyperchloremia in parvoviral gastroenteritis (Jacobs et al. 1980; Heald et al. 1986). Presumably, vomiting plays a more important role than does diarrhea in the acid-base and electrolyte disturbances of dogs with parvoviral gastroenteritis.

TABLE 10-2. **Electrolyte Composition of Luminal Fluid at the End of Individual Segments of the Gastrointestinal Tract**

Segment End	Na+ (mEq/L)	K+ (mEq/L)	HCO$_3^-$ (mEq/L)	Cl- (mEq/L)
Duodenum	60	15	15	60
Jejunum	140	6	30	100
Ileum	140	8	70	60
Colon	40	90	30	15*

Source: Sleisinger MH and Fordtran JS (eds): *Gastrointestinal Diseases*, 3rd ed. Philadelphia, WB Saunders Co., p. 258, 1983.

*The large anion gap in luminal fluid at the end of the colon is due to the presence of organic anions resulting from bacterial metabolism. These organic anions represent functional base loss in the stool, because they could have been metabolized in the body to yield HCO$_3^-$.

RENAL TUBULAR ACIDOSIS

Renal tubular acidosis (RTA) is characterized by hyperchloremic metabolic acidosis caused by either decreased HCO$_3^-$ reabsorption (proximal RTA) or defective acid excretion (distal RTA) in the presence of a normal glomerular filtration rate (GFR). RTA is uncommonly recognized in small animal practice.

DISTAL RENAL TUBULAR ACIDOSIS

In *distal (classic or type 1) RTA*, the urine cannot be maximally acidified because of impaired hydrogen ion secretion in the collecting ducts, and urine pH is typically above 6.0, despite moderately to markedly decreased plasma HCO$_3^-$ concentration. Increased urine pH (>6.0) in the presence of acidosis is the hallmark of distal RTA. Urinary tract infection by a urease-positive organism (e.g., *Proteus* sp., *Staphylococcus aureus*) must be ruled out before considering distal RTA. Urinary net acid excretion is decreased, but bicarbonaturia is usually mild because urinary HCO$_3^-$ concentration is 1 to 3 mEq/L in the pH range 6.0 to 6.5. Nephrolithiasis (usually calcium phosphate stones), nephrocalcinosis (resulting from alkaline urine pH and decreased urinary citrate concentration), bone demineralization (resulting from loss of bone buffer stores during chronic acidosis), and urinary potassium wasting with hypokalemia are features of distal RTA in human patients. Urinary fractional excretion of HCO$_3^-$

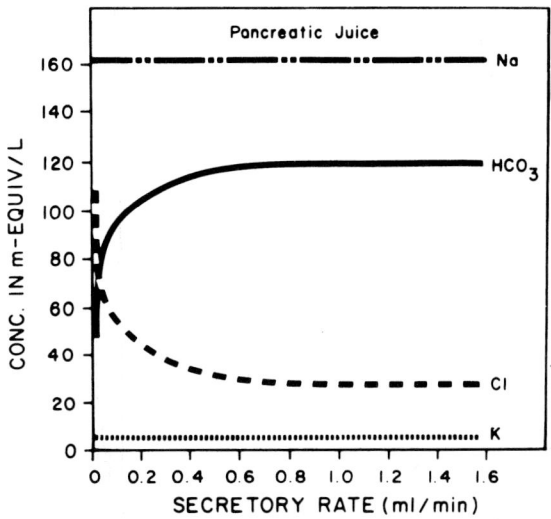

FIGURE 10-3. Influence of secretory rate on electrolyte composition of canine pancreatic juice. Note the inverse relationship between Cl^- and HCO_3^- concentrations and the relatively constant concentrations of Na^+ and K^+. (From Cohen JJ and Kassirer JP: *Acid-Base.* Boston, Little, Brown, & Co., p. 135, 1982.)

is normal (<5%) in distal RTA when plasma HCO_3^- concentration is increased to normal by alkali administration.

A diagnosis of distal RTA may be confirmed by an ammonium chloride tolerance test during which urine pH is monitored (using a pH meter) before and at hourly intervals for 5 h after oral administration of 0.2 g/kg NH_4Cl. Under such conditions, the urine pH of normal dogs decreased to a minimum value of 5.16 at 4 h after administration of ammonium chloride (Shaw 1989). Dogs in this study also developed systemic acidosis (pH approximately 7.22 and HCO_3^- approximately 14 mEq/L at 2 h after ammonium chloride administration). The amount of alkali required to correct the acidosis in human patients with distal RTA is variable but typically less than that required in proximal RTA. The required dosage of alkali in distal RTA may be as little as 1 mEq/kg/day (i.e., that required to offset daily endogenous acid production) or more than 2 to 4 mEq/kg/day. A combination of potassium and sodium citrate (depending on potassium balance) may be the preferred source of alkali (Rose 1994b).

PROXIMAL RENAL TUBULAR ACIDOSIS

In *proximal (type 2) RTA*, renal reabsorption of HCO_3^- is markedly reduced and urinary fractional excretion of HCO_3^- is increased (>15%) when plasma HCO_3^- concentration is increased to normal. Bicarbonaturia is absent and urine pH is appropriately low when metabolic acidosis is present and plasma HCO_3^- concentration is decreased, because distal acidifying ability is intact. When plasma HCO_3^- concentration is decreased, the filtered load of HCO_3^- is reduced and almost all of the filtered HCO_3^- is reabsorbed in the distal tubules, despite the presence of the proximal tubular defect. Thus, proximal RTA can be viewed as a "self-limiting" disorder in which plasma HCO_3^- stabilizes at a lower than normal concentration after the filtered load falls sufficiently that distal HCO_3^- reabsorption can maintain plasma HCO_3^- at a new but lower steady-state concentration.

Other abnormalities of proximal tubular function typically accompany impaired HCO_3^- reabsorption in proximal RTA, and these include defects in glucose, phosphate, sodium, potassium, uric acid, and amino acid reabsorption. This combination of proximal tubular defects is known as Fanconi's syndrome. Serum potasssium concentration is usually normal in affected human patients at the time of diagnosis, but alkali therapy may precipitate hypokalemia and aggravate urinary potassium wasting, presumably by increasing distal delivery of sodium and HCO_3^-.

The diagnosis of proximal RTA is made by finding an acid urine pH (<5.5–6.0) in the presence of hyperchloremic metabolic acidosis and normal GFR but an increased urine pH (>6.0) and increased urinary fractional excretion of HCO_3^- (>15%) after plasma HCO_3^- concentration has been increased to normal by alkali administration. If present, the detection of other defects in proximal tubular function (e.g., glucosuria with normal blood glucose concentration) establishes the diagnosis. Correction of metabolic acidosis by alkali therapy is more difficult in proximal RTA than in distal RTA because of the marked bicarbonaturia that occurs when plasma HCO_3^- concentration is increased to normal. Alkali dosages in excess of 10 mEq/kg/day may be required to correct the plasma HCO_3^- concentration, and such therapy may result in frank hypokalemia. Thus, potassium citrate may be the preferred source of alkali.

Multiple renal tubular reabsorptive defects resembling Fanconi's syndrome have been reported in young basenji dogs (Easley and Breitschwerdt 1976; Bovee et al. 1978a, 1978b; Bovee et al. 1979). Clinical findings included polyuria, polydipsia, weight loss, dehydration, and weakness. Affected dogs had abnormal fractional reabsorption of glucose, bicarbonate, phosphate, sodium, potassium, and urate and they had isolated cystinuria or generalized aminoaciduria. The renal tubular disorder in affected basenji dogs is thought to be due to a metabolic or membrane defect affecting sodium movement or increased back leak or cell-to-lumen flux of amino acids. In one study, brush border membranes isolated from basenji dogs with Fanconi's syndrome had decreased sodium-dependent glucose transport but no abnormality of cystine uptake despite the observed reabsorptive defect for cystine (McNamara et al. 1989). Defective urinary concentrating ability leads to isosthenuria or hyposthenuria and GFR may be normal initially but decreased later in the course of the disease. Hypokalemia has also been observed late in the course of the disease (Easley and Breitschwerdt 1976). Death usually results from acute renal failure and papillary necrosis or acute pyelonephritis. A distinctive renal lesion is hyperchromatic karyomegaly of renal tubular cells.

Fanconi's syndrome has been observed sporadically in other breeds (MacKenzie and van den Broek 1982; McEwan and Macartney 1987; Padrid 1988; Escolar et al. 1993; Settles and Schmidt 1994) and has been reported in association with administration of some drugs (Meyer 1977; Brown et al. 1986a; Bark and Perk 1995). In one case, Fanconi's syndrome developed in association with

TABLE 10-3. **Clinical Features of Proximal and Distal Renal Tubular Acidosis**

Clinical Feature	Proximal RTA	Distal RTA
Hypercalciuria	Yes	Yes
Hyperphosphaturia	Yes	Yes
Urinary citrate	Normal	Decreased
Bone disease	Less severe	More severe
Nephrocalcinosis	No	Yes
Nephrolithiasis	No	Yes (calcium phosphate)
Hypokalemia	Mild	Mild to severe
Potassium wasting	Worsened by NaHCO$_3$	Improved by NaHCO$_3$
Alkali required for treatment	>10 mEq/kg/day	<3 mEq/kg/day
Other defects of proximal tubular function*	Yes	No
Reduction in plasma HCO$_3^-$	Moderate	Variable (can be severe)
FE$_{HCO_3^-}$ at normal plasma HCO$_3^-$ concentration†	>15%	<5%
Urine pH during acidemia	<5.5	>6.0
Urine pH after NH$_4$Cl	<5.5	>6.0

*Decreased fractional reabsorption of sodium, potassium, phosphate, urate, glucose, and amino acids
†FE, Fractional excretion.

primary hypoparathyroidism and resolved after treatment with calcium and calcitriol (Freeman et al. 1994). Rickets in growing children and osteomalacia in adults are features of Fanconi's syndrome in human patients that are usually not observed in affected dogs. However, congenital Fanconi's syndrome and renal dysplasia were associated with histologic features of rickets in two Border terriers (Darrigrand-Haag et al. 1996). The skeletal abnormalities in one of the affected dogs resolved after treatment with calcitriol and potassium phosphate.

In one report, an 8-year-old female German shepherd dog had hyperchloremic metabolic acidosis, polyuria, polydipsia, isosthenuria, glucosuria with normal blood glucose concentration, and alkaline urine pH (7.46) after oral administration of NH$_4$Cl (DiBartola and Leonard 1982). The metabolic acidosis was unresponsive to NaHCO$_3$ administration at dosages up to 4 mEq/kg/day. This dog appeared to have distal (type 1) RTA and renal glucosuria. In another case of apparent distal RTA, a 5-year-old mixed breed dog was presented for evaluation of anorexia and was determined to have alkaline urine pH with hyperchloremic metabolic acidosis (Polzin et al. 1982). In another report, an 8-year-old female German shepherd dog was presented for polyuria, polydipisia, weight loss, and lethargy (Bovee 1984). It had a normal GFR, metabolic acidosis, hyposthenuria, and intermittent glucosuria. Fractional reabsorption of sodium, glucose, and HCO$_3^-$ was decreased but reabsorption of chloride, phosphate, potassium, urate, and amino acids was normal. The dog gained weight and its clinical signs were reversed after treatment with NaHCO$_3$ at approximately 10 mEq/kg/day. This dog appeared to have proximal (type 2) RTA.

Distal RTA has been reported in two cats with pyelonephritis caused by *Escherichia coli* (Drazner 1980; Watson et al. 1986). Clinical signs included polyuria, polydipsia, anorexia, lethargy, enlarged kidneys, and isosthenuria. In one cat, urine pH was 5.0 at the time pyelonephritis was first diagnosed but distal RTA was documented at a later time by the presence of hyperchloremic metabolic acidosis, alkaline urine pH, and failure to lower urine pH after oral administration of NH$_4$Cl (Drazner 1980).

Findings were similar for the other cat, but hyperphosphaturia and persistent hypokalemia also were detected (Watson et al. 1986). Distal RTA and hepatic lipidosis were reported in another cat without urinary tract infection (Brown et al. 1986b). The clinical features of proximal (type 2) and distal (type 1) RTA are summarized in Table 10-3.

Hyporeninemic hypoaldosteronism, characterized by hyperkalemia with decreased plasma renin and aldosterone concentrations, occurs in some human patients, notably those with diabetes mellitus who also have mild to moderate renal insufficiency (DeFronzo 1980). The hyperchloremic metabolic acidosis observed in these patients has been called *type 4 RTA*. This syndrome has not been characterized in veterinary medicine but should be considered in dogs and cats with hyperkalemia and mild to moderate hyperchloremic metabolic acidosis after hypoadrenocorticism has been ruled out by an adrenocorticotropic hormone (ACTH) response test. The diagnosis may be established by finding an inappropriately decreased plasma aldosterone concentration in the presence of hyperkalemia.

CARBONIC ANHYDRASE INHIBITORS

Carbonic anhydrase inhibitors such as acetazolamide (Diamox) decrease proximal tubular reabsorption of HCO$_3^-$ in the kidney by noncompetitive inhibition of luminal and cellular carbonic anhydrase. Hypokalemia is due to increased sodium delivery to the distal nephron and its reabsorption there in exchange for potassium. As hyperchloremic metabolic acidosis develops, the filtered load of HCO$_3^-$ decreases and the effect of carbonic anhydrase inhibitors on HCO$_3^-$ reabsorption is limited. Acetazolamide given at 7 to 10 mg/kg t.i.d. causes self-limiting hyperchloremic metabolic acidosis, mild to moderate hypokalemia, and mild hypocalcemia in dogs (Rose and Carter 1979; Haskins et al. 1981). The effects of acetazolamide were greatest after 3 days of administration and blood chemistry results stabilized after 5 days of administration (Rose and Carter 1979). Acetazolamide is used most commonly in small animal practice for the treatment of glaucoma.

AMMONIUM CHLORIDE

Administration of NH_4Cl is equivalent to administration of HCl because the NH_4^+ is converted in the liver to urea and H^+. Ammonium chloride has been used commonly as a urinary acidifier in dogs and cats. A study of cats receiving 800 mg of NH_4Cl per day as powder or tablet showed that venous blood pH and HCO_3^- concentrations were decreased to values at the lower end of the normal range (Senior et al. 1986). A combination product supplying 580 mg each of NH_4Cl and D,L-methionine had a more marked effect on venous blood pH and HCO_3^- concentrations than that observed with 800 mg of NH_4Cl alone, but results were still within the reported normal range (Senior et al. 1986). In another study of cats, NH_4Cl at 300 mg/kg/day did not significantly alter venous blood pH, Pco_2, or HCO_3^- concentration but 400 mg/kg/day significantly decreased blood HCO_3^- concentration during the course of the study (Finco et al. 1986). Ammonium chloride at a dosage of 535 mg/kg/day administered to dogs over 6 days caused hyperchloremic metabolic acidosis and was associated with hypokalemia, presumably related to increased aldosterone secretion (Magner et al. 1988). In another study of dogs, NH_4Cl at 200 mg/kg/day reduced urine pH to approximately 5.0 and produced mild metabolic acidosis without change in serum potassium concentration (Schober 1996).

In young, growing, and adult dogs, addition of NH_4Cl to the diet leads to demineralization of bone (Jaffe et al. 1932; Burnell 1971). Chronic acid feeding has also been reported to affect bone metabolism in cats. Diets containing 3% NH_4Cl slowed growth of young cats, decreased blood pH and HCO_3^- concentrations, and lowered urine pH. Urinary calcium excretion increased in these cats, and bone demineralization was observed on histologic examination of caudal vertebrae (Buffington et al. 1989). Adult cats fed 1.5% NH_4Cl for 6 months developed hyperchloremic metabolic acidosis and negative balance for calcium and potassium (Ching et al. 1989), but no significant changes in trabecular bone remodeling or bone mineral density were found (Ching et al. 1990). In one study, administration of NH_4Cl to cats fed a potassium-restricted diet resulted in hypokalemia, possibly by reducing gastrointestinal absorption of potassium (Dow et al. 1990). Results of these studies indicate that NH_4Cl should be used with caution and blood gases should be monitored during therapy.

INFUSION OF CATIONIC AMINO ACIDS

Metabolism of cationic amino acids (e.g., lysine, arginine, histidine) results in production of H^+ as the NH_4^+ from these amino acids is converted to urea in the liver. For this reason, amino acid–containing fluids used in total parenteral nutrition can contribute to hyperchloremic metabolic acidosis. Other contributing factors are the presence of sulfur-containing amino acids (e.g., methionine, cysteine) in the fluid as well as development of hypophosphatemia during refeeding, which may reduce renal excretion of titratable acid.

POSTHYPOCAPNIC METABOLIC ACIDOSIS

During compensation for chronic respiratory alkalosis, renal net acid excretion decreases with consequent reduction in plasma HCO_3^- and increase in plasma Cl^- concentrations. When the stimulus for hyperventilation is removed and Pco_2 increases, pH decreases because it requires 1 to 3 days for the kidneys to increase net acid excretion and increase plasma HCO_3^- concentration. Until this occurs, a state of "posthypocapnic" metabolic acidosis exists. Recovery is spontaneous as long as sodium and phosphate are available in the diet to allow the appropriate increase in renal net acid excretion (Gougoux et al. 1975).

DILUTIONAL ACIDOSIS

Dilutional acidosis refers to a decrease in plasma HCO_3^- concentration that occurs when extracellular volume is expanded using an alkali-free chloride-containing solution such as 0.9% NaCl. The high chloride concentration of 0.9% NaCl and the highly resorbable nature of the chloride ion in the renal tubules contribute to the decrease in plasma HCO_3^- concentration and increase in Cl^- concentration. Dilutional acidosis can be corrected by substitution of a solution with a lower chloride concentration (e.g., lactated Ringer's solution, 0.45% NaCl).

HYPOADRENOCORTICISM

Aldosterone increases renal tubular lumen negativity by enhancing sodium reabsorption in the collecting duct and secondarily increases hydrogen ion secretion. It also directly stimulates H^+ secretion by increasing the activity of the luminal H^+-ATPase pump in the medullary collecting duct. These effects allow urinary excretion of H^+ and K^+ when distal delivery of sodium is decreased. Deficiency of aldosterone in hypoadrenocorticism results in metabolic acidosis and hyperkalemia. Metabolic acidosis of variable severity is common in dogs with hypoadrenocorticism (Melian and Peterson 1996; Peterson et al. 1996). In one study, uncompensated metabolic acidosis was found in 43%, compensated metabolic acidosis in 25%, mixed metabolic acidosis and respiratory alkalosis in 11%, and normal acid-base balance in 21% of 28 dogs with hypoadrenocorticism that had blood gas analysis performed (Melian and Peterson 1996). In one study of 10 cats with hypoadrenocorticism, 3 were reported to have decreased serum total CO_2 concentrations (Peterson et al. 1989). Treatment of hypoadrenocorticism includes volume expansion with 0.9% NaCl and replacement of deficient mineralocorticoids and glucocorticoids.

Disorders Associated with an Increased Anion Gap

ETHYLENE GLYCOL INGESTION

Ethylene glycol (EG) is an organic solvent (molecular mass 62 daltons) used in commercial antifreeze solutions. Ingestion of antifreeze by dogs and cats is a common cause of oliguric acute renal failure in small animal practice and mortality exceeds 80% in affected animals (Grauer and Thrall 1982; Thrall et al. 1984; Connally et al. 1996). Ethylene glycol itself is not toxic, but it is converted in the liver to several metabolites that cause

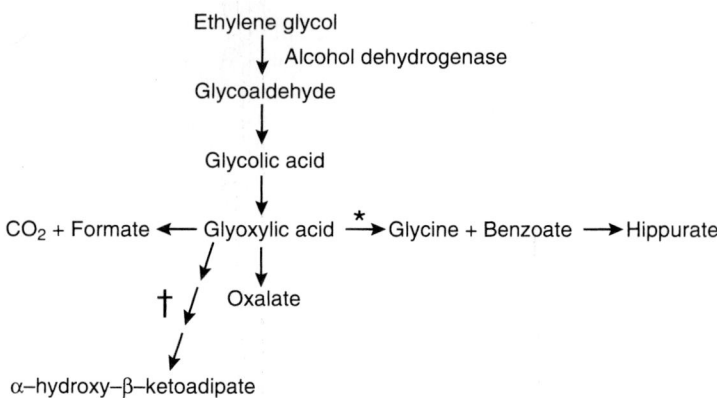

FIGURE 10–4. Metabolism of ethylene glycol.

* Pyridoxine is a cofactor for this reaction.
† Thiamine is a cofactor for this reaction.

severe metabolic acidosis and acute renal failure (Fig. 10–4). It is rapidly absorbed from the gastrointestinal tract and is undetectable in plasma of dogs 48 h after administration (Nunamaker et al. 1971; Sanyer et al. 1973).

PATHOPHYSIOLOGY

Ethylene glycol is first metabolized in the liver to glycoaldehyde by alcohol dehydrogenase. Glycoaldehyde uncouples oxidative phosphorylation and may contribute to neurologic signs observed early in the course of intoxication. Subsequent steps in metabolism produce glycolic and glyoxylic acids. Glycolic acid is primarily responsible for the severe metabolic acidosis that occurs in animals poisoned by EG (Clay and Murphy 1977). Renal tubular injury results from glycoaldehyde, glycolic acid, and glyoxylic acids and calcium oxalate crystals are deposited within renal tubules. The observation of these birefringent crystals in the presence of acute tubular nephrosis confirms the diagnosis of EG intoxication.

Vomiting, polydipsia, and polyuria may occur soon after ingestion of EG, but these signs are often not detected by owners of poisoned animals. Within 12 h of ingestion, neurologic signs (e.g., lethargy, ataxia, stupor, seizures, coma) may develop. Cardiac and pulmonary manifestations (e.g., tachypnea, tachycardia) occur 12 to 24 h after ingestion but are rarely detected in clinical cases. Oxalate crystals may be detected in the urine as early as 3 to 6 h after ingestion of EG (Dial et al. 1994a, 1994b). Renal failure occurs in dogs as early as 24 to 48 h after ingestion and is manifested by anorexia, lethargy, vomiting, and oliguria or anuria (Grauer et al. 1984). In cats, azotemia may develop within 12 to 24 h after ingestion of EG (Dial et al. 1994a). Unfortunately, most dogs and cats with EG poisoning are presented for veterinary attention after renal failure has already developed.

A severe normochloremic (i.e., high anion gap) metabolic acidosis occurs within 3 h of EG ingestion and persists for at least 24 h (Grauer et al. 1984; Thrall et al. 1984; Dial et al. 1994a, 1994b). Serum hyperosmolality and osmolal gap peak 1 to 6 h after ingestion and persist for 12 to 24 h (Grauer et al. 1984; Dial et al. 1994a, 1994b), but the osmolal gap may be normal in animals presented later in the course of the disease (Thrall et al. 1984). Calcium oxalate dihydrate crystals ("Maltese cross" or "envelope" forms) may be observed in the urine, but calcium oxalate monohydrate crystals ("picket fence" or "dumbbell" forms) are observed more commonly. Calcium oxalate dihydrate crystals are occasionally found in the urine of normal dogs and cats, whereas calcium oxalate monohydrate crystals are rarely seen except in animals that have ingested EG (Thrall et al. 1984; Dial et al. 1994a) (Fig. 10–5). Crystals previously referred to as hippurates actually are calcium oxalate monohydrate crystals (Kramer et al. 1984; Thrall et al. 1985). Other laboratory findings include azotemia, isosthenuria, hypocalcemia, hyperphosphatemia, and hyperglycemia (Thrall et al. 1984). Hyperphosphatemia observed very early in the course of EG intoxication (3–12 h after ingestion) is probably due to the high phosphorus content of rust-retardant antifreeze preparations (Dial et al. 1994b; Connally et al. 1996). Hyperechogenicity of the renal cortex is observed on renal ultrasonography as early as 5 h after ingestion of EG (Adams et al. 1989).

TREATMENT

The response to treatment depends on the amount of EG ingested and the amount of time that elapses before treatment. In early studies, dogs that ingested <10 mL/kg EG were saved if treated within 2 to 4 h of ingestion (Beckett and Shields 1971; Nunamaker et al. 1971; Sanyer et al. 1973) and cats survived up to 6 mL/kg EG if treated within 4 h (Penumarthy and Oehme 1974). Treatment consists of inducing vomiting with apomorphine or performing gastric lavage with activated charcoal if ingestion has been recent (<8 h before presentation). Severe hypocalcemia is corrected with calcium gluconate and $NaHCO_3$ is administered to combat metabolic acidosis. An $NaHCO_3$ dosage of 1 to 2 mEq/kg may be used empirically. Calcium gluconate and $NaHCO_3$ must not be given simultaneously, because calcium carbonate crystals form and the solution becomes turbid. An attempt to stimulate urine production with furosemide (2–4 mg/kg) or mannitol (1 g/kg) is recommended but is usually futile.

Alcohol dehydrogenase has greater affinity for ethanol than EG. For this reason, 20% ethanol has been adminis-

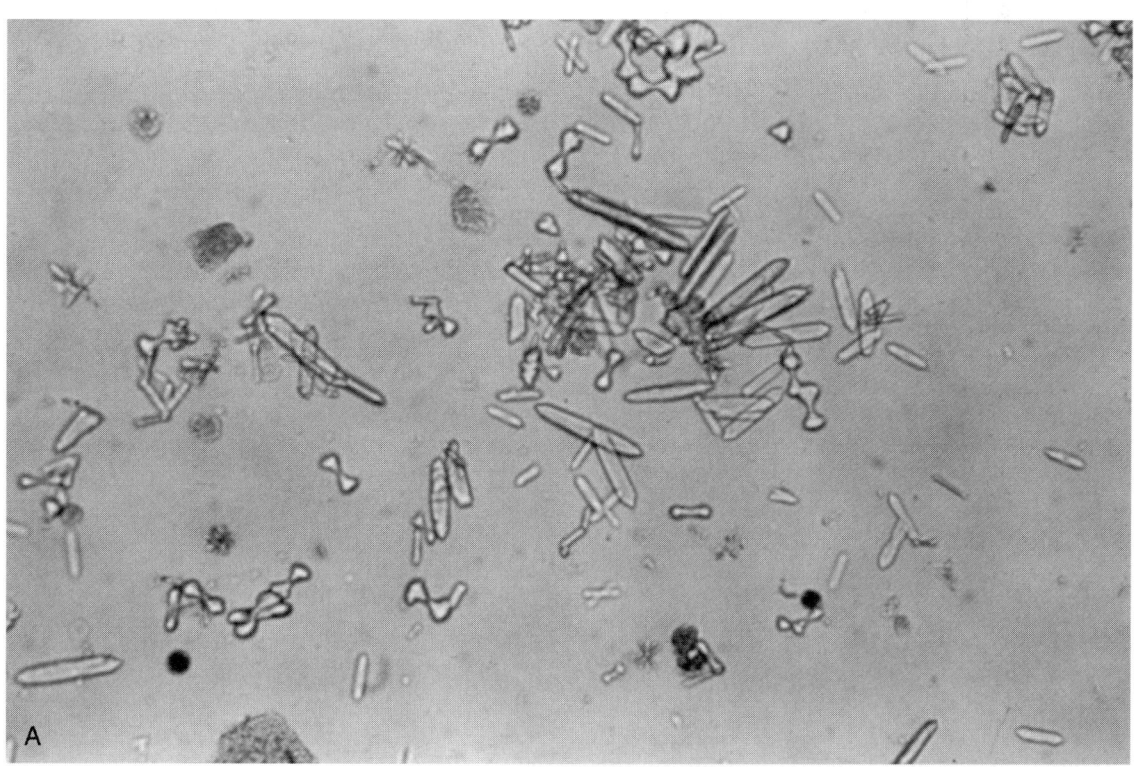
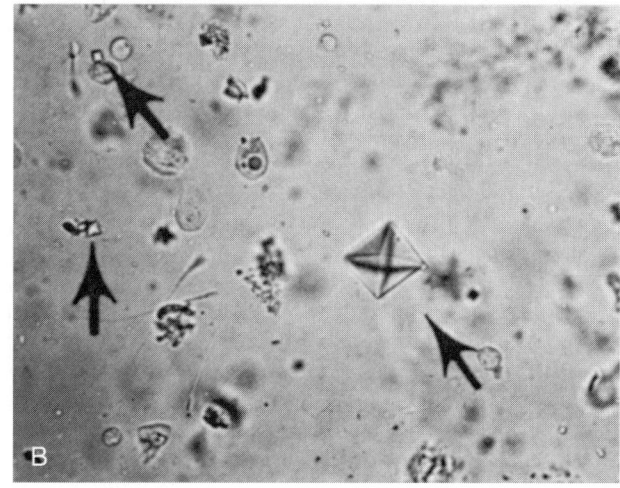

FIGURE 10-5. Photomicrographs of (A) calcium oxalate monohydrate and (B) dihydrate crystals in urine sediment. (From Chew DJ and DiBartola SP: Diagnosis and pathophysiology of renal disease. In Ettinger SJ: *Textbook of Veterinary Internal Medicine.* Philadelphia, WB Saunders, p. 1907, 1989.)

tered intravenously to affected dogs at a dosage of 5.5 mL/kg q4h for five treatments and then q6h for four additional treatments (Grauer and Thrall 1986). Cats are treated with 20% ethanol at a dosage of 5 mL/kg q6h for five treatments and then q8h for four additional treatments. This treatment is unlikely to be of benefit if more than 12 to 24 h has elapsed since ingestion of EG. 4-Methylpyrazole (Antizol) is a pharmacologic inhibitor of alcohol dehydrogenase that has become available to treat dogs with EG toxicosis (Dial et al. 1989, 1994b). In dogs, it is superior to ethanol because it does not cause central nervous system (CNS) depression, but it must be administered within 8 h of EG ingestion. The dosage of 4-methylpyrazole used in dogs with EG intoxication is 20 mg/kg IV, followed by 15 mg/kg IV at 12 and 24 h and 5 mg/kg IV at 36 h (Dial et al. 1989, 1994b; Connally et al. 1996). Unfortunately, 4-methylpyrazole is not efficacious in EG-intoxicated cats unless administered at the same time as the EG is consumed. The observed lack of effectiveness of 4-methylpyrazole in EG-intoxicated cats may be related to a shorter half-life of EG in cats (2–5 h) compared with dogs (8–10 h) and more rapid development of acute renal failure in cats or to decreased efficacy of 4-methylpyrazole as an inhibitor of alcohol dehydrogenase in cats (Dial et al. 1994a). Thiamine promotes conversion of glyoxylate to glycine and pyridoxine promotes conversion of glyoxylate to α-hydroxy-β-ketoadipate (see Fig. 10–4). These vitamins may be administered to promote alternative pathways of glyoxylate metabolism, but efficacy has not been demonstrated for such treatment. In one study, all nonazotemic dogs treated with 4-methylpyrazole within 2 to 8.5 h after EG ingestion survived, whereas only 1 of 21 azotemic dogs treated 8.5 to 38 h after ingestion survived (Connally et al. 1996).

Peritoneal dialysis is necessary if the animal is in anuric or oliguric renal failure at the time of presentation. Early dialysis may also be helpful to remove toxic intermediate metabolites. Despite dialysis, affected dogs may progress to end-stage renal disease and become dialysis dependent. The prognosis for survival in adult dogs and cats with anuric or oliguric acute renal failure caused by EG intoxication is unfortunately very poor (Thrall et al. 1984; Connally et al. 1996).

SALICYLATE INTOXICATION

Aspirin (acetylsalicylic acid) is hydrolyzed to salicylic acid ($pK_a' = 3.0$) in the liver. Salicylate intoxication is uncommon in small animal practice and is an example of a mixed acid-base disturbance characterized by metabolic acidosis and respiratory alkalosis. Salicylate intoxication in anesthetized, spontaneously breathing dogs resulted in a mixed respiratory alkalosis and metabolic acidosis (Silva et al. 1986). The stimulation of ventilation is due to a direct effect of salicylate on the medullary respiratory center. Salicylate also uncouples oxidative phosphorylation in mitochondria, and the associated disturbances in carbohydrate metabolism lead to metabolic acidosis characterized by an increased anion gap associated with accumulation of lactic acid, ketoacids, and other organic acids. Salicylate usually makes a minor contribution to the observed increase in unmeasured anions.

Gastric lavage with activated charcoal should be performed if ingestion occurred less than 6 to 12 h before admission. Administration of $NaHCO_3$ promotes removal of salicylate from tissues and enhances its urinary excretion by the mechanism of *diffusion trapping*. Alkalinization of ECF and urine increases the proportion of drug present in the ionized form and thus favors diffusion of more nonionized salicylic acid from cells into ECF and urine, where it can be trapped as the poorly diffusible ionized form. An attempt should be made to maintain urine pH above 7.5 during alkaline diuresis with $NaHCO_3$, especially if metabolic acidosis is the predominant acid-base disturbance. Alkalinization should be carried out with caution, if at all, when respiratory alkalosis is the predominant acid-base disturbance. Glucose infusion is recommended to prevent reduction in CNS glucose concentration. Hypokalemia may develop during treatment as a result of $NaHCO_3$ administration and diuresis, and parenteral fluids should be supplemented with potassium as needed.

DIABETIC KETOACIDOSIS

PATHOPHYSIOLOGY

Overproduction of acetoacetic acid ($pK_a' = 3.58$) and β-hydroxybutyrate ($pK_a' = 4.70$) by the liver occurs in diabetes mellitus because of a deficiency of insulin and relative excess of glucagon. An increase in glucagon and decrease in insulin shift the liver from its normal role in esterification of fatty acids into triglycerides to β-oxidation of fatty acids into ketoacids. At the normal pH of ECF (7.40), these organic acids are completely dissociated and the hydrogen ions that are released titrate HCO_3^- and other body buffers. Acetone is formed by the nonenzymatic decarboxylation of acetoacetate and does not contribute additional fixed acid. The pathophysiology and treatment of diabetic ketoacidosis are discussed in detail in Chapter 17.

Metabolic acidosis is common in dogs and cats with diabetic ketoacidosis. In one series, mean plasma HCO_3^- concentration in 72 dogs with diabetic ketoacidosis was approximately 11 mEq/L at the time of diagnosis with a range of 4 to 20 mEq/L, whereas the mean HCO_3^- concentration in 20 affected cats was 13 mEq/L with a range of 8 to 22 mEq/L (Feldman and Nelson 1996a). In an early study of dogs with diabetes mellitus, mean plasma HCO_3^- concentration was 13.7 mEq/L in eight survivors (range, 9.3–21.0 mEq/L) and 18.1 mEq/L in five nonsurvivors (range, 13.4–30.2 mEq/L) (Ling et al. 1977). In another study of dogs with diabetic ketoacidosis, mean arterial pH and HCO_3^- concentration were 7.201 (range, 6.986–7.395) and 11.1 mEq/L (range, 4.1–19.7 mEq/L) before treatment and 7.407 ± 0.053 and 18.2 ± 0.7 mEq/L 24 h after treatment (Macintire 1993). Only three dogs (those with pH < 7.1) received sodium bicarbonate treatment. Metabolic acidosis with median pH of 7.14 (range, 7.04–7.24) and HCO_3^- concentration of 10 mEq/L (range, 6–15 mEq/L) was found in 25 of 33 cats evaluated by venous blood gas analysis in a survey of cats with diabetic ketoacidosis (Bruskiewicz et al. 1997). Cats with HCO_3^- concentrations below 14 mEq/L received bicarbonate supplementation of their fluids. In another series of diabetic cats, median total CO_2 was 13 mEq/L in ketoacidotic cats and 15 mEq/L in nonketoacidotic cats (Crenshaw and Peterson 1996).

The nitroprusside reagent (e.g., Acetest) detects only ketone (–C=O) groups (e.g., acetoacetate, acetone). The concentration of β-hydroxybutyrate typically exceeds that of acetoacetate in uncontrolled diabetic ketoacidosis, and the dipstick reaction underestimates the degree of ketonuria. This problem can be overcome by adding a few drops of hydrogen peroxide to urine, which nonenzymatically converts β-hydroxybutyrate to acetoacetate (Narins et al. 1982). When insulin is administered and metabolism of ketones proceeds, there is a shift toward acetoacetate and the dipstick reaction transiently becomes more strongly positive. This possibility should be recognized by the clinician and should not cause concern. The increase in unmeasured anions (as reflected in the anion gap) gives a rough estimate of the concentration of ketoanions in serum. This estimate is inaccurate, however, if lactic acidosis develops because lactate is also an unmeasured anion.

To some extent, the anions of these ketoacids are excreted in the urine along with sodium and potassium for electroneutrality. These organic anions are lost from the body and cannot be metabolized to HCO_3^- after correction of diabetic ketoacidosis with insulin therapy. Their loss thus contributes to depletion of body buffer and cation stores. Osmotic diuresis is induced by hyperglycemia and also contributes to the whole-body cation deficit. The extent of impairment in renal function may determine whether patients with diabetic ketoacidosis have an increased anion gap metabolic acidosis or hyperchloremic metabolic acidosis at the time of presentation. Patients with severe volume depletion have an increased anion gap because of retention of ketoanions, whereas those without volume depletion have hyperchloremia as a result of increased urinary excretion of the sodium and potassium salts of ketoanions and retention of chloride (Adrogue et al. 1982, 1984).

TREATMENT

The best treatment for the acidosis of uncontrolled diabetes mellitus is fluid therapy and insulin. Insulin administration allows glucose utilization by skeletal muscle and adipose tissue, decreases hepatic glucose production, prevents lipolysis and ketogenesis, and permits peripheral metabolism of ketoacids. Several regimens for administration of insulin to ketoacidotic dogs and cats have been described (Feldman and Nelson 1996b). The particular protocol of insulin administration is probably less crucial to the ultimate outcome than the individualized care provided by the veterinarian during management of the diabetic animal.

Several factors may contribute to a delay in the repair of the HCO_3^- deficit in patients with diabetic ketoacidosis (Harrington and Cohen 1982b). Ketoacid anions that have been excreted in the urine are lost to the body and cannot be metabolized to HCO_3^-. After treatment with fluids and insulin, recovery may be faster in patients with a high anion gap, because the retained ketoanions are metabolized, yielding HCO_3^- (Adrogue et al. 1982, 1984). Thus, withholding alkali may be more rational for diabetic patients with high-anion-gap metabolic acidosis than for those with hyperchloremic metabolic acidosis. Dilutional acidosis may occur if extracellular fluid volume (ECFV) is expanded with alkali-free solutions such as 0.9% saline. If hyperventilation persists, it may impair renal reabsorption of HCO_3^- and renal acid excretion may require several days to become fully augmented.

The use of $NaHCO_3$ to treat diabetic ketoacidosis is highly controversial and clear benefits of its use have not been demonstrated in human patients. For example, there was no difference in recovery (based on rate of decrease of blood glucose and ketone concentrations and rate of increase of blood or cerebrospinal fluid (CSF) pH or HCO_3^- concentration) when $NaHCO_3$ was or was not administered to human patients with diabetic ketoacidosis who presented with blood pH values in the range 6.90 to 7.14 (Morris et al. 1986). In another study, treatment with $NaHCO_3$ actually delayed resolution of ketosis in diabetic ketoacidosis (Okuda et al. 1996).

There are several theoretical arguments against the use of $NaHCO_3$ in diabetic ketoacidosis. Acidosis in the CNS may develop after $NaHCO_3$ administration. The blood-brain barrier is permeable to CO_2 but less permeable to the charged HCO_3^- ion. If $NaHCO_3$ is administered, pH increases in ECF as the HCO_3^-/PCO_2 ratio increases, and compensatory hyperventilation decreases somewhat. As a result, PCO_2 increases and CO_2 diffuses into the CNS. Bicarbonate diffusion into CNS, however, lags behind that of CO_2. During this time, the HCO_3^-/PCO_2 ratio and pH in the CNS may decrease. This has been referred to as *paradoxical CNS acidosis* (Posner and Plum 1967). The frequency of occurrence of this complication and its clinical significance are uncertain (Kreisberg 1978).

The pathophysiology of diabetic ketoacidosis also affects oxygen delivery to tissues. Chronic acidosis shifts the oxygen-hemoglobin dissociation curve to the right, thus enhancing delivery of oxygen to the tissues. On the other hand, phosphorus deficiency in diabetes decreases red cell 2,3-diphosphoglycerate concentration and causes a shift of the oxygen-hemoglobin dissociation curve back to the left. Correction of acidosis with $NaHCO_3$ shifts the curve farther to the left and potentially decreases oxygen delivery to tissues. Administration of insulin and fluid therapy, however, also lead to correction of the acidosis and should have a similar effect on the oxygen-hemoglobin dissociation curve.

Overzealous therapy with $NaHCO_3$ may contribute to late development of metabolic alkalosis because insulin promotes metabolism of retained ketoacid anions to HCO_3^-. This excess HCO_3^- should be readily excreted in the urine if renal function is adequate. Other potentially detrimental effects of $NaHCO_3$ therapy include aggravation of hyperosmolality as a consequence of the obligatory sodium load, tetany resulting from a sudden decrease in ionized serum calcium concentration, and precipitation of severe hypokalemia as extracellular potassium ions move into cells during administration of insulin and correction of acidosis. For all these reasons, $NaHCO_3$ is not used unless severe acidosis (pH < 7.1–7.2) is present and then only in small amounts (see section on treatment of metabolic acidosis).

UREMIC ACIDOSIS

PATHOPHYSIOLOGY

The metabolic acidosis of chronic renal failure is usually mild to moderate in severity (plasma HCO_3^- concentration, 12–15 mEq/L) and may be hyperchloremic early in the course of the disease process (Widmer et al. 1979). Later in the course of the disease, the anion gap increases because of retention of phosphates, sulfates, and organic anions. Acid-base status is usually well preserved in chronic renal failure until GFR falls to 10 to 20% of normal. In retrospective studies of small animal patients with chronic renal failure, plasma HCO_3^- concentrations were below 16 mEq/L in 40% of dogs with chronic renal failure caused by amyloidosis (DiBartola et al. 1989) and below 15 mEq/L in 63% of cats with chronic renal failure of various causes (DiBartola et al. 1987). A high anion gap was observed in 43% of affected dogs (>25 mEq/L) and in 19% of affected cats (>35 mEq/L) in these studies. In acute renal failure, there has been insufficient time for the kidneys to adapt to the disease state, and the metabolic acidosis of acute renal failure is usually more severe than that observed in chronic renal failure. Complications such as sepsis and marked tissue catabolism may contribute to the severity of metabolic acidosis in acute renal failure.

Delivery of HCO_3^- from the proximal tubules to the distal nephron is increased in chronic renal failure (Warnock 1988). In dogs with experimentally induced unilateral renal disease, renal HCO_3^- reabsorption was not different in the diseased and control kidneys, but bicarbonaturia developed when the normal kidney was removed and the contralateral diseased kidney was forced to function in a uremic environment (Morrin et al. 1962b). The osmotic diuresis characteristic of uremia may thus contribute to the increased delivery of HCO_3^- to the distal tubules. Increased parathyroid hormone concentration as a result of renal secondary hyperparathyroidism does not seem to have important adverse effects on HCO_3^- reabsorption in experimentally induced renal disease in dogs (Arruda et al. 1976; Schmidt et al. 1976; Schmidt and Gavellas 1977). The ability to lower urine pH maximally is preserved in chronic renal failure.

The main method by which the diseased kidney responds to chronic retention of fixed acid is by enhanced renal ammoniagenesis. Total ammonium excretion falls during progressive chronic renal disease, but ammonium excretion is observed to be markedly increased when expressed per 100 mL GFR or per remnant nephron (Dorhout-Mees et al. 1966; Sabatini 1983). On a per-nephron basis, the diseased kidney can increase its ammonium excretion three- to fivefold (Simpson 1971; Welbourne et al. 1972; Warnock 1988). This adaptive mechanism seems to be fully expended when the GFR falls below 20% of normal. At this point, the diseased kidneys can no longer effectively cope with the daily fixed acid load and a new steady state is established at a lower than normal plasma HCO_3^- concentration. The relatively mild decrease in plasma HCO_3^- concentration that is observed in chronic renal failure has been attributed to the contribution of the large reservoir of buffer (e.g., calcium carbonate) in bone. The capacity of the skeleton to buffer the amount of acid that accumulates in long-standing chronic renal failure, however, has been questioned (Oh 1991). The decrease in total ammonium excretion that occurs in chronic renal failure may be counterbalanced by decreased urinary excretion of organic anions (e.g., citrate, lactate, pyruvate, ketoanions) (Cohen et al. 1997). Metabolism of these retained organic anions would result in a net gain of HCO_3^- that would offset the decreased excretion of H^+ in the form of NH_4^+.

The amount of phosphate buffer available in urine in chronic renal failure is relatively fixed and likely to be at its maximum because of hyperphosphatemia and the effects of increased plasma parathyroid hormone concentration (Simpson 1971; Sabatini 1983). Furthermore, phosphorus binders and dietary phosphorus restriction are commonly used to treat chronic renal failure and actually may limit the amount of phosphate that can contribute to titratable acidity. When expressed on a per-nephron basis, however, titratable acidity is increased in chronic renal failure (Morrin et al. 1962a).

TREATMENT

Whether or not to treat well-compensated, mild to moderate metabolic acidosis in adult patients with chronic renal failure is controversial. The potential benefits of such treatment include minimizing potential depletion of bone buffers, preventing the catabolic effects of uremic acidosis on muscle protein, preventing tubulointerstitial damage resulting from complement activation by ammonia, and improving the patient's ability to combat a superimposed acidotic crisis (e.g., acute diarrhea) (Rose 1994c). Thus, treatment with oral $NaHCO_3$ at a dosage of 0.5 to 1.0 mEq/kg/day or an amount sufficient to maintain plasma HCO_3^- concentration at 15 mEq/L or above is reasonable if the patient can tolerate the associated sodium load. One teaspoon of baking soda contains 5 g of $NaHCO_3$ (1.3 g of which is sodium). An advantage of using calcium carbonate (e.g. Tums, Os-Cal) as a phosphorus binder in chronic renal failure is that this compound can serve as both a source of alkali and a source of calcium, if small amounts of calcitriol (2–3 ng/kg/day) are also provided. The patient should be monitored for development of hypercalcemia when calcium carbonate and calcitriol are administered concurrently.

LACTIC ACIDOSIS

Lactic acidosis is characterized by an accumulation of lactate in body fluids and a plasma lactate concentration above 5 mEq/L (Madias 1986). The pK_a' of lactic acid is 3.86 and it is completely dissociated at the normal pH of ECF (7.40). Lactic acidosis has been divided into two categories (Table 10–4) (Cohen and Woods 1976; Kreisberg 1984; Hindman 1990). In type A (hypoxic) lactic acidosis, mitochondrial function is normal but O_2 delivery to tissues is inadequate. In type B (nonhypoxic) lactic acidosis, there is adequate O_2 delivery to tissues but defective mitochondrial oxidative function and abnormal carbohydrate metabolism. Inborn errors of metabolism affecting gluconeogenesis and mitochondrial oxidative function are documented to cause type B lactic acidosis in humans. Defects in mitochondrial oxidative function are called mitochondrial myopathies and are caused by hereditary defects in specific mitochondrial enzyme sys-

TABLE 10–4. Causes of L-Lactic Acidosis*

Type A: Hypoxic
Increased oxygen demand
    Severe exercise
    Convulsions
Decreased oxygen availability
    Reduced tissue perfusion
        Cardiac arrest, cardiopulmonary resuscitation
        Shock
        Hypovolemia
        Left ventricular failure
        Low cardiac output
        Acute pulmonary edema
    Reduced arterial oxygen content
        Hypoxemia ($P_{O_2} \leq 30$ mm Hg)
        Extremely severe anemia (packed cell volume < 10%)

Type B: Nonhypoxic
Drugs and toxins
    Phenformin
    Salicylates
    Ethylene glycol
    Many others (see Madias 1986)
Diabetes mellitus
Liver failure
Neoplasia (e.g., lymphosarcoma)
Sepsis
Renal failure
Hypoglycemia
Hereditary defects
    Mitochondrial myopathies
    Defects in gluconeogenesis

*D-Lactic acidosis occurs with short bowel syndrome in human beings and has been observed in cats fed propylene glycol (Christopher et al. 1989, 1990).

tems. A number of case reports suggest that similar defects occur in dogs (Houlton and Herrtage 1980; Vijayasarathy et al. 1994; Olby et al. 1997). Pyruvate dehydrogenase deficiency is suspected to occur in Clumber spaniels (Herrtage and Houlton 1979; Jarvinen and Sankari 1996). This discussion focuses on type A (hypoxic) lactic acidosis.

NORMAL PHYSIOLOGY

Lactate is a metabolic end product. Its production allows regeneration of cytosolic nicotinamide adenine dinucleotide (NAD^+) during anaerobic metabolism and its ultimate fate is reoxidation back to pyruvate:

$$CH_3COCOO^- + NADH + H^+ \underset{\text{lactate dehydrogenase}}{\rightleftharpoons} CH_3CHOHCOO^- + NAD^+$$
(pyruvate) (lactate)

The equilibrium of this reaction is far to the right, and the normal ratio of lactate to pyruvate is 10:1. The main determinants of cytosolic lactate concentration are the concentration of pyruvate and the $NADH/NAD^+$ ratio, both of which are affected by mitochondrial oxidative function.

Pyruvate is produced in the cytosol by anaerobic glycolysis (Embden-Meyerhof pathway). Under aerobic conditions, NADH is oxidized to NAD^+ in the mitochondria and pyruvate enters the mitochondria for conversion to acetylcoenzyme A (CoA) and utilization in the tricarboxylic acid (Krebs) cycle, or it is converted to oxaloacetate and used for gluconeogenesis in the liver and renal cortex. Under anaerobic conditions (e.g., tissue hypoxia), oxidative pathways in the mitochondria are disrupted and NAD^+ must be replenished by reduction of pyruvate to lactate in the cytosol. Thus, lactate accumulation is the price to be paid for maintaining energy production under anaerobic conditions.

At rest, skin, red cells, brain, skeletal muscle, and gut all produce lactate. During tissue hypoxia, skeletal muscle and gut become the major producers of lactate. The liver and kidney are the main consumers of lactate, using it for gluconeogenesis (primarily in the liver) or oxidizing it to CO_2 and water. Protons are consumed when lactate is metabolized:

Gluconeogenesis
$$2CH_3CHOHCOO^- + 2H^+ \rightarrow C_6H_{12}O_6$$

Oxidative metabolism
$$CH_3CHOHCOO^- + H^+ + 3O_2 \rightarrow 3CO_2 + 3H_2O$$

Both of these reactions require normal mitochondrial oxidative function. The protons are actually consumed when ATP is synthesized from ADP and when NADH is oxidized to NAD^+ in the mitochondria (Kreisberg 1984; Madias 1986). Protons are released by hydrolysis of ATP to ADP and by reduction of NAD^+ to NADH, reactions that occur mainly in the cytosol. The protons do not actually arise from dissociation of lactic acid because the anion lactate is the predominant metabolite at normal hepatocyte intracellular pH (pH_i = 7.00–7.20). Thus, lactic acidosis really reflects imbalance between ATP hydrolysis and synthesis and between reduction and oxidation of NAD^+. The protons produced during anaerobic glycolysis are buffered by bicarbonate and nonbicarbonate buffers. Protons are consumed and the buffers replenished when lactate is metabolized to glucose or oxidized to CO_2 and water.

PATHOPHYSIOLOGY

Lactic acidosis occurs when production of lactate by muscle and gut exceeds its utilization by liver and kidney. Both pathways of lactate utilization depend on intact mitochondrial oxidative function, and clinical settings characterized by tissue hypoxia are the most common causes of lactic acidosis (see Table 10–4). Hepatic uptake of lactate is reduced when arterial PO_2 decreases to approximately 30 mm Hg (Tashkin et al. 1972). Severe acidosis further impairs hepatic uptake of lactate and the liver eventually becomes a producer rather than a consumer of lactate (Lloyd et al. 1973).

In an experimental model of hypoxic lactic acidosis (type A) induced by ventilating dogs with 8% O_2, lactate concentration was > 5 mEq/L, pH < 7.2, HCO_3^- concentration < 12 mEq/L, PO_2 < 30 mm Hg, and hepatocyte pH_i < 7.00 (Arieff and Graf 1987). When a similar degree of acidosis was created by infusing lactic acid into dogs with normal PO_2, hepatocyte pH_i remained > 7.00 and hepatic extraction of lactate (as a percentage of the delivered load) was approximately three times higher than that observed in the hypoxic animals. Hypoxemia reduces hepatic O_2 uptake and hepatocyte pH_i decreases, presumably as a result of CO_2 accumulation within cells. This study demonstrated that impaired hepatic extraction of lactate is related to decreased hepatic O_2 uptake and pH_i but not to arterial pH. During severe hypoxia, increased lactate production by gut and muscle and decreased hepatic extraction of lactate lead to progressive lactic acidosis.

CLINICAL FEATURES

Lactic acidosis may occur in several clinical settings, especially those associated with poor perfusion and tissue hypoxia (e.g., cardiac arrest and cardiopulmonary resuscitation, shock, left ventricular failure). The clinician should strongly consider the possibility of lactic acidosis in such settings (see Table 10–4). Usually, lactic acidosis results from accumulation of the L isomer of lactate. D-Lactic acidosis, characterized by the accumulation of the D isomer, is rare but has been reported in human patients with "short-bowel syndrome" in whom gut bacteria metabolize glucose to D-lactate. D-Lactic acidosis has also been observed in cats fed propylene glycol (Christopher et al. 1989, 1990).

Lactic acidosis should be suspected whenever there is an unexplained increase in unmeasured anions (i.e., an unexplained increase in the anion gap). Confirmation requires measurement of plasma lactate concentration, but this has not been performed commonly in small animal practice. Care should be taken to avoid vascular stasis when collecting venous blood for lactate determinations, and blood samples should be centrifuged immediately after collection to avoid a spurious increase in lactate concentration related to anaerobic glycolysis by red cells.

Lactate concentrations in dogs have been reported in many experimental studies (Cain and Dunn 1964; Cohen et al. 1964; Takano 1966; Kazemi et al. 1969; Gennari et al. 1972; Tashkin et al. 1972; Hornbein and Pavlin 1975; Pavlin and Hornbein 1975; Madias et al. 1980; Honer and Jennings 1983; Fine et al. 1984; Jennings and Davidson 1984; Maskrey and Jennings 1985; Graham et al. 1986; Musch et al. 1986; Evans 1987; Hetenyi et al. 1988; Mathias et al. 1988; Ilkiw et al. 1989; Vail et al. 1990a, 1990b). From results of these studies, normal plasma lactate concentrations in dogs are expected to be less than 2 mEq/L. Control plasma lactate concentrations in cats were 1.46 mEq/L in one study (Atkins et al. 1985).

Racing caused venous lactate concentrations in greyhounds to increase from 0.57 to 28.93 mEq/L, but lactate concentrations returned to 0.53 mEq/L at 3 h after exercise (Ilkiw et al. 1989). Arterial pH decreased from 7.365 to 6.997 and returned to 7.372 at 3 h after exercise, while HCO_3^- concentration decreased from 21.1 to 3.1 mEq/L and returned to 20.5 mEq/L at 3 h after exercise. Plasma potassium concentration does not increase in response to organic acidoses as it does in acute mineral acidoses (Adrogue and Madias 1981). In the racing greyhounds, there was no change in plasma potassium concentration despite severe lactic acidosis.

CARDIAC ARREST AND CARDIOPULMONARY RESUSCITATION

Oxygen delivery to and CO_2 removal from tissues are dependent on adequate tissue perfusion. Cardiac arrest is an extreme example of impaired tissue perfusion. During cardiopulmonary resuscitation (CPR), reduced tissue perfusion and reduced O_2 delivery cause anaerobic metabolism and lactic acidosis. In dogs, lactate concentrations increased linearly during the time between cardiac arrest and the onset of CPR (Carden et al. 1985). Lactate concentrations increased progressively during closed-chest CPR in dogs (Carden et al. 1987) and remained stable but did not decrease during 30 min of open-chest CPR (Carden et al. 1985). In this model, closed-chest CPR did not provide adequate tissue perfusion and O_2 delivery to halt anaerobic metabolism.

During CPR, arterial blood gases reflect alveolar-arterial gas exchange whereas mixed venous blood gases reflect tissue acid-base status and oxygenation (Mathias et al. 1988). Respiratory alkalosis develops in arterial blood as a result of mechanical ventilation, whereas respiratory acidosis develops in venous blood because of poor tissue perfusion and impaired transport of accumulated CO_2 to the lungs. In one study of human patients undergoing CPR, average arterial pH was 7.41, whereas average mixed venous pH was 7.15 (Weil et al. 1986). Arterial PCO_2 averaged 32 mm Hg and mixed venous PCO_2 74 mm Hg, whereas arterial and venous HCO_3^- concentrations were similar.

Closed-chest CPR, initiated after 6 min of cardiac arrest, was studied in dogs (Sanders et al. 1988). Sodium bicarbonate (2 mEq/kg) was administered after 20 min of cardiac arrest. Administration of $NaHCO_3$ increased both arterial and venous pH. Before $NaHCO_3$, arterial PCO_2 was approximately 40 mm Hg and with CPR it decreased to 20 mm Hg as a result of mechanical ventilation. After $NaHCO_3$, arterial PCO_2 increased to 30 mm Hg. Venous PCO_2 was nearly 50 mm Hg, and it slowly increased during 30 min of cardiac arrest to 60 mm Hg in untreated dogs. Bicarbonate treatment caused venous PCO_2 to increase transiently to 100 mm Hg, and it decreased to 70 mm Hg at 10 min after $NaHCO_3$ administration. The pH of CSF was not changed by $NaHCO_3$ administration.

The normal arteriovenous pH gradient in dogs is 0.01 to 0.04 (Martin et al. 1985; Bergman and Harris 1988; Adrogue et al. 1989). Reduced cardiac output increases arteriovenous pH and PCO_2 gradients as a result of arterial hypocapnia and venous hypercapnia (Weil et al. 1986; Bergman and Harris 1988; Mathias et al. 1988; Adrogue et al. 1989). The ventilation-to-perfusion ratio is increased because of decreased pulmonary blood flow, accounting for the observed arterial hypocapnia. Venous hypercapnia results from anaerobic metabolism and a greater than normal addition of CO_2 to venous blood from hypoperfused tissues and diminished CO_2 excretion in the lungs because of pulmonary hypoperfusion. These increases in arteriovenous pH and PCO_2 gradients occur only if pulmonary ventilation continues. Respiratory arrest abolishes arteriovenous pH and PCO_2 gradients (Adrogue et al. 1989). In summary, arterial PCO_2 is not an accurate reflection of CO_2 removal from tissues during CPR, and analysis of mixed venous PCO_2 is recommended (Martin et al. 1985; Weil et al. 1986; Bergman and Harris 1988; Mathias et al. 1988; Adrogue et al. 1989).

During CPR and ventilation with 100% O_2, arterial PO_2 may be normal, but tissue perfusion is low (20–25% of normal) (Hindman 1990). After $NaHCO_3$ administration, additional CO_2 is produced, and venous hypercapnia persists if ventilation is inadequate. Improving tissue perfusion is much more important during CPR than is $NaHCO_3$ administration. Effective cardiac compression and adequate perfusion allow delivery of O_2 to and removal of CO_2 from tissues. On the other hand, tissue acidosis is aggravated and pH_i decreased by $NaHCO_3$ administration if the CO_2 generated cannot be removed from the tissues by the lungs. The increase in tissue CO_2 decreases pH_i because CO_2 diffuses more rapidly into cells than does the charged HCO_3^-, thereby lowering the intracellular HCO_3^-/PCO_2 ratio. Intracellular acidosis of the myocardium leads to impaired cardiac contractility, decreased cardiac output, and aggravation of lactic acidosis. Thus, the main goals of CPR are to provide adequate tissue perfusion by effective cardiac compression and to ventilate the patient with 100% O_2. In one study of short (5 min) and prolonged (15 min) cardiac arrest in dogs, $NaHCO_3$ administration improved acidosis without a significant increase in PCO_2 (Vukmir et al. 1995). The authors concluded that $NaHCO_3$ may be useful to reverse the acidosis of cardiac arrest if ventilation is adequate and $NaHCO_3$ is administered in a reasonable therapeutic window.

LYMPHOSARCOMA IN DOGS

Dogs with lymphosarcoma had higher lactate concentrations than control animals, and their lactate concentrations increased significantly 30 min after administration of 500 mg/kg dextrose (Vail et al. 1990b). Blood lactate concentrations were higher before and 1 h after infusion of lactated Ringer's solution in dogs with lymphosarcoma as compared with control animals (Vail et al. 1990a). Blood lactate concentration returned to baseline during the second hour of the 6-h infusion. The authors concluded that dogs with stage III or IV lymphosarcoma may have abnormal carbohydrate metabolism and a transient inability to handle lactate loads. Tumors may produce increased amounts of lactate as a result of excessive anaerobic metabolism and possibly as a result of less than normal hepatic extraction of lactate.

TREATMENT

The outcome of lactic acidosis depends on the severity and reversibility of the underlying disease process responsible for the acid-base disturbance. If treatment of lactic acidosis is to be successful, prompt diagnosis and correction of the underlying disease state are crucial. Tissue perfusion and oxygen delivery should be improved by aggressive fluid therapy to expand ECFV. Ventilation with O_2 should be considered if the patient's spontaneous ventilation is inadequate. Infections should be treated with appropriate antimicrobial agents, and cardiac output should be improved, if necessary, by administration of inotropic agents. If the underlying disease cannot be corrected, the prognosis for patients with lactic acidosis is very poor. If the underlying disease can be corrected, the accumulated lactate is metabolized, yielding an equivalent amount of HCO_3^-, and the acidosis is reversed.

When the pH of the patient's blood falls below 7.1 to 7.2, administration of alkali is justified to prevent the detrimental effects of severe acidosis on the cardiovascular system (e.g., impaired myocardial contractility, impaired cardiovascular responsiveness to catecholamines, increased susceptibility to ventricular arrhythmias). Small doses of $NaHCO_3$ should be administered to increase the patient's pH to 7.2 (Madias 1986; Hindman 1990; Adrogue and Madias 1998).

Approximately 10 to 15% of administered $NaHCO_3$ is converted immediately to CO_2 (Hindman 1990). It is essential that ventilation increase to allow removal of accumulated CO_2 from the body. It is probably safe to administer $NaHCO_3$ if the patient can reasonably be expected to increase ventilation spontaneously. If not, administration of $NaHCO_3$ may be detrimental. In any case, $NaHCO_3$ should be administered slowly to minimize the increase in mixed venous P_{CO_2}.

The volume of distribution (V_d) of administered HCO_3^- is variable, depending on the severity of the acidosis (Adrogue et al. 1983). Thus, there is no simple way to calculate the dosage of $NaHCO_3$ required to increase the pH to 7.2. Volumes of distribution of 0.21 and 0.5 have been recommended for calculation of the bicarbonate space (Hindman 1990; Adrogue and Madias 1998). Sodium bicarbonate should be used cautiously and only in amounts necessary to increase the pH to 7.2. It should be administered slowly over several minutes to a few hours, and at least 30 min should be allowed to elapse after the infusion before judging its effect (Adrogue and Madias 1998).

The use of $NaHCO_3$ in lactic acidosis is controversial (Stacpoole 1986; Narins and Cohen 1987). Using the canine model of hypoxic lactic acidosis described above (Arieff and Graf 1987), affected dogs were left untreated, treated with 2.5 mEq/kg $NaHCO_3$, or treated with 2.5 mEq/kg 1 M NaCl (Graf et al. 1985b, 1985c). Animals treated with bicarbonate showed a greater decrease in pH and HCO_3^- concentration and higher lactate concentration than the other groups. Gut lactate production was greater in dogs that received $NaHCO_3$ than in dogs that received NaCl, and portal vein P_{CO_2} was higher in the group that received $NaHCO_3$. Arterial blood pressure and cardiac output declined in the untreated group and the group that received $NaHCO_3$ but were higher in the group that received NaCl. Increased portal vein P_{CO_2} and hepatic accumulation of lactate presumably caused hepatocyte pH_i to decrease. The ability of the liver to extract lactate depends on adequate hepatic blood flow and normal hepatocyte pH_i, both of which are decreased in this model. During hypoxia ($P_{O_2} <$ 30 mm Hg), the liver is unable to increase its lactate extraction, despite an increased load delivered from the ischemic gut. The investigators concluded that use of $NaHCO_3$ during lactic acidosis may not be effective and may even be detrimental.

Dichloroacetate (DCA) stimulates the enzyme pyruvate dehydrogenase, which converts pyruvate to acetyl CoA (Crabb et al. 1981). In the canine model of hypoxic lactic acidosis described before (Arieff and Graf 1987), DCA was compared with NaCl (Graf et al. 1985a). Dichloroacetate increased pH and HCO_3^- concentration and maintained a constant lactate concentration, whereas NaCl treatment was associated with a decrease in pH and HCO_3^- concentration and an increase in lactate concentration. Hepatic lactate extraction increased with DCA, while liver and muscle accumulation of lactate decreased. Muscle pH_i increased with DCA, but neither treatment changed arterial blood pressure or cardiac output. Dichloroacetate was also studied in a cardiac arrest model in dogs (Sheikh et al. 1986). This study compared DCA, DCA and $NaHCO_3$, $NaHCO_3$, and no treatment. Bicarbonate treatment increased arterial pH, but DCA did not. Dichloroacetate did not decrease lactate concentration or increase pH in either the peripheral circulation or CNS. Thus, there are conflicting results regarding the usefulness of DCA in canine models of lactic acidosis.

Carbicarb is an equimolar mixture of Na_2CO_3 and $NaHCO_3$ that limits the generation of CO_2 during the buffering process:

$$Na_2CO_3 + H_2O + CO_2 \rightarrow 2HCO_3^- + 2Na^+$$

Some of the HCO_3^- generated from this reaction, however, can buffer H^+ released from nonbicarbonate buffers and generate CO_2 in the presence of carbonic anhydrase:

$$2HCO_3^- + 2H^+ \rightarrow 2H_2CO_3 \rightarrow 2H_2O + 2CO_2$$

In the canine model of hypoxic lactic acidosis described earlier (Arieff and Graf 1987), 2.5 mEq/kg Carbicarb was compared with 2.5 mEq/kg $NaHCO_3$ (Bersin and Arieff 1988). Arterial pH increased after administration of Carbicarb but decreased after $NaHCO_3$. Mixed venous P_{CO_2} was unchanged after Carbicarb administration but increased after $NaHCO_3$. Arterial lactate concentration increased after administration of $NaHCO_3$ but stablized after Carbicarb whereas lactate utilization by gut, muscle, and liver improved with Carbicarb but decreased after NaHCO₃. Hepatocyte pH$_i$ increased after Carbicarb and decreased after NaHCO₃. Arterial blood pressure decreased to a lesser extent and cardiac output stabilized with Carbicarb, whereas cardiac output decreased with NaHCO₃. It was concluded that Carbicarb had a beneficial effect on myocardial contractility. Myocardial contractility may decrease after NaHCO₃ administration as a result of increased venous PCO_2 and decreased myocardial pH$_i$. Decreased cardiac output follows and leads to decreased blood flow and decreased O₂ delivery to gut, muscle, and liver, resulting in decreased lactate utilization and increased production. Carbicarb improved arterial pH without impairing myocardial contractility, presumably because it did not increase venous PCO_2. This study suggests that Carbicarb is superior to NaHCO₃ in the treatment of lactic acidosis in dogs.

In another study, Carbicarb was compared with sodium bicarbonate and hypertonic saline in a canine model of hemorrhagic shock (Benjamin et al. 1994). All dogs received identical sodium loads. Groups that received Carbicarb and sodium bicarbonate experienced similar increases in serum bicarbonate, but arterial PCO_2 increased more in bicarbonate-treated dogs than in those treated with Carbicarb. Hemodynamics, oxygen delivery, and oxygen consumption improved in all three groups and these effects were attributed to the sodium load. Carbicarb, NaHCO₃, and NaCl were compared in a model of hypoxic lactic acidosis in anesthetized, mechanically ventilated dogs (Rhee et al. 1993). Carbicarb increased arterial pH, base excess, and cardiac index without an increase in lactate. Bicarbonate increased PCO_2 but no adverse effects of NaHCO₃ on hemodynamics or intracellular pH were detected.

A sodium-free 0.3 N solution of tromethamine (THAM) is another CO₂-consuming alkalinizing agent that is capable of buffering both nonvolatile (H⁺) and volatile (H₂CO₃ derived from CO₂) acid. Tromethamine and sodium bicarbonate had similar buffering ability when evaluated in dogs with experimentally induced metabolic acidosis (Moon et al. 1997). Dogs treated with tromethamine did not experience the transient hypernatremia and hypercapnia that were observed in bicarbonate-treated dogs.

Treatment of Metabolic Acidosis

The main goal in treatment of metabolic acidosis is prompt diagnosis and specific treatment of the underlying cause of the acid-base disorder. Correction of the underlying disease that is responsible for the patient's metabolic acidosis may be all that is necessary (e.g., fluids and insulin in diabetic ketoacidosis). In some instances, however, the underlying disease cannot be corrected (e.g., chronic renal failure) and alkali therapy must be considered.

In general, administration of NaHCO₃ should be reserved for clinical settings in which the patient's blood pH is less than 7.1 to 7.2, and NaHCO₃ should be administered only in amounts necessary to increase the pH to 7.2. Therapy with sodium bicarbonate is less likely to be harmful in animals with simple hyperchloremic metabolic acidosis (normal anion gap) because of the absence of unmeasured organic anions. In patients with normochloremic metabolic acidosis (increased anion gap), unmeasured organic anions (e.g., ketoacids, lactate) are present and can be metabolized to HCO₃⁻ during recovery. Administration of NaHCO₃ in such a setting may result in late development of metabolic alkalosis. This complication should not be serious if renal function is normal, because the kidneys can excrete the excess HCO₃⁻.

Severe acidosis may lead to life-threatening cardiovascular complications (e.g., impaired cardiac contractility, impaired pressor response to catecholamines, sensitization to ventricular arrhythmias) (Mitchell et al. 1972). Thus, if blood pH is less than 7.1 to 7.2, judicious treatment with NaHCO₃ is justified. The aim of therapy should be to increase the patient's pH to 7.2 ([H⁺] = 63 nEq/L), at which point the risk of life-threatening hemodynamic complications is reduced.

For example, consider a 10-kg dog with pH 7.000, [H⁺] = 100 nEq/L, [HCO₃⁻] = 6 mEq/L, and PCO_2 = 25 mm Hg. We assume that normal values are pH 7.387, [H⁺] = 41 nEq/L, [HCO₃⁻] = 21 mEq/L, and PCO_2 = 36 mm Hg and that the normal compensatory respiratory response to metabolic acidosis is a 0.7 mm Hg decrement in PCO_2 per 1.0 mEq/L decrement in [HCO₃⁻]. How much NaHCO₃ must be administered to increase the dog's pH to 7.200 ([H⁺] = 63 nEq/L)? This may be determined using the Henderson equation:

$$[H^+] = \frac{24 P_{CO_2}}{[HCO_3^-]}$$

Thus, the desired [HCO₃⁻] would be 24(25)/63 or 9.5 mEq/L if we assume that the PCO_2 will not change. However, alveolar hyperventilation is likely to subside somewhat as the acidemia is partially corrected. If we assume that the PCO_2 will increase to 28 mm Hg, the required [HCO₃⁻] is 24(28)/63 or 10.7 mEq/L. Thus, we want to increase the dog's [HCO₃⁻] to 9.5 to 10.7 mEq/L.

We still must determine how much NaHCO₃ to administer. This can be calculated using the formula

$$mEq\ HCO_3^- = V_d \times weight\ (kg) \times HCO_3^-\ deficit\ per\ L$$

where V_d is the volume of distribution for HCO₃⁻. The volume of distribution of HCO₃⁻, however, varies inversely with the initial HCO₃⁻ concentration and changes for at least 90 min after HCO₃⁻ administration to dogs (Adrogue et al. 1983). In this study, dogs with chronic metabolic acidosis and initial plasma HCO₃⁻ concentrations of 10 mEq/L were given 5 mEq/kg NaHCO₃ and had average V_d values of 60% at 30 min and 76% at 90 min. This increase in V_d represents distribution of administered HCO₃⁻ from extracellular to intracellular sites. Bicarbonate distributes to ECF within 15 min and to intracellular and bone buffers within 2 to 4 h (Rose 1994d). Thus, it is impossible to assign a single value for the V_d of NaHCO₃ administered to dogs with metabolic acidosis. Any dosage recommendations must be considered only rough guidelines to treatment.

The dogs in this study (Adrogue et al. 1983) had ECFVs equal to approximately 24.5% of body weight as measured by radiosulfate space. If we arbitrarily choose 0.5, a value approximately twice ECFV,

$$HCO_3^- \text{ (mEq)} = 0.5 \times 10 \times (9.5-6) = 17.5 \text{ mEq}$$

or

$$HCO_3^- \text{ (mEq)} = 0.5 \times 10 \times (10.7-6) = 23.5 \text{ mEq}$$

Thus, the desired amount of $NaHCO_3$ is between 17.5 and 23.5 mEq. The $NaHCO_3$ should be administered over the first few hours of therapy and blood gases reevaluated before making a decision about additional alkali administration. This amount of $NaHCO_3$ represents a dose of 1.7 to 2.3 mEq/kg and an empirical dose of 2 mEq/kg could safely have been used.

In patients with severe acidosis, any additional small reduction in plasma HCO_3^- concentration represents a large percentage change and can markedly increase $[H^+]$ (and reduce pH) (Rose 1994e). For example, consider a normal dog with pH 7.387, $[H^+] = 41$ nEq/L, $P_{CO_2} = 36$ mm Hg, and $[HCO_3^-] = 21$ mEq/L that sustains a peracute reduction in $[HCO_3^-]$ of 2 mEq/L (new $[HCO_3^-] = 19$ mEq/L) before respiratory compensation can develop. The new $[H^+]$ can be calculated from the Henderson equation as $24(36)/19 = 45$ nEq/L (pH 7.347). This represents a 0.04 U change in pH and a 4 nEq/L change in $[H^+]$. Now consider a dog with pH 7.102, $[H^+] = 79$ nEq/L, $P_{CO_2} = 23$ mm Hg, $[HCO_3^-] = 7$ mEq/L that sustains a peracute reduction in $[HCO_3^-]$ of 2 mEq/L (new $[HCO_3^-] = 5$ mEq/L) before respiratory compensation can develop. The dog's new $[H^+]$ is $24(23)/5 = 110$ nEq/L (pH 6.959). This represents a 0.14 U change in pH and a 31 nEq/L change in $[H^+]$. This change in $[H^+]$ is almost eight times greater than that observed in the previous example. Thus, a small change in $[HCO_3^-]$ has a much more dramatic effect on $[H^+]$ and pH when the initial $[HCO_3^-]$ concentration is very low. For this reason, patients with very low plasma HCO_3^- concentrations and pH values less than 7.1 to 7.2 should be treated promptly with small amounts of $NaHCO_3$ to increase their pH to the hemodynamically safe value of 7.2.

Potential complications of $NaHCO_3$ therapy include volume overload caused by administered sodium, tetany resulting from decreased serum ionized calcium concentration caused by increased binding of calcium to plasma proteins, decreased O_2 delivery to tissues because of increased affinity of hemoglobin for O_2, paradoxical CNS acidosis as hyperventilation abates and CO_2 diffuses into CSF, late development of alkalosis as metabolism of organic anions (e.g. ketoanions, lactate) replenishes body HCO_3^- stores, and hypokalemia as potassium ions enter and H^+ ions exit intracellular fluid in response to alkalinization of ECF (Hartsfield 1981).

▶ Metabolic Alkalosis

Metabolic alkalosis is characterized by a primary increase in plasma HCO_3^- concentration, decreased $[H^+]$, increased pH, and a secondary or adaptive increase in P_{CO_2}. Metabolic alkalosis was the third most common acid-base disturbance in dogs and cats in one study (Cornelius and Rawlings 1981).

Metabolic alkalosis can be caused by loss of chloride-rich fluid from the body via either the gastrointestinal tract or kidneys or by chronic administration of alkali. In the normal animal, renal excretion of exogenously administered alkali is effective and it is difficult to create metabolic alkalosis by administration of alkali unless there is some factor preventing renal HCO_3^- excretion. Most cases of metabolic alkalosis in small animal practice are caused either by vomiting of stomach contents or by administration of diuretics. In a review of 962 dogs evaluated by blood gas determinations, 20 (2%) were found to be alkalemic (Robinson and Hardy 1988). Of these 20 dogs, 13 had metabolic alkalosis and 7 had respiratory alkalosis. Of the 13 dogs with metabolic alkalosis, 10 had a history of gastrointestinal disease.

Classification of Metabolic Alkalosis

Patients with metabolic alkalosis may be divided into two groups (Harrington and Kassirer 1982c, Jacobson 1989a, 1989b; Rose 1994f; Toto and Alpern 1996). One group has ECFV depletion and avid renal retention of sodium and chloride. These patients respond to chloride administration and are said to have *chloride-responsive metabolic alkalosis*. The other group has normal or increased ECFV and all sodium chloride ingested on a daily basis is excreted in the urine. These patients do not respond to chloride administration and are said to have *chloride-resistant metabolic alkalosis*.

In most instances of chloride-responsive metabolic alkalosis, the chloride concentration of the fluid lost from the body is greater than that of the ECF, so there has been a disproportionate loss of chloride. For example, the chloride concentration of gastric fluid is approximately 150 mEq/L, whereas serum chloride concentration is approximately 110 mEq/L in the dog and 120 mEq/L in the cat. Chloride-responsive metabolic alkalosis is much more common in small animal practice than is chloride-resistant metabolic alkalosis.

Development of Chloride-Responsive Metabolic Alkalosis

The pathophysiology of chloride-responsive metabolic alkalosis can be understood by considering the events associated with selective removal of gastric HCl (Needle et al. 1964; Kassirer and Schwartz 1966a, 1966b). Loss of H^+ from the stomach is associated, milliequivalent for milliequivalent, with an increase in the concentration of HCO_3^- in ECF. Plasma HCO_3^- concentration and the filtered load of HCO_3^- in the kidneys increase. Natriuresis, kaliuresis, suppression of net acid excretion with bicarbonaturia, increased urine flow rate, and renal water loss follow, but bicarbonaturia is transient and insufficient to return plasma HCO_3^- concentration to normal (Needle et al. 1964). These events occurred without any change in GFR in a study of dogs made alkalotic by hemofiltration and replacement of ECF with a solution containing HCO_3^- as the only anion (Borkan et al. 1987). The abatement of bicarbonaturia was thought to be due to renal sodium avidity, engendered by the volume deficit that developed as a result of the initial natriuresis and diuresis. Renal sodium avidity is thus established and contributes to perpetuation of the alkalosis and development of a potassium deficit as long as chloride intake remains deficient. These events constitute the *development phase* of chloride-responsive metabolic alkalosis.

Probably the most important factors in the *maintenance phase* of chloride-responsive metabolic alkalosis are ECFV depletion and the chloride deficit, two factors that are difficult to separate experimentally (Cohen 1968; Jacobson and Seldin 1983; Harrington 1984; Sabatini and Kurtzman 1984; Norris and Kurtzman 1988). Other factors that contribute to perpetuation of metabolic alkalosis are the effects of aldosterone and the potassium deficit. Aldosterone concentration is increased by ECFV depletion and results in increased distal Na^+-H^+ and Na^+-K^+ exchange. This results in perpetuation of alkalosis and development of a potassium deficit. Potassium depletion leads to a transcellular shift of H^+ from extracellular to intracellular fluid in exchange for potassium ions. When this shift occurs in renal tubular cells, it decreases intracellular pH and enhances H^+ secretion by the renal tubular cells, further aggravating the alkalosis. Hypokalemia also stimulates renal ammoniagenesis, presumably through stimulation of glutaminase via decreased intracellular pH. The increase in renal ammonium excretion enhances renal acid excretion and contributes to increased plasma HCO_3^- concentration. Hypokalemia also may decrease GFR through glomerular hemodynamic changes and may directly impair chloride reabsorption in the distal nephron, resulting in enhanced lumen electronegativity and facilitation of H^+ secretion into tubular fluid.

Response of the Body to Metabolic Alkalosis

The body's response to metabolic alkalosis is the reverse of its response to administration of a mineral acid such as HCl. The kidney is more effective in excreting an alkaline load than an acid load, provided the subject is not sodium avid and sufficient chloride is provided.

ACUTE BUFFER RESPONSE

In an early study of the buffer response to alkali, nephrectomized dogs were given 20 mEq/kg $NaHCO_3$ with a resultant increase in plasma HCO_3^- concentration to approximately 60 mEq/L (Swan et al. 1955). Of the administered HCO_3^-, almost one-third (32%) was titrated by intracellular buffers. Of this 32%, 4% was converted to carbonic acid by H^+ from lactic acid released into ECF from cells. Increased intracellular pH enhances cellular production of lactic acid by stimulation of phosphofructokinase. Approximately 2% entered red cells in exchange for chloride (so-called chloride shift), and 26% was titrated by H^+ released from intracellular proteins and phosphates while sodium and potassium ions entered cells to maintain electroneutrality. By comparison, approximately 50% of a mineral acid load is handled by intracellular buffers (Swan and Pitts 1955; Schwartz et al. 1957).

Approximately two-thirds (68%) of the HCO_3^- load was confined to ECF. In response to the increase in pH, plasma proteins buffered 1% of this HCO_3^-. That is,

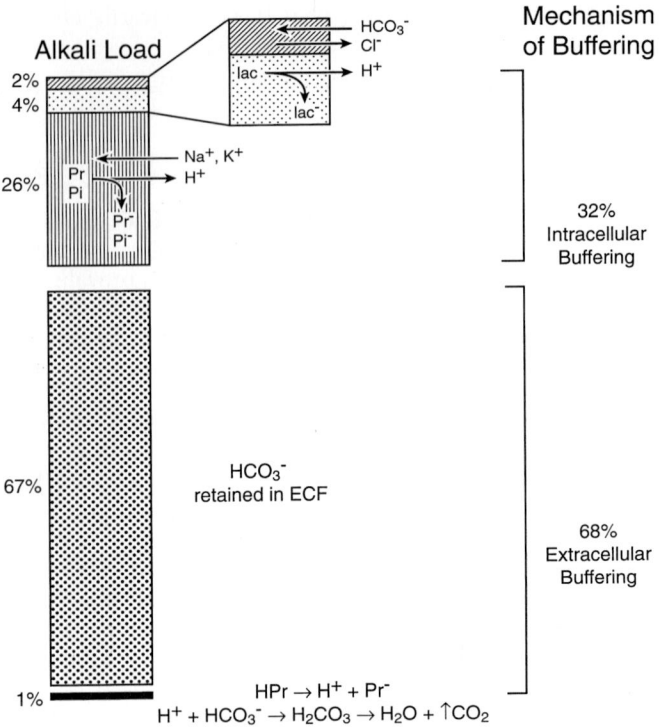

FIGURE 10-6. Distribution of buffer response to a fixed alkaline load. (Drawing by Tim Vojt. Adapted from Pitts RF: *Physiology of the Kidney and Body Fluids*, 2nd ed. Chicago, Year Book Medical Publishers, p. 173, 1968.)

plasma proteins released hydrogen ions in numbers sufficient to convert 1% of the infused HCO_3^- to carbonic acid. The remaining 67% was retained in the ECF compartment and contributed to the observed increase in plasma HCO_3^- concentration. These buffer reactions are summarized in Figure 10-6.

RESPIRATORY RESPONSE TO METABOLIC ALKALOSIS

The decrease in $[H^+]$ that accompanies chronic metabolic alkalosis stimulates chemoreceptors and is responsible for the observed decrease in alveolar ventilation. Secondary or adaptive alveolar hypoventilation protects pH in the presence of increased plasma HCO_3^- concentration (Fig. 10-7). A review of studies of dogs with experimentally induced metabolic alkalosis suggests that for each 1.0 mEq/L increase in plasma HCO_3^- concentration there is an adaptive 0.55 to 0.77 mm Hg increase in P_{CO_2} (Chazan et al. 1969; Penman et al. 1972; Madias et al. 1980; Madias et al. 1984; Borkan et al. 1987). This adaptive hypoventilation is associated with some degree of hypoxemia. Arterial P_{O_2} decreased to 60 to 70 mm Hg in dogs made alkalotic by feeding a diet with a chloride deficit and administering furosemide (Penman et al. 1972).

The ventilatory response to metabolic alkalosis is usually considered to be less marked than the response to metabolic acidosis (i.e., a 0.6 mm Hg increase in P_{CO_2} for each 1 mEq/L increase in plasma HCO_3^- concentration in metabolic alkalosis as compared with a 1.2 mm Hg decrease in P_{CO_2} for each 1 mEq/L decrease in plasma

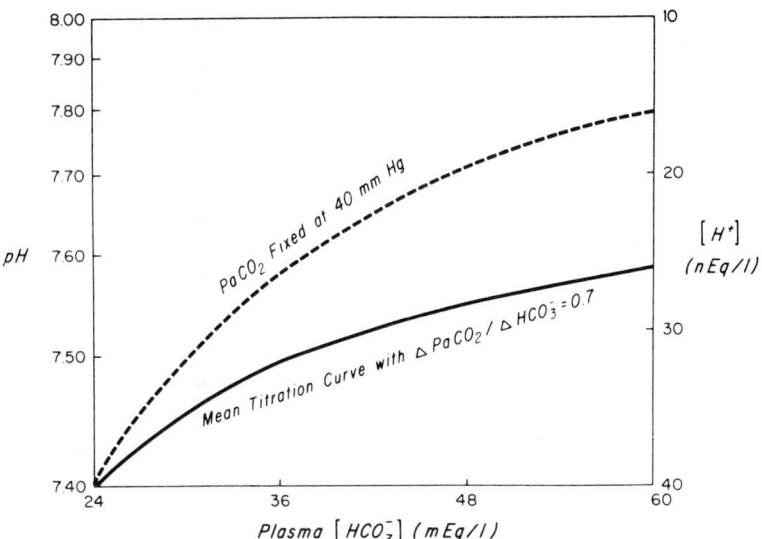

FIGURE 10-7. Beneficial effect of respiratory adaptation on [H+] and pH. (From Harrington JT and Kassirer JP: Metabolic alkalosis. In Cohen JJ and Kassirer JP: *Acid-Base*. Boston, Little, Brown & Co, p. 237, 1982.)

HCO_3^- concentration in metabolic acidosis). This view has been challenged by a study of the ventilatory response of dogs to HCl acidosis and metabolic alkalosis induced by diuretics, removal of gastric acid, or mineralocorticoid administration (Madias et al. 1984). The ventilatory responses to all of these experimental acid-base disturbances were not significantly different from one another and it was concluded that an average change of 0.74 mm Hg P_{CO_2} can be expected for each 1.0 mEq/L change of plasma HCO_3^- concentration of metabolic origin. In one study, the respiratory compensation for metabolic alkalosis ranged from 0.4 to 0.6 mm Hg increment in P_{CO_2} for each 1 mEq/L increment in HCO_3^- for arterial, mixed venous, and jugular venous samples in dogs made alkalotic by the administration of furosemide (Ilkiw et al. 1991). As a rule, 1 mEq/L increase in plasma HCO_3^- concentration is expected to be associated with an adaptive 0.7 mm Hg increase in P_{CO_2} in dogs with metabolic alkalosis.

RENAL RESPONSE TO METABOLIC ALKALOSIS

In the normal animal, the kidneys rapidly and effectively excrete administered alkali. Metabolic alkalosis persists only if renal excretion of HCO_3^- is impaired. This may occur if there is reduced GFR (decreased filtered load of HCO_3^-), a continued high rate of alkali administration, or some stimulus for the kidneys to retain sodium in the presence of a relative chloride deficit. In most dogs and cats with metabolic alkalosis, a combination of renal sodium avidity and diminished chloride availability is responsible for perpetuation of the alkalosis. A potassium deficit and hypokalemia develop as the kidneys increase Na^+-K^+ exchange in the distal nephron.

When sodium, chloride, and water are removed in proportion to their concentrations in ECF, sodium avidity develops but alkalosis does not (Harrington and Kassirer 1982d). When the sodium deficit in an alkalotic animal is repaired by infusing a fluid identical in composition to the alkalotic ECF, metabolic alkalosis is corrected by selective retention of chloride (Cohen 1968). This occurs even when the filtered load of chloride is kept constant during the infusion of fluid (Cohen 1970). Thus, both sodium avidity and decreased chloride availability seem to be necessary for the perpetuation of metabolic alkalosis.

Potassium deficiency does not cause alkalosis but rather is a result of the alkalotic state. In fact, isolated potassium deficiency in dogs leads to mild metabolic acidosis (Burnell and Dawbron 1970; Burnell et al. 1974). When potassium retention is prevented but sodium chloride is supplied, alkalosis is corrected despite a persisting potassium deficit (Atkins and Schwartz 1962; Needle et al. 1964; Kassirer and Schwartz 1966a). If potassium is supplied but chloride is not, alkalosis cannot be corrected (Kassirer et al. 1965). Administration of potassium chloride leads to complete correction of both alkalosis and the potassium deficit.

The renal response to hypercapnia in metabolic alkalosis was studied in normal unanesthetized dogs made alkalotic by dietary chloride restriction and administration of ethacrynic acid (Madias et al. 1980). Adaptive hypercapnia was allowed to develop and then prevented by exposure to hypoxia. During development of metabolic alkalosis, serum sodium concentration remained unchanged but serum chloride, potassium, and phosphorus concentrations decreased while lactate and unmeasured anion (i.e., anion gap) concentrations increased. With hypercapnia, plasma HCO_3^- concentration was maintained at 7.7 mEq/L above control values, whereas without hypercapnia it was maintained at 4.5 mEq/L above control values. Thus, approximately 60% of the increase in plasma HCO_3^- concentration was due to the renal response to chloride and volume depletion, whereas 40% of the increase could be attributed to adaptive hypercapnia. This response appeared to be a direct effect of P_{CO_2} on renal acid excretion and HCO_3^- reabsorption and was not related to any change in extracellular pH because the degree of alkalemia remained unchanged throughout the experiment. This portion of the increase in plasma HCO_3^- concentration (40%) may be considered maladaptive because it contributes to a higher extracellular pH. When metabolic alkalosis persists, this indiscriminate renal response to hypercapnia results in a further increase

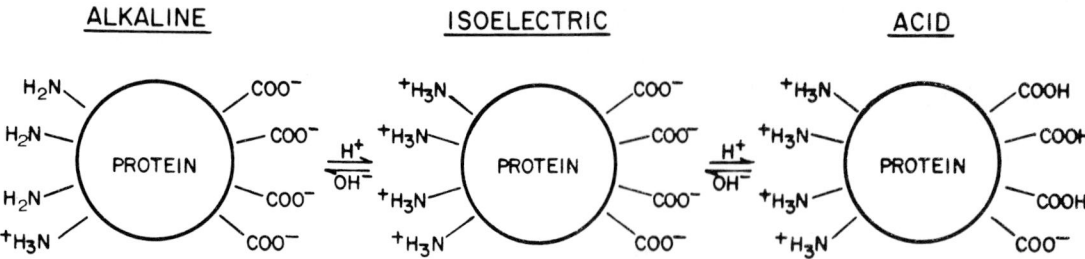

FIGURE 10–8. Effect of alkalosis and acidosis on the charge of plasma proteins. (Modified from Pitts RF: *Physiology of the Kidney and Body Fluids*, 2nd ed. Chicago, Year Book Medical Publishers, p. 186, 1974.)

in plasma HCO_3^- concentration and abrogates the original beneficial effect of the increased plasma HCO_3^- concentration on extracellular pH.

Clinical Features of Metabolic Alkalosis

The clinical features of dogs and cats with metabolic alkalosis are usually those of the underlying disease process. Neurologic signs have been reported in human patients with severe metabolic alkalosis and include agitation, disorientation, stupor, and coma (Harrington and Kassirer 1982e). Muscle twitching and seizures may occur but have been observed rarely in dogs with severe metabolic alkalosis.

Clinical signs may also result from the accompanying potassium depletion. Signs of potassium depletion include muscle weakness of varying severity, cardiac arrhythmias, alterations in renal function (e.g., defective concentrating ability), and gastrointestinal motility disturbances (e.g., ileus). These complications are discussed in Chapter 5.

Muscle twitching may occur as a result of decreased serum ionized calcium concentration because alkalosis increases the number of negative charges on proteins, allowing more calcium ions to be bound (Fig. 10–8). Serum ionized calcium concentration decreases and may account for neuromuscular irritability by rendering the resting potential of cells less negative (Fig. 10–9). Administration of a single dose (4 mEq/kg) of sodium bicarbonate to normal cats resulted in a 10% decrease in serum ionized calcium concentration and an 8% decrease in serum total calcium concentration. These changes persisted for 3 h, but no clinical signs were observed (Chew et al. 1989).

Metabolic alkalosis shifts the oxygen-hemoglobin dissociation curve to the left (Bohr effect) and impairs oxygen release from hemoglobin. This effect probably is not clinically significant because an increase in red cell 2,3-diphosphoglycerate concentration occurs after 6 to 8 h of metabolic alkalosis and results in a shift of the curve back to the right (Bellingham et al. 1971).

Diagnosis of Metabolic Alkalosis

Specific clinical manifestations of metabolic alkalosis have not been reported in dogs and cats. The clinician must have a high index of suspicion for this disorder when presented with an animal having compatible clinical signs, usually chronic vomiting of stomach contents. Thus, an accurate history is the key to suspecting the diagnosis. Metabolic alkalosis can also be suspected from the results of routine serum biochemical tests. Blood gas analysis should be performed if decreased serum chloride and potassium concentrations are observed and total CO_2 content is increased. Blood gas analysis allows the clinician to determine whether primary metabolic alkalosis is present and whether the magnitude of respiratory compensation is as predicted (see earlier). The concentration of unmeasured anions (i.e., anion gap) in metabolic alkalosis may increase because of loss of hydrogen ions from nonbicarbonate buffers. The increased anion gap is due primarily to increased numbers of negative charges on proteins and due partially to the increase in plasma protein concentration that occurs as a consequence of ECFV depletion (Adrogue et al. 1978).

Urine pH is low during the maintenance phase of metabolic alkalosis because of enhanced distal Na^+-H^+

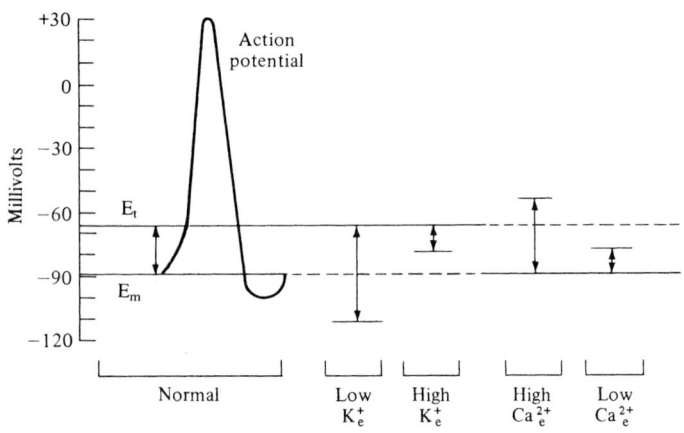

FIGURE 10–9. Effect of hypocalcemia on the resting potential (E_m) of cells. The height of the arrows is equal to the difference between the resting and threshold potentials and represents the excitability of the cell membrane. (From Rose BD: *Clinical Physiology of Acid-Base and Electrolyte Disorders*, 3rd ed. New York, McGraw-Hill Co., p. 704, 1989.)

exchange and reabsorption of all filtered HCO_3^-. Urine pH, however, is alkaline during development of and recovery from metabolic alkalosis. Thus, urinary pH is of little diagnostic significance in metabolic alkalosis.

Causes of Metabolic Alkalosis

Metabolic alkalosis can be caused by continuous administration of alkali, disproportionate loss of chloride (chloride-responsive alkalosis), or excessive mineralocorticoid effect (chloride-resistant alkalosis). In some instances, the mechanism of metabolic alkalosis is unknown, and these examples are classified as miscellaneous. Most dogs with gastric dilatation-volvulus have metabolic acidosis or normal blood gas values at presentation (Muir 1982; Wingfield et al. 1982), but, uncommonly, metabolic alkalosis and hypokalemia have been reported (Kagan and Schaer 1983). The causes of metabolic alkalosis are listed in Table 10–5 and the pathophysiology of the major types of metabolic alkalosis is considered further here.

CHLORIDE-RESPONSIVE METABOLIC ALKALOSIS

Chronic vomiting of stomach contents and administration of diuretics are the most common causes of chloride-responsive metabolic alkalosis in dogs and cats.

ADMINISTRATION OF ALKALI

Acute administration of 4 mEq/kg $NaHCO_3$ to normal unanesthetized cats resulted in mild increases in venous blood pH and HCO_3^- concentration lasting 180 min (Chew et al. 1991). A slight decrease in serum chloride concentration persisted for 30 min, whereas a mild increase in P_{CO_2} persisted for 60 min. A solution of $NaHCO_3$ (6.6 mEq/L) infused over 30 min into anesthetized dogs caused transient increases in arterial P_{CO_2}, pH, base excess, and standard bicarbonate concentration (Hartsfield et al. 1981). Prompt renal excretion of administered $NaHCO_3$ presumably prevented any persistent change in acid-base values in these acute studies. Renal acid excretion decreases, urine pH increases, and administered $NaHCO_3$ is excreted within hours. There is an acute increase in carbonic acid and P_{CO_2} as body buffers release H^+ to combine with the administered HCO_3^-. The excess $NaHCO_3$ is excreted in the urine, increased ventilation occurs in response to increased P_{CO_2}, and acid-base balance is restored to normal.

When alkali is administered chronically, plasma HCO_3^- concentration becomes a function of the daily dosage administered but returns to normal within a few days after alkali administration is discontinued. If alkali is given to subjects rendered sodium avid by prior dietary salt restriction, smaller dosages of alkali result in greater increases in plasma HCO_3^- concentration than are observed when higher alkali dosages are used in subjects receiving normal amounts of dietary salt.

Sources of alkali other than $NaHCO_3$ may also contribute to metabolic alkalosis. Such organic anions include lactate that has accumulated during lactic acidosis, ketoacids in uncontrolled diabetes mellitus, and citrate in banked blood or that administered in an attempt to prevent recurrence of calcium oxalate urolithiasis. These organic anions yield HCO_3^- when metabolized:

$$Anion^- + O_2 \rightarrow HCO_3^- + CO_2 + H_2O$$

Often, this reaction serves to replace the HCO_3^- titrated during development of the acidosis (e.g., lactic acidosis, diabetic ketoacidosis). If $NaHCO_3$ has been administered during treatment, however, metabolism of the organic anion after correction of the acidosis can result in metabolic alkalosis. If renal function is normal and volume depletion is not present, the kidneys promptly excrete the excess HCO_3^- and restore normal acid-base balance.

Usually, administration of nonabsorbable alkali (e.g., aluminum hydroxide used as a phosphorus binder in patients with renal failure) does not cause metabolic alkalosis. Neutralization of H^+ by $Al(OH)_3$ in the stomach results in the net addition of HCO_3^- to ECF. Combination of Al^{3+} with HCO_3^- secreted by the pancreas produces insoluble $Al_2(CO_3)_3$ in the duodenum and there is no net increase in HCO_3^- ions in ECF. If, however, $Al(OH)_3$ is administered concurrently with a cationic exchange resin (e.g., polysytrene sulfonate), the resin can bind Al^{3+}, leaving HCO_3^- secreted by the pancreas to be reabsorbed in the small intestine, thus resulting in alkalinization of ECF. When renal failure is present, the kidneys have reduced capacity to excrete retained HCO_3^- and metabolic alkalosis could result. This sequence of events is most likely to occur in an animal with oliguric renal failure that is treated concurrently with $Al(OH)_3$ for hyperphosphatemia and with polystyrene sulfonate for hyperkalemia.

GASTRIC FLUID LOSS

The H^+ and Na^+ concentrations of gastric fluid are inversely related to one another whereas the K^+ concentration is relatively stable (approximately 10 mEq/L). The Cl^- concentration is very high (approximately 150 mEq/L) and remains remarkably constant even when hypochloremia develops. Subtracting the sum of the Na^+ and K^+ concentrations of gastric fluid from the Cl^- concentration yields an approximation of the H^+ concentration. The composition of gastric fluid is compared with that of other body fluids in Figure 10–10. When a dog or cat

TABLE 10–5. Causes of Metabolic Alkalosis

Chloride responsive
Vomiting of stomach contents
Diuretic therapy
Posthypercapnia

Chloride resistant
Primary hyperaldosteronism
Hyperadrenocorticism

Alkali administration
Oral administration of sodium bicarbonate or other organic anions (e.g., lactate, citrate, gluconate, acetate)
Oral administration of cation exchange resin with nonabsorbable alkali (e.g., phosphorus binder)

Miscellaneous
Refeeding after fasting
High-dose penicillin
Severe potassium or magnesium deficiency

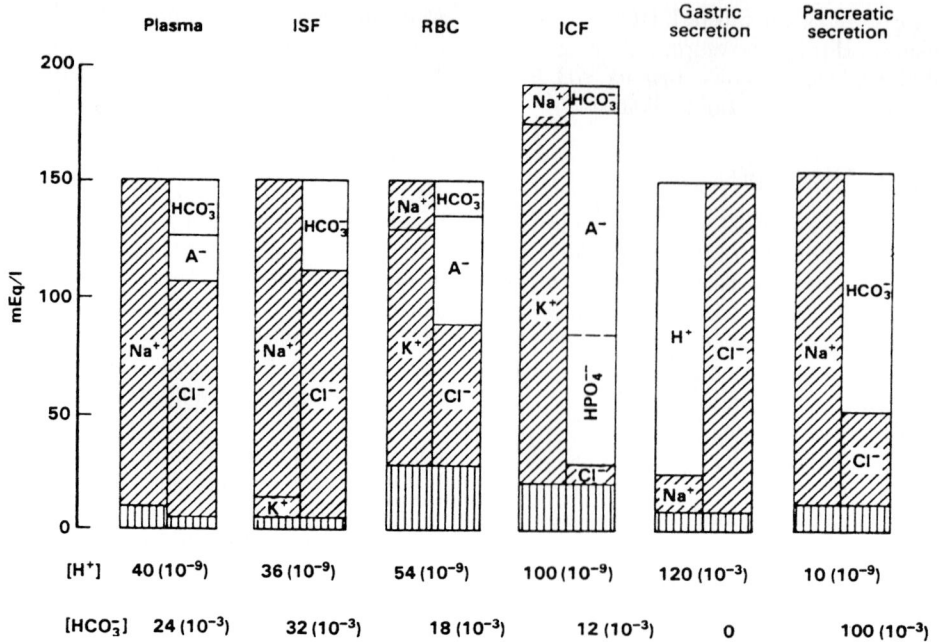

FIGURE 10-10. Comparison of electrolyte composition of gastric juice to other body fluids using Gamblegrams. Strong ions are crosshatched. (From Jones NL: *Blood Gases and Acid-Base Physiology*, 2nd ed. New York, Thieme Medical Publishers, p. 133, 1987.)

vomits stomach contents, water is lost along with large amounts of HCl and small amounts of potassium and sodium.

The H^+ produced during gastric acid secretion originates from the dissociation of carbonic acid; thus, an equal number of HCO_3^- ions are generated in ECF. In the normal animal, gastric acid secretion does not disturb acid-base balance because the increase in ECF HCO_3^- concentration that accompanies parietal cell H^+ secretion is balanced by pancreatic HCO_3^- secretion in the duodenum, and Cl^- secreted into the stomach is recaptured lower in the gastrointestinal tract. When stomach contents are lost, H^+ and Cl^- are removed from this system and HCO_3^- secreted into the duodenum by the pancreas is no longer titrated by gastric H^+ but is reabsorbed farther down in the gastrointestinal tract in place of Cl^-. The normal relationship between gastric and pancreatic secretions in the gastrointestinal tract is shown in Figure 10-11. Continued loss of gastric fluid can result in marked increases in plasma HCO_3^- concentration, and chronic vomiting of stomach contents is the most common cause of metabolic alkalosis in small animal practice.

In studies of gastric alkalosis, experimental subjects are rendered sodium avid by feeding a low-salt diet. Gastric fluid is then continuously removed by nasogastric suction and fluid and electrolyte losses other than HCl are quantitatively replaced (Needle et al. 1964; Kassirer and Schwartz 1966a, 1966b). The effects of repeated gastric drainage over 3 days on plasma HCO_3^- and chloride concentrations and on potassium, sodium, and chloride balance in experimental dogs are shown in Figure 10-12. Note that the resulting metabolic alkalosis is corrected by provision of NaCl despite a progressively negative potassium balance. In the clinical setting, persistent

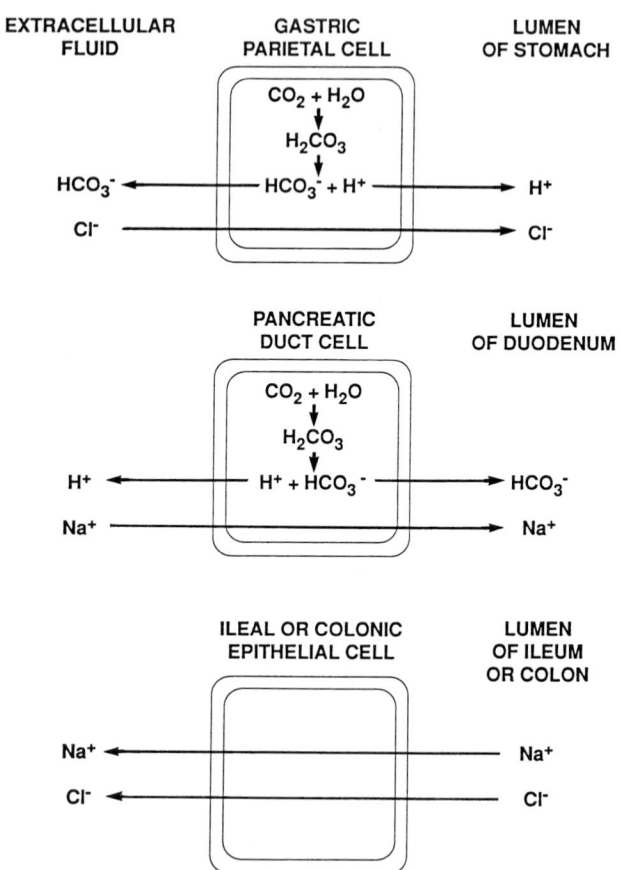

FIGURE 10-11. Normal relationship between gastric and pancreatic secretions in the gastrointestinal tract. (Modified from Guyton AC: *Textbook of Medical Physiology*, 7th ed. Philadelphia, WB Saunders Co., pp. 775-779, 1986.)

aldosterone concentrations before and after administration of ACTH, normal plasma renin activity, hyperchloremia, and normal total CO_2 content (23 mEq/L) (Breitschwerdt et al. 1985). Alkalosis was not observed at any time during hospitalization despite repeated blood gas evaluation. Grossly, there was a 3-mm nodule on the adrenal gland and histologically, hyperplasia of the zona glomerulosa was observed. Three other dogs with weakness and hypokalemia were observed to have adrenal tumors (one adenoma and two adenocarcinomas) (Feldman and Nelson 1996c). Very high plasma aldosterone concentrations were documented in two of these dogs.

HYPERADRENOCORTICISM

Metabolic alkalosis occurs in approximately one-third of human patients with Cushing's syndrome (Harrington and Kassirer 1982f). It is more common in patients with adrenocortical carcinoma and in those with ectopic production of ACTH by a nonadrenal malignancy than in those with pituitary-dependent hyperadrenocorticism. The frequency of metabolic alkalosis and serum electrolyte disturbances in dogs with hyperadrenocorticism is uncertain. Often, serum sodium and potassium concentrations are normal in dogs with hyperadrenocorticism. This may reflect the fact that 80 to 85% of dogs with hyperadrenocorticism have pituitary-dependent disease. In a large group of dogs with hyperadrenocorticism, 21 of 52 (40%) dogs had increased serum sodium concentrations and 25 of 52 (48%) had decreased serum potassium concentrations (Ling et al. 1979). The relative frequency of pituitary- and adrenal-dependent disease was not reported in this study. In another study, mild hypernatremia and hypokalemia were observed occasionally in dogs with hyperadrenocorticism, and total CO_2 content was increased in 33% of affected dogs (Peterson 1984). In another report, hypokalemia was found in only 5% of dogs with pituitary-dependent hyperadrenocorticism but in 45% of those with adrenocortical neoplasia (Meijer 1980). A high rate of secretion of cortisol and other corticosteroids such as desoxycorticosterone and corticosterone in patients with adrenocortical malignancies could be responsible for hypernatremia, hypokalemia, and metabolic alkalosis in adrenal-dependent hyperadrenocorticism.

MISCELLANEOUS

Large doses of penicillin, ampicillin, or carbenicillin administered as a sodium salt can lead to hypokalemia and metabolic alkalosis in human patients. The drug may increase lumen electronegativity in the distal nephron by acting as a nonresorbable anion and enhancing Na^+-H^+ and Na^+-K^+ exchange. "Refeeding" alkalosis can occur in human patients when glucose is administered after prolonged fasting. The mechanism for this type of alkalosis is unknown. These types of metabolic alkalosis have not been reported in the veterinary literature.

Treatment of Metabolic Alkalosis

Acid-base disturbances are secondary phenomena. Diagnosis and definitive treatment of the responsible disease process are integral to the successful resolution of acid-base disorders. It must be remembered, however, that alkalosis persists until chloride is replaced if vomiting of stomach contents or diuretic administration is responsible for the metabolic alkalosis. The goal of treatment in chloride-responsive metabolic alkalosis is to replace the chloride deficit while providing sufficient potassium and sodium to replace existing deficits. Definitive treatment of the underlying disease process (e.g., removal of a gastric foreign body) prevents recurrence of the metabolic alkalosis.

Patients with chronic pulmonary disease that have hypoxemia and hypercapnia are at greater risk from metabolic alkalosis than others, because superimposition of metabolic alkalosis can further reduce ventilation and lead to worsening of hypoxemia. Thus, metabolic alkalosis should be treated appropriately if present and avoided if not present. Giving oxygen to patients with metabolic alkalosis should also be avoided if possible because this may impair ventilation and further aggravate hypercapnia.

Potassium without chloride (e.g., potassium phosphate) corrects neither the alkalosis nor the potassium deficit because administered potassium is excreted in the urine. A chloride salt must be given for alkalosis to be resolved and potassium retention to occur. Provision of chloride as either the sodium or potassium salt corrects chloride-responsive metabolic alkalosis. This therapy allows the kidneys to reabsorb the sodium the body requires with chloride to maintain electroneutrality. Thus, an NaCl solution (0.45 or 0.9%) with added KCl is the fluid of choice for dogs and cats with chloride-responsive metabolic alkalosis. It is best to use solutions containing both NaCl and KCl because affected animals typically have been sick long enough to develop clinically significant potassium deficits. Administering 0.9% NaCl without KCl can cause diuresis and increased urinary excretion of potassium, thus worsening any potassium deficit. As shown in Figure 10–12, provision of NaCl corrects metabolic alkalosis induced in dogs by gastric drainage, but the potassium deficit persists unless potassium is provided. A few days may be required to restore normal electrolyte and acid-base balance but, in nearly all instances, these measures are sufficient to resolve the alkalosis. In human patients with severe metabolic alkalosis or in those with severely impaired renal function, HCl or arginine HCl has been used for rapid correction of metabolic alkalosis, but there is no report of the use of these compounds in animals with metabolic alkalosis and their use is not recommended.

Cimetidine, ranitidine, or famotidine may be considered as adjunctive therapy if gastric losses are ongoing because this approach reduces gastric acid secretion. For the patient with heart failure receiving loop diuretics, oral KCl administration is the best way to provide chloride without sodium and prevent further retention of fluid and aggravation of edema. Even in the presence of sodium avidity, provision of chloride lessens Na^+-H^+ and Na^+-K^+ exchange at distal nephron sites and prevents development of alkalosis when loop diuretics are used. Simultaneous use of distal blocking agents such as spironolactone, triamterene, or amiloride may also be considered. These drugs work in the principal cells of the cortical collecting tubule and impair Na^+-H^+ and Na^+-K^+ exchange by inhibiting aldosterone-sensitive sodium channels. In metabolic alkalosis caused by chronic administration of alkali, discontinuation of the source of alkali results in correction of the alkalosis over a few days, provided that renal function is normal.

Chloride-resistant metabolic alkalosis is uncommon in comparison with chloride-responsive metabolic alkalosis. When present, its successful treatment requires that the underlying disease be diagnosed and treated before alkalosis can be resolved. Cases of chloride-resistant metabolic alkalosis are rare in veterinary medicine.

REFERENCES

Adams WH, Toal RL, Walker MA, et al.: Early renal ultrasonographic findings in dogs with experimentally induced ethylene glycol nephrosis. Am J Vet Res 50:1370, 1989.

Adrogue HJ and Madias NE: Changes in plasma potassium concentration during acute acid base disturbances. J Clin Invest 71:456, 1981.

Adrogue HJ and Madias NE: Management of life-threatening acid-base disorders. N Engl J Med 338:26, 1998.

Adrogue HJ, Brensilver J, and Madias NE: Changes in the plasma anion gap during chronic metabolic acid-base disturbances. Am J Physiol 235:F291, 1978.

Adrogue HJ, Brensilver J, Cohen J, et al.: Influence of steady-state alterations in acid-base equilibrium on the fate of administered bicarbonate in the dog. J Clin Invest 71:867, 1983.

Adrogue HJ, Eknoyan G, and Suki WK: Diabetic ketoacidosis: Role of the kidney in the acid-base homeostasis re-evaluated. Kidney Int 25:591, 1984.

Adrogue HJ, Rashad MN, Gorin AB, et al.: Arteriovenous acid-base disparity in circulatory failure: Studies on mechanism. Am J Physiol 257:F1087, 1989.

Adrogue HJ, Wilson H, Boyd AE, et al.: Plasma acid-base patterns in diabetic ketoacidosis. N Engl J Med 307:1603, 1982.

Arieff AI and Graf H: Pathophysiology of type A hypoxic lactic acidosis in dogs. Am J Physiol 253:E271, 1987.

Arruda JAL, Carrasquillo T, Cubria A, et al.: Bicarbonate reabsorption in chronic renal failure. Kidney Int 9:481, 1976.

Atkins CE, Tyler R, and Greenlee P: Clinical, biochemical, acid-base, and electrolyte abnormalities in cats after hypertonic sodium phosphate enema administration. Am J Vet Res 46:980, 1985.

Atkins EL and Schwartz WB: Factors governing correction of the alkalosis associated with potassium deficiency: The critical role of chloride in the recovery process. J Clin Invest 41:218, 1962.

Bark H and Perk R: Fanconi syndrome associated with amoxicillin therapy in the dog. Canine Pract 20:19, 1995.

Beckett SD and Shields RP: Treatment of acute ethylene glycol (antifreeze) poisoning in the dog. J Am Vet Med Assoc 158:472, 1971.

Bellingham AJ, Detter JC, and Lenfant C: Regulatory mechanisms of hemoglobin oxygen affinity in acidosis and alkalosis. J Clin Invest 50:700, 1971.

Benjamin J, Oropello JM, Abalos AM, et al.: Effects of acid-base correction on hemodynamics, oxygen dynamics, and resuscitability in severe canine hemorrhagic shock. Crit Care Med 22:1616, 1994.

Bergman KS and Harris BH: Arteriovenous pH difference—A new index of perfusion. J Pediatr Surg 23:1190, 1988.

Bersin RM and Arieff AL: Improved hemodynamic function during hypoxia with Carbicarb, a new agent for the management of acidosis. Circulation 77:227, 1988.

Borkan S, Northrup TE, Cohen JJ, et al.: Renal response to metabolic alkalosis induced by isovolemic hemofiltration in the dog. Kidney Int 32:322, 1987.

Bovee KC: *Characterization and Treatment of Isolated Renal Tubular Acidosis in a Dog*. Washington, DC, American College of Veterinary Internal Medicine, p. 48, 1984.

Bovee KC, Joyce T, Reynolds R, et al.: The Fanconi syndrome in basenji dogs: A new model for renal transport defects. Science 201:1129, 1978a.

Bovee KC, Joyce T, Reynolds R, et al.: Spontaneous Fanconi syndrome in the dog. Metabolism 27:45, 1978b.

Bovee KC, Joyce T, Blazer-Yost B, et al.: Characterization of renal defects in dogs with a syndrome similar to Fanconi syndrome in man. J Am Vet Med Assoc 174:1094, 1979.

Breitschwerdt EB, Meuten DJ, Greenfield CL, et al.: Idiopathic hyperaldosteronism in a dog. J Am Vet Med Assoc 187:841, 1985.

Brown SA, Rackich PM, Barsanti JA, et al.: Fanconi syndrome and acute renal failure associated with gentamicin therapy in a dog. J Am Anim Hosp Assoc 22:635, 1986a.

Brown SA, Spyridakis LK, and Crowell WA: Distal renal tubular acidosis and hepatic lipidosis in a cat. J Am Vet Med Assoc 189:1350, 1986b.

Bruskiewicz KA, Nelson RW, Feldman EC, et al.: Diabetic ketosis and ketoacidosis in cats: 42 cases (1980–1995). J Am Vet Med Assoc 211:188, 1997.

Buffington CA, Cook NE, Rogers QR, et al.: The role of diet in feline struvite urolithiasis syndrome. In Burger IH and Rivers JPW (eds): Nutrition of the Dog and Cat. London, Cambridge University Press, p. 357, 1989.

Burnell JM: Changes in bone sodium and carbonate in metabolic acidosis and alkalosis in the dog. J Clin Invest 50:327, 1971.

Burnell JM and Dawbron JK: Acid-base parameters in potassium depletion in the dog. Am J Physiol 218:1583, 1970.

Burnell JM, Teubner EJ, and Simpson DP: Metabolic acidosis accompanying potassium deprivation. Am J Physiol 227:329, 1974.

Cain SM and Dunn JE: Transient arterial lactic acid changes in unanesthetized dogs at 21,000 feet. Am J Physiol 206:1437, 1964.

Carden DL, Martin GB, Nowak RM, et al.: Lactic acidosis as a predictor of downtime during cardiopulmonary arrest in dogs. Am J Emerg Med 3:120, 1985.

Carden DL, Martin GB, Nowak RM, et al.: Lactic acidosis during closed-chest CPR in dogs. Ann Emerg Med 16:1317, 1987.

Chazan JA, Appleton FM, London AM, et al.: Effects of chronic metabolic acid-base disturbances on the composition of cerebrospinal fluid in the dog. Clin Sci 36:345, 1969.

Chew DJ, Leonard M, and Muir WW: Effect of sodium bicarbonate infusions on ionized calcium and total calcium concentrations in serum of clinically normal cats. Am J Vet Res 50:145, 1989.

Chew DJ, Leonard M, and Muir WW: Effect of sodium bicarbonate infusion on serum osmolality, electrolyte concentrations, and blood gas tensions in cats. Am J Vet Res 52:12, 1991.

Ching SV, Fettman MJ, Hamar DW, et al.: The effect of chronic dietary acidification using ammonium chloride on acid-base and mineral metabolism in the adult cat. J Nutr 119:902, 1989.

Ching SV, Norrdin RW, Fettman MJ, et al.: Trabecular bone remodeling and bone mineral density in the adult cat during chronic dietary acidification with ammonium chloride. J Bone Miner Res 5:547, 1990.

Christopher MM, Perman V, White JG, et al.: Propylene glycol–induced Heinz body formation and D-lactic acidosis in cats. Prog Clin Biol Res 319:69, 1989.

Christopher MM, Eckfeld JH, and Eaton JW: Propylene glycol ingestion causes D-lactic acidosis. Lab Invest 62:114, 1990.

Clark DD, Chang BS, Garella SG, et al.: Secondary hypocapnia fails to protect "whole body" intracellular pH during chronic HCl-acidosis in the dog. Kidney Int 23:336, 1983.

Clay KL and Murphy RC: On the metabolic acidosis of ethylene glycol intoxication. Toxicol Appl Pharmacol 39:39, 1977.

Cohen JJ: Correction of metabolic alkalosis by the kidney after isometric expansion of extracellular fluid. *J Clin Invest* 47:1181, 1968.

Cohen JJ: Selective chloride retention in repair of metabolic alkalosis without increasing filtered load. *Am J Physiol* 218:165, 1970.

Cohen JJ, Brackett NC, and Schwartz WB: The nature of the carbon dioxide titration curve in the normal dog. *J Clin Invest* 43:777, 1964.

Cohen JJ, Madias NE, Wolf CJ, et al.: Regulation of acid-base equilibrium in chronic hypocapnia: Evidence that the response of the kidney is not geared to the defense of extracellular [H^+]. *J Clin Invest* 57:1483, 1976.

Cohen RD and Woods RA: *Clinical and Biochemical Aspects of Lactic Acidosis*. London, Blackwell Scientific, 1976.

Cohen RM, Feldman GM, and Fernandez PC: The balance of acid, base and charge in health and disease. *Kidney Int* 52:287, 1997.

Connally HE, Thrall MA, Forney SD, et al.: Safety and efficacy of 4-methylpyrazole for treatment of suspected or confirmed ethylene glycol intoxication: 107 cases (1983–1995). *J Am Vet Med Assoc* 209:1880, 1996.

Cornelius LM and Rawlings CA: Arterial blood gas and acid base values in dogs with various diseases and signs of disease. *J Am Vet Med Assoc* 178:992, 1981.

Crabb DW, Young EA, and Harris RA: The metabolic effects of dichloroacetate. *Metab Clin Exp* 30:1024, 1981.

Crenshaw KL and Peterson ME: Pretreatment clinical and laboratory evaluation of cats with diabetes mellitus: 104 cases (1992–1994). *J Am Vet Med Assoc* 209:943, 1996.

Darrigrand-Haag RA, Center SA, Randolph JF, et al.: Congenital Fanconi syndrome associated with renal dysplasia in 2 Border terriers. *J Vet Intern Med* 10:412, 1996.

DeFronzo RA: Hyperkalemia and hyporeninemic hypoaldosteronism. *Kidney Int* 17:118, 1980.

DeSousa RC, Harrington JT, Ricanati ES, et al.: Renal regulation of acid-base equilibrium during chronic administration of mineral acid. *J Clin Invest* 53:465, 1974.

Dial SM, Thrall M, and Hamar DW: 4-Methylpyrazole as treatment for naturally acquired ethylene glycol intoxication in dogs. *J Am Vet Med Assoc* 195:73, 1989.

Dial SM, Thrall MAH, and Hamar DW: Comparison of ethanol and 4-methylpyrazole as treatments for ethylene glycol intoxication in cats. *Am J Vet Res* 55:1771, 1994a.

Dial SM, Thrall MAH, and Hamar DW: Efficacy of 4-methylpyrazole for treatment of ethylene glycol intoxication in dogs. *Am J Vet Res* 55:1762, 1994b.

DiBartola SP and Leonard PO: Renal tubular acidosis in a dog. *J Am Vet Med Assoc* 180:70, 1982.

DiBartola SP, Rutgers HC, Zack PM, et al.: Clinicopathologic findings associated with chronic renal disease in cats: 74 cases (1973–1984). *J Am Vet Med Assoc* 190:1196, 1987.

DiBartola SP, Tarr MJ, Parker AT, et al.: Clinicopathologic findings in dogs with renal amyloidosis: 59 cases (1976–1986). *J Am Vet Med Assoc* 195:358, 1989.

Dorhout-Mees EJ, Machado M, Slatopolsky E, et al.: The functional adaptation of the diseased kidney. III. Ammonium excretion. *J Clin Invest* 45:289, 1966.

Dow SW, Fettman MJ, Smith KR, et al.: Effects of dietary acidification and potassium depletion on acid-base balance, mineral metabolism and renal function in adult cats. *J Nutr* 120:569, 1990.

Drazner FH: Distal renal tubular acidosis associated with chronic pyelonephritis in a cat. *Calif Vet* 34:15, 1980.

Easley JR and Breitschwerdt EB: Glucosuria associated with renal tubular dysfunction in three basenji dogs. *J Am Vet Med Assoc* 168:938, 1976.

Eger CE, Robinson WF, and Huxtable CRR: Primary aldosteronism (Conn's syndrome) in a cat: A case report and review of comparative aspects. *J Small Anim Pract* 24:293, 1983.

Escolar E, Perezalenza D, Diaz M, et al.: Canine Fanconi syndrome. *J Small Anim Pract* 34:567, 1993.

Evans GO: Plasma lactate measurements in healthy beagles. *Am J Vet Res* 48:131, 1987.

Feldman EC and Nelson RW: *Canine and Feline Endocrinology and Reproduction*. Philadelphia, WB Saunders Co., p. 400, 1996a.

Feldman EC and Nelson RW: *Canine and Feline Endocrinology and Reproduction*. Philadelphia, WB Saunders Co., p. 411, 1996b.

Feldman EC and Nelson RW: *Canine and Feline Endocrinology and Reproduction*. Philadelphia, WB Saunders Co., p. 262, 1996c.

Finco DR, Barsanti JA, and Brown SA: Ammonium chloride as a urinary acidifier in cats: Efficacy, safety, and rationale for its use. *Mod Vet Pract* 67:537, 1986.

Fine A, Brosnan JT, and Herzberg GR: Release of lactate by the liver in metabolic acidosis in vivo. *Metabolism* 33:393, 1984.

Freeman LM, Breitschwerdt EB, Keene BW, et al.: Fanconi's syndrome in a dog with primary hypoparathyroidism. *J Vet Intern Med* 8:349, 1994.

Gennari FJ, Goldstein MB, and Schwartz WB: The nature of the renal adaptation to chronic hypocapnia. *J Clin Invest* 51:1722, 1972.

Gougoux A, Kaehny WD, and Cohen JJ: Renal adaptation to chronic hypocapnia: Dietary constraints in achieving H^+ retention. *Am J Physiol* 229:1330, 1975.

Graf H, Leach W, and Arieff AI: Effects of dichloroacetate in the treatment of hypoxic lactic acidosis in dogs. *J Clin Invest* 76:919, 1985a.

Graf H, Leach W, and Arieff AI: Evidence for a detrimental effect of bicarbonate therapy in hypoxic lactic acidosis. *Science* 227:754, 1985b.

Graf H, Leach W, and Arieff AI: Metabolic effects of sodium bicarbonate in hypoxic lactic acidosis in dogs. *Am J Physiol* 249:F630, 1985c.

Graham TE, Barclay JK, and Wilson BA: Skeletal muscle lactate release and glycolytic intermediates during hypercapnia. *J Appl Physiol* 60:568, 1986.

Grauer GF and Thrall MA: Ethylene glycol (antifreeze) poisoning in the dog and cat. *J Am Anim Hosp Assoc* 18:492, 1982.

Grauer GF and Thrall MA: Ethylene glycol (antifreeze) poisoning. In Kirk RW (ed): *Current Veterinary Therapy IX*. Philadelphia, WB Saunders Co., p. 206, 1986.

Grauer GF, Thrall MA, Henre BA, et al.: Early clinicopathologic findings in dogs ingesting ethylene glycol. *J Am Vet Med Assoc* 45:2299, 1984.

Harrington JT: Metabolic alkalosis. *Kidney Int* 26:88, 1984.

Harrington JT and Cohen JJ: Metabolic acidosis. In Cohen JJ and Kassirer JP (eds): *Acid-Base*. Boston, Little, Brown & Co., p. 128, 1982a.

Harrington JT and Cohen JJ: Metabolic acidosis. In Cohen JJ and Kassirer JP (eds): *Acid-Base*. Boston, Little, Brown & Co., p. 157, 1982b.

Harrington JT and Kassirer JP: Metabolic alkalosis. In Cohen JJ and Kassirer JP (eds): *Acid-Base*. Boston, Little, Brown & Co., p. 227, 1982c.

Harrington JT and Kassirer JP: Metabolic alkalosis. In Cohen JJ and Kassirer JP (eds): *Acid-Base*. Boston, Little, Brown & Co., p. 232, 1982d.

Harrington JT and Kassirer JP: Metabolic alkalosis. In Cohen JJ and Kassirer JP (eds): *Acid-Base*. Boston, Little, Brown & Co., p. 240, 1982e.

Harrington JT and Kassirer JP: Metabolic alkalosis. In Cohen JJ and Kassirer JP (eds): *Acid-Base*. Boston, Little, Brown & Co., p. 280, 1982f.

Hartsfield SM: Sodium bicarbonate and bicarbonate precursors for treatment of metabolic acidosis. *J Am Vet Med Assoc* 179:914, 1981.

Hartsfield SM, Thurmon JC, Corbin JE, et al.: Effects of sodium acetate, bicarbonate and lactate on acid-base status in anesthetized dogs. *J Vet Pharmacol Ther* 4:51, 1981.

Haskins SC, Munger RJ, Helphrey MG, et al.: Effect of acetazolamide on blood acid-base and electrolyte values in dogs. *J Am Vet Med Assoc* 179:914, 1981.

Heald RD, Jones BD, and Schmidt DA: Blood gas and electrolyte concentrations in canine parvoviral enteritis. *J Am Anim Hosp Assoc* 22:745, 1986.

Herrtage ME and Houlton JE: Collapsing Clumber spaniels. *Vet Rec* 105:334, 1979.

Hetenyi G, Paradis H, and Kucharczyk J: Glucose and lactate turnover and gluconeogenesis in chronic metabolic acidosis and alkalosis in normal and diabetic dogs. *Can J Physiol Pharmacol* 66:140, 1988.

Hindman BJ: Sodium bicarbonate in the treatment of subtypes of acute lactic acidosis: Physiologic considerations. *Anesthesiology* 72:1064, 1990.

Honer WG and Jennings DB: PCO_2 modulation of ventilation and HCO_3^- buffer during chronic metabolic acidosis. *Respir Physiol* 54:241, 1983.

Hornbein TF and Pavlin EG: Distribution of H^+ and HCO_3^- between CSF and blood during respiratory alkalosis in dogs. *Am J Physiol* 228:1149, 1975.

Houlton JE and Herrtage ME: Mitochondrial myopathy in the Sussex spaniel. *Vet Rec* 106:206, 1980.

Ilkiw JE, Davis PE, and Church DB: Hematologic, biochemical, blood gas, and acid base values in greyhounds before and after exercise. *Am J Vet Res* 50:583, 1989.

Ilkiw JE, Rose RJ, and Martin ICA: A comparison of simultaneous collected arterial, mixed venous, jugular venous and cephalic venous blood samples in the assessment of blood gas and acid base status in dogs. *J Vet Intern Med* 5:294, 1991.

Jacobs RM, Weiser MG, Hall RL, et al.: Clinicopathologic findings of canine parvoviral enteritis. *J Am Anim Hosp Assoc* 16:809, 1980.

Jacobson HR: Chloride-responsive metabolic alkalosis. In Seldin DW and Gebisch G (eds): *The Regulation of Acid-Base Balance.* New York, Raven Press, p. 431, 1989a.

Jacobson HR: Chloride-resistant metabolic alkalosis. In Seldin DW and Gebisch G (eds): *The Regulation of Acid-Base Balance.* New York, Raven Press, p. 459, 1989b.

Jacobson HR and Seldin DW: On the generation, maintenance, and correction of metabolic alkalosis. *Am J Physiol* 245:F425, 1983.

Jaffe HC, Bodansky A, and Chandler JP: Ammonium chloride decalcification as modified by calcium intake: The relationship between generalized osteoporosis and osteitis fibrosa. *J Exp Med* 56:823, 1932.

Jarvinen A-K and Sankari S: Lactic acidosis in a Clumber spaniel. *Acta Vet Scand* 37:119, 1996.

Jennings DB and Davidson JSD. Acid-base and ventilatory adaptations in conscious dogs during chronic hypercapnia. *Respir Physiol* 58:377, 1984.

Kagan KG and Schaer M: Gastric dilatation and volvulus in a dog—A case justifying electrolyte and acid-base assessment. *J Am Vet Med Assoc* 182:703, 1983.

Kassirer JP and Schwartz WB: Correction of metabolic alkalosis in man without repair of potassium deficiency: A reevaluation of the role of potassium. *Am J Med* 38:19, 1966a.

Kassirer JP and Schwartz WB: The response of normal man to selective depletion of hydrochloric acid. Factors in the genesis of persistent gastric alkalosis. *Am J Med* 40:10, 1966b.

Kassirer JP, Berkman PM, Lawrenz DR, et al.: The critical role of chloride in the correction of hypokalemic alkalosis in man. *Am J Med* 38:172, 1965.

Kazemi H, Valenca LM, and Shannon DC: Brain and cerebrospinal fluid lactate concentration in respiratory acidosis and alkalosis. *Respir Physiol* 6:178, 1969.

Kramer JW, Bistline D, Sheridan P, et al.: Identification of hippuric acid crystals in the urine of ethylene glycol–intoxicated dogs and cats. *J Am Vet Med Assoc* 184:584, 1984.

Kreisberg RA: Diabetic ketoacidosis: New concepts and trends in pathogenesis and treatment. *Arch Intern Med* 88:681, 1978.

Kreisberg RA: Pathogenesis and management of lactic acidosis. *Annu Rev Med* 35:181, 1984.

Lemieux G, Lemieux C, Duplessis S, et al.: Metabolic characteristics of cat kidney: Failure to adapt to metabolic acidosis. *Am J Physiol* 259:R277, 1990.

Ling GV, Lowenstine LJ, Pulley LT, et al.: Diabetes mellitus in dogs: A review of initial evaluation, immediate and long-term management, and outcome. *J Am Vet Med Assoc* 170:521, 1977.

Ling GV, Stabenfeldt GH, Comer KM, et al.: Canine hyperadrenocorticism: Pretreatment clinical and laboratory evaluation of 117 cases. *J Am Vet Med Assoc* 174:1211, 1979.

Lloyd MH, Iles RA, Simpson BR, et al.: The effect of simulated metabolic acidosis on intracellular pH and lactate metabolism in the isolated perfused rat liver. *Clin Sci* 45:543, 1973.

Lowance DC, Garfinkel HB, Mattern WD, et al.: The effect of chronic hypotonic volume expansion on the renal regulation of acid-base equilibrium. *J Clin Invest* 51:2928, 1972.

Macintire DK: Treatment of diabetic ketoacidosis in dogs by continuous low-dose intravenous infusion of insulin. *J Am Vet Med Assoc* 202:1266, 1993.

MacKenzie CP and van den Broek A: The Fanconi syndrome in a whippet. *J Small Anim Pract* 23:469, 1982.

Madias NE: Lactic acidosis. *Kidney Int* 29:752, 1986.

Madias NE and Zelman SJ: The renal response to chronic mineral acid feeding: A re-examination of the role of systemic pH. *Kidney Int* 29:667, 1986.

Madias NE, Schwartz WB, and Cohen JJ: The maladaptive renal response to secondary hypocapnia during chronic HCl acidosis in the dog. *J Clin Invest* 60:1393, 1977.

Madias NE, Adrogue HJ, and Cohen JJ: Maladaptive renal response to secondary hypercapnia in chronic metabolic alkalosis. *Am J Physiol* 238:F283, 1980.

Madias NE, Bossert WH, and Adrogue HJ: Ventilatory response to chronic metabolic acidosis and alkalosis in the dog. *J Appl Physiol* 56:1640, 1984.

Madias NE, Wolf CJ, and Cohen JJ: Regulation of acid-base equilibrium in chronic hypercapnia. *Kidney Int* 27:538, 1985.

Magner PO, Robinson L, Halperin RM, et al.: The plasma potassium concentration in metabolic acidosis: A re-evaluation. *Am J Kidney Dis* 11:220, 1988.

Marsh JD, Margolis TI, and Kim D: Mechanism of diminished contractile response to catecholamines during acidosis. *Am J Physiol* 254:H20, 1988.

Martin GB, Carden DL, Nowak RM, et al.: Comparison of central venous and arterial pH and PCO_2 during open chest CPR in the canine model. *Ann Emerg Med* 14:529, 1985.

Maskrey M and Jennings DB: Ventilation and acid-base balance in awake dogs exposed to heat and CO_2. *J Appl Physiol* 58:549, 1985.

Mathias DW, Clifford PS, and Klopfenstein HS: Mixed venous blood gases are superior to arterial blood gases in assessing acid-base status and oxygenation during acute cardiac tamponade in dogs. *J Clin Invest* 82:833, 1988.

McEwan NA and Macartney L: Fanconi's syndrome in a Yorkshire terrier. *J Small Anim Pract* 28:737, 1987.

McNamara PD, Rea CT, Bovee KC, et al.: Cystinuria in dogs: Comparison of the cystinuric component of the Fanconi syndrome in basenji dogs to isolated cystinuria. *Metabolism* 38:8, 1989.

Meijer JC: Canine hyperadrenocorticism. In Kirk RW (ed): *Current Veterinary Therapy VII.* Philadelphia, WB Saunders Co., p. 975, 1980.

Melian C and Peterson ME: Diagnosis and treatment of naturally-occurring hypoadrenocorticism in 42 dogs. *J Small Anim Pract* 37:268, 1996.

Meyer DJ: Temporary remission of hypoglycemia in a dog with an insulinoma after treatment with streptozotocin. *Am J Vet Res* 38:1201, 1977.

Mitchell JH, Wildenthal K, and Johnson RL: The effects of acid-base disturbances on cardiovascular and pulmonary function. *Kidney Int* 1:375, 1972.

Moon PE, Gabor L, Gleed RD, et al.: Acid-base, metabolic, and hemodynamic effects of sodium bicarbonate or tromethamine administration in anesthetized dogs with experimentally induced metabolic acidosis. *Am J Vet Res* 58:771, 1997.

Morrin PAF, Bricker NS, Kime SW, et al.: Observations on the acidifying capacity of the experimentally diseased kidney of the dog. *J Clin Invest* 41:1297, 1962a.

Morrin PAF, Gedney WB, Newmark LN, et al.: Bicarbonate reabsorption in the dog with experimental renal disease. *J Clin Invest* 41:1303, 1962b.

Morris LR, Murphy MB, and Kitabchi AE: Bicarbonate therapy in severe diabetic ketoacidosis. *Ann Intern Med* 105:836, 1986.

Muir WW: Acid-base and electrolyte disturbances in dogs with gastric-dilatation volvulus. *J Am Vet Med Assoc* 181:229, 1982.

Musch TI, Friedman DB, Haidet GC, et al.: Arterial blood gases and acid-base status of dogs during graded dynamic exercise. *J Appl Physiol* 61:1914, 1986.

Narins RG and Cohen JJ: Bicarbonate therapy for organic acidosis: The case for its continued use. *Ann Intern Med* 106:615, 1987.

Narins RG, Jones ER, Stom MC, et al.: Diagnostic strategies in disorders of fluid, electrolyte and acid base homeostasis. *Am J Med* 72:496, 1982.

Needle MA, Kaloyandies GJ, and Schwartz WB: The effects of selective depletion of hydrochloric acid on acid base and electrolyte equilibrium. *J Clin Invest* 43:1836, 1964.

Norris SH and Kurtzman NA: Does chloride play an independent role in the pathogenesis of metabolic alkalosis? *Semin Nephrol* 8:101, 1988.

Nunamaker DM, Medway W, and Berg P: Treatment of ethylene glycol poisoning in the dog. *J Am Vet Med Assoc* 159:310, 1971.

Oh MS: Irrelevance of bone buffering to acid-base homeostasis in chronic metabolic acidosis. *Nephron* 59:7, 1991.

Okuda Y, Adrogue HJ, Field JB, et al.: Counterproductive effects of sodium bicarbonate in diabetic ketoacidosis. *J Clin Endocrinol Metab* 81:314, 1996.

Olby NJ, Chan KK, Targett MP, et al.: Suspected mitochondrial myopathy in a Jack Russell terrier. *J Small Anim Pract* 38:213, 1997.

Orchard CH and Kentish JC: Effects of changes of pH on the contractile function of cardiac muscle. *Am J Physiol* 258:C967, 1990.

Padrid P: Fanconi syndrome in a mixed breed dog. *Mod Vet Pract* 69:162, 1988.

Pavlin EG and Hornbein TF: Distribution of H^+ and HCO_3^- between CSF and blood during respiratory acidosis. *Am J Physiol* 228:1145, 1975.

Penman RW, Luke RF, and Jarboe TM: Respiratory effects of hypochloremic alkalosis and potassium depletion in the dog. *J Appl Physiol* 33:170, 1972.

Penumarthy L and Oehme FW: Treatment of ethylene glycol toxicosis in cats. *Am J Vet Res* 36:209, 1974.

Peterson M: Hyperadrenocorticism. *Vet Clin North Am* 14:731, 1984.

Peterson ME, Greco DS, and Orth DN: Primary hypoadrenocorticism in ten cats. *J Vet Intern Med* 3:55, 1989.

Peterson ME, Kintzer PP, and Kass PH: Pretreatment clinical and laboratory findings in dogs with hypoadrenocorticism—225 cases (1979–1993). *J Am Vet Med Assoc* 208:85, 1996.

Polzin DJ, Stevens JB, and Osborne CA: Clinical evaluation of the anion gap in evaluation of acid-base disorders in dogs. *Compend Contin Educ Pract Vet* 4:102, 1982.

Posner J and Plum F: Spinal fluid pH and neurologic symptoms in systemic acidosis. *N Engl J Med* 277:605, 1967.

Rhee KH, Toro LO, McDonald GG, et al.: Carbicarb, sodium bicarbonate, and sodium chloride in hypoxic lactic acidosis. *Chest* 104:913, 1993.

Robinson EP and Hardy RM Clinical signs, diagnosis, and treatment of alkalemia in dogs: 20 cases (1982–1984). *J Am Vet Med Assoc* 192:943, 1988.

Rose BD: *Clinical Physiology of Acid-Base and Electrolyte Disorders*. New York, McGraw-Hill Book Co., p. 542, 1994a.

Rose BD: *Clinical Physiology of Acid-Base and Electrolyte Disorders*. New York, McGraw-Hill Co., p. 588, 1994b.

Rose BD: *Clinical Physiology of Acid-Base and Electrolyte Disorders*. New York, McGraw-Hill Co., p. 564, 1994c.

Rose BD: *Clinical Physiology of Acid-Base and Electrolyte Disorders*. New York, McGraw-Hill Co., p. 591, 1994d.

Rose BD: *Clinical Physiology of Acid-Base and Electrolyte Disorders*. New York, McGraw-Hill Co., p. 589, 1994e.

Rose BD: *Clinical Physiology of Acid-Base and Electrolyte Disorders*. New York, McGraw-Hill Book Co., p. 515, 1994f.

Rose RJ and Carter J: Some physiological and biochemical effects of acetazolamide in the dog. *J Vet Pharmacol Ther* 2:215, 1979.

Sabatini S: The acidosis of chronic renal failure. *Med Clin North Am* 67:845, 1983.

Sabatini S and Kurtzman NA: The maintenance of metabolic alkalosis: Factors which decrease bicarbonate excretion. *Kidney Int* 25:357, 1984.

Sanders AB, Otto CW, Kern KB, et al.: Acid-base balance in a canine model of cardiac arrest. *Ann Emerg Med* 17:667, 1988.

Sanyer JL, Oehme FW, and McGavin MD: Systematic treatment of ethylene glycol toxicosis in dogs. *Am J Vet Res* 34:527, 1973.

Schmidt RW and Gavellas G: Bicarbonate reabsorption in dogs with experimental renal disease: Effects of proportional reduction of sodium or phosphate intake. *Kidney Int* 12:393, 1977.

Schmidt RW, Bricker NS, and Gavellas G: Renal bicarbonate reabsorption in experimental uremia in the dog. *Kidney Int* 10:287, 1976.

Schober KE: Investigation into intraerythrocytic and extraerythrocytic acid-base and electrolyte changes after long-term ammonium chloride administration in dogs. *Am J Vet Res* 57:743, 1996.

Schwartz WB, Orning KJ, and Porter R: The internal distribution of hydrogen ions with varying degrees of metabolic acidosis. *J Clin Invest* 36:373, 1957.

Schwartz WB, Hays RM, Pak A, et al.: Effects of chronic hypercapnia on electrolyte and acid-base equilibrium. II. Recovery, with special reference to the influence of chloride intake. *J Clin Invest* 40:1238, 1961.

Senior DF, Sundstrom DA, and Wolfson BB: Effectiveness of ammonium chloride as a urinary acidifier in cats fed a popular brand of canned cat food. *Feline Pract* 16:24, 1986a.

Senior DF, Sundstrom DA, and Wolfson BB: Testing the effects of ammonium chloride and DL-methionine on the urinary pH of cats. *Vet Med* 81:88, 1986b.

Settles EL and Schmidt D: Fanconi syndrome in a Labrador retriever. *J Vet Intern Med* 8:390, 1994.

Shaw DH: Acute response of urine pH following ammonium chloride administration to dogs. *Am J Vet Res* 50:1829, 1989.

Sheikh A, Fleisher G, Delgado-Paredes C, et al.: Effect of dichloroacetate in the treatment of anoxic lactic acidosis in dogs. *Crit Care Med* 14:970, 1986.

Shull RM: The value of anion gap and osmolal gap determinations in veterinary medicine. *Vet Clin Pathol* 7:12, 1978.

Silva PRM, Fonseca-Costa A, Zin WA, et al.: Respiratory and acid-base parameters during salicylic intoxication in dogs. *Braz J Med Biol Res* 19:279, 1986.

Simpson DP: Control of hydrogen ion homeostasis and renal acidosis. *Medicine (Baltimore)* 50:503, 1971.

Stacpoole PW: Lactic acidosis: The case against bicarbonate therapy. *Ann Intern Med* 105:276, 1986.

Straus E, Johnson GF, and Yalow RS: Canine Zollinger-Ellison syndrome. *Gastroenterology* 72:380, 1977.

Swan RC and Pitts RF: Neutralization of infused acid by nephrectomized dogs. *J Clin Invest* 34:205, 1955.

Swan RC, Axelrod DR, Seip M, et al.: Distribution of sodium bicarbonate infused into nephrectomized dogs. *J Clin Invest* 34:1795, 1955.

Takano N: Blood lactate accumulation and its causative factors during passive hyperventilation in dogs. *Jpn J Physiol* 16:481, 1966.

Tashkin DP, Goldstein PJ, and Simmons DH: Hepatic lactate uptake during decreased liver perfusion. *Am J Physiol* 223:968, 1972.

Thrall MA, Grauer GF, and Mero KN: Clinicopathologic findings in dogs and cats with ethylene glycol intoxication. *J Am Vet Med Assoc* 184:37, 1984.

Thrall MA, Dial SM, and Winder DR: Identification of calcium oxalate monohydrate crystals by X-ray diffraction in urine of ethylene glycol–intoxicated dogs. *Vet Pathol* 22:625, 1985.

Toto RD and Alpern RJ: Metabolic acid-base disorders. In Kokko JP and Tannen RL (eds): *Fluids and Electrolytes*. Philadelphia, WB Saunders Co., p. 201, 1996.

Vail DM, Ogilvie GK, Fettman MJ, et al.: Exacerbation of hyperlactatemia by infusion of lactated Ringer's solution in dogs with lymphoma. *J Vet Intern Med* 4:228, 1990a.

Vail DM, Ogilvie GK, Wheeler SL, et al.: Alterations in carbohydrate metabolism in canine lymphoma. *J Vet Intern Med* 4:8, 1990b.

Valtin H and Gennari FJ: *Acid-Base Disorders: Basic Concepts and Management*. Boston, Little, Brown & Co., 1987.

Vijayasarathy C, Giger U, Prociuk U, et al.: Canine mitochondrial myopathy associated with reduced mitochondrial messenger RNA and altered cytochrome *c* oxidase activities in fibroblasts and skeletal muscle. *Comp Biochem Physiol* 109:887, 1994.

Vukmir RB, Bircher NG, Radovsky A, et al.: Sodium bicarbonate may improve outcome in dogs with brief or prolonged cardiac arrest. *Crit Care Med* 23:515, 1995.

Warnock DG: Uremic acidosis. *Kidney Int* 34:278, 1988.

Watson ADJ, Culvenor JA, Middleton DJ, et al.: Distal renal tubular acidosis in a cat with pyelonephritis. *Vet Rec* 119:65, 1986.

Weil MH, Rackow EC, Trevino R, et al.: Difference in acid-base state between venous and arterial blood during cardiopulmonary resuscitation. *N Engl J Med* 315:153, 1986.

Welbourne T, Weber M, and Bank N: The effect of glutamine administration on urinary ammonium excretion in normal subjects and patients with renal disease. *J Clin Invest* 51:1852, 1972.

Widmer B, Gerhard RE, Harrington JT, et al.: Serum electrolyte and acid-base composition: The influence of graded degrees of chronic renal failure. *Arch Intern Med* 139:1099, 1979.

Wingfield WE, Twedt DC, Moore RW, et al.: Acid-base and electrolyte values in dogs with acute gastric dilatation-volvulus. *J Am Vet Med Assoc* 180:1070, 1982.

CHAPTER 11

Respiratory Acid-Base Disorders

HELIO AUTRAN DE MORAIS   STEPHEN P. DiBARTOLA

Metabolic processes normally produce approximately 15,000 mmol of CO_2 each day. Carbon dioxide produced in the tissues readily penetrates cellular membranes and equilibrium is achieved rapidly between intracellular and extracellular compartments. After reaching the plasma, CO_2 diffuses rapidly into red blood cells. Within red blood cells, in the presence of carbonic anhydrase activity, CO_2 and H_2O combine to form H_2CO_3, which, under physiologic conditions, dissociates into H^+ and HCO_3^- ions. The HCO_3^- ions diffuse from the red cells into plasma in exchange for Cl^- ions from plasma ("chloride shift") (Fig. 11–1). Most of the CO_2 (81%) produced in tissues is transported to the lungs in this fashion. A small amount (8%) is transported dissolved in plasma, and some (11%) is transported combined with certain amino groups of hemoglobin, forming carbaminohemoglobin (Valtin and Gennari 1987).

The H^+ ions formed as a result of carbonic anhydrase activity in red blood cells and those released during the formation of carbaminohemoglobin combine primarily with hemoglobin. The small amount of H^+ formed by dissociation of carbonic acid in plasma combines with phosphate and plasma proteins. The addition to venous blood of CO_2 from body tissues is responsible for the observation that venous blood pH is slightly lower and the carbon dioxide tension (PCO_2) and HCO_3^- concentrations are higher than those in the arterial blood.

▶ PCO_2 and Alveolar Ventilation

The lungs are the only route for CO_2 elimination. Carbon dioxide diffuses efficiently across the alveolar capillary-wall so that the alveolar CO_2 tension is essentially the same in the alveoli ($PACO_2$) and arteries ($PaCO_2$). In the steady state, $PaCO_2$ is inversely proportional to alveolar ventilation. As a result, measurement of a patient's $PaCO_2$

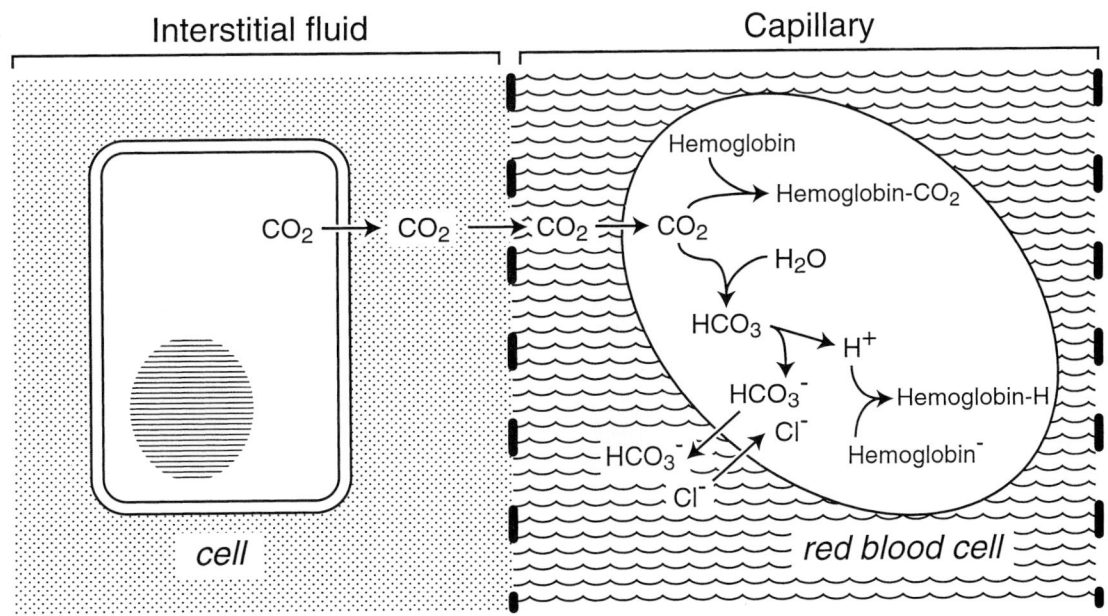

FIGURE 11–1. The chloride shift. Increased CO_2 from cell metabolism leaves plasma and enters red blood cells, where it combines with hemoglobin and forms carbaminohemoglobin. The largest amount of CO_2 inside red blood cells, however, is hydrated to form carbonic acid, which dissociates into bicarbonate and hydrogen ions. Bicarbonate diffuses out of the red blood cells into plasma in exchange for chloride ions.

provides the clinician with direct information about the adequacy of alveolar ventilation. Hypercapnia (increased $PaCO_2$) indicates alveolar hypoventilation and hypocapnia (decreased $PaCO_2$) indicates alveolar hyperventilation.

In the normal animal, alveolar ventilation is controlled by chemoreceptors that detect alterations in $[H^+]$ and O_2 delivery and translate these changes into appropriate compensatory adjustments in respiratory rate and tidal volume. The main physiologic stimuli for ventilation are CO_2-induced increases in $[H^+]$ and hypoxemia. Central chemoreceptors in the brain stem medulla respond primarily to CO_2-induced alterations in $[H^+]$, whereas peripheral chemoreceptors in the aortic arch and carotid arteries respond primarily to decreased oxygen delivery.

Normally, hypercapnia is the main stimulus for ventilation with alveolar ventilation increasing in a linear fashion with increasing PCO_2. Hypoxemia does not stimulate ventilation until PO_2 decreases to less than 60 mm Hg. The response of the central chemoreceptors to CO_2 is damped in chronic hypercapnia, and hypoxemia becomes the major stimulus for ventilation in this setting. The apparent lack of sensitivity may be related to the compensatory increase in plasma HCO_3^- concentration that occurs in chronic hypercapnia. A given increase in PCO_2 causes a smaller increment in $[H^+]$ at a higher HCO_3^- concentration as compared with a lower one. Thus, the normal compensatory increase in HCO_3^- protects extracellular $[H^+]$ but in doing so limits stimulation of alveolar ventilation and potentially aggravates hypoxemia and hypercapnia. Other factors that may alter ventilation include voluntary cerebrocortical influences, drugs, toxins, and nociceptive receptors in the lung.

▶ Alveolar-Arterial Oxygen Difference

In animals with hypoxemia or hypercapnia, the alveolar-arterial oxygen difference ($[A-a]$ O_2 gradient) may be useful in differentiating intrinsic pulmonary disease from extrapulmonary disorders in determining the underlying cause of abnormal blood gas results. Hypoxemic patients with normal $(A-a)$ O_2 usually have normal pulmonary function and the hypoxemia is a result of hypoventilation or decreased inspired oxygen tension (PIO_2). The $(A-a)$ O_2 gradient represents the difference (in mm Hg) between alveolar PO_2 (PAO_2) and arterial PO_2 (PaO_2) and can be estimated clinically as

$$(A-a)\ O_2\ \text{gradient} = (150 - 1.25\ PaCO_2) - PaO_2$$

(see the Appendix for the derivation of the $(A-a)$ O_2 gradient formula).

In a normal dog with $PaO_2 = 100$ mm Hg and $PaCO_2 = 36$ mm Hg, the $(A-a)$ O_2 gradient is 5 mm Hg. Values below 15 to 25 mm Hg are generally considered normal (DiBartola and de Morais, 1992).

Clinical Implications

Hypoxia can be caused by hypoventilation, decreased PIO_2, diffusion impairment across the alveolar-arterial membrane, ventilation-perfusion (V-Q) mismatch, or right-to-left shunt. Hypoxemic patients with abnormal $(A-a)$ O_2 usually have abnormal lung function or a right-to-left shunt (Fig. 11–2).

HYPOVENTILATION

The prevailing PAO_2 is determined by the balance between removal of O_2 by the blood and replenishment of O_2 by alveolar ventilation. If alveolar ventilation is abnormally low, PAO_2 and PaO_2 decrease and $PACO_2$ and $PaCO_2$ increase. The $(A-a)$ O_2 gradient therefore does not change. Deviations from the idealized $(A-a)$ O_2 gradient indicate concurrent V-Q mismatch or right-to-left-shunting. Clinically, the most important causes of hypoventilation are central nervous system disease, respiratory

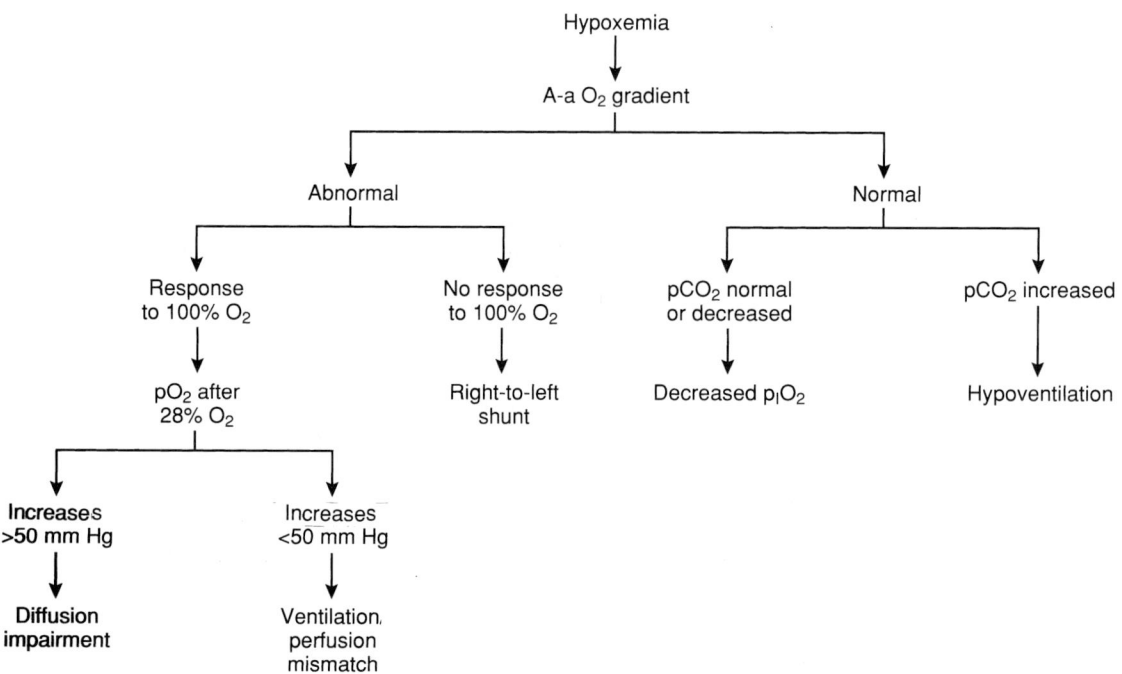

FIGURE 11–2. Algorithm depicting the clinical approach to the patient with hypoxemia.

depressant drugs, neuromuscular diseases affecting the respiratory muscles, chest wall injury, upper airway obstruction, and severe diffuse pulmonary disease.

DECREASED P_{IO_2}

A decrease in P_{IO_2} may result from a decrease in barometric pressure (P_B), usually associated with residence at high altitudes. It may also occur with improper anesthetic technique (e.g., administration of N_2O without O_2). As a result of the decrease in P_{IO_2}, decreases in P_{AO_2} and P_{aO_2} occur. In this setting, there is an increase in alveolar ventilation secondary to hypoxemia, which in turn decreases P_{aCO_2}. The (A−a) O_2 difference remains within normal limits because of the concomitant decrease in P_{IO_2} (see Appendix).

DIFFUSION IMPAIRMENT

Diffusion impairment occurs whenever there is inadequate equilibration of O_2 tension between the alveoli and capillary blood. In the normal individual at rest, capillary O_2 tension rapidly reaches that of the alveoli. Consequently, it is possible to have a diffusion impairment that is detectable only as hypoxemia during exercise. Diffusion impairment may occur earlier in the course of chronic pulmonary disease than V-Q mismatch, but most small animal patients with clinical signs apparent to their owners usually have both V-Q mismatch and diffusion impairment by the time they are brought to the veterinarian. Diffusion impairment may be due to thickening of the alveolar capillary wall (e.g., diffuse pulmonary interstitial disease), loss of alveolar surface area (e.g., emphysema), or loss of capillary surface area (e.g., vasculitis).

VENTILATION-PERFUSION MISMATCH

Ventilation-perfusion mismatch is common in patients with pulmonary disease. It occurs in areas of the lung where there is lack of ventilation or perfusion resulting in inefficient gas exchange. Ventilation-perfusion mismatch may occur as a result of increased airway resistance (e.g., asthma, bronchitis), decreased compliance (e.g., pulmonary fibrosis), increased compliance (e.g., emphysema), or vascular disease (e.g., pulmonary embolism). The severity of V-Q mismatch can be assessed using the (A−a) O_2 gradient. An increase in the gradient can be caused by both abnormally low and abnormally high V-Q ratios in the lungs. Patients with V-Q mismatch are usually hypoxemic but have normal or decreased P_{aCO_2}. Their hypoxemia can be corrected by increasing the fraction of inspired oxygen (F_{IO_2}) by use of 100% O_2. A P_{aO_2} of approximately 500 mm Hg is expected in a normal animal breathing 100% O_2.

RIGHT-TO-LEFT SHUNT

In patients with right-to-left shunting, some blood enters the systemic arterial circulation without previously passing through ventilated areas of the lungs. A small amount of right-to-left shunting is present in normal animals. Pathologic right-to-left shunting can be caused by alveolar collapse (i.e., atelectasis), filling of alveoli with fluid (e.g., pulmonary edema), alveolar consolidation (e.g., pneumonia), and extrapulmonary shunts (e.g., congenital cardiac anomalies). Patients with right-to-left shunting have decreased P_{aO_2} with normal or decreased P_{aCO_2} because mixed venous blood is being added directly to arterial blood without the occurrence of gas exchange in alveoli. The P_{aO_2} of patients with right-to-left shunting fails to increase to normal even after breathing 100% O_2 (Table 11–1). An algorithm for the clinical approach to the patient with hypoxemia is presented in Figure 11–2.

TABLE 11–1. Theoretical Effect of Breathing 21% and 100% Oxygen on Mean P_{O_2} Values in Alveolar Gas, Arterial Blood, and Mixed Venous Blood

F_{IO_2}	Ideal Gas Exchange		V-Q Mismatch		Right-to-Left Shunt	
	21%	100%	21%	100%	21%	100%
P_{O_2} (venous)	40	51	40	51	40	42
P_{O_2} (alveolar)	101	673	106	675	114	677
P_{O_2} (arterial)	101	673	89	673	59	125
(A − a) P_{O_2} gradient	0	0	17	2	55	552

Source: Murray JF: Gas exchange and oxygen transport. In Murray JF: *The Normal Lung*. Philadelphia, WB Saunders Co., p. 194, 1986.

▶ Overview of Respiratory Acid-Base Disorders

The P_{CO_2} of blood is an important determinant of the prevailing acidity of body fluids because it determines their carbonic acid concentration. The P_{CO_2} is one of the independent variables in the control of acid-base balance. Increases in P_{CO_2} cause a decrease in pH (respiratory acidosis), whereas decreases in P_{CO_2} increase pH (respiratory alkalosis).

Changes in the CO_2 tension of blood can have dramatic effects on pH (and [H^+]) yet have insignificant effects on plasma HCO_3^- concentration. This may occur even though changes in CO_2 tension cause equimolar changes in H^+ and HCO_3^- concentrations. The greater effect on pH occurs because the H^+ concentration of body fluids is measured in nEq/L whereas the HCO_3^- concentration is measured in mEq/L. Given concentrations of 40 nEq/L for [H^+] (pH 7.40) and 24 mEq/L for HCO_3^-, there are approximately 600,000 HCO_3^- ions for each H^+ ion. Without the benefit of body buffers, a sudden increase in P_{CO_2} from 40 to 80 mm Hg would increase the [H^+] from 40 to 80 nEq/L (a pH change from 7.400 to 7.095). At the same time, the HCO_3^- concentration would increase from 24.0 to 24.000040 mEq/L, a difference that would be undetectable.

Metabolic Compensation

Primary changes in P_{CO_2} generate adaptive responses to maintain arterial pH close to normal. This adaptive response is reflected by a change in HCO_3^-. In respiratory acid-base disorders, this change occurs in two phases. The first phase represents titration of nonbicarbonate buffers. These reactions begin within 15 min and an acute steady state is rapidly established. The second phase reflects renal adaptation and consists of changes in electrolyte and net acid excretion and Cl^- and HCO_3^- reabsorption. These events occur over 2 to 5 days and a chronic steady state is established with extracellular pH returning toward normal.

ACUTE ADAPTIVE RESPONSE

Increases in P_{CO_2} cause CO_2 to diffuse into the cells. The CO_2 diffuses across cell membranes almost immediately, causing an increase in P_{CO_2} and a decrease in pH intracellularly. Intracellular buffers play a critical role in hypercapnia, handling 97% of the H^+ ion load in acute hypercapnia in dogs (Giebisch et al. 1955). Only 3% of the H^+ load is handled by extracellular buffers, primarily plasma proteins. The acute compensatory increase in HCO_3^- concentration observed in cases of respiratory acidosis results from bicarbonate ions produced intracellularly leaving the cells in exchange for chloride ions (chloride shift). These changes are summarized in Figure 11–3.

During decreases in P_{CO_2}, CO_2 leaves the cells to achieve a new equilibrium point, causing intracellular alkalosis. The final response is almost the opposite of that observed during acute hypercapnia. Chloride ions leave red blood cells in exchange for HCO_3^-, causing a decrease in plasma HCO_3^- concentration. As in respiratory acidosis, intracellular phosphates and proteins are the major buffers in the initial adaptive response to acute hypocapnia. The tissue buffer response to severe acute hypocapnia has been studied in nephrectomized dogs (Giebisch et al. 1955). Extracellular buffering by release of H^+ from plasma proteins constituted only 1% of the response and intracellular buffering accounted for the remaining 99%. These changes are summarized in Figure 11–4.

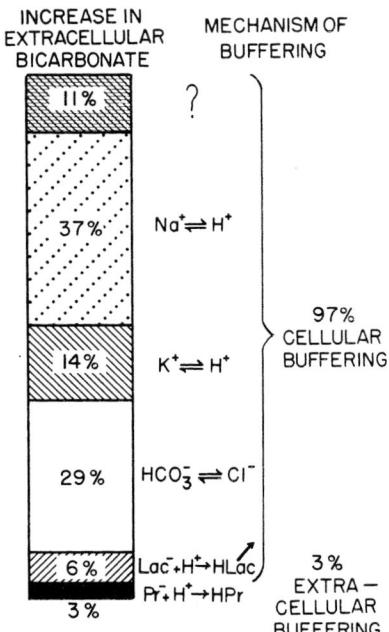

FIGURE 11–3. Mechanisms of buffering CO_2 in respiratory acidosis in the dog. (From Pitts RF: *Physiology of the Kidney and Body Fluids,* 2nd ed. Chicago, Year Book Medical Publishers, p. 175, 1968.)

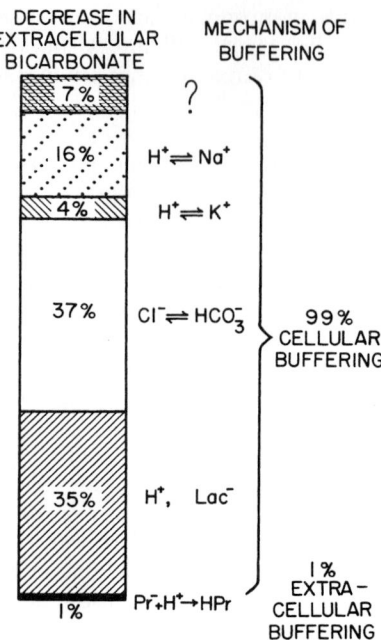

FIGURE 11–4. Mechanisms of buffering CO_2 in respiratory alkalosis in the dog. (From Pitts RF: *Physiology of the Kidney and Body Fluids,* 2nd ed. Chicago, Year Book Medical Publishers, p. 176, 1968.)

CHRONIC ADAPTIVE RESPONSE

When the inspired concentration of CO_2 is increased and maintained at a new level in dogs, it takes 2 to 5 days for renal compensation to stabilize plasma HCO_3^- at a higher concentration (Polak et al. 1961; Schwartz et al. 1965; Jennings and Davidson 1984; van Ypersele de Strihou et al. 1962). The increase in P_{CO_2} in chronic respiratory acidosis causes intracellular H^+ to increase in the renal tubular cells, resulting in stimulation of net acid excretion (primarily as $NH_4^+Cl^-$) (Rose 1989). Chloruresis, negative chloride balance, enhanced fractional and absolute bicarbonate reabsorption, and enhanced net acid excretion are typically associated with the renal response to chronic respiratory acidosis (Galla and Luke 1988). The chloride lost in the urine decreases the urine strong ion difference (SID) because it is accompanied by NH_4^+ rather than sodium ions and increases the plasma SID and consequently HCO_3^-. Hypochloremia is a common finding in dogs with experimentally induced chronic hypercapnia (Madias et al. 1985; Polak et al. 1961; Schwartz et al. 1965; van Ypersele de Strihou et al. 1962). The increase in plasma HCO_3^- concentration is accompanied by a reciprocal decrease in serum chloride concentration, indicating that the kidney increases the proportion of HCO_3^- and decreases the proportion of chloride that it reabsorbs with sodium during adaptation to chronic hypercapnia. This increases SID and consequently increases HCO_3^- concentration. This mechanism is shown schematically in Figure 11–5. A new steady state is reached when the increased filtered load of HCO_3^- resulting from the increased plasma concentration of HCO_3^- is balanced by increased renal reabsorption of HCO_3^-. During recovery from chronic hypercapnia, chloride restriction hampers the return of plasma HCO_3^- concentration to normal. Thus, the kidney must be pro-

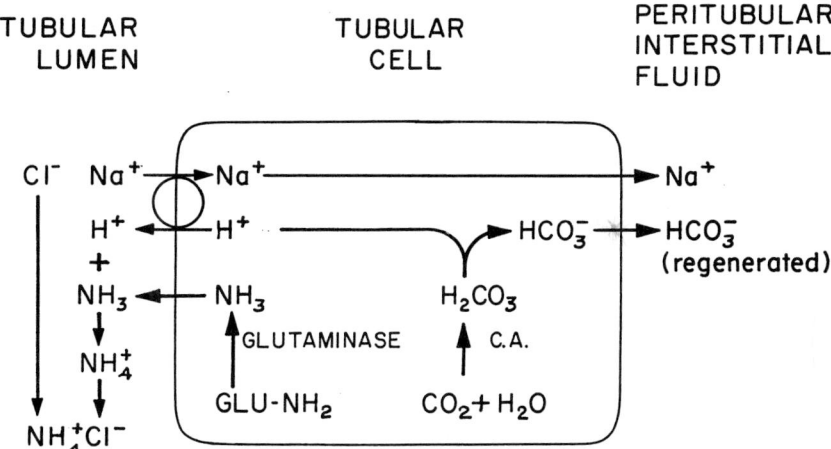

FIGURE 11-5. Diagram showing how HCO_3^- ions are reabsorbed during Na^+-H^+ exchange in the renal tubular cells and how NH_4^+ is excreted in tubular fluid.

vided with chloride during recovery so that it can preferentially reabsorb chloride with sodium, excrete excess HCO_3^- in the urine, and reestablish normal SID in the plasma.

The renal response to sustained hypocapnia is accomplished by a decrease in net acid excretion and is usually complete within 3 days. When P_{CO_2} is decreased abruptly, HCO_3^- excretion increases transiently, urine pH increases, and titratable acid excretion decreases. Within 24 h, half of the reduction in plasma HCO_3^- is a consequence of decreased renal NH_4^+ and titratable acid excretion. The increase in chloride reabsorption decreases plasma SID and consequently HCO_3^- and is responsible for the hyperchloremia observed in dogs with experimentally induced chronic hypocapnia (Gennari et al. 1972). As plasma HCO_3^- concentration decreases, the filtered load of HCO_3^- decreases and urine pH returns to normal. When P_{CO_2} is decreased slowly, most of the reduction in plasma HCO_3^- concentration results from decreased NH_4^+ excretion by the kidneys.

Decreased H^+ ion secretion reduces sodium reabsorption in exchange for H^+ ions in the renal tubules. The decrease in net acid excretion by the kidneys in chronic hypocapnia is accompanied by a reciprocal increase in urinary excretion of cations, usually sodium. This response differs from that observed in chronic hypercapnia, wherein the increase in net acid excretion is accompanied by a parallel increase in urinary excretion of chloride. The increased urinary loss of sodium causes a small decrease in plasma volume when hypocapnia is sustained. This decrease in net acid excretion was accompanied by an increase in urinary excretion of sodium in dogs receiving a normal diet and by an increase in the urinary excretion of potassium in dogs receiving a low-salt diet. In dogs with the normal diet, serum chloride concentration increased significantly and there was a slight increase in the concentration of unmeasured anions. There were no significant changes in serum sodium or potassium concentrations (Gennari et al. 1972).

▶ Respiratory Acidosis

Respiratory acidosis results from a primary increase in P_{CO_2} in the blood. It is synonymous with the term primary hypercapnia and is characterized by increased P_{CO_2}, increased $[H^+]$, decreased pH, and a compensatory increase in HCO_3^- concentration in blood. In the authors' experience, this is a relatively uncommon acid-base disorder in small animals.

Carbon dioxide accumulation is caused by alveolar hypoventilation. In the presence of normal pulmonary function, it is impossible for increased CO_2 production to result in hypercapnia. Hypoxemia typically occurs earlier in the course of pulmonary disease than does hypercapnia, because CO_2 is approximately 20 times more diffusible than O_2. Also, as ventilation increases in response to disease and hypoxemia is ameliorated, CO_2 removal is improved but O_2 delivery is not because hemoglobin is 80 to 90% saturated at P_{O_2} above 60 mm Hg.

Adaptive increases in plasma HCO_3^- concentration occur in two phases. The acute phase begins within the first 15 min of exposure to hypercapnia. In dogs, the expected metabolic compensation for acute respiratory acidosis is an increase of 1.5 mEq/L for each 10 mm Hg increase in P_{CO_2} (de Morais and DiBartola 1991). A compensatory increase of 0.7 mEq/L in HCO_3^- for each 10 mm Hg increase in P_{CO_2} was found in anesthetized cats (Hampson et al. 1987). These cats, however, were exposed to different levels of CO_2 for only 15 min at each level, and this may account to some extent for the minimal compensation observed. The chronic compensation reflects renal adaptation and consists of increased net acid excretion and increased HCO_3^- reabsorption. In dogs, metabolic compensation for chronic respiratory acidosis results in an increase in HCO_3^- of 3.5 mEq/L for each 10 mm Hg increase in P_{CO_2} (de Morais and DiBartola 1991). The expected compensation in cats with chronic respiratory acidosis is not known.

Clinical Features of Respiratory Acidosis

Clinical signs in animals with respiratory acidosis reflect the underlying disease process responsible for hypercapnia rather than hypercapnia itself. Specific clinical signs have not been recognized and reported in dogs and cats, but chronic experimentally induced hypercapnia has been shown to increase ventilation markedly in dogs (Jennings and Davidson 1984). The clinician should have a high

TABLE 11-2. Causes of Respiratory Acidosis

Airway obstruction
    Aspiration (e.g., foreign body, vomitus)
Respiratory center depression
    Neurologic disease (e.g., brain stem, high cervical spinal cord lesion)
    Drugs (e.g., narcotics, sedatives, barbiturates, inhalation anesthetics)
Cardiopulmonary arrest
Neuromuscular defects
    Myasthenia gravis
    Tetanus
    Botulism
    Polyradiculoneuritis
    Polymyositis
    Tick paralysis
    Hypokalemic periodic paralysis in Burmese cats
    Hypokalemic myopathy in cats
    Drug-induced (succinylcholine, pancuronium, aminoglycosides with anesthetics, organophosphates)
Restrictive defects
    Diaphragmatic hernia
    Pneumothorax
    Pleural effusion
    Hemothorax
    Chest wall trauma
    Pulmonary fibrosis
    Pyothorax
Pulmonary disease
    Respiratory distress syndrome
    Pneumonia
    Severe pulmonary edema
    Diffuse metastatic disease
    Smoke inhalation
    Pulmonary thromboembolism
    Chronic obstructive pulmonary disease
    Pulmonary fibrosis
Inadequate mechanical ventilation

---

index of suspicion when presented with an animal suffering from a disorder likely to be associated with respiratory acidosis (Table 11–2). Factors likely to influence the clinical signs include the magnitude and rapidity of onset of hypercapnia, severity of acidemia, and extent of hypoxemia.

In acute hypoventilation, hypoxemia is the immediate threat to life, and a laboratory diagnosis of acute hypercapnia is often not made in small animal practice. Causes of acute hypercapnia include cardiopulmonary arrest, acute airway obstruction, and anesthesia with inadequate ventilation (see Table 11–2). An acutely compromised patient dies of hypoxemia before hypercapnia can become severe. Abrupt cessation of ventilation is fatal within 4 min, whereas severe hypercapnia would not develop for 10 to 15 min in such a setting (Madias and Cohen 1982b). Many dogs and cats presented to veterinarians for evaluation have been ill long enough to develop a chronic steady state (i.e., 2–5 days) and their blood gas values reflect adaptation to chronic hypercapnia as described earlier.

Diagnosis of Respiratory Acidosis

Clinical evaluation of the patient is not reliable in making a diagnosis of respiratory acidosis. The clinician must have a high index of suspicion based on the patient's underlying disease process and must establish the diagnosis by arterial blood gas evaluation. Hypercapnia with acidemia is diagnostic of respiratory acidosis, whereas hypercapnia with a normal pH or alkalemia suggests a mixed acid-base disorder (see Chapter 12). Knowledge of the normal ventilatory response to metabolic alkalosis in dogs aids the clinician in ruling out a simple acid-base disorder with normal respiratory compensation. The normal compensation for respiratory acidosis does not return extracellular pH to normal and a pH value less than 7.35 would be expected in primary respiratory acidosis.

Causes of Respiratory Acidosis

Respiratory acidosis can result from any disease process that interferes with neurologic control of ventilation, the mechanics of ventilation, or alveolar gas exchange. The causes of respiratory acidosis are listed in Table 11–2.

Treatment of Respiratory Acidosis

The most effective treatment for respiratory acidosis consists of rapid diagnosis and elimination of the underlying cause of alveolar hypoventilation. Airway obstruction should be identified promptly and relieved. Medications that depress ventilation should be discontinued, if possible. Pleurocentesis should be performed to remove fluid or air when pleural effusion or pneumothorax is present. Often, it is not possible to remove the underlying cause of hypercapnia in patients with chronic pulmonary disease, but appropriate treatment of the underlying disease should be carried out. If necessary, ventilatory assistance must be provided. Arterial blood gases must be monitored frequently to verify that the mechanical ventilator is adjusted properly so as to prevent either inadequate or excessive alveolar ventilation.

Oxygen therapy may be lifesaving in patients with acute hypercapnia. In patients with chronic hypercapnia, however, the central chemoreceptors become progressively insensitive to the effects of retained CO_2 and hypoxemia becomes the main drive for ventilation. Increasing the concentration of inspired O_2 by O_2 therapy can decrease ventilation in this setting and aggravate hypercapnia. If oxygen is administered, Po_2 should not be increased above 60 mm Hg because the hypoxic drive for ventilation remains adequate up to this level. On the other hand, small increments of Po_2 can be helpful because the slope of the sigmoidal oxygen-hemoglobin dissociation curve is steep in the region of Po_2 between 20 and 60 mm Hg (Fig. 11–6). Blood Pco_2 must be decreased slowly in patients with chronic hypercapnia. In human patients, rapid decreases in Pco_2 can result in cardiac arrhythmias, decreased cardiac output, and reduced cerebral blood flow (Madias and Cohen 1982a). Also, a sudden decrease in blood Pco_2 may result in rapid diffusion of CO_2 from cerebrospinal fluid into blood, thus quickly increasing the cerebrospinal fluid pH.

Therapy with $NaHCO_3$ is usually not indicated in respiratory acidosis. Administration of $NaHCO_3$ decreases $[H^+]$ and ventilatory drive, thus worsening hypoxemia. For this reason, $NaHCO_3$ administration should be

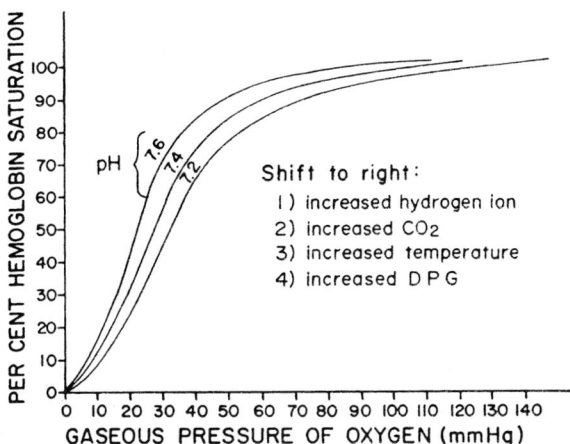

FIGURE 11-6. Shift of the oxygen-hemoglobin dissociation curve to the right by increases in (1) hydrogen ions, (2) CO_2, (3) temperature, or (4) 2,3-diphosphoglycerate. (From Guyton AC: *Textbook of Medical Physiology*, 7th ed. Philadelphia, WB Saunders Co., p. 498, 1986.)

avoided. Administration of a parenteral solution with adequate amounts of chloride facilitates recovery from chronic hypercapnia and prevents the development of metabolic alkalosis after P_{CO_2} has returned to normal. Dogs recovering from chronic hypercapnia and receiving a low-salt diet had persistently increased plasma HCO_3^- concentrations (Schwartz et al. 1961). Addition of sodium chloride or potassium chloride to the diet allowed full correction of the acid-base disturbance. Provision of sufficient chloride allows the kidney to reabsorb sodium in conjunction with chloride and excrete the HCO_3^- retained during compensation for chronic hypercapnia.

▶ Respiratory Alkalosis

Respiratory alkalosis results from a primary decrease in P_{CO_2} in the blood. It is synonymous with the term primary hypocapnia and is characterized by decreased P_{CO_2}, decreased $[H^+]$, increased pH, and a compensatory decrease in HCO_3^- concentration in blood. It was the least commonly encountered of the four primary acid-base disturbances in one report (Cornelius and Rawlings 1981). In this study, however, 24 mm Hg was considered the lower limit of normal for P_{CO_2}, and this may have caused some dogs with respiratory alkalosis to be considered normal. In the authors' experience, respiratory alkalosis is a relatively common acid-base disorder, occurring more often than metabolic alkalosis and respiratory acidosis.

Overview of Respiratory Alkalosis

Primary hypocapnia occurs whenever the magnitude of alveolar ventilation exceeds that required to eliminate the CO_2 produced by metabolic processes in the tissues. Primary hyperventilation can result from hypoxemia (stimulation of peripheral chemoreceptors), pulmonary disease without hypoxemia (stimulation of pulmonary nociceptive receptors), or direct stimulation of the central medullary respiratory center (Table 11-3). Overzealous mechanical ventilation can also produce primary hypocapnia. A compensatory decrease in the HCO_3^- concentration of body fluids follows and minimizes the decrease in $[H^+]$. This compensatory response occurs in two phases. A compensatory decrease of 2.5 mEq/L in HCO_3^- concentration for each 10 mm Hg decrease in P_{CO_2} is expected in dogs with acute respiratory alkalosis (de Morais and DiBartola 1991). Similar results were obtained with anesthetized cats (Hampson et al. 1987). No data are available on compensation in cats with chronic respiratory alkalosis. During chronic respiratory alkalosis in dogs, a 5.5 mEq/L decrease in HCO_3^- is expected for each 10 mm Hg decrease in P_{CO_2} (de Morais and DiBartola 1991). This represents effective compensation and the pH is usually normal or near normal in dogs with chronic respiratory alkalosis. In this setting, abnormal P_{CO_2} and HCO_3^- with normal pH may not be the result of a mixed acid-base disorder.

Clinical Features of Respiratory Alkalosis

Clinical signs directly attributable to hypocapnia have not been recognized and reported in dogs and cats. In humans, clinical signs such as light-headedness, confusion, paresthesias of the extremities, tightness of the chest,

TABLE 11-3. Causes of Respiratory Alkalosis

Hypoxemia (stimulation of peripheral chemoreceptors by decreased oxygen delivery)
  Right-to-left shunting
  Decreased P_{IO_2} (e.g., residence at high altitude)
  Congestive heart failure
  Severe anemia
  Hypotension
  Pulmonary diseases causing ventilation-perfusion inequality
    Pneumonia
    Pulmonary embolism
    Pulmonary fibrosis
    Pulmonary edema
    Acute pulmonary distress syndrome
Pulmonary disease (stimulation of nociceptive receptors independent of hypoxemia)
  Pneumonia
  Pulmonary embolism
  Interstitial lung disease
  Pulmonary edema
  Acute respiratory distress syndrome
Central nervous system–mediated hypocapnia (direct stimulation of medullary respiratory center)
  Liver disease
  Gram-negative sepsis
  Drugs
    Salicylate intoxication
    Progesterone
    Xanthines (e.g., aminophylline)
  Recovery from metabolic acidosis
  Central neurologic disease
    Trauma
    Tumor
    Infection
    Inflammation (e.g., granulomatous meningoencephalitis)
    Cerebrovascular accident
  Exercise
  Heatstroke
Mechanical ventilation

and circumoral numbness have been reported in acute respiratory alkalosis (Gennari and Kassirer 1982a). Clinical signs are much less likely to occur in chronic than in acute respiratory alkalosis because extracellular pH deviates much less from normal in chronic hypocapnia. Many dogs with chronic respiratory alkalosis have tachypnea as the only clinical abnormality. Central neurologic signs in acute hypocapnia may result from reduced cerebral blood flow caused by the increased cerebral vascular resistance that occurs in acute hypocapnia.

The effects of acute hypocapnia on blood pressure and cardiac output are markedly different in awake and anesthetized subjects. Cardiac output and blood pressure decrease in anesthetized but not in awake subjects. The observed difference may be related in part to the fact that anesthetized subjects may not develop an adequate reflex tachycardia. In anesthetized dogs subjected to acute hypocapnia, blood pressure decreased because of a decrease in cardiac output with a less than normal compensatory increase in total peripheral resistance and heart rate remained unchanged (Little and Smith 1964; Muir et al. 1990). Chronic hypocapnia is associated with a predictable progression of cardiovascular effects, but these effects typically have been studied in subjects who were also hypoxemic (e.g., studies of residence at high altitudes) and many of the observed effects may have been a consequence of hypoxemia (Gennari and Kassirer 1982b). The clinical signs observed in dogs and cats with respiratory alkalosis are usually due to the underlying disease process and not to the respiratory alkalosis itself.

Diagnosis of Respiratory Alkalosis

Although tachypnea may be observed, clinical signs are inadequate to make a diagnosis of respiratory alkalosis. The clinician should have a high index of suspicion when presented with an animal suffering from a disease process likely to be associated with respiratory alkalosis (see Table 11–3). The historical and physical findings must be correlated with arterial blood gas analysis to make the diagnosis. Blood pH is often high in acute respiratory alkalosis because plasma HCO_3^- concentration falls only slightly in acute hypocapnia. In dogs with chronic hypocapnia, pH increases only slightly because of the compensatory decrease in plasma HCO_3^- concentration resulting from renal adaptation. Thus, severe alkalemia occurs only in acute hypocapnia.

Causes of Respiratory Alkalosis

Causes of respiratory alkalosis include hypoxemia, pulmonary disease with or without hypoxemia, direct stimulation of the medullary respiratory center, and overzealous mechanical ventilation. The specific causes of respiratory alkalosis are listed in Table 11–3. Unexplained respiratory alkalosis in human patients may be a useful clue to the presence of gram-negative sepsis (Simmons et al. 1960; Blair 1971; Mazzara et al. 1974). Pulmonary edema can also cause respiratory alkalosis by decreasing compliance and stimulating ventilation, but metabolic acidosis and respiratory acidosis are more commonly observed in human patients. Dogs have good collateral ventilation, however, and hypercapnia occurs only in fulminant pulmonary edema (Ware and Bonagura 1988). Acute respiratory distress syndrome can be associated with respiratory alkalosis in dogs (Parent et al. 1996). Respiratory alkalosis can occur during recovery from metabolic acidosis because hyperventilation persists for 24 to 48 h after correction of metabolic acidosis.

When PO_2 decreases below 60 mm Hg, the peripheral chemoreceptors mediate an increase in the rate and depth of breathing. The effect of the resulting hypocapnia and decreased $[H^+]$ on the central chemoreceptors is to damp this initial hyperventilation. As renal compensation occurs, plasma HCO_3^- concentration decreases and $[H^+]$ increases, thus removing the central inhibition of further hyperventilation. A steady state emerges when the peripherally mediated hypoxemic drive to ventilation is balanced by the central effect of the alkalemia resulting from renal adaptation to hypocapnia. If PCO_2 is held constant in the presence of hypoxemia (as may occur in patients with pulmonary disease), the damping effect of hypocapnia does not occur and a lesser degree of hypoxemia may stimulate ventilation.

Some pulmonary diseases can cause hypocapnia independent of hypoxemia. This effect results from afferent vagal signals that stimulate ventilation. The receptors involved are stretch receptors and two distinct types of nociceptive receptors (Gennari and Kassirer 1982c; Rose 1989). The stretch receptors are located in the smooth muscle of the tracheobronchial tree. The two nociceptive receptors are irritant receptors in the epithelial lining of small airways and juxtacapillary receptors (so-called J receptors) lining capillaries in the pulmonary interstitium. The irritant receptors respond to irritant substances and local inflammation in small airways and the juxtacapillary receptors respond to interstitial edema, fibrosis, or pulmonary capillary congestion. The nociceptive receptors are probably responsible for the hyperventilation in pulmonary disease that occurs independent of hypoxemia.

Treatment of Respiratory Alkalosis

Treatment must be aimed at removal of the underlying disorder responsible for the hypocapnia. No other therapy is likely to be effective. Hypocapnia itself is not a major threat to the well-being of the patient and the underlying disease responsible for hypocapnia should receive primary therapeutic attention.

REFERENCES

Arieff AI and Graf H: Pathophysiology of type A hypoxic lactic acidosis in dogs. *Am J Physiol* 253:E271–E276, 1987.

Blair E: Acid-base balance in bacteremic shock. *Arch Intern Med* 127:731–739, 1971.

Cornelius LM and Rawlings CA: Arterial blood gas and acid base values in dogs with various diseases and signs of disease. *J Am Vet Med Assoc* 178:992–995, 1981.

de Morais HSA and DiBartola SP: Ventilatory and metabolic compensation in dogs with acid-base disturbances. *J Vet Emerg Crit Care* 1(2):39–49, 1991.

DiBartola SP and de Morais HAS: Respiratory acid-base disorders. In DiBartola SP: *Fluid Therapy in Small Animal Practice*. Philadelphia, WB Saunders Co., pp. 258–275, 1992.

Galla JH and Luke RG: Chloride transport and disorders of acid-base balance. *Annu Rev Physiol* 50:141–158, 1988.

Gennari FJ and Kassirer JP: Respiratory alkalosis. In Cohen JJ and Kassirer JP: *Acid-Base*. Boston, Little, Brown & Co., pp. 357–361, 1982a.

Gennari FJ and Kassirer JP: Respiratory alkalosis. In Cohen JJ and Kassirer JP: *Acid-Base*. Boston, Little, Brown & Co., p. 359, 1982b.

Gennari FJ and Kassirer JP: Respiratory alkalosis. In Cohen JJ and Kassirer JP: *Acid-Base*. Boston, Little, Brown & Co., pp. 367–368, 1982c.

Gennari FJ, Goldstein MB, and Schwartz WB: The nature of the renal adaptation to chronic hypocapnia. *J Clin Invest* 51:1722–1730, 1972.

Giebisch G, Berger L, and Pitts RF: The extrarenal response to acute acid-base disturbances of respiratory origin. *J Clin Invest* 34:231–245, 1955.

Hampson NB, Jöbsis-Vandler Vliet FF and Piantadosi CA: Skeletal muscle oxygen availability during respiratory acid-base disturbances in cats. *Respir Physiol* 70:143–158, 1987.

Jennings DB and Davidson JSD: Acid-base and ventilatory adaptations in conscious dogs during chronic hypercapnia. *Respir Physiol* 58:377–393, 1984.

Jones NL: *Blood Gases and Acid-Base Physiology*. New York, Thieme Medical Publishers, pp. 23–24, 1987.

Little RC and Smith SW: Cardiovascular response to acute hypocapnia due to overbreathing. *Am J Physiol* 206:1025–1030, 1964.

Madias NE and Cohen JJ: Respiratory acidosis. In Cohen JJ and Kassirer JP: *Acid-Base*. Boston, Little, Brown & Co., p. 332, 1982a.

Madias NE and Cohen JJ: Respiratory acidosis. In Cohen JJ and Kassirer JP: *Acid-Base*. Boston, Little, Brown & Co., p. 324, 1982b.

Madias NE, Wolf CJ, and Cohen JJ: Regulation of acid-base equilibrium in chronic hypercapnia. *Kidney Int* 27:538–543, 1985.

Mazzara JT, Ayres SM, and Grace WJ: Extreme hypocapnia in the critically ill patient. *Am J Med* 56:450–456, 1974.

Muir WW, Wagner AE, and Buchanan C: Effects of acute hyperventilation on serum potassium in the dog. *Vet Surg* 19:83–87, 1990.

Murray JF: Gas exchange and oxygen transport. In Murray JF: *The Normal Lung*. Philadelphia, WB Saunders Co., p. 194, 1986.

Parent C, King LG, Van Winkle TJ, and Walker LM: Respiratory function and treatment in dogs with acute respiratory distress syndrome: 19 cases (1985–1993). *J Am Vet Med Assoc* 208:1428–1433, 1996.

Polak A, Haynie GD, Hays RM, et al.: Effects of chronic hypercapnia on electrolyte and acid-base equilibrium. I. Adaptation. *J Clin Invest* 40:1223–1237, 1961.

Rose BD: *Clinical Physiology of Acid-Base and Electrolyte Disorders*, 3rd ed. New York, McGraw-Hill, p. 584, 1989.

Schwartz WB, Hays RM, Polak A, et al.: Effects of chronic hypercapnia on electrolyte and acid-base equilibrium. II. Recovery, with special reference to the influence of chloride intake. *J Clin Invest* 40:1238–1249, 1961.

Schwartz WB, Brackett NC, and Cohen JJ: The response of extracellular hydrogen ion concentration to graded degrees of chronic hypercapnia: The physiologic limits of the defense of pH. *J Clin Invest* 44:291–301, 1965.

Simmons DH, Nicoloff J, and Guze LB: Hyperventilation and respiratory alkalosis as signs of gram-negative septicemia. *J Am Med Assoc* 174:2196–2199, 1960.

Valtin H and Gennari FJ: *Acid Base Disorders: Basic Concepts and Clinical Management*. Boston, Little, Brown & Co., pp. 7–10, 1987.

van Ypersele de Strihou C, Gulyassy PF, and Schwartz WB: Effects of chronic hypercapnia on electrolyte and acid-base equilibrium. III. Characteristics of the adaptive and recovery process as evaluated by provision of alkali. *J Clin Invest* 41:2246–2253, 1962.

Ware WA and Bonagura JD: Pulmonary edema. In Fox PR (ed): *Canine and Feline Cardiology*. New York, Churchill Livingstone, pp. 205–217, 1988.

APPENDIX TO CHAPTER 11
Alveolar-Arterial Oxygen Difference Equation

The (A−a) O_2 gradient represents the difference (in mm Hg) between alveolar PO_2 (PAO_2) and arterial PO_2 (PaO_2),

$$(A-a)\ O_2\ \text{gradient} = PAO_2 - PaO_2$$

PAO_2 cannot be measured clinically, and it is considered to be equal to the difference between the inspired PO_2 (PIO_2) and the alveolar PCO_2 (i.e., $PAO_2 = PIO_2 - PaCO_2$). Carbon dioxide is readily diffusible and $PACO_2$ is, therefore, equal to $PaCO_2$. With a respiratory quotient (R) of 0.8, 125 molecules of O_2 are utilized for each 100 molecules of CO_2 produced. The respiratory quotient is a function of cellular metabolism. It is approximately 1.0 when carbohydrate is the sole energy source and 0.7 when fat is the sole energy source. In fasting patients, the respiratory quotient is approximately 0.8 (Jones 1987). The simplified alveolar-air equation can, therefore, be rewritten as ($PAO_2 = PIO_2 - 1.25\ PaCO_2$), where the factor 1.25 (the reciprocal of 0.8) is the respiratory quotient and adjusts the equation to reflect the differences in production of CO_2 and O_2.

The PIO_2 in a patient breathing room air (fraction of inspired O_2 or $FIO_2 = 21\%$) at sea level (barometric pressure or $PB = 760$ mm Hg) and with normal body temperature (pulmonary water pressure or $PH_2O = 47$ mm Hg) equals approximately 150 mm Hg. In this setting, the alveolar-air equation can be written as

$$PAO_2 = 150 - 1.25 PaCO_2$$

To obtain the alveolar-arterial oxygen gradient, measured PaO_2 is subtracted from estimated PAO_2:

$$(A-a)\ O_2\ \text{gradient} = (150 - 1.25 PaCO_2) - PaO_2$$

CHAPTER 12

Mixed Acid-Base Disorders

HELIO AUTRAN DE MORAIS

A patient will have as many diseases as he/she pleases.
Anonymous

A *mixed* acid-base disturbance is characterized by the presence of two or more separate primary acid-base abnormalities occurring in the same patient. An acid-base disturbance is said to be *simple* if it is limited to the primary disturbance and the expected compensatory response. Table 12–1 shows a classification of mixed acid-base disorders.

Recognition of a mixed acid-base disorder is important from a diagnostic and a therapeutic point of view. It permits early detection of complications (e.g., the presence of metabolic acidosis and respiratory alkalosis in a dog with parvovirus gastroenteritis may indicate sepsis), provides orientation for treatment (e.g., $NaHCO_3$ is contraindicated in the majority of patients with metabolic acidosis and respiratory acidosis), and allows detection of complications associated with therapy (e.g., a patient with chronic respiratory acidosis that develops metabolic alkalosis after treatment with diuretics experiences further compromise of ventilation by the metabolic process).

TABLE 12–1. Classification of Mixed Acid-Base Disorders

A. Disorders with neutralizing effects on pH
  1. Mixed respiratory-metabolic disorders
     a. Respiratory acidosis and metabolic alkalosis
     b. Respiratory alkalosis and metabolic acidosis
  2. Mixed metabolic disorders
     a. Metabolic acidosis and metabolic alkalosis
B. Disorders with additive effects on pH
  1. Mixed respiratory-metabolic disorders
     a. Respiratory acidosis and metabolic acidosis
     b. Respiratory alkalosis and metabolic alkalosis
  2. Mixed metabolic disorders
     a. Normal plus high-anion-gap metabolic acidosis
     b. Mixed high-anion-gap metabolic acidosis
     c. Mixed normal-anion-gap metabolic acidosis
C. Triple disorders
  a. Metabolic acidosis, metabolic alkalosis, and respiratory acidosis
  b. Metabolic acidosis, metabolic alkalosis, and respiratory alkalosis

In approaching mixed acid-base disturbances, a proper understanding of the terms acidosis, alkalosis, acidemia, and alkalemia is crucial. *Acidosis* and *alkalosis* refer to the pathophysiologic processes that cause net accumulation of acid or alkali in the body, whereas *acidemia* and *alkalemia* refer specifically to the pH of extracellular fluid. In acidemia, the extracellular fluid pH is less than normal and the [H^+] higher than normal. In alkalemia, the extracellular fluid pH is higher than normal and the [H^+] lower than normal. For example, a patient with chronic respiratory alkalosis may have a blood pH value that is within the normal range. Such a patient has alkalosis but does not have alkalemia.

▶ Compensation

The definition of a simple acid-base disturbance includes both the primary process causing changes in carbon dioxide tension (P_{CO_2}) or [HCO_3^-] and the compensatory mechanisms affecting these measurements. Consequently, lack of appropriate compensation is evidence of a mixed acid-base disorder. Unfortunately, the magnitude of expected compensation in a given clinical situation is not known with certainty, and data for dogs have been derived mainly from experiments using normal dogs (de Morais and DiBartola 1991). Little is known about the expected compensation in cats with simple acid-base disturbances. The reader is referred to Chapters 9, 10, and 11 for further discussion of compensation.

Respiratory Compensation in Metabolic Processes

Metabolic acidosis is characterized by an increase in [H^+], a decrease in serum [HCO_3^-] and blood pH, and a decrease in P_{CO_2} related to secondary hyperventilation. The expected decrease in P_{CO_2} in dogs with metabolic acidosis may be estimated as 0.7 mm Hg for each 1 mEq/L decrease in [HCO_3^-] (de Morais and DiBartola, 1991).

Metabolic alkalosis is characterized by a decrease in [H^+], an increase in serum [HCO_3^-] and blood pH, and an increase in P_{CO_2} related to compensatory hypoventilation. As a rule, a 1.0 mEq/L increase in plasma [HCO_3^-] is expected to be associated with an adaptive 0.7 mm Hg increase in P_{CO_2} in dogs with metabolic alkalosis (de Morais and DiBartola 1991).

Time is an important consideration when assessing compensation. Even in the experimental setting where sudden changes in [HCO_3^-] can be achieved, the respiratory response to acute metabolic acidosis in human beings occurs more slowly, and it often takes 12 to 24 h for the maximal respiratory compensation to develop (Pierce et al. 1970). Thus, using the formulas within the first 24 h of onset of metabolic acidosis may lead to underestimation of the ventilatory response and the erroneous assumption that a mixed metabolic and respiratory acidosis is present.

Little is known about ventilatory compensation in cats with metabolic acidosis or alkalosis. In one study in which cats were chronically fed a diet containing NH_4Cl, significant decreases in pH and [HCO_3^-] were observed, but there was no change in P_{CO_2} (Ching et al. 1989). Similar results were obtained in another study in which cats were also made acidotic with NH_4Cl (Lemieux et al. 1990). The latter study also showed that, contrary to what happens in dogs and human beings, the feline kidney is apparently unable to adapt to metabolic acidosis and does not increase production of ammonia or glucose from glutamine during acidosis. On the basis of these studies, cats may not compensate for metabolic acidosis to the same extent as dogs and human beings, if they compensate at all. Thus, formulas for dogs or human beings should not be extrapolated for use in cats. The clinical finding of metabolic acidosis and normal P_{CO_2} in a cat should not be interpreted as evidence of a mixed process until more data are available about respiratory compensation in cats.

Metabolic Compensation in Respiratory Processes

Respiratory acidosis is the acid-base disorder resulting from a primary increase in P_{CO_2} in the blood. It is synonymous with *primary hypercapnia* and is characterized by increased P_{CO_2}, increased [H^+], decreased pH, and a compensatory increase in [HCO_3^-] in blood. *Respiratory alkalosis* is the acid-base disorder resulting from a primary decrease in P_{CO_2} in the blood. It is synonymous with the term *primary hypocapnia* and is characterized by decreased P_{CO_2}, decreased [H^+], increased pH, and a compensatory decrease in [HCO_3^-] in blood.

Adaptive changes in plasma [HCO_3^-] occur in two phases. In respiratory acidosis the first phase represents titration of nonbicarbonate buffers, whereas in respiratory alkalosis the first phase represents release of H^+ from nonbicarbonate buffers within cells. This response is completed within 15 min.

The second phase reflects renal adaptation and consists of increased net acid excretion and increased HCO_3^- reabsorption (decreased Cl^- reabsorption) in respiratory acidosis and a decrease in net acid excretion in respiratory alkalosis. Renal adaptation requires 2 to 5 days for a chronic steady state to be established (Polak et al. 1961; Schwartz et al. 1965; Gennari et al. 1972).

A compensatory increase of 0.15 mEq/L in [HCO_3^-] for each 1 mm Hg increase in P_{CO_2} should be expected in dogs with acute respiratory acidosis, whereas a 0.25 mEq/L decrease in [HCO_3^-] for each 1 mm Hg decrease in P_{CO_2} should be expected in dogs with acute respiratory alkalosis (de Morais and DiBartola 1991). The compensation during acute respiratory acidosis is approximately 60% of the response in acute respiratory alkalosis.

In anesthetized, artificially ventilated cats made hypercapnic by exposure to increasing CO_2 levels, the average compensatory increase in [HCO_3^-] was 0.07 mEq/L for each 1 mm Hg increase in P_{CO_2} (Hampson et al. 1987). These cats, however, were exposed to different levels of CO_2 for only 15 min at each level, and this may be responsible to some extent for the minimal compensation observed. In the same study, hyperventilation was induced and maintained for 30 min at each level. The [HCO_3^-] decreased an average 0.26 mEq/L for each 1 mm Hg decrease in P_{CO_2}, a value similar to that obtained for dogs.

In dogs with chronic respiratory acidosis, serum [HCO_3^-] increases 0.35 mEq/L for each 1 mm Hg increase in P_{CO_2} (de Morais and DiBartola 1991). In dogs with chronic respiratory alkalosis a decrease of 0.55 mEq/L in [HCO_3^-] is expected for each 1 mm Hg decrease in P_{CO_2} (Adams and Polzin 1989; de Morais and DiBartola 1991). It is interesting to note that even in severe chronic respiratory alkalosis, the pH is usually normal. The normalization of pH in a clinical setting may, however, take longer than 5 to 7 days. In human beings with sustained respiratory alkalosis, the pH may not return to normal for 2 weeks or more (Narins and Emmett 1980).

When analyzing secondary changes in a given disturbance, it is important to remember that (1) with the exception of chronic respiratory alkalosis, compensation does not return the pH to normal; (2) overcompensation does not occur; and (3) sufficient time must elapse for compensation to reach a steady state, at which time the formulas in Table 12–2 can be used. Respiratory compensation is similar in metabolic acidosis and alkalosis, but the metabolic compensation in respiratory acidosis is only 60% of that achieved in respiratory alkalosis.

TABLE 12–2. **Compensatory Response in Simple Acid-Base Disturbances in Dogs**

Disturbance	Clinical Guide for Compensation	
Metabolic acidosis	Each 1 mEq/L ↓ HCO_3^-	P_{CO_2} ↓ by 0.7 mm Hg
Metabolic alkalosis	Each 1 mEq/L ↑ HCO_3^-	P_{CO_2} ↑ by 0.7 mm Hg
Respiratory acidosis		
Acute	Each 1 mm Hg ↑ P_{CO_2}	HCO_3^- ↑ by 0.15 mEq/L
Chronic	Each 1 mm Hg ↑ P_{CO_2}	HCO_3^- ↑ by 0.35 mEq/L
Respiratory alkalosis		
Acute	Each 1 mm Hg ↓ P_{CO_2}	HCO_3^- ↓ by 0.25 mEq/L
Chronic	Each 1 mm Hg ↓ P_{CO_2}	HCO_3^- ↓ by 0.55 mEq/L

From de Morais HSA and DiBartola SP: Ventilatory and metabolic compensation in dogs with acid-base disturbances. *J Vet Emerg Crit Care* 1:39–49, 1991.

▶ Clinical Approach

The first step is a careful history to search for clues that may lead the clinician to suspect the presence of acid-base disorders, followed by a complete physical examination. Urinalysis, routine serum chemistries, and electrolyte concentrations are useful, but confirmation of a mixed acid-base disorder requires blood gas analysis.

Using blood gas analysis, a mixed acid-base disorder should be suspected when inappropriate compensation for the primary disorder is demonstrated. If the patient's P_{CO_2} in a metabolic process or $[HCO_3^-]$ in a respiratory process differs from the calculated compensation by more than 2 mm Hg or 2 mEq/L, the compensation is not appropriate (Adams and Polzin 1989; de Morais and DiBartola 1991). However, a more conservative approach (using ±3 instead of ±2) may be advisable for patients with primary metabolic acidosis because experimentally there is a wide range of change in P_{CO_2} (0.5–1.1 mm Hg) for each 1 mEq/L decrease in $[HCO_3^-]$ (de Morais and DiBartola 1991). The expected compensation can be estimated using the formulas presented in Table 12–2.

An example illustrates how these formulas can be utilized. Consider a dog that presents with diarrhea and hypoadrenocorticism-like syndrome (HLS) (DiBartola et al. 1985) that has the following arterial blood gas values: pH = 7.38, $[HCO_3^-]$ = 15 mEq/L, and P_{CO_2} = 26 mm Hg. Assuming P_{CO_2} = 36 mm Hg and $[HCO_3^-]$ = 21 mEq/L as average normal values, the expected compensation can be estimated:

$$P_{CO_2\ expected} = 36 + [(15 - 21) \times 0.7] \pm 3 = 31.8 \pm 3$$

Thus, this patient has a P_{CO_2} that is lower than expected, indicating the presence of respiratory alkalosis in addition to metabolic acidosis.

Some useful guidelines for detecting a mixed process when first looking at the blood gas results are the following (Bia and Thier 1981):

1. The presence of a normal pH (with abnormal P_{CO_2} and/or $[HCO_3^-]$) usually implies a mixed process (with the exception of chronic respiratory alkalosis).
2. A pH change in a direction opposite to that predicted for the known primary disorder requires the diagnosis of a mixed disturbance.
3. P_{CO_2} and $[HCO_3^-]$ changing in opposite directions implies a mixed disorder.
4. Values in the expected compensatory range do not prove that there is only one disturbance but only provide support for this possibility, if consistent with the remaining clinical data.

To avoid overdiagnosing mixed disturbances, the clinician should ask two questions when considering a patient with inappropriate compensation: (1) Has there been enough time for the compensatory changes to reach a steady state? If not, the diagnosis of a mixed disturbance should not be made until the necessary time has elapsed. (2) Were there any technical problems in the collection, handling, or analysis of the blood sample that may have been responsible for the results? Table 12–3 lists some potential problems that may lead to the misdiagnosis of mixed acid-base disorders.

TABLE 12–3. Potential Problems That May Lead to Misdiagnosing Mixed Acid-Base Disorders

Use of venous blood
    Local metabolism may affect P_{CO_2}
    Normal values for compensation were established using arterial blood
Too much heparin (>10% of total volume)
    Decreases $[HCO_3^-]$ and P_{CO_2}
Storage of sample for more than 20 min
    Increases P_{CO_2} and decreases pH
Errors in calculation of $[HCO_3^-]$

The *anion gap* (AG) is a helpful tool in the differentiation between hyperchloremic and high-AG metabolic acidoses. Chemically, there is no AG because the electroneutrality law must be maintained. The AG is actually the difference between the unmeasured anions (UA^-) and unmeasured cations (UC^+)—see below. Following the electroneutrality law, we obtain

$$([Na^+] + [K^+] + [UC^+]) - ([Cl^-] + [HCO_3^-] + [UA^-])$$

or

$$\begin{aligned} AG &= ([Na^+] + [K^+]) - ([Cl^-] + [HCO_3^-]) \\ &= ([UA^-] - [UC^+]) \end{aligned}$$

Thus, every time there is a decrease in HCO_3^-, either Cl^- or UA^- must increase to maintain electroneutrality. In metabolic acidosis, every time HCO_3^- is replaced by Cl^-, the difference ($[UA^-] - [UC^+]$) and consequently the AG remain the same (hyperchloremic, or normal AG, acidosis). When HCO_3^- is replaced by UA^-, the difference ($[UA^-] - [UC^+]$) and the AG increase while $[Cl^-]$ remains the same (normochloremic, or high-AG, acidosis).

Except for some relatively uncommon circumstances, an increase in the AG implies accumulation of organic acids in the body (Narins and Emmett 1980). Although a decrease in the AG also may occur, disorders characterized by a decrease in the AG are rare (Gabow 1985). Hypoalbuminemia is probably the most important cause of a decrease in the AG, and each decrease of 1 g/dL in albumin concentration has been associated with a decrease of 3 mEq/L in the AG (McAuliffe et al. 1986).

Plasma $[Cl^-]$ and $[HCO_3^-]$ have a tendency to change in opposite directions in metabolic alkalosis and hyperchloremic acidosis, whereas sodium concentration tends to remain normal in acid-base disturbances unless the primary disorder also affects sodium concentration. The difference between the sodium and chloride concentrations ($[Na^+] - [Cl^-]$) is useful in the assessment of metabolic disturbances not associated with an increase in UA^-. Normally, $[Na^+] - [Cl^-]$ is approximately 36 mEq/L in dogs and cats. An increase in this value (usually caused by hypochloremia) is an indication of metabolic alkalosis, and a decrease is an indication of hyperchloremic acidosis (Stewart 1981). The $[Na^+] - [Cl^-]$ used in conjunction with the AG is useful in estimating the presence of a mixed metabolic process (Table 12–4).

TABLE 12-4. **Use of the Anion Gap (AG) in Combination with [Na⁺] − [Cl⁻] to Assess Metabolic Disorders***

	Normal AG	High AG
↓ [Na⁺] − [Cl⁻]	Hyperchloremic acidosis	Hyperchloremic acidosis and ↑ unmeasured anion acidosis
Normal [Na⁺] − [Cl⁻]	Normal	↑ Unmeasured anion acidosis
↑ [Na⁺] − [Cl⁻]	Metabolic alkalosis	Metabolic alkalosis and ↑ unmeasured acidosis

*Metabolic compensation in chronic respiratory acid-base disturbances can also change [Na⁺] − [Cl⁻] by changing [Cl⁻] (hypochloremia and increased [Na⁺] − [Cl⁻] in chronic respiratory acidosis and hyperchloremia and decreased [Na⁺] − [Cl⁻] in chronic respiratory alkalosis).

A stepwise approach should be followed for all patients with suspected mixed acid-base disorders (Fig. 12-1):

1. Perform electrolyte and blood gas analysis.
2. Calculate [HCO_3^-] to rule out laboratory error.
3. Determine pH and the nature of the primary disorder.
4. Calculate the AG.
5. Calculate the [Na⁺]−[Cl⁻].
6. Calculate the expected compensation (see Table 12-2).
7. Compare the AG with [Na⁺]−[Cl⁻] (see Table 12-4).
8. Consider other laboratory data (e.g., creatinine, glucose).
9. Correlate clinical and laboratory findings.
10. Plan individualized therapy.

▶ Mixed Acid-Base Disturbances

Disorders with Neutralizing Effects on pH

Patients with mixed disorders composed of primary problems with an offsetting effect on pH may be presented with normal, low, or high pH. When pH is abnormal, however, because of the counterbalancing effect of the second primary disorder, changes tend not to be pronounced. Table 12-5 shows examples of potential causes of counterbalancing mixed acid-base disorders.

RESPIRATORY ACIDOSIS AND METABOLIC ALKALOSIS

This is an uncommon clinical situation and, in human medicine, usually occurs in patients with chronic lung disease who develop vomiting or are treated with diuretics (Bia and Thier 1981). Dogs with gastric dilatation-volvulus (GDV) also can present with metabolic alkalosis caused by loss of gastric acid and respiratory acidosis resulting from diaphragmatic compression caused by the distended stomach (Adams and Polzin 1989). The P_{CO_2} and [HCO_3^-] are high, and pH tends to be normal or only slightly abnormal. Treatment should be directed at correcting the underlying disease process. No treatment

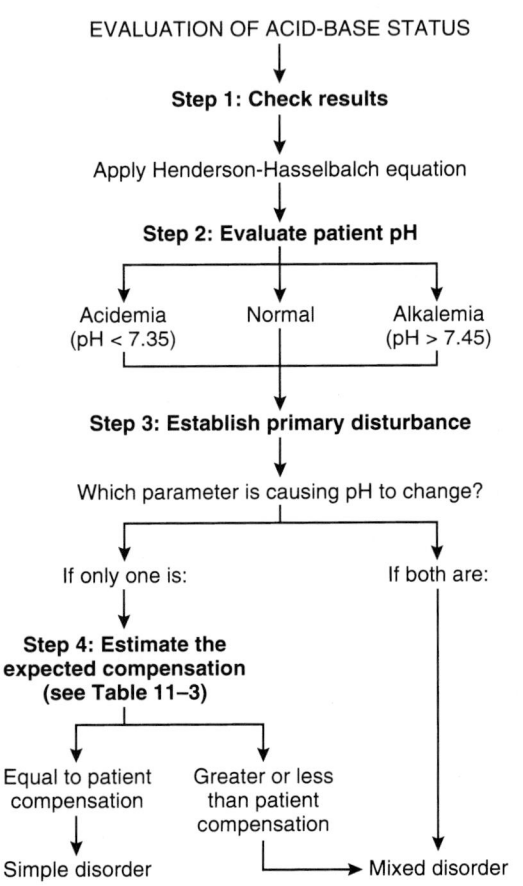

FIGURE 12-1. Algorithm for evaluation of acid-base status in patients with suspected mixed acid-base disorders.

TABLE 12-5. **Examples of Potential Causes of Counterbalancing Mixed Acid-Base Disorders**

A. Respiratory alkalosis and metabolic acidosis
  1. Hypoadrenocorticism-like syndrome in dogs with gastrointestinal disease
  2. Septic shock
  3. Salicylate toxicity
  4. Heat stroke
  5. Gastric dilatation-volvulus
  6. Liver disease (RTA and impaired metabolism of lactate)
  7. Pulmonary edema
  8. Parvovirus gastroenteritis and septicemia
  9. Severe exercise
  10. Acute tumor lysis syndrome
  11. Acute respiratory distress syndrome
  12. Cardiopulmonary resuscitation (only in arterial blood)
B. Respiratory acidosis and metabolic alkalosis
  1. Pulmonary edema and diuretics
  2. Gastric dilatation-volvulus
C. Metabolic acidosis and metabolic alkalosis
  1. Gastric dilatation-volvulus
  2. Renal failure with vomiting
  3. Vomiting and diarrhea
  4. Vomiting and lactic acidosis
  5. Renal failure and diuretics
  6. Diabetic ketoacidosis with vomiting
  7. NaHCO₃ therapy in diabetic ketoacidosis
  8. Liver disease (hypoproteinemia, diuretics, vomiting, RTA, and impaired metabolism of lactate)

is necessary to correct pH (Bia and Thier 1981). Patients with chronic pulmonary disease that have hypoxemia and hypercapnia are at greater risk from metabolic alkalosis than are others because superimposition of metabolic alkalosis can further reduce ventilation and lead to worsening of hypoxemia (Rose 1989). Therefore, metabolic alkalosis should not be overlooked if the patient has a chronic lung disease.

RESPIRATORY ALKALOSIS AND METABOLIC ACIDOSIS

Many clinical situations can lead to this mixed disorder, usually with high-AG metabolic acidosis. These patients have low Pco_2 and low $[HCO_3^-]$, and their pH tends to be nearly normal. It is important to remember that chronic respiratory alkalosis is the only simple acid-base disturbance potentially characterized by a normal pH. Thus, in the presence of a normal pH, low Pco_2, and low $[HCO_3^-]$, the clinician must decide whether the patient has simple respiratory alkalosis or metabolic acidosis associated with respiratory alkalosis. In this situation, the history can provide important clues. The presence of hypoxemia or increased arterial-alveolar oxygen difference suggests that the patient has a chronic respiratory alkalosis. The AG is also helpful in diagnosis because the majority of metabolic acidoses associated with respiratory alkalosis are of the high-AG type.

Dogs with HLS can be presented with metabolic acidosis and respiratory alkalosis, but the reason is not known (DiBartola et al. 1985). Dogs with early septic shock are usually presented with respiratory alkalosis that later in the course of the illness is complicated by lactic acidosis (Hauptman and Tvedten 1986; Goodwin and Schaer 1990). Sepsis complicating any disease known to cause metabolic acidosis can result in development of this mixed disturbance. Exercise can also cause a mixed disorder that begins with respiratory alkalosis. In mild exercise (35% of maximum O_2 consumption), there is a mild respiratory alkalosis (Musch et al. 1986). When dogs are maximally exercised, lactic acidosis is superimposed on the initial respiratory alkalosis (Musch et al. 1986; Ilkiw et al. 1989). Dogs with heatstroke are also presented initially with respiratory alkalosis and later develop mixed respiratory alkalosis and metabolic acidosis (Schall 1980).

Gastric dilatation-volvulus complex has been associated with respiratory alkalosis and metabolic acidosis in dogs (Muir 1982), in which the respiratory alkalosis may be the result of pain (Muir 1982) or septicemia (Adams and Polzin 1989). Patients with liver disease may develop a wide variety of acid-base disturbances. Metabolic acidosis has been associated with liver disease in dogs (Cornelius and Rawlings 1981). Hyperventilation is common and appears to be multifactorial (Center 1989). Human patients with chronic active hepatitis may develop renal tubular acidosis (RTA), and patients with cirrhosis demonstrate enhanced proximal renal tubular sodium reabsorption that may limit distal H^+ secretion (Better et al. 1972) and lead to hyperchloremic acidosis. At the same time, net lactic acid production may be accelerated in some patients with liver disease, because liver disease can diminish liver uptake and metabolism of lactate (Narins and Emmett 1980).

Pulmonary edema may cause respiratory alkalosis by decreasing compliance and stimulating ventilation (Aberman and Fulop 1972). As discussed earlier, lactic acidosis can complicate pulmonary edema, particularly when associated with low-output heart failure. Salicylate toxicity in dogs and cats causes hyperventilation initially, but metabolic acidosis then develops (Oehme 1986). The hyperventilation associated with salicylate toxicity is caused by central stimulation, and only a small portion of the hyperventilation can be attributed to hyperthermia (Silva et al. 1986). In human patients with salicylate intoxication, metabolic acidosis is due to accumulation of organic acids, including lactate and ketoacids (Rose 1989). This may also be true in small animals (Oehme 1986). One dog with acute tumor lysis syndrome was presented with alkalemia, respiratory alkalosis, high AG, and normal $[Na^+] - [Cl^-]$ (Laing and Carter 1988). The $[HCO_3^-]$ was in the range expected for chronic respiratory alkalosis, but the disease was believed to be acute in nature. Severe babesiosis in dogs may lead to mixed metabolic acidosis and respiratory alkalosis. Affected dogs had severe hypoxemia and the acid-base disturbances were corrected after blood transfusion (Leisewitz et al. 1996).

Special considerations apply to cardiopulmonary resuscitation. Arterial blood gases may indicate respiratory alkalosis, because gas exchange is occurring in blood that traverses the pulmonary circulation. Mixed venous Pco_2 has been shown to be significantly higher than arterial Pco_2 during cardiopulmonary resuscitation in dogs (Lippert et al. 1988). In this setting, arterial values reflect the adequacy of ventilatory support, whereas mixed venous values may correlate better with tissue pH (Weil et al. 1986).

In patients with mixed metabolic acidosis and respiratory alkalosis, pH tends to be normal, and specific treatment to correct pH is not necessary (Bia and Thier 1981). Treatment should be directed at the underlying causes of the metabolic acidosis and respiratory alkalosis.

METABOLIC ACIDOSIS AND METABOLIC ALKALOSIS

This mixed disorder is usually seen in patients with long-standing metabolic acidosis (e.g., chronic renal failure, uncomplicated ketoacidosis, or diarrhea) that begin vomiting. Depending on the relative severity of the two opposing disorders, pH and $[HCO_3^-]$ can be increased, normal, or decreased. Recognition of both disturbances in this setting is important because treatment of one without attention to the other permits the unattended abnormality to emerge unopposed. Alternatively, this mixed metabolic disorder can begin as metabolic alkalosis with subsequent development of severe volume depletion resulting in hypoperfusion and lactic acidosis. Remember, however, that a high AG in metabolic alkalosis may result not only from lactic acidosis but also from pH-induced changes in the electronegative net charge of plasma proteins (Madias et al. 1979).

When metabolic acidosis is of the high-AG type, the diagnosis is suggested by a high AG and increased $[Na^+] - [Cl^-]$. When metabolic acidosis is of the normal-AG type, the diagnosis is more difficult, because these disturbances have offsetting effects on $[HCO_3^-]$ and $[Cl^-]$. Serum electrolytes and blood gases may be within the normal range in this setting. The history and physical examination are essential for the diagnosis of a combination of hyperchloremic metabolic acidosis and metabolic alkalosis (Narins and Emmett 1980).

Concurrent vomiting and diarrhea are potential causes of mixed hyperchloremic acidosis and metabolic alkalosis. Dogs with parvovirus gastroenteritis can present with metabolic alkalosis, metabolic acidosis, or normal blood gas results (the latter suggesting a mixed disorder) (Heald et al. 1986). Overzealous administration of $NaHCO_3$ to patients with metabolic acidosis can also result in this mixed disorder in veterinary medicine (Robinson and Hardy 1988). Another disease that can present with metabolic acidosis, metabolic alkalosis, or a combination of both is GDV (Muir 1982; Wingfield et al. 1982; Kagan and Schaer 1983). In this disease, loss of gastric acid causes metabolic alkalosis, whereas metabolic acidosis is believed to result from lactic acid accumulation (Muir 1982; Wingfield et al. 1982). The pH is usually normal in mixed metabolic acidosis and metabolic alkalosis, and treatment of stable patients should be directed at resolving the underlying disease processes. For patients with GDV, more aggressive therapy is necessary (i.e., relief of gastric distention and treatment of shock).

Disorders with Additive Effects on pH

Mixed disorders composed of primary problems with an additive effect on pH always involve an abnormal pH. Depending on the combination of primary problems, the pH can be dangerously high or low and requires immediate attention. Table 12–6 shows examples of potential causes of additive mixed acid-base disorders.

RESPIRATORY ACIDOSIS AND METABOLIC ACIDOSIS

This combination of acid-base disturbances may occur in a variety of settings, including HLS in dogs with gastrointestinal disease (DiBartola et al. 1985); cardiopulmonary arrest; and severe pulmonary edema, especially when associated with low cardiac output, low tissue perfusion, and lactic acidosis. In most of these situations, metabolic acidosis is a result of lactic acid accumulation. There is an additive effect lowering the pH if the normal compensation for the metabolic acidosis is impaired because of pulmonary disease. The $[HCO_3^-]$ is low, P_{CO_2} is normal or high, and the resultant pH can be dangerously low. A mild form of mixed metabolic and respiratory acidosis can be seen in dogs undergoing gastrointestinal endoscopy (Jergens et al. 1995).

The association between respiratory acidosis and metabolic acidosis has been observed in a dog with HLS, but the cause of respiratory acidosis was unclear (DiBartola et al. 1985). Metabolic acidosis in these patients could be due to diarrhea or dilutional acidosis because some of them have severe hyponatremia, hypochloremia, hyperkalemia, and normal AG (DiBartola et al. 1985). Lactic acidosis may also be contributory because some affected patients have signs compatible with hypovolemia (DiBartola et al. 1985). The venom of the scorpion *Leiurus quinquestriatus* may cause severe metabolic and respiratory acidosis in dogs (Tarasiuk et al. 1994).

Dogs, cats, and human patients with cardiopulmonary arrest typically develop lactic acidosis because of low cardiac output and hypoventilation (Weil et al. 1986; Lippert et al. 1988; Nakakimura et al. 1990). During resuscitation, however, arterial blood gases may indicate a normal pH with mixed metabolic acidosis and respiratory alkalosis and not reflect the ongoing marked reduction in mixed venous and tissue pH. Mixed venous blood should be used for analysis in this setting (Weil et al. 1986).

Patients with pulmonary edema may develop hypoxemia and lactic acidosis (Ware and Bonagura 1988). The situation is worse in patients in which pulmonary edema is secondary to heart failure. Low cardiac output compromises tissue perfusion, worsening the lactic acidosis (Narins and Emmett 1980). Dogs in septic shock usually demonstrate a respiratory alkalosis and metabolic acidosis. Later in the course of the disease process, however, patients may develop respiratory acidosis because of ventilation-perfusion (V-Q) mismatch (Hauptman and Tvedten 1986; Goodwin and Schaer 1990).

Dogs with GDV can also be presented with metabolic acidosis caused by lactic acidosis and respiratory acidosis resulting from diaphragmatic compression by the distended stomach (Muir 1982). Two dogs with acute tumor lysis syndrome were reported to have metabolic and res-

TABLE 12–6. Examples of Potential Causes of Additive Mixed Acid-Base Disorders

A. Respiratory acidosis and metabolic acidosis
 1. Hypoadrenocorticism-like syndrome in dogs with gastrointestinal disease
 2. Cardiopulmonary arrest
 3. Severe pulmonary edema
 4. Thoracic trauma with hypovolemic shock
 5. Low-cardiac-output heart failure with pulmonary edema
 6. Advanced septic shock (V-Q mismatch)
 7. Gastric dilatation-volvulus
 8. Acute tumor lysis syndrome
 9. Acute respiratory distress syndrome
 10. Gastrointesttinal endoscopy*
B. Respiratory alkalosis and metabolic alkalosis
 1. Gastric dilatation-volvulus
 2. Hyperadrenocorticism with pulmonary thromboembolism
 3. Respirator-induced mixed alkalosis (correction of P_{CO_2} too rapidly)
 4. Congestive heart failure and diuretics
 5. Hepatic disease and diuretics, vomiting, or hypoproteinemia
 6. Parvovirus gastroenteritis and septicemia
C. Normal plus high-anion-gap metabolic acidosis
 1. Renal failure
 2. NH_4Cl therapy and renal failure
 3. Resolving diabetic ketoacidosis
 4. Diarrhea complicating high-AG acidosis
 5. Liver disease (RTA and impaired metabolism of lactate)
D. Mixed high-anion-gap metabolic acidosis
 1. Diabetic ketoacidosis and renal failure
 2. Diabetic ketoacidosis and lactic acidosis
 3. Ethylene glycol intoxication with lactic acidosis
 4. Uremic acidosis and other high AG acidosis
E. Mixed normal-anion-gap metabolic acidosis
 1. Marked volume depletion (type 1 RTA) and diarrhea (e.g., chronic active hepatitis and diarrhea or cirrhosis with ascites and diarrhea)?
 2. Diarrhea and parenteral nutrition

*pH is usually only slightly acidemic and most patients do not require treatment.

piratory acidosis (Laing and Carter 1988). With one of these animals, however, insufficient time may have elapsed for full ventilatory compensation to be established. Metabolic acidosis with high AG occurred and was assumed to be the result of lactic acid accumulation (Laing and Carter 1988), but lactate concentrations were not determined. All patients had substantial lung lesions at necropsy.

Systemic pH is very low in patients with combined metabolic and respiratory acidosis, and specific therapy must be initiated quickly to correct acidemia and support ventilation (Bia and Thier 1981). In patients in which lactic acidosis is the cause of metabolic acidosis, tissue hypoxia is the most likely underlying cause, and therapeutic measures should be taken to augment oxygen delivery to the tissues (Madias 1986). $NaHCO_3$ is known to increase Pco_2 in dogs (Hartsfield et al. 1981) and human beings (Jones 1987) and must be used cautiously in situations in which the patient cannot excrete the CO_2 generated by $NaHCO_3$ administration (Nishikawa, 1993). Patients should not receive $NaHCO_3$ unless their pH is below the hemodynamically critical level (pH < 7.10–7.20) (Madias 1986). In this situation, small titrated doses of $NaHCO_3$ are used as a temporizing measure to achieve a pH compatible with cardiovascular responsiveness (pH ≥ 7.20) while attempts to improve oxygenation are continued (Hindman 1990). Carbicarb (an equimolar mixture of Na_2CO_3 and $NaHCO_3$) and dichloroacetate may be useful, especially for patients with lactic acidosis, but more clinical data are needed before their use can be advocated.

RESPIRATORY ALKALOSIS AND METABOLIC ALKALOSIS

This mixed disorder is commonly present in human patients with hepatic failure or those with congestive heart failure and pulmonary edema who are treated with diuretics. These patients have low Pco_2, high $[HCO_3^-]$, and high pH, and their alkalemia may be severe. Similar clinical conditions also occur in small animal medicine, but severe alkalemia is not common. Mixed respiratory and metabolic alkalosis was not observed in a study of 20 dogs with alkalemia identified among 962 dogs for which blood gas analysis was performed (Robinson and Hardy 1988). In dogs with experimental metabolic alkalosis, superimposition of chronic respiratory alkalosis causes a decrease in $[HCO_3^-]$, sufficient not only to prevent development of significant alkalemia but also to offset entirely the effect of hypocapnia on plasma $[H^+]$ (Madias et al. 1990).

Mixed respiratory and metabolic alkalosis is more likely to occur with chloride-responsive metabolic alkalosis (e.g., vomiting, diuretics) than with chloride-resistant metabolic alkalosis because the latter condition is rare in veterinary medicine. Overzealous administration of $NaHCO_3$ to patients with respiratory alkalosis and metabolic acidosis is another potential cause of this mixed disorder (Russo 1983). Chloride-responsive alkalosis persists until chloride is replaced. Patients with respiratory acidosis and a compensatory increase in $[HCO_3^-]$ may develop mixed respiratory and metabolic alkalosis if Pco_2 is lowered too rapidly while $[HCO_3^-]$ remains high (Narins and Emmett 1980). The GDV complex can also be associated with this mixed disorder in dogs (Adams and Polzin 1989). The goal of treatment in chloride-responsive metabolic alkalosis is to replace the chloride deficit while providing sufficient potassium and sodium to replace existing deficits. Definitive treatment of the underlying disease process prevents recurrence of the metabolic alkalosis.

Chloride-resistant metabolic alkalosis is observed in human patients with hyperadrenocorticism. Approximately 33% of dogs with hyperadrenocorticism have an increase in total CO_2 concentration (Peterson 1984). Dogs with hyperadrenocorticism may develop pulmonary thromboembolism (Burns et al. 1981; King et al. 1985; LaRue and Murtaugh 1990), and patients with thromboembolism can be presented with hypoxemia and hypocapnia (LaRue and Murtaugh 1990). The combination of hyperadrenocorticism with pulmonary thromboembolism could potentially be associated with mixed respiratory and metabolic alkalosis or metabolic acidosis if hypoxia is severe enough to cause lactic acidosis. Despite this possibility, three animals for which arterial blood gas data were available demonstrated only a simple disorder (Burns et al. 1981).

NORMAL AND HIGH-ANION-GAP METABOLIC ACIDOSIS

This mixed disorder is usually seen in patients with renal failure, in the resolving phase of ketoacidosis, or in patients with high-AG acidosis that develop diarrhea. The pH and $[HCO_3^-]$ are low, and the diagnosis is suggested by a high AG and decreased $[Na^+] - [Cl^-]$.

Human patients with chronic renal failure (serum creatinine concentration of 2–4 mg/dL) initially develop hyperchloremic acidosis. With progression of the disease (serum creatinine concentration of 4–14 mg/dL), metabolic acidosis progresses, but the further decrease in total CO_2 is associated with an increase in UA^- while hyperchloremia remains unchanged (Widmer et al. 1979). Human patients with advanced renal failure, however, may sometimes have a simple acid-base disorder, either hyperchloremic or high-AG acidosis (Wallia et al. 1986; Ray et al. 1990). Patients with diabetes mellitus may have a mixed high-AG and hyperchloremic acidosis because of development of diarrhea or in the resolving phase of the ketoacidotic crisis (Wallia et al. 1986; Ray et al. 1990). Hyperchloremia in the recovery phase develops for at least three reasons: (1) large volumes of saline are administered, (2) KCl is infused in large doses, and (3) ketones are lost in the urine and NaCl is reabsorbed by the kidneys (Narins and Emmett 1980). As discussed earlier, human patients with chronic hepatic disease may have enhanced proximal renal tubular sodium reabsorption that may limit distal H^+ secretion (Better et al. 1972). This may lead to hyperchloremic acidosis, decreased lactate metabolism, and development of a high-AG acidosis. The treatment in this situation should be directed at the primary disorder responsible for metabolic acidosis. Treatment with $NaHCO_3$ may be necessary for selected patients, but it should be used cautiously because ultimately the metabolism of previously accumulated organic anions generates additional HCO_3^- (Rose 1989).

MIXED HIGH-ANION-GAP METABOLIC ACIDOSIS

Two different causes of high-AG metabolic acidosis may coexist in the same patient, and this is usually a result of lactic or uremic acidosis superimposed on another cause of high-AG acidosis. The pH and $[HCO_3^-]$ are low in affected patients, and the AG is high with normal $[Na^+]-[Cl^-]$. If blood gases and serum electrolytes alone are assessed, it is not possible to differentiate between simple and mixed high-AG metabolic acidosis. Serum creatinine concentration, blood urea nitrogen (BUN), and plasma lactate concentration must be measured to confirm the presence of this mixed disorder (Narins and Emmett 1980).

Patients with ketoacidosis may develop lactic acidosis because of decreased tissue perfusion or impaired lactate utilization caused by decreased insulin activity. In this circumstance, lactic acidosis promotes conversion of acetoacetate to β-hydroxybutyrate, which does not react with nitroprusside in the urinalysis dipstrip reagent pad, thereby masking the ketoacidosis (Narins and Emmett 1980). It has been suggested that adding a few drops of hydrogen peroxide to the urine specimen would nonenzymatically convert β-hydroxybutyrate to acetoacetate, which would then be detected by the nitroprusside reagent (Narins et al. 1982). This method, however, has been shown to be ineffective in converting β-hydroxybutyrate to acetoacetate (Christopher et al. 1991).

Treatment in this mixed disorder should be directed toward resolving the primary disorder causing metabolic acidosis and toward stabilizing the patient. Treatment of lactic acidosis was discussed earlier in this chapter and in Chapter 10. As in other forms of high-AG metabolic acidosis, treatment with $NaHCO_3$ should be avoided because metabolism of accumulated organic anions generates HCO_3^- (Rose 1989). The intial goal for patients with severe acidosis is to increase the systemic pH to 7.20 (Rose 1989).

MIXED NORMAL-ANION-GAP METABOLIC ACIDOSIS

This is a rare disorder in veterinary medicine because the only clinical situation that commonly causes hyperchloremic acidosis is diarrhea. The pH and $[HCO_3^-]$ are decreased in these patients, and the AG is normal with low $[Na^+]-[Cl^-]$. Parenteral nutrition in patients with diarrhea could cause a mixed hyperchloremic acidosis because of addition of cationic amino acids (e.g., lysine HCl, arginine HCl). If the disease causing diarrhea is also causing volume depletion (e.g., hepatic disease with ascites), sodium reabsorption in the proximal renal tubule is enhanced, diminishing sodium delivery to the distal nephron and consequently limiting distal H^+ secretion (Better et al. 1972), and a mixed disorder may result. Treatment should be directed toward resolving the primary disease responsible for the acidosis. Treatment with $NaHCO_3$ should be used only if pH is below 7.20 or the $[HCO_3^-]$ is less than 12 mEq/L.

Triple Disorders

METABOLIC ACIDOSIS, METABOLIC ALKALOSIS, AND RESPIRATORY ACIDOSIS OR ALKALOSIS

Triple disorders occur whenever a respiratory disturbance complicates a mixed metabolic acidosis and metabolic alkalosis. The pH and $[HCO_3^-]$ may be normal, decreased, or increased, and PCO_2 is greater than expected when the mixed metabolic disturbance is complicated by respiratory acidosis and lower than expected when it is complicated by respiratory alkalosis. Some potential causes of triple acid-base disorders are listed in Table 12–7. Patients with low-output heart failure treated with diuretics may develop lactic acidosis and hypochloremic alkalosis. If such a patient develops interstitial pulmonary edema, there is a decrease in compliance and stimulation of ventilation causes PCO_2 to fall and respiratory alkalosis to develop (Aberman and Fulop 1972). With increasing severity of the edema, hypoventilation with respiratory acidosis may occur (Aberman and Fulop 1972). Dogs have good collateral ventilation, however, and hypercapnia occurs only in fulminant pulmonary edema (Ware and Bonagura 1988).

Patients with GDV can present with metabolic alkalosis and lactic acidosis (Muir 1982; Wingfield et al. 1982; Kagan and Schaer 1983). These patients can also develop respiratory alkalosis because of a pain-induced increase in ventilation (Muir 1982) or septicemia (Adams and Polzin 1989). Respiratory acidosis can also develop if ventilation is impaired by a grossly overdistended stomach (Muir 1982). Other potential causes of triple disorders are outlined in Table 12–7. The treatment of triple disorders should be directed at stabilizing the patient's clinical condition and resolving the underlying disease process. In the majority of these cases, the metabolic acidosis is due to lactic acid accumulation; therefore, the principles discussed under mixed respiratory acidosis with lactic acidosis are valid here.

▶ Treatment

When treating mixed acid-base disorders, two points are important (Bia and Thier 1981; Emmett and Narins 1987). First, the aim of therapy is to return the pH to normal; therefore the systemic pH of the patient must always be considered. For example, if a dog has a pH of 7.35 and $[HCO_3^-]$ of 12 mEq/L, no attempts should be made to correct this relatively normal pH. Second, do not overlook the second disorder. The effect that treating one disorder has on the second disorder must be anticipated, and both processes ought to be assessed simultaneously. The potential complications of treatment should also be anticipated (e.g., overshoot metabolic alkalosis after $NaHCO_3$ treatment), and iatrogenic mixed acid-base disorders should be avoided (e.g., administration of drugs that suppress ventilation in patients with metabolic acido-

TABLE 12–7. Examples of Potential Causes of Triple Disorders

A. Metabolic acidosis, metabolic alkalosis, and respiratory acidosis
  1. Low-output heart failure with pulmonary edema and diuretics
  2. Gastric dilatation-volvulus
B. Metabolic acidosis, metabolic alkalosis, and respiratory alkalosis
  1. Low-output heart failure with pulmonary edema and diuretics
  2. Gastric dilatation-volvulus
  3. Liver disease (hypoproteinemia, RTA, impaired metabolism of lactate, and hyperventilation)
  4. Parvovirus gastroenteritis (vomiting, diarrhea, and septicemia)

sis). The reader is referred to chapters on the individual acid-base disorders for further discussion of treatment (Chapters 10 and 11). Bear in mind, however, that mixed disturbances that have additive effects on pH (e.g., respiratory and metabolic acidosis) require more aggressive therapy than those with neutralizing effects (e.g., respiratory alkalosis and metabolic acidosis).

REFERENCES

Aberman A and Fulop M: The metabolic and respiratory acidosis of acute pulmonary edema. *Ann Intern Med* 76:173–178, 1972.

Adams LG and Polzin DJ: Mixed acid-base disorders. *Vet Clin North Am Small Anim Pract* 19:307–326, 1989.

Adrogué HJ and Madias NE: Changes in plasma potassium concentration during acute acid-base disturbances. *Am J Med* 71:456–471, 1981.

Adrogué HJ, Brensilver J, and Madias NE: Changes in plasma anion gap during chronic metabolic acid-base disturbances. *Am J Physiol* 235:F291–F297, 1978.

Adrogué HJ, Wilson H, Boyd AE III, et al.: Plasma acid-base patterns in diabetic ketoacidosis. *N Engl J Med* 307:1603–1610, 1982.

Adrogué HJ, Brensilver J, Cohen JJ, et al.: Influence of steady-state alterations in acid-base equilibrium on the fate of administered bicarbonate in the dog. *J Clin Invest* 71:867–883, 1983.

Adrogué HJ, Chap Z, Ishida T, et al.: Role of the endocrine pancreas in the kalemic response to acute metabolic acidosis in conscious dogs. *J Clin Invest* 75:798–808, 1985.

Badrick T and Hickman P: Anion gap (letter). *Lancet* 1:157, 1989.

Battle DC, Hizon M, Cohen E, et al.: The use of the urinary anion gap in the diagnosis of hyperchloremic metabolic acidosis. *N Engl J Med* 318:594–599, 1988.

Bercovici M, Chen CB, Goldstein MB, et al.: Effect of acute changes in the $Paco_2$ on acid-base parameters in normal dogs and dogs with metabolic acidosis or alkalosis. *Can J Physiol Pharmacol* 61:166–173, 1983.

Bersin RM and Arieff AI: Improved hemodynamic function during hypoxia with Carbicarb, a new agent for the management of acidosis. *Circulation* 77:227–233, 1988.

Better O, Goldschmid Z, Chaimowitz C, et al.: Defect in urinary acidification in cirrhosis. *Arch Intern Med* 130:77–82, 1972.

Bia M and Thier SO: Mixed acid-base disturbances: A clinical approach. *Med Clin North Am* 65:347–361, 1981.

Bleich HL, Berkman PM, and Schwartz WB: The response of cerebrospinal fluid composition to sustained hypercapnia. *J Clin Invest* 43:11–16, 1964.

Brice AG and Welch HG: Effect of respiratory alkalosis on skeletal muscle metabolism in the dog. *J Appl Physiol* 58:658–664, 1985.

Brimioulle S, Lejeune P, Vachiery J-L, et al.: Effects of acidosis and alkalosis on hypoxic vasoconstriction in dogs. *Am J Physiol* 258:H347–H353, 1990.

Brown SA, Spyridakis LK, and Crowell WA: Distal renal tubular acidosis and hepatic lipidosis in a cat. *J Am Vet Med Assoc* 189:1350–1352, 1986.

Bureau M and Bouverot P: Blood and CSF acid-base changes, and rate of ventilatory acclimatization of awake dogs to 3,550 m. *Respir Physiol* 24:203–216, 1975.

Burnell JM, Villami MF, Uyeno BT, et al.: The effect in humans of extracellular pH change on the relationship between serum potassium concentration and intracellular potassium. *J Clin Invest* 35:935–939, 1956.

Burns MG, Kelly AB, Hornof WJ, et al.: Pulmonary artery thrombosis in three dogs with hyperadrenocorticism. *J Am Vet Med Assoc* 178:388–393, 1981.

Bushinsky DA, Coe FL, Katzenberg C, et al.: Arterial Pco_2 in chronic metabolic acidosis. *Kidney Int* 22:311–314, 1982.

Cain SM and Dunn JE II: Transient arterial lactic acid changes in unanesthetized dogs at 21,000 feet. *Am J Physiol* 206:1437–1440, 1964.

Center SA: Pathophysiology and laboratory diagnosis of liver disease. In Ettinger SJ (ed): *Textbook of Veterinary Internal Medicine: Diseases of Dog and Cat*, 3rd ed. Philadelphia, WB Saunders Co., pp. 1421–1478, 1989.

Ching SV, Fettman MJ, Hamar DW, et al.: The effect of chronic dietary acidification using ammonium chloride on acid-base and mineral metabolism in the adult cat. *J Nutr* 119:902–915, 1989.

Christopher M, Periera J, Brigmon R, et al.: Automated determination of β-hydroxybutyrate for the assessment of ketoacidosis. *Proceedings American College of Veterinary Internal Medicine*, New Orleans, p. 903, 1991.

Clark DD, Chang BS, Garella SG et al.: Secondary hypocapnia fails to protect "whole-blood" intracellular pH during chronic HCl-acidosis in the dog. *Kidney Int* 23:336–341, 1983.

Cohen JJ, Brackett NC, and Schwartz WB: The nature of the carbon dioxide titration curve in the normal dog. *J Clin Invest* 43:777–786, 1964.

Cohen JJ, Madias NE, Wolf CJ et al.: Regulation of acid-base equilibrium in chronic hypocapnia: Evidence that the response of the kidney is not geared to the defense of extracellular [H^+]. *J Clin Invest* 57:1483–1489, 1976.

Cornelius LM and Rawlings CA: Arterial blood gas and acid-base values in dogs with various diseases and signs of disease. *J Am Vet Med Assoc* 178:992–995, 1981.

de Morais HSA and DiBartola SP: Ventilatory and metabolic compensation in dogs with acid-base disturbances. *J Vet Emerg Crit Care* 1:39–49, 1991.

DeSousa RC, Harrington JT, Ricanati ES, et al.: Renal regulation of acid-base equilibrium during chronic administration of mineral acid. *J Clin Invest* 53:465–476, 1974.

DiBartola SP, Chew DJ, and Jacobs G: Quantitative urinalysis including 24-hour protein excretion in the dog. *J Am Anim Hosp Assoc* 16:537–546, 1980.

DiBartola SP, Johnson SE, Davenport DJ, et al.: Clinicopathologic findings resembling hypoadrenocorticism in dogs with primary gastrointestinal disease. *J Am Vet Med Assoc* 187:60–63, 1985.

DiNubile MJ: The increment in the anion gap: Overextension of a concept. *Lancet* 2:951–953, 1988.

DuBose TD Jr: Clinical approach to patients with acid-base disorders. *Med Clin North Am* 67:799–813, 1983.

Elkinton JR: Clinical disorders of acid-base regulation. A survey of seventeen years' diagnostic experience. *Med Clin North Am* 50:1352–1363, 1966.

Emmett M and Narins RG: Mixed acid-base disorders. In Maxwell MH, Kleeman CR, and Narins RG (eds): *Clinical Disorders of Fluid and Electrolyte Metabolism*, 4th ed. New York, McGraw-Hill, pp. 743–758, 1987.

Fencl V: Acid-base balance in cerebral fluids. In American Physiological Society (ed): *Handbook of Physiology: Respiratory System*. Bethesda, MD, American Physiological Society, pp. 115–140, 1986.

Fulop M: Serum potassium in lactic acidosis and ketoacidosis. *N Engl J Med* 300:1087–1089, 1979.

Gabow PA: Disorders associated with altered anion gap. *Kidney Int* 27:472–483, 1985.

Gabow PA, Kachny WD, Fennessey PV, et al.: Diagnostic importance of an increased serum anion gap. *N Engl J Med* 303:854–858, 1980.

Gennari FJ, Goldstein MB, and Schwartz W: The nature of the renal adaptation to chronic hypocapnia. *J Clin Invest* 51:1722–1730, 1972.

Giebisch G, Berger L, Pitts R, et al.: The extrarenal response to acute acid-base disturbances of respiratory origin. *J Clin Invest* 34:231–245, 1955.

Goldstein MB, Bear R, Richardson RMA, et al.: The urine anion gap: A clinical useful index of ammonium excretion. *Am J Med Sci* 292:198–202, 1986.

Goodkin DA, Krishna GG, and Narins RG: The role of the anion gap in detecting and managing mixed metabolic acid-base disorders. *Clin Endocrinol Metab* 13:333–349, 1984.

Goodwin J-K and Schaer M: Septic shock. *Vet Clin North Am Small Anim Pract* 19:1239–1258, 1990.

Graf H, Leach W, and Arieff AI: Effects of dichloroacetate in the treatment of hypoxic lactic acidosis in dogs. *J Clin Invest* 76:919–923, 1985a.

Graf H, Leach W, and Arieff AI: Evidence of a detrimental effect of bicarbonate therapy in hypoxic lactic acidosis. *Science* 227:754–756, 1985b.

Halperin ML and Bun-Chen C: Influence of acute hyponatremia on renal ammoniagenesis in dogs with chronic metabolic acidosis. *Am J Physiol* 258:F328–F332, 1990.

Halperin ML, Vinay P, Gougoux A, et al.: Regulation on the maximum rate of renal ammoniagenesis in the acidotic dog. *Am J Physiol* 248:F607–F615, 1985.

Hampson NB, Jöbsis-VandlerVliet FF, and Piantadosi CA: Skeletal muscle oxygen availability during respiratory acid-base disturbances in cats. *Respir Physiol* 70:143–158, 1987.

Hansen JE and Simmons DH: A systematic error in the determination of blood P_{CO_2}. *Am Rev Respir Dis* 115:1061–1063, 1977.

Hartsfield SM, Thurmon JC, Corbin JE, et al.: Effects of sodium acetate, bicarbonate, and lactate on acid-base status in anesthetized dogs. *J Vet Pharmacol Ther* 4:51–61, 1981.

Hauptman JG and Tvedten H: Osmolal and anion gaps in dogs with acute endotoxic shock. *Am J Vet Res* 47:1617–1619, 1986.

Heald RD, Jones BD, and Schmidt DA: Blood gas and electrolyte concentrations in canine parvoviral enteritis. *J Am Anim Hosp Assoc* 22:745–748, 1986.

Hindman BJ: Sodium bicarbonate in the treatment of subtypes of acute lactic acidosis: Physiologic considerations. *Anesthesiology* 72:1064–1076, 1990.

Hulter HN, Toto RD, Sebastian A, et al.: Effect of extracellular fluid volume depletion on renal regulation of acid-base and potassium equilibrium during prolonged mineral acid administration. *J Lab Clin Med* 103:854–868, 1984.

Hutchison AS, Ralston SH, Dryburgh FJ, et al.: Too much heparin: Possible source of error in blood gas analysis. *Br Med J* 287:1131–1132, 1983.

Ilkiw JE, Davis PE, and Church DB: Hematological, biochemical, blood-gas, and acid-base values in greyhounds before and after exercise. *Am J Vet Res* 50:583–586, 1989.

Jennings DB and Davidson JSD: Acid-base and ventilatory adaptation in conscious dogs during chronic hypercapnia. *Respir Physiol* 58:377–393, 1984.

Jergens AE, Riedesel DH, Ries PA, et al.: Cardiopulmonary responses in healthy dogs during endoscopic examination of the gastrointestinal tract. *Am J Vet Res* 56:215–220, 1995.

Jones NL: *Blood Gases and Acid-Base Physiology*, 2nd ed. New York, Thieme Medical Publishers, 1987.

Kagan KG and Schaer M: Gastric dilatation and volvulus in a dog—A case justifying electrolyte and acid-base assessment. *J Am Vet Med Assoc* 183:703–705, 1983.

Kazemi H, Shannon DC, and Carvallo-Gil E: Brain CO_2 buffering capacity in respiratory acidosis and alkalosis. *J Appl Physiol* 22:241–246, 1967.

Kazemi H, Valenca LM, and Shannon DC: Brain and cerebrospinal fluid lactate concentration in respiratory acidosis and alkalosis. *Respir Physiol* 6:178–186, 1969.

King RR, Mauderly JL, Hahn FF, et al.: Pulmonary function studies in a dog with pulmonary thromboembolism associated with Cushing's disease. *J Am Anim Hosp Assoc* 21:555–562, 1985.

Laing EJ and Carter RF: Acute tumor lysis syndrome following treatment of canine lymphoma. *J Am Anim Hosp Assoc* 24:691–696, 1988.

LaRue MJ and Murtaugh RJ: Pulmonary thromboembolism in dogs: 47 cases (1986–1987). *J Am Vet Med Assoc* 197:1368–1372, 1990.

Leisewitz AL, Guthrie AJ, and Berry WL: Evaluation of the effect of whole-blood transfusion on the oxygen status and acid-base balance of *Babesia canis* infected dogs. *J S Afr Vet Assoc* 67:20–26, 1996.

Leith DE: The new acid-base: Power and simplicity. *Proceedings American College Veterinary Internal Medicine*, Washington, DC, pp. 449–455, 1990.

Lemieux G, Kiss A-L, Lemieux C, et al.: Renal tubular biochemistry during acute and chronic metabolic alkalosis in the dog. *Kidney Int* 27:908–918, 1985.

Lemieux G, Lemieux C, Duplessis S, et al.: Metabolic characteristics of cat kidney: Failure to adapt to metabolic acidosis. *Am J Physiol* 259:R277–R281, 1990.

Lippert AC, Evans AT, White BC, et al.: The effect of resuscitation technique and pre-arrest state of oxygenation on blood-gas values during cardiopulmonary resuscitation in dogs. *Vet Surg* 17:283–290, 1988.

Lowance DC, Garfinkel HB, Mattern WD, et al.: The effect of chronic hypotonic volume expansion on the renal regulation of acid-base equilibrium. *J Clin Invest* 51:2928–2940, 1972.

Madias NE: Lactic acidosis. *Kidney Int* 29:752–774, 1986.

Madias NE and Zelman SJ: The renal response to chronic mineral acid-feeding: A reexamination of the role of systemic pH. *Kidney Int* 29:667–674, 1986.

Madias NE, Schwartz WB, and Cohen JJ: The maladaptive renal response to secondary hypocapnia during chronic HCl acidosis in the dog. *J Clin Invest* 60:1393–1401, 1977.

Madias NE, Ayus C, and Adrogué HJ: Increased anion gap in metabolic alkalosis: The role of plasma protein equivalency. *N Engl J Med* 300:1421–1423, 1979.

Madias NE, Adrogué HJ, and Cohen JJ: Maladaptive renal response to secondary hypercapnia in chronic metabolic alkalosis. *Am J Physiol* 238:F283–F289, 1980.

Madias NE, Bossert WH, and Adrogué HJ: Ventilatory response to chronic metabolic acidosis and alkalosis in the dog. *J Appl Physiol* 56:1640–1646, 1984.

Madias NE, Wolf CJ, and Cohen JJ: Regulation of acid-base equilibrium in chronic hypercapnia. *Kidney Int* 27:538–543, 1985.

Madias NE, Cohen JJ, and Adrogué HJ: Influence of acute and chronic respiratory alkalosis on preexisting chronic metabolic alkalosis. *Am J Physiol* 258:F479–F485, 1990.

Madiedo G, Sciacca R, and Hause L: Air bubbles and temperature effect on blood gas analysis. *J Clin Pathol* 33:864–867, 1980.

Magner PO, Robinson L, Halperin RM, et al.: The plasma potassium concentration in metabolic acidosis: A re-evaluation. *Am J Kidney Dis* 11:220–224, 1988.

Maskrey M and Jennings DB: Ventilation and acid-base balance in awake dogs exposed to heat and CO_2. *J Appl Physiol* 58:549–557, 1985.

McAuliffe JJ, Lind LJ, Leith DE, et al.: Hypoproteinemic alkalosis. *Am J Med* 81:86–90, 1986.

Muir WW III: Acid-base and electrolyte disturbances in dogs with gastric dilatation-volvulus. *J Am Vet Med Assoc* 181:229–231, 1982.

Muir WW III, Wagner AE, and Buchanan C: Effects of acute hyperventilation on serum potassium in the dog. *Vet Surg* 19:83–87, 1990.

Musch TI, Friedman DB, Haidet GC, et al.: Arterial blood gases and acid-base status of dogs during graded dynamic exercise. *J Appl Physiol* 61:1914–1919, 1986.

Nakakimura K, Fleischer JE, Drummond JC, et al.: Glucose administration before cardiac arrest worsens neurologic outcome in cats. *Anesthesiology* 72:1005–1011, 1990.

Nanji A and Blank D: Spurious increases in the anion gap due to exposure of serum to air (letter). *N Engl J Med* 307:190, 1982.

Narins RG and Emmett M: Simple and mixed acid-base disorders: A practical approach. *Medicine (Baltimore)* 59:161–187, 1980.

Narins RG, Jones ER, Stom MC, et al.: Diagnostic strategies in disorders of fluid, electrolyte, and acid-base homeostasis. *Am J Med* 72:496–506, 1982.

Natelson S: On the significance of the expression, "anion gap." *Clin Chem* 29:283–284, 1983.

Nattie EE, Edwards WH, and Marin-Padilla M: Newborn puppy cerebral acid-base regulation in experimental asphyxia and recovery. *J Appl Physiol* 56:1178–1186, 1984.

Nishikawa T: Acute haemodynamic effect of sodium bicarbonate in canine respiratory or metabolic acidosis. *Br J Anaesth* 70:196–200, 1993.

Oehme FW: Aspirin and acetaminophen. In Kirk RW (ed): *Current Veterinary Therapy IX.* Philadelphia, WB Saunders Co., pp. 188–190, 1986.

Orringer CE, Eustage JC, Wunsch CD, et al.: Natural history of latic acidosis after grand-mal seizures: A model for the study of an anion-gap acidosis not associated with hyperkalemia. *N Engl J Med* 297:796–799, 1977.

Oster JR, Perez GO, and Vaamonde CA: Relationship between blood pH and potassium and phosphorus during acute metabolic acidosis. *Am J Physiol* 4:F345–F351, 1978.

Oster JR, Perez GO, Castro A, et al.: Plasma potassium response to acute metabolic acidosis induced by mineral and non-mineral acids. *Miner Electrolyte Metab* 4:28–36, 1980.

Oster JR, Perez GO, and Materson BJ: Use of anion gap in clinical medicine. *South Med J* 81:229–237, 1988.

Parent C, King LG, Van Winkle TJ, and Walker LM: Respiratory function and treatment in dogs with acute respiratory distress syndrome: 19 cases (1985–1993). *J Am Vet Med Assoc* 208:1428–1433, 1996.

Peterson ME: Hyperadrenocorticism. *Vet Clin North Am Small Anim Pract* 14:731–749, 1984.

Pierce NF, Fedson DS, Brigham KL, et al.: The ventilatory response to acute base deficit in humans. Time course during development and correction of metabolic acidosis. *Ann Intern Med* 72:633–645, 1970.

Polak A, Haynie GD, Hays RM, et al.: Effects of chronic hypercapnia on electrolyte and acid-base equilibrium. I. Adaptation. *J Clin Invest* 40:1223–1237, 1961.

Polzin DJ and Osborne CA: Anion gap—Diagnostic and therapeutic applications. In Kirk RW (ed): *Current Veterinary Therapy IX.* Philadelphia, WB Saunders Co., pp. 52–59, 1986.

Polzin DJ, Stevens JB, and Osborne CA: Clinical application of the anion gap in evaluation of acid-base disorders in dogs. *Compend Contin Educ Pract Vet* 4:1021–1033, 1982.

Ray S, Piraino B, Chong TK, et al.: Acid excretion and serum electrolyte patterns in patients with advanced chronic renal failure. *Miner Electrolyte Metab* 16:355–361, 1990.

Robertson SA: Simple acid-base disorders. *Vet Clin North Am Small Anim Pract* 19:289–306, 1989.

Robinson EP and Hardy RM: Clinical signs, diagnosis, and treatment of alkalemia in dogs: 20 cases (1982–1984). *J Am Vet Med Assoc* 7:943–949, 1988.

Rose BD: *Clinical Physiology of Acid-Base and Electrolyte Disorders*, 3rd ed. New York, McGraw-Hill, 1989.

Rose RJ and Carter J: Some physiological and biochemical effects of acetazolamide in the dog. *J Vet Pharmacol Ther* 2:215–221, 1979.

Russo EA: Iatrogenic metabolic alkalosis with respiratory alkalosis in a dog with patent ductus arteriosus. *J Am Vet Med Assoc* 183:889–892, 1983.

Schall WD: Heat stroke. In Kirk RW (ed): *Current Veterinary Therapy VII.* Philadelphia, WB Saunders Co., pp. 195–197, 1980.

Schwartz WB, Brackett NC, and Cohen JJ: The response of extracellular hydrogen ion concentration to graded degrees of chronic hypercapnia: The physiologic limits of defense of pH. *J Clin Invest* 44:291–301, 1965.

Shaw D: The relationship between urine ammonium excretion and urine anion gap in dogs (abstract). *J Vet Intern Med* 5:130, 1991.

Siggaard-Andersen O, Astrup RG, Bates RG, et al.: Report of ad hoc committee on acid-base terminology. *Ann N Y Acad Sci* 133:251–258, 1966.

Silva PRM, Fonseca-Costa A, Zin WA, et al.: Respiratory and acid-base parameters during salicylic intoxication in dogs. *Braz J Med Biol Res* 19:279–286, 1986.

Simmons DH and Avedon M: Acid-base alterations and plasma potassium concentration. *Am J Physiol* 197:319–325, 1959.

Stewart PA: Independent and dependent variables of acid-base control. *Respir Physiol* 33:9–26, 1978.

Stewart PA: *How to Understand Acid-Base.* New York, Elsevier, 1981.

Swan RC and Pitts RF: Neutralization of infused acid by nephrectomized dogs. *J Clin Invest* 34:205–212, 1954.

Tarasiuk A, Sofer S, Huberfeld SI, and Scharf SM: Hemodynamic effects following injection of venom from the scorpion *Leiurus quinquestriatus*. *J Crit Care* 9:134–140, 1994.

van Ypersele de Strihou C, Gulyassy PF, and Schwartz WB: Effects of chronic hypercapnia on electrolyte and acid-base equilibrium. III. Characteristics of the adaptive and recovery process as evaluated by provision of alkali. *J Clin Invest* 41:2246–2253, 1962.

Wallia R, Greenberg A, Piraino B, et al.: Serum electrolyte patterns in end-stage renal disease. *Am J Kidney Dis* 8:98–104, 1986.

Ware WA and Bonagura JD: Pulmonary edema. In Fox PR (ed): *Canine and Feline Cardiology.* New York, Churchill Livingstone, pp. 205–217, 1988.

Weil MH, Rackow EC, Trevino R, et al.: Difference in acid-base state between venous and arterial blood during cardiopulmonary resuscitation. *N Engl J Med* 315:153–156, 1986.

Widmer B, Gerhardt RE, Harrington JT, et al.: Serum electrolyte and acid-base composition: The influence of graded degrees of chronic renal failure. *Arch Intern Med* 139:1099–1102, 1979.

Willard MD: Disorders of potassium homeostasis. *Vet Clin North Am Small Anim Pract* 19:241–263, 1989.

Wilson EA and Green RA: Clinical analysis of mixed acid-base disturbances. *Compend Contin Educ Pract Vet* 7:S364–S371, 1985.

Wingfield WE, Twedt DC, Moore RW, et al.: Acid-base and electrolyte values in dogs with acute gastric dilatation-volvulus. *J Am Vet Med Assoc* 180:1070–1072, 1982.

SECTION 4

Fluid Therapy

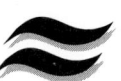

CHAPTER 13

Introduction to Fluid Therapy

STEPHEN P. DiBARTOLA

> *She had apparently reached the last moments of earthly existence, and now nothing could injure her—indeed, so entirely was she reduced, that I feared I should be unable to get my apparatus ready ere she expired. Having inserted a tube into the basilic vein, cautiously—anxiously, I watched the effects; ounce after ounce was injected, but no visible change was produced. Still persevering, I thought she began to breathe less laboriously, soon the sharpened features, and sunken eye, and fallen jaw, pale and cold, bearing the manifest impress of death's signet, began to glow with returning animation; the pulse which had long ceased, returned to the wrist; at first small and quick, by degrees it became more and more distinct, fuller, slower, and firmer, and in the short space of half an hour, when six pints had been injected, she expressed in a firm voice that she was free from all uneasiness, actually became jocular, and fancied that all she needed was a little sleep; her extremities were warm, and every feature bore the aspect of comfort and health.*
>
> Thomas Latta, describing the first use of intravenous fluid therapy in a human patient with cholera in a letter to the Lancet, 1832.

Fluid therapy is supportive. The underlying disease process that caused the fluid, electrolyte, and acid-base disturbances in the patient must be diagnosed and treated appropriately. Normal homeostatic mechanisms allow the clinician considerable margin for error in fluid therapy, provided that the heart and kidneys are normal. This is fortunate, because estimation of the patient's fluid deficit is difficult and may be quite inaccurate. The purpose of this chapter is to provide an overview of the principles of fluid therapy. The composition and distribution of body fluids are discussed in Chapter 1 and the technical aspects of vascular access are discussed in Chapter 14. In formulating and implementing a fluid therapy plan, six questions should be considered (Muir and DiBartola 1983; DiBartola 1985):

1. Is fluid therapy indicated?
2. What type of fluid should be given?
3. By what route should the fluid be given?
4. How rapidly should the fluid be given?
5. How much fluid should be given?
6. When should fluid therapy be discontinued?

▶ Is Fluid Therapy Indicated?

For medical patients, the answer to this question depends on an assessment of the animal's state of hydration. For surgical patients, there are additional indications for fluid therapy, such as maintenance of venous access for emergencies and establishment of diuresis to maintain renal perfusion during anesthesia (see Chapter 15). The hydration status of the animal is estimated by careful evaluation of the history, physical examination findings, and the results of a few simple laboratory tests (Finco 1972a; Cornelius 1980).

In its most narrow sense, dehydration refers to loss of pure water. The term dehydration, however, is usually used to include hypotonic, isotonic, and hypertonic fluid losses. The type of dehydration is classified by the tonicity of the fluid remaining in the body (e.g., a hypotonic loss would result in hypertonic dehydration). Isotonic and hypotonic losses are most common in small animal practice. Isotonic fluid loss can result in volume depletion and nonosmotic stimulation of antidiuretic hormone (ADH) release, thus preventing effective excretion of consumed water and resulting in hypotonic dehydration. Types of dehydration are depicted in Figure 3–1 and are discussed in detail in Chapter 3.

Fluid Balance

Normal sources of fluid input are water consumed in food, water that is drunk, and water produced in the body as a result of metabolism. Nutrient oxidation produces approximately 0.1 g of water per kilocalorie of energy released (Anderson 1982). Maintenance water and electrolyte needs parallel caloric expenditure (Harrison et al. 1960; Haskins 1984, 1988), and normal daily losses of water and electrolytes include respiratory, fecal, and urinary losses. Estimated daily caloric and water requirements for dogs and cats are shown in Tables 13–1 and 13–2 (Haskins 1988) and in Figure 13–1 (Harrison et al. 1960). Respiratory loss of fluid can be important in dogs, because panting has been adapted for thermoregulation in this species. Normally, cutaneous losses are unimportant in dogs and cats because eccrine sweat glands are limited to the foot pads and do not play an important role in thermoregulation. Sympathetic stimulation as a result of heat stress in the cat may result in increased secretion of saliva, and a small volume of fluid may be lost by this route.

In disease states, decreased fluid intake results from anorexia, and increased fluid loss may occur through urinary (e.g., polyuria) and gastrointestinal (e.g., vomiting, diarrhea) routes. Other less common routes of loss include skin (e.g., extensive burns), respiratory tract, and salivary secretions, as described before. Third-space loss of fluid occurs when effective circulating volume is decreased, but the fluid lost remains in the body. Examples include intestinal obstruction, peritonitis, pancreatitis, and effusions or hemorrhage into body cavities. Decreased fluid intake and increased loss often coexist (e.g., anorexia, vomiting, and polyuria in a uremic animal).

History

Historical information about the route of fluid loss may suggest the patient's electrolyte and acid-base derangements. The time period over which fluid losses have occurred and an estimate of their magnitude should be determined. Information about food and water consumption, gastrointestinal losses (e.g., vomiting, diarrhea), urinary losses (i.e., polyuria), and traumatic losses (e.g., blood loss, extensive burns) should be obtained from the owner. Excessive insensible water losses (e.g., increased panting, fever) and third-space losses may be determined from the history and physical examination. In addition, the clinician's knowledge of the suspected disease can aid in predicting the composition of the fluid lost (e.g., vomiting caused by pyloric obstruction leads to loss of hydrogen, chloride, potassium, and sodium ions and development of metabolic alkalosis, whereas small-bowel diarrhea typically leads to loss of bicarbonate, chloride, sodium, and potassium ions and development of metabolic acidosis) (Table 13–3).

TABLE 13–1. Daily Water and Calorie Requirements for the Dog*

Body Weight (kg)	Total kcal/day or Water mL/day	/kg	/h
1	132	132	6
2	214	107	9
3	285	95	12
4	348	87	15
5	407	81	17
6	463	77	19
7	515	74	21
8	566	71	24
9	615	68	26
10	662	66	28
11	707	64	29
12	752	63	31
13	795	61	33
14	837	60	35
15	879	59	37
16	919	57	38
17	959	56	40
18	998	55	42
19	1037	55	43
20	1075	54	45
21	1112	53	46
22	1149	52	48
23	1185	52	49
24	1221	51	51
25	1256	50	52
26	1291	50	54
27	1326	49	55
28	1360	49	57
29	1394	48	58
30	1427	48	59
35	1590	45	66
40	1746	44	73
45	1896	42	79
50	2041	41	85
55	2182	40	91
60	2319	39	97
70	2583	37	108
80	2836	35	118
90	3080	34	128
100	3316	33	138

Source: Haskins SC: A simple fluid therapy planning guide. *Semin Vet Med Surg (Small Anim)* 3:232, 1988.
*132 kcal/kg$^{0.75}$; Nutritional requirements of the dog. National Research Council, Bethesda, MD, 1985.

TABLE 13–2. Daily Water and Calorie Requirements for the Cat*

Body Weight (kg)	Total kcal/day or Water mL/day	/kg	/h
1.0	80	80	3
1.5	108	72	5
2.0	135	67	6
2.5	159	64	7
3.0	182	61	8
3.5	205	58	9
4.0	226	57	9
4.5	247	55	10
5.0	268	53	11

Source: Haskins SC: A simple fluid therapy planning guide. *Semin Vet Med Surg (Small Anim)* 3:232, 1988.
*80 kcal/kg$^{0.75}$; Nutritional requirements of the cat. National Research Council, Bethesda, MD, 1987.

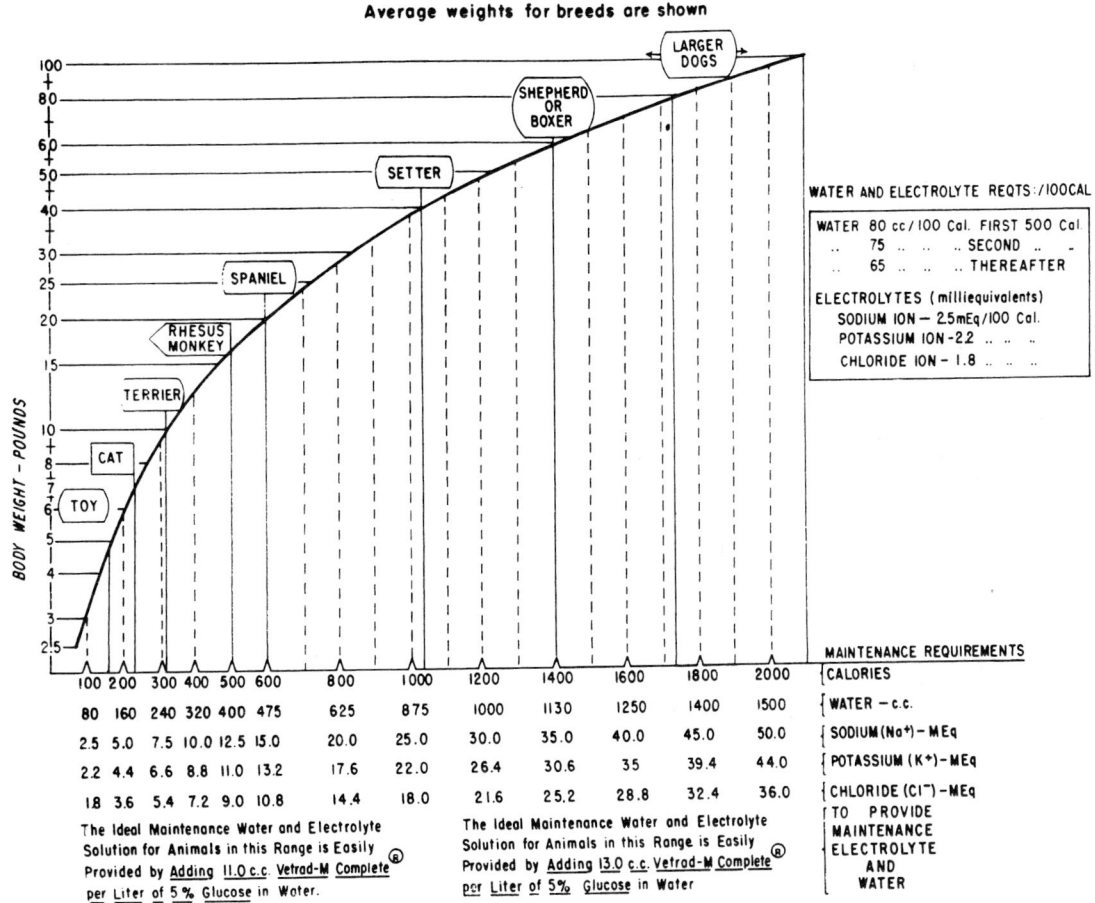

FIGURE 13-1. Daily water, calorie, and electrolyte requirements for dogs and cats. (From Harrison JB, Sussman HH, and Pickering DE: Fluid and electrolyte therapy in small animals. *J Am Vet Med Assoc* 137:638, 1960.)

Physical Examination

The physical findings associated with fluid losses of 5 to 15% of body weight vary from no clinically detectable changes (5%) to signs of hypovolemic shock and impending death (15%) (Table 13–4) (Harrison et al. 1960; Finco 1972a; Cornelius 1980). The clinician may estimate the hydration deficit by evaluating skin turgor or pliability, the moistness of the mucous membranes, the position of the eyes in their orbits, heart rate, the character of peripheral pulses, capillary refill time, and extent of peripheral venous distention (e.g., inspection of jugular veins). A decrease in the volume of the interstitial compartment leads to decreased skin turgor and dryness of the mucous membranes. A decrease in plasma volume leads to tachycardia, alterations in peripheral pulses, and collapse of peripheral veins. The fluid deficit in a given patient is difficult to determine with accuracy because of the subjectivity of skin turgor evaluation and the possibility of undetected ongoing (contemporary) losses. Thus, a crude clinical estimate of hydration status and the patient's response to fluid administration become important tools in evaluating the extent of dehydration that was present and in formulating ongoing fluid therapy.

Skin turgor is dependent on the amount of subcutaneous fat and elastin as well as on interstitial volume. Detection of dehydration by skin turgor is dependent on the animal's skin turgor before dehydration developed, the position of the animal (e.g., standing, recumbent) when the skin is checked, the site used for evaluation, and the amount of subcutaneous fat (Hardy and Osborne 1979). Skin pliability should be tested over the lumbar region with the dog in a standing position. When evaluated by skin turgor, obese animals may appear well hydrated owing to excessive subcutaneous fat despite being dehydrated. On the other hand, emaciated animals and older animals may appear more dehydrated than they actually are owing to lack of subcutaneous fat and elastin. A false impression of dehydration may also occur with persistent panting, which may dry the oral mucous membranes.

Signs of hypovolemic shock appear when dehydration becomes severe (12–15% of body weight) or when there has been an acute and severe loss of extracellular fluid. These signs include lassitude, cool extremities, tachycardia, rapid and weak pulses, and prolonged capillary refill time. The urinary bladder should be small in a dehydrated animal with normal renal function. A large, urine-filled bladder in a severely dehydrated patient indicates failure of the normal renal concentrating mechanism.

Body weight recorded on a serial basis is the best indicator of hydration status, especially when fluid loss has been acute and previous body weight has been recorded. Loss of 1 kg of body weight indicates a fluid deficit of 1 L. Unfortunately, previous body weight is

TABLE 13-3. Potential Fluid, Electrolyte, and Acid-Base Disturbances in Various Diseases and Suggested Crystalloid Solutions

Abnormality	Type of Dehydration	Electrolyte Balance	Acid-Base Status	Fluid Therapy
Simple dehydration, stress, exercise	Hypertonic	—	—	Half strength or balanced electrolyte solution; 5% dextrose solution
Heat stroke	Hypertonic	K^+ variable; Na^+ variable	Metabolic acidosis	Half strength electrolyte solution followed by balanced electrolyte solution
Anorexia	Isotonic	K^+ loss	Mild metabolic acidosis	Balanced electrolyte solution; KCl
Starvation	Isotonic	K^+ loss	Mild metabolic acidosis	Half strength or balanced electrolyte solution; KCl; calories
Vomiting	Isotonic or hypertonic	Na^+, K^+, and Cl^- loss	Metabolic alkalosis; metabolic acidosis chronically	Ringer's solution; 0.9% saline with KCl supplementation
Diarrhea	Isotonic or hypertonic	Na^+ loss; K^+ loss chronically	Metabolic acidosis	Balanced electrolyte solution; HCO_3^-; KCl (if chronic)
Diabetes mellitus	Hypertonic	K^+ loss	Metabolic acidosis	Balanced electrolyte solutions; KCl
Hyperadrenocorticism	Isotonic	K^+ loss	Occasionally mild metabolic alkalosis	Balanced electrolyte solutions; KCl
Hypoadrenocorticism	Isotonic or hypertonic	Na^+ loss; K^+ retention	Metabolic acidosis	0.9% saline followed by balanced electrolyte solutions
Urethral obstruction	Isotonic or hypertonic	K^+ retention; Na^+, Cl^- variable	Metabolic acidosis	0.9% saline followed by balanced electrolyte solutions; KCl postobstruction
Acute renal failure	Isotonic or hypertonic (with vomiting)	K^+ retention; Na^+, Cl^- variable	Metabolic acidosis	Balanced electrolyte solutions
Chronic renal failure	Isotonic or hypertonic (with vomiting)	Na^+, K^+, Cl^- variable	Metabolic acidosis	Balanced electrolyte solutions
Congestive heart failure	Plethoric (Na^+, H_2O retention early); hypotonic chronically	Na^+ retention (but dilutional hyponatremia)	Metabolic acidosis (chronically)	5% dextrose solution
Hemorrhagic shock	Isotonic		Metabolic acidosis	Balanced electrolyte solutions; blood
Endotoxic shock	Isotonic		Metabolic acidosis	Balanced electrolyte solutions; 0.9% saline

Source: Muir WW and DiBartola SP: Fluid therapy. In Kirk RW: *Current Veterinary Therapy VIII*. Philadelphia, WB Saunders Co., p 31, 1983.

often unknown in animals presented for treatment. Records from previous routine hospital visits, however, may provide this information. Loss of weight in chronic diseases includes loss of muscle mass as well as fluid loss. An anorexic animal may lose 0.1 to 0.3 kg of body weight per day per 1000 kcal energy requirement (Finco 1977). Losses in excess of this amount indicate fluid loss. Another factor that must be considered in evaluating body weight is the possibility of third-space loss. Fluid lost into a third space does not decrease body weight (Haskins 1988).

Laboratory Findings

The hematocrit or packed cell volume (PCV), total plasma protein concentration (TPP), and urine specific gravity (USG) are simple laboratory tests that can aid in the evaluation of hydration. It is important to obtain these values before initiating fluid therapy. The PCV and TPP should be evaluated together to minimize errors in interpretation. The PCV and TPP increase with all types of fluid losses excluding hemorrhage, whereas serum sodium concentration increases, decreases, or remains unchanged depending on the loss (e.g., hypotonic, hypertonic, isotonic). The effects of the different types of dehydration on the serum sodium concentration are discussed in Chapter 3. Table 13-5 shows possible interpretations of various combinations of PCV and TPP values. The PCV alone may be an unreliable indicator of hemoconcentration in water-deprived dogs, and although TPP increases, test results may not be above the upper limit of the normal range (Hardy and Osborne 1979). The USG before fluid therapy is helpful in the preliminary evaluation of renal function. Urine specific gravity should be high (>1.045) in a dehydrated dog or cat if renal function is normal. This may not be true if other disorders affecting renal concentrating ability, such as medullary washout of solute, are present. Furthermore, previous administration of corticosteroids or furosemide can decrease urinary concentrating ability. After fluid therapy has been initiated, USG falls into the isosthenuric range if rehydration has been achieved.

▶ What Type of Fluid Should Be Given?

A fluid is said to be *balanced* if its composition resembles that of extracellular fluid (e.g., lactated Ringer's solution)

TABLE 13-4. Physical Findings in Dehydration

Percent Dehydration	Clinical Signs
<5	Not detectable
5–6	Subtle loss of skin elasticity
6–8	Definite delay in return of skin to normal position
	Slight prolongation of capillary refill time
	Eyes possibly sunken in orbits
	Possibly dry mucous membranes
10–12	Tented skin stands in place
	Definite prolongation of capillary refill time
	Eyes sunken in orbits
	Dry mucous membranes
	Possibly signs of shock (tachycardia, cool extremities, rapid and weak pulses)
12–15	Definite signs of shock
	Death imminent

Source: Muir WW and DiBartola SP: Fluid therapy. In Kirk RW: *Current Veterinary Therapy VIII*. Philadelphia, WB Saunders Co., p 33, 1983.

and *unbalanced* if it does not (e.g., normal saline). Fluid preparations may be further classified as crystalloids or colloids. *Crystalloids* are solutions containing electrolyte and nonelectrolyte solutes capable of entering all body fluid compartments (e.g., 5% dextrose, 0.9% saline, lactated Ringer's solution). *Colloids* are large-molecular-weight substances that are restricted to the plasma compartment and include plasma, dextrans, and hydroxyethyl starch (hetastarch).

Colloids may be used in patients with shock and in those with severe hypoalbuminemia (i.e., albumin <1.5 g/dL). A major limitation to the use of plasma as a colloid is the rapid disappearance of albumin from the vascular space. Dextrans are polymers of glucose that have average molecular weights of 40,000 (dextran 40) or 70,000 (dextran 70). Their use in humans has been associated with coagulopathies. Hetastarch has a molecular weight of 69,000. In humans, coagulopathies have also been associated with the use of hetastarch. The main advantages of colloids are that more of the administered solution remains in the plasma compartment and there is less risk of edema. Colloids are discussed in detail in Chapter 23.

Crystalloid solutions are equally effective at expanding the plasma compartment, but 2.5 to 3.0 times as much crystalloid solution must be given (compared with a colloid solution) because the crystalloid is distributed to other sites (e.g., interstitial compartment, intracellular compartment) (Virgilio et al. 1979; Monafo 1981; Moss et al. 1981). Pulmonary capillaries are normally more permeable to protein, resulting in a higher interstitial concentration of protein and more resistance to leakage of fluid from capillaries (Rose 1994a). Peripheral edema is more likely to occur after crystalloid administration because muscle and subcutaneous capillaries are less permeable to protein.

Crystalloid solutions can be classified as *replacement* or *maintenance* solutions. The composition of *replacement solutions* (e.g., lactated Ringer's) resembles that of extracellular fluid (Fig. 13–2). *Maintenance solutions* contain less sodium (40–60 mEq/L) and more potassium (15–30 mEq/L) than replacement fluids. A simple maintenance solution can be formulated by mixing one part 0.9% NaCl with two parts 5% dextrose and adding 20 mEq KCl per liter of final solution. The approximate composition of such a fluid would be 51 mEq/L sodium, 20 mEq/L potassium, 71 mEq/L chloride, and 33.5 g/L dextrose. It would provide 133 kcal/L and have an osmolality of 328 mOsm/kg. An alternative maintenance solution may be made by mixing one part lactated Ringer's solution with two parts 5% dextrose and adding 20 mEq KCl per liter of final solution. This solution has the following approximate composition: 43 mEq/L sodium, 21 mEq/L potassium, 56 mEq/L chloride, 1 mEq/L calcium, 9 mEq/L lactate and 33.5 g/L dextrose. It would provide 133 kcal/L and have an osmolality of 317 mOsm/kg. If preferred, the clinician can achieve a similar effect by alternating administration of 5% dextrose in water with 0.9% saline or lactated Ringer's solution in a 2:1 ratio throughout a 24-h period.

Another commonly employed crystalloid is 5% dextrose. Administering 5% dextrose is equivalent to giving water because the glucose is oxidized to CO_2 and water. In fact, the main reason for giving 5% dextrose is to replace a pure water deficit. Except in very small animals, administration of 5% dextrose cannot be relied upon to maintain daily caloric needs because 5% dextrose contains only 200 kcal/L. Consider a normal, active 10-kg dog. Its maintenance energy requirement (MER) is approximately 740 kcal:

MER (kcal) = 60 × body weight (kg) + 140

To provide this number of kilocalories from 5% dextrose (200 kcal/L), almost 4 L of fluid must be administered

TABLE 13-5. Interpretation of Hematocrit and Total Plasma Protein Concentrations

PCV (%)	Total Plasma Proteins (g/dL)	Interpretation
Increased	Increased	Dehydration
Increased	Normal or decreased	Splenic contraction
		Polycythemia
		Dehydration with preexisting hypoproteinemia
Normal	Increased	Normal hydration with hyperproteinemia
		Anemia with dehydration
Decreased	Increased	Anemia with dehydration
		Anemia with preexisting hyperproteinemia
Decreased	Normal	Nonblood loss anemia with normal hydration
Normal	Normal	Normal hydration
		Dehydration with preexisting anemia and hypoproteinemia
		Acute hemorrhage
		Dehydration with secondary compartment shift
Decreased	Decreased	Blood loss
		Anemia and hypoproteinemia
		Overhydration

Source: Muir WW and DiBartola SP: Fluid therapy. In Kirk RW: *Current Veterinary Therapy VIII*. Philadelphia, WB Saunders Co., p 34, 1983.

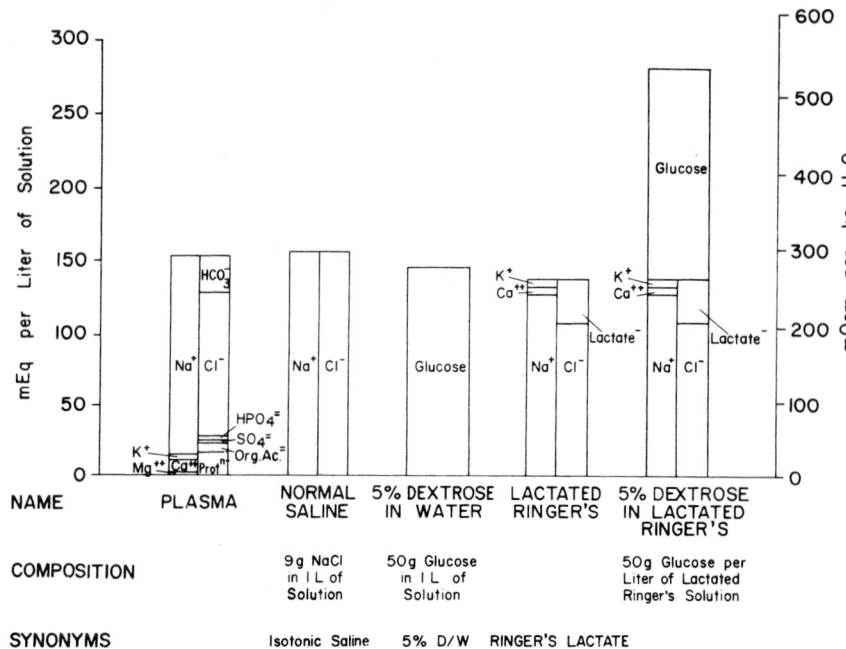

FIGURE 13-2. Comparison of electrolyte composition of plasma to that of commonly used crystalloid solutions. (From Muir WW and DiBartola SP: Fluid therapy. In Kirk RW: *Current Veterinary Therapy VIII.* Philadelphia, WB Saunders Co., p. 30, 1983.)

per day. Such a volume is almost seven times more than the daily maintenance requirement for fluid in this dog (see later). Administration of 4 L of 5% dextrose over a 24-h period would initiate a diuresis that would impair utilization of the administered dextrose and cause increased urinary losses of electrolytes.

The veterinary practitioner can manage most animals requiring fluid therapy with a limited number of crystalloid and additive solutions. The most useful crystalloid solutions for routine use are a balanced replacement solution such as Ringer's or lactated Ringer's solution, 0.9% saline, and 5% dextrose in water. The solute composition of these fluids is compared with that of extracellular fluid in Figure 13–2, and the electrolyte composition of several commercially available solutions is summarized in Table 13–6.

Supplementation of crystalloid solutions with KCl may be necessary when losses have included large amounts of potassium. An empirical scale has been devised to estimate the amount of potassium to add to parenterally administered fluids (Table 13–7) (Greene and Scott 1975). This protocol has not been evaluated experimentally in dogs or cats but has been used effectively in these species at the Ohio State University Veterinary Teaching Hospital over the past 20 years. Potassium supplementation is discussed in Chapter 5.

Other additive solutions include 50% dextrose, calcium chloride, calcium gluconate, potassium phosphate, 8.4% sodium bicarbonate, and water-soluble B vitamins. Thiamine supplementation may be particularly important in cats, because their requirement for this vitamin may be higher than that of dogs. Phosphate is rarely used as an additive but is required in patients with diabetic ketoacidosis during insulin therapy (Willard et al. 1987). Phosphate supplementation is discussed in Chapter 7. Theoretically, sodium bicarbonate should not be added to solutions containing calcium (e.g., Ringer's or lactated Ringer's solution) because of the risk of forming insoluble calcium carbonate crystals. Despite this concern, no adverse consequences have been observed when small amounts of sodium bicarbonate have been added to lactated Ringer's solution (Haskins 1984, 1988).

When additives are used, the clinician must keep in mind that the final osmolality of the fluid may be higher than anticipated. The final osmolality may be approximated by adding the number of milliequivalents per liter of electrolyte and millimoles per liter of nonelectrolyte solutes found in the solution. The final osmolality of the solution may also differ depending on how the solution was formulated. For example, if 500 mL of lactated Ringer's solution is mixed with 500 mL of 5% dextrose to create a replacement solution with 2.5% dextrose, the resulting solution has an approximate osmolality of 275 mOsm/kg (virtually the same as that of lactated Ringer's solution). On the other hand, if 50 mL of 50% dextrose is added to 1 L of lactated Ringer's solution, the resulting solution contains 2.5% dextrose but has an approximate osmolality of 391 mOsm/kg, which is substantially higher.

The choice of fluid to administer is dependent on the nature of the disease process and the composition of the fluid lost. The clinician should attempt to replace losses with a fluid that is similar in volume and electrolyte composition to that which has been lost from the body (see Table 13–3). If clinical assessment of hydration status is suggestive of hypovolemia, a replacement fluid (e.g., lactated Ringer's solution) should be administered rapidly. If there are no clinical signs of hypovolemia, the hydration deficit and maintenance needs may be combined and administered over the next 24 h.

Persistent vomiting caused by pyloric obstruction would be expected to result in losses of hydrochloric acid, potassium, sodium, and water, potentially producing hypokalemia, hypochloremia, and metabolic alkalosis. The initial fluid of choice in this setting is 0.9% NaCl with 20

TABLE 13-6. Electrolyte Composition of Commercially Available Fluids

Fluid	Glucose* (g/L)	Na+ (mEq/L)	Cl− (mEq/L)	K+ (mEq/L)	Ca²⁺ (mEq/L)	Mg²⁺ (mEq/L)	Buffer† (mEq/L)	Osmolarity (mOsm/L)	Cal/L	pH
Dextrose and Electrolyte Solution Composition										
5% dextrose	50	0	0	0	0	0	0	252	170	4.0
10% dextrose	100	0	0	0	0	0	0	505	340	4.0
2.5% dextrose in 0.45% NaCl	25	77	77	0	0	0	0	280	85	4.5
5% dextrose in 0.45% NaCl	50	77	77	0	0	0	0	406	170	4.0
5% dextrose in 0.9% NaCl	50	154	154	0	0	0	0	560	170	4.0
0.45% NaCl	0	77	77	0	0	0	0	154	0	5.0
0.9% NaCl	0	154	154	0	0	0	0	308	0	5.0
3% NaCl	0	513	513	0	0	0	0	1026	0	5.0
Ringer's solution	0	147.5	156	4	4.5	0	0	310	0	5.5
Ringer's lactated solution	0	130	109	4	3	0	28 (L)	272	9	6.5
2.5% dextrose in Ringer's lactated solution	25	130	109	4	3	0	28 (L)	398	94	5.0
5% dextrose in Ringer's lactated solution	50	130	109	4	3	0	28 (L)	524	179	5.0
2.5% dextrose in half-strength Ringer's lactated solution	25	65.5	55	2	1.5	0	14 (L)	263	89	5.0
Normosol-M in 5% dextrose‡	50	40	40	13	0	3	16 (A)	364	175	5.5
Normosol-R‡	0	140	98	5	0	3	27 (A) 23 (G)	296	18	6.4
Plasma-Lyte§	0	140	103	10	5	3	47 (A) 8 (L)	312	17	5.5
Plasma-Lyte M in 5% dextrose§	50	40	40	16	5	3	12 (A) 12 (L)	376	178	5.5
Plasma	1	145	105	5	5	3	24 (B)	300	—	7.4
Additives and Special Solutions										
20% mannitol	200 (M)	0	0	0	0	0	0	1099	—	
7.5% NaHCO₃	0	893	0	0	0	0	893	1786	0	
8.4% NaHCO₃	0	1000	0	0	0	0	1000 (B)	2000	0	
10% CaCl₂	0	0	2720	0	1360	0	0	4080	0	
14.9% KCl	0	0	2000	2000	0	0	0	4000	0	
50% dextrose	500	0	0	0	0	0	0	2780	1700	4.2

Source: Chew DJ and DiBartola SP: *Manual of Small Animal Nephrology and Urology.* New York, Churchill-Livingstone, p. 308, 1986.
*All glucose, with one exception: M, mannitol.
†Buffers used: A, acetate; B, bicarbonate; G, gluconate; L, lactate.
‡CEVA Laboratories. Overland Park, Kansas.
§Travenol Laboratories, Deerfield, Illinois.

to 30 mEq KCl per liter. Except in the case of vomiting of stomach contents, lactated Ringer's is a good first choice for fluid therapy while awaiting laboratory results. Normal saline (0.9% NaCl) is less ideal because it is not a balanced solution. It contains chloride in greater concentration than body fluids (154 mEq/L versus 110 mEq/L in dogs and 120 mEq/L in cats), and, as a result of displacement of bicarbonate with chloride in extracellular fluid and initiation of natriuresis, it has a mild acidifying effect (Rose 1979). Fluids should be stored at room temperature or preferably warmed to body temperature in a 37°C water bath or incubator before use (Finco 1972b). This warming eliminates any decrease in body temperature that might otherwise occur during administration (Finco 1972b; Cornelius et al. 1978). Examples of fluid therapy in specific diseases are listed in Table 13-3.

In one study, five different solutions were administered to unanesthetized dogs over a 1-h period: 0.9% NaCl, 0.9% NaCl with 5% dextrose, lactated Ringer's solution, Normosol-R, and Normosol-R with 2% dextran (Rose 1979). The approximate composition of these fluids is presented in Table 13-8. The fluids were warmed to body temperature and no decreases in rectal temperature were observed. Laboratory parameters were measured after 1 h of infusion. Fluids were administered at 76 mL/kg/h except for Normosol-R with dextran, which was administered at a rate of 31.5 mL/kg/h.

TABLE 13-7. Sliding Scale for Potassium Supplementation

Serum Potassium (mEq/L)	mEq KCl to add to 250 mL Fluid	Maximal Fluid Infusion Rate* (mL/kg/h)
<2.0	20	6
2.1–2.5	15	8
2.6–3.0	10	12
3.1–3.5	7	16

Source: Muir WW and DiBartola SP: Fluid therapy. In Kirk RW: *Current Veterinary Therapy VIII.* Philadelphia, WB Saunders Co., p 38, 1983.
*SO AS NOT TO EXCEED 0.5 mEq/kg/h.

TABLE 13-8. Composition of Fluids Administered to Awake Dogs

Solution	Na (mmol/L)	K (mmol/L)	Ca (mmol/L)	Mg (mmol/L)	Cl (mmol/L)	Lactate (mmol/L)	Acetate (mmol/L)	Gluconate (mmol/L)	Glucose (mmol/L)	pH
0.9% sodium chloride	154				154					5.4
0.9% sodium chloride plus 5% dextrose	154				154				277.5	4.2
Hartmann's solution*	131	5	2		112	28				6.3
Normosol-R	140	5		1.5	98		27	23		5.7
Normosol-R plus 2% dextran	140	5		1.5	98		27	23		6.4

Source: Rose RJ: Some physiological and biochemical effects of the intravenous administration of five different electrolyte solutions in the dog. *J Vet Pharmacol Ther* 2:281, 1979.
*Lactated Ringer's solution.

Most of the fluids increased heart rate, diastolic arterial pressure, and central venous pressure (CVP), and all of them decreased hematocrit, hemoglobin, and total protein concentrations by 21 to 25%. All solutions except for Normosol-R and Normosol-R with 2% dextran caused an increase in serum chloride concentration, and the saline solutions decreased pH and bicarbonate concentration. All solutions except Normosol-R caused a decrease in serum potassium concentration. The causes of the decreased serum potassium concentrations in these dogs presumably included dilution and increased distal tubular flow rate with enhanced urinary excretion of potassium. The presence of 5% dextrose in two of the solutions resulted in significantly lower serum potassium concentrations, suggesting movement of potassium into cells with glucose.

Serum sodium concentrations were similar despite differences in the sodium concentrations of the various fluids, demonstrating effective natriuresis in normal dogs receiving sodium-containing crystalloid solutions. Serum chloride concentration increased with administration of the saline solutions containing 154 mEq/L chloride, and mild metabolic acidosis developed. Serum chloride concentration also increased slightly with administration of lactated Ringer's solution (112 mEq/L chloride), but there was no change in acid-base balance. The increased serum chloride concentration and alterations in acid-base balance could have resulted from decreased reabsorption of bicarbonate with sodium in the kidney during natriuresis and decreased strong ion difference (Stewart 1981, 1983). Expansion acidosis is an unlikely explanation because all fluids administered presumably expanded the extracellular fluid volume.

Anions such as acetate, gluconate, and lactate are added to crystalloid solutions as a source of base because their oxidative metabolism in the body yields bicarbonate. The alkalinizing effect of the metabolism of these anions and that of citrate is as follows:

Acetate

$$NaC_2H_3O_2 + 2O_2 \rightarrow CO_2 + H_2O + Na^+HCO_3^-$$

Citrate

$$K_3C_6H_5O_7 + 4\tfrac{1}{2}O_2 \rightarrow 3CO_2 + 3H_2O + 3K^+HCO_3^-$$

Gluconate

$$NaC_6H_{11}O_7 + 5\tfrac{1}{2}O_2 \rightarrow 5CO_2 + 5H_2O + Na^+HCO_3^-$$

Lactate

$$NaC_3H_5O_3 + 3O_2 \rightarrow 2CO_2 + 2H_2O + Na^+HCO_3^-$$

Most lactate is produced in muscle and gut and metabolized to either glucose (via cytosolic gluconeogenesis) or CO_2 and water (via mitochondrial oxidation) in the liver. Normally, gluconeogenesis predominates. Acetate is metabolized primarily in muscle. The alkalinizing effect of these anions is delayed because of the requirement for metabolism. In one study, equivalent doses of acetate, bicarbonate, and lactate had similar alkalinizing effects in anesthetized dogs 45 min after infusion (Hartsfield et al. 1981). The effect of bicarbonate occurred earliest because metabolism was not necessary.

Lactate was originally introduced for the treatment of acidosis because of technical difficulties in preparation of bicarbonate solutions suitable for intravenous use (Schwartz and Waters 1962; Cohen and Simpson 1975). These technical difficulties have been overcome, but crystalloid solutions containing lactate as a source of base (e.g., lactated Ringer's solution) are still widely used for fluid therapy in clinical practice. Most patients treated with lactate-containing replacement solutions respond well, probably as a result of extracellular fluid volume expansion and improved tissue perfusion.

Whether it is converted to glucose or oxidized to CO_2 and water, the metabolism of lactate consumes hydrogen ions and has an alkalinizing effect:

Gluconeogenesis

$$2CH_3CHOHCOO^- + 2H^+ \rightarrow C_6H_{12}O_6$$

Oxidative metabolism

$$CH_3CHOHCOO^- + H^+ + 3O_2 \rightarrow 3CO_2 + H_2O$$

There has been some concern that lactate in lactated Ringer's solution may be harmful to patients with poor tissue perfusion and severe metabolic acidosis (pH < 7.1–7.2). Administration of lactate as a salt cannot contribute directly to metabolic acidosis. Rather, the ability of the liver to metabolize lactate and the potentially detrimental effect of lactate on myocardial contractility have been debated. During severe hypoxia, increased lactate production in gut and muscle and decreased hepatic extraction of lactate led to progressive lactic acidosis. In moderate metabolic acidosis, administration of lactated Ringer's solution is probably beneficial because any tendency toward lactate accumulation is likely to be offset by improved hepatic perfusion and oxygen delivery as a result of extracellular fluid volume expansion.

Crystalloid solutions with preservatives must be avoided in cats. Benzoic acid derivatives (e.g., benzyl alcohol, methylparaben, propylparaben, ethylparaben) are added to some solutions for their antimicrobial effect. Clinical signs in cats receiving fluids with such preservatives have included behavioral changes, hypersalivation, ataxia, muscle fasciculations, seizures, dilated nonresponsive pupils, coma, and death (Bedford and Clark 1972; Ryan 1982; Cullison et al. 1983). Young cats may be at increased risk for these complications.

▶ By What Route Should Fluids Be Given?

The route of fluid therapy depends on the nature of the clinical disorder, its severity, and its duration.

Intravenous

The intravenous route is preferred when the patient is very ill, when there has been severe fluid loss, or when the fluid loss has been acute. This route is also used during anesthesia to maintain renal perfusion and vascular access for emergencies. The intravenous route provides rapid dispersion of water and electrolytes and allows precise dosage. A large volume can be given rapidly, and hypertonic fluids can be given safely via a large vein. This route requires vascular access and close monitoring during infusion to avoid complications such as overhydration, infection, thrombosis, phlebitis, embolism, and impaired fluid delivery (e.g., obstruction of the catheter by a change in the patient's limb position).

The veins available for vascular access include the jugular, cephalic, lateral saphenous, and femoral veins. There are advantages and disadvantages of each, but the jugular vein is most useful because it allows delivery of large volumes, administration of hypertonic or potentially irritating solutions, measurement of CVP, and repeated venous blood sampling. The cephalic vein is also commonly used, but fluid delivery can be hindered by flexion of the elbow, and extremely hypertonic or irritating solutions should not be used. Intravenous catheters should be removed and a new catheter placed in a different vein every 72 h to avoid complications. The types of catheters used and their placement are discussed in Chapter 14.

Subcutaneous

The subcutaneous route is convenient for maintenance fluid therapy in small dogs and cats. The subcutaneous space in dogs and cats can accommodate relatively large volumes of fluid, and potassium can be used in concentrations up to 30 to 35 mEq/L without irritation (Finco 1977). Approximately 10 mL/kg or 50 to 200 mL may be administered per site (Schaer 1989). Fluid is administered under the skin along the back from the area of the scapulae to the lumbar region. Volume overload is unlikely to occur when fluids are administered by the subcutaneous route, and it is a useful transitional route when the animal is being weaned from intravenous fluid therapy. Furthermore, the subcutaneous route can be used by some owners to give fluids at home to animals with chronic disease problems (e.g., chronic renal failure).

The subcutaneous route is not adequate for patients with acute and severe losses (e.g., shock) and is not recommended in extremely dehydrated or hypothermic animals because peripheral vasoconstriction may reduce absorption and dispersion of the administered fluid in these settings. The volume that may be given is limited by skin elasticity, and this route is not useful in larger animals requiring large volumes of fluids. Irritating or hypertonic solutions must not be used by the subcutaneous route; only isotonic fluids are recommended. The subcutaneous administration of 5% dextrose in water should be avoided because equilibration of extracellular fluid with a pool of electrolyte-free solution may lead to temporary aggravation of electrolyte imbalance.

Oral

The oral route is the most physiologic and fluids with a wide variety of compositions may be given. Oral fluid therapy is useful for administering hypertonic fluids with high caloric density. Fluid can be administered rapidly with minimal side effects, and caloric needs can be met. This route should not be used, however, in the presence of gastrointestinal dysfunction (e.g., vomiting, diarrhea). The oral route is also inadequate in animals that have had acute or extensive fluid losses, because dispersion and utilization of the administered fluid and electrolytes are not sufficiently rapid. In anorexic animals without vomiting or diarrhea, fluid can be administered by the oral route using a number of different techniques (e.g., nasogastric tube, pharyngostomy tube, gastrostomy tube).

Intraperitoneal

Intraperitoneal administration of fluid allows rapid absorption of large volumes. Only isotonic fluids can be used because administration of hypertonic fluids results in further contraction of the extracellular compartment as water enters the peritoneal space by osmosis. Peritonitis is also a potential complication of this route. The intraperitoneal route is not employed commonly except to perform peritoneal dialysis as described in Chapter 25.

Intraosseous (Intramedullary)

The intraosseous, or intramedullary, route is useful in very young or small animals in which venous access is difficult. The procedure has been available for many years (Corley 1963) and has received renewed attention (Fiser 1989; Garvey 1989; Otto et al. 1989). This route provides rapid vascular access via bone marrow sinusoids and medullary venous channels and allows rapid dispersion of fluid. The bone marrow does not collapse when the patient is hypovolemic, and access to the marrow is easier and more rapidly achieved than performing a venous cutdown. Sites that can be used for intraosseous administration of fluid include the tibial tuberosity, trochanteric fossa of the femur, wing of the ilium, and greater tubercle of the humerus. The periosteum should be anesthetized by infiltration with 1% lidocaine solution to avoid pain during needle placement. The potential risks include osteomyelitis and pain on administration of fluid. Pain, however, was not observed clinically in two studies (Garvey 1989; Otto et al. 1989).

▶ How Fast May Fluids Be Given?

The flow of fluids through a catheter is governed by Poiseuille's law:

$$\text{Flow} = \frac{\pi(P_1 - P_2)r^4}{8\eta L}$$

where $P_1 - P_2$ represents the pressure differential on the fluid, η is the viscosity of the fluid, r is the radius of the catheter, and L is the length of the catheter. Thus, the diameter of the catheter is of primary importance in establishing a rapid rate of flow. The choice of catheter length is sometimes affected by factors other than flow rate (e.g., use of jugular catheters to monitor CVP). In a study of gravity flow of lactated Ringer's solution, in vivo flow rates averaged 7% less than in vitro flow rates, presumably because of tissue pressure (Fulton and Hauptman 1991). Fluid flow rate increased by 50% when the pressure differential was increased by raising the fluid bag from 0.91 to 1.75 m. Flow rate increased linearly with increasing catheter radius rather than geometrically as predicted by Poiseuille's law.

The rate of fluid administration is dictated by the magnitude and rapidity of the fluid loss. Acute, severe losses in patients with hypotension or shock demand rapid replacement. When necessary, fluids can be given safely at a rate of one blood volume per hour (i.e., 80–90 mL/kg/h in dogs or 50–55 mL/kg/h in cats) (Finco 1972b). Fluids administered at 90 mL/kg/h did not cause pulmonary edema in normal dogs and cats (Cornelius et al. 1978; Bjorling and Rawlings 1983).

Anesthetized cats receiving lactated Ringer's solution at a rate of 225 mL/kg over 1 h developed serous nasal discharge, chemosis, ascites, diarrhea, and fluid exudation from catheter sites. At necropsy, these cats had ascites, pancreatic edema, and accumulation of free fluid in the trachea. Body temperature decreased and CVP and left atrial pressure increased in cats receiving 225 mL/kg/h, whereas hematocrit, total protein concentration, and colloidal osmotic pressure decreased in cats receiving both 90 and 225 mL/kg/h (Bjorling and Rawlings 1983).

Lactated Ringer's solution was administered to unanesthetized, dehydrated dogs at rates of 90, 225, and 360 mL/kg over 1 h (Cornelius et al. 1978). At rates of 90 and 225 mL/kg/h, some dogs had serous nasal discharge, mild coughing, and slight chemosis. At 360 mL/kg/h, marked serous nasal discharge, restlessness, coughing, dyspnea, pulmonary crackles, ascites, polyuria, chemosis, protrusion of eyes, and diarrhea were observed. These signs resolved when fluid administration was discontinued. Hematocrit, TPP, and serum potassium concentration decreased during fluid administration. In this study, body temperature decreased despite the fact that fluids were warmed to 37°C. Serum sodium concentration remained unchanged, but pulse rate, respiratory rate, and systemic arterial pressure increased slightly. Pulmonary capillary wedge pressure (PWP) and CVP increased, and these measurements correlated well with one another. It was concluded that lactated Ringer's solution at 90 mL/kg/h was tolerated safely. Central venous pressure should be monitored if fluids must be administered at rates in excess of 90 mL/kg/h.

Contemporary losses must also be considered when adjusting the rate of fluid administration. Severe ongoing losses (e.g., vomiting and diarrhea in a patient with acute gastroenteritis) may necessitate rapid administration to keep pace with contemporary fluid loss. When fluids are given rapidly, it is necessary to monitor cardiovascular and renal function.

It is usually not necessary or desirable to replace the hydration deficit rapidly in chronic disease states. Instead, the hydration deficit may be calculated, the daily maintenance requirement of fluid added to this, and the total volume administered over 24 h (Schall 1982). This approach allows adequate time for equilibration of fluid and electrolytes with the intracellular compartment and avoids potential complications (e.g., edema or effusion related to increased hydrostatic pressure, diuresis and loss of administered electrolytes in urine). It is the method most commonly employed for medical patients at the Ohio State University Veterinary Teaching Hospital. An alternative approach is to replace the hydration deficit over the first 4 to 8 h of treatment, followed by maintenance therapy.

Whenever possible, fluid deficits should be replaced before anesthesia and surgery. During the induction and maintenance of anesthesia, prevention of hypovolemia and maintenance of renal perfusion are essential. Induction of a diuresis in this setting may be an important factor in the prevention of intraoperative acute renal failure. A basal fluid administration rate of 5 to 10 mL/kg/h is recommended during anesthesia and surgery. During major surgery (e.g., exploratory laparotomy, thoracotomy), fluid administration at twice this basal rate is recommended. Fluid therapy during anesthesia and surgery is discussed in more detail in Chapter 15.

Most administration sets designed for adult human patients deliver 10 to 20 drops per mL, whereas pediatric administration sets deliver 60 drops per mL (Schall 1982). This information is used to calculate the drip rate:
Adult administration set:

$$\text{mL/h} \times 1 \text{ h}/60 \text{ min} \times 10 \text{ drops/mL}$$

or

$$(\text{mL/h})/6 = \text{drops/min}$$

Pediatric administration set:

$$\text{mL/h} \times 1 \text{ h}/60 \text{ min} \times 60 \text{ drops/mL}$$

or

$$\text{mL/h} = \text{drops/min}$$

Fluid orders should be written so that the volume to be administered is recorded as mL/day, mL/h, and drops/

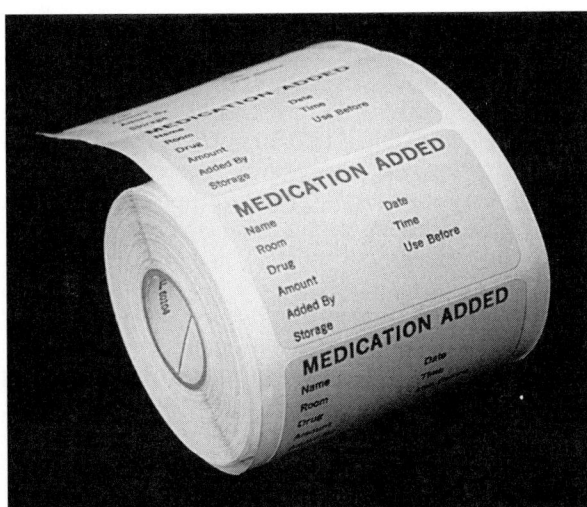

FIGURE 13-3. Adhesive label for fluid additives. (From Chew DJ: Parenteral fluid therapy. In Sherding RG [ed]: *The Cat: Diseases and Clinical Management.* New York, Churchill Livingstone, p. 50, 1989.)

min. This allows personnel to detect errors in calculations. The clinician should not assume that the animal has received the volume of fluid ordered, and the volume actually received should be noted in the record by nursing personnel. All additives should be clearly listed on the bottle, and adhesive labels for this purpose are available (Fig. 13-3). A strip of adhesive tape can be attached to the bottle and marked appropriately to provide a quick visual estimate of the volume of fluid received (Fig. 13-4). In the Buretrol system, a reservoir allows a predetermined volume of fluid to be delivered over a given time period (Fig. 13-5). This approach prevents infusion of excessive volumes of fluid to small animals. Infusion pumps are available for clinical use (e.g., IVAC, Flow Guard 8000) and provide a highly accurate record of the volume infused (Fig. 13-6). These pumps also have alarm systems that can alert personnel when flow is obstructed. The technical aspects of fluid therapy are discussed in detail in Chapter 14.

▶ How Much Fluid Should Be Given?

The purpose of fluid therapy is to increase tissue perfusion, repair fluid deficits, supply daily fluid needs, and replace ongoing losses. It has been emphasized that "the aim of therapy is not to administer fluids but to induce positive fluid balance" (Rose 1994b).

Components of Fluid Therapy

The initial assessment of hydration determines the volume of fluid needed to replace the *hydration deficit (replacement requirement)* (Harrison et al. 1960; Finco 1972c). The hydration deficit is calculated as the percentage dehydration (estimated by physical examination) times the patient's body weight in kilograms. The resultant value is the fluid deficit in liters. This calculation underestimates the fluid requirement in hypovolemic shock, wherein the amount of fluid required for treatment may be two to four times the amount of blood lost because of vasodilatation and increased volume of distribution of administered fluid.

Coincident with or after replacement of the animal's hydration deficit, the *maintenance fluid requirement* must be administered (Harrison et al. 1960; Finco 1972c). The maintenance fluid requirement is the volume needed per day to keep the animal in balance (i.e., no net change in body water). It has been suggested that daily fluid requirements (mL/kg/day) parallel energy requirements (kcal/kg/day) (Harrison et al. 1960; Haskins 1984, 1988).

The *basal energy requirement* (BER) is that of a resting animal in a thermoneutral environment 12 to 18 h after eating (Kleiber 1975). In dogs, BER is not a linear function of body weight but rather is related to body surface area by the following equation (Abrams 1977):

$$BER \ (kcal/day) = 97W^{0.655}$$

where W is body weight in kg. This relationship is plotted in Figure 13-7 so that BER may be determined from body weight.

The *maintenance energy requirement* (MER) is that of a moderately active adult animal in a nonthermoneutral environment. The MER in sedentary animals is approximately 1.5 to 2.0 BER. The energy (and presumably fluid) requirements of hospitalized animals are probably somewhat higher than the BER. Animals in catabolic states (e.g., starvation, hyperthyroidism, extensive burns), however, have higher energy (and presumably fluid) requirements.

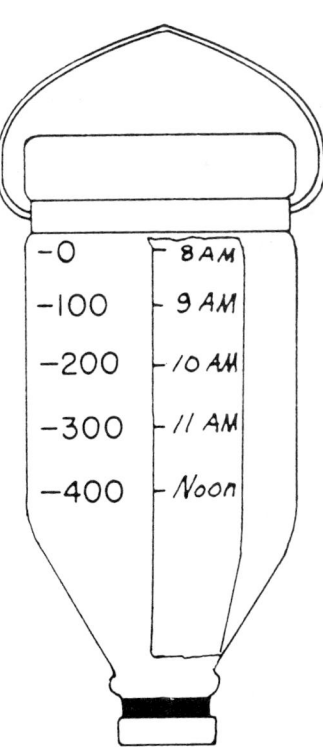

FIGURE 13-4. Use of labeled adhesive tape to monitor rate of fluid administration. (From Chew DJ: Parenteral fluid therapy. In Sherding RG [ed]: *The Cat: Diseases and Clinical Management.* New York, Churchill Livingstone, p. 54, 1989.)

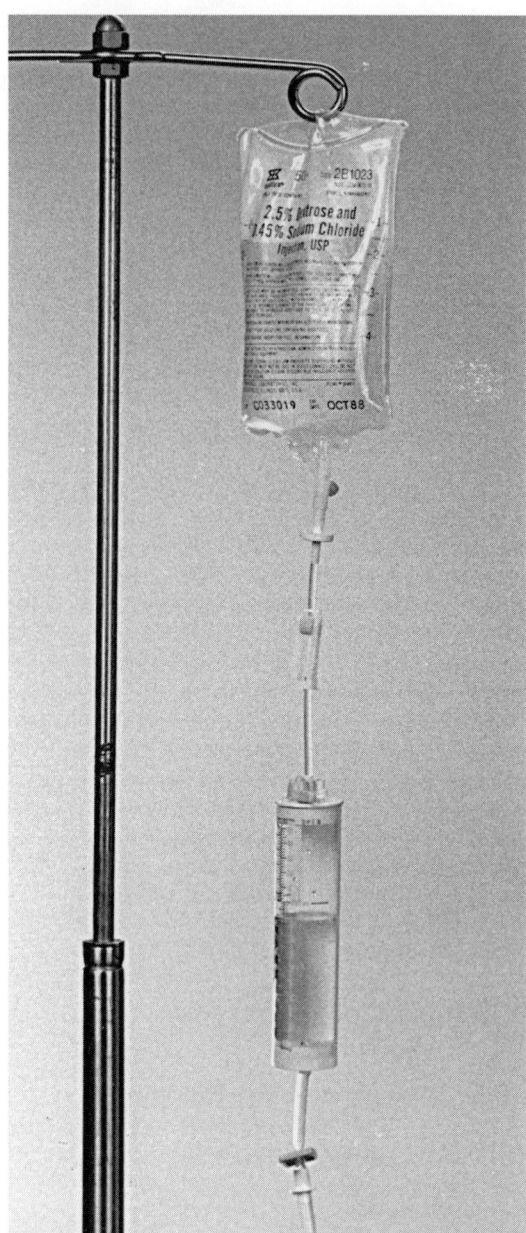

FIGURE 13-5. Buretrol device. (From Chew DJ: Parenteral fluid therapy. In Sherding RG [ed]: *The Cat: Diseases and Clinical Management.* New York, Churchill Livingstone, p. 53, 1989.)

cats is typically estimated as 40 to 60 mL/kg/day (Chew 1977; Chew et al. 1991). Large dogs are prescribed the lower limit (40 mL/kg/day) and cats and small dogs the upper limit (60 mL/kg/day) of this range (Chew 1989). Approximately two-thirds (27–40 mL/kg/day) of the maintenance requirement represents *sensible* (i.e., easy to measure) losses of fluid (urine output) and one-third (13–20 mL/kg/day) represents *insensible* (i.e., difficult to measure) losses (primarily fecal and respiratory water loss). Thus, daily maintenance for a 10-kg dog might be 600 mL, with 400 mL representing sensible loss and 200 mL insensible loss. When estimating the hydration deficit, calculating maintenance needs, and combining these volumes of fluid for delivery over 24 h, the information in

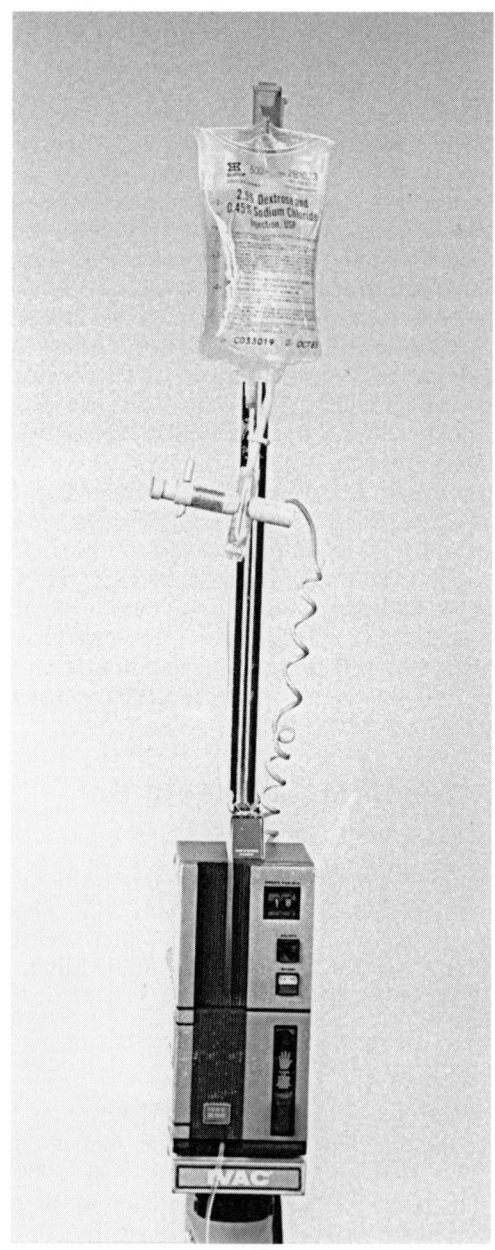

FIGURE 13-6. Fluid infusion pump. (From Chew DJ: Parenteral fluid therapy. In Sherding RG [ed]: *The Cat: Diseases and Clinical Management.* New York, Churchill Livingstone, p. 54, 1989.)

In domestic cats, the relationship of basal heat production to body weight is almost linear because of the small size and relatively narrow normal range of body weight in this species (McDonald et al. 1984). On the basis of available data, BER in cats may be estimated as 50 to 60 kcal/kg/day and MER as 70 to 80 kcal/kg/day. The question remains, however, whether daily energy requirements actually approximate daily fluid requirements. Daily fluid requirements of anorexic dogs and cats in a hospital environment and the relationship of these fluid requirements to the daily urinary solute load are areas deserving future clinical study.

At the Ohio State University Veterinary Teaching Hospital, the maintenance fluid requirement for dogs and

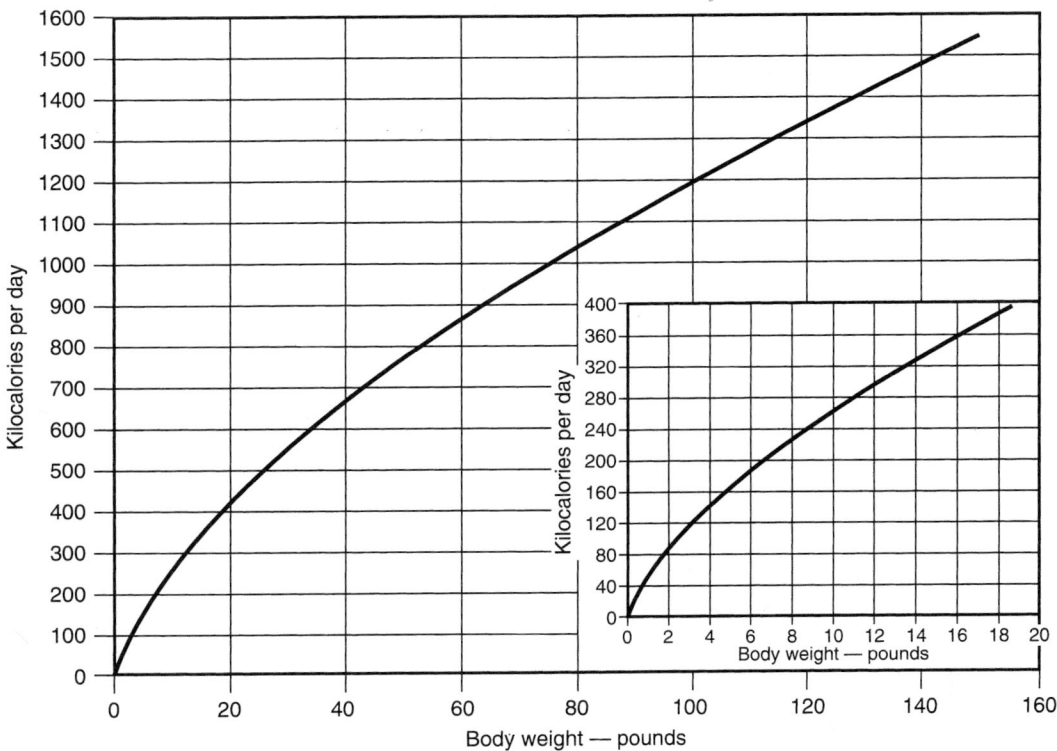

FIGURE 13-7. Basal energy rate as a function of body weight in pounds.

Table 13-9 can be used to determine quickly the rate of fluid administration (assuming that 60 mL/kg/day represents the maintenance rate).

In addition to the hydration deficit (replacement requirement) and maintenance requirement, *contemporary (ongoing) losses* must be considered. These are not always easily determined or quantitated in small animals but can be very important in fluid therapy. An attempt should be made to estimate ongoing losses, which may include losses related to vomiting, diarrhea, polyuria, large wounds or burns, drains, peritoneal or pleural losses, panting, fever, and blood loss. During surgical procedures, careful attention should be given to the amount of blood lost, drying of exposed tissues, and effusions removed by suction. Blood lost at surgery should be estimated and 3 mL of crystalloid solution administered for each milliliter of blood lost. Each 4 × 4 in. gauze sponge, when saturated with blood, represents a blood loss of 15 mL (Muir and DiBartola 1983). Contemporary losses must be estimated and carefully replaced along with the maintenance volume of fluid. Table 13-10 summarizes the components of fluid therapy and their calculation.

Failure to Achieve Rehydration

Repeated assessment of the patient by observation of clinical signs and determinations of body weight, urine output, PCV, TPP, and USG is mandatory in making appropriate readjustments of fluid therapy. Reasons for

TABLE 13-9. **Maintenance and Dehydration Fluid Volume Requirements***

Maintenance (M) + Dehydration (%)	mL/kg/day	Factor × Maintenance
M + 1	70	1.17
M + 2	80	1.33
M + 3	90	1.50
M + 4	100	1.67
M + 5	110	1.83
M + 6	120	2.00
M + 7	130	2.17
M + 8	140	2.33
M + 9	150	2.50
M + 10	160	2.67

Source: Chew DJ, Kohn CW, and DiBartola SP: Disorders of fluid balance and fluid therapy. In Fenner WR (ed): *Quick Reference to Veterinary Medicine*, 2nd ed. Philadelphia, JB Lippincott, p. 570, 1991.
*Maintenance defined as 60 mL/kg/day.

TABLE 13-10. **Calculation of Replacement Requirement (Hydration Deficit)**

1. Hydration deficit (replacement requirement)
   a. Body weight (lbs) × % dehydration as a decimal × 500* = deficit in milliliters
   b. Body weight (kg) × % dehydration as a decimal = deficit in liters
2. Maintenance requirement (40–60 mL/kg/day)
   a. Sensible losses (urine output): 27–40 mL/kg/day
   b. Insensible losses (fecal, cutaneous, respiratory): 13–20 mL/kg/day
3. Contemporary (ongoing) losses (e.g., vomiting, diarrhea, polyuria)

Source: Muir WW and DiBartola SP: Fluid therapy. In Kirk RW: *Current Veterinary Therapy VIII*. Philadelphia, WB Saunders Co., p. 35, 1983.
*500 mL = 1 lb.

failure to achieve satisfactory rehydration include calculation errors, underestimation of the initial hydration deficit, contemporary losses larger than first appreciated (e.g., vomiting, diarrhea), infusion of fluid at an excessively rapid rate with consequent diuresis and obligatory urinary loss of fluid and electrolytes, administered fluid not reaching the extracellular compartment (e.g., technical problems with the intravenous catheter, third-space loss), sensible losses larger than appreciated (e.g., polyuria), and insensible losses larger than appreciated (e.g., panting, fever). Failure to achieve successful hydration is an indication to increase the volume of fluid administered if renal and cardiovascular function are adequate. As a rule, the daily fluid volume may be increased by an amount equivalent to 5% of body weight if the initial infusion fails to restore hydration. Finally, the possibility must be considered that the animal was not dehydrated at presentation (e.g., abnormal skin turgor related to old age or emaciation). This should be considered if the animal does not gain weight despite several days of fluid therapy.

▶ Monitoring Fluid Therapy

It is important to remember that the hydration deficit as estimated by history and physical examination is only an *estimate*, and fluid therapy must be tailored to physical (e.g., body weight) and laboratory (e.g., PCV, TPP) findings over the first few days of fluid therapy.

Physical and Laboratory Findings

A complete physical examination, including evaluation of skin turgor and careful thoracic auscultation, should be performed once or twice daily for animals receiving fluid therapy. Hematocrit, TPP, and body weight should be monitored. Serial body weight is the single most important parameter to follow. Animals receiving continuous fluid therapy should be weighed once or twice daily *using the same scale*. A gain or loss of 1 kg can be considered an excess or deficit of 1 L of fluid, because lean body mass is not quickly gained or lost. A dehydrated patient should gain weight as rehydration is achieved, and afterward weight should remain relatively constant. However, weight increases without restoration of effective circulating volume in patients with severe third-space losses.

Urine Output

The clinician must observe the animal's urine output after fluid therapy has begun. Oliguria should be strongly suspected in patients with acute renal failure, especially those with possible ethylene glycol ingestion.

Urine output should be monitored when fluids are administered intravenously at a rapid rate and renal function is in question. Normal urine output is 1 to 2 mL/kg/h. As the patient becomes rehydrated, physiologic oliguria should resolve, and urine output should increase while USG decreases. If oliguria that was present at admission persists after the hydration deficit has been replaced, it is prudent to divide daily fluid therapy into six 4-h intervals if the status of renal function is uncertain. The calculated insensible volume plus a volume equal to the urine output of the previous 4 h is administered over each 4-h period (known as measuring "ins and outs"). The risk of overhydration is minimized, and fluid therapy keeps pace with urine output even if oliguria is present when this technique is used. If oliguria persists, an increase in the daily fluid volume by an amount equal to 5% of body weight is justified on the assumption that the initial clinical estimate of dehydration was inaccurate. If oliguria does not respond to mild volume expansion, administration of increased volumes of fluid may result in pulmonary edema.

Central Venous Pressure

Measurement of CVP with a jugular catheter positioned at the level of the right atrium allows the cardiovascular response to fluid administration to be monitored. Normal CVP is 0 to 3 cm H_2O. Central venous pressure increases from below normal into the normal range when fluids are administered to a dehydrated animal. A progressive increase in CVP above normal during fluid therapy is an indication to decrease the rate of fluid administration or to stop fluid therapy temporarily. A sudden increase in CVP may indicate failure of the cardiovascular system to handle the fluid load effectively and could result in pulmonary edema caused by left-sided heart failure. In addition to the volume of fluid administered, other factors that may affect CVP include heart rate, vascular capacity, and cardiac contractility. A reduction in any of these three parameters could cause an increase in CVP.

The Frank-Starling curve (Fig. 13–8) relates stroke volume (SV) to left ventricular end-diastolic pressure (LVEDP). If there is no obstruction across the mitral valve, left atrial pressure (LAP) should equal LVEDP, a measure of cardiac function. Pulmonary capillary wedge pressure (PWP) measured with a Swan-Ganz catheter is an estimate of LAP. Generally, there is a direct relationship between right atrial pressure (RAP) and LAP. Thus,

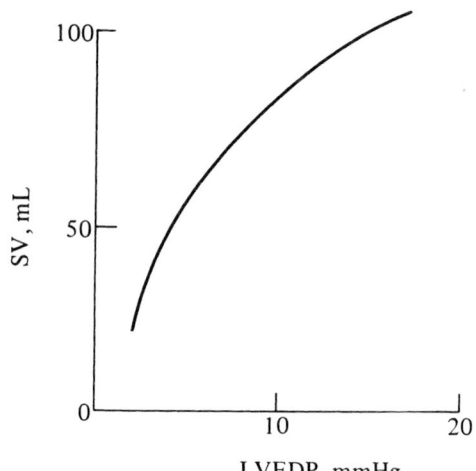

FIGURE 13–8. Frank-Starling law of the heart relating stroke volume (SV) to left ventricular end-diastolic pressure (LVEDP). (From Rose BD: *Clinical Physiology of Acid-Base and Electrolyte Disorders*, 3rd ed. New York, McGraw-Hill, p. 369, 1989, with permission of the McGraw-Hill Companies.)

measuring CVP gives an indirect indication of LVEDP. Without cardiac dysfunction, CVP correlates well with PWP and LAP. In one study (Cornelius et al. 1978), pulmonary artery diastolic pressure and PWP increased before CVP in dogs receiving an infusion of lactated Ringer's solution.

Complications of Fluid Therapy

Signs of overhydration occur when fluid is administered too rapidly. These may include serous nasal discharge, chemosis, restlessness, shivering, tachycardia, cough, tachypnea, dyspnea, pulmonary crackles and edema, ascites, polyuria, exophthalmos, diarrhea, and vomiting (Cornelius et al. 1978). Expected laboratory abnormalities include a reduction in PCV and TPP and an increase in body weight.

When the intravenous route is chosen for fluid therapy, the clinician has made a commitment to careful, aseptic catheter placement and proper maintenance (see Chapter 14). The animal should be checked daily for cleanliness of the catheter site, local pain or swelling, fever, or cardiac murmurs. If any of these signs are observed, the catheter should be removed, its tip cultured, the patient started on appropriate antibiotic therapy, and a new catheter placed in another vein. Even in the absence of complications, the catheter should be removed and an alternative site chosen every 72 h (Schall 1982; Haskins 1984). Complications related to catheter placement include bacterial endocarditis, thrombophlebitis, thromboembolism, and migration of a catheter fragment. When not in use, the catheter should be irrigated with a small volume (<1 mL) of a solution containing 5 U of heparin per milliliter of 0.9% NaCl ("heparinized saline"). The complications of fluid therapy are discussed further in Chapter 14.

▶ When Should Fluid Therapy Be Discontinued?

Ideally, fluid therapy is discontinued when hydration is restored and the animal can maintain fluid balance on its own by oral intake of food and water. As the animal recovers, fluid therapy is usually tapered by decreasing the volume of fluid administered by 25 to 50% per day. During this period, therapy may be changed from the intravenous to the subcutaneous route when possible, based on the volume of fluid to be given each day. If an animal remains anorexic for more than 3 to 5 days, enteral or parenteral nutritional therapy must be considered. Parenteral nutrition is discussed in Chapter 22.

REFERENCES

Abrams JT: The nutrition of the dog. In Rechcigl M (ed): *CRC Handbook Series in Nutrition and Food. Section G: Diets, Culture Media, and Food Supplements*. Boca Raton, FL, CRC Press, p. 1, 1977.

Anderson RS: Water balance in the dog and cat. *J Small Anim Pract* 23:588, 1982.

Bedford PGC and Clark EGC: Experimental benzoic acid poisoning in the cat. *Vet Rec* 90:53, 1972.

Bjorling DE and Rawlings CA: Relationship of intravenous administration of Ringer's lactate solution to pulmonary edema in halothane-anesthetized cats. *Am J Vet Res* 44:1000, 1983.

Chew DJ: Fluid therapy in dogs and cats with renal failure. *Kal Kan Symposium for the Treatment of Diseases of the Dog and Cat*, Columbus, p. 29, 1977.

Chew DJ: Parenteral fluid therapy. In Sherding RG (ed): *The Cat: Diseases and Management*. New York, Churchill Livingstone, p. 35, 1989.

Chew DJ, Kohn CW, and DiBartola SP: Disorders of fluid balance and fluid therapy. In Fenner WR (ed): *Quick Reference to Veterinary Medicine*. Philadelphia, JB Lippincott, p. 561, 1991.

Cohen RD and Simpson R: Lactate metabolism. *Anesthesiology* 43:661, 1975.

Corley EA: Intramedullary transfusion in small animals. *J Am Vet Med Assoc* 142:1005, 1963.

Cornelius LM: Fluid therapy in small animal practice. *J Am Vet Med Assoc* 176:110, 1980.

Cornelius LM, Finco DR, and Culver DH: Physiologic effects of rapid infusion of Ringer's lactate solution into dogs. *Am J Vet Res* 39:1185, 1978.

Cullison RF, Menard PD, and Buck WB: Toxicosis in cats from the use of benzyl alcohol in lactated Ringer's solution. *J Am Vet Med Assoc* 182:61, 1983.

DiBartola SP: Disorders of fluid, acid-base, and electrolyte balance. In Sherding RG (ed): *Medical Emergencies (Contemporary Issues in Small Animal Practice)*. New York, Churchill Livingstone, p. 137, 1985.

Finco DR: Fluid therapy—Detecting deviations from normal. *J Am Anim Hosp Assoc* 8:155, 1972a.

Finco DR: General guidelines for fluid therapy. *J Am Anim Hosp Assoc* 8:166, 1972b.

Finco DR: A scheme for fluid therapy in the dog and cat. *J Am Anim Hosp Assoc* 8:178, 1972c.

Finco DR: Fluid therapy. In Kirk RW (ed): *Current Veterinary Therapy VI*. Philadelphia, WB Saunders Co., p. 8, 1977.

Fiser DH: Intraosseous infusion. *N Engl J Med* 322:1579, 1989.

Fulton RB and Hauptman JG: In vitro and in vivo rates of fluid flow through catheters in peripheral veins of dogs. *J Am Vet Med Assoc* 198:1622, 1991.

Garvey MS: Fluid and electrolyte balance in critical patients. *Vet Clin North Am Small Anim Pract* 19:1021, 1989.

Greene RW and Scott RC: Lower urinary tract disease. In Ettinger SJ (ed): *Textbook of Veterinary Internal Medicine*. Philadelphia, WB Saunders Co., p. 1572, 1975.

Hardy RM and Osborne CA: Water deprivation test in the dog: Maximal normal values. *J Am Vet Med Assoc* 174:479, 1979.

Harrison JB, Sussman HH, and Pickering DE: Fluid and electrolyte therapy in small animals. *J Am Vet Med Assoc* 137:637, 1960.

Hartsfield SM, Thurmon JC, Corbin JE, et al.: Effects of sodium acetate, bicarbonate and lactate on acid-base status in anesthetized dogs. *J Vet Pharmacol Ther* 4:51, 1981.

Haskins SC: Fluid and electrolyte therapy. *Compend Contin Educ Pract Vet* 6:244, 1984.

Haskins SC: A simple fluid therapy planning guide. *Semin Vet Med Surg* 3:227, 1988.

Kleiber M: *The Fire of Life*. Huntington, NY, Robert E. Krieger Publishing Co., 1975.

McDonald ML, Rogers QR, and Morris JG: Nutrition of the domestic cat, a mammalian carnivore. *Annu Rev Nutr* 4:521, 1984.

Monafo W: Expensive salt water. *Surgery* 89:525, 1981.

Moss GS, Lowe RJ, Jilek J, et al: Colloid or crystalloid in the resuscitation of hemorrhagic shock: A controlled clinical trial. *Surgery* 89:434, 1981.

Muir WW and DiBartola SP: Fluid therapy. In Kirk RW (ed): *Current Veterinary Therapy VIII*. Philadelphia, WB Saunders Co., p. 28, 1983.

Otto CM, McCal-Kauffman G, and Crowe DT: Intraosseus infusion of fluids and therapeutics. *Compend Contin Educ Pract Vet* 11:421, 1989.

Rose BD: *Clinical Physiology of Acid Base and Electrolyte Disorders*. New York, McGraw-Hill, p. 455, 1994a.

Rose BD: *Clinical Physiology of Acid Base and Electrolyte Disorders*. New York, McGraw-Hill, p. 409, 1994b.

Rose RJ: Some physiological and biochemical effects of the intravenous administration of five different electrolyte solutions in the dog. *J Vet Pharmacol Ther* 2:279, 1979.

Ryan CP: Toxicity associated with lactated Ringer's solution containing preservatives. *J Am Vet Med Assoc* 12:7, 1982.

Schaer M: General principles of fluid therapy in small animal medicine. *Vet Clin North Am Small Anim Pract* 19:203, 1989.

Schall WD: General principles of fluid therapy. *Vet Clin North Am* 12:453, 1982.

Schwartz WB and Waters WC: Lactate versus bicarbonate. *Am J Med* 32:831, 1962.

Stewart PA: *How to Understand Acid-Base*. New York, Elsevier, 1981.

Stewart PA: Modern quantitative acid-base chemistry. *Can J Physiol Pharmacol* 61:1444, 1983.

Virgilio RW, Rice CL, Smith DE, et al.: Crystalloid versus colloid resuscitation: Is one better? *Surgery* 85:129, 1979.

Willard MD, Zerbe CA, Schall WD, et al.: Severe hypophosphatemia associated with diabetes mellitus in six dogs and one cat. *J Am Vet Med Assoc* 190:1007, 1987.

CHAPTER 14

Technical Aspects of Fluid Therapy
CATHETERS AND MONITORING OF FLUID THERAPY

BERNIE HANSEN

Fluid therapy is an indispensable component of veterinary medical practice. As veterinary emergency and critical care practice has become more sophisticated, there has been increased interest in identifying optimal techniques of fluid therapy delivery. Nevertheless, there have been only a few reports of clinical studies comparing therapies or identifying complications in veterinary patients, and many of the principles described in this chapter are based on interpretation of human medical practice. Whenever possible, the guidelines offered here are based on clinical studies in veterinary patients, experimental work using animal models, the author's personal experience, and a bit of common sense.

▶ Routes of Fluid Administration

The most frequently used routes of parenteral therapy are intravenous, intraosseous, and subcutaneous. Intraperitoneal administration of fluids is potentially hazardous and offers no significant advantages over other routes; therefore it is not discussed further. The route of parenteral fluid administration is chosen on the basis of the underlying disorder and its severity, therapeutic goals, fluid composition, and characteristics of the patient including species, size, age, and accessibility of veins.

Subcutaneous

Subcutaneous administration is a convenient and inexpensive route of maintenance fluid therapy. The volume administered at any single site is limited by the distensibility of subcutaneous tissue. Therefore, fluids are usually administered in the subcutaneous space over the dorsal neck and cranial trunk, where loose connective tissue is abundant. The fluid should be warmed to body temperature before administration to limit the patient's discomfort and enhance local blood flow and absorption. The skin should be cleansed with a cotton ball and alcohol to remove debris from the surface. Fluid may be administered with a syringe and 22 gauge needle in small animals or by gravity flow with a fluid administration set through a 20 to 18 gauge needle in larger animals.

The composition of fluid administered subcutaneously should be comparable to that of extracellular fluid. Fluids devoid of electrolytes (e.g., 5% dextrose in water) should not be used, because electrolyte equilibration into a subcutaneous pool of this fluid may precede significant absorption and transiently aggravate electrolyte imbalances. Fluids can be supplemented with potassium at a concentration up to 40 mEq/L; higher concentrations of potassium are painful and damaging to tissues. Some dogs and cats have limited distensibility of their subcutaneous tissues and rapid administration of even small volumes of fluid creates a hard, painful mass easily detected by palpation. Peripheral vasoconstriction in hypovolemic animals may limit absorption of fluids and prevents successful use of the subcutaneous route. Other potential complications include infection resulting in subcutaneous cellulitis and skin necrosis from caustic or hypertonic fluids or fluids administered under high pressure into an unyielding subcutaneous space.

Intravenous

Intravenous administration is the route of choice when blood volume expansion is desired. It is clearly superior to subcutaneous administration for any critically ill patient with poor perfusion of tissues. Indications for vein cannulation include administration of fluids, drugs, total parenteral nutrition, blood products, intravenous anesthetics, and provision of easy venous access for emergencies.

Intraosseous

Intraosseous fluid administration provides access to the vascular space via the capillary beds of the medullary vascular system. It is an excellent alternative to the intravenous route in animals in which vascular access is technically difficult because of circulatory collapse or peripheral venous thrombosis. This route is best suited for rapid, short-term administration of fluids, blood products, or drugs in emergency situations.

Intravenous Catheters

Catheter products currently available include wing-tip needle, over-the-needle, through-the-needle, venous cutdown, and special-purpose catheters (Fig. 14–1, Table 14–1). Selection of a particular product depends on factors including operator experience, availability, cost, and patient's requirements.

The catheters most often used for routine fluid administration are the over-the-needle and through-the-needle types. Smaller diameter catheters made of soft material are less traumatic to veins than large or stiff catheters. For routine maintenance therapy, the smallest gauge catheter that provides adequate flow should be used. If rapid administration of fluid is required, the largest gauge size possible should be used (Table 14–2). The maximal fluid flow rate increases as the radius of the catheter lumen is increased. For small catheters (20–14 gauge), this relationship is linear, whereas for larger catheters, flow rate increases geometrically with size and is proportional to the lumen radius raised to the fourth power (r^4) (Fulton and Hauptman 1991). Short over-the-needle catheters are preferred for rapid intravenous access in emergencies because they can be inserted rapidly and are available in sizes up to 8.5 French.

Winged Needle Catheters

Winged needle catheters are designed for short-term administration of fluid or drugs into a peripheral vein. They are available in needle sizes of 27 to 16 gauge and with various lengths of plastic tubing connecting the needle to a Luer adapter. Plastic wings at the needle hub facilitate handling and securing the needle. The risk of needle puncture of the vessel wall and subsequent extravasation is high because the sharp needle bevel is left exposed within the lumen of the vein. Therefore, these catheters are best used only for single infusions of nonirritating drugs or fluids under direct supervision. They are usually positioned in the cephalic vein, where there is less risk of displacement by movement of the patient. They must be located sufficiently distal to the elbow that joint flexion wil not displace the needle through the vessel wall.

Over-the-Needle Catheters

Over-the-needle catheters are well suited for rapid insertion into peripheral veins. The wide range of available gauge sizes allows flexibility in vein selection and maximal flow rates. Some are designed for arterial and small-vein cannulation (Arrow Radial Artery catheter, Arrow International) and incorporate a wire guide stylet that

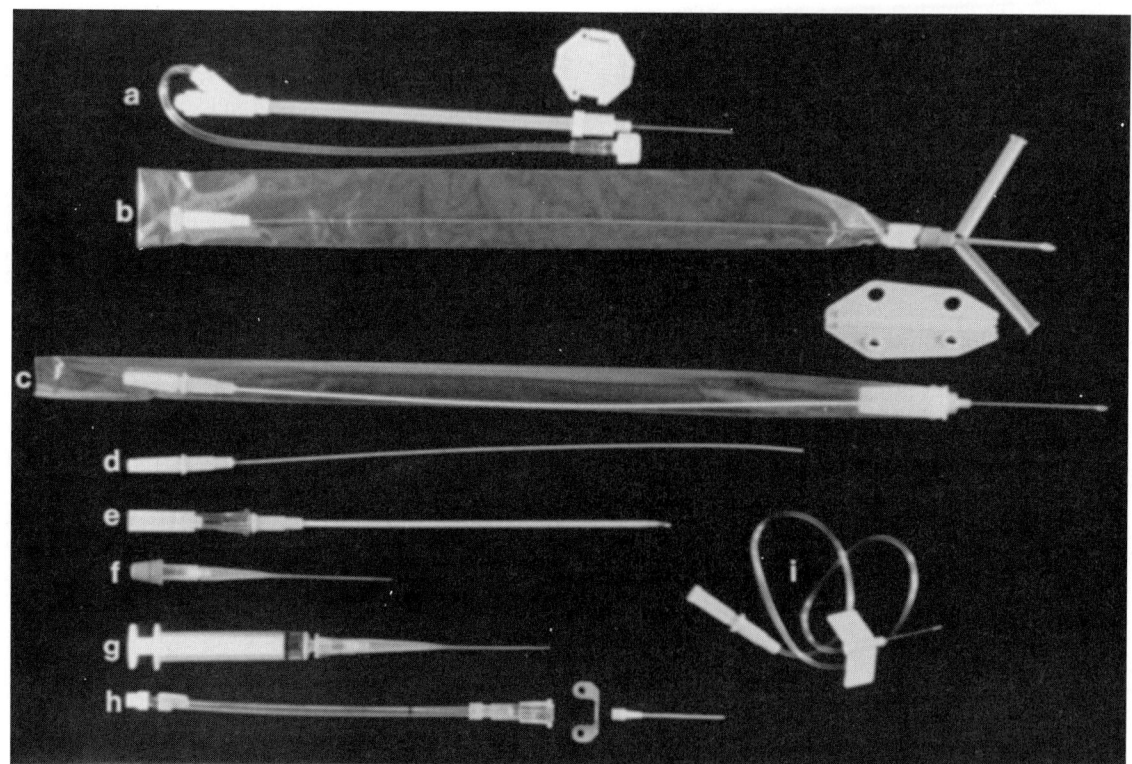

FIGURE 14–1. Examples of different intravenous catheter styles. (A) I.V. Intrafusor (through-the-needle with needle guard), Sorenson Division, Abbott Critical Care. (B) Venocath intravenous catheter (through-the-needle with needle guard), Abbott Laboratories. (C) Intracath intravenous catheter (through-the-needle with needle guard), Becton-Dickinson. (D) Cutdown catheter, Becton-Dickinson. (E) Angiocath radiopaque Teflon catheter (over-the-needle), Becton-Dickinson. (F) Sovereign indwelling catheter (over-the-needle), Sherwood Medical. (G) Argyle Medicut (over-the-needle), Sherwood Medical. (H) Arrow radial artery catheterization set (over-the-needle with wire guide stylet), Arrow International Inc. (I) E-Z Set infusion set (winged needle), Becton-Dickinson.

TABLE 14–1. Intravenous Catheters

Product	Gauges	Material	Radiopaque*	Manufacturer†
Wing-Tip Catheters				
Butterfly	16–25	Needle	U	Abbott Critical Care
Miniset	19–27	Needle	U	Baxter
E-Z Set	16–27	Needle	U	Becton-Dickinson & Co.
Minicath	19–25	Needle	U	Becton-Dickinson & Co.
Short Over-the-Needle Catheters (0.75–6 in.)				
Clear-cath	14–24	Teflon	S	Abbott Critical Care
Abbocath-T	14–24	Teflon	U	Abbott Laboratories
Twin-Cath‡	16–18	Polyurethane	U	Arrow
Arrow Artery Catheterization Sets§	14–22	Teflon	U	Arrow
Quick-Cath	14–24	Teflon	U	Baxter
Flash-Cath	14–24	Teflon	S	Baxter
A-Cath	14–24	Teflon	U	CharterMed
Cathlon IV	14–22	Teflon	N, U, S	Critikon
Jelco	14–24	Teflon	U, S	Critikon
Intima	18–24	Polyurethane	N	Becton-Dickinson & Co.
Angiocath	10–24	Teflon	U	Becton-Dickinson & Co.
Novalon	14–24	Teflon	U	Becton-Dickinson & Co.
Insyte	14–24	Polyurethane	S	Becton-Dickinson & Co.
Streamline	18–26‖	Elastomeric hydrogel	U	Menlo Care
Sovereign	14–22	Polypropylene	N	Sherwood
Sovereign Special	16–20	Polypropylene	N	Sherwood
Argyle Medicut	12–22	Polypropylene	N	Sherwood
Argyle 14 cm Medicut	10–16	Polypropylene	N	Sherwood
Long Over-the-Needle Catheters (6–36 in.)				
Centrasil	16	Silicone elastomer	U	Baxter
E-Z Cath	14–18	Teflon	U	Becton-Dickinson & Co.
Through-the Needle Catheters (6–36 in.)				
IV Intrafusor	15–21	Polyvinyl chloride	S	Abbott Critical Care
Venocath	16–18	Teflon	S	Abbott Laboratories
I-Cath	16–22	Polyvinyl chloride	S	CharterMed
Intracath	16–22	Polyurethane	U	Becton-Dickinson & Co.
Landmark	No. 20–24‖	Elastomeric hydrogel	U	Menlo Care
Argyle Intramedicut	14–20	Polyvinyl chloride	S	Sherwood

*N, Nonradiopaque; S, radiopaque striped; U, uniformly radiopaque.
†Abbott Critical Care Systems, 1212 Terra Bella Ave, Mountain View, CA 94043
  Abbott Laboratories, 100 Abbott Park Rd, Abbott Park, IL 60064
  Arrow International, Inc., Hill and George Avenues, Reading, PA 19610
  Baxter Healthcare Corporation, Alternate Care division, 1425 Lake Cooke Road, Deerfield, IL 60015
  Becton-Dickinson & Co., 1 Becton Dr, Franklin Lakes, NJ 07417
  CharterMed, Inc., 70 Oberlin Avenue North, Lakewood, NJ 08701
  Critikon, In., P.O. Box 31800, Tampa, FL 33631-3800
  Menlo Care, Inc., 1350 Willow Road, Menlo Park, CA 94025
  Sherwood Medical, 1915 Olive Street, St. Louis, MO 63103
‡ Double-lumen catheter.
§ Guide wire assists difficult venous catheterization.
‖ Streamline and Landmark catheters expand two gauge sizes in situ.

facilitates placement. Multilumen catheters (Arrow Twin Cath, Arrow International) allow infusion of incompatible solutions through a single catheter. Over-the-needle catheters are useful for short procedures such as anesthesia and for intravenous fluid administration for 48 h (longer in some patients). These catheters are usually positioned in the cephalic, accessory cephalic, medial and lateral saphenous, or femoral veins. Any accessible superficial vein may be satisfactory (e.g., ear veins in rabbits or dogs with pendulous ears).

There are several disadvantages associated with over-the-needle catheters. They may fray or splinter at the tip during insertion and cause excessive injury to the vein with a high risk of thrombosis. They are difficult to secure adequately and may slide in and out of the skin during a patient's movement. This action facilitates entry of skin surface bacteria through the catheter wound and into the vein. When they are located in distal limb veins, fluid flow through these catheters is often affected by limb position (e.g., elbow flexion often stops gravity flow of fluids through a cephalic vein catheter). Most brands of these catheters are composed of stiff materials and are

TABLE 14-2. Suggested Intravenous Catheter Gauges

Weight	Jugular Vein (Through-the Needle)	Limb Vein (Over-the-Needle)
Maintenance Therapy		
<5 kg	22	24–20
5–15 kg	22–19	22–18
>15 kg	19–16	20–18
Resuscitation		
<5 kg	22–19	22–18
5–15 kg	19–16	18–14
>15 kg	16–14	16–10

not suited for extended dwell periods in an external jugular vein or in veins that cross a joint where motion enhances catheter-induced vessel trauma.

Catheters inserted over a guide wire are a variation of the over-the-needle catheter. These products are designed mainly for pulmonary arterial and central venous catheterization in humans and are available in a variety of lengths. The guide wire technique allows central vein access via insertion into peripheral veins that might not be successfully cannulated otherwise. Silicone elastomer catheters (Centrasil, Baxter; others) are particularly well suited for long-term central venous catheterization in animals receiving total parenteral nutrition. These catheters are not routinely used in small animal practice, however, and are not discussed further.

Through-the-Needle Catheters

Through-the-needle catheters are long (6–36 in.) and are often used to gain deep or central venous access from peripheral sites. The catheter tip may be positioned in a large central vein with rapid blood flow, allowing safe administration of viscous or hypertonic solutions. They are usually used to cannulate the external jugular and saphenous veins. It is often difficult to thread these catheters past the elbow and axillary regions of the forelimb, and they are of limited usefulness in cephalic veins. The rate of fluid flow through a deep or central venous catheter is not affected by body position and movement. Multiple blood samples may be withdrawn easily from these catheters. They may be anchored securely to the skin and tunneled extensively through subcutaneous tissue and are therefore less likely to conduct surface bacteria into a vein than are shorter catheters. Small-vein cannulation is often more difficult than with over-the-needle catheterization, and the risk of catheter or air embolization during catheterization is greater.

▶ Catheter Composition

Catheter composition affects handling characteristics during insertion and influences the potential for thrombosis and phlebitis. Widely used catheter materials include polyvinyl chloride (PVC), polyethylene, polypropylene, polyurethane, silicon elastomer (Silastic), tetrafluoroethylene (TFE Teflon), fluoroethylenepropylene (FEP Teflon), and elastomeric hydrogel (Table 14–3). These materials are chemically inert, but leaching of plasticizers and stabilizing agents from some plastics probably contributes to the development of phlebitis, especially in small veins with low blood flow (Spilezewski et al. 1988; Otto 1990; Wistbacka and Nuutinen 1985). Silicone elastomer catheters are the most chemically inert, whereas PVC, polypropylene, and polyethylene are the most reactive. Teflon and polyurethane are intermediate in reactivity. Catheter thrombogenicity is related not only to chemical reactivity but also to the stiffness of the material and the smoothness of its surface (Hecker and Scandrett 1985; Di Costanzo et al. 1988). Teflon is the stiffest material; polypropylene, PCV, and polyethylene are more flexible. Stiff catheters are easier to pass through the skin and subcutaneous tissues but are more prone to kinking and more likely to damage vessel walls and cause thrombophlebitis. Polyurethane elastomer (Vialon, Arrow International; others) and silicone elastomer catheters are much softer and more flexible. Silicone elastomer catheters are so flexible that they are difficult to introduce into a vein without a stylet or guide wire. Elastomeric hydrogel (Aquavene, Menlo Care) is as stiff as Teflon during insertion but hydrates with plasma water after insertion. Within 30 min, this material softens to the consistency of silicone.

Many brands of catheters are made radiopaque by the addition of heavy metal salts (barium or bismuth) to the plastic. When mixed uniformly into the material, these salts increase the roughness of the catheter surface and increase the risk of thrombosis (Hecker and Scandrett 1985). If embedded within the wall of the catheter, or if the catheter is coated with another, less thrombogenic material (e.g., siliconized PVC), this risk is lower. Heparin coating may significantly reduce catheter thrombus formation (Solomon et al. 1987), but this is available mainly on human central venous catheters that are poorly suited for use in dogs and cats.

Some manufacturers have developed antibiotic-coated catheters that appear to reduce the risk of catheter-associated sepsis. Examples of antiseptics either coated onto or impregnated into catheters include minocycline-rifampin and chlorhexidine–silver sulfadiazine (Raad et al. 1996; Maki et al. 1997).

▶ Vein Selection

Catheter site selection depends on several factors including operator experience, accessibility, therapeutic goals,

TABLE 14-3. Catheter Materials

Material	Reactivity	Stiffness	Thrombogenicity
Teflon	+ +	+ + + +	+ +
Polyether-based polyurethane	+	+ +	+
Polyester-based polyurethane	+ +	+ + +	+ +
Polyvinyl chloride	+ + + +	+ + +	+ + +
Polyethylene	+ + +	+ + +	+ + +
Polypropylene	+ + +	+ + +	+ + +
Silicone elastomer	+	+	+

Relative values for each material: +, minimal; + +, mild; + + +, moderate; + + + +, high.

risk of infection, risk of damage to the catheter, and risk of thrombosis.

Accessibility

Peripheral vein cannulation is most often performed in the cephalic and accessory cephalic veins of the thoracic limbs and the lateral saphenous vein of the pelvic limbs. Other suitable veins include the medial saphenous and (in some cats) the femoral veins and the ear veins in dogs with pendulous ears. In animals with poor tissue perfusion caused by hypovolemia, some of these veins may fill poorly with blood and are difficult to visualize. In this setting, the saphenous veins may be superior because the relatively thin skin overlying them allows better visualization and control over catheter insertion. Catheterization may be facilitated by the vascular access procedures described in the following sections.

Therapeutic Goals

Short-term administration of fluids may be accomplished using any vein, and choice of vein in this setting depends primarily on operator experience and catheter design. Central venous catheterization is preferred in patients that require long-term fluid administration or parenteral nutrition, administration of hypertonic solutions or irritating drugs, frequent blood sampling, or central venous pressure monitoring. Central venous access is most easily accomplished by cannulation of the external jugular, saphenous, or femoral veins. The right external jugular is preferred over the left because this vein joins the cranial vena cava in a straighter line through the brachycephalic trunk than does the left, facilitating catheter passage into the cranial vena cava.

Risk of Infection

The risk of infection is increased in the presence of bandage contamination. Catheters inserted into peripheral veins that are likely to be soiled by vomiting, diarrhea, or urine pose a greater threat. Therefore, the saphenous and femoral veins are not ideal choices in animals with diarrhea or polyuria, and the cephalic vein is not a good choice in an animal with frequent vomiting. There is a greater threat of infection of catheters inserted through a cutdown incision or through skin that is wounded or infected. Unhealthy skin is therefore avoided, and catheters inserted through emergency cutdown incisions are removed as soon as possible.

Risk of Damage to the Catheter

Catheters located in limb veins are particularly accessible to the animal's teeth, and some animals chew at and damage or remove the catheter. Catheters located in an ear vein may prompt scratching and head shaking that eventually dislodge the device. Some form of restraint such as an Elizabethan collar may be necessary to prevent damage to catheters located at these sites. The risk of catheter damage is considerably lower when the jugular vein is used and bandaged adequately. Surprisingly, most dogs and cats do not disturb properly positioned, carefully bandaged intravenous catheters. Animals that chew or scratch at their catheters frequently do so because of excessive irritation. Catheters and bandages that were tolerated initially and subsequently provoke chewing or scratching should be carefully inspected for evidence of tightness, wetness, or infection.

Risk of Thrombosis

There is a risk of thrombosis whenever a vein is cannulated. Thrombosis is more likely in small veins with low blood flow or when a catheter is inserted through a vein that traverses a mobile joint. Some diseases such as vasculitis and autoimmune hemolytic anemia are complicated by increased risk of serious thrombosis and pulmonary thromboembolism (Klein et al. 1989). Intravenous catheterization in these animals is probably accompanied by a higher risk of clinically significant thrombosis than in other diseases. It may be advisable to avoid central venous catheterization in these animals and rely instead on peripheral vein cannulation with short, soft, small-diameter catheters that are removed as soon as possible. Cats with aortic saddle thrombi have poor blood flow to their pelvic limbs and devitalization of those tissues. Pelvic limb vein catheterization in these animals is associated with a high risk of venous thrombosis and infection and must be avoided.

▶ Catheter Placement

Skin Preparation

Except when immediate venous access is required, strict aseptic technique should be used for skin preparation and catheter insertion. If chronic use of an intravenous catheter is anticipated, the skin is prepared as for any surgical procedure.

1. A wide clip centered on the intended venipuncture site is performed.
2. The operator washes his or her hands and dons a clean examination glove on the dominant hand.
3. Local anesthesia with subcutaneous lidocaine often facilitates catheterization. Although some animals react to the transient sting of injected lidocaine, this is often less stressful than the sensation produced by a large-gauge catheter being forced through the skin. Local anesthesia also provides the option of making a facilitation incision at the venipuncture site (see the following). If local anesthesia is desired, the skin is wiped once with an alcohol-soaked cotton ball and the venipuncture site is anesthetized with 0.1 to 0.5 mL of lidocaine administered subcutaneously. Doing this before the sterile scrub allows time for anesthesia to develop before catheter insertion. By mixing eight to nine parts of lidocaine with one to two parts of sodium bicarbonate solution, much of the sting of lidocaine is eliminated. This should be done immediately before administration of the block, because bringing the pH of lidocaine up to a physiologic range greatly shortens its shelf life.

4. The skin is cleaned with cotton balls or gauze sponges and the surgical scrub of choice for at least 2 min. Frequent changing of the cotton balls or sponges facilitates removal of surface debris. The following antiseptic agents are useful:
   a. Chlorhexidine gluconate (Hibiclens, Solvahex). These products contain 4% chlorhexidine and are active against a broad spectrum of gram-positive and gram-negative bacteria. The activity of chlorhexidine is not diminished by the presence of organic matter such as blood and is not appreciably degraded by alcohol. There is considerable residual activity after a single application. Chlorhexidine solutions should not be used on cats because of the risk of stomatitis and esophagitis if the patient ingests any residual solution.
   b. Povidone-iodine (Betadine, Xenodine). This formulation of iodine supplies the antiseptic activity of iodine in a form that is less irritating and less staining than iodine or tincture of iodine. The antiseptic activity is reduced in the presence of organic matter, and this formulation is more likely to cause skin irritation than is chlorhexidine (Osuna et al. 1990a, 1990b). It is the preferred antiseptic for use on cats.
   c. Two percent iodine, tincture of iodine. Iodine is bactericidal at very low concentrations. In the absence of organic matter, a 1% solution kills most surface bacteria within seconds. It discolors hair and skin and frequently causes skin irritation.
   d. Ethyl alcohol, isopropyl alcohol. These agents are typically used as 70% solutions. By themselves, they are erratic germicidal agents and require wet contact for at least 2 min. Hence, they are not particularly useful antiseptics (Burrows 1982). They are commonly used to remove excess surgical scrub from the prepared skin site during catheterization. The germicidal activities of iodine, povidone-iodine, and chlorhexidine are increased in the presence of ethyl alcohol. There appears to be no advantage to using isopropyl alcohol over sterile saline as a final rinse to remove residual antiseptic soap (Osuna et al. 1990b). Isopropyl alcohol causes vasodilatation at the site of application and may promote cutaneous bleeding during venipuncture. This effect may be even more pronounced when using rubbing alcohols, some of which have added rubefacients.
5. Residual scrub solution is removed from the skin and surrounding hair with cotton balls or gauze sponges soaked in alcohol, sterile water, or sterile saline solution.
6. If desired, the skin may be painted with a povidone-iodine solution or an iodine solution. The solution is allowed to dry before catheter insertion.

Percutaneous Catheterization

WINGED NEEDLE CATHETERS

MATERIALS NEEDED (Fig. 14–2)

a. Appropriate catheter
b. 2 clean latex examination gloves
c. 1 roll 1 in. white tape
d. 1 catheter injection cap or catheter "T" piece
e. Syringe with heparinized saline solution, 1 to 2 IU/mL
f. Single dose of povidone-iodine ointment applied on a sterile gauze sponge

▶▶▶ PROCEDURE

1. The venipuncture site is prepared as just described.
2. The operator washes his or her hands and dons clean examination gloves.
3. The catheter is flushed with heparinized saline to purge air from the system. The syringe is then disconnected from the tubing and the catheter held by its "wings" in the dominant hand. To prevent fluid from draining out of the system, the tubing is held coiled in the same hand with the Luer end held level with the needle tip.
4. After an assistant occludes the vein, it is stabilized by tensing the skin slightly with the opposite hand. Neither the needle shaft nor the skin at the intended point of insertion is touched.
5. The catheter is held by the plastic wings with the bevel facing up and is pushed through the skin and into the vein (see Fig. 14–2A). There are two technique options:
   a. Direct puncture: The vein is visualized and the needle tip is positioned directly over the vein and pointed in the same direction as blood flow. While holding the needle at a 30° angle with respect to the long axis of the vein, the needle is advanced through the skin and vessel wall in a single rapid motion.
   b. Indirect method: The vein is visualized and the needle enters the skin slightly to either side of the vein. The needle is pushed through the skin at a 45° angle and is then advanced subcutaneously for 0.5 cm (1/4 in.) parallel to the vein. At that point the needle is redirected at a shallower angle into the vein.
6. Blood flows into the catheter tubing when the vein is entered. The needle is advanced fully into the vein. The risk of penetrating the vessel wall is minimized by lifting the needle slightly as it is advanced (see Fig. 14–2A).
7. The assistant releases the vein.
8. The syringe with heparinized saline is attached to the tubing and the catheter is filled with solution. Alternatively, an intravenous fluid line is attached if immediate fluid administration is desired. The skin near the end of the catheter is observed for any evidence of extravasation at the start of the infusion.
9. The wing tabs are laid flat on the skin surface and a single piece of white tape is wrapped over the wings and around the limb. This tape should be applied snugly but not tightly enough to occlude the vein. The point of entry is not covered by the tape.
10. The gauze sponge with antiseptic ointment is applied to the skin penetration site and is secured to the limb with a second piece of 1 in. white tape.
11. The tubing is coiled and the Luer end is secured to

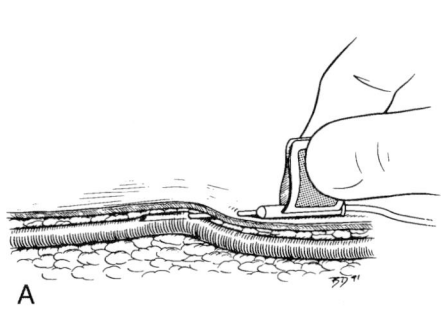
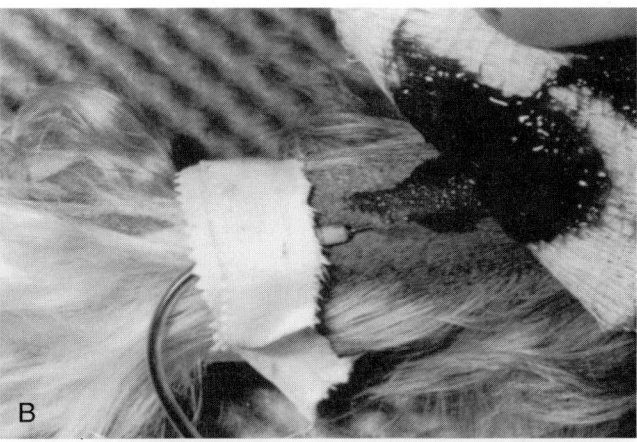
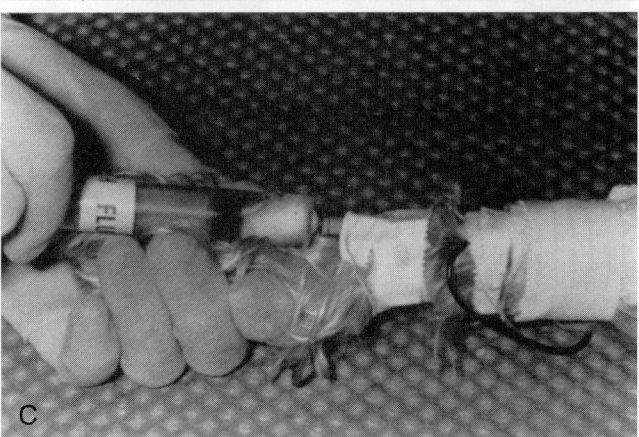

FIGURE 14–2. *(A)* Catheterization of a superficial vein with a winged needle catheter. The shaft of the needle is lifted up against the superficial wall of the vessel and is held parallel to its long axis as the needle is advanced. This maneuver prevents accidental penetration of the deep wall of the vessel. The needle bevel helps prevent inadvertent penetration of the superficial wall of the vessel. *(B)* The catheter is anchored with white tape, and a guaze with povidone-iodine ointment is applied to the point of insertion. *(C)* The gauze is held with another strip of white tape, the catheter tubing is coiled, and the Luer end of the catheter tubing is anchored to the limb with a separate piece of tape. This tape relieves tension on the catheter when the Luer end is manipulated. A final successful aspiration confirms proper needle positioning.

the limb (see Fig. 14–2B) with another piece of tape. This coil helps prevent movement of the catheter if traction is applied to the tubing (see Fig. 14–2C).

OVER-THE-NEEDLE STYLE CATHETERS

MATERIALS NEEDED (Fig. 14–3)

a. Appropriate catheter
b. 2 clean latex examination gloves
c. 1 roll 1 in. waterproof white tape
d. 1 roll each of appropriately sized stretch gauze, stretch bandaging material, and cast padding
e. 1 catheter injection cap or catheter T piece
f. Syringe with heparinized saline solution, 1 to 2 IU/mL
g. Sterile gauze sponges
h. Single dose of povidone-iodine ointment

All materials are arranged ready for use on a clean tray or Mayo stand (see Fig. 14–3A):

a. Antiseptic ointment applied onto a gauze sponge
b. Syringe with heparinized saline attached to T piece and air flushed out
c. Catheter opened and ready for use
d. Tape strips made as needed

▶▶▶ PROCEDURE

1. The venipuncture site is prepared as described before.
2. The operator washes his or her hands and dons clean examination gloves.
3. A small incision through the skin facilitates insertion of large-gauge catheters (18 gauge and larger) or placement of the catheter through tough skin (see the following). The techniques for direct and indirect insertion are the same as noted before. Indirect catheterization is preferred as this forms a subcutaneous tunnel between the point of entry through the skin and the point of entry into the vein that serves as a barrier to bacterial migration.
4. An assistant restrains the animal and occludes the proximal vein. The catheter is grasped firmly at the junction of the needle and catheter hubs, ensuring that the catheter does not loosen and partially slide off the needle during manipulation. The skin is never touched at the point of insertion, nor is the catheter shaft. The needle bevel is directed up during the procedure. The needle is advanced, first subcutaneously, then into the vein. Penetration of the vein often is heralded by a distinct "pop" as the needle punctures the tough vessel wall and by the flow of blood into the needle hub (see Fig. 14–3B).
5. The needle and catheter are advanced *as a unit* for another 3 to 5 mm. This ensures that both the needle and catheter tips are within the lumen of the vein. During this maneuver the needle shaft is held as parallel to the long axis of the vein as practical, and the catheter tip is lifted away from the deep wall of the vein (as described for winged needle catheterization). Once the catheter tip has entered the vessel, the operator grasps the catheter hub with one hand,

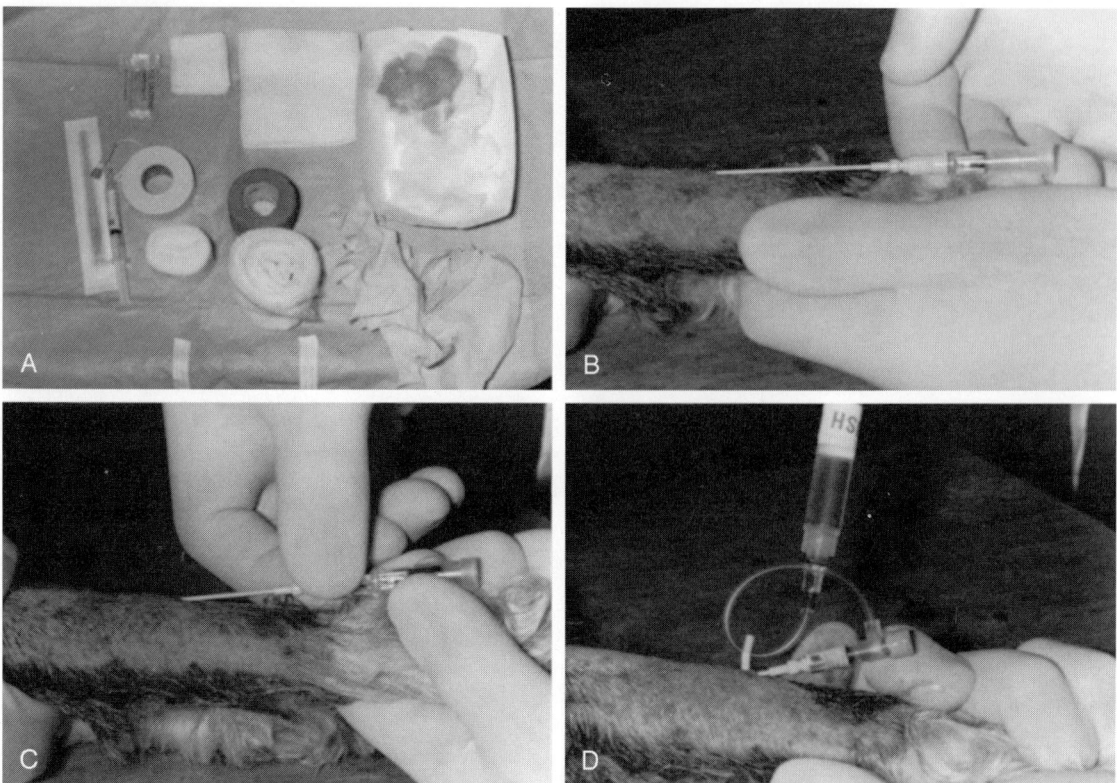

FIGURE 14-3. (A) Materials for over-the-needle catheterization arranged on a tray ready for use. (B) Placement in a cephalic vein. The vein has just been penetrated by the needle tip, and blood flow into the clear needle hub is visible. The needle and catheter are advanced together as a unit a few more millimeters into the vein. (C) Advancing the catheter. Accidental displacement due to patient movement is avoided by firmly gripping the limb with the same hand used to hold the needle hub. The catheter hub is grasped with the other hand, and the catheter is advanced off the needle and up the vein. (D) The catheter is in place. The needle has been withdrawn and set aside, and a T piece, previously filled with heparinized saline solution, is attached. Blood is purged from the catheter by injecting 1 to 2 mL of solution while watching for evidence of extravasation.

the needle hub with the other, and slides the catheter off the needle and into the lumen of the vein (see Fig. 14–3C). If the catheter material is very soft and flexible, an alternative technique is to retract the needle 5 mm back into the catheter and advance the catheter and needle in unison all the way into the vein.

6. The assistant releases the vein and the needle is withdrawn.
7. The catheter injection cap or T piece is attached and the catheter flushed with heparinized saline solution (see Fig. 14–3D).
8. Any blood or fluid on the catheter hub and surrounding skin is cleaned off with sterile gauze sponges.
9. If a cephalic or lateral saphenous vein is cannulated, the catheter hub is wrapped with a strip of 1/2 or 1 in. white tape and this strip is extended around the limb. The tape should be pressed tightly onto the catheter hub but loosely anchored to the limb (see Fig. 14–3E). The goal is to secure it to the limb yet avoid wrapping it too tightly. When cannulating the medial saphenous or femoral vein (or any vein at a large, flat surface), the catheter hub is anchored to the skin with a suture. A single loop of suture material is placed through the skin under the catheter hub and loosely tied with a square knot. The free ends of this suture are then tied tightly around the catheter hub with a surgeon's knot. This suturing technique provides a secure anchor without putting excessive tension on the skin.
10. The point of insertion is covered with antiseptic ointment on a sterile gauze sponge.
11. If the catheter is to remain in place for more than 6 h, it should be covered with a short, light bandage that extends 6 to 12 cm above and below the point of insertion (see later) (see Fig. 14–3F and G).

THROUGH-THE-NEEDLE-CATHETERS

MATERIALS NEEDED (Fig. 14–4)

a. Appropriate catheter (premeasure the desired length)
b. 2 clean latex examination gloves
c. 00 or 000 monofilament nylon, needle holders, suture scissors, 22 gauge needle
d. 1 roll 1 in. waterproof white tape
e. 1 roll each of appropriately sized stretch gauze and cast padding
f. 1 catheter injection cap or catheter T piece
g. Syringe with heparinized saline solution, 1 to 2 IU/mL

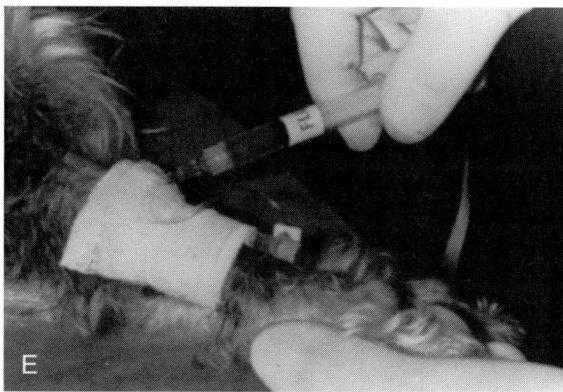
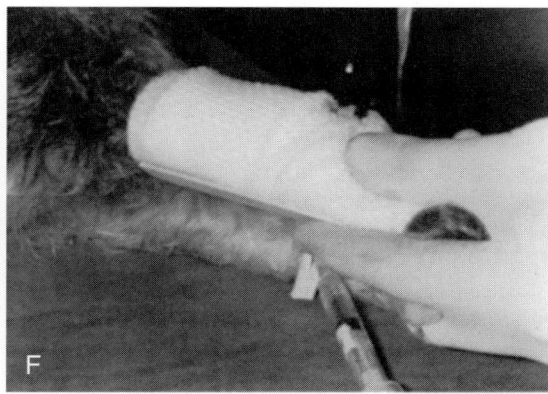
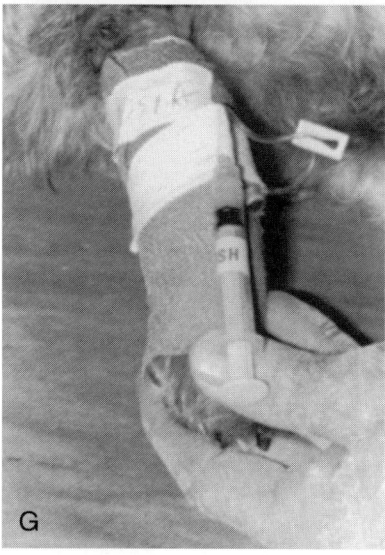

FIGURE 14-3 *Continued. (E)* The catheter hub is anchored to the limb with 1 in. white tape wrapped loosely around the limb. The tape is pressed firmly on the catheter hub, wrapped completely around the limb, and adhered back onto itself. Another tape strip holds a sterile gauze with povidone-iodine ointment over the point of insertion in the skin. *(F)* A thick layer of cast padding has been applied to the limb. Because the catheter hub is near the carpus, a tongue depressor splint is incorporated between the cast padding and elastic gauze to immobilize the joint. *(G)* The completed bandage. White tape is used to anchor the Luer end of the T piece to the bandage. Another piece of tape labeled with the date, time, and operator initials has been applied.

    h. Sterile gauze sponges
    i. Single dose of povidone-iodine ointment
    j. Tube of cyanoacrylate adhesive (Superglue)

All materials are arranged ready for use on a clean tray or Mayo stand (see Fig. 14-4A):

1. Antiseptic ointment applied onto a gauze sponge.
2. Syringe with heparinized saline attached to T piece and air flushed out
3. Catheter opened and ready for use
4. Tape strips made as needed

▶▶▶ PROCEDURE

1. The venipuncture site is prepared as described before.
2. The operator washes his or her hands and dons clean examination gloves.
3. As with over-the-needle catheters, a small skin incision facilitates insertion of large-gauge catheters and eases access through tough skin. The techniques for direct and indirect insertion are the same as noted before. Indirect insertion is preferred as this forms a subcutaneous tunnel between the point of entry through the skin and the point of entry through the vein that serves as a barrier to bacterial migration. The skin at the point of insertion is never touched, nor are the needle shaft and catheter.
4. Proper positioning is critical for successful cannulation of the external jugular vein. In animals with thin skin and large, easily distended veins the procedure is easily accomplished with the animal restrained in lateral recumbency. In this position, the external jugular vein is usually located directly lateral to the trachea. Sternal recumbency or a sitting position is preferred in animals that resist being restrained on their side and in those with thick skin or small, poorly distensible veins. In both the sternal and sitting positions, the animal should be held with its pelvic limbs directed away from the side chosen for venipuncture (see Fig. 14-4B). This maneuver makes the neck more convex on that side and reduces the depth of the jugular furrow. An assistant elevates the head, and the nose is initially held in a horizontal position and directed away from the intended site at a 30 to 45° angle with the median plane. If the animal has abundant loose skin on the neck, elevation of the nose tenses the skin and facilitates identification of the vein. It is helpful to experiment with different head and nose positions until the optimal position is found. If the operator is right handed, the vein is occluded at the thoracic inlet with the thumb of the left hand and the left index finger is used to palpate the vein. The puncture site should be 1 to 2 cm (about 1/2 to 3/4 in.) lateral to the vein and in the cranial half of the neck.

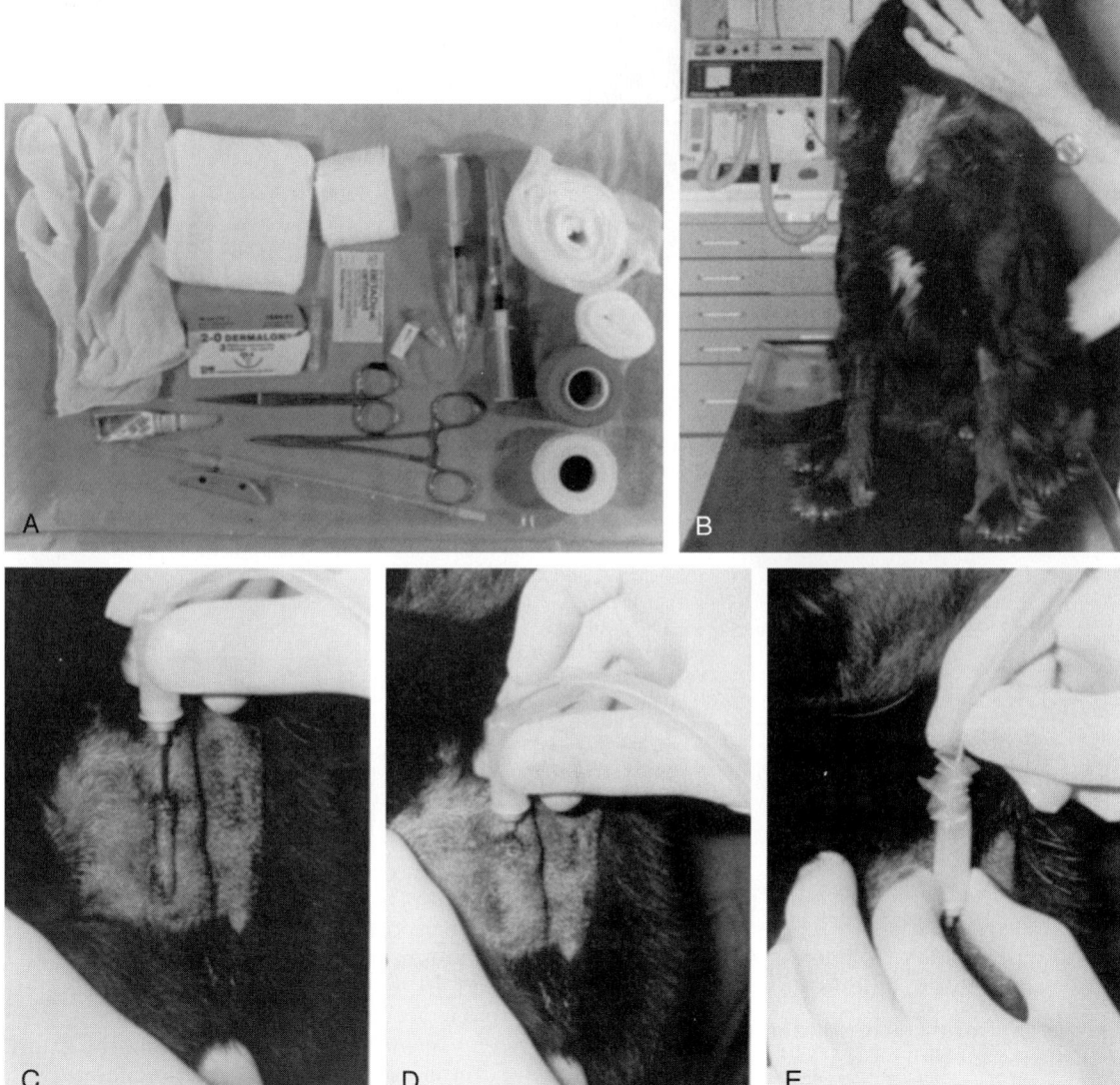

FIGURE 14-4. *(A)* Materials needed for through-the-needle catheter placement are arranged on a tray ready for use. Materials include disposable examination gloves, gauze sponges, povidone-iodine ointment, heparinized saline solution attached to a connector T piece, cast padding, stretch gauze, Vetrap, 1 in. white tape, through-the-needle catheter, suture material, needle holders, scissors, and cyanoacrylic adhesive. *(B)* Proper positioning of a dog for catheterization of the right external jugular vein. Note that the assistant stands to the dog's left, the rear limbs are pointed slightly to the left, and the head is held back with the nose nearly level. This position helps make the jugular furrow shallow and the vein more easily identified. *(C)* Following penetration of the skin, the needle is advanced subcutaneously, parallel to the vein, for approximately 2 cm. *(D)* The needle is then directed into the vein and reflux of blood ("flashback") is seen in the catheter lumen. *(E)* The needle is stabilized with one hand while the catheter is advanced through its protective sheath with the other.

5. The catheter should be fully retracted and not visible at the needle bevel. The device is grasped firmly at the hub of the needle and the skin is penetrated with the bevel of the needle facing away from the skin surface. When possible, the needle is advanced subcutaneously parallel to the vein for at least 2 cm (3/4 in.) before introduction into the vein (see Fig. 14-4C). Penetration of the vein is usually heralded by a distinct pop as the needle punctures the tough wall of the vessel. A flashback of blood entering the needle hub is usually, but not always, seen (see Fig. 14-4D). The catheter is then advanced (see Fig. 14-4E).

6. If successful venipuncture is suspected but no flashback is observed, the operator may try advancing the catheter through the needle. If the catheter is not easily advanced, it is likely that the catheter has entered subcutaneous tissue. In that case, the catheter and needle are withdrawn in unison. The catheter

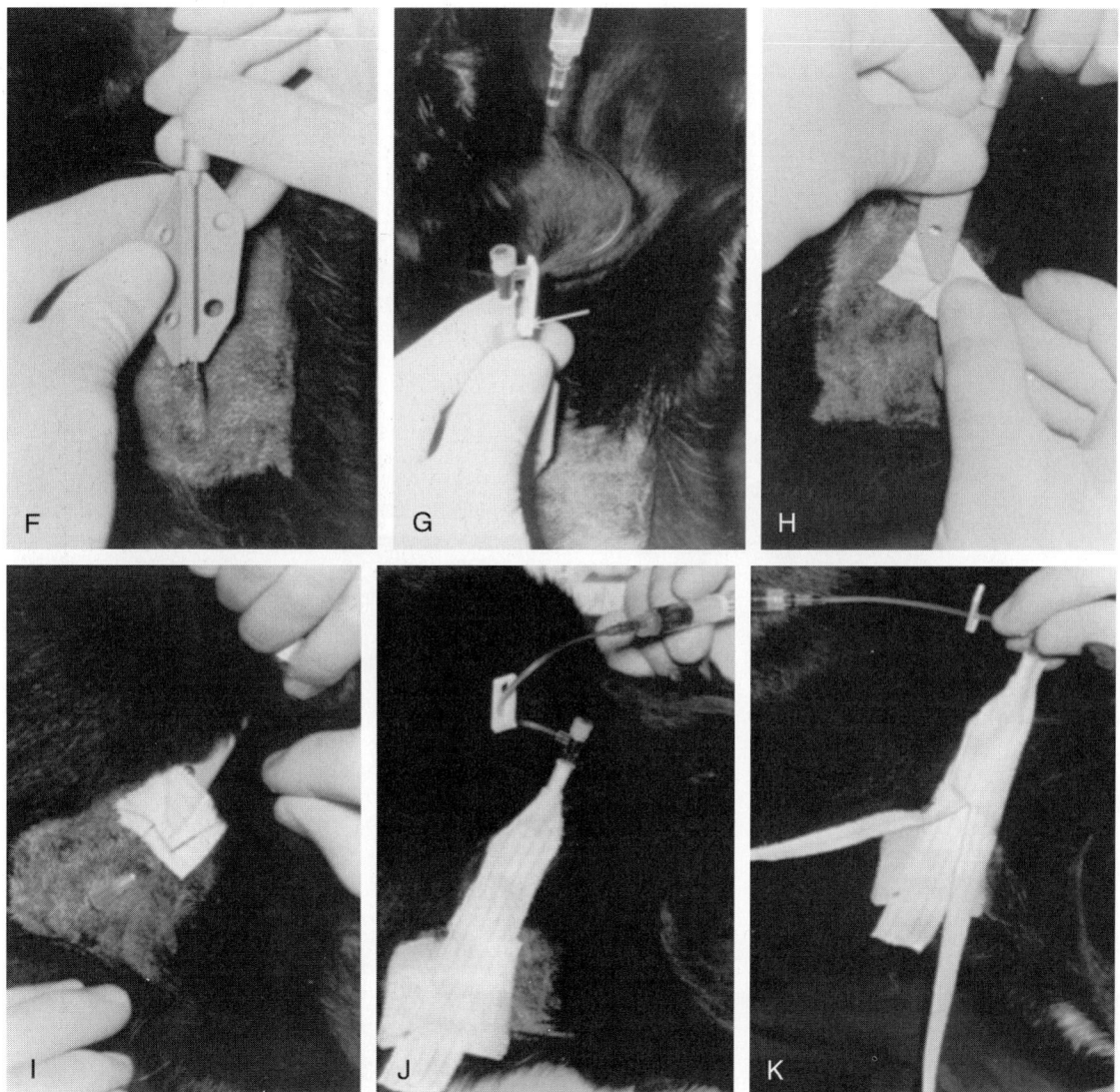

FIGURE 14–4 *Continued. (F)* The catheter needle and proximal catheter shaft are enclosed in a plastic guard. *(G)* A T piece (previously attached to a 3 mL syringe and filled with heparinized saline) has been attached to the catheter. Air is aspirated from the catheter until blood begins to enter the syringe. The syringe is held vertically to trap all air bubbles in the syringe. The catheter is then purged of blood by injecting 1 to 2 mL of the heparinized saline. If desired, a drop of cyanoacrylic adhesive is applied to the joint between the needle hub and catheter hub (arrow) and the two are pressed together. *(H)* The catheter is withdrawn 1 to 2 cm and dried with a sterile gauze sponge, and the needle guard is positioned in the desired final orientation (i.e., pointed dorsally at a right angle to the long axis of the cervical spine). A piece of waterproof white tape is then folded over the exposed catheter and the end of the needle guard to prevent kinking of the catheter tubing. *(I)* Two sutures are placed through the tape and anesthetized skin to anchor the catheter securely. Threading the suture through a preplaced needle is often easier than using a swedged-on needle. *(J)* A 2 × 2 sterile gauze sponge with povidone-iodine ointment has been applied at the point of insertion, and a strip of white tape has been applied over the assembly. This tape is firmly pressed onto the catheter Luer hub, the needle guard, and the anchoring tape; thus it holds the catheter to the anchored tape and keeps the gauze in place. *(K)* A long strip of 1 in. white tape has been split lengthwise up to the last 3 in. The unsplit end is firmly pressed over the catheter assembly. One-half is wrapped loosely around the dog's neck, traveling dorsally on the ipsilateral side. The other half is wrapped in the opposite direction. This tape loosely (but securely) anchors the catheter to the dog's neck.

Illustration continued on following page

should not be pulled back through the needle until the needle is withdrawn because of the risk of shearing on the needle bevel. The needle and catheter are inspected for damage; if none is present, another attempt is made. This and any subsequent attempts are made through the original skin wound.

7. Because the needle forms a hole in the vessel wall that is larger in diameter than the catheter, postcatheterization hemorrhage is occasionally a problem. This can be minimized by holding the venipuncture site above the level of the heart to reduce venous pressure, such by performing jugular vein cannulation with the

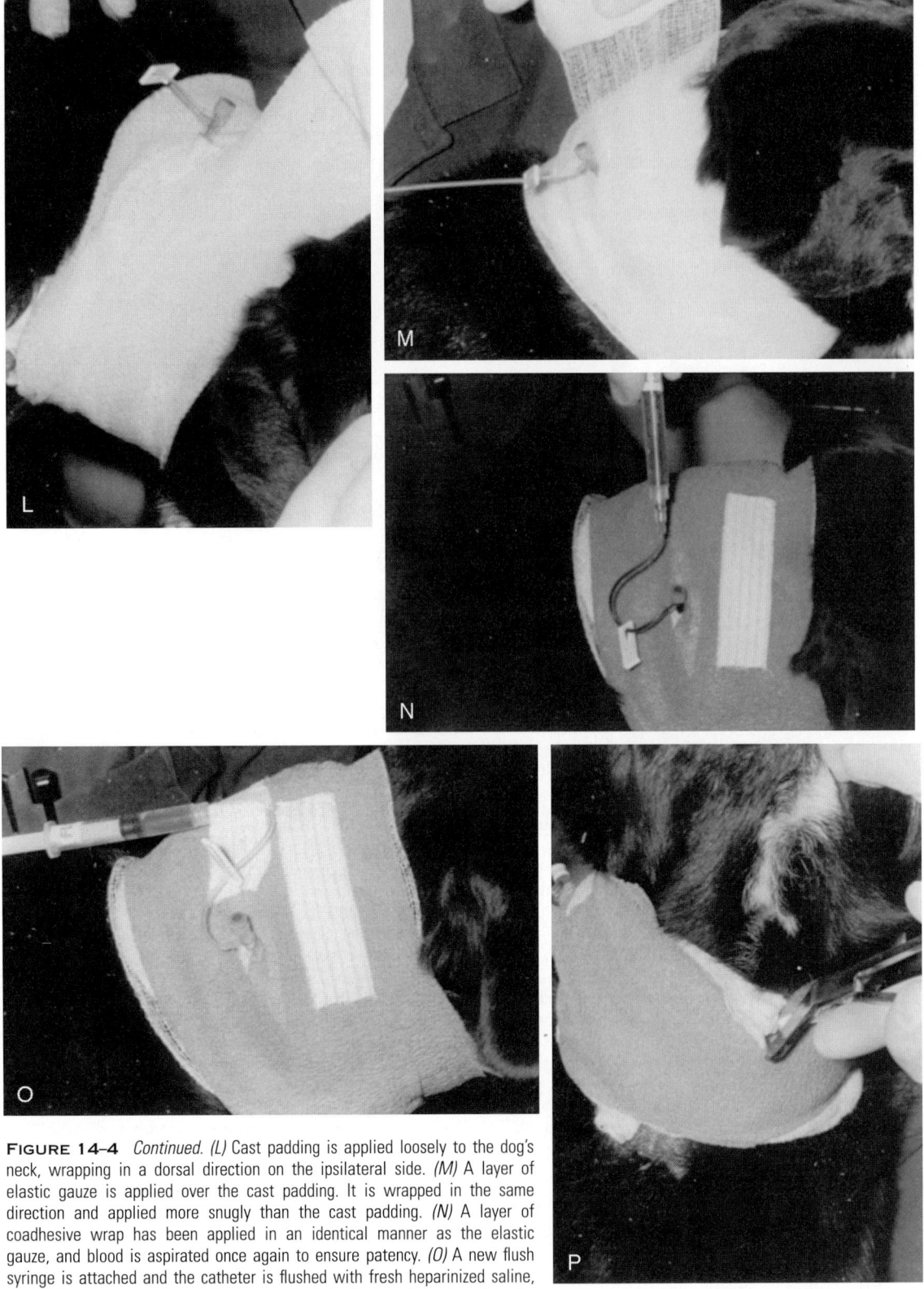

FIGURE 14–4 *Continued.* *(L)* Cast padding is applied loosely to the dog's neck, wrapping in a dorsal direction on the ipsilateral side. *(M)* A layer of elastic gauze is applied over the cast padding. It is wrapped in the same direction and applied more snugly than the cast padding. *(N)* A layer of coadhesive wrap has been applied in an identical manner as the elastic gauze, and blood is aspirated once again to ensure patency. *(O)* A new flush syringe is attached and the catheter is flushed with fresh heparinized saline, the T piece is clamped, and the Luer end of the T piece is anchored to the bandage with white tape. *(P)* The ventral aspect of the bandage is examined with the dog's head held in a mildly flexed position. If the bandage appears tight, it may be partially cut as shown here to relieve tension.

animal in a sitting position. Accurate needle positioning minimizes laceration of the vein, and rapid application of a sterile dressing and bandage provides direct compression.

8. Depending on the brand of catheter used, the needle is split off the catheter or is covered with a plastic needle guard as directed by the manufacturer (see Fig. 14–4F).
9. The T piece or catheter injection cap is attached to the Luer hub. The syringe with heparinized saline solution is then attached to the T piece or, if an injection cap is used, the cap is penetrated 1 to 2 mm with a needle attached to the syringe. Air is aspirated from the catheter and patency is confirmed by successful aspiration of blood. The catheter then is filled with heparinized saline solution (see Fig. 14–4G).
10. The catheter is withdrawn 1 to 2 cm (1/2–3/4 in.) from the skin and dried with a sterile gauze sponge. A 2.5 to 5 cm (1–2 in.) butterfly of waterproof white tape is wrapped around the catheter and needle guard and is sutured to the skin at points on both sides of the catheter within 0.5 cm (0.2 in.) of the penetration site. This piece of tape should bridge the needle guard and the exposed portion of catheter to where it enters the skin (see Fig. 14–4H and I). Through-the-needle catheters frequently fail because of kinking at the point of exit from the needle guard or the point of entry into the skin. The tape prevents this by forming a protective "sandwich" around the catheter as it exits the needle guard or hub.
11. The point of insertion is covered with the antiseptic-treated gauze sponge.
12. The Luer connection at the junction of the needle and catheter hubs is dried with a sterile gauze sponge and a drop of cyanoacrylate adhesive may be applied to the surfaces before forcing them together. Alternatively, this connection may be bridged with a strip of tape (see Fig. 14–4J).
13. The catheter is anchored with a strip of white tape (see Fig. 14–4K). If a jugular vein is cannulated, the tape is anchored to the base of the needle guard and then wrapped up the neck in a dorsal direction on the ipsilateral side to help prevent the catheter from slipping ventrally later. The goal is to secure the catheter to the skin, not to wrap it on tightly.
14. Cast padding, stretch gauze, and elastic bandage material are applied, wrapping dorsally on the ipsilateral side in the case of a jugular vein catheter. While wrapping the catheter bandage, the limb or neck is held in a natural position (partially flexed limb or nose pointed down) to prevent binding (see Fig. 14–4L through P).

Vascular Access Procedures

These techniques aid catheterization when direct percutaneous access is difficult. They are especially helpful in emergencies when cannulation with a large-gauge catheter is required (Crowe 1988, 1990; Haskins 1988).

PERCUTANEOUS FACILITATION PROCEDURE

A small incision is made through the skin at the intended point of entry directly over or just to the side of the vein. This incision is easily made with the bevel edge of an 18 gauge needle or with a number 11 blade. In the conscious patient, local anesthesia is administered with subcutaneous lidocaine at least 2 min before the procedure is performed. The needle or blade is held like a pencil and the skin is incised to the subcutis for up to several millimeters in length, creating a wound large enough for the catheter to pass through. This incision reduces the resistance encountered as the catheter traverses the skin and provides greater control of the venipuncture when compared with forcing the catheter through unbroken skin.

MINICUTDOWN PROCEDURE

This approach is the same as the facilitation procedure, but the incision is sufficiently extended so that the vessel's sides and superficial surface are visible. The vessel may be catheterized directly or may be carefully dissected free of surrounding tissue, elevated from the wound, incised with the bevel of a 20 gauge needle, and catheterized. Entry into the vein is facilitated by use of a disposable catheter spade introducer (Catheter Introducer, Becton-Dickinson) or a bent hypodermic needle. This procedure is best done on any superficial vessel that has not been previously traumatized by percutaneous attempts. It is a rapid, reliable technique in emergency situations when direct percutaneous catheterization is difficult because of vascular collapse. However, it is frequently difficult to maintain sterility during insertion and the catheter should be removed as soon as possible.

EMERGENCY CUTDOWN PROCEDURE

An emergency cutdown is used to cannulate a limb vein when attempts at percutaneous catheterization have failed or are likely to fail in a patient that requires immediate venous access. *This is an essential skill for emergency clinicians that should be applied to any patient requiring immediate venous access.* The preferred vein is the lateral saphenous (because the thin skin overlying this vein facilitates access), but the same technique may be used for access to the cephalic or medial saphenous veins. With practice, the operator should be able to obtain vascular access within 30 to 60 seconds.

If time permits, the hair is clipped and the skin cleaned. This step may be omitted in patients requiring immediate access. Conscious animals may require local anesthesia with 1 to 2% lidocaine/bicarbonate. A 0.5 to 1.5 in. incision is made with a number 11 Bard-Parker blade parallel to, but not directly over, the vein. The incision is made just cranial (lateral saphenous) or lateral (cephalic) to the vein. The wound is retracted to expose the vein, and a closed, curved tip mosquito forceps is then pushed down directly on the vein. The jaws are opened to bluntly strip perivascular fascia away from the vein. The forceps are lifted from the wound, the jaws are closed, and the step is repeated three to five times. Aggressive pressure directly on the vein is necessary to strip away the fascia effectively. This is critical to allow rapid, reliable access to the vein lumen in the next step. Then the jaws of the forceps are closed and the instrument tip is passed under the vein and advanced so that the vein is stretched over the handles at the fingerholds.

A small venotomy incision is made with the blade, and a disposable catheter introducer is inserted completely into the wound. A large-bore over-the-needle catheter is inserted into the venotomy, with the needle pulled back from the tip of the catheter.

Once the tip of the catheter is in the vein, the introducer is removed and the forceps are pulled toward the paw to straighten and stretch the vein. The catheter is advanced off the needle, the needle withdrawn, and an intravenous fluid line connected directly to the catheter. The wound edges are then drawn together, and the entire area is wrapped with white tape to close the wound temporarily, protect it from contamination, and secure the catheter–fluid line to the limb. When the patient has been stabilized, an elective, sterile catheter should be inserted into a different limb and the cutdown catheter removed.

To remove the catheter, the tape is removed and the wound liberally flushed with a sterile irrigant solution. Sterile 4 × 4 in. gauze sponges are held over the area and the catheter is withdrawn. Firm pressure applied over the area for 2 to 3 min usually prevents continuous hemorrhage. The sponges are then removed and the wound carefully irrigated some more. If the venotomy incision continues to bleed, partial or complete ligation may be necessary. The proximal two-thirds to three-fourths of the skin incision is closed using monofilament nylon, leaving the distal section free to drain. The wound is covered with a light dressing that is changed at least daily until healing is advanced, usually 3 to 5 days.

ELECTIVE CUTDOWN PROCEDURE

This surgical procedure should be performed under sterile conditions. Conscious animals are anesthetized or sedated with an opioid analgesic and a tranquilizer (e.g., oxymorphone 0.05 to 0.10 mg/kg and acepromazine 0.05 mg/kg intravenously). Local anesthesia with lidocaine is administered if needed. The skin over the intended vein is prepared and draped. A long (2.5–5 cm; 1–2 in.) incision is made through the skin slightly to one side of and parallel to the vessel. The vein is identified and dissected free with fine curved strabismus scissors and hemostats. If a hematoma from previous percutaneous attempts at catheterization is present, the vein is difficult to locate. The vein usually lies at the center of the hematoma and is visible as a longitudinal off-white band coursing through it (Haskins 1988). The vein is stretched over the closed handles of a mosquito forceps and a small venotomy incision is made between the two handles. The vein is catheterized as described in the preceding section.

The wound is irrigated and the skin is closed around the catheter. If the catheter is to remain in place for a long time, as for parenteral nutrition, the catheter should be tunneled subcutaneously 2 to 20 cm (1–8 in.) and exit a sterile site at a convenient location. This subcutaneous tunnel serves as a barrier to bacterial migration along the catheter wall.

INTRAOSSEOUS VASCULAR ACCESS

This route is useful for emergency administration of fluids, blood products, and drugs to animals in which rapid vascular access is difficult because of vascular collapse or small size of the patient (Fiser 1990; Otto et al. 1989). The most commonly used sites include the intertrochanteric fossa of the femur, the wing of the ilium, the tibial tuberosity, the medial surface of the proximal tibia 1 to 2 cm (1/2–3/4 in.) distal to the tibial tuberosity, and the greater tubercle of the humerus.

MATERIALS NEEDED (Fig. 14–5A)

a. 2% lidocaine injection
b. Number 11 scalpel blade
c. Needle: 16–20 gauge bone marrow needle (dogs, cats)
   18–22 gauge spinal needle (cats, young dogs)
   18–25 gauge hypodermic needle (neonates of any species)
   Commercial intraosseous needle (Cook intraosseous infusion needle, Cook Critical Care)
d. 12 mL syringe
e. Heparinized saline solution in a 3 to 6 mL syringe
f. Antiseptic ointment on a sterile gauze sponge
g. Limb stocking material
h. Bandaging material

▶▶▶ PROCEDURE

1. The site is clipped and prepared aseptically when conditions permit. In the conscious animal, the skin and periosteum are anesthetized with lidocaine.
2. A stab incision is made through the skin with the blade and the needle is introduced into the wound and advanced to the periosteum. The needle is seated into the cortex by pushing the needle lightly into the bone while rotating it about its long axis back and forth over 30° turns.
3. When the needle is seated in the cortex, the pressure applied to it is increased and it is rotated and forced through the cortex. A sudden loss of resistance is often felt as the cortex is breached.
4. The position of the needle may be tested by flicking it with a finger. If the needle is firmly seated in bone, it will not wobble when struck. When the limb is moved, the needle should move solidly with the bone.
5. The 12 mL syringe is used to apply vacuum. If the needle tip is within the bone marrow, some marrow elements should enter the syringe. The needle is then flushed with heparinized saline solution. Little or no resistance should be felt. Fluid delivered by gravity flow should flow freely (Fig. 14–5B). If it fails to do so, the needle is rotated 90 to 180° to move the bevel edge away from the inner cortex. The fluid infusion is begun and the surrounding tissue is frequently palpated and observed for any evidence of fluid leakage from the bone. Leakage usually occurs when the needle has penetrated the opposite cortex and the tip is outside the bone or when excessive rocking motion was used during insertion, leaving a large hole in the cortical bone surrounding the needle through which fluid escapes.

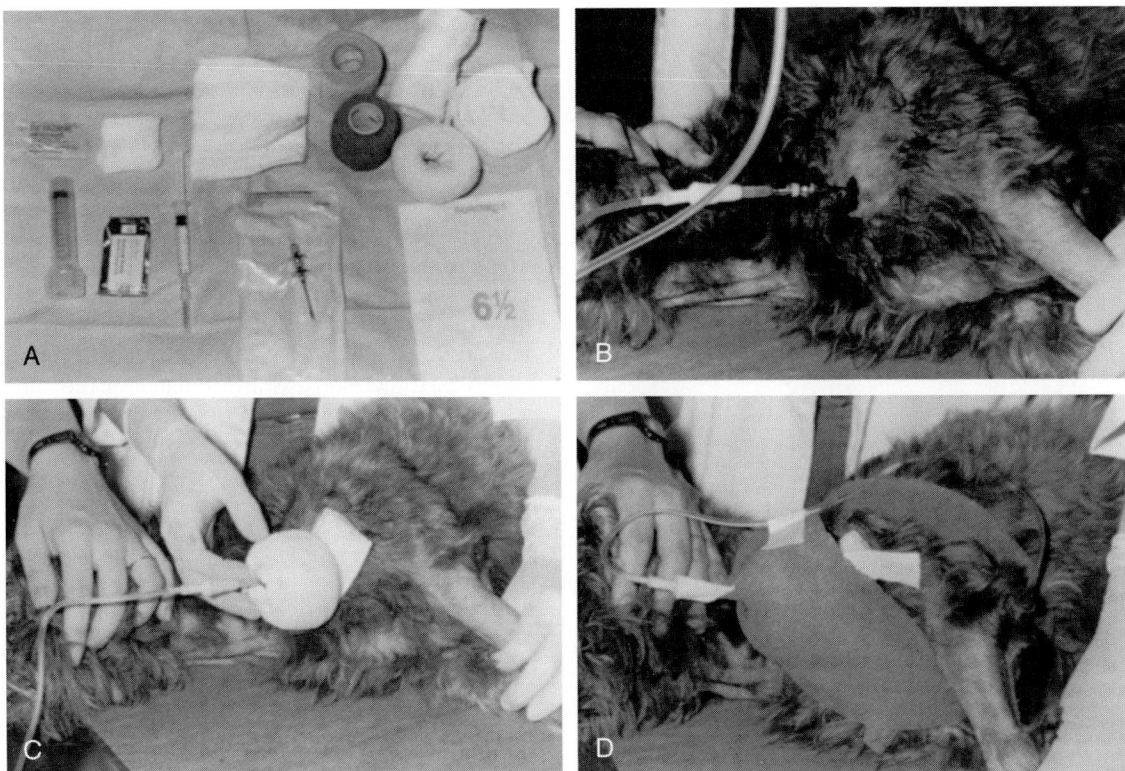

FIGURE 14–5. (A) Materials used for placement of an intraosseous needle catheter arranged on a tray and ready for use. (B) A bone marrow needle has been placed in the greater tubercle of the humerus, and a fluid administration set is attached if immediate administration of fluids is required. (C) The needle is bandaged in place if it is to remain in place for an extended period. The administration set is temporarily disconnected and a "doughnut" of sterile limb stocking material is placed around the bone marrow needle. This roll should be thick enough to extend past the needle hub. (D) The catheter and limb stocking material are bound firmly to the dog with bandage material.

6. When the needle is properly positioned, it is anchored by passing a suture through the periosteum and tying it to the hub of the needle or to a tape butterfly secured to the hub. The entry site is covered with antiseptic ointment. A "doughnut" of limb stocking material is placed around the needle. It should be thick enough to be level with the top of the needle hub (Fig. 14–5C). The padding is then secured to the patient with bandaging material (Fig. 14–5D).

Bandaging

All intravenous catheters must be secured adequately to the body. Catheters left in place for over 6 h should be covered with a sterile dressing and a bandage that provides protection against traction, damage, and contamination. The bandage should be heavy enough to protect the catheter but should not be completely occlusive so that moisture can evaporate from the skin and dressing. The point of entry should be covered with povidone-iodine ointment on a sterile gauze sponge. Povidone-iodine is preferred over triple-antibiotic ointments, which have been shown to support growth of fungi and resistant bacteria (Norden 1969; Zinner et al. 1969). Catheters used for short procedures may be dressed with a small amount of ointment at the entry site and secured to the neck or limb with white tape. White tape is inelastic and must be wrapped loosely (with the neck or limb held in a natural position) to prevent binding, venous occlusion, and edema. Additional stability is achieved by suturing the catheter hub to the skin before wrapping. The catheter should be anchored securely enough to minimize any in-and-out movement through the skin. This allows the skin to close around the catheter and form a natural barrier to bacterial migration. Interestingly, there is little evidence from human patients that any type of dressing reduces the incidence of catheter infection compared with catheters left exposed and kept clean and dry.

If the catheter is to remain in place for longer periods, a layer of cast padding thick enough to provide some physical support to the entire bandage is applied. A layer of stretch gauze may be wrapped around the padding; this should be applied snugly enough to create a firm unit of material but not tightly enough to occlude venous return. The outermost layer may be an adhesive (Elastikon, Johnson & Johnson) or coadhesive (Vetrap, 3M Animal Care Products) bandaging material. This material is also wrapped on snugly but not tightly enough to occlude venous return. If the animal is prone to peripheral edema, a limb bandage may be extended distally to the paw. This is not routinely necessary, however, in an ambulatory animal with a properly applied catheter bandage. A heavy full-limb bandage may be used (with or without a rigid splint) if the indwelling catheter crosses a joint. Immobilization of the joint in this setting helps reduce endothelial trauma and may help prevent venous thrombosis secondary to mechanical injury by the catheter.

▶ Catheter Maintenance

The need for an intravenous catheter should be reviewed daily and the catheter removed when it is no longer therapeutically necessary. Until then, the vein and the limb or face should be examined three times daily for evidence of infection or edema. Regional lymph nodes should be palpated for signs of swelling or tenderness. If any evidence of inflammation or thrombosis is found, the catheter should be removed. If the bandage is too tight, it should be loosened or completely replaced. When distal edema is evident, the culprit is usually white tape that was applied too tightly.

Over-the-needle catheters are routinely removed after 48 h when practical. The dressing covering a through-the-needle catheter should be routinely replaced at 48 to 72 h or more frequently if it appears wet or soiled. At this time the skin and vein are examined and palpated for evidence of inflammation or thrombosis. If either is suspected, the catheter is removed. If the catheter and vein appear in good condition, the skin surrounding the entry site is cleansed with an antiseptic scrub and cotton balls. Disruption of the entry wound or any in-and-out movement of the catheter through the wound is avoided. The skin is allowed to dry completely, fresh antiseptic ointment on a sterile gauze is applied, and the catheter is rewrapped. Percutaneously inserted through-the-needle catheters are routinely removed after 4 days; however, they may be safely left in place for longer periods if they were inserted using a long subcutaneous tunnel and are carefully maintained (Mathews et al. 1996). If intravenous therapy is to be continued, a new catheter is inserted before the old one is removed whenever possible. Intraosseous catheters are removed when they are no longer needed, when fluid begins leaking into surrounding tissue, or by 48 h, whichever comes first. Surgically inserted catheters made of inert materials and with long subcutaneous tunnels may be left in place for periods ranging from days to months.

Catheters should be flushed periodically with heparinized solution to reduce the risk of clot formation. No objective studies have addressed this issue in veterinary patients, but several studies of human patients suggest that heparin solutions provide some protection against catheter occlusion. For example, the patency of indwelling intravenous catheters used in human obstetric patients is better maintained with a dilute heparin flush (100 IU/mL, q6h) than with saline (Meyer et al. 1995). On the basis of human practice and observations of veterinary patients, catheters that are not being used may be filled once daily with undiluted heparin (1000 IU/mL). Catheters used for intermittent administration of drugs should be flushed with diluted heparin (1000 U/10–500 mL) in 0.9% saline immediately after drug administration. If intravenous fluids are administered continuously, periodic flushing may be unnecessary. Frequent flushing with higher concentrations of heparin in cats and small dogs may produce systemic anticoagulation and should be avoided.

Sterility of the infusion system must be maintained. Only new sterile administration sets should be attached to a new catheter and disconnections are made only when essential. The patient's end of the administration tubing is anchored to the catheter bandage with a piece of white tape to relieve traction and prevent separation of the Luer connection to the catheter. All intravenous tubing and containers are changed every 48 to 72 h or sooner if contamination is suspected. Injection ports should be cleaned carefully with 70% isopropanol before needle puncture. Injection caps are replaced if they are observed to leak or if they have been penetrated more than approximately 20 times.

▶ Complications of Intravenous Therapy

Extravasation

Extravasation of fluid and infiltration of surrounding tissue occur when a catheter is displaced out of the vein. Needle catheters and stiff plastic catheters are more likely to perforate the vessel wall than softer polyurethane or silicone catheters. Extravasation at a peripheral vein site is heralded by swelling and tenderness. Cooling of the skin over the catheter tip may be palpated if room temperature fluids are being administered. If the intravenous solution contains irritating drugs such as thiobarbiturates or thiacetarsamide, swelling may be accompanied by increasing pain, heat, redness, and induration followed by necrosis and sloughing of skin and perivascular tissues. Signs of central venous extravasation may be absent until large quantities of fluid are administered. Complications of central venous extravasation include mediastinal or pleural fluid accumulation resulting in dyspnea. This may be documented by evaluation of physical signs, thoracic radiographs, and fluid analysis. Penetration of the right atrium may occur with a catheter positioned too deeply in the chest, resulting in accumulation of blood and fluid in the pericardial sac and cardiac tamponade.

Extravasation of a short catheter at a peripheral site may be detected early by frequent inspection of the vein. Catheter positioning and patency should be evaluated before injecting any irritating substance. This may be accomplished by aspirating blood and administering a test injection of sterile saline while observing the perivascular area. To aspirate blood without disconnecting a fluid administration line, the fluid container is lowered below the level of the catheter tip. Gravity flow pulls blood back until it is visible at the catheter hub or administration set tubing. Other recommendations to minimize the risk of extravasation include the following: (1) avoid winged needle catheters for prolonged infusions, (2) use the smallest and softest catheter that will perform adequately, (3) select a large vein at a location well away from a joint, and (4) limit movement of peripheral vein catheters located near joints by immobilizing the limb with a heavy bandage or splint.

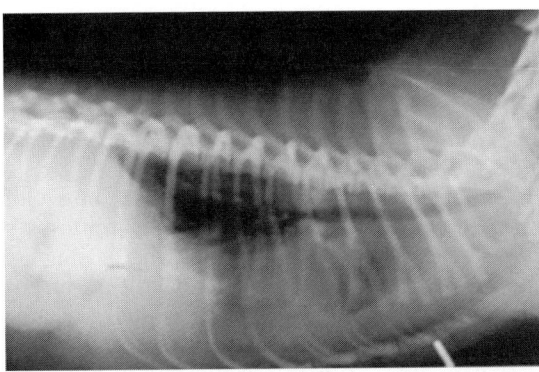

FIGURE 14-6. Lateral thoracic radiograph of a dog with right atrial and cranial vena caval thrombosis that developed following catheterization of the external jugular veins. Thrombosis resulted in anterior caval syndrome with edema of the head, neck, and forelimbs, and pleural effusion.

Thrombosis

Thrombosis is a common complication of indwelling catheters. Catheters left in place for more than a few hours are covered with a fibrin sheath and platelets. This sheath strips away from the catheter surface during catheter removal and either is incorporated in the vessel wall or embolizes the pulmonary arteries. When small in mass, these emboli usually go unnoticed. Another, potentially more damaging type of thrombus usually forms at contact points between the catheter and the vessel wall (Borow and Crowley 1985). Endothelial injury at these points results in local inflammation and thrombus formation. These thrombi are more likely to develop when stiff or reactive catheter materials are used, on long catheters that cross a joint, and on catheters with frayed tips. Mural thrombi may grow progressively and eventually obliterate the vessel lumen. Complications of these thrombi may be both obvious and serious (Figs. 14-6 and 14-7) (Di Costanzo et al. 1988; Solomon et al. 1987; Wistbacka and Nuutinen 1985).

Thrombophlebitis

Thrombophlebitis may be caused by mechanical, chemical, or infectious processes at the catheter site. Damage to the endothelial lining of the vein initiates both inflammation (phlebitis) and thrombus formation on the vessel wall. Early signs of thrombophlebitis include tenderness and erythema of the skin over the vessel and palpable induration of the vessel itself. If left untreated, these early signs progress and the vessel may become completely thrombosed. This is recognized as severe hardening of the vessel and may be accompanied by complete occlusion and inability to infuse fluids. Purulent discharge may be noted from the catheter site. Systemic signs of inflammation including fever and leukocytosis may be present, although some animals develop severe local reactions in the absence of systemic signs.

Mechanical damage is minimized by selecting small catheters and large veins; by using soft, inert catheter materials; and by securely anchoring the catheter to the skin to minimize in-and-out motion. If an indwelling catheter crosses a joint, the limb should be immobilized to limit trauma to the vascular endothelium. Irritating drugs should be administered after adequate dilution and only into veins with high blood flow rates to minimize local endothelial injury. Hypertonic solutions should be administered only into central veins wherever possible.

Infection

Any intravenous catheter supports infection. The majority of catheter-related infections are probably caused by migration of bacteria from the skin along the external surface of the catheter wall into the vein. In human beings receiving intravenous fluid therapy, infection arising from contamination of the catheter hub and fluid administration set connections is comparatively less likely if sterile technique is strictly followed (Cercenado et al. 1990). Veterinary patients that chew, disconnect, and defecate on their administration sets are probably at higher risk for this source of contamination. The prevalence of positive bacteriologic cultures from catheters at the time of removal ranged from 10.7 to 26% in three small surveys of veterinary patients (Mathews et al. 1996; Lippert et al. 1988; Burrows 1982).

Signs of infection may be identical to those of thrombophlebitis. There is normally a small (1–5 mm) diameter zone of inflammation surrounding the skin puncture site, and inflammation extending beyond this range is suspect (Haskins 1988). Systemic signs including fever and leukocytosis may develop in bacteremic animals. Some may develop organ infection at remote sites (endocarditis, abscessation), and some develop sepsis syndrome or septic shock or even die (Burrows 1982). Other animals, however, develop catheter-related bacteremia with minimal clinical signs. Catheter infection should always be suspected in animals developing clinical evidence of infection while an indwelling catheter is present.

If catheter infection is suspected, the catheter should be removed immediately. Bacteriologic culture of the catheter tip assists in the diagnosis of catheter infection. Before removal, the skin is scrubbed with antiseptic solution and carefully cleaned with alcohol. When the alcohol has dried, the catheter is removed aseptically and the catheter tip cut off with a sterile blade and dropped into a tube of culture medium broth for bacteriologic

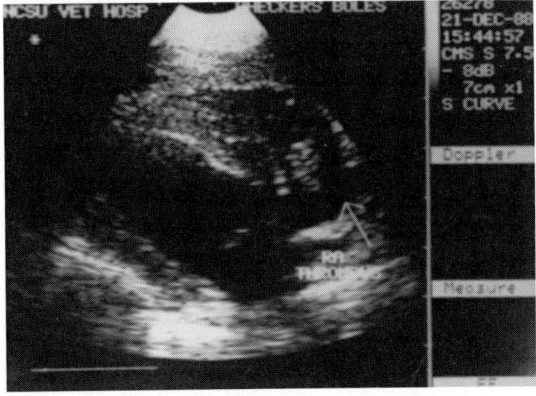

FIGURE 14-7. Two-dimensional echocardiogram of the same dog as in Figure 14-6, demonstrating a large thrombus (arrow) in the right atrial lumen.

evaluation. If the catheter is suspected to be the cause of infection in a bacteremic animal but the catheter cannot be easily replaced (e.g., catheters inserted surgically in animals with limited venous access), differential bacteriologic culture may be performed. In this procedure, cultures are performed on blood drawn simultaneously through a peripheral vein and through the catheter. In human beings, if the catheter blood sample demonstrates a sevenfold increase in identical bacterial colonies compared with the peripheral vein blood culture, the catheter is probably the source of the bacteremia (Fan et al. 1989).

Prevention of infection is assisted by using sterile technique during catheterization, tunneling the catheter subcutaneously before venipuncture, avoiding tubing disconnections, proper maintenance of the catheter dressing, and careful management of injection ports and fluid containers (Timsit et al. 1996; Mathews et al. 1996). Antibiotic therapy does not appear to alter the risk of catheter infection but is used to treat infections after catheter removal.

Catheter Embolism

Catheter embolism occurs when a fragment of the catheter becomes free and is carried by blood flow until it lodges in the heart or a pulmonary artery. This may occur in any of the following circumstances:

1. The catheter is accidentally cut during bandage removal.
2. A through-the-needle catheter is advanced, then pulled back into the needle shaft and sheared off by the needle bevel.
3. The needle within an over-the-needle catheter is partially withdrawn and then reinserted while the catheter tip is still within the vein. If the flexible catheter tip is bent to the side, the needle catches on the catheter shaft and amputates the end of the catheter.
4. The catheter shaft disconnects from the catheter hub.

If catheter amputation is observed, a tourniquet is immediately applied proximal to the venipuncture site to hold the embolus and prevent further migration. If the catheter is made of radiopaque material, the area is radiographed to identify the embolus position and it is removed surgically if possible. Long fragments that have migrated to the right ventricle may be removed with a transvenous loop snare under fluoroscopic guidance (Fox et al. 1985).

Catheter embolization is best prevented by careful technique during catheter insertion and removal. A misplaced catheter is never withdrawn while the needle is left in place; instead, the catheter and needle are withdrawn together as a unit.

Air Embolism

Air embolism may occur whenever a catheter is within a vein. The risk of air embolism is highest during insertion of central venous catheters. When the catheter enters the thoracic cavity, the catheter tip is exposed to negative intrathoracic pressure and air embolism occurs if the free end of the catheter is exposed to the atmosphere. This risk may be higher in dogs with extrathoracic airway obstruction (e.g., brachycephalic breeds) because increased inspiratory effort can produce markedly negative intrathoracic pressure. Air embolism during catheterization is avoided by completing the procedure and sealing the Luer end as rapidly as possible.

Air embolism may also result from disconnections or the presence of air within the fluid administration system. The risk of air embolism is higher when using vented fluid administration sets. This risk may be reduced substantially by using collapsible plastic containers and non-vented administration sets. The practice of injecting air into glass containers to increase the rate of fluid delivery is extremely hazardous and should be avoided.

Small air emboli are trapped in the pulmonary vasculature and usually go unnoticed. Larger emboli markedly increase pulmonary vascular resistance and cause respiratory distress and pulmonary edema (Hall et al. 1988). A slow infusion of air into the vascular space of dogs increases pulmonary artery and central venous pressures and produces a progressive fall in arterial blood pressure. Ultimately, arterial blood pressure is markedly reduced and cardiovascular collapse occurs. Administration of a bolus of air produces an air lock in the right ventricular outflow tract and circulatory obstruction.

The best treatment for air embolism is to aspirate the air immediately from the right atrium and ventricle if a central venous catheter is in place. If this is not possible, the animal is positioned in left lateral recumbency to trap gas in the right ventricular apex and allow blood to flow through the right ventricular outflow tract. Standard cardiopulmonary resuscitation procedures are instituted if the animal develops respiratory or cardiac arrest (Thayer et al. 1980).

Exsanguination

Exsanguination is possible whenever the catheter or administration tubing is disconnected by the unobserved animal. Metal floor grates pose a unique threat: they can snag and separate tubing connection sites, and during the resulting hemorrhage, blood dripping to the cage floor underneath the grate may be difficult to see. Disconnections are particularly likely in dogs that change position frequently. Blood loss may be most severe through cephalic vein catheters when an animal is in sternal recumbency with its elbows flexed. Anchoring the patient's end of the administration tubing to the catheter bandage helps prevent disconnection at the catheter. The junctions between tubing extension pieces may be covered with white tape to prevent disconnections at these points. Use of Luer-Lok connections (as opposed to slip-Luer connections) also helps to reduce the likelihood of an accidental disconnection.

▶ Fluid Administration and Monitoring

The many different types of available fluid administration sets and connection devices offer considerable flexibility in intravenous fluid administration (Fig. 14–8). Multiple-

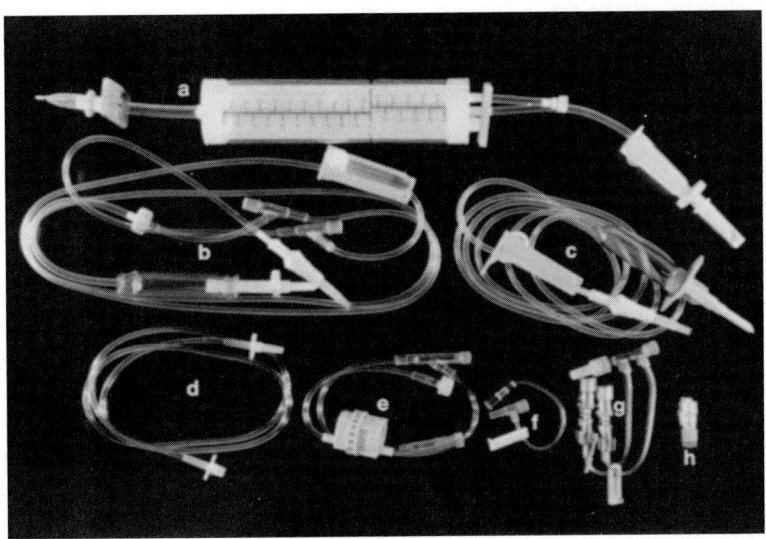

FIGURE 14-8. Samples of various fluid therapy disposable equipment. *(A)* 150 mL valveless burette (Buretrol, Baxter Healthcare). *(B)* Solution administration set (Continu-Flo, Travenol), 2.1 m long, with check valve, adjustable clamp, and two injection ports. *(C)* Solution administration set (basic solution set, Baxter Healthcare), 1.8 m long. *(D)* IV extension tubing (Pharmaseal extension tube, Baxter Healthcare), 84 cm long. *(E)* Calibrated flow regulator (Dial-A-Flo regulator IV extension set, Abbott Laboratories, Inc.). *(F)* 13 cm extension set with T piece (Abbott Hospitals, Inc.). *(G)* Double T connector (Medex Inc., Hilliard, Ohio). *(H)* Jelco intermittent injection cap (Critikon).

port flow connectors allow simultaneous infusion of compatible solutions through a single catheter. In-line volume control sets (Buretrol, Baxter Healthcare) permit accurate delivery of small volumes of fluids. A variety of different tubing lengths, diameters, and connections allow many different configurations and combinations of fluids to be delivered to a single catheter. Fluid administration sets are available from several manufacturers. The two basic types are vented and nonvented; these are available in several lengths. All administration sets utilize an in-line drip chamber to estimate the rate of flow. Depending on the brand, the drip sizes are calibrated so that 1 mL = 10, 15, 20, or 60 drops. Drops per minute are calculated from the formula

$$\text{Drops per minute} = \frac{\text{total infusion volume} \times \text{drops/mL}}{\text{total infusion time (min)}}$$

For example, to administer 2000 mL over 24 h using a Baxter basic solution set (10 drops = 1 mL):

$$\frac{2000 \text{ mL} \times 10 \text{ drops/mL}}{1440 \text{ min}} = 14 \text{ drops/min}$$

The rate of flow is regulated by tightening or releasing the intravenous tubing clamp while watching and counting the drip rate. Fluid administration rate may also be controlled by in-line flow regulators (Stat 2 Pumpette, ConMed Corp.) or, more accurately, by electronic fluid pumps or rate controllers. In-line flow regulators are calibrated tubing clamps. Accurate use of these devices depends on unimpeded flow through short catheters 20 gauge or larger and on maintaining a constant height of about 75 cm (30 in.) between the drip chamber and the level of the heart.

Two types of fluid pumps are available: rate-consistent pumps, which are used when fluids must be given at a constant rate, and volumetric pumps, which deliver specific volumes of fluid over a desired unit of time (Figs. 14–9 through 14–11). The rate-consistent type of fluid pump is useful for drug infusions when a constant flow rate is important, whereas the volumetric pumps are used to deliver prescribed volumes of fluid accurately over time. Many volumetric pumps require a dedicated administration set with an in-line calibrated cassette that determines the volume delivered per cycle. Some models use a photoelectric drip detector that attaches to the administration set drip chamber. All pumps deliver fluid at the desired rate and do so under pressure. This pressure can overcome resistance to flow from viscous solutions, filters, and tubing kinks. It also increases the risk to the patient in the case of extravasation, as fluid is pumped into the perivascular tissues under pressure. To prevent this, some models are equipped with pressure-monitoring circuitry and can be adjusted to produce an alarm at preset values. Pumps marketed specifically for use in animals are available (e.g., Vet/IV, Sensor Devices).

Electronic flow controllers depend on gravity for flow and use drip sensors to measure the rate of administration (Fig. 14–12). The drip sensor output is directed to a feedback loop that regulates the degree of occlusion of administration set tubing that is threaded through mechanical jaws. These devices do not add any pressure to the system and the infusion pressure depends on the height of the solution container above the catheter. Consequently, these devices do not work well with animals that move frequently or when flow is restricted by positional catheters.

Intravenous solution containers should be numbered consecutively and clearly labeled with the date, time, and patient's name. Any additives should be clearly identified as to type, quantity added, date and time added, and by whom. A calibrated timing label is applied to the container and is used to monitor the rate of flow over time (Fig. 14–13). All patients receiving intravenous fluid therapy should be weighed at least daily. Abnormal fluid losses through the urinary tract, nasogastric suction, or cavity drainage should be measured and replaced with equal volumes of appropriate intravenous replacement fluids at frequent intervals. Fluid losses in animals with vomiting or diarrhea may be monitored by routine weighing of soiled cage papers. The weight of a dry cage paper is subtracted from the measured weight, and the difference (in grams) is converted to milliliters of water

300 TECHNICAL ASPECTS OF FLUID THERAPY

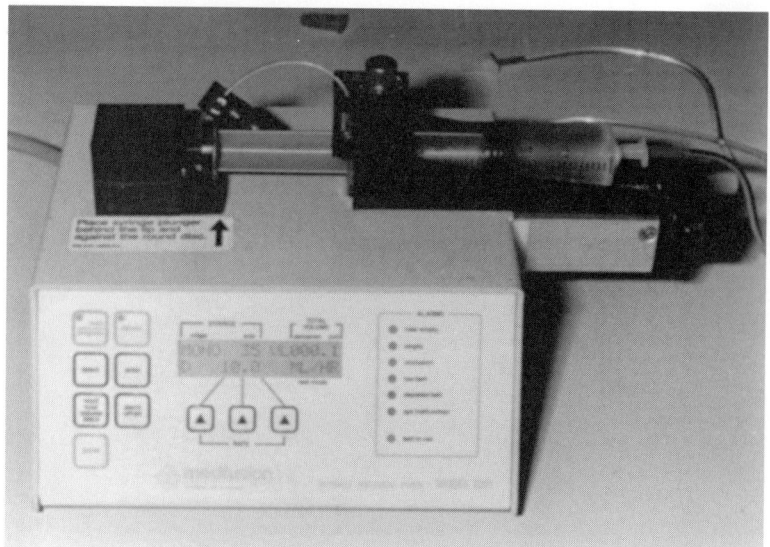

FIGURE 14-9. Example of a syringe pump. Syringe pumps are ideal for constant-rate infusions of drugs to any size animal and for administration of intravenous fluids to very small animals.

and replaced with appropriate intravenous replacement fluid. Daily monitoring of the PCV and total plasma solids helps assess the extracellular fluid compartment volume. Measurement of urine specific gravity in animals capable of concentrating their urine assists in detection of inadequate circulating blood volume (in animals being treated for shock or extracellular fluid losses) or inadequate administration of water (in animals receiving maintenance fluid therapy).

▶ Central Venous Pressure Monitoring

Central venous pressure (CVP) measurement is a useful diagnostic procedure for the management of fluid therapy, particularly in critically ill animals. The CVP is the blood

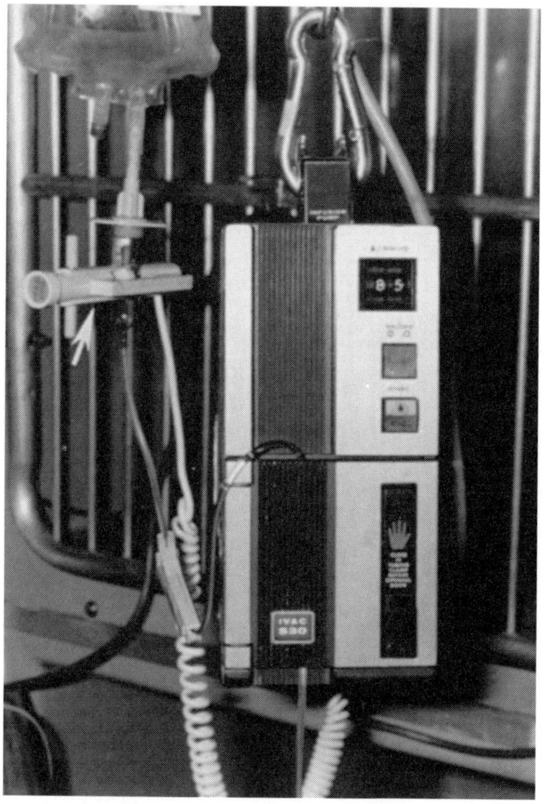

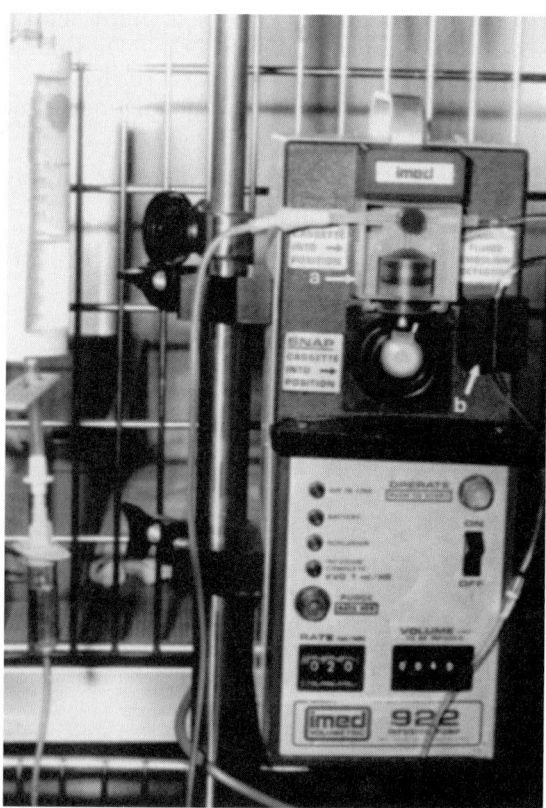

FIGURE 14-10. Example of a rate-consistent peristaltic pump. The device uses a drip sensor clamped to the administration tubing drip chamber (arrow), and the delivery rate is set as drops per minute.

FIGURE 14-11. Example of a volumetric pump. The fluid administration set is plugged into a (A) sterile disposable calibrated cassette that serves as both pump piston and measuring device. The machine settings include rate in milliliters per hour and total volume to be delivered. An in-line air bubble detector (B) interrupts the infusion if air is sensed within the tubing.

pressure within the intrathoracic portions of the cranial or caudal vena cava. Central venous pressure is measured clinically for two reasons: (1) to gain information about cardiac function and (2) to gain information about intravascular blood volume. The CVP is only slightly higher than the right atrial pressure (RAP), and the two terms, CVP and RAP, are often used interchangeably.

The CVP (or RAP) affects, and is affected by, cardiac output. Right atrial pressure is quantitatively similar to the pressure in the right ventricle at the end of diastole. As RAP and right ventricular end-diastolic pressure (EDP) increase, right ventricular end-diastolic volume (EDV) increases. The relationship between ventricular EDP and EDV is not linear (Fig. 14–14). At low ventricular volumes, an increase in EDV does not increase ventricular EDP significantly. At high ventricular volumes when the limit of ventricular distention is reached, small increases in EDV increase both ventricular EDP and atrial pressure substantially. Clinically, if EDV is increased by administration of intravenous fluids, there is little initial increase in EDP (steep portion of curve, Fig. 14–14) until the limit of ventricular expansion is reached. At that point, administration of more fluids no longer increases EDV substantially, but EDP and atrial pressure rise rapidly (plateau portion of curve, Fig. 14–14).

Ventricular EDV is an important determinant of stroke volume and cardiac output. The relationship between EDV and stroke volume is nearly linear in normal animals; as EDV increases, stroke volume and cardiac output increase according to the Frank-Starling law of

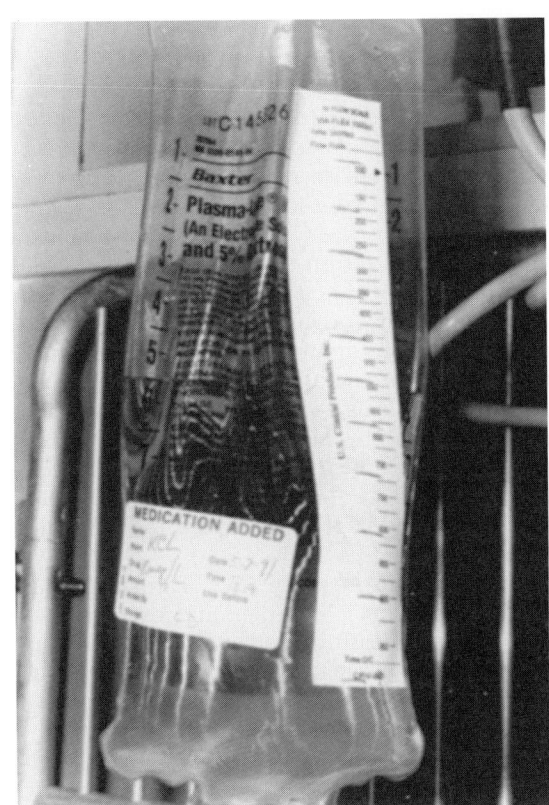

FIGURE 14–13. A properly labeled intravenous solution set.

the heart. In many situations (e.g., shock states) it is desirable to increase both stroke volume and cardiac output maximally to optimize oxygen transport to tissues. This is accomplished most effectively by increasing ventricular EDV. End-diastolic volume is not easily measured clinically. However, atrial pressure can be monitored to make inferences about likely changes in ventricular vol-

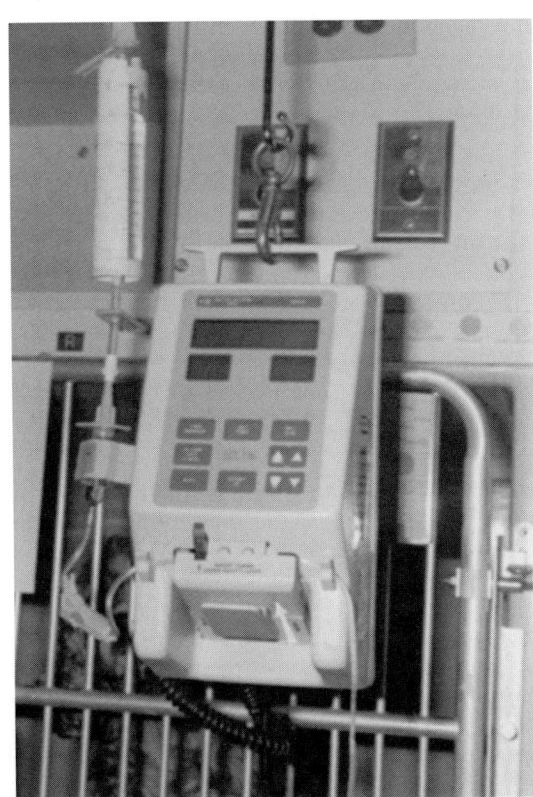

FIGURE 14–12. Example of an electronic fluid rate controller. The device depends upon gravity to drive the flow of fluid, and the drip rate is controlled by mechanical jaws (arrow).

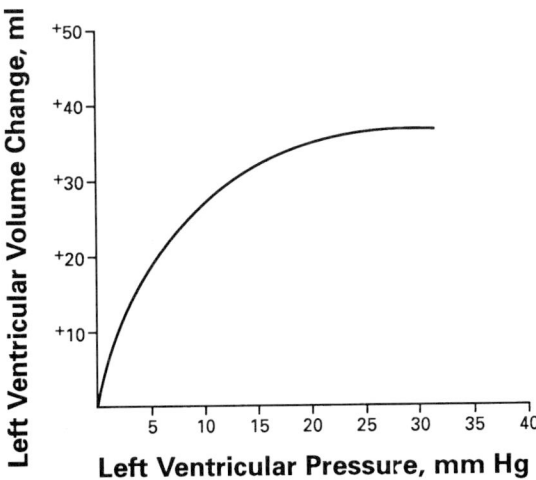

FIGURE 14–14. Graph depicting the relationship between left ventricular diastolic pressure and left ventricular volume gain in the dog. As pressure increases, diastolic volume increases rapidly until the limit of ventricular distention is reached. At that point, even large increases in pressure will not increase ventricular volume substantially.

ume. Just as the relationship between RAP and EDV is not linear, the relationship between RAP and cardiac output is not linear (Fig. 14–15). At low pressures, a small increase in RAP generates a large increase in cardiac output. At higher pressures, a large increase in RAP does not substantially increase cardiac output (plateau phase of Frank-Starling curve, Fig. 14–15).

As stated earlier, the CVP also reflects venous blood volume and venous return to the heart. The vascular bed is able to accommodate changes in volume with minimal changes in pressure. If a fluid challenge is rapidly administered, both venous return to the heart and CVP rise. Within minutes, circulatory reflexes and stress relaxation of large-capacity veins return venous pressure and flow toward normal. If the intravascular volume is reduced, the CVP falls rapidly. If intravascular volume is high relative to cardiac performance and capacitance vessels are already distended to their limits, the CVP may fall slowly or not at all.

The relationship between CVP, cardiac output, and the vascular system is complex and dynamic. Consequently, a single measurement of CVP does not predict cardiac output or vascular blood volume. Although there is a general trend for animals with reduced blood volume to have a low CVP, a dog or cat could experience lethal blood loss and yet have a normal CVP. Nevertheless, *repeated* measurements during fluid therapy can give important clues about the compliance of these systems. When these results are interpreted in light of other clinical findings, valuable information about hemodynamic status is obtained.

Measurement

A central venous catheter must be in place. The catheter tip should ideally reside within the thorax at or near the

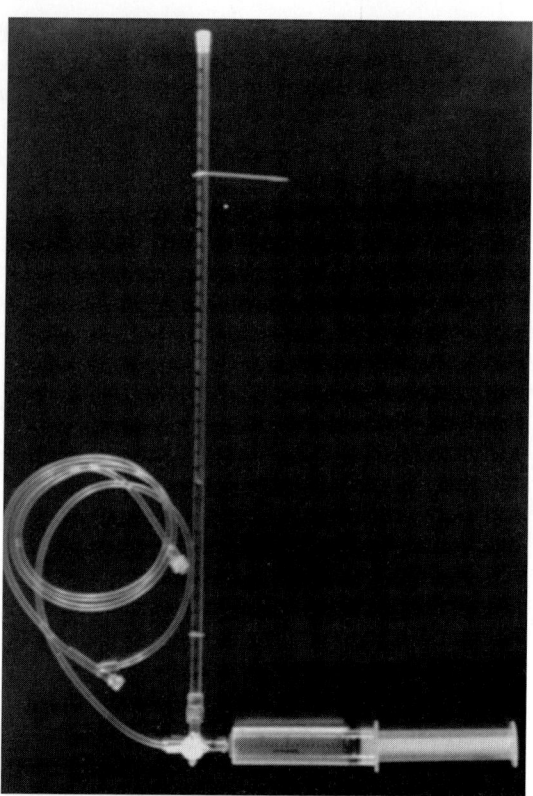

FIGURE 14–16. An example of a central venous pressure manometer (Medex) complete with stopcock, syringe, and patient tubing.

right atrium. A catheter placed in the lateral saphenous vein and positioned so that the tip resides in the caudal vena cava may be an acceptable substitute in cats (Machon et al. 1995). Materials necessary for CVP measurement using a water manometer include (Fig. 14–16):

a. Central venous catheter in place
b. Water manometer (Pharmaseal manometer tray, American Pharmaseal Company; Medex manometer set, Medex Inc.)
c. One 30 in. IV extension tubing set if needed
d. Three-way stopcock if needed
e. 20 mL syringe filled with saline solution
f. 20 gauge needle

The manometer and tubing are primed with saline solution and the column is filled to a level well above the anticipated CVP of the patient. The animal is positioned in sternal or lateral recumbency, with lateral recumbency preferred. The stopcock at the bottom of the manometer should rest on the table or cage floor. When the stopcock is turned to connect the column of saline with the catheter, the hydrostatic pressure in the column forces fluid through the catheter. The saline column continues to fall until the hydrostatic pressure of the column reaches equilibrium with the hydrostatic pressure of the blood at the end of the catheter. When it has reached equilibrium and has stopped falling, the height of the saline column above the catheter tip, expressed as centimeters of water, reflects the blood pressure within the vessel at the catheter tip. Therefore, it is important to know approximately where the catheter tip lies in relation to the manometer

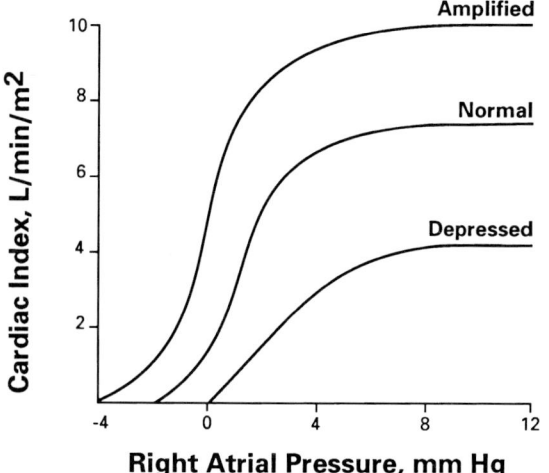

FIGURE 14–15. Family of Starling curves plotting the relationship of right atrial pressure (RAP) (or right ventricular end-diastolic pressure) with cardiac index (CI). In the normal heart, small increments in RAP within the normal range (0–4 mm Hg) yield large increases in CI. This response is augmented in dogs with endogenous sympathetic cardiac stimulation or in dogs receiving inotropic drugs ("amplified" curve) and is depressed in dogs with myocardial failure ("depressed" curve).

fluid column. When the animal is in lateral recumbency, the cranial vena cava lies near the midline, and the sternum is a good reference point. In sternal recumbency, the cranial vena cava is approximately level with the point of the shoulder (scapulohumeral) joint.

When the appropriate external anatomic landmark is found, the manometer column is positioned with the stopcock resting on the table surface immediately next to the landmark and the centimeter mark nearest that point is labeled. This mark is now the *zero reference point* on the manometer, and all subsequent measurements are read as the distance from that mark. Measurements can be made with the manometer located anywhere nearby that is convenient, as long as the stopcock rests on the same horizontal surface as the animal (Fig. 14–17). If the animal is in a cage, the manometer may be taped to the wall of the cage and used there.

When obtaining a CVP measurement, rhythmic fluctuations in the height of the saline column meniscus are usually seen. These oscillations are due to two factors: Large ones occur with respiration, and smaller ones occur with each heartbeat. Fluctuations in the column synchronized with respirations are usually easily seen. As the patient inhales, the intrathoracic pressure drops and CVP falls; the reverse occurs during exhalation. These excursions are exaggerated in animals with upper airway obstruction and are reversed by positive-pressure ventilation. With regard to the cardiac cycle, CVP rises steadily until atrial contraction, jumps up a bit during atrial contraction, and then falls rapidly at the beginning of diastole (Fig. 14–18). The response of the fluid column in the manometer is too slow to show all of the peaks and valleys of these pressure changes accurately. When using a water column manometer, the best method is to measure the CVP just before inspiration and at the lowest diastolic swing. This value correlates best with real CVP (Clayton 1988).

If the rhythmic fluctuations are absent, malpositioning of the catheter should be suspected: either it is too short or too long and the tip is not within the thoracic cavity, or the tip is butted up against a vessel wall or the right atrial wall. Obstruction of the catheter tip can be confirmed by aspirating blood from the catheter: blood flows rapidly and with little resistance if it is floating freely within the lumen of the vessel. A high CVP or the presence of large fluctuations synchronous with the heartbeat suggests that the catheter tip is in the lumen of the right ventricle; if this is the case, it should be partially withdrawn to the proper level.

Water manometers tend to overestimate CVP by 0.5 to 5 cm H_2O; this overestimation varies from patient to patient and from measurement to measurement in the same patient, even when positioning is done as carefully as possible (Clayton 1988). This variation can be important when following a critically ill animal that requires aggressive fluid support and in animals that are hyperventilating, dyspneic, or being treated with positive-pressure ventilation. A calibrated electronic pressure transducer connected to the catheter with a short, stiff tube is more accurate in these patients.

Interpretation

Measurement of CVP in animals during fluid challenge yields important information about cardiovascular status (Table 14–4). As intravenous fluids are administered and the intravascular blood volume expands, venous return and CVP begin to rise. A rapid infusion of 20 mL/kg crystalloid or 5 mL/kg colloid into a euvolemic animal with normal cardiac function results in a modest increase in CVP (2–4 cm H_2O) that returns to baseline within 15 min. A minimal increase or no increase in CVP implies that the vascular volume is markedly reduced. A CVP that rises and returns to baseline rapidly (<5 min) implies that there is reduced vascular volume and that the initial volume load has been accommodated by rapid changes in vasomotor tone. A large increase in CVP (>4 cm H_2O) implies reduced cardiac compliance or increased venous blood volume or both. A slow (15 min) return toward baseline indicates that blood volume is close to normal. A very prolonged return to baseline (>30 min) suggests that the intravascular blood volume is elevated relative to cardiac performance.

When treating a dog or cat with noncardiogenic shock,

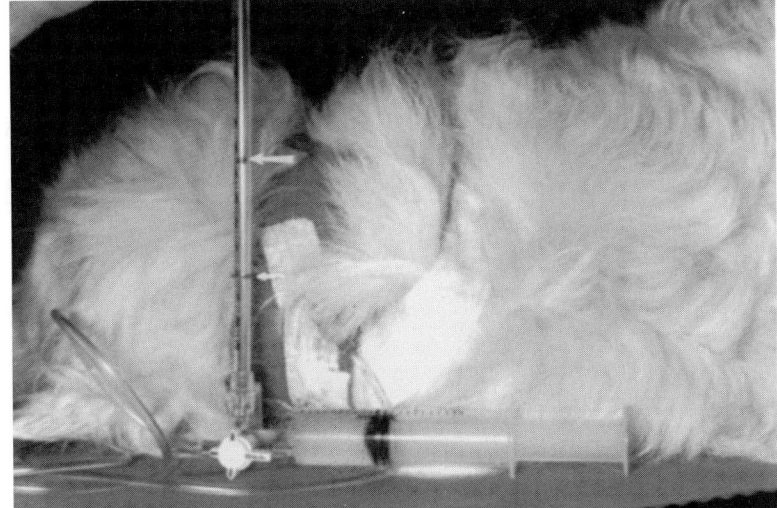

FIGURE 14–17. Measurement of central venous pressure (CVP) using a saline column manometer. The dog is positioned in lateral recumbency, and the manometer rests on the table surface. The location of the patient's midline was estimated to be level with the "0" on the column, and a marker ring has been slid to that point (small arrow). The saline column stopped falling, and the ball (large arrow) floating at the top of the saline column rests at 4.5 cm at the end of expiration. Therefore, this patient's CVP is read as 4.5 − 0 = 4.5 cm.

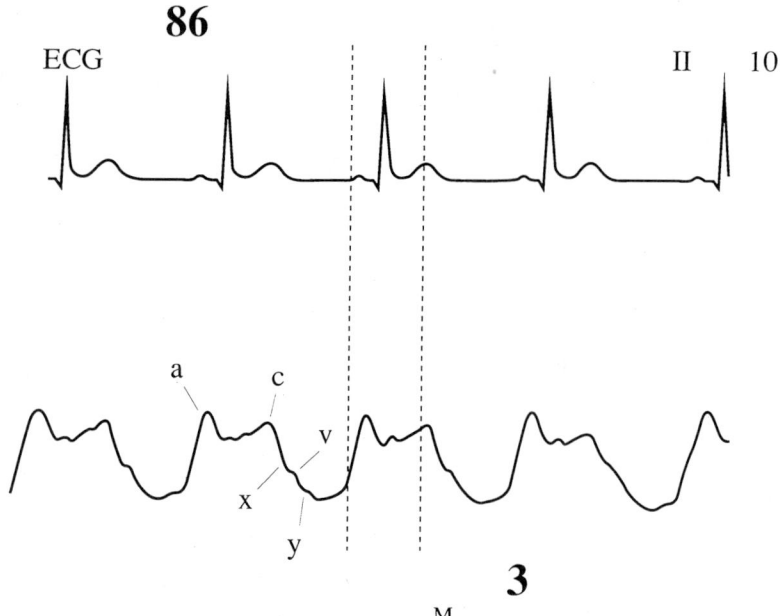

FIGURE 14-18. Tracing from a photograph of a patient monitor screen with simultaneous display of the electrocardiogram (top) and CVP (bottom). The CVP trace is characterized by the positive a-, c-, and v-waves and by the two negative depressions called the x- and y-descents. The a-wave represents the increase in RAP and CVP during atrial contraction, the c-wave represents the slight increase in atrial pressure as the tricuspid valve bulges into the right atrium during early ventricular contraction, and the v-wave represents the increase in pressure that occurs as blood flows into the atrium while the tricuspid valve is still closed. The x-descent corresponds to the period of ventricular ejection when blood is emptied from the heart. The y-descent represents the drop in atrial pressure that follows opening of the tricuspid valve and rapid blood flow into the ventricle. The mean CVP is 3 mm Hg, and the ECG-derived heart rate is 86 beats/min.

an immediate therapeutic goal might be to administer an intravenous fluid challenge rapidly enough to raise the CVP significantly, by about 2 to 4 cm H_2O, within the first few minutes of therapy. The rate of fall of the CVP is then observed to make inferences about venous return relative to cardiac performance. If the CVP returns to baseline rapidly, another fluid challenge is administered and the process is repeated. If necessary, repeated fluid boluses may be given until the CVP reaches 5 to 10 cm H_2O (or 3–7 mm Hg if using a pressure transducer) and

TABLE 14-4. Possible Interpretations of CVP Measurement with Volume Challenge*

CVP	Initial Increase†	Return to Baseline	Cardiac Status	Vascular Volume	Cardiac Output
Below normal	+	Rapid	Normal	Reduced	Low
			Hyperdynamic	Reduced	Low to normal
	+ to ++	Moderate	Depressed	Reduced	Very low
			Hyperdynamic	Normal	High
Normal	+ to ++	Rapid	Normal	Reduced	Low to normal
	++	Moderate	Normal	Normal	Normal
			Hyperdynamic	Normal	High
	++	Slow	Normal	Elevated	High
			Hyperdynamic	Elevated	Very high
	+++	Rapid	Depressed	Reduced	Very low
	+++	Moderate	Depressed	Normal	Low
	+++	Slow	Depressed	Elevated	Low to normal
Above normal	++	Moderate	Normal	Elevated	High
			Hyperdynamic	Elevated	Very high
	+++	Moderate	Depressed	Reduced	Very low
	+++	Slow	Depressed	Normal	Low
			Depressed	Elevated	Low to normal

Source: Otto CW: Central venous pressure monitoring. In Blitt CD (ed): *Monitoring in Anesthesia and Critical Care Medicine.* New York, Churchill Livingstone, pp. 169–210, 1990.
*Approximately 5 mL/kg colloid solution IV or 20 mL/kg crystalloid solution IV.
† +, Minimal; ++, moderate; +++, large.

takes 10 to 15 min to fall. In that setting, it is likely that blood volume and venous return are nearly optimal relative to cardiac performance and that further increases in CVP are unlikely to yield significant increases in cardiac output. In animals with normal right heart function and pleural and intraabdominal pressures, the CVP should not be pushed higher than about 10 to 12 mm Hg. When that pressure is reached, it is likely that pulmonary venous pressure is above 12 to 15 mm Hg (assuming that the left and right ventricles are functioning symmetrically), increasing the likelihood of pulmonary edema. When this limit has been reached, giving more fluids will not help cardiac output at all (because it will no longer increase EDV) but will only make the patient congested. If there is a need to increase cardiac output further, positive inotropic agents such as dobutamine and/or peripheral vasodilator drugs such as nitroprusside are administered.

Central venous pressure monitoring is also useful in less critical situations. When administering fluids to an animal with oliguria or congestive heart failure, the CVP can be used to monitor therapy and help prevent inadvertent overadministration of fluids. In that setting, the baseline CVP is measured before fluid therapy is begun and subsequently measured at intervals frequent enough to minimize the risk of fluid overload, usually every 2 to 8 h. During chronic (slow) fluid administration, significant increases in CVP may not occur until the venous system's volume capacity has been reached; therefore, any observed increase should be carefully evaluated.

Central venous pressure measurement can be used in a variety of situations to assist in diagnosis and optimal fluid therapy management. It is important to obtain CVP measurements in as technically precise a manner as possible and to obtain consecutive measurements with the patient in the same position each time. As with any monitoring tool, CVP measurements must be interpreted in light of other diagnostic findings and the pitfall of relying too heavily on a single test must be avoided.

REFERENCES

Borow M and Crowley JG: Evaluation of central venous catheter thrombogenicity. *Acta Anaesthiol Scand Suppl* 81:59–64, 1985.

Burrows CF: Inadequate skin preparation as a cause of intravenous catheter–related infection in the dog. *J Am Vet Med Assoc* 180:747–749, 1982.

Cercenado E, Ena J, Rodríguez-Créixems M, et al.: A conservative procedure for the diagnosis of catheter-related infections. *Arch Intern Med* 150:1417–1420, 1990.

Clayton DG: Inaccuracies in manometric central venous pressure measurement. *Resuscitation* 16:221–230, 1988.

Crowe DT: Practical life-saving surgical procedures involving the cardiovascular system. VECCS, *Proceedings of the First International Emergency and Critical Care Symposium*, pp. 32–37, 1988.

Crowe DT: Vascular surgery procedures for emergency and critical care patients. VECCS, *Proceedings of the Second International Emergency and Critical Care Symposium*, pp. 291–301, 1990.

Di Costanzo J, Sastre B, Choux R, et al.: Mechanism of thrombogenesis during total parenteral nutrition: role of catheter composition. *J Parenter Enter Nutr* 12:190–194, 1988.

Fan ST, Teoh-Chan CH, and Lau KF: Evaluation of central venous catheter sepsis by differential quantitative blood culture. *Eur J Clin Microbiol Infect Dis* 8:142–144, 1989.

Fiser DH: Intraosseous infusion. *N Engl J Med* 322:1579–1581, 1990.

Fox PR, Sos TA, and Bond BR: Nonsurgical removal of a catheter embolus from the heart of a dog. *J Am Vet Med Assoc* 187:275–276, 1985.

Fulton RB and Hauptman JG: In vitro and in vivo rates of fluid flow through catheters in peripheral veins of dogs. *J Am Vet Med Assoc* 198:1622–1624, 1991.

Hall JE, Hofman WF, and Ehrhart IC: Venous occlusion pressure and vascular permeability in the dog lung after air embolization. *J Appl Physiol* 65:34–40, 1988.

Haskins SC: Emergency anesthesia and critical care procedures. VECCS, *Proceedings of the First International Emergency and Critical Care Symposium*, pp. 153–157, 1988.

Hecker JF and Scandrett LA: Roughness and thrombogenicity of the outer surfaces of intravascular catheters. *J Biomed Mater Res* 19:381–395, 1985.

Klein MK, Dow SW, and Rosychuk RA: Pulmonary thromboembolism associated with immune-mediated hemolytic anemia in dogs: Ten cases (1982–1987). *J Am Vet Med Assoc* 195:246–250, 1989.

Lippert AC, Fulton RB, and Parr AM: Nosocomial infection surveillance in a small animal intensive care unit. *J Am Anim Hosp Assoc* 24:627–636, 1988.

Machon RG, Raffe MR, and Robinson EP: Central venous pressure measurements in the caudal vena cava of sedated cats. *J Vet Emerg Crit Care* 5:121–129, 1995.

Maki DG, Stolz SM, Wheeler S, et al: Prevention of central venous catheter–related bloodstream infection by use of an antiseptic-impregnated catheter. A randomized, controlled trial. *Ann Intern Med* 127:257–266, 1997.

Mathews KA, Brooks MJ, and Vallient AE: A prospective study of intravenous catheter contamination. *J Vet Emerg Crit Care* 6:33–43, 1996.

Meyer BA, Little CJ, Thorp JA, et al.: Heparin versus normal saline as a peripheral line flush in maintenance of intermittent intravenous lines in obstetric patients. *Obstet Gynecol* 85:433–436, 1995.

Norden CW: Application of antibiotic ointment to the site of venous catheterization—A controlled trial. *J Infect Dis* 120:611–615, 1969.

Osuna DJ, DeYoung DJ, and Walker RL: Comparison of three skin preparation techniques in the dog. Part 1: Experimental trial. *Vet Surg* 19:14–19, 1990a.

Osuna DJ, DeYoung DJ, and Walker RL: Comparison of three skin preparation techniques. Part 2: Clinical trial in 100 dogs. *Vet Surg* 19:20–23, 1990b.

Otto CM, Kaufman GM, and Crowe DT: Intraosseous infusion of fluids and therapeutics. *Compend Contin Educ Pract Vet* 11:421–430, 1989.

Otto CW: Central venous pressure monitoring. In Blitt CD (ed): *Monitoring in Anesthesia and Critical Care Medicine*. New York, Churchill Livingstone, pp. 169–210, 1990.

Raad I, Darouiche R, Hachem R, et al.: The broad-spectrum activity and efficacy of catheters coated with minocycline and rifampin. *J Infect Dis* 173:418–424, 1996.

Solomon DD, Arnold WL, Martin ND, et al.: An in vivo method for the evaluation of catheter thrombogenicity. *J Biomed Mater Res* 21:43–57, 1987.

Spilezewski KL, Anderson JM, Schaap RN, et al.: In vivo biocompatibility of catheter materials. *Biomaterials* 9:253–256, 1988.

Thayer GW, Carrig CB, and Evans AT: Fatal venous air embolism associated with pneumocystography in a cat. *J Am Vet Med Assoc* 176:643–645, 1980.

Timsit JF, Sebille V, Farkas JC, et al.: Effect of subcutaneous tunneling on internal jugular catheter–related sepsis in critically ill patients: A prospective randomized multicenter study. *JAMA* 276:1416–1420, 1996.

Wistbacka JO and Nuutinen LS: Catheter-related complications of total parenteral nutrition (TPN): A review. *Acta Anaesthiol Scand* 29:84–88, 1985.

Zinner SH, Denny-Brown BC, Braun P, et al.: Risk of infection with intravenous catheters: Effect of application of antibiotic ointment. *J Infect Dis* 120:616–619, 1969.

CHAPTER 15

Perioperative Management of Fluid Therapy

PETER J. PASCOE

The normal mechanisms of fluid homeostasis are disturbed when an animal undergoes anesthesia and surgery. Consequently, animals should receive fluids during the perioperative period to maintain proper fluid balance. Anesthetized animals should receive fluids:

1. To establish and maintain venous access. A minimal rate of fluid administration is necessary (e.g., 3 mL/h) and will ensure rapid access to the circulation in the event of an emergency in the perioperative period.
2. To counter the physiologic changes that are associated with anesthetics. Most of the drugs and techniques that are used to anesthetize animals have some effect on the circulation.
3. To replace fluids lost during anesthesia and surgery. During the procedure, the animal cannot drink and its metabolic rate is reduced (decreased production of metabolic water). At the same time, the animal continues to produce urine, salivate, secrete fluid into the gastrointestinal tract, and lose water by evaporation from the respiratory tract. The aim should be at least to replace the expected insensible fluid losses.
4. To correct fluid losses caused by disease and to replace ongoing losses attributed to the procedure. The volume of fluid lost or gained depends on the type of surgical procedure, the skill of the surgeon, the preoperative state of the animal, and the equipment used by the anesthetist. Trauma and surgery are associated with increased secretion of antidiuretic hormone (ADH) and additional secretion may occur as a result of hypotension or hypovolemia. Other stress hormones (e.g., cortisol, catecholamines, renin) released during the procedure also may play a role in upsetting normal fluid homeostasis and warrant perioperative fluid therapy.

▶ Preoperative Preparation of the Patient

The animal's fluid balance should be as close to normal as possible before anesthesia. Almost all anesthetics have some effects on circulatory and renal function, and it is important that the patient's circulating volume be optimal so that these effects are not exacerbated. Disturbances that require attention may be classified by their urgency. Some can be corrected acutely (e.g., hypovolemia), some require more time to correct (e.g., hypernatremia), and a few require completion of the procedure before correction of the problem can occur (e.g., hypervolemia associated with acute renal failure in a patient being prepared for hemodialysis).

Changes in Vascular Volume

HYPOVOLEMIA

Hypovolemia may be due to fluid loss directly from the vascular space (e.g., hemorrhage), a more general loss (e.g., dehydration), or changes in vascular tone. In all cases, fluid should be given to replace the loss. For a simple loss in which the composition of the vascular space is relatively normal, the loss can be replaced effectively using an isotonic crystalloid, a hypertonic crystalloid, an artificial colloid, or a blood product. The fluid used depends on the severity of the loss and the financial resources of the client. Acute blood loss of up to 30% of blood volume can be replaced adequately using a crystalloid solution (assuming normal hematocrit and total protein concentration before therapy), whereas a loss of 50% of blood volume or more will probably require blood component therapy and possibly additional crystalloid or colloid support. Occasionally, fluid therapy is not sufficient, and surgical management is required to stop bleeding (e.g., ruptured vena cava). In these instances, it is crucial to have one or more large gauge venous catheters in place in an attempt to keep pace with the loss. In cats and dogs <5 kg, it usually is feasible to place an 18 gauge catheter in the jugular vein. In many dogs of 5 to 15 kg it is feasible to place a 16 gauge catheter in a cephalic vein whereas in dogs >15 kg a 14 gauge catheter normally may be placed. After the catheter has been placed, the animal should be anesthetized using a technique that induces minimal disturbances in volume status and cardiovascular function. Some investigators advocate withholding fluids from trauma patients with major vessel rupture before surgical intervention. In one study of human patients, a marginal benefit was demonstrated using this approach (Bickell et al. 1994). It is likely to be a realistic approach only when blood loss is rapid and surgery is required immediately. In patients with major blood loss but no central vessel rupture, it is more appropriate to replace the volume deficit before anesthetizing the animal.

If the patient is expected to lose a large volume of blood during an anticipated elective surgery, the animal can donate blood in advance so as to have autologous blood available. The animal can donate one unit of blood and then return 3 weeks later, at which time the first unit of blood can be returned to the animal and two units of blood drawn. This procedure can be repeated to collect several units from the same animal. This approach usually is not possible because of the lead time needed to complete these multiple collections. Another alternative in an animal with relatively normal hematocrit and total protein concentration is to collect blood immediately before surgery (10–15% of estimated blood volume) and replace it with three times the volume of crystalloid. The expectation is that the animal will lose less protein and red cell volume during the surgery because of hemodilution, and the collected blood will be available for transfusion when it is needed after surgery. These approaches have been evaluated in human medicine and have been found to be very expensive and to provide little benefit to the patient (Kanter et al. 1996; Clugston et al. 1995; Brecher and Rosenfeld 1994; Goodnough et al. 1994). Nevertheless, the American Society of Anesthesiologists (ASA) published guidelines for the use of packed red cells including the following statements (Practice Guidelines, 1996):

1. When appropriate, preoperative autologous blood donation, intraoperative and postoperative blood recovery, acute normovolemic hemodilution and measures to decrease blood loss (deliberate hypotension and pharmacologic agents) may be beneficial.
2. The indications for transfusion of autologous RBC may be more liberal than for allogeneic RBC because of the lower (but still significant) risks associated with the former.

HYPERVOLEMIA

Hypervolemia is likely to be either iatrogenic or the result of oliguric renal failure or heart failure. In the former situation, it may simply be sufficient to monitor the patient carefully until its fluid volume status has normalized. In the case of oliguric renal failure, it is difficult to reduce the blood volume without dialysis. The primary risk of hypervolemia is related to hypertension and an increase in myocardial work, which could lead to failure in a heart with marginal reserve. Hypervolemia also may lead to pulmonary edema, in which case the circulating volume should be reduced by administration of a diuretic (if renal function is normal) or by phlebotomy if necessary.

Changes in Content

Occasionally, changes in vascular volume do not affect the composition of blood, but in many cases changes in composition also occur and require attention.

ANEMIA

The major concern with anemic patients is the supply of oxygen to the tissues after the animal has been anesthetized with drugs that may impair cardiovascular function. In the chronically anemic animal, some compensation already has occurred to facilitate delivery of oxygen to the tissues. This compensation usually occurs as a result of an increase in cardiac output and a change in the affinity of hemoglobin for oxygen. When the animal is anesthetized, especially using drugs such as alpha$_2$ agonists or inhalants, cardiac output is decreased which reduces the delivery of oxygen to the tissues. Administration of 100% oxygen increases the amount of oxygen in solution (0.3 mL per 100 mL of blood per 100 mm Hg pressure) but this effect provides little compensation for the decline in cardiac output. Figure 15–1 illustrates the relationship between hemoglobin concentration and cardiac index assuming a constant saturation of hemoglobin (99%) to deliver oxygen at a given rate (15 mL/kg/min). The second line shows the same relationship for a PaO_2 of 500 mm Hg assuming a hemoglobin saturation of 100%. In acute anemia, the animal may have been able to increase cardiac output, but there has not been sufficient time for changes in hemoglobin affinity to occur and the delivery of oxygen is likely to be decreased further. What is a "critical" hematocrit value? Many human patients are anesthetized and survive with hemoglobin concentrations as low as 3 to 4 g/dL. (Asao et al. 1997; Carson et al. 1988), but anesthesia is not recommended in this situation unless great care is taken to ensure that the patient has adequate cardiovascular reserve and unless techniques can be used that minimize reduction in cardiac output. The ASA guidelines are based on the available literature in human medicine (Practice Guidelines, 1996). The ASA recommendations for use of packed red cells include the following:

1. Transfusion is rarely indicated when the hemoglobin is >10 g/dL and is almost always indicated when it is <6 g/dL, especially when the anemia is acute.
2. The determination of whether intermediate hemoglobin concentrations (6–10 g/dL) justify or require RBC transfusion should be based on the patient's risk for complications of inadequate oxygenation.
3. The use of a single hemoglobin "trigger" for all patients and other approaches that fail to consider all important physiologic and surgical factors affecting oxygenation are not recommended.

Although hemoglobin concentration is reported on the complete blood count, it is more common for veterinarians to evaluate the hematocrit, which usually is approximately three times the hemoglobin concentration (g/dL). A scoring system for the rational use of packed red blood cells (RBCs) in dogs was developed in an attempt to decrease unnecessary use (Kerl and Hohenhaus 1993). This scoring system, however, did not account for blood transfusions under conditions of rapid blood loss and failure to maintain blood pressure. It is important to assess anemic dogs and cats carefully and to assess the likelihood of blood loss during the procedure. A dog with a hematocrit of 18% and a healthy cardiovascular system about to undergo a noninvasive diagnostic procedure may

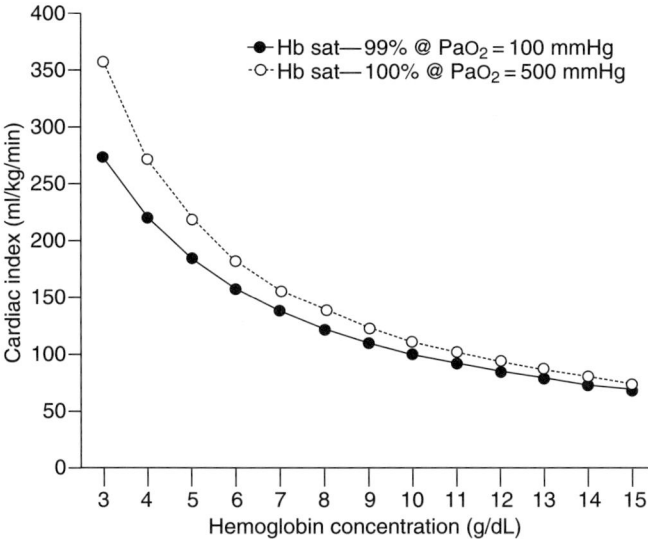

FIGURE 15-1. The graph indicates the alteration in cardiac index needed to provide an oxygen delivery of 15 mL/kg/min when the PaO_2 is increased from 100 to 500 mm Hg, assuming that hemoglobin saturation increases from 99 to 100%. Note that the increased PaO_2 begins to make a difference only when the hemogloblin decreases below about 5 g/dL.

be a candidate for anesthesia without prior transfusion. A patient with the same hematocrit but with significant mitral regurgitation and about to undergo an exploratory laparotomy for an undefined abdominal mass would be more likely to require a preoperative blood transfusion.

POLYCYTHEMIA

Patients with polycythemia are at risk for complications because of the increased viscosity of their blood. High viscosity increases myocardial work and may lead to inadequate flow in some capillary beds, especially if the animal becomes hypotensive (Baer et al. 1987). The hematocrit should be reduced to at least 65% by removal of blood and replacement with an isotonic crystalloid before the polycythemic patient is anesthetized. Animals with polycythemia caused by chronic hypoxia (e.g., tetralogy of Fallot) must be monitored carefully for signs of inadequate oxygen delivery when such hemodilution is undertaken.

HYPOPROTEINEMIA

Many drugs given during anesthesia are highly protein bound, and hypoproteinemia may result in a greater fraction of the anesthetic being available. More profound depression thus may occur from a given dose in the hypoproteinemic patient. Most drugs bind to albumin, and it is this fraction of the proteins that is of greatest importance. If, however, the drug is titrated to effect, the increased free fraction of drug is accounted for by close monitoring of anesthetic induction. Thus, concerns about hypoproteinemia are greater when using intramuscular injection or bolus dose techniques.

Hypoproteinemia also may affect the balance between hydrostatic and colloid oncotic pressure, leading to increased loss of fluid from the capillaries. This effect is of particular concern to the anesthetist because it may increase the likelihood of pulmonary edema formation.

Clinically, this effect is of limited importance unless there is a strong possibility that left atrial pressure is increased (e.g., low oncotic pressure in an animal with mitral regurgitation).

HYPERPROTEINEMIA

Increased plasma protein concentration is of concern only as a sign of hypovolemia. In normally hydrated dogs and cats with hyperproteinemia, it is the globulins that are increased, and this fraction has less impact on protein binding of drugs and oncotic pressure than does albumin. However, hyperproteinemia may be a cause of pseudohyponatremia if the total protein concentration excedes 10 g/dL.

HYPONATREMIA

Rapid correction of hyponatremia may be necessary to treat cerebral edema (usually only when serum sodium is <130 mEq/L). With acute hyponatremia, rapid correction may not cause any complications in the brain, but with chronic hyponatremia a rapid change in serum sodium concentration can lead to an osmotic demyelination syndrome or myelinolysis occurring one to several days after therapy (O'Brien et al. 1994; Laureno and Karp 1997). In both acute and chronic situations the rate of change should be approximately 0.5 to 1 mEq/h unless the patient is manifesting signs of cerebral edema, in which case initial therapy with 3% saline may be used to increase serum sodium concentration by 5 to 6 mEq/L over 2 to 3 h. Ideally, hyponatremia should be corrected before surgery but, given the required time frame, this is not always possible. The anesthetist must therefore be prepared to monitor changes in serum sodium concentration carefully in order to prevent myelinolysis. It may be necessary to administer a diuretic to facilitate excretion of free water. See Chapter 3 for more information.

HYPERNATREMIA

Rapid correction of hypernatremia can lead to acute cerebral edema. If the patient is severely hypovolemic, it is important to correct that deficit using a solution with a sodium concentration similar to that of the patient. If the animal is not severely dehydrated and the serum sodium exceeds 165 mEq/L, correction should proceed slowly to achieve a rate of change of 0.5 to 1 mEq/h using 0.45% NaCl or 5% dextrose. In dogs, administration of 5% dextrose at 3.7 mL/kg/h should decrease the serum sodium concentration by 1 mEq/h. Hypernatremia may increase the minimum alveolar concentration of inhalants and a higher dose may be required to maintain anesthesia (Tanifuji and Eger 1978).

HYPOKALEMIA

Hypokalemia can lead to muscle weakness, cardiac arrhythmias, hypotension, and renal insufficiency with associated metabolic acidosis in dogs and cats. In patients with mild hypokalemia but no clinical signs and no identifiable underlying cause, it probably is unnecessary to treat the animal. The patient with hypokalemia that is likely to have a whole-body deficit of potassium should be treated to correct this deficit if possible. The usual recommendation is to correct the deficit at a maximal rate of 0.5 mEq/

kg/h, although higher rates can be used if a severe deficit of total body potassium is suspected (up to 1.0 mEq/kg/h). If the hypokalemic patient must be anesthetized, it is important to monitor for cardiac arrhythmias and to recognize that the heart will be refractory to class I antiarrhythmic drugs (e.g., quinidine, procainamide, lidocaine) and more sensitive to the toxic effects of digitalis glycosides. Hypotension may occur because there is a decrease in systemic vascular resistance possibly related to decreased sensitivity to angiotensin II (Galvez et al. 1977). The pressor response to norepinephrine is normal. If muscle relaxants are to be used, it is prudent to start with a dose that is 30 to 50% lower than the normal dose and titrate the final dose, to effect. Care should be taken administering glucose, sodium bicarbonate or beta$_2$ agonists because they tend to decrease serum potassium concentration. If a potassium-supplemented solution is to be used during anesthesia to correct the deficit, it should be used in conjunction with a solution containing a normal concentration of potassium (4–5 mEq/L) and the two solutions should be clearly labeled. If the animal requires a bolus of fluid during anesthesia, the solution with normal potassium concentration should be used, thus reducing the risk of iatrogenic hyperkalemia. Solutions containing more than 60 mEq/L of potassium should be given by a central vein.

HYPERKALEMIA

Hyperkalemia also is associated with muscle weakness and cardiac arrhythmias. If these signs are present, it is crucial to reduce the effects of hyperkalemia even though it is not possible to reduce total body potassium content without treating the primary condition (e.g., oliguric renal failure, urethral obstruction). Animals with moderate hyperkalemia (6–7 mEq/L) are more likely to develop arrhythmias during anesthesia even if they have not demonstrated electrocardiographic abnormalities earlier. Therapy for hyperkalemia includes administration of calcium to alter the threshold potential of cells, sodium bicarbonate to alter the flux of potassium across the cell membrane, and glucose to facilitate movement of potassium into cells. Insulin may be used with glucose to avoid hyperglycemia but the blood glucose concentration must be monitored. Beta-adrenergic agonists such as albuterol and salbutamol have been used to manage hyperkalemia and their activity may be enhanced with the use of insulin (Allon and Copkney 1990; Lens et al. 1989). One study in dogs documented the effect of epinephrine and ritodrine in reducing hyperkalemia (Follett et al. 1990). After the animal is anesthetized, ventilation should be monitored and controlled if necessary because hypercapnia may decrease pH and facilitate potassium efflux from cells. Depolarizing muscle relaxants (e.g., succinylcholine) should be avoided because they may cause release of potassium from cells. Nondepolarizing relaxants should be used cautiously (50–70% of the normal dose) to avoid prolonged effects. The patient should be monitored carefully by electrocardiography and frequent measurements of serum glucose, potassium, and ionized calcium concentrations and acid-base status. See Chapter 5 for more information.

HYPOCALCEMIA

Decreased calcium concentrations are associated with increased neuromuscular excitability. In the heart, this may manifest itself as a prolonged QT interval and other arrhythmias (ventricular premature contractions, ventricular fibrillation). As with the other electrolytes, the rate of change is an important factor in the type of clinical signs seen. It is important to treat a patient with hypocalcemia and clinical signs before anesthesia. This can be achieved rapidly while the electrocardiogram is monitored for signs of overly rapid correction (bradycardia). Hyperthermia associated with hypocalcemic seizure activity also should be treated before anesthesia. Hypocalcemic patients are at increased risk from the toxic manifestations of digoxin therapy, and this risk should be taken into consideration when preparing cardiac patients for anesthesia.

HYPERCALCEMIA

Signs of muscle weakness also may be seen with hypercalcemia but arrhythmias are relatively uncommon. Cardiovascular manifestations when they do occur include bradycardia with prolonged PR interval, wide QRS complex, and shortened QT interval. Hypercalcemia is difficult to treat acutely and usually requires treatment for at least 24 h before anesthesia. See Chapter 6 for more information.

HYPEROSMOLALITY

Hyperosmolality usually is associated with hypernatremia, hyperglycemia, ketoacidosis, uremia, or the presence of exogenous toxins (e.g., ethylene glycol). In some cases it may be impossible to reverse the hyperosmolar state adequately before anesthesia because therapy (e.g., hemodialysis) may require an invasive procedure. Hyperosmolality may be associated with disruption of the blood-brain barrier leading to greater uptake of some drugs (Zunkeler et al. 1996). This is unlikely to affect most anesthetics because they readily cross the blood-brain barrier normally. The hyperosmolar state associated with hypernatremia may increase the dose of inhalant required for anesthesia (Tanifuji and Eger 1978).

HYPOOSMOLALITY

This invariably is associated with an excess of free water and hyponatremia and should be managed as described before.

HYPOGLYCEMIA

Hypoglycemia in an awake patient usually is manifested by somnolence progressing to coma. In the anesthetized animal, there may be no outward signs, and unless blood glucose concentration is being monitored it is unlikely that hypoglycemia would be detected. Hence, it is important to recognize and manage hypoglycemia preoperatively. Most animals regulate their blood glucose concentration closely, but this may not be the case in very young animals, those with insulinomas, and animals with portosystemic shunts. It usually is unnecessary to remove very young animals from their dam until the time of premedication if they are receiving a liquid diet only. If they have been orphaned or are ill and have not been taking in fluids, it is best to check blood glucose concentration before anesthesia and treat accordingly. If blood is difficult to obtain, the animal can be given some oral glucose in the form of Karo syrup or some other clear dextrose-containing fluid (Faggella and Aronsohn 1993). Intraoperatively, it may be best to use a 2.5 to 5% glucose solution intravenously. Postoperatively, these patients should be monitored carefully or given additional Karo syrup until they can return to their previous feeding regimen. Animals with insulinomas can have resting blood glucose concentrations of 30 to 40 mg/dL and may be tolerating these low glucose concentrations quite well. If exogenous glucose is administered as a bolus to an animal with hyperinsulinism, massive release of insulin may trigger a hypoglycemic crisis. It therefore is important to use relatively dilute solutions of glucose and administer them as an infusion rather than as a bolus. We typically administer 2.5% glucose to these patients the night before surgery at 1 to 1.5 times the normal maintenance rate. Intraoperatively, blood glucose concentration is monitored carefully and glucose infusions continued as necessary. After the tumor is removed, blood glucose concentration usually returns rapidly to the normal range. Animals with portosystemic shunts may become hypoglycemic and glucose supplementation may be needed in the perioperative period. In one retrospective series, 2 of 13 dogs with portosystemic shunts were reported to have developed hypoglycemia intraoperatively (Komtebedde et al. 1991).

HYPERGLYCEMIA

Hyperglycemia typically occurs in diabetic dogs and cats and in stressed cats. Hyperglycemia itself may not be dangerous but if blood glucose concentration exceeds 400 mg/dL it may contribute to a hyperosmolar diuresis with subsequent dehydration. With diabetic animals, it is ideal if anesthesia can be postponed until blood glucose concentration can be better regulated. If this is not feasible, the animal should be treated with insulin and glucose to stabilize blood-glucose between 200 and 300 mg/dL. In patients with brain trauma or those suffering from focal or global brain ischemia during surgery, hyperglycemia may be detrimental to neurologic outcome (Wass and Lanier 1996; Sieber and Traystman 1992; Sieber 1997; Shapira et al. 1995; Feldman et al. 1995). In animal models, blood glucose concentrations as low as 150 to 200 mg/dL have been shown to have negative effects on outcome, but the threshold for cerebral damage seems to be approximately 200 mg/dL (Sieber and Traystman 1992; Li et al. 1995). In a study of dogs, dextrose administration was associated with greater renal damage after an ischemic insult than lactated Ringer's solution (Moursi et al. 1987). It is thought that increased intracellular glucose contributes to lactic acidosis in the cell, decreasing the chance of cell survival.

METABOLIC ACIDOSIS

Dogs and cats generally tolerate moderate acidosis reasonably well. However, severe acidosis is likely to lead to reduced activity of enzyme systems in the body with subsequent alterations in energy production and metabolism of drugs. Acidosis also may alter the activity of some anesthetic drugs because more of the unionized active form of anionic drugs is available at lower pH values. In patients with acidosis arising from insufficient oxygen delivery to tissues because of inadequate circulating volume, correction of the volume deficit may reverse acidosis without need for further therapy. Dogs and cats with diabetic ketoacidosis rarely require exogenous alkali if fluid therapy and insulin administration are managed appropriately. In cases in which the underlying condition is difficult to reverse (e.g., hypoxemia related to airway pathology, heart failure, pheochromocytoma), it is important to manage the acidosis before anesthesia. This is normally done using sodium bicarbonate (see Chapter 10 for more information). Sodium bicarbonate usually is available as an 8.4% solution with 1 mEq bicarbonate per mL and an osmolality of 2000 mOsm/L. In animals that are hyperosmolar or hypernatremic, it may be advisable to dilute bicarbonate to an isosmotic solution to prevent further exacerbation of the animal's condition. An osmolality of 300 mOsm/L can be achieved by diluting 1.5 mL of the 8.4% solution in 8.5 mL of sterile water. Sodium bicarbonate also should not be administered through the same IV line as catecholamines because it inactivates them (Table 15–1). Care should be taken when administering sodium bicarbonate to patients with respiratory depression because it increases the production of CO_2. If the animal is unable to increase its ventilation in response to increased production of CO_2 there may be little overall change in pH.

TABLE 15–1. **Compatibility of Intravenous Solutions with Other Drugs That Might Be Administered During Anesthesia**

Solution	Comments
5% dextrose	The pH of the solution ranges from 3.5 to 6.5, so alkaline solutions may precipitate.
Lactated Ringer's	Slightly acidic and contains calcium. Do not administer with blood products. Sodium bicarbonate may also react with the calcium and form calcium carbonate.
Acetated polyionic	If it contains no calcium, can be used with blood products and sodium bicarbonate.
Sodium chloride 0.9%	Usually slightly acidic but is compatible with most intravenous solutions. May cause precipitation if added to mannitol.
Sodium bicarbonate	Alkaline solution—incompatible with dobutamine, dopamine, isoproterenol, norepinephrine, and epinephrine. May react with calcium in solution (e.g., lactated Ringer's, acetated Ringer's, some polygelatins).
Dextrans	Slightly acidic—may degrade acid-labile drugs and may form drug complexes but appear to be compatible with most intravenous solutions.
Hetastarch	May be incompatible with some antibiotics—crystals formed with amikacin, cefamandole, cefoperazone, and tobramycin.
Polygelatins	Some preparations contain calcium and these should not be used with blood products or sodium bicarbonate.
Blood and plasma	Do not administer through the same line as calcium salts.

METABOLIC ALKALOSIS

Conditions that cause metabolic alkalosis may be associated with a high mortality rate, and 10 of 20 dogs with primary alkalemia died in one study (Robinson and Hardy 1988). Induction of anesthesia in an alkalotic patient may be associated with an increased dose requirement because of a decreased amount of unionized drug. In most cases, management of metabolic alkalosis requires the administration of chloride-containing solutions. This normally is achieved using 0.9% NaCl supplemented with KCl. Mild alkalosis may be caused by hypoalbuminemia, and correction of serum albumin concentration may be sufficient to correct the alkalosis.

Changes in Distribution

DEHYDRATION

Dehydration reduces vascular volume and results in changes in the volume of the intracellular space. The type and extent of change in the various compartments depend on the type of fluid lost. With pure water loss, volume contraction occurs in the intracellular compartment, whereas with hypotonic dehydration an increase in the volume of the intracellular compartment may occur. With hypotonic loss, it is relatively simple to replace the circulating volume, but it takes longer to replenish the volume lost from the rest of the body. These concepts are discussed further in Chapter 3.

PERIPHERAL EDEMA

Peripheral edema usually is a reflection of poor circulation, leaky capillaries, or low oncotic pressure. Peripheral edema may have little impact on the course of anesthesia and surgery, but edema in certain locations may make induction and maintenance of anesthesia difficult for the anesthetist. If the limbs are edematous, it may be difficult to achieve venous or arterial access. In such cases, it may be necessary to use the jugular vein to place an intravenous catheter because the neck usually is less affected than are the limbs. Occasionally, dogs suffer damage to or occlusion of the jugular veins that can be associated with edema of the head and neck, potentially including the airway. Great care should be taken when intubating affected animals because the affected tissue often is very fragile. It may be necessary to create a tracheostomy if the upper airway becomes obstructed and there is no way to improve venous drainage. Therapy aimed at improving local (e.g., hot packs, massage) and general (e.g., positive inotropes) circulation or increasing colloid oncotic pressure may reduce peripheral edema.

PULMONARY EDEMA

Pulmonary edema is of great concern to the anesthetist because it impairs gas exchange in the lungs and potentially reduces uptake of inhaled anesthetics. Formation of edema in the pulmonary circulation is a result of increased hydrostatic pressure, decreased colloid oncotic pressure, or damage to the endothelium allowing leakage of fluid. Increased hydrostatic pressure may be caused by absolute (e.g., volume overload) or relative (e.g., redistribution of blood to the pulmonary circulation) hypervolemia, increased pulmonary venous pressure (e.g., left ventricular failure, mitral regurgitation), or increased pulmonary flow (e.g., left-to-right shunt, anemia). Volume overload should be treated with diuretics or phlebotomy as described earlier (hypervolemia). In animals with left ventricular failure or mitral regurgitation, the aim of therapy is to promote forward flow by using vasodilators or positive inotropes. In the acute setting, dobutamine is a suitable positive inotrope because it increases myocardial contractility while tending to decrease systemic vascular resistance. Nitroprusside or nitroglycerin can be used to decrease peripheral vascular resistance and can be titrated to effect. Ideally, therapy should be monitored using a catheter that allows measurement of pulmonary capillary wedge pressure.

A decrease in colloid oncotic pressure rarely causes pulmonary edema acutely in dogs and cats, but it is important to take low colloid oncotic pressure into account when designing an anesthetic regimen because pulmonary edema may occur with smaller increases in pulmonary hydrostatic pressure. Both ketamine and large doses of oxymorphone have been shown to increase pulmonary vascular pressures (Copland et al. 1987; Haskins et al. 1985). If it is thought that low colloid oncotic pressure is contributing to pulmonary edema, therapy should be instituted to increase colloid oncotic pressure (e.g., plasma, dextrans, hetastarch, polygelatins). In the case of pulmonary edema related to leaky membranes, therapy should be aimed at reducing pulmonary vascular pressure (e.g., nitroprusside, diuretics) and providing supportive care for the animal. Supportive care involves provision of oxygen, suction of froth from the airway, and institution of positive-pressure ventilation if necessary. Mechanical ventilation may improve gas exchange in patients with pulmonary edema. Positive pressure ventilation with the addition of positive end-expiratory pressure (PEEP) or continuous positive airway pressure (CPAP) may not reduce lung water but may increase access to previously collapsed regions of the lung and may increase the capacity of the interstitium to hold fluid.

PLEURAL FLUID

Pleural fluid acts as a space-occupying lesion and impairs ventilation. In most cases, pleural fluid should be drained before anesthetizing the animal. If there appears to be a continuous air leak from the lung, it is best to place a chest drain before anesthesia or place a large-gauge catheter (e.g., 14 gauge) that can be aspirated rapidly to remove any accumulated air. In cases of hemothorax, blood is defibrinated during its residence in the pleural space. Accumulated blood can be aspirated from the pleural space and given back to the animal intravenously without providing additional anticoagulants. Autotransfusion should only be performed if there is minimal risk of bacterial contamination of the blood and no risk of the blood containing cancer cells that could metastasize to other areas of the body. The blood should be passed through a filter to remove clots before it is autotransfused. Cats with pleuritis appear to be in great pain and often are very fractious. It may be beneficial to provide sedation and analgesia (e.g., oxymorphone) as well as oxygen before attempting to drain the chest.

PERITONEAL FLUID

A large volume of fluid in the abdomen can increase intraabdominal pressure (so-called abdominal compartment syndrome) and should be drained before anesthesia if feasible. Abdominal compartment syndrome is associated with a number of physiologic changes including hypoventilation with reduced pulmonary compliance; tachycardia; low cardiac output; and increased central venous, mean pulmonary artery, and pulmonary capillary wedge pressure. In the abdomen the increased pressure reduces urine output and decreases blood flow to the abdominal wall and the splanchnic vascular beds. Intraabdominal hypertension also may increase intracranial pressure with a decrease in cerebral perfusion pressure (Ivatury et al. 1997).

Drainage of the abdomen usually is achieved by placing a catheter in the abdominal cavity and draining the fluid with a syringe. It is helpful if the catheter has additional side holes cut in it before insertion so that there is less likelihood of the catheter being obstructed by the omentum. Most affected animals have greater respiratory distress lying on their back, and the catheter usually is inserted with the animal on its side. The author usually places the catheter about halfway between the last rib and the ischium, 1 to 4 in. off the midline. Draining fluid in this manner can take a long time, but this is actually advantageous because rapid removal can result in mesenteric vasodilatation and cardiovascular collapse (Ivatury et al. 1997). In the case of hemoabdomen, the blood may have been defibrinated but it is best to collect it in an anticoagulant (e.g., heparin, citrate). Collected blood should be used only if there is no gross contamination of the abdomen and no risk of neoplasia. The blood should be passed through a filter to remove clots before it is autotransfused. In cases of massive trauma, it may be better to leave the blood in the abdomen until the surgeon is ready to stop the bleeding. Although the accumulated blood may compromise ventilation during this time, the increased intraabdominal pressure may reduce the rate of hemorrhage.

INCREASED INTRACRANIAL PRESSURE

Increased intracranial pressure (ICP) requires careful management in terms of fluid balance. The cranial vault is a relatively fixed cavity and any accumulated fluid tends to increase the pressure. An increase in the fluid content of the brain or in the volume of blood or cerebrospinal fluid in the cranial vault promotes an increase in ICP. In situations in which the cause is medically reversible (e.g., hyponatremia), therapy should be carried out before anesthesia. In cases in which the diagnosis or treatment requires anesthesia, the preoperative assessment of the patient must include a detailed examination of fluid balance. Animals with an acute increase in ICP caused by trauma also may be hypovolemic because of other injuries. Judicious use of hypertonic resuscitation fluids is appropriate for these patients because such fluids promote a reduction in ICP while restoring circulating volume (Zornow and Prough 1995). Patients with chronically increased ICP often have had decreased food and water intake for some time and may have been treated with diuretics to reduce ICP. Consequently such patients often are dehydrated and may have electrolyte disturbances. Whenever possible, preoperative assessment should include examination of the animal for signs of dehydration, an assessment of the cause of increased ICP, an evaluation of renal function, and measurement of serum electrolytes, hematocrit, total proteins, osmolality, and colloid oncotic pressure. If the animal clearly is dehydrated, it should be given fluids before anesthesia to increase its circulating volume. If plasma osmolality is <320 mOsm/kg, it may be beneficial to treat the animal with mannitol (0.25–1 g/kg).

INCREASED INTRAOCULAR PRESSURE

Patients with glaucoma often are treated similarly to patients with a raised ICP (i.e., diuretics) but they also are given carbonic anhydrase inhibitors (e.g., dichlorphenamide, Daranide), which can cause metabolic acidosis over the course of 12 to 24 h. Although correction of the acidosis may not be essential in many of these animals, treatment with sodium bicarbonate may decrease the risk associated with anesthesia. The combination of dehydration and acidosis may significantly reduce the dose of thiopental required for induction and care should be taken to titrate this drug to effect in these patients.

AGE

As animals get older, body water and cardiovascular reserve decrease. These changes make older animals more susceptible to fluid overload in the perioperative period. Geriatric patients admitted to the hospital several days before anesthesia and surgery may not have been drinking well (i.e., low tolerance for a new environment) and may be dehydrated.

PREGNANCY

Pregnancy is associated with many changes in fluid balance. In women, the typical changes associated with pregnancy include hyponatremia; decreased blood urea nitrogen and creatinine concentrations; respiratory alkalosis; decreased serum calcium, magnesium, and protein concentrations; and decreased hematocrit. Similar changes have been documented in dogs. Serum protein concentrations tend to decrease during pregnancy, with the most marked change being a decrease in serum albumin concentration (Cairoli et al. 1980). Hematocrit decreases (Allard et al. 1989), with a proportionately greater decrease with increasing numbers of fetuses (Kaneko et al. 1993). The pregnant dog has a decreased baroreceptor response to hypotension (Brooks and Keil 1994b) and is more susceptible to hypotension with blood loss (Brooks and Keil 1994a). Thus, the pregnant animal may be more susceptible to the negative circulatory effects of anesthetics and may require an increased volume of fluids during a surgical procedure. In bitches and queens that have been in labor for some time, dehydration and endotoxemia also may be present and add to circulatory instability. Affected patients may benefit from fluid therapy before anesthesia.

Changes in Function

CARDIOVASCULAR DISEASE

If the heart is failing, it may not tolerate an increased fluid load. Increased preload in this setting may not result in increased cardiac output because of changes in the Frank-Starling curve. Conversely, even a failing heart does not function optimally if preload is allowed to decrease too much. In a prospective study of human patients, it was found that the frequency of postoperative heart failure was highest in patients who had received less than 500 mL/h of fluids intraoperatively (Charlson et al. 1991). The most common cause of congestive heart failure in dogs is mitral insufficiency. This condition is characterized by excessive retrograde flow with an increasing volume load on the heart. Treatment often involves use of vasodilators (e.g., nitroglycerin, hydralazine, and angiotensin converting enzyme inhibitors) to decrease afterload and diuretics and salt restriction to decrease circulating volume. Consequently, cardiac patients have the potential to be hypovolemic. The diagnosis of relative hypovolemia in these patients is based on clinical signs such as skin turgor, mucous membrane color, capillary refill time, and jugular venous distention. Evaluation of renal function (including urine output) may assist in deciding whether the animal is adequately hydrated. Thoracic radiographs can be used to help assess pulmonary venous distention (i.e., lack of pulmonary venous distention implies lower left atrial pressure and hence lack of excessive preload). The most useful measurement in these patients is pulmonary capillary wedge pressure (PCWP). Pulmonary capillary wedge pressure is obtained by inserting a balloon-tipped catheter into the pulmonary vein from either the jugular or femoral vein. Such invasive monitoring certainly is warranted in some cardiac patients and provides the best guide to fluid therapy. If the animal has right-sided heart failure, monitoring central venous pressure (CVP) provides similar information. In one study, use of CVP or PCWP was associated with more aggressive fluid therapy (>500 mL/h), which in turn was associated with a lower risk of postoperative congestive heart failure (Charlson et al. 1991). In the past, it has been recommended that fluids containing low concentrations of sodium be administered to cardiac patients (e.g., 0.45% saline in 2.5% dextrose). Most of these patients have an increase in total body sodium and an increase in total body water. The latter tends to exceed the former, and affected patients may be hyponatremic (Anand et al. 1989). Thus, it seems illogical to give a solution that contains additional free water. If such a patient is hypovolemic, it would be more appropriate to use a balanced electrolyte solution. If the patient is not hypovolemic, it already has excessive volume and fluids may not be needed.

In other myocardial diseases, it also is important to assess the patient preoperatively for signs of dehydration and heart failure (e.g., distended jugular veins, slow jugular emptying, jugular pulses, ascites, pulmonary edema, pleural effusion). Invasive monitoring as described earlier may be necessary to optimize fluid therapy during anesthesia and surgery. Blood may flow best at a hematocrit of 25 to 30%, but it may be necessary to maintain higher values in order to maintain optimal tissue oxygenation. If an animal in heart failure also is anemic, consideration should be given to preloading the animal with packed red cells in order to optimize oxygen delivery.

COAGULATION DEFECTS

Any coagulation defect that is likely to increase intraoperative blood loss should be corrected before surgery if possible. If an animal has a known coagulation defect (e.g., hemophilia, hepatic failure, coumarin poisoning, von Willebrand's disease), it should be given fresh frozen plasma, cryoprecipitate, fresh plasma or fresh whole blood, and vitamin K in the case of coumarin poisoning. These treatments should be given within a few hours of surgery because the half-lives of most clotting factors are relatively short. Although fresh frozen plasma and fresh plasma may have sufficient clotting factors to reverse the coagulation defect, such therapy often fails in animals with severe defects. In Doberman pinschers with von Willebrand's disease, fresh frozen plasma (450 mL) did not decrease buccal mucosal bleeding time despite an increase in von Willebrand's factor, whereas cryoprecipitate reversed the defect successfully (Ching et al. 1994). Therapy with plasma from donors receiving desamino d-arginine vasopressin (DDAVP) may be more effective than plasma from untreated donors. Cryoprecipitate is prepared from a number of donors and therefore has the potential to provide greater antigenic stimulation or transmit disease. Cryoprecipitate contains 10 to 20 times the normal amount of clotting factors and can be given in a small volume. Thus, it may be useful in animals in which volume overload may be a concern (e.g., Doberman pinschers with von Willebrand's disease and cardiomyopathy). The author has not used cryoprecipitate and has successfully managed dogs with von Willebrand's disease using fresh frozen plasma in mildly affected dogs or by treating both the plasma donor and recipient with DDAVP (1 µg/kg subcutaneously) in more severely affected dogs.

Animals with thrombocytopenia or dysfunctional platelets may require platelet infusion before surgery. Platelet life span in immune-mediated thrombocytopenia is considerably shortened, and platelet infusions may be effective for only a matter of hours. Although it is commonplace for platelet-rich plasma to be prepared for affected people, this is relatively rare in veterinary medicine. Platelet preparations have a short half-life (12–24 h) and so they generally are prepared for individual patients in veterinary medicine. Consequently, most patients that are thrombocytopenic or have platelet dysfunction are treated with fresh whole blood. The amount of blood needed (TV) depends on the platelet count of the patient (P_E), the platelet count of the donor blood (P_D), the target platelet count (P_T), and the blood volume (BV) of the patient:

$$BV \times P_E + TV \times P_D = (BV + TV) \times P_T$$

Note: Volumes must be expressed in the same units (i.e., blood volume in µL if platelet count is per µL or platelet count/L if blood volume is in L.)

The ASA guidelines for infusion of platelets are as follows (Practice Guidelines, 1996):

1. Prophylactic platelet transfusion is rarely indicated when thrombocytopenia is due to increased platelet destruction (e.g., idiopathic thrombocytopenic purpura).

2. Prophylactic platelet transfusion is rarely indicated when thrombocytopenia is due to decreased platelet production when the platelet count is greater than 100×10^9/L and is usually indicated when the platelet count is below 50×10^9/L. The determination of whether patients with intermediate platelet counts ($50–100 \times 10^9$/L) require therapy should be based on the risk of bleeding.
3. Surgical and obstetric patients with microvascular bleeding usually require platelet transfusion if the platelet count is less than 50×10^9/L and rarely require therapy if it is greater than 100×10^9/L. With intermediate platelet counts ($50–100 \times 10^9$/L), the determination should be based on the patient's risk for more significant bleeding.
4. Operative procedures ordinarily associated with insignificant blood loss may be undertaken in patients with platelet counts less than 50×10^9/L.
5. Platelet transfusion may be indicated despite an apparently adequate platelet count if a known platelet dysfunction and microvascular bleeding are present.

Patients with disseminated intravascular coagulation (DIC) may need surgical intervention to correct the initiating cause of the DIC. Restoration of circulating volume with fresh whole blood or fresh frozen plasma is the mainstay of preoperative therapy for patients with DIC. If heparin is used, it should be given at a dosage that does not cause significant prolongation of bleeding time (e.g., 75 IU/kg q8h subcutaneously). If heparin is added to the blood or plasma (same dosage) the activated partial thromboplastin time (APTT) should be determined before surgery to ensure that it is not excessively prolonged (i.e., not more than twice normal).

RENAL DISEASE
Patients with chronic renal insufficiency are at risk for having their disease exacerbated by the hemodynamic changes during anesthesia and surgery. Affected animals should be managed carefully during the perioperative period. They should be allowed access to water up until the time of premedication. Any dehydration present should be corrected before anesthesia.

Patients with severe oliguric renal insufficiency are of concern because they have severely limited ability to excrete an extra fluid load and may already be hypervolemic and hypertensive. If possible, it is advantageous in these animals to monitor CVP as a guide to fluid therapy. Monitoring CVP provides information on how well the heart is able to pump the existing circulating volume and allows the anesthetist to watch the response to fluid therapy in the perioperative period.

HEPATIC DISEASE
Mild hepatic insufficiency rarely causes significant disturbances in fluid balance but significant alterations occur as the severity of hepatic injury progresses. The liver synthesizes many proteins, and hypoalbuminemia and deficiencies of clotting factors may occur as hepatic insufficiency progresses. These alterations are managed as described earlier. Blood ammonia concentrations are increased in patients with portosystemic shunts and in those with hepatic failure. Consequently, it is important not to administer additional ammonia by the use of stored blood products that may have increased ammonia content.

Endocrine Disease
DIABETES INSIPIDUS
Animals with diabetes insipidus must be monitored carefully during the preoperative period to be sure they continue to drink water. Animals with complete central diabetes insipidus can become markedly dehydrated within a matter of hours (5% dehydration may occur after 4 h of water deprivation). Consequently, affected animals should have access to water until the time of premedication.

HYPERADRENOCORTICISM
Animals with hyperadrenocorticism are polyuric and polydipsic and should have access to water until the time of premedication. Some dogs with hyperadrenocorticism have mildly increased serum sodium and mildly decreased serum potassium concentrations, but these rarely are of sufficient magnitude to be of concern. Animals with hyperadrenocorticism tend to be hypertensive, which may exacerbate underlying cardiac disease (e.g., mitral regurgitation) and they may have increased sensitivity to vasoconstrictive drugs. In addition, they bruise easily and special care should be taken when placing IV catheters. If the affected animal is being anesthetized for major surgery, hypercoagulability and increased risk of pulmonary thromboembolism are concerns. Prophylactic therapies for hypercoagulability may include the use of heparin, plasma, and hetastarch.

HYPOADRENOCORTICISM
Hyponatremia, hypochloremia, hyperkalemia, hypovolemia, hypoglycemia, metabolic acidosis, and azotemia commonly are associated with hypoadrenocorticism. These abnormalities are associated with hypotension and decreased sensitivity to positive inotropes and vasoconstrictive drugs. The fluid of choice for management of these animals is 0.9% NaCl, which tends to correct all of the preceding abnormalities except the hypoglycemia and metabolic acidosis, which should be monitored during therapy and corrected as necessary by administration of glucose and sodium bicarbonate. Hypotension can be especially difficult to manage in these patients intraoperatively and steroid replacement should be started before induction of anesthesia.

DIABETES MELLITUS
In controlled diabetes, there rarely is any major concern about fluid balance preoperatively. The animal's normal feeding regimen and insulin dose are used on the day before surgery. On the morning of surgery, the animal receives half its daily dose of insulin and blood glucose concentration is monitored throughout the procedure. The animal is treated with glucose and/or insulin as determined by serial blood glucose measurements. Animals with uncontrolled diabetes may be dehydrated and may require fluid therapy before anesthesia.

HYPOTHYROIDISM

Patients with hypothyroidism rarely have any electrolyte disturbances but can be hypotensive and have a poor response to positive inotropes and vasoconstrictors. If possible, the animal should be adequately treated for hypothyroidism for at least 1 to 2 weeks before it is anesthetized.

HYPERTHYROIDISM

Animals with hyperthyroidism tend to be in a hyperdynamic state and are at risk for fatal, catecholamine-mediated arrhythmias when anesthetized. It is best if the animal is treated with an agent that antagonizes the action of thyroxine (e.g., methimazole) for at least 2 weeks before anesthesia (Peterson 1984).

Access to the Circulation

The technical aspects of fluid administration are covered in Chapter 14. In the perioperative period, access to the circulation via the intravenous (IV) or intraosseous (IO) route should be available so that fluids can be given rapidly should the need arise. As discussed earlier, the diameter of the catheter should be sufficient to allow fluids to be administered rapidly enough for the expected deficits. It also is important that the connections to the animal be set up carefully and that they are secure. If the fluid line becomes disconnected with the animal draped for surgery, it may not be detected quickly and the animal may experience significant blood loss from the catheter. When the patient is prepared for a surgical procedure, the anesthetist should make sure to set up the fluid lines so that an injection port is accessible without the need to reach under the drapes. Also, the animal should be positioned in such a way that the fluids can flow easily. Drugs added to the fluids and administered through the same line must be compatible (see Table 15–1). If an animal will be receiving several drugs, it may be necessary to create additional access sites in order to prevent incompatible drugs from being administered through the same line. Consideration also must be given to the site of access. In cats undergoing declawing of the front paws, it is advisable to place the catheter in the hind leg so that it does not interfere with the surgery. In patients in which the caudal vena cava is to be occluded during surgery, it is important to have the catheter in the forelimb or neck so that fluids reach the remaining circulation during the occlusion. In an emergency in an anesthetized animal with no venous access, the most visible vessel usually is the sublingual vein. This vein can be catheterized rapidly if necessary.

Thermodynamic Considerations

Infusion of fluids into the body at temperatures less than normal body temperature requires that the animal warms the fluid and this effect cools the animal. If we assume that the specific heat of water (and most of the crystalloid solutions used in fluid therapy) is 1 kcal/kg/°C, it would cost the animal 18 kcal to raise the temperature of 1 L of fluid from 20 to 38°C. If the specific heat of the body is 0.83 kcal/kg/°C, 1 L of fluid at 20°C would cool a 21.7-kg dog by 1°C (Gentilello and Moujaes 1995). Stated in another way, a fluid infusion rate of 10 mL/kg/h at 20°C would cost the patient 0.18 kcal/h and would tend to cool the body by approximately 0.2°C/h. These losses are relatively minor in comparison with the body heat lost via radiation but may become more significant when massive fluid volumes are required or the infused fluid is much colder (e.g., stored blood products).

Effects of Anesthesia

Some drugs may alter sympathetic activity and thus affect blood volume and the distribution and excretion of body fluids. Acepromazine is a potent alpha$_1$ antagonist and even low dosages of the drug (0.001 mg/kg) induce this effect. In the healthy patient, this effect is associated with minor decreases in arterial blood pressure and hematocrit (Coulter et al. 1981). In an animal with increased sympathetic tone, however, the administration of acepromazine may result in profound hypotension. Acepromazine also is a dopamine antagonist and may inhibit the effect of dopamine to increase renal blood flow. Such an effect has been demonstrated with chlorpromazine, but no studies have been carried out with acepromazine (Brotzu 1970). The alpha$_2$ agonists have profound effects on the circulation and on renal function. In dogs and cats, administration of these drugs, even at low doses, causes a significant decrease in cardiac output (40–60%). They also have a direct effect on the kidney, the end result of which is significant diuresis (urine output increases 3- to 10-fold). The mechanism for this effect appears to be related to antagonism of ADH, and this dehydrating effect may be even more significant in a patient that is avidly conserving water. The opioids have a variety of actions. The mu agonists (e.g., morphine, oxymorphone, meperidine) have an antidiuretic effect, whereas the kappa agonists (e.g., butorphanol, pentazocine, nalbuphine) tend to promote diuresis. The antidiuresis associated with the mu agonists may be the result of stimulation of ADH release. Release of ADH may be stimulated in the awake patient but there is a reduction in the release of ADH in anesthetized patients receiving large doses of potent opioids (causing a reduced stress response) (de Lange et al. 1982). The dissociative drugs (e.g., ketamine, tiletamine) tend to decrease urine output despite increases in cardiac output and blood pressure (Fischer et al. 1979). These drugs also tend to decrease baroreceptor responses, and this may be important in the anesthetized patient with relative hypovolemia that undergoes changes in body position.

Drugs that are used for the induction and maintenance of anesthesia all tend to decrease urine output, mainly through their hemodynamic effects (Ishihara et al. 1978). Thiopental has been shown to alter renal sodium resorption leading to increased sodium and water losses in dogs (Gagnon et al. 1982), but in human patients there is either no change or a decrease in urine output (Ishihara et al. 1978). Thiopental also decreases hematocrit (which may be significant in an anemic patient) but it has little effect on plasma volume (Usenik and Cronkite 1965). Propofol causes hypotension if given rapidly, and it may cause some reduction in glomerular filtration rate and urine flow (Petersen et al. 1996). In normal sheep, there was minimal effect on renal function but there was a significant detrimental effect during sepsis (Booke et al. 1996). Etomidate preserves circulation better than most other drugs administered IV for induction but it may alter renal function by virtue of the base in which it is constituted. Etomidate usually is supplied in propylene glycol, which can induce renal failure if enough is given. This would be unlikely with an induction dose of the drug, but continuous infusion might be associated with nephrotoxicity from the propylene glycol or the hemolysis that is likely to occur. Severe renal insufficiency was reported in dogs after an infusion of etomidate (Moon 1994). All of the inhalants are associated with a decrease in renal function, but this effect can be prevented to some extent by preloading the animals with fluids. Methoxyflurane has long been associated with nephrotoxicity in people, but this effect has not been reported in dogs and cats. There is some concern that sevoflurane can react with soda lime or baralime, releasing a polyvinyl compound (Compound A) that is nephrotoxic.

Positive-pressure ventilation has been associated with changes in renal function. A reduction in urine output occurs with the institution of positive-pressure ventilation, with CPAP or PEEP (Kaczmarczyk 1994). The techniques of PEEP and CPAP increase CVP, mean pulmonary artery pressure, and PCWP (Matsumura et al. 1983). The increase in CVP tends to increase renal vein pressure, which may alter interstitial pressure within the kidney (Rossaint et al. 1993). The use of intermittent positive-pressure ventilation (IPPV) and PEEP or CPAP is associated with an increase in ADH secretion, but it is likely that increased renal interstitial pressure has a more important effect because the decrease in urine output can be seen without changes in ADH (Rossaint et al. 1992).

Regional anesthetic techniques also may result in volume-responsive hypotension. This is particularly true with epidural or intrathecal techniques. In people, the spinal cord ends at vertebral level L1-2 and it is necessary to inject enough drug to extend high into the thoracic region in order to block enough spinal segments for abdominal surgery. As a result, there is a significant block of sympathetic outflow from the thoracic and lumbar spinal cord segments, which can result in hypotension. In the dog, the cord ends at vertebral level L6-7 and in the cat the cord ends at S1-2. Thus, it is feasible to achieve an effective abdominal block in dogs and cats without a significant loss of sympathetic tone. Still, hypotension can occur with this technique, and the animal should be monitored accordingly.

▶ Monitoring Fluid Therapy

Determining the best fluid regimen and judging the adequacy of therapy are dependent on monitoring the patient. Unfortunately, clinical signs are a crude guide at best, and technology has not provided techniques to monitor all of the necessary information. Nevertheless, we can obtain a reasonable amount of information and integrate it into a picture that helps guide our therapy.

Monitoring Changes in Volume

Methods for monitoring intravascular volume are not available in routine practice. Most of the techniques that have been used in the laboratory involve dye dilution and require sophisticated measuring techniques and calculations to determine intravascular volume. Even if such information was available, it is unlikely that absolute values for vascular volume would be of much use because it is unlikely that a normal volume measurement for the animal in question would be available before the procedure. Trends over time, however, may be helpful. Devices that measure changes in blood volume are available on sophisticated hemodialysis machines and provide a guide to therapy in situations in which blood volumes can change rapidly. In general, however, changes in blood volume must be inferred from clinical signs.

Loss of skin turgor is a helpful sign when present, but in many animals skin turgor changes little until volume depletion is severe (Hardy and Osborne 1979). Radiographic signs of hypovolemia include microcardia and a decrease in the size of the caudal vena cava and pulmonary vessels. Capillary refill time is used to monitor the microcirculation and, if prolonged, implies poor tissue perfusion. Poor tissue perfusion may be the result of hypovolemia, heart failure, vasoconstriction, or endotoxemia. This clinical sign recently has been examined carefully in humans and was found to be a poor predictor of volume status (Schriger and Baraff 1991). Capillary refill time is significantly affected by body temperature and ambient temperature (Gorelick et al. 1993; Baraff 1993). Also, capillary refill time can appear normal immediately after cardiac arrest. In dogs and cats, it is usual to use the mucous membranes of the mouth for testing capillary refill, and this technique may avoid some of the changes occurring in people as a result of alterations in ambient temperature because the temperature of the mouth remains relatively constant. The ability to assess capillary refill time accurately is affected by the presence of pigment in the mucous membranes of some animals, making it impossible to obtain a result in these individuals.

Heart rate increases in response to hypovolemia but is a nonspecific sign. In anesthetized animals that develop unexplained tachycardia, the author often gives a fluid bolus to determine whether or not the animal is hypovolemic. A decreased heart rate after fluid infusion without resumption of tachycardia is indicative of preexisting hypovolemia.

Low CVP, PCWP, and systemic blood pressure all can imply low circulating volume but also can change for other reasons. The CVP and PCWP probably are better measurements of volume status because they are affected by cardiac preload, which is largely dependent on blood volume. In dogs and cats receiving IPPV and direct arterial pressure monitoring, systolic pressure may vary because of the effect of intrathoracic pressure changes on venous return. Although not totally predictable, significant decreases in systolic pressures associated with ventilation are indicative of hypovolemia (assuming ventilation pressure is 10–20 cm H_2O). In one study, the systolic pressure variation was approximately 6% with a 5% loss of blood volume and increased linearly to approximately 11% with 30% loss of blood volume (Perel et al. 1987). Systolic pressure variation was much less in hypotension without hypovolemia (Pizov et al. 1988).

Cardiac output tends to decrease with hypovolemia,

but this is a relatively nonspecific change because cardiac output also decreases with increased systemic vascular resistance or myocardial failure. Evaluation of cardiac output in conjunction with pressure measurements allows the clinician to interpret volume status more readily. Determination of cardiac output and PCWP requires placement of a thermistor and pressure port in the pulmonary artery with sophisticated and expensive equipment. Placement of these catheters in small patients (<5 kg) is particularly difficult and makes it virtually impossible to obtain such readings in a clinical setting.

Urine output decreases with hypovolemia but also decreases with hypotension or low cardiac output. If urine output remains relatively normal, it is unlikely that the animal is hypovolemic. Measurement of urine volume requires time, and it is difficult to obtain accurate measurements at shorter time intervals than every hour. Consequently, measurement of urine volume cannot be used to monitor acute changes in circulating volume. The only available method for the measurement of urine output involves the insertion of a urinary catheter, and this involves some risk of introducing a urinary tract infection (UTI) (Palacios et al. 1995; Rebollo et al. 1996; Stamm 1978; Wenzel et al. 1976). The risk of UTI with catheterization is greater in female than in male dogs (Biertuempfel and Ling 1981). If monitoring urine output is necessary, a sterile urinary catheter should be inserted aseptically and immediately connected to a closed drainage system (Lees 1996). The reservoir of the urinary collection system should be maintained below the level of the patient. If the animal is being moved, it is best to clamp the drainage system so that urine cannot reflux up the tubing into the bladder. The urinary catheter should be left in the patient for the shortest duration possible because the risk of a UTI increases with every day the catheter is left in place. Ideally, the animal should not receive antibiotics while the catheter is in place (unless UTI already has been diagnosed) because use of antibiotics increases the likelihood of antibiotic-resistant UTI. Withholding antibiotics may not be feasible in a surgical setting and it is important to monitor for development of UTI using urinalysis and urine culture.

Monitoring Changes in Composition

Blood samples must be obtained to monitor changes in the composition of the blood. The results of sodium, potassium, chloride, calcium, bicarbonate, pH, carbon dioxide tension (Pco_2), Po_2, osmolality, colloid oncotic pressure, hematocrit, protein, glucose, urea, and creatinine determinations may affect fluid therapy decisions. When a patient requires monitoring of the composition of blood, it is important to determine how blood samples are to be obtained intraoperatively. It often is difficult to obtain samples from peripheral venous catheters (particularly in small patients) and other sites must be used. Samples can be obtained from the jugular vein with relative ease and a jugular catheter should be placed if several samples are likely to be required. If it is not necessary to measure CVP, a short IV catheter can be used (1.5 to 2 in.). Also useful in the anesthetized patient are the lingual veins. These vessels usually are readily accessible during anesthesia and can be sampled several times without the insertion of a catheter. All of these measurements can be obtained using such samples but care must be taken with interpretation of Po_2. Single arterial samples can be obtained from the lingual, femoral, ulnar, auricular, or dorsal pedal arteries. If several samples will be required and it is advisable to know the Pao_2, an arterial catheter should be placed. In most dogs and cats, the most accessible vessel for this purpose is the dorsal pedal artery over the metatarsal area. If this vessel is inaccessible (e.g., bilateral tibial fractures) or cannot be catheterized, it is feasible to use the other vessels mentioned. If a femoral arterial catheter is placed, it is necessary to be careful because it is relatively easy for such catheters to pull out of the vessel while still attached to the skin. Unless a long stiff catheter has been placed in the femoral artery, it is not advisable to allow the animal to recover with the catheter still in place. The ulnar artery is difficult to catheterize because the shape of the leg makes it difficult to approach the site at a narrow enough angle. The auricular arteries are useful in dogs with large ears (e.g., spaniels, dachshunds) and can be used in the postoperative period, although there is some risk of ischemia with prolonged catheterization. A catheter can be placed in the lingual artery after induction of anesthesia but it must be removed before the end of surgery and the vessel held off for 15 min after the catheter has been removed to prevent the formation of a sublingual hematoma. Care must be taken when flushing auricular and lingual arterial catheters to prevent the injection of air because air could be introduced into the carotid arteries, resulting in air embolism of the cerebral arteries.

The electrocardiogram is used to presumptively identify changes in electrolyte concentrations. The electrocardiogram is useful in this regard because the magnitude of electrocardiographic changes is dependent both on the rate of change and on the actual serum concentration of electrolyte.

Monitoring Changes in Distribution

Dehydration is monitored using the clinical signs described earlier. The presence or absence of peripheral edema and ascites should be readily apparent. In some cases, it may be helpful to measure limb or abdominal circumference to determine whether the fluid accumulation is increasing or decreasing. Measuring the size of the abdomen is particularly difficult but still may be of use in individual patients. An indelible marker can be used to identify the site of measurement for future reference, and thus improve accuracy. Pleural fluid accumulation can be monitored only by thoracic radiography or by draining the fluid on an intermittent or continuous basis.

Intracranial pressure can be measured and can play a crucial role in the management of patients with increased ICP. The catheter is inserted into the cranial vault and attached to a measuring device. The simplest approach is to use a fluid-filled catheter, which can provide sensitive measurements of ICP and also allow measurement of intracranial compliance. The latter can be helpful because it can provide an estimate of the risk of brain herniation.

A fiber-optic catheter that measures pressure indirectly can be inserted directly into the brain. The objective measurement of intraocular pressure with a Schiøtz or applanation tonometer may help guide fluid therapy in cases with high intraocular pressure.

▶ Intraoperative Fluid Management

Intraoperative fluid management depends on

a. How well the patient has been prepared beforehand
b. How much fluid loss occurs normally (insensible loss)
c. How much fluid loss occurs because of the equipment used (e.g., dry gas causes greater water loss than humidified gas)
d. Changes in vascular tone and cardiac output
e. The amount and nature of the tissue exposed during surgery
f. The amount of blood lost

In most patients, crystalloid solutions are used first with colloids and blood products being added as required.

Crystalloids

The anesthetized animal has ongoing fluid losses of approximately $132 \times BW^{0.75}$ mL/day for the dog and $80 \times BW^{0.75}$ mL/day for the cat, where BW is body weight in kg. It is likely that losses will be less than predicted by these formulas because the metabolic rate of most anesthetized animals is less than in the awake resting state. A maintenance solution would be appropriate merely to replace this loss. However, it is expected that fluid losses will increase under anesthesia because of increased loss from the respiratory tract and that there will be changes in hemodynamics that will require fluid therapy (see earlier). Consequently, it has been traditional to use isotonic replacement solutions during anesthesia and expect that any excess sodium will be excreted by the kidneys in the postoperative period. Replacement solutions do not contain high concentrations of potassium and can be given rapidly if necessary without risk of potassium toxicity.

The rate of administration often is set arbitrarily at 10 mL/kg/h. This rate of administration is based on research in humans in the 1960s suggesting that this rate was appropriate for losses occurring during major abdominal surgery. The author has used this approach in many dogs and cats with few adverse effects. In the original studies, blood volume was measured using radioactive tracers (Shires et al. 1961; Virtue et al. 1965). These techniques are accurate in a steady state but may not be accurate when volumes are changing during fluid infusion. Later studies evaluated the dilution of hemoglobin or albumin or the change in blood water content to assess acute changes in blood volume (Svensén and Hahn 1997; Ståhle et al. 1997; Hahn et al. 1997). These studies were performed in healthy human volunteers and may not apply to anesthetized animals. They do, however, provide some useful information. In one study (Hahn et al. 1997), infusions were carried out at different rates using two different volumes. The interstitial fluid space is roughly twice the volume of the intravascular space, and isotonic replacement solutions redistribute, leaving approximately 33% of the infused volume in the vascular space. In this study, the volume retained in the vascular space 15 min after the end of the infusion was approximately 20% and it was approximately 15% after 30 min, indicating rapid redistribution of crystalloid solutions. In another study, slightly different results were obtained for the volumes of distribution. Using albumin gave the highest volume of distribution, followed by blood hemoglobin, and finally blood water (Svensén and Hahn 1997). Albumin may be lost into the interstitium more rapidly during fluid administration, and this may account for the different volumes measured. The volume of distribution for the balanced electrolyte solution was similar to the expected plasma volume but only 50 to 70% of the expected volume for the interstitial space. Regions of the interstitial space with poor blood supply or rigid structure (e.g., bone) may be less likely to take up fluid, and this may account for the difference in calculated volumes.

The authors proposed that these data could be used to calculate infusion rates that would expand the plasma compartment (bolus) and maintain it at this volume (infusion). To increase blood volume by 5% the patient would receive 36 mL/kg/h for 20 min and an ongoing infusion of 15 mL/kg/h (Svensén and Hahn 1997). In another study, nomograms were presented for men and women showing the infusion rate and time required to achieve specific blood volume expansion and the infusion rate required to maintain this expansion (Hahn and Svensén 1997). Whether these data apply to anesthetized animals is uncertain, but the results suggest that a fluid rate of 10 mL/kg/h is relatively conservative.

In a study of healthy dogs undergoing elective ovariohysterectomy or castration, the rate of polyionic fluid administration was examined to determine how it affected hematocrit, total protein concentration, glucose concentration, and systolic blood pressure (Gaynor et al. 1996). The authors tested an acetated polyionic solution given at 0, 5, 10, and 15 mL/kg/h for 1 to 2 h. They saw no differences among groups, suggesting that there was no advantage to fluid therapy for these cases. Cardiac output and renal function were not evaluated and so it is not possible to say whether fluids affected these functions. Crystalloid fluid administration at 11 mL/kg/h for 60 min to halothane-anesthetized cats did not result in any changes in packed cell volume or total protein concentration (Bjorling and Rawlings 1983). These cats had undergone thoracotomy for placement of catheters and did not start the study with normal values (PCV = 25%, total proteins = 4.9 g/dL, colloid oncotic pressure = 10.2 mm Hg) and thus may be regarded as similar to compromised animals in a clinical situation.

Even after deciding that 10 mL/kg/h of an isotonic fluid is a good starting point for intraoperative fluid therapy, a decision still must be made about which solution to use. Common crystalloids available include normal saline (0.9% NaCl), a lactated polyionic fluid (lactated Ringer's solution), an acetated polyionic fluid (e.g., acetated Ringer's, Normosol-R, Plasma-Lyte 148, Isolyte S, Polyionic R), or 5% dextrose in water, saline, or polyionic solutions.

NORMAL SALINE

Normal saline is used widely as a replacement solution intraoperatively. It is the solution of choice for patients with hypercalcemia or hypochloremic alkalosis. This solution contains higher amounts of chloride than plasma and tends to decrease the strong ion difference, leading to acidosis. In classical terms, it dilutes the concentration of bicarbonate and provides large amounts of chloride for reabsorption from the glomerular filtrate, thus leading to hyperchloremic acidosis. The degree of acidosis is not likely to be a problem in the healthy patient but may exacerbate acidosis in a compromised patient.

LACTATED RINGER'S SOLUTION (HARTMANN'S SOLUTION)

Lactated Ringer's solution (LRS) is a balanced electrolyte solution containing lactate that contributes to the correction of acidosis and is the author's fluid of choice for most anesthetized patients. Potential disadvantages of this solution are as follows:

a. It contains calcium and because blood products generally are stored using a compound that chelates calcium, it is not ideal to administer LRS through the same intravenous line as blood products. A 1:10 mixture of blood and LRS resulted in clot formation within 2 min at 37°C (Ryden and Oberman 1975) (see Table 15–1).
b. It contains less sodium than plasma, which could lead to greater loss of fluid into the intracellular compartment, which in turn may be detrimental in patients with cerebral edema. In models of traumatic brain injury, infusion of lactated Ringer's was associated with an increase in ICP (Zornow et al. 1989; Ramming et al. 1994). In a model of closed-head trauma in rats, use of LRS did not affect neurologic outcome or formation of brain edema (Feldman et al. 1995).
c. It contains lactate, which mostly is metabolized in the liver (approximately 56% of normal lactate metabolism occurs in the liver). Infusion of LRS was not associated with an increase in blood lactate concentrations (Didwania et al. 1997) even when there was significant impairment of hepatic function (Goldstein and MacLean 1972). Hepatic removal of lactate, however, is a saturable process and infusion of lactate in patients with severe hyperlactatemia (>9 mmol/L) may result in an increase in blood lactate concentration (Naylor et al. 1984). However, at concentrations of lactate above 9 mmol/L the peripheral tissues remove more lactate than the liver and peripheral metabolism of lactate is not saturable (Naylor et al. 1984). In clinical patients with initial lactate concentrations above 10 mmol/L, infusion of LRS and other volume support was always associated with a decrease in blood lactate concentrations (Canizaro et al. 1971). Some patients with cancer may be hyperlactatemic and have increased ability to recycle lactate to glucose (Waterhouse 1974). In some patients with cancer cachexia, concern has been expressed that the metabolism of lactate consumes energy and thus lactated solutions should not be used. It has been shown that dogs with lymphoma have a transient inability to cope with the lactate load imposed by infusion of LRS (Vail et al. 1990). Although this may be valid in unusual cases, the amount of lactate provided with LRS at 10 mL/kg/h is approximately 36% of the basal production or utilization rate (Adrogue et al. 1996) and it is likely that the negative effect is transient.

The metabolism of lactate is either by gluconeogenesis or by oxidation and in both instances hydrogen ions are consumed. It takes approximately 30 min for this alkalinizing effect to be accomplished (Hartsfield et al. 1981). The alkalinizing effect is not as great as that seen with acetate (about 50%) and this may be due to the presence in LRS of D-lactate, which is not readily metabolized in dogs (Hartsfield et al. 1981).

ACETATED POLYIONIC SOLUTIONS

Acetate is thought to be metabolized rapidly throughout the body, and the alkalinizing effect of this solution is more readily available. As with lactate, the effect takes approximately 30 min to be evident (Hartsfield et al. 1981). In some commercial solutions, gluconate also is used. There is little information on the effects of gluconate but it does appear to cause a slight increase in pH (Kirkendol et al. 1980). Acetated Ringer's suffers from the same disadvantage as LRS in terms of its sodium content. Many of the commercial solutions are calcium free and can be given through the same line as blood products. The main disadvantage of solutions containing acetate is the vasodilatation that can occur with rapid administration (Iseki et al. 1980; Graefe et al. 1978). In a normal healthy patient, a bolus of acetated polyionic solution usually results in an increase in heart rate but little change in blood pressure (Saragoca et al. 1985), but in a patient that is already hypovolemic dramatic decreases in blood pressure can be seen (Fig. 15–2). Acetate-containing solutions also are contraindicated in patients with diabetic ketoacidosis.

5% DEXTROSE

Five percent dextrose in water contains no electrolytes, and when the dextrose is metabolized only water remains. Five percent dextrose may be the solution of choice for patients that have suffered from pure water loss, but it is rarely indicated as the prime replacement solution during anesthesia and surgery. Apart from the fact that the volume of distribution of the 5% dextrose is likely to be larger than that of a balanced electrolyte solution (which would result in a diminished ability to maintain circulating volume) (Roberts et al. 1985), the glucose itself may be detrimental under certain circumstances. In both acute renal and acute cerebral injury, high concentrations of glucose may be detrimental (Moursi et al. 1987; Li et al. 1995; Lam et al. 1991). Concentrations of glucose over

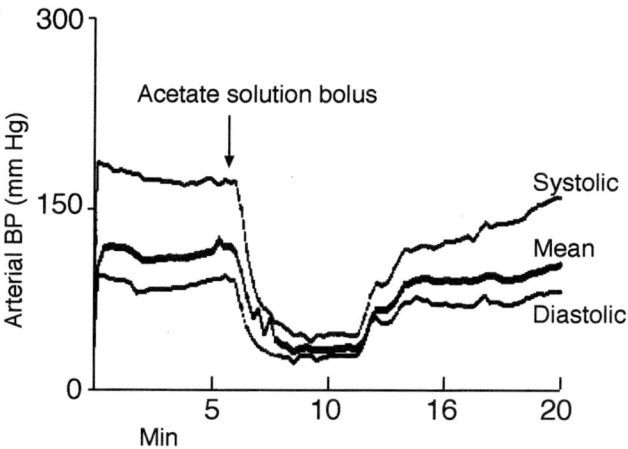

FIGURE 15-2. Administration of an acetated solution (Plasmalyte 148) to a 16-kg dog being anesthetized for cataract surgery. The 50-mL bolus was given before the start of surgery. Hypotension occurred and the dog was given 0.5 μg/kg of epinephrine IV when the mean pressure had leveled off at 33 mm Hg (about 10 min).

200 mg/dL may be of concern in cerebral ischemia (Li et al. 1995; Lam et al. 1991).

2.5% DEXTROSE IN HALF-STRENGTH IONIC SOLUTION

Dextrose (5%) can be mixed with any of the preceding ionic solutions in a 1:1 ratio to halve the ionic strength. Such solutions may be of use in the management of patients with hypernatremia. These solutions are designed to increase the free-water content of the body and it is important to monitor electrolyte concentrations to ensure that excessive dilution does not occur.

HYPERTONIC SOLUTIONS

These solutions may provide rapid resuscitation in the preoperative period but are seldom used intraoperatively. They may be needed in special circumstances such as for an animal with rapid hemorrhage when blood products are unavailable, an animal with a high intracranial pressure, or a patient with hyponatremia. Most of these solutions have very high sodium concentrations and it is important to monitor serum sodium concentrations before and after their administration. Maintenance with an isotonic crystalloid usually is required after administration of these solutions. See Chapter 24 for more information about hypertonic solutions.

Colloids

Dextrans, hetastarch, polygelatins, and plasma are the main colloid solutions available. They are used to correct hypovolemia, provide colloid oncotic pressure, and, in the case of fresh frozen plasma, provide clotting factors. The synthetic colloids are polydisperse colloids that, by definition, contain particles of several different molecular weights. In the past, the average molecular weight (M_w) of such solutions was described but this approach favors the high-molecular-weight particles. It now is common to describe the solution according to the number molecular weight (M_n), which is the total weight of all the molecules divided by the number of molecules. In the case of dextran 70, the M_w is 70,000 but the M_n is 41,000 (Table 15-2). Use of M_n allows recognition of the smaller molecular weight particles in the solution. The terms have clinical significance because the oncotic pressure exerted by the solution depends on the number of particles present, whereas the duration of effect depends on the size of the particles present. The duration of effect of a colloid is short if the particles rapidly leak through the endothelium.

DEXTRANS

The dextran molecule is a linear polysaccharide produced by certain strains of *Leuconostoc* bacteria growing in sucrose-containing media. Dextrans are supplied in low- and high-molecular-weight forms (dextran 40 and 70, respectively) with plasma half-lives estimated at 1 to 3 and 2 to 6 h (Thompson et al. 1970). In dogs with normal renal function, 70% of a dose of dextran 40 and 40% of a dose of dextran 70 are excreted unchanged in the urine within 24 h. The remaining molecules are metabolized slowly to glucose by dextranase in the liver. Some of these molecules may be present in the body weeks after their administration. The plasma volume expansion achieved per gram of dextran is roughly the same, regardless of molecular weight (approximately 20–25 mL water/g dextran) (Hint 1971). Clinically, however, dextran 40 has a greater concentration per milliliter and provides greater plasma volume expansion initially.

Concerns about the use of dextrans include effects on hemostasis and allergic reactions. Dextrans tend to prolong bleeding times by interfering with fibrin clot formation, reducing factor VIII and von Willebrand's factor, diluting clotting factors, and interfering with platelet function. In dogs, rapid infusion of dextran 70 caused a decrease in von Willebrand's factor antigen and factor VIII activity and increases in activated partial thromboplastin time (APTT) and buccal mucosal bleeding time (Concannon et al. 1992). Dextrans and hetastarch also alter the structure of the fibrin clot, giving it a weaker, more chaotic appearance (Gollub and Schaefer 1968). These effects suggest that dextrans may not be the best choice for fluid therapy when major surgery is planned. Clinically, it seems that infusions of dextrans have been associated with increased bleeding, but no studies have documented increased blood loss when dextrans have been used. Allergic reactions have been reported in human patients, but the frequency appears to be less than 0.1% and such reactions have not been reported in dogs or cats.

In humans, dextran 40 has been used to reduce the occurrence of deep vein thrombosis. This effect is thought to be due to decreased viscosity of blood after dextran administration. There also is some evidence that low-molecular-weight dextrans alter red cell aggregation and decrease clumping of red cells in the microcirculation. Use of dextran 70 also reduced the frequency of fatal postoperative pulmonary embolism from 2.0 to 0.35%. In these studies, dextrans were given on the day of surgery. The only common conditions in dogs and cats complicated by pulmonary thromboembolism are hyperadrenocorticism and the nephrotic syndrome, and the use of

TABLE 15–2. Physicochemical Properties of the Artificial Colloids

Colloid	M_w	M_n	Colloid (g/L)	pH	Relative Viscosity	Na (mmol/L)	Cl (mmol/L)	Ca (mmol/L)	K (mmol/L)	Osmolality (mOsm/L)	Colloid Oncotic Pressure (mm Hg)
Dextran 40, NaCl	40,000	26,000	100	3.5–7	5.1–5.4	154	154	0	0	310	NM* (Tønnessen et al. 1993)
Dextran 40, dextrose	40,000	26,000	100	3–7		0	0	0	0	255	NM (Tønnessen et al. 1993)
Dextran 70, NaCl	70,000	41,000	60	5.1–5.7	3.4–4	154	154	0	0	310	59 (Tønnessen et al. 1993)
Hetastarch	450,000	69,000	60	5.5		154	154	0	0	310	29–32 (Tønnessen et al. 1993)
Pentastarch	264,000	63,000	100	5.0		154	154	0	0	326	40
Oxypolygelatin (Vetaplasma, Gelifundol)	30,000	23,300	55			145	100	2	0	200	45–47
Succinylated gelatin (Gelofusine)	35,000	22,600	40	7.4		154	125	0.4	0.4	279	465?
Urea-linked gelatin (Haemaccel)	35,000	24,500	35	7.2–7.3	1.7–1.8	145	145	6.26	5.1	310	NM (Tønnessen et al. 1993) 25.5–28.5 (Evans et al. 1996)

* NM, Not measurable because of diffusion of smaller molecules.

dextrans has not been investigated in these settings in veterinary medicine.

A number of reports have linked dextrans to renal failure. This complication has been attributed to increased viscosity of the glomerular filtrate associated with early excretion of low-molecular-weight particles (Kurnik et al. 1991; Zwaveling et al. 1989). Experimental studies of dogs identified changes in proximal tubular cells but no effect on renal function. Affected human patients have received large doses of dextrans and have had an associated increase in oncotic pressure. Treatment by exchange transfusion to lower oncotic pressure has been successful, suggesting that the renal changes are not structural but functional (Zwaveling et al. 1989). There are no reports of renal failure after dextran administration in dogs or cats.

HETASTARCH

Hetastarch is a synthetic polymer of glucose (amylopectin) that closely resembles glycogen and contains predominantly α-1,4 linkages. Hydroxyethyl groups are added to the molecule with a substitution ratio of 0.5 to 0.7 (i.e., 50–70% of the glucose molecules have hydroxyethyl groups attached), which makes the molecule more water soluble and slows hydrolysis by amylase. The commercially available preparation of hetastarch has an average molecular weight (M_w) of 450,000 with a number molecular weight (M_n) of 69,000 making it the largest of the colloid molecules available. The smaller molecules (molecular weight <59,000) are excreted by the kidneys or pass through the vascular endothelium into the interstitial space. Molecules that reach the interstitial space are taken up by macrophages and slowly metabolized by cellular lysozymes. The larger molecules are slowly broken down by α-amylases. Dogs have approximately three times as much amylase as do humans and hetastarch is broken down faster. In dogs, 31.5% of administered hetastarch was excreted in the urine and 38% remained in plasma after 24 h (Thompson et al. 1970). The half-life of hetastarch in humans varies with time after administration and dose (e.g., the half-life is 1.5–3.6 days during the first 3 days after administration and 13–17 days between 7 and 42 days after administration). After three consecutive daily doses, the excretion of 41 to 46% of hetastarch took 168 h, compared with 48 h after a single dose. This dependence on time and dose has not been demonstrated in dogs (Smiley 1992). In hypoalbuminemic dogs, the administration of hetastarch was associated with an increase in colloid oncotic pressure and a reduction in peripheral edema in most treated patients. There was no apparent correlation between the dose of hetastarch or the change in colloid oncotic pressure and resolution of edema. A few dogs showed prolongation of APTT and a decrease in platelet numbers, but it was unclear whether this effect was due to the hetastarch treatment. Some dogs with abnormal hemostasis before treatment actually became normal after treatment (Smiley and Garvey 1994). In another trial using hetastarch in 30 hypoalbuminemic dogs, there was an increase in colloid oncotic pressure with the administration of 7.7 to 43.9 mL/kg but this effect lasted less than 12 h. It was suggested that maintenance of colloid oncotic pressure would require additional hetastarch or administration of other colloids (Moore and Garvey 1996).

As with dextrans, there has been concern about the effect of hetastarch on coagulation (Strauss 1981). In early experiments in dogs, infusion of 10 mL/kg was not associated with blood loss or any change in bleeding time. With infusions of 20 to 30 mL/kg, however, bleeding time and quantity of blood lost increased. These effects were more pronounced with dextrans than with hetastarch (Karlson et al. 1967). The factor VIII complex consistently is decreased after hetastarch administration and it is advised that hetastarch not be given to dogs with known or suspected von Willebrand's disease (Smiley 1992). In a study in which very large doses (110–120 mL/kg) of hetastarch were used, prolonged bleeding times were identified. Platelets appeared swollen and shiny and had decreased adhesion (Lewis et al. 1966). Clots were friable and had weak tensile strength. These effects were presumably due to more than just hemodilution, and these findings should be borne in mind when using hetastarch at the time of surgery. Studies in humans undergoing surgery have not documented any increase in blood loss associated with the administration of hetastarch (Vogt et al. 1996; Beyer et al. 1997). The author has not seen increased bleeding tendency in dogs given hetastarch, but the dose used has not exceeded 20 mL/kg.

Hetastarch administration increases plasma volume by 71 to 172% of the administered volume and generally increases plasma volume by at least the volume administered (Smiley 1992). In this regard, hetastarch is about equivalent to dextran 70 but has a slightly longer duration of action. In one study in dogs, 25 mL/kg of dextran 70 or hetastarch gave an almost identical increase in plasma volume compared with the volume infused (approximately 140%), but at 12 h the dextran effect had decreased to 18% whereas the hetastarch effect had decreased to 38%. By 24 h, the dextran effect had further decreased to 1% whereas hetastarch still caused a 16% increase in plasma volume compared with the volume infused (Thompson et al. 1970). The incidence of anaphylactoid reactions with hetastarch use in people is similar to that recorded for dextrans. Whereas antibodies to dextrans have been found in humans, no antibodies to hetastarch have been found in dogs, cats, or humans even after chronic use. The frequency of life-threatening reactions appears to be lower for hetastarch than for other colloids (Smiley 1992). No anaphylactoid reactions to hetastarch have been reported in dogs or cats.

PENTASTARCH

Pentastarch is a less substituted hydroxyethyl starch (substitution ratio 0.45) with a lower molecular weight. It has a shorter half-life (2.5 h) and is more rapidly hydrolyzed than hetastarch. About 70% of the pentastarch is excreted within 24 h and 80% is excreted within 1 week. As with the comparison of dextran 40 and 70, the higher concentration of this solution may lead to a greater initial increase in plasma volume, but the duration of expansion is shorter than for hetastarch. Pentastarch is thought to have limited effects on coagulation (Strauss et al. 1988). In trials in humans it has been shown to be equivalent to albumin in efficacy when used in different clinical settings

(Nagy et al. 1993; London et al. 1989, 1992). It has become available in the United States and is the most expensive of the artificial colloids.

GELATIN SOLUTIONS

Gelatin solutions are prepared by degradation of bovine collagen and come in several forms. The process involves exposure of the raw material to hydrochloric acid for several days, to saturated calcium hydroxide for several weeks, and finally to a temperature of at least 138°C. The three currently used preparations are oxypolygelatin (Vetaplasma), succinylated gelatin (Gelofusine), and urea-linked gelatin (Haemaccel). Oxypolygelatin has become available in the United States and the other two forms have been used extensively in Europe. The main advantages of these solutions are that they have lower molecular weights than the other colloids (and hence are excreted rapidly), they appear to be minimally antigenic, and they have minimal effects on coagulation (Lundsgaard-Hansen and Tshirren 1978). In one report, the use of over 79,000 units of succinylated gelatin in humans was summarized (Lundsgaard-Hansen and Tshirren 1978). The infusion of a solution of succinylated gelatin was associated with an increase in plasma volume equal to or approximately 10% less than the volume infused; hence there is little risk of volume overload. Of the infused volume, approximately 50% was present in the circulation after 4 to 5 h, although it has been stated that the plasma half-life is approximately 8 h (Lundsgaard-Hansen and Tshirren 1978). The plasma half-life of oxypolygelatin is 2 to 4 h. The majority of the gelatin is excreted by the kidneys, with 71% of the urea-linked gelatin and 62% of the succinylated gelatin being found in the urine in people within 24 h. In chimpanzees, 66% of a dose of oxypolygelatin was found in the urine within 24 h. Mechanisms for the metabolism of the remaining molecules are not well defined but it is thought that they are metabolized by proteolytic enzymes in the liver with some of the end products being excreted in the feces (approximately 15% of the total dose) (Lundsgaard-Hansen and Tshirren 1978).

Anaphylactoid reactions to gelatin solutions are rare. It is uncertain whether these reactions represent an immunologic response or are due to histamine release. An overall incidence of allergic reactions to gelatins was reported to be 0.115% with the highest incidence being reported for oxypolygelatin (0.617%) (Ring and Messmer 1977). In this report, it was also noted that the severity of the reactions was greater with the gelatins than with other colloids (0.038% vs. 0.008% for dextrans and 0.006% for hetastarch). In a study of the release of histamine associated with use of urea-linked gelatin in anesthetized patients, a 26% incidence of histamine release was reported with 4 of 57 patients exhibiting life-threatening signs (Lorenz et al. 1994). Patients with malignant disease were twice as likely to release histamine and were seven times more likely to have a life-threatening episode. Pretreatment of patients with histamine blockers (both H_1 and H_2) reduced the incidence of clinical signs to 0% (Lorenz et al. 1994). The gelatin solution (500 mL) in this study was given over 20 min (approximately 20–25 mL/kg/h), and it has been recommended that these solutions be administered slowly.

In the early reports of gelatin infusion, minimal effects on coagulation were identified (Lundsgaard-Hansen and Tshirren 1978). Subsequent studies however, showed that the effects are somewhat similar to those observed with other colloids but of lesser magnitude. An increase in bleeding time was recorded in healthy people and in trauma victims (Evans et al. 1996; de Jonge et al. 1998) and was attributed to a decrease in von Willebrand's factor activity (de Jonge et al. 1998). In studies using thromboelastography to measure the dynamics of clot formation, dilution with gelatins resulted in more rapid onset of clot formation, more rapid strengthening of the clot, and some decrease in the maximal strength obtained (Mortier et al. 1997; Egli et al. 1997). In both of these studies, gelatin was compared with hydroxyethyl starch and the latter induced greater changes than did the gelatin solution. In one study, 50% dilution with dextran 40 prolonged most coagulation parameters to such an extent as to be unmeasurable (Mortier et al. 1997). In a clinical study examining the use of gelatin as a priming solution before cardiopulmonary bypass, ristocetin-induced platelet agglutination was significantly impaired, and this effect was not corrected by the use of aprotinin as compared with the control group (albumin prime) (Tabuchi et al. 1995). There also was a direct correlation between postoperative blood loss and the amount of gelatin used during the operation with the greatest blood loss occurring in patients receiving more than 3.5 L of gelatin (approximately 45 mL/kg) (Tabuchi et al. 1995). In another study evaluating human patients undergoing orthopedic surgery, no major differences were noted between patients receiving similar volumes of 6% hetastarch or 3% gelatin (<33 mL/kg/day) for colloid replacement (Beyer et al. 1997). Despite these findings, gelatin infusions often are given rapidly to veterinary patients before or during surgery with little evidence of adverse effects on coagulation or histamine release.

PLASMA PROTEIN

Plasma protein is available either as a fresh or frozen preparation or as liquid or frozen plasma that has been harvested during the collection and storage of blood. Fresh plasma may be prepared so that it contains platelets (platelet-rich plasma) and clotting factors. It must be used within 4 h of preparation because of the risk of bacterial contamination at the recommended room temperature storage. Fresh frozen plasma contains clotting factors, which are destroyed if the unit has been thawed for more than 8 h, but contains no platelets. Fresh frozen plasma can be used in any situation in which blood volume must be expanded, hematocrit is within an acceptable range, and no allergic reaction to foreign protein is anticipated. If there is no major concern about dilution of existing clotting factors, the stored form of the plasma can be used. The infusion of plasma tends to increase colloid oncotic pressure and increase both serum albumin and globulin concentrations. The main concerns about the use of plasma intraoperatively are cost and the potential for allergic reactions. Commercially, plasma is more expensive than any of the other colloids except pentastarch, but its use is justified in animals with marginal coagulation (e.g., use of fresh frozen plasma in a patient with low plasma protein concentration related to hepatic dysfunction) or in surgical cases in which there is concern about dilutional coagulopathy. Life-threatening allergic reactions to plasma infusions are not common, but urticaria may be observed. The author has not seen any episodes of profound hypotension associated with plasma infusions but has seen considerable swelling of the head and limbs develop. If such a reaction occurs, the plasma infusion should be stopped immediately and the animal treated with antihistamines (H_1 and H_2 blockers). Corticosteroids also may be administered if warranted by the severity of the reaction. This type of therapy rarely reverses the clinical signs but may prevent exacerbation of the condition. A note should be made in the patient's medical record to ensure that it does not receive infusions of plasma products in the future. In dogs and cats with portosystemic shunts, there is concern about the ammonia content of stored plasma because it tends to increase with time. Clinical signs of encephalopathy in these patients are related in part to blood ammonia concentration, and it is advisable not to burden them with an additional source of ammonia.

PACKED RED BLOOD CELLS

Packed red cells are used primarily in patients with low hematocrits before surgery or in patients that are likely to have low tolerance for a decreased hematocrit that develops during surgery (e.g., a patient with minimal cardiovascular reserve). It is advisable to crossmatch both dogs and cats before transfusion. Crossmatching requires some time, and it is important to plan for the use of packed red cells by having the crossmatch results available before the animal requires transfusion. The indications for packed red cells are given in the earlier section on anemia. Administration of packed red cells can be difficult because of the viscosity of the solution and can be facilitated by diluting the cells with warm normal saline, by using adult rather than pediatric administration sets, and by using the largest venous access possible (ideally >20 gauge). Smaller needles (<20 gauge) tend to impede the flow of the blood and may lead to hemolysis if external pressure is applied for the administration.

WHOLE BLOOD

Ideally, whole blood is used when the animal needs all of the components present in whole blood. Practically, whole blood often is used because it is more convenient than individual component therapy. Fresh whole blood contains all of the normal clotting factors as well as active platelets. Clotting factors and platelets deteriorate within the first 24 h and stored whole blood is ineffective at restoring normal coagulation. Whole blood typically is used in patients that are bleeding actively or have already lost a large volume of blood and are likely to become severely hemodiluted if other fluids are used. Some concern has been expressed about the effect of blood transfusion on immune function. A beneficial effect was first noticed in renal transplant patients. Patients who had received blood transfusions in association with renal transplantation were less likely to reject the grafted organ (Opelz et al. 1973). Additional studies in human patients showed an increased frequency of infections in patients receiving homogeneic blood transfusions (Duffy and Neal 1996). These included wound infections, urinary tract infections (Koval et al. 1997), and respiratory tract infections, and the frequency of infection increased with the number of units of blood received (Tartter 1994). Patients receiving their own blood did not have such an increase in infection rate, and studies have focused on reducing the white cell count in transfused blood to determine whether this will alter the infection rate (Blajchman 1997). This approach seems to have met with success, but further analysis is required before its efficacy is understood (Houbiers et al. 1997). Another effect of immunosuppression caused by blood transfusions is its effect on cancer development. In several animal models, allogeneic infusions have been associated with increased tumor growth, but the results of studies in humans are not clear (Francis and Shenton 1981; Rusthoven 1994). Leukocyte removal before transfusion may reduce the effect on cancer growth (Blajchman et al. 1993). To date, no studies in veterinary medicine have addressed these issues.

Another concern with the administration of blood products is that citrate present in stored blood will decrease the availability of calcium in the recipient. In normal humans, the amount of citrate found in one unit of blood (approximately 32 mg/kg) can be metabolized in 3 to 5 min without the person developing hypocalcemia. The rate of metabolism of citrate, however, decreases with decreased hepatic perfusion (e.g., shock), decreased hepatic function, and hypothermia. In these settings, plasma citrate concentration may increase rapidly. This effect is of concern mainly when blood is given rapidly (>30 mL/kg/h) and calcium salts may be given when rapid transfusion of blood or plasma is required (Abbott 1983). Calcium must be given through a separate IV line because it may cause the transfused blood to clot in the line if it is given concurrently. If serum ionized calcium concentration can be measured, sufficient calcium should be given to return ionized calcium to normal, but the animal should be treated only if serum ionized calcium concentration is decreased. If blood is not being given rapidly or is not needed on a continuous basis, it rarely is necessary to administer calcium because the serum calcium concentration will be corrected rapidly by the animal (Abbott 1983) by changes in parathyroid hormone concentration as well as by mobilization of calcium stores in the body (Silberstein et al. 1986).

Stored blood usually is kept at 4°C and is more likely to cause arrhythmias and decreased cardiac output if administered without being warmed first. A 250 mL unit of blood at 4°C requires 7.2 kcal of heat to warm it to 38°C. Stated differently, an infusion of 25 to 30 mL/kg of blood at 4°C can decrease body temperature by as much as 1°C. Given these facts, it is best if blood can be warmed before it is given. This can be achieved by placing the blood in warm water (up to 42°C but no higher) before infusion or by running the blood through a warming device as it is being infused. Warming can be as simple as running the line through a container of warm water or as sophisticated as using a device specifically designed to heat blood safely as it is being infused. The effectiveness of these techniques depends on the length of line exposed to the heat and the rate of infusion. Most of the commercial devices that are designed for this purpose require the addition of an extra length of line that conforms to the heating device. Such devices further increase the cost of blood or blood component therapy.

HEMOGLOBIN SOLUTIONS

Various hemoglobin solutions have been tested over the years but only one has been licensed for veterinary use. Oxyglobin is an ultrapure glutaraldehyde polymerized hemoglobin of bovine origin made up in a modified lactated Ringer's solution. This hemoglobin solution has a P50 (oxygen tension at 50% saturation) of 35 mm Hg, a molecular weight of 64 to 500 kilodaltons and a colloid oncotic pressure of approximately 20 mm Hg (Paradis 1997). It comes as a purple colored solution and contains 13 mg/dL of hemoglobin. The solution may be stored at room temperature and has a shelf life of 24 months. This latter feature makes it an attractive product for veterinarians who use canine or feline blood infrequently and who do not have access to blood donors of known status. When given to a patient, it acts as a colloidal solution but has the added advantage of providing oxygen-carrying capacity. It can be given intraoperatively in any situation where blood would normally be used except in circumstances requiring clotting factors or platelets. Administration leads to jaundice and hematuria in many patients and interference with a number of biochemical tests (e.g., sodium, potassium, chloride, blood urea) may occur (Callas et al. 1997). Monitoring the patient by use of pulse oximetry reflects changes in arterial hemoglobin saturation (Hughes et al. 1996) but measurement of hematocrit alone no longer provides an accurate indication of hemoglobin content. Measurement of total protein concentration using a refractometer also will be affected due to the presence of free hemoglobin. The recommended rate of administration for Oxyglobin is 10 mL/kg/h, but higher rates of infusion have been used in many animals suffering from acute hypovolemia. Although there are promising clinical anecdotes about the use of this product, limited scientific information about its safety and efficacy in patients is available at the present time.

▶ Postoperative Fluid Management

The patient will continue to lose fluids over time and may have decreased food and water intake after surgery. Consequently, it is essential to consider fluid therapy in the postoperative period. The choice of fluid is governed by factors similar to those used before and during surgery. A main factor to consider is when the animal is likely to be able to regulate its own fluid balance. With minor surgical procedures, this may be almost immediately after surgery, but with procedures in which recovery is slow or oral intake is contraindicated, it is necessary to continue fluid therapy. Continuing fluid therapy may be particularly important in geriatric patients because they often are unwilling to drink in the hospital environment and may be at greater risk because of marginal renal function.

REFERENCES

Abbott TR: Changes in serum calcium fractions and citrate concentrations during massive blood transfusions and cardiopulmonary bypass. *Br J Anaesth* 55:753–759, 1983.

Adrogue HJ and Tannen RL: Ketoacidosis, hyperosmolar states, and lactic acidosis. In Kokko JP and Tannen RL (eds): *Fluids and Electrolytes*, 3rd ed. Philadelphia, WB Saunders Co., pp. 643–674, 1996.

Allard RL, Carlos AD, and Faltin EC: Canine hematological changes during gestation and lactation. *Companion Anim Pract* 19:3–6, 1989.

Allon M and Copkney C: Albuterol and insulin for treatment of hyperkalemia in hemodialysis patients. *Kidney Int* 38:869–872, 1990.

Anand IS, Ferrari R, Kalra GS, et al.: Edema of cardiac origin. Studies of body water and sodium, renal function, hemodynamic indexes, and plasma hormones in untreated congestive cardiac failure. *Circulation* 80:299–305, 1989.

Asao Y, Hirasaki A, Matsushita M, et al.: [A patient who recovered successfully from severe anemia which continued for one hour]. *Masui* 46:700–703, 1997.

Baer RW, Vlahakes GJ, Uhlig PN, et al.: Maximum myocardial oxygen transport during anemia and polycythemia in dogs. *Am J Physiol* 252:H1086–H1095, 1987.

Baraff LJ: Capillary refill: Is it a useful clinical sign? *Pediatrics* 92:723–724, 1993.

Beyer R, Harmening U, Rittmeyer O, et al.: Use of modified fluid gelatin and hydroxyethyl starch for colloidal volume replacement in major orthopaedic surgery. *Br J Anaesth* 78:44–50, 1997.

Bickell WH, Wall MJ, Pepe PE, et al.: Immediate versus delayed fluid resuscitation for hypotensive patients with penetrating torso injuries. *N Engl J Med* 331:1105–1109, 1994.

Biertuempfel P and Ling G: Urinary tract infection resulting from catheterization in healthy adult dogs. *J Am Vet Med Assoc* 178:989–991, 1981.

Bjorling DE and Rawlings CA: Relationship of intravenous administration of Ringer's lactate solution to pulmonary edema in halothane-anesthetized cats. *Am J Vet Res* 44:1000–1006, 1983.

Blajchman M: Allogeneic blood transfusions, immunomodulation, and postoperative bacterial infection: Do we have the answers yet? *Transfusion* 37:121–125, 1997.

Blajchman M, Bardossy L, Carmen R, et al.: Allogeneic blood transfusion–induced enhancement of tumor growth: Two animal models showing amelioration by leukodepletion and passive transfer using spleen cells. *Blood* 81:1880–1882, 1993.

Booke M, Armstrong C, Hinder F, et al.: The effects of propofol on hemodynamics and renal blood flow in healthy and in septic sheep, and combined with fentanyl in septic sheep. *Anesth Analg* 82:738–743, 1996.

Brecher M and Rosenfeld M: Mathematical and computer modeling of an acute normovolemic hemodilution. *Transfusion* 34:176–179, 1994.

Brooks VL and Keil LC: Hemorrhage decreases arterial pressure sooner in pregnant compared with nonpregnant dogs: Role of baroreflex. *Am J Physiol* 266:H1610–H1619, 1994a.

Brooks VL and Keil LC: Changes in the baroreflex during pregnancy in conscious dogs: Heart rate and hormonal responses. *Endocrinology* 135:1894–1901, 1994b.

Brotzu G: Inhibition by chlorpromazine of the effects of dopamine on the dog kidney. *J Pharm Pharmacol* 22:664–667, 1970.

Cairoli F, Colombo G, and Arrighi S: Variazioni di alcune componenti ematiche nella cagna di razza beagle durante la gravidanza ed il puerperio. *Clin Vet* 103:267–283, 1980.

Callas DD, Clark TL, Moreira PL, et al.: In vitro effects of a novel hemoglobin-based oxygen carrier on routine chemistry, therapeutic drug, coagulation, hematology, and blood bank assays. *Clin Chem* 43:1744–1748, 1997.

Canizaro PC, Prager MD, and Shires GT: The infusion of Ringer's lactate solution during shock. Changes in lactate, excess lactate, and pH. *Am J Surg* 122:494–501, 1971.

Carson JL, Poses RM, Spence RK, et al.: Severity of anaemia and operative mortality and morbidity. *Lancet* 1:727–729, 1988.

Charlson M, MacKenzie C, Gold J, et al.: Risk for postoperative congestive heart failure. *Surg Gynecol Obstet* 172:95–104, 1991.

Ching YNLH, Meyers KM, Brassard JA, et al.: Effect of cryoprecipitate and plasma on plasma von Willebrand factor mulitmers and bleeding time in Doberman pinschers with type-I von Willebrand's disease. *Am J Vet Res* 55:102–110, 1994.

Clugston P, Fitzpatrick D, Kester D, et al.: Autologous blood use in reduction mammaplasty: Is it justified? *Plast Reconstr Surg* 95:824–828, 1995.

Concannon KT, Haskins SC, and Feldman BF: Hemostatic defects associated with two infusion rates of dextran 70 in dogs. *Am J Vet Res* 53:1369–1375, 1992.

Copland VS, Haskins SC, and Patz JD: Oxymorphone: Cardiovascular pulmonary and behavioral effects in dogs. *Am J Vet Res* 48:1626–1630, 1987.

Coulter DB, Whelan SC, and Wilson RC: Dermination of blood pressure by indirect methods in dogs given acetylpromazine maleate. *Cornell Vet* 71:76–84, 1981.

de Jonge E, Levi M, Berends F, et al.: Impaired haemostasis by intravenous administration of a gelatin-based plasma expander in human subjects. *Thromb Haemost* 79:286–290, 1998.

de Lange S, Boscoe MJ, Stanley TH, et al.: Antidiuretic and growth hormone responses during coronary artery surgery with sufentanil-oxygen and alfentanil-oxygen anesthesia in man. *Anesth Analg* 61:434–438, 1982.

Didwania A, Miller J, Kassel D, et al.: Effect of intravenous lactated Ringer's solution infusion on the circulating lactate concentration: Part 3. Results of a prospective, randomized, double-blind, placebo-controlled trial. *Crit Care Med* 25:1851–1854, 1997.

Duffy G and Neal K: Differences in post-operative infection rates between patients receiving autologous and allogeneic blood transfusion: A meta-analysis of published randomized and non-randomized studies. *Transfus Med* 6:325–328, 1996.

Egli GA, Zollinger A, Seifert B, et al.: Effect of progressive haemodilution with hydroxyethyl starch, gelatin and albumin on blood coagulation. *Br J Anaesth* 78:684–689, 1997.

Evans PA, Garnett M, Boffard K, et al.: Evaluation of the effect of colloid (Haemaccel) on the bleeding time in the trauma patient. *J R Soc Med* 89:101P–104P, 1996.

Faggella AM and Aronsohn MG: Anesthetic techniques for neutering 6- to 14-week-old kittens. *J Am Vet Med Assoc* 202:56–62, 1993.

Feldman Z, Zachari S, Reichenthal E, et al.: Brain edema and neurological status with rapid infusion of lactated Ringer's or 5% dextrose solution following head trauma. *J Neurosurg* 83:1060–1066, 1995.

Fischer D, Omlor D, and Kreuscher D: Influence of ketamine anaesthesia on renal and cardiovascular functions in mongrel dogs. *Int Urol Nephrol* 11:271–277, 1979.

Follett DV, Loeb RG, Haskins SC, et al.: Effects of epinephrine and ritodrine in dogs with acute hyperkalemia. *Anesth Analg* 70:400–406, 1990.

Francis DM and Shenton BK: Blood transfusion and tumour growth: Evidence from laboratory animals. *Lancet* 2:871, 1981.

Gagnon JA, Felipe L, and Nelson LD: Influence of thiopental anesthesia on renal sodium and water excretion in the dog. *Am J Physiol* 243:F265–F270, 1982.

Galvez OG, Bay WH, Roberts BW, et al.: The hemodynamic effects of potassium deficiency in the dog. *Circ Res* 40(suppl 1):I-11–I-16, 1977.

Gaynor JS, Wertz EM, Kesel LM, et al.: Effect of intravenous administration of fluids on packed cell volume, blood pressure, and total protein and blood glucose concentrations in healthy halothane-anesthetized dogs. *J Am Vet Med Assoc* 208:2013–2015, 1996.

Gentilello LM and Moujaes S: Treatment of hypothermia in trauma victims: Thermodynamic considerations. *J Intensive Care Med* 10:5–14, 1995.

Goldstein SM and MacLean LD: Ringer's lactate infusion with severe hepatic damage: Effect on arterial lactate level. *Can J Surg* 15:318–321, 1972.

Gollub S and Schaefer C: Structural alteration in canine fibrin produced by colloid plasma expanders. *Surg Gynecol Obstet* 127:783–793, 1968.

Goodnough L, Grishaber J, Monk T, et al.: Acute preoperative hemodilution in patients undergoing radical prostatectomy: A case study analysis of efficacy. *Anesth Analg* 78:932–937, 1994.

Gorelick MH, Shaw KN, and Baker MD: Effect of ambient temperature on capillary refill in healthy children. *Pediatrics* 92:699–702, 1993.

Graefe U, Milutinovich J, Follette WC, et al.: Less dialysis-induced morbidity and vascular instability with bicarbonate in dialysate. *Ann Intern Med* 88:332–336, 1978.

Hahn RG and Svensén C: Plasma dilution and the rate of infusion of Ringer's solution. *Br J Anaesth* 79:64–67, 1997.

Hahn RG, Drobin D, and Ståhle L: Volume kinetics of Ringer's solution in female volunteers. *Br J Anaesth* 78:144–148, 1997.

Hardy RM and Osborne CA: Water deprivation test in the dog: Maximal normal values. *JAMA* 174:479–483, 1979.

Hartsfield SM, Thurmon JC, Corbin JE, et al.: Effects of sodium acetate, bicarbonate and lactate on acid-base status in anaesthetized dogs. *J Vet Pharmacol Ther* 4:51–61, 1981.

Haskins SC, Farver TB, and Patz JD: Ketamine in dogs. *Am J Vet Res* 46:1855–1860, 1985.

Hint H: Relationships between the chemical and physicochemical properties of dextrans and its pharmacological effects. In Derrick JR and Guest MR (eds): *Dextrans. Current Concepts of Basic Actions and Clinical Applications*. Springfield, IL, Charles C Thomas, pp. 3–26, 1971.

Houbiers JG, van de Velde CJ, vande Watering LM, et al.: Transfusion of red cells is associated with increased incidence of bacterial infection after colorectal surgery: A prospective study. *Transfusion* 37:126–134, 1997.

Hughes GS, Francom SF, Antal EJ, et al.: Effects of a novel hemoglobin-based oxygen carrier on percent saturation as determined with arterial blood gas analysis and pulse oximetry. *Ann Emerg Med* 27:164–169, 1996.

Iseki K, Onoyama K, Maeda T, et al.: Comparison of hemodynamics induced by conventional acetate hemodialysis, bicarbonate hemodialysis and ultrafiltration. *Clin Nephrol* 14:294–298, 1980.

Ishihara H, Ishida K, Oyama T, et al.: Effects of general anaesthesia and surgery on renal function and plasma ADH levels. *Can Anaesth Soc J* 25:312–318, 1978.

Ivatury RR, Diebel L, Porter JM, et al.: Intra-abdominal hypertension and the abdominal compartment syndrome. *Surg Clin North Am* 77:783–800, 1997.

Kaczmarczyk G: Pulmonary-renal axis during positive-pressure ventilation. *New Horiz* 2:512–517, 1994.

Kaneko M, Nakayama H, Igarashi N, et al.: Relationship between the number of fetuses and the blood constituents of beagles in late pregnancy. *J Vet Med Sci* 55:681–682, 1993.

Kanter M, van Maanen D, Anders K, et al.: Preoperative autologous blood donations before elective hysterectomy. *JAMA* 276:798–801, 1996.

Karlson KE, Garzon AA, Shaftan GW, et al.: Increased blood loss associated with administration of certain plasma expanders: Dextran 75, dextran 40, and hydroxyethyl starch. *Surgery* 62:670–678, 1967.

Kerl ME and Hohenhaus AE: Packed red blood cell transfusions in dogs: 131 cases 1989. *J Am Vet Med Assoc* 202:1495–1499, 1993.

Kirkendol PL, Starrs J, and Gonzalez FM: The effect of acetate, lactate, succinate and gluconate on plasma pH and electrolytes in dogs. *Trans Am Soc Artif Intern Organs* 26:323–327, 1980.

Komtebedde J, Forsyth SF, Breznock EM, et al.: Intrahepatic portosystemic venous anomaly in the dog: Perioperative management and complications. *Vet Surg* 20:37–42, 1991.

Koval K, Rosenberg A, Zuckerman J, et al.: Does blood transfusion increase the risk of infection after hip fracture? *J Orthop Trauma* 11:260–265, 1997.

Kurnik BR, Singer F, and Groh WC: Case report: Dextran-induced acute anuric renal failure. *Am J Med Sci* 302:28–30, 1991.

Lam AM, Winn HR, Cullen BF, et al.: Hyperglycemia and neurological outcome in patients with head injury. *J Neurosurg* 75:545–551, 1991.

Laureno R and Karp B: Myelinolysis after correction of hyponatremia. *Ann Intern Med* 126:57–62, 1997.

Lees G: Use and misuse of indwelling urethral catheters. *Vet Clin North Am Small Anim Pract* 26:499–505, 1996.

Lens XM, Montoliu J, Cases A, et al.: Treatment of hyperkalaemia in renal failure: Salbutamol v. insulin. *Nephrol Dial Transplant* 4:228–232, 1989.

Lewis JH, Szeto ILF, Bayre WL, et al.: Severe hemodilution with hydroxyethyl starch and dextrans. *Arch Surg* 93:941–950, 1966.

Li LPA, Shamloo M, Katsura Ki, et al.: Critical values for plasma glucose in aggravating ischaemic brain damage: Correlation to extracellular pH. *Neurobiol Dis* 2:97–108, 1995.

London M, Ho J, Triedman J, et al.: A randomized clinical trial of 10% pentastarch low molecular weight hydroxyethyl starch versus 5% albumin for plasma volume expansion after cardiac operations. *J Thorac Cardiovasc Surg* 97:785–797, 1989.

London M, Franks M, Verrier E, et al.: The safety and efficacy of ten percent pentastarch as a cardiopulmonary bypass priming solution. A randomized clinical trial. *J Thorac Cardiovasc Surg* 104:284–296, 1992.

Lorenz W, Duda D, Dick W, et al.: Incidence and clinical importance of perioperative histamine release: Randomized study of volume loading and antihistamines after induction of anaesthesia. *Lancet* 343:933–940, 1994.

Lundsgaard-Hansen P and Tshirren B: Modified fluid gelatin as a plasma substitute. *Prog Clin Biol Res* 19:227–257, 1978.

Matsumura LK, Ajzen H, Chacra AR, et al.: Effect of positive pressure breathing on plasma antidiuretic hormone and renal function in dogs. *Braz J Med Biol Res* 16:261–270, 1983.

Moon PF: Acute toxicosis in two dogs associated with etomidate–propylene glycol infusion. *Lab Anim Sci* 44:590–594, 1994.

Moore LE and Garvey MS: The effect of hetastarch on serum colloid oncotic pressure in hypoalbuminemic dogs. *J Vet Intern Med* 10:300–303, 1996.

Mortier E, Ongenae M, De Baerdemaeker L, et al.: In vitro evaluation of the effect of profound haemodilution with hydroxyethyl starch 6%, modified fluid gelatin 4% and dextran 40 10% on coagulation profile measured by thromboelastography. *Anaesthesia* 52:1061–1064, 1997.

Moursi M, Rising CL, Zelenock GB, et al.: Dextrose administration exacerbates acute renal ischemic damage in anesthetized dogs. *Arch Surg* 122:790–794, 1987.

Nagy K, Davis J, Duda J, et al.: A comparison of pentastarch and lactated Ringer's solution in the ressucitation of patients with hemorrhagic shock. *Circ Shock* 40:289–294, 1993.

Naylor JM, Kronfeld DS, Freeman DE, et al.: Hepatic and extrahepatic lactate metabolism in sheep: Effects of lactate loading and pH. *Am J Physiol* 247:E747–E755, 1984.

O'Brien D, Kroll R, Johnson G, et al.: Myelinolysis after correction of hyponatremia in two dogs. *J Vet Intern Med* 8:40–48, 1994.

Opelz G, Sengar DP, Mickey MR, et al.: Effect of blood transfusions on subsequent kidney transplants. *Transplant Proc* 5:253–259, 1973.

Palacios A, Martainez M, Costela J, et al.: [Postoperative infection and anesthesia: Analysis of various risk factors.] *Rev Esp Anestesiol Reanim* 42:87–90, 1995.

Paradis NA: Dose-response relationship between aortic infusions of polymerized bovine hemoglobin and return of circulation in a canine model of ventricular fibrillation and advanced cardiac life support. *Crit Care Med* 25:476–483, 1997.

Perel A, Pizov R, and Cotev S: Systolic pressure variation is a sensitive indicator of hypovolemia in ventilated dogs subjected to graded hemorrhage. *Anesthesiology* 67:495–502, 1987.

Petersen J, Shalmi M, Christensen S, et al.: Comparison of the renal effects of six sedating agents in rats. *Physiol Behav* 60:759–765, 1996.

Peterson ME: Feline hyperthyroidism. *Vet Clin North Am Small Anim Pract* 14:809–826, 1984.

Pizov R, Ya'ari Y, and Perel A: Systolic pressure variation is greater during hemorrhage than during sodium nitroprusside–induced hypotension in ventilated dogs. *Anesth Analg* 67:170–174, 1988.

Practice Guidelines for blood component therapy: A report by the American Society of Anesthesiologists Task Force on Blood Component Therapy. *Anesthesiology* 84:732–747, 1996.

Ramming S, Shackford SR, Zhuang J, et al.: The relationship of fluid balance and sodium administration to cerebral edema formation and intracranial pressure in a porcine model of brain injury. *J Trauma* 37:705–713, 1994.

Rebollo M, Bernal J, Llorca J, et al.: Nosocomial infections in patients having cardiovascular operations: A multivariate analysis of risk factors. *J Thorac Cardiovasc Surg* 112:908–913, 1996.

Ring J and Messmer K: Incidence and severity of anaphylactoid reactions to colloid volume substitutes. *Lancet* 1:466–469, 1977.

Roberts JP, Roberts JD, Skinner C, et al.: Extracellular fluid deficit following operation and its correction with Ringer's lactate: A reassessment. *Ann Surg* 202:1–8, 1985.

Robinson EP and Hardy RM: Clinical signs, diagnosis, and treatment of alkalemia in dogs: 20 cases (1982–1984). *J Am Vet Med Assoc* 192:943–949, 1988.

Rossaint R, Jorres D, Nienhaus M, et al.: Positive end-expiratory pressure reduces renal excretion without hormonal activation after volume expansion in dogs. *Anesthesiology* 77:700–708, 1992.

Rossaint R, Krebs M, Forther J, et al.: Inferior vena caval pressure increase contributes to sodium and water retention during PEEP in awake dogs. *J Appl Physiol* 75:2484–2492, 1993.

Rusthoven JJ: Blood transfusion and cancer: Clinical studies. In Singal DP (ed): *Immunological Effects of Blood Transfusion*. Boca Raton, FL, CRC Press, pp. 85–110, 1994.

Ryden SE and Oberman HA: Compatibility of common intravenous solutions with CPD blood. *Transfusion* 15:250–255, 1975.

Saragoca MA, Bessa AM, Mulinari RA, et al.: Sodium acetate, an arterial vasodilator: Haemodynamic characterisation in normal dogs. *Proc Eur Dialysis Transplant Assoc Euro* 21:221–224, 1985.

Schriger DL and Baraff LJ: Capillary refill—Is it a useful predictor of hypovolemic states? *Ann Emerg Med* 20:601–605, 1991.

Shapira Y, Artru AA, Qassam N, et al.: Brain edema and neurologic status with rapid infusion of 0.9% saline or 5% dextrose after head trauma. *J Neurosurg Anesthesiol* 7:17–25, 1995.

Shires T, Williams J, and Brown F: Acute changes in extracellular fluids associated with major surgical procedures. *Ann Surg* 154:803–810, 1961.

Sieber FE: The neurologic implications of diabetic hyperglycemia during surgical procedures at increased risk for brain ischemia. *J Clin Anesth* 9:334–340, 1997.

Sieber FE and Traystman RJ: Special issues: Glucose and the brain. *Crit Care Med* 20:104–114, 1992.

Silberstein LE, Naryshkin S, Haddad JJ, et al.: Calcium homeostasis during therapeutic plasma exchange. *Transfusion* 26:151–155, 1986.

Smiley LE: The use of hetastarch for plasma expansion. *Probl Vet Med* 4:652–667, 1992.

Smiley LE and Garvey MS: The use of hetastarch as adjunct therapy in 26 dogs with hypoalbuminemia: A phase two clinical trial. *J Vet Intern Med* 8:195–202, 1994.

Stamm W: Infections related to medical devices. *Ann Intern Med* 89:764–769, 1978.

Strauss R, Stansfield C, Henriksen R, et al.: Pentastarch may cause fewer effects on coagulation than hetastarch. *Transfusion* 28:257–260, 1988.

Strauss RG: Review of the effects of hydroxyethyl starch on the blood coagulation system. *Transfusion* 21:299–302, 1981.

Ståhle L, Nilsson A, and Hahn RG: Modeling the volume of expandable body fluid spaces during i.v. fluid therapy. *Br J Anaesth* 78:138–143, 1997.

Svensén C and Hahn RG: Volume kinetics of Ringer solution, dextran 70 and hypertonic saline in male volunteers. *Anesthesiology* 87:204–212, 1997.

Tabuchi N, de Haan J, Gallandat Huet RC, et al.: Gelatin use impairs platelet adhesion during cardiac surgery. *Thromb Haemost* 74:1447–1451, 1995.

Tanifuji Y and Eger EI: Brain sodium, potassium, and osmolality: Effects on anesthetic requirement. *Anesth Analg* 57:404–410, 1978.

Tartter PI: Blood transfusion and bacterial infections: Clinical studies. In Singal DP (ed): *Immunological Effects of Blood Transfusion.* Boca Raton, FL, CRC Press, pp. 111–126, 1994.

Thompson WL, Fukushima T, Rutherford RB, et al.: Intravascular persistence, tissue storage, and excretion of hydroxyethyl starch. *Surg Gynecol Obstet* 131:965–972, 1970.

Tønnessen T, Tølløfsrud S, Kongsgaard UE, et al.: Colloid osmotic pressure of plasma replacement fluids. *Acta Anaesthesiol Scand* 37:424–426, 1993.

Usenik EA and Cronkite EP: Effects of barbiturate anesthesia on leukocytes in normal and splenectomized dogs. *Anesth Analg* 44:167–170, 1965.

Vail DM, Ogilvie GK, Fettman MJ, et al.: Exacerbation of hyperlactatemia by infusion of lactated Ringer's solution in dogs with lymphoma. *J Vet Intern Med* 4:228–232, 1990.

Virtue RW, LeVine DS, and Aikawa JK: Fluid shifts during the surgical period: RISA and S35 determinations following glucose, saline or lactate infusion. *Ann Surg* 163:523–528, 1965.

Vogt NH, Bothner U, Lerch G, et al.: Large-dose administration of 6% hydroxyethyl starch 200/0.5 total hip arthroplasty: Plasma homeostasis, hemostasis, and renal function compared to use of 5% human albumin. *Anesth Analg* 83:262–268, 1996.

Wass CT and Lanier WL: Glucose modulation of ischemic brain injury: Review and clinical recommendations. *Mayo Clin Proc* 71:801–812, 1996.

Waterhouse C: Lactate metabolism in patients with cancer. *Cancer* 33:66–71, 1974.

Wenzel R, Osterman C, and Hunting K: Hospital-acquired infections. II. Infection rates by site, service and common procedures in a university hospital. *Am J Epidemiol* 104:645–651, 1976.

Zornow MH and Prough DS: Fluid management in patients with traumatic brain injury. *New Horiz* 3:488–498, 1995.

Zornow MH, Scheller MS, and Shackford SR: Effect of a hypertonic lactated Ringer's solution on intracranial pressure and cerebral water content in a model of traumatic brain injury. *J Trauma* 29:484–488, 1989.

Zunkeler B, Carson RE, Olson J, et al.: Hyperosmolar blood-brain barrier disruption in baboons: An in vivo study using positron emission tomography and rubidium-82. *J Neurosurg* 84:494–502, 1996.

Zwaveling JH, Meulenbelt J, van Xanten NH, et al.: Renal failure associated with the use of dextran-40. *Neth J Med* 35:321–326, 1989.

CHAPTER 16

Fluid and Electrolyte Disturbances in Gastrointestinal, Pancreatic, and Hepatic Disease

KENNETH W. SIMPSON   SHARON A. CENTER   NICHOLE BIRNBAUM

The gastrointestinal tract (GIT) is extremely well adapted to the task of assimilating a wide variety of nutrients and absorbs approximately 99% of the fluid presented to it (Fig. 16–1) (Burrows 1983). Most of the fluid absorbed in the GIT each day is derived from endogenous secretions. Exogenous fluid in the form of food and water constitutes 30 to 50 mL/kg/day, and endogenous secretions from the salivary glands, stomach, pancreas, liver, and small intestine represent two to three times this volume or 1.5 to 2 blood volumes (7% of body weight) (see Fig. 16–1). Considering this massive flux of fluid into the GIT, it is easy to see why fluid loss from or sequestration by the GIT can alter the electrolyte and acid-base status of the patient. The causes and consequences of fluid loss or sequestration are not uniform and depend on the region of the GIT involved. For example, gastric outflow obstruction is often associated with metabolic alkalosis and hypokalemia caused by loss of chloride and potassium in gastric secretions, whereas diarrhea may cause metabolic acidosis and hypokalemia because of loss of bicarbonate and potassium in the feces.

▶ Normal Physiology of the Gastrointestinal Tract

Absorption and Secretion of Water and Electrolytes

STOMACH
Unstimulated acid secretion by the stomach in dogs and cats is minimal (e.g., <0.04 mmol/kg$^{0.75}$/h in the dog) (Happe and De Bruijne 1982). The "acid pump" or H$^+$, K$^+$-adenosinetriphosphatase (H$^+$, K$^+$-ATPase) is located in tubulovesicles within the cytoplasm of parietal cells (Sachs 1994). In the stimulated state, H$^+$, K$^+$-ATPase and KCl transporters are incorporated in the parietal cell canalicular membrane. Hydrogen ions derived from the ionization of water within the parietal cells are transported into the gastric lumen in exchange for potassium ions. Potassium and chloride transporters in the canalicular membrane allow luminal transfer of potassium and chloride ions. Carbonic anhydrase catalyzes the combination of OH$^-$ with CO$_2$ to form HCO$_3^-$, which diffuses into the blood (so-called alkaline tide). Acid secretion in dogs has been estimated at 30 mL/kg/day (Burrows 1983). Stimulation with pentagastrin results in a rapid increase in fluid and hydrogen ion secretion, with pH rapidly declining to less than 1.0. Acid secretion in dogs reaches a peak of 28 mL/kg$^{0.75}$/h or 4.1 mmol HCl/kg$^{0.75}$/h. Potassium transport reaches a peak of 0.34 mmol/kg$^{0.75}$/h and sodium transport a peak of 0.09 mmol/kg$^{0.75}$/h (Happe and De Bruijne 1982). The concentrations of K$^+$ (10–20 mEq/L) and Cl$^-$ (120–160 mEq/L) in gastric juice are higher than those of plasma (approximately 4 mEq/L and 110 mEq/L, respectively, in the dog).

Acid secretion by parietal cells is regulated by a variety of neurochemical and neurohumoral stimuli (Soll and Berglindh 1994, Lloyd and Debas 1994). Luminal peptides, digested protein, acetylcholine, and gastrin-releasing peptide stimulate gastrin secretion from G cells and cause histamine release from enterochromaffin-like cells (Fig. 16–2). Histamine is also released from mast cells. Acetylcholine and gastrin can also directly stimulate parietal cells. Somatostatin acts to decrease gastrin, histamine, and acid secretion. Acid secretion can be decreased by blocking H$_2$ (e.g., cimetidine, ranitidine, famotidine), gastrin (e.g., proglumide), and acetylcholine (e.g., atropine) receptors and by inhibiting adenyl cyclase (e.g., prostaglandin E analogues) and H$^+$, K$^+$-ATPase (e.g., omeprazole). Somatostatin directly decreases gastric acid and gastrin secretion.

PANCREAS
The exocrine pancreas plays a major role in the digestion of food. It secretes enzymes that digest a wide variety of foodstuffs and bicarbonate, which serves to solubilize secreted enzymes and neutralize gastric acid so that optimal enzyme activity is maintained. Pancreatic secretions

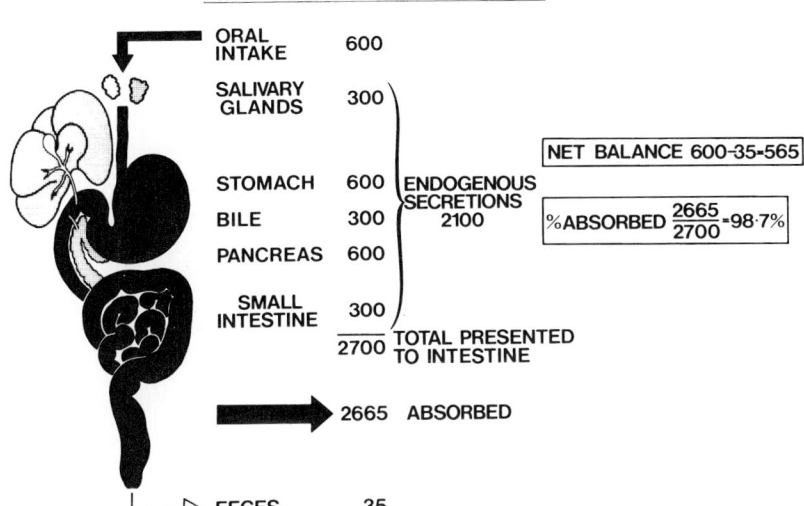

FIGURE 16–1. Normal canine intestinal water balance. Of a total volume of about 3 L of fluid presented to the intestine of a 20-kg dog each day, only about 20% comes from the diet; the remainder comes from the endogenous secretions of the gastrointestinal tract. Most of this fluid is resorbed and only a fraction of it appears in the feces. A decrease in absorption or, less commonly, an increase in secretion results in an increase in fecal water content and diarrhea. (From Burrows CF: Chronic diarrhea in the dog. *Vet Clin North Am* 13:521, 1983.)

also play an important role in the absorption of cobalamin (vitamin B_{12}) and in the regulation of the bacterial flora of the small intestine, and they directly influence small intestinal function by modifying certain enzymes on the intestinal brush border and exerting trophic effects on the mucosa.

Histologically, the pancreas is composed of many secretory lobules that contain acinar cells. These secretory acini are drained by a branching ductular system that is lined by a variety of epithelial cells. The acini and ducts are surrounded by a dense network of capillaries, nerves, and lymphatics.

Pancreatic acinar cells are responsible for the synthesis of digestive enzymes, whereas the cells lining the ductular system are the major source of fluid and electrolyte secretion. The electrolyte composition of pancreatic secretion changes in response to stimulation. At low rates of secretion, the chloride concentration exceeds that of bicarbonate, whereas at higher rates the bicarbonate concentration is higher than the chloride concentration (Fig.

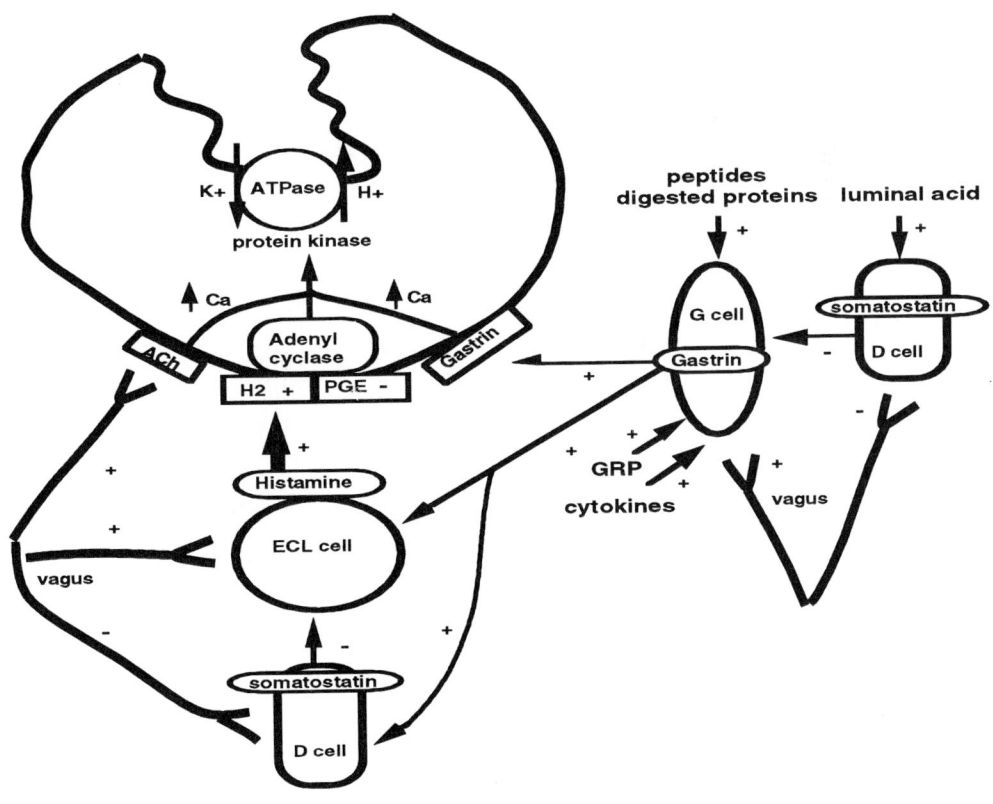

FIGURE 16–2. Regulation of gastric acid secretion.

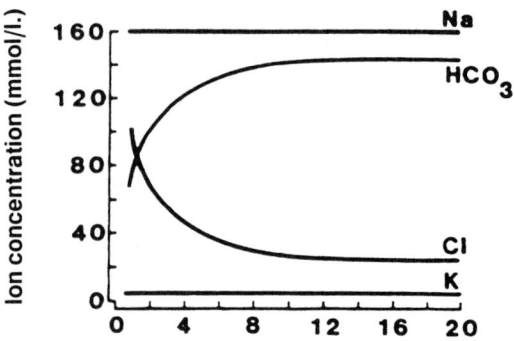

FIGURE 16-3. Ionic composition of pancreatic juice secreted at different flow rates in the anesthetized cat in response to secretin. (From Argent BE and Case RM: Pancreatic ducts: Cellular mechanism and control of bicarbonate. In Johnson LR [ed]: *Physiology of the Gastrointestinal Tract*, 3rd ed. New York, Raven Press, p. 1473, 1994.)

quantitatively most important. Pancreatic secretion occurs not only in response to a meal but also cyclically throughout the day. Peaks in interdigestive secretion are accompanied by an increase in biliary secretion and intestinal motility. These cycles are thought to be mediated by motilin and may serve an intestinal housekeeping function by flushing digestive products, cell debris, and bacteria along the intestinal tract. Inhibition of exocrine pancreatic secretion has not been studied as extensively as stimulation, but glucagon and somatostatin appear to decrease pancreatic secretion.

INTESTINE

Net absorption of fluid and electrolytes in the intestine reflects a balance between absorption and secretion, and the final outcome in the healthy intestine represents a victory for absorption. The ability of the intestine to absorb fluid and electrolytes varies according to site. In a 20-kg dog, approximately 2.70 L of fluid (oral intake, stomach juice, saliva, pancreatic juice, and bile) is presented to the small intestine each day. Approximately 1.35 L is absorbed in the jejunum, 1 L in the ileum, and 300 mL in the colon, with 50 mL remaining in the feces (Strombeck 1996). From these figures it can be calculated that the jejunum absorbs 50%, the ileum 75%, and the colon 90% of the fluid presented to the intestinal tract (Fig. 16–5). The progressive increase in absorptive efficiency along the intestinal tract is a function of enterocyte pore size, membrane potential difference, and the type of transport processes associated with each intestinal segment (Moseley 1996; Chang and Rao 1994; Sellin 1998). Whereas the jejunal epithelium is "leaky" and transfers a large amount of fluid (isotonic absorption), the tight epithelial junctions of the distal colon allow a high transepithelial voltage gradient to develop and net solute transfer occurs against this gradient (Sellin 1998).

16–3). In the stimulated cat pancreas, the HCO_3^- concentration increases from 70 to 145 mEq/L and the Cl^- concentration decreases from 100 to 30 mEq/L. Concentrations of Na^+ and K^+ in pancreatic secretions are similar to those of plasma. The concentrations of electrolytes also change within the pancreatic ductular system. A decrease in Cl^- concentration from the intralobular ducts to the main ducts is thought to arise through the exchange of Cl^- for HCO_3^-. Secretin is the principal mediator of pancreatic fluid and electrolyte secretion (Fig. 16–4) and is released in response to acidification of the proximal small intestine. Secretin and cholecystokinin have synergistic effects on fluid and electrolyte secretion. Bicarbonate is responsible for solubilizing zymogens within the pancreatic ductular system and neutralizing gastric acid in the duodenum to provide an optimal pH for pancreatic enzyme activity. Pancreatic duct cells also produce intrinsic factor, which is a protein necessary for the absorption of cobalamin (vitamin B_{12}).

Classically, the pancreatic response to a meal has been divided into cephalic, gastric, and intestinal phases. Under normal feeding conditions, these phases overlap and occur simultaneously, but the intestinal phase appears to be

The absorption of water is passive in the small and large intestines and follows the transport of solutes across the intestinal epithelium (Chang and Rao 1994). Passive absorption of water or electrolytes can be transcellular (i.e., through the cytoplasm of the cells) or paracellular (i.e., via the lateral intercellular spaces and tight junctions

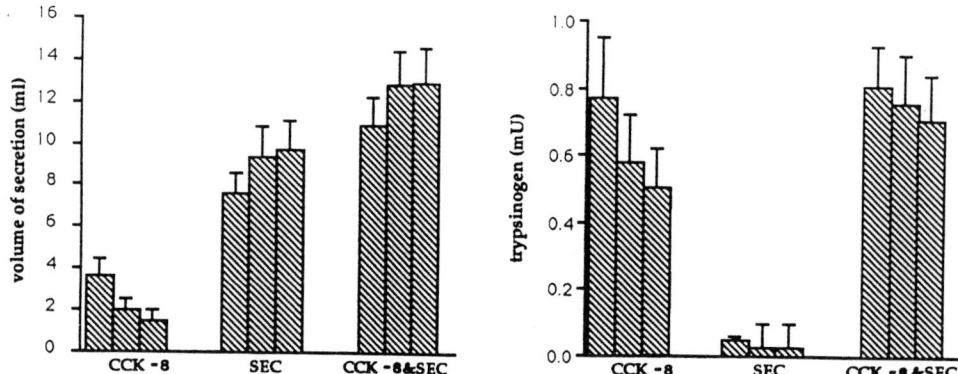

FIGURE 16-4. Output of trypsinogen and fluid in pancreatic juice during intravenous infusion of cholecystokinin (CCK-8), secretin (Sec), and CCK-8 and Sec together. Data (means ± SE) for eight dogs are expressed as total output per 15 min during 45-min infusion periods. Order of secretagogues was varied, and there was a 15-min rest period between secretagogues. (From Simpson KW, Alpers DH, DeWille J, et al.: Cellular localization and hormonal regulation of pancreatic intrinsic factor secretion in dogs. *Am J Physiol* 265:G178–G188, 1993.)

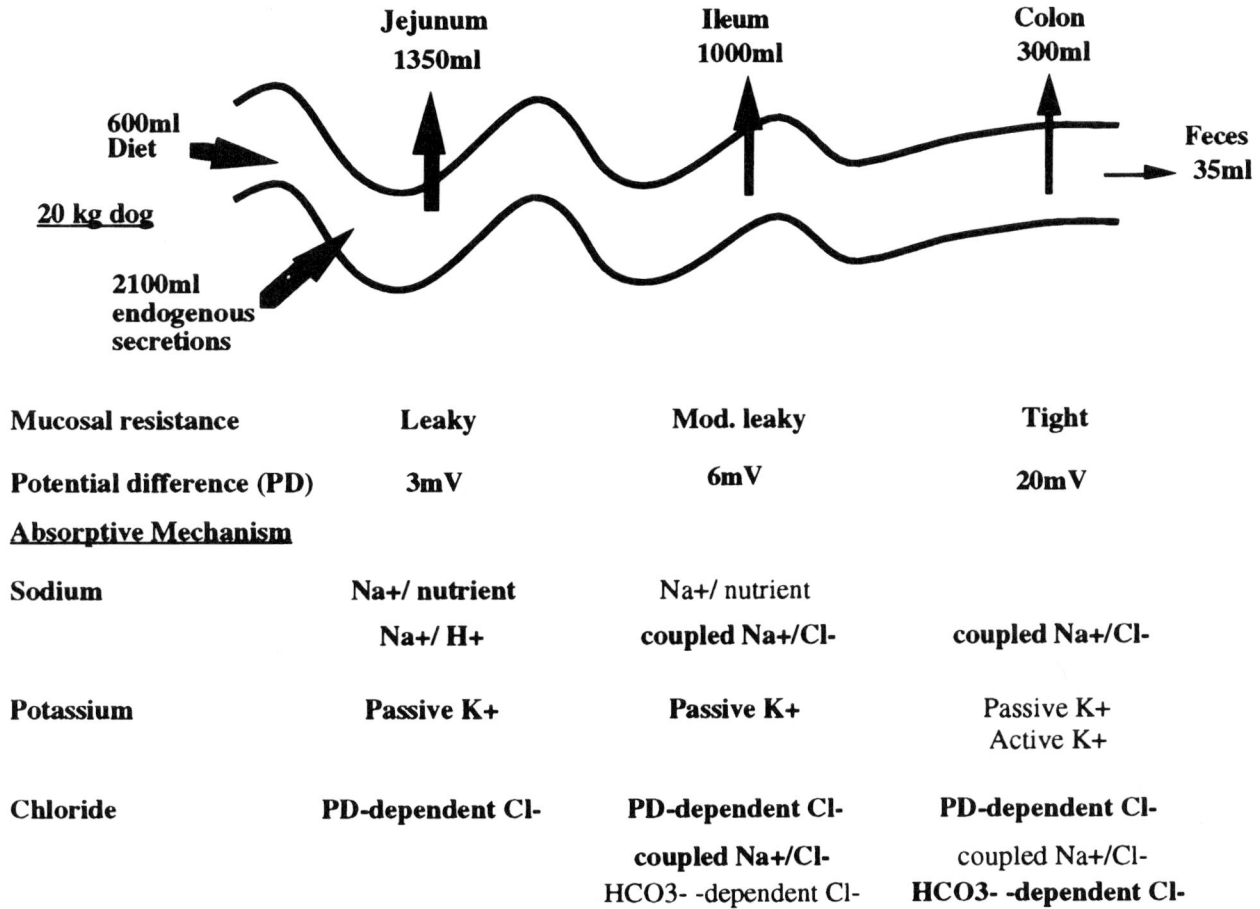

FIGURE 16-5. Fluid and electrolyte absorption in the gastrointestinal tract. (Adapted from Sellin 1998; Burrows 1983; Chang and Rao 1994.)

between enterocytes), and transfer occurs down a chemical or electrical gradient (e.g., passive transport of Na^+ and Cl^- in the jejunum and ileum).

Active transport involves transport against a concentration gradient and requires energy input (e.g., Na^+ transport driven by the Na^+, K^+ pump). The Na^+, K^+-ATPase is present in all enterocytes (Fig. 16–6 mechanism A; see also Fig. 16–5) and maintains the electrochemical Na^+ gradient required not only for net transepithelial Na^+ movement but also for the transport of many other solutes (Sellin 1998). Solvent drag is the term used to describe solute movement secondary to water flow (e.g., NaCl transport in the jejunum via the paracellular route). The relative importance of each transport system is site dependent (see Figs. 16–5 and 16–6), and the location of the enterocyte in the villus or crypt is also important: villus enterocytes absorb whereas crypt enterocytes secrete.

JEJUNUM

Because of the high permeability of the jejunum, passive transport processes make a major contribution to overall Na^+ and Cl^- movement in this segment of the intestinal tract. The luminal membranes of the epithelial cells in this region contain sodium-dependent transporters for hexose sugars and amino acids (see Figs. 16–5 and 16–6, mechanism B). Sodium enters the epithelial cell down its concentration gradient and is the driving force for accumulation of the nutrient intracellularly. Glucose and glutamine supply energy. Sodium is then extruded from the cell at the basolateral membrane by Na^+, K^+-ATPase while the hexose sugar or amino acid diffuses out of the cell at the basolateral membrane down a favorable concentration gradient. Therefore, Na^+, K^+-ATPase drives net absorption of both Na^+ and the sugar or amino acid. Proteins that function as Na^+-H^+ exchangers are present in the luminal membranes of the enterocytes in the jejunum and allow absorbed Na^+ to be exchanged for intracellular H^+ (see Figs. 16–5 and 16–6, mechanism C). This exchange is driven by both the electrochemical gradient for Na^+ and a pH gradient that results from a moderately acidic intracellular environment (Sellin 1998). As Na^+ is extruded at the basolateral membrane by Na^+, K^+-ATPase, HCO_3^- also moves out of the cell, resulting in net absorption of sodium bicarbonate. Although Na^+-nutrient absorption and Na^+-HCO_3^- absorption occur in the jejunum as already described, solvent drag–mediated Na^+ absorption secondary to monosaccharide absorption is the major mechanism for Na^+ absorption in this segment.

Movement of K^+ in the intestinal tract follows its electrochemical gradient and, in general, secretion pre-

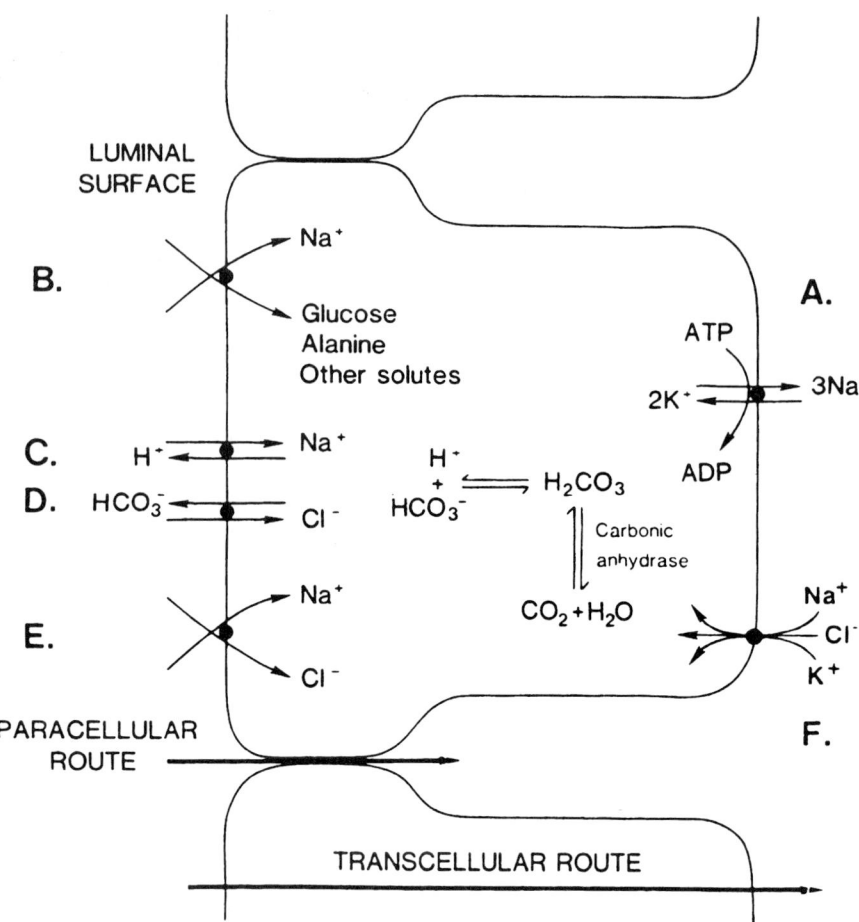

FIGURE 16-6. Summary of membrane transport processes present in different regions of the small intestine. Absorptive mechanisms: all enterocytes (A), jejunum (B), and ileum (B–E). Secretory mechanisms (F). (From Moseley RH: Fluid and electrolyte disorders and gastrointestinal disease. In Kokko JP and Tannen RL: *Fluid and Electrolytes*. Philadelphia, WB Saunders Co., p. 680, 1996.)

dominates (Sellin 1998). In the small intestine, most K^+ secretion is passive and results from the generation of a lumen-negative potential difference across the epithelium (Sellin 1998). This negative potential difference attracts K^+ into the intestinal lumen, and consequently the concentration of K^+ is always higher in intestinal contents than in plasma. In the jejunum, solvent drag created by glucose and amino acid transport causes passive absorption of Cl^- and HCO_3^-.

ILEUM

The predominant form of Na^+ absorption in the ileum is neutral NaCl absorption (see Figs. 16–5 and 16–6, mechanisms C and D or E) with some contribution by Na^+-nutrient absorption (see Figs. 16–5 and 16–6, mechanism B). The contents of the ileum and colon are normally alkaline (Edmonds 1974, Strombeck 1996). Solvent drag–mediated passive absorption of Cl^- and HCO_3^- does not occur in the ileum and colon, but a Cl^--HCO_3^- exchange mechanism is present. The exact mechanism of HCO_3^- secretion in duodenal, ileal, and colonic enterocytes is unknown but is thought to involve both electrogenic and electroneutral components and discrete apical and basolateral transporters (Sellin 1998).

COLON

Absorption of Na^+ in the colon is achieved against a large electrochemical gradient (see Fig. 16–5) and is principally a result of active Na^+ transport (Fordtran 1967). Colonic Na^+ absorption is also influenced by mineralocorticoids (e.g., aldosterone). Mineralocorticoids increase the activity of Na^+ channels in the luminal membranes of colonic epithelial cells and may increase Na^+, K^+-ATPase in the basolateral membranes. The colonic epithelium contains K^+ channels and is capable of active potassium transport. Absorption of potassium is thought to be accomplished by means of a K^+-ATPase with characteristics similar to those of both basolateral membrane Na^+, K^+-ATPase and parietal cell H^+, K^+-ATPase (Binder and Sandle 1994). The concentration of K^+ in colonic contents is high because of the high potential difference generated and can approach 90 mEq/L (Fordtran 1967). Active K^+ secretion is mediated by Na^+, K^+-ATPase or by Na^+- K^+-$2Cl^-$ cotransport. Aldosterone and cyclic AMP (cAMP) increase apical K^+ conductance and stimulate secretion of K^+ (see Fig. 16–5) (Binder and Sandle 1994). Colonic absorption is important in small-intestinal disease because the colon may compensate for fluid losses associated with small-bowel dysfunction. Alternatively, patients with small-bowel dysfunction may present with signs of large-bowel disease. This is thought to result from impairment of colonic absorption or stimulation of colonic secretion by products of abnormal small-intestinal function such as hydroxylated fatty acids or deconjugated bile acids.

The primary anions in the colon are short-chain fatty acids, which are generated by bacterial metabolism of carbohydrate and protein (Sellin 1998). These short-chain fatty acids include acetate, propionate, and butyrate, which are the preferred metabolic substrates for colonic cells. They are known to stimulate Na^+, water, and K^+ absorption by the colon, but the exact mechanism of this process has not been defined (Ruppin et al. 1980).

Intestinal secretion is a function of villus crypt cells. It is thought to be caused by the electrogenic transport of Cl^- across the basolateral membrane into the enterocyte (see Fig. 16–6, mechanism F) and Cl^- efflux through Cl^- channels in the microvillus membrane into the intestinal lumen (Fig. 16–7).

Control of Absorption and Secretion of Water and Electrolytes

Control of absorption and secretion is an autonomous process that is regulated by the neurocrine systems located in the submucosal plexus (Cooke 1989; Cooke and Reddix 1994; Moseley 1996; Sellin 1998). Acetylcholine and vasoactive intestinal polypeptide (VIP) are the major mediators of gastrointestinal secretion, whereas norepinephrine, somatostatin, and opioids are the principal regulators of absorption. At the cellular level, acetylcholine and VIP cause an increase in intracellular calcium and cAMP that inhibits neutral NaCl absorption and facilitates transcellular Cl^- efflux. Many bacterial agents exert their effects by increasing the intracellular concentration of cAMP in enterocytes. Norepinephrine, somatostatin, and opioids lower intracellular cAMP and calcium concentrations and stimulate neutral NaCl absorption (see Fig. 16–7).

Volume status and intestinal blood flow also influence ion transport. Systemic volume expansion results in an increase in intestinal secretion, whereas volume contraction results in adrenergic stimulation and increased absorption (Chang and Rao 1994). Osmotic forces are also important in the regulation of electrolyte and fluid transport. Luminal osmolality is normally maintained close to plasma osmolality (Chang and Rao 1994). After intake of hypertonic foods and liquids, rapid equilibration is accomplished by movement of water into the intestinal lumen. In particular, the duodenum and upper jejunum are subject to major fluid shifts. As intestinal chyme moves distally, absorptive processes steadily decrease luminal Na^+, Cl^-, and water. Osmotic diarrhea results if nonabsorbable solutes such as disaccharides remain in the lumen. Increased fluid absorption in the colon can compensate to some extent for fluid lost into the lumen of the small bowel, but eventually colon absorptive capacity is overwhelmed. Cations such as magnesium and anions such as sulfate are poorly absorbed and can also lead to osmotic diarrhea.

In response to inflammation, the number of immune cells in the lamina propria increases. Inflammation can lead to mucosal ulceration, exudation of protein, motility dysfunction, and loss of absorptive surface area, all of which can result in intestinal fluid loss. Many secretagogues associated with inflammation have been identified. Adenosine, serotonin, and histamine have both direct effects on epithelial cells and indirect effects via neural pathways. Other secretagogues include oxidants (e.g., superoxides, hydrogen peroxide, and OH^- released from neutrophils) that stimulate Cl^- secretion, cytokines (e.g., interleukin-1, interleukin-3), arachidonic acid, platelet-activating factor, substance P, kallikreins, and bradykinin (Sellin 1998). *Escherichia coli* heat-labile enterotoxin and enterotoxins produced by *Vibrio cholerae*, *Salmonella* sp., *Campylobacter jejuni*, *Pseudomonas aeruginosa*, and *Shigella* sp. activate adenylate cyclase, producing cAMP and augmenting secretion in the intestine (Hamer and Gorbach 1998) (see Fig. 16–7). The eicosanoids, especially the lipoxygenase metabolites of arachidonic acid, are central to the secretory response associated with inflammation. Kinins stimulate secretion in both the small and large intestines, where they stimulate production of prostaglandin E_2 (Musch et al. 1982).

Acid-base balance may also affect intestinal electrolyte transport. In the rat, metabolic acidosis is a potent stimulus for ileal Na^+ absorption (possibly in exchange for H^+), whereas metabolic alkalosis decreases Na^+ absorption but increases HCO_3^- secretion (Chang and Rao 1994).

▶ Pathophysiology of the Gastrointestinal Tract

Vomiting

Vomiting is a reflex act that is initiated by stimulation of the vomiting center in the medulla. The vomiting center can be stimulated directly or indirectly via the chemoreceptor trigger zone (CTZ), which is situated in the area postrema (Fig. 16–8). The blood-brain barrier is limited at this point, enabling blood-borne substances such as toxins or drugs to stimulate the CTZ. Neurologic input

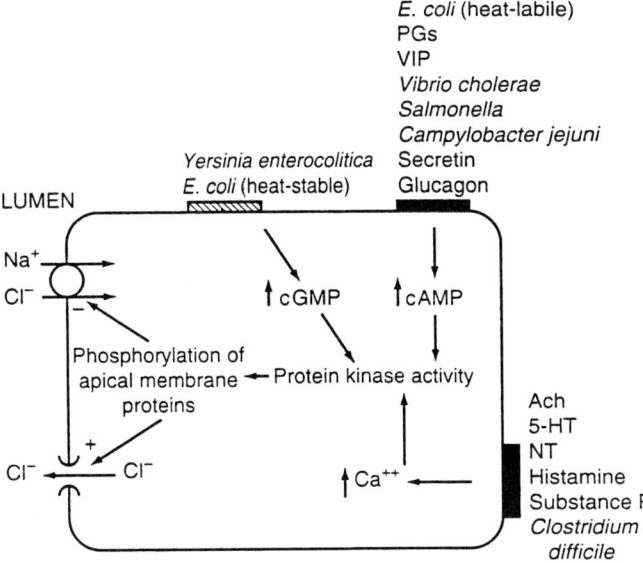

FIGURE 16–7. Role of intracellular messengers cGMP, cAMP, and Ca^{2+} on NaCl absorption and Cl^- secretion by small intestine epithelium. Increases in messenger-specific protein kinase activity result in phosphorylation of specific brush border membrane phosphoproteins that alter ion movement. PGs, Prostaglandins; VIP, vasoactive intestinal polypeptide; Ach, acetylcholine; 5-HT, serotonin; NT, neurotensin. (From Moseley RH: Fluid and electrolyte disorders and gastrointestinal disease. In Kokko JP and Tannen RL: *Fluid and Electrolytes*. Philadelphia, WB Saunders, p. 681, 1996.)

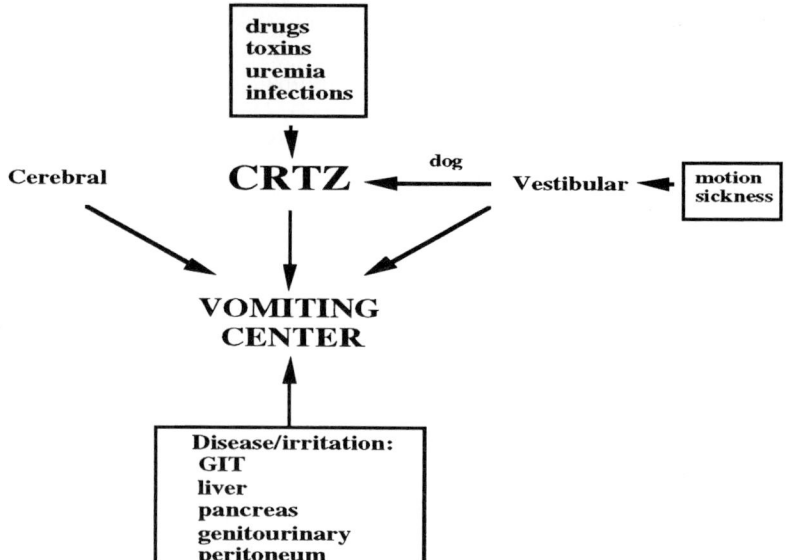

Figure 16-8. Initiation of vomiting. CRTZ, Chemoreceptor trigger zone.

from the vestibular nucleus can also stimulate the CTZ in the dog or the vomiting center. Disease or irritation of the GIT, abdominal organs, or peritoneum and cerebral diseases can directly stimulate the vomiting center via visceral receptors and vagal afferents.

Once the vomiting center is adequately stimulated, a series of visceral events is initiated. This sequence of events includes inhibition of proximal gastrointestinal motility, a retrograde power contraction in the small intestine, and antral relaxation, which enables transfer of intestinal contents to the stomach. These events are followed by moderate-amplitude contractions in the gastric antrum and intestine and shortening of the intraabdominal esophagus. Dilatation of the cardia and lower esophageal sphincter enables transfer of gastric contents to the esophagus during retching and vomiting. Retching often precedes vomiting and is characterized by rhythmic inspiratory movements against a closed glottis. Negative intrathoracic pressure during retching prevents expulsion of esophageal contents. During vomiting, the abdominal muscles contract and intrathoracic and intraabdominal pressures are positive, resulting in forceful expulsion of gastric contents from the mouth.

Vomiting is associated with a wide range of disease processes and, when frequent or severe, can have major effects on fluid, electrolyte, and acid-base balance. The consequences of vomiting depend to some extent on the cause. Vomiting of gastric and intestinal contents usually involves loss of fluid containing Cl^-, K^+, Na^+, and HCO_3^-, and dehydration is accompanied to a variable extent by hypochloremia, hypokalemia, and hyponatremia (Cornelius and Rawlings 1981; Twedt and Grauer 1982). Metabolic acidosis is generally more common than metabolic alkalosis in dogs with gastrointestinal disease (Cornelius and Rawlings 1981).

With obstruction of the gastric outflow tract or proximal duodenum, loss of Cl^- can exceed that of HCO_3^-, and hypochloremia, hypokalemia, and metabolic alkalosis result (Cornelius and Rawlings 1981; Twedt and Grauer 1982; Robinson and Hardy 1988). Metabolic alkalosis is self-perpetuating because of increased renal reabsorption of $NaHCO_3$ in the presence of volume, chloride, and potassium depletion (Rose 1984). These metabolic disturbances arise as a result of preferential conservation of volume at the expense of extracellular pH. The renal reabsorption of almost all filtered HCO_3^- and the exchange of sodium for hydrogen ions in the distal tubule promote an acidic urine pH despite extracellular alkalemia (so-called paradoxical aciduruia) (Van Slyke and Evans 1947; Rose 1984).

Metabolic alkalosis in patients with gastrointestinal signs is not invariably associated with outflow obstruction and has been encountered in dogs with parvovirus enteritis and acute pancreatitis (Heald et al. 1986). Diseases characterized by hypersecretion of acid, such as gastrinoma, may also be associated with metabolic alkalosis and aciduria. Basal gastric acid secretion in two dogs with gastrin-producing tumors (1.7 and 2.7 mmol/h/kg$^{0.75}$ HCl) was maximal in the unstimulated state (Simpson and Dykes 1997). In this situation, hypochloremia, hypokalemia, metabolic alkalosis, and dehydration are probably due to gastric hypersecretion of acid (Simpson and Dykes 1997).

Diarrhea

The pathomechanisms in patients with diarrhea include increased intestinal secretion, decreased intestinal absorption, rapid transit of intestinal contents, and mesenteric, vascular, or lymphatic disease (Ooms and Degryse 1986).

Secretory agents include neuropeptides of the enteric system (found in neuroendocrine tumors), cholinergic agonists, gastrointestinal hormones, bacterial enterotoxins, deconjugated bile acids, and hydroxy fatty acids (Ooms and Degryse 1986). Secretory diarrhea results when prosecretory stimulation overwhelms absorptive forces. Secretory diarrhea is manifested by increased colonic secretion of sodium-rich fluid. Volume depletion resulting from sodium and water loss stimulates antidiuretic hormone release, which in turn stimulates water retention by the kidneys and dilutional hyponatremia.

Decreased intestinal absorption may result from decreased intestinal surface area as a consequence of damage by infectious agents (e.g., parvovirus), cellular infiltration, or surgery. Damage to the intestinal epithelial barrier may also increase intestinal permeability, disrupting paracellular and transcellular absorptive pathways. An increase in the osmolality of intestinal contents may also decrease absorption. Specific causes of osmotic diarrhea include overeating, sudden dietary change, osmotic laxative ingestion, maldigestion, or malabsorption. Absorption of water and electrolytes is retarded by accumulation of nonabsorbable solutes in the gut lumen, and there is net water movement from plasma to the gut lumen. In osmotic diarrhea, the concentration of sodium in the stool may remain below that of plasma, leading to water loss in excess of sodium, dehydration, and hypernatremia, especially when water intake is inadequate (Fordtran 1967). This finding has been observed in dogs and people with hepatic encephalopathy (HE) treated with lactulose (Nelson et al. 1983). Intestinal absorption may also be affected by diseases that cause increased venous pressure, lymphatic pressure, decreased interstitial osmotic pressure (hypoalbuminemia), and increased epithelial permeability. Disorders of intestinal motility result in decreased intestinal fluid absorption because of decreased contact time between luminal contents and the enterocytes.

An understanding of these pathomechanisms is useful in identifying the pathophysiology and establishing appropriate treatment of patients with diarrhea, but diarrhea caused by only one mechanism is rare in clinical practice. For example, a dog with inflammatory bowel disease may have decreased intestinal absorption caused by decreased surface area, increased mucosal permeability, increased intraluminal osmotic forces, and decreased interstitial osmotic forces coupled with rapid transit of intestinal contents and increased intestinal secretion.

FLUID AND ELECTROLYTE ABNORMALITIES IN DIARRHEA

The fluid and electrolyte abnormalities associated with diarrhea include volume depletion, hyponatremia or hypernatremia, hypokalemia, and metabolic acidosis (Cornelius and Rawlings 1981; Twedt and Grauer 1982; Moseley 1996). The metabolic acidosis that develops is characterized by hyperchloremia and a normal anion gap caused by loss of diarrheal fluid with relatively low chloride and high bicarbonate concentrations. Serious electrolyte and acid-base abnormalities are relatively uncommon in patients with diarrhea as a sole complaint. When diarrhea is severe and protracted or is accompanied by vomiting, acid-base and electrolyte disturbances are more likely, but it is difficult to predict which abnormalities will be present. For example, decreased total CO_2 concentrations were identified in less than 17% of 134 dogs with parvovirus enteritis in one study (Jacobs et al. 1980), whereas metabolic alkalosis and hypochloremia were more common than metabolic acidosis in another study of dogs with parvovirus enteritis (Heald et al. 1986).

Hypoadrenocorticism should be ruled out whenever hyperkalemia and hyponatremia are present, but up to 26% of dogs with hypoadrenocorticism may have normal mineralocorticoid function and normal Na/K ratios (Lifton et al. 1996). Therefore, a history of intermittent signs of gastrointestinal disease may warrant an adrenocorticotropic hormone stimulation test despite a normal Na/K ratio. Clinicopathologic findings in dogs with primary gastrointestinal disease may mimic those of hypoadrenocorticism with Na/K ratios below 27:1 and metabolic acidosis (DiBartola et al. 1985; Malik et al. 1990). Gastrointestinal diseases reported to mimic primary hypoadrenocorticism include trichuriasis, ancylostomiasis, salmonellosis, and perforated duodenal ulcer. Postulated mechanisms of these electrolyte derangements include metabolic acidosis secondary to volume depletion and fecal loss of bicarbonate with subsequent translocation of potassium from intra- to extracellular fluid. Selective aldosterone deficiency does not appear to be responsible for hyperkalemia and hyponatremia in dogs with trichuriasis that have laboratory abnormalities that mimic those of hypoadrenocorticism (Graves et al. 1994). Hypocalcemia and hypomagnesemia occur uncommonly in veterinary patients with diarrhea.

Normal stool water contains a higher concentration of potassium than sodium (Fordtran 1967). As stool volumes increase in human patients with diarrhea, there is a progressive increase in the sodium and chloride concentrations and a decrease in potassium concentration and the electrolyte composition of the stool approaches that of plasma (Fordtran 1967). In cases of diarrhea, there is a linear relationship between fluid and sodium loss (Fordtran 1967). In human patients, measurements of fecal electrolyte concentrations and osmolality are used to calculate an osmolality gap, which aids in the differentiation of osmotic and secretory diarrhea. The osmolality, sodium concentration, and potassium concentration of feces from four normal cats were reported as 622 to 927 mOsm/kg, 27 to 57 mEq/L, and 19 to 46 mEq/L, respectively (Gregory et al. 1990). Stool normally contains high concentrations of potassium, and fecal potassium loss can become severe in protracted diarrheal states (Fordtran 1967). Stimulation of the renin-aldosterone axis as a result of volume depletion has been suggested as one potential cause of potassium loss (Moseley 1996).

Dogs with gastrin-secreting tumors may be presented for evaluation of intermittent or profuse watery diarrhea, vomiting, and weight loss. In this setting, diarrhea and vomiting are probably a result of the increased volume and acidity of gastric secretions, which cause gastrointestinal ulceration and destruction of pancreatic enzymes (Simpson and Dykes 1997). The high concentrations of gastrin may also adversely affect intestinal function.

In humans, profuse watery intermittent or fulminant diarrhea can be caused by tumors secreting VIP (VIPomas) (Krejs 1987). The majority of these tumors are located in the pancreas, although the VIPoma syndrome has been associated with tumors at a number of other sites in humans. Additional findings include severe hypokalemia, metabolic acidosis, and occasionally hypochlorhydria. The profound secretory diarrhea results from the stimulatory action of VIP on intestinal secretion. The VIPoma syndrome differs from gastrinoma in that patients with VIPoma have normal serum gastrin concentrations and lack gastric acid hypersecretion and secondary upper GIT ulceration.

▶ Management of Disorders of the Gastrointestinal Tract

Overview of Fluid Therapy for Vomiting and Diarrhea

Correction of volume, electrolyte, and acid-base disturbances is an essential part of the management of patients with vomiting and diarrhea. The most appropriate type, route, and rate of fluid replacement are chosen on the basis of the patient's hydration, tissue perfusion, and electrolyte and acid-base status. The presence of anemia or hypoalbuminemia and the potential for continuing fluid loss through vomiting, diarrhea, fever, and compensatory hyperventilation associated with metabolic acidosis must also be taken into account. Minimal evaluation of the patient with gastrointestinal disease should include determination of body temperature, heart rate, skin turgor, capillary refill time, packed cell volume (PCV), total protein concentration, urine specific gravity, and urine pH as well as serum concentrations of sodium, potassium, chloride, total CO_2, and glucose. Measurement of blood gases, blood pressure (central venous and arterial), and urine output are required for optimal care of patients with severe gastrointestinal disease.

Oral fluid therapy may be useful for patients with diarrhea that can tolerate oral intake. Subcutaneous administration of an isotonic balanced electrolyte solution may be sufficient to correct mild (≤5%) fluid deficits but is insufficient for patients with moderate (5–10%) or severe (>10%) dehydration. For patients with moderate to severe dehydration, inadequate oral intake, electrolyte imbalance, or signs of hypovolemic or endotoxic shock, intravenous fluid administration is necessary.

The rate of fluid administration depends on the presence or absence of shock, the extent of dehydration, and the presence of cardiac or renal disease that may predispose the patient to volume overload. Patients with a history of vomiting that are mildly dehydrated are usually responsive to crystalloids (e.g., lactated Ringer's solution or 9% NaCl) at a rate that provides maintenance needs and replaces existing deficits and ongoing losses over a 24-h period. Patients with signs of shock require more aggressive support. The volume deficit can be replaced with crystalloids at an initial rate of 60 to 90 mL/kg/h, which is then tailored to maintain tissue perfusion and hydration. Central venous pressure monitoring and evaluation of urine output are necessary for patients with severe gastrointestinal disease, especially those with third-space losses of fluid into the gut or peritoneum. Colloids and hypertonic solutions can also be used to reduce the amount of crystalloid required (e.g., 5 mL/kg of 7% NaCl in 6% dextran IV, 10–20 mL/kg/day of degraded gelatin [Haemaccel] IV). Colloids are also useful in hypoproteinemic patients. Endotoxic shock is a common complication of severe gastrointestinal disease. Warning signs of endotoxemic shock include fever or subnormal body temperature, tachycardia, increased respiratory rate, slow capillary refill time, hyperemic or pale mucous membranes, transient leukopenia followed by leukocytosis with a left shift and toxic neutrophils, low-normal central venous pressure, and bounding pulses. Patients with endotoxic shock must be treated aggressively with fluid therapy, broad-spectrum antibiotics, glucocorticoids, oxygen, glucose, and bicarbonate as indicated (Haskins 1990).

The effect of vomiting and diarrhea on acid-base balance is difficult to predict, and therapeutic intervention to correct acid-base imbalance should be based on blood gas analysis. Patients with normal acid-base status or mild metabolic acidosis may be given lactated Ringer's solution at a rate sufficient to correct fluid deficits and provide for maintenance and ongoing losses over a 24-h period. Potassium depletion may be a consequence of prolonged diarrhea, vomiting, or anorexia, but most polyionic replacement fluids contain only small amounts of potassium. Consequently, KCl is usually added to parenteral fluids and adjusted on the basis of serum potassium concentrations. When severe metabolic acidosis is present (pH < 7.1, HCO_3^- < 10 mEq/L), sodium bicarbonate (1 mEq/kg) can be given. Care should be taken to rule out respiratory acidosis before administering sodium bicarbonate and to administer it slowly and in small amounts (0.5 mEq/kg over 15 min) to prevent cerebrospinal fluid acidosis, aggravation of hypokalemia, or hypocalcemia. Additional bicarbonate supplementation is based on repeated blood gas analyses. Metabolic alkalosis usually responds to correction of the volume, chloride, and potassium deficits with 0.9% NaCl supplemented with KCl administered intravenously.

Diagnostic investigations should initially focus on ruling out upper gastrointestinal obstruction. Administration of antisecretory drugs (e.g., H_2 antagonists) may limit chloride efflux into gastric juice. When acid hypersecretion is present or suspected, it is best managed by administration of a proton pump inhibitor (e.g., omeprazole at 0.2–0.7 mg/kg q24h). Somatostatin analogs may also be useful to control gastric acid hypersecretion (e.g., octreotide at 2–20 μg/kg SQ q8h) (Simpson and Dykes 1997).

Other symptomatic treatments considered initially in patients with vomiting and diarrhea are nothing by mouth and antiemetics or antacids when vomiting persists. Prophylactic use of antibiotics (e.g., cephalosporins, ampicillin) may be warranted in animals with shock and suspected gastrointestinal barrier dysfunction. Analgesia can be provided by using opioids (e.g., buprenorphine at 0.0075–0.01 mg/kg IM).

ORAL REHYDRATION SOLUTIONS

The rationale for use of oral rehydration solutions (ORSs) is the coupled transport of sodium with glucose or other actively transported small organic molecules and hence the promotion of water absorption (Curran 1960; Farthing 1988). These cotransport processes often remain relatively unaffected in acute infectious (e.g., bacterial, viral) cases of diarrhea (Thillainayagam et al. 1998). In secretory diarrhea, the epithelium maintains its absorptive capacity and cotransport processes that are important for the success of oral rehydration therapy (Thillainayagam et al. 1998). With certain viral causes of diarrhea (e.g., rotaviral infection in children), patchy epithelial damage may allow oral rehydration to be of benefit (Sack et al. 1978; Santosham et al. 1982). A balanced ORS has a carbohydrate-to-sodium ratio of 1:1 to 2:1, potassium, chloride, an alkali source, and an osmolality between 250 and 310 mOsm/kg. The ideal formula still remains controversial (Sladen and Dawson 1969; Thillainayagam et al. 1998). Alkali sources such as bicarbonate and citrate also enhance the absorption of water and electrolytes (Sladen et al. 1968).

Clinical trials of ORSs containing complex carbohydrates or glucose polymers in place of glucose have resulted in decreased volume and duration of diarrhea. A potential explanation for the beneficial effect of such solutions is that glucose polymer molecules contain more glucose residues without delivering a high osmotic load to the intestinal lumen. Much of the breakdown of the polymer occurs at the epithelial surface, and the smaller molecules do not accumulate in the intestinal lumen. The relative hypotonicity of glucose polymer solutions may be the major contributor to their efficacy (Thillainayagam et al. 1998).

In children, oral electrolyte solutions can be used to treat mild to severe dehydration even in the presence of vomiting as long as the patient is able to swallow small amounts frequently (Avery and Snyder 1990). A volume equal to the amount that would be given intravenously is appropriate. Reports of the effectiveness of ORSs in veterinary patients are limited, but favorable results have been reported in the treatment of uncomplicated acute gastroenteritis in dogs and cats with Pedialyte at a daily dosage of 150 mL/kg body weight until a bland diet could be reintroduced (Romatowski 1985). Commercial solutions such as Pedialyte are readily available but usually contain too much glucose and too little sodium and carry some risk of hypertonic diarrhea (Romatowski 1985). A more physiologic solution recommended by the World Health Organization contains 90 mEq/L sodium, 20 mEq/L potassium, 80 mEq/L chloride, 30 mEq/L bicarbonate, and 111 mmol/L glucose. Such a solution can be prepared by adding 3.5 g NaCl, 2.5 g $NaHCO_3$, 1.5 g KCl, and 20 g glucose to 1 L water (Romatowski 1985).

PATIENT MONITORING

For stable patients, minimal monitoring includes regular assessment of vital signs and fluid and electrolyte balance. In patients with systemic abnormalities, monitoring should be more aggressive and should include vital signs, weight, PCV, total protein concentration, fluid intake and output, blood pressure (central venous and arterial), and determination of serum concentrations of electrolytes and glucose, acid-base status, platelets, and coagulation status.

Protein-Losing Enteropathy

Hypoproteinemia characterized by a decrease in both albumin and globulin is often associated with gastrointestinal disease or blood loss. When total protein or albumin concentrations decrease to less than 4.0 g/dL or 1.5 g/dL, respectively, some type of natural or synthetic colloid replacement can be instituted to avoid interstitial fluid accumulation and pulmonary edema (Tobias and Schertel 1992). Benefit from colloid administration is often short lived because colloids are rapidly lost into the gut. The short duration of effect and the expense of colloids have resulted in the use of colloids for brief support, whereas long-term treatment is focused on the underlying cause of the protein loss.

Gastric Dilatation and Volvulus

Gastric dilatation and gastric dilatation-volvulus (GDV) are life-threatening conditions that are frequently accompanied by severe hypovolemic shock. Hypovolemic shock arises as a consequence of impaired venous return caused by obstruction of the caudal vena cava by gastric distention. Devitalization of the gastric wall, splenic torsion, congestion of abdominal viscera, and endotoxic shock further exacerbate the hypovolemic crisis.

A variety of acid-base and electrolyte disturbances have been observed in dogs with GDV (Muir 1982; Wingfield et al. 1982). Metabolic acidosis and hypokalemia were the most common abnormalities in one study, occurring in 15 of 57 and 16 of 57 dogs, respectively (Muir 1982). Metabolic acidosis is probably due to decreased tissue perfusion, anaerobic metabolism, and accumulation of lactic acid (Muir 1982). Metabolic alkalosis may also occur as a result of vomiting or sequestration of acid in the stomach (Muir 1982). Either respiratory acidosis or respiratory alkalosis may be observed and reflect hypoventilation or hyperventilation, respectively. The variety of acid-base and electrolyte abnormalities in dogs with GDV dictates that fluid therapy be individualized on the basis of blood gas analysis and serum electrolyte concentrations.

Gastric decompression and fluid therapy are the most important emergency treatments for dogs with GDV. Fluid therapy has traditionally consisted of shock doses (60–90 mL/kg/h) of lactated Ringer's solution given via large-gauge catheters into the cephalic or jugular veins. Experimental studies that have compared crystalloids (60 mL/kg 0.9% NaCl followed by 20 mL/kg/h) with hypertonic saline (5 mL/kg 7% NaCl in 6% dextran followed by 0.9% NaCl 20 mL/kg/h) in dogs with GDV-induced shock indicated that hypertonic saline maintains better myocardial performance, higher heart rate, and lower systemic vascular resistance than crystalloid alone (Allen et al. 1991). The resuscitative dose of hypertonic saline was delivered in 5 to 10 min as compared with an hour for the crystalloid. Potassium and bicarbonate are best administered on the basis of blood gas and electrolyte measurements.

Acute Pancreatitis

Acute pancreatitis is a potentially life-threatening condition affecting dogs and cats (Hill and Van Winkle 1993; Simpson 1993, 1997; Simpson et al. 1994; Hess et al. 1998). Clinical abnormalities are highly variable and in dogs range from mild dehydration and vomiting to shock, hemorrhagic diathesis, and death. Anorexia, lethargy, and weight loss are the most common clinical signs in cats with pancreatitis. The severity of clinical signs is thought to reflect the severity of pancreatitis (i.e., mild edematous versus severe necrotizing or suppurative) and the presence of systemic complications such as shock, pancreatic infection and necrosis, sepsis, and disseminated intravascular coagulation.

The cause of acute pancreatitis in dogs and cats usually remains undetermined. Regardless of the initiating cause, active pancreatic enzymes (e.g., trypsin, phospholipase, collagenase, elastase) and inflammatory mediators (e.g., kallikreins, kinins, free radicals, complement components, thromboplastins) are released in an active form into the pancreatic tissues and blood vessels. Activated factor XII (Hageman's factor) and trypsin appear to be largely responsible for activation of the coagulation, fibrinolytic, kinin, and complement cascades. Pancreatic defense mechanisms limit trypsinogen activation within the pancreas, and circulating α_1-antitrypsin and α_2-macroglobulin bind to active enzymes and prevent systemic damage (Ohlsson 1971; Simpson et al. 1995; Melgarejo et al. 1996).

When these defense systems are overwhelmed, increased pancreatic capillary permeability leads to fluid loss into the pancreas and abdomen, a decline in pancreatic blood flow, and an increase in the local concentrations of pancreatic enzymes and inflammatory mediators. Large numbers of leukocytes migrate to the inflamed pancreas and serve as a continued source of free radicals, inflammatory mediators, and enzymes. This vicious, self-perpetuating cycle can ultimately lead to thrombosis of pancreatic blood vessels and pancreatic necrosis. Bacterial translocation from the GIT may cause endotoxic shock, pancreatic necrosis and infection, or pancreatic abscess formation. Systemic complications such as impaired cardiovascular (e.g., hypovolemic shock, myocardial damage), hematologic (e.g., disseminated intravascular coagulation), respiratory (e.g., pleural effusion), hepatic (e.g., hepatic parenchymal damage, biliary stasis), renal (e.g., glomerular and tubular damage), and metabolic (lipemia, hypocalcemia, diabetes mellitus, hypoproteinemia) function may develop. In experimental pancreatitis, death ensues when α_2-macroglobulin is depleted (Ohlsson 1971).

Many electrolyte and acid-base disturbances have been reported in dogs and cats with acute pancreatitis. Hypokalemia, hypoglycemia, hyponatremia, hypochloremia, hypocalcemia, hypoalbuminemia, and azotemia have been reported (Duffel 1975; Owens et al. 1975; Schaer 1979; Hill and Van Winkle 1993; Simpson 1997; Hess et al. 1998). Hyperkalemia, hypernatremia, and hypercalcemia have been observed less commonly. Hypokalemia, hypochloremia, and hyponatremia are probably consequences of increased loss of these electrolytes in vomitus or diarrhea, decreased oral intake, and transcellular shifts. Concomitant diabetes mellitus also contributes. Hypoproteinemia is more common in dogs with acute pancreatitis than in cats and is thought to be a consequence of intra- and peripancreatic exudation of albumin. Hypoalbuminemia also contributes to the hypocalcemia observed in dogs with pancreatitis (Meuten et al. 1982), and hypoalbuminemia and decreased total serum calcium concentration were among the few clinicopathologic changes noted in cats with experimentally induced acute pancreatitis (Kitchell et al. 1986). Hypocalcemia, however, is not always attributable to hypoalbuminemia and did not account for the hypocalcemia observed in 30% of 40 cats with naturally occurring fatal pancreatitis (Hill and Van Winkle 1993).

Additional mechanisms that may decrease serum total calcium concentration in acute pancreatitis include alteration of the parathyroid-calcium axis and sequestration of calcium in the pancreas and other tissues (Rattner et al. 1990; Izquierdo et al. 1985; Bhattacharya et al. 1985, 1988). Hypercalcemia has been reported in dogs with acute pancreatitis (Hess et al. 1998). The clinical relevance of this finding remains unclear because serum total calcium concentrations were corrected for albumin and ionized calcium concentrations were not measured (Peoples 1988). Hyperglycemia and glucosuria are especially frequent in cats with pancreatitis, but ketonuria is infrequent, suggesting that stress may be a more common cause for these abnormalities than diabetes mellitus. However, mild diabetes mellitus or recrudescence of a previous diabetic state may occur in cats with acute pancreatitis. Azotemia is usually present and is often prerenal or renal in origin. Some studies report a high frequency of concurrent pancreatitis and nephritis (Duffel 1975; Macy 1989), whereas others (Hill and Van Winkle 1993; Simpson 1997) do not. Clarification of a possible relationship between pancreatitis and renal disease awaits future studies. Acid-base abnormalities in dogs and cats with acute pancreatitis usually consist of metabolic acidosis, but metaboic alkalosis may also be observed (Hess et al. 1998).

Medical management of acute pancreatitis is usually initiated before the diagnosis is confirmed and is based on presenting clinical findings and laboratory abnormalities (e.g., PCV, urinalysis, and total protein, blood urea nitrogen, glucose, sodium, and potassium concentrations). See the information given earlier about fluid therapy for vomiting and diarrhea. Hypovolemia and dehydration are evaluated and corrected by intravenous administration of fluids. The type of fluid chosen should be based on serum electrolytes (e.g., sodium, potassium, chloride, total CO_2) to restore normal electrolyte and acid-base balance. Hypocalcemia is usually not of clinical concern and requires no specific treatment. If hypoglycemia is present, dextrose (2.5 to 5%) is added to the fluids. Insulin therapy is initiated if hyperglycemia, glucosuria, and ketonuria are present. Stress hyperglycemia should be ruled out when ketonuria is absent.

Other symptomatic treatments initially considered include nothing by mouth and antiemetics or antacids when vomiting is persistent. Centrally acting antiemetics such as metaclopramide or phenothiazine derivatives are indicated for patients with intractable vomiting. Prophylactic use of antibiotics (i.e., cephalosporins or ampicillin alone or in combination with enrofloxacin or amikacin) may be warranted for patients with shock, fever, diabetes mellitus, or hemorrhagic diarrhea or vomitus. Analgesia can be provided by using opioids (e.g., buprenorphine at 0.0075–0.01 mg/kg IM).

After a diagnosis of pancreatitis is confirmed, fluid therapy is continued and more specific therapy may be employed. The majority of dogs with acute pancreatitis respond to fluid therapy and nothing by mouth for 48 h. More specific therapy is usually reserved for dogs that do not respond to fluid therapy or that have signs of disseminated intravascular coagulation. In contrast to dogs, cats with acute pancreatitis are more commonly presented with anorexia than vomiting, but episodes of pancreatic inflammation appear to be more protracted. No treatment regimens for pancreatitis have been critically evaluated in dogs or cats with naturally occurring pancreatitis.

Specific therapy in humans consists of preventing further pancreatitis from developing and limiting the local and systemic consequences of pancreatitis. Therapy aimed at inhibiting pancreatic secretion (e.g., glucagon, somatostatin) or intracellular activation of proteases (e.g., gabexate mesylate) that has been beneficial in ameliorating experimental pancreatitis has shown little benefit in the treatment of clinical patients. This lack of success may be related to the timing of therapy in relation to the development of pancreatitis. Therapy in experimental pancreatitis is usually initiated before or shortly after induction of pancreatitis, whereas most clinical patients are not presented until 24 to 48 h after the onset of pancreatitis. These findings have led to more therapeutic emphasis on limitation of damage, including limiting the effects of inflammatory mediators or pancreatic enzymes and maintaining pancreatic perfusion.

The systemic effects of pancreatitis may be ameliorated in experimental animals by maintaining adequate pancreatic microcirculation and protease-antiprotease balance. The pancreatic microcirculation in dogs with experimental pancreatitis was maintained more effectively by use of dextran-containing solutions than by use of crystalloids (Horton et al. 1989; Klar et al. 1990). The pancreatic microcirculation of cats with experimental pancreatitis was maintained by low-dose dopamine infusion (5 μg/kg/min) (Karanjia et al. 1990). Natural protease inhibitors contained in plasma help restore protease-antiprotease balance when administered in large volumes (Cuschieri et al. 1983). For this reason, it may be beneficial to administer fresh frozen plasma (10–20 mL/kg) to dogs with pancreatitis. Administration of fresh frozen plasma may also be beneficial for management of disseminated intravascular coagulation or other coagulopathies. Heparin administration (75–150 IU/kg SQ q8h) may be warranted in the early stages of acute pancreatitis to delay development of disseminated intravascular coagulation. Heparin may also clear lipemia, which is a frequent finding in acute pancreatitis. Clearing of lipemia facilitates performance and interpretation of serum biochemistry tests. Oral pancreatic enzyme extracts have been reported to reduce pain in humans with chronic pancreatitis but are less likely to be effective in dogs because dogs do not appear to have a protease-mediated negative feedback system.

Small-Bowel Obstruction

Intestinal obstruction can be classified as acute or chronic, partial or complete, and simple or strangulated. The cause of obstruction may be extraluminal compression, intramural thickening, or an intraluminal mass. The most common extraluminal cause of obstruction is intussusception (Wilson and Burt 1974). Intestinal neoplasia is the most common intramural cause of obstruction in veterinary patients, but hematoma, focal granulomas related to feline infectious peritonitis, inflammatory bowel disease, stricture, and phycomycosis are also observed (Moore and Carpenter 1984a, 1984b; Harvey et al. 1996). Foreign objects such as peach pits, toys, and fishhooks are common causes of intraluminal obstruction in dogs, whereas string linear foreign objects (frequently anchored under the tongue) are common in cats. The adverse effects of intestinal obstruction are a consequence of fluid loss into the GIT, proliferation of intestinal bacteria, and inflammation of the intestine (Cullen et al. 1997). Intestinal perforation further exacerbates the clinical situation and is common with linear foreign objects and intestinal neoplasia.

Vomiting would be expected to be a major feature of intestinal obstruction. Complete intestinal obstruction in dogs, however, is frequently not associated with vomiting (Shields 1965; Lantz 1981). Clinical signs are more often related to marked loss of fluid and electrolytes into the intestine. Bowel distention causes a steady decline in intestinal absorptive capacity and an increase in the secretion of sodium, potassium, and albumin into the lumen (Lantz 1981). With complete obstruction of the ileum, there is a gradual increase in the secretion of sodium, potassium, and water into the obstructed bowel, which can reach 13 mL/min after 60 h of obstruction (Shields 1965). Metabolic acidosis is a consequence of bicarbonate loss, dehydration, and starvation (Lantz 1981). Stagnated luminal contents and impaired motility provide a favorable environment for the proliferation of bacteria and the elaboration of bacterial toxins. Anoxia and devitalization of the bowel wall allow translocation of bacteria and toxins transmurally and then systemically. If untreated, potentially fatal endotoxemic shock can develop. Partial obstruction, especially of the distal small intestine, can be associated with chronic diarrhea and weight loss caused by intestinal stasis, and affected animals may have a history of responding to antibiotic treatment.

Physical findings range from mild dehydration to signs of septic shock and depend on the severity of fluid loss, fluid shifts, and intestinal compromise caused by obstruction. Shock and abdominal pain are often the predominant findings with strangulated obstructions such as intestinal volvulus, incarcerated obstructions, and intussusception.

Fluid therapy should be instituted on the basis of clinical findings and initial laboratory findings. Fluid shifts can be severe, and close monitoring of central venous pressure, PCV, total protein concentration, urine output, acid-base status, and electrolyte concentrations is often initiated to detect and correct changes in fluid balance. Hypochloremia and hypokalemia are frequent in patients with intestinal obstruction. Metabolic alkalosis suggests upper duodenal obstruction. Fluid balance and electrolyte abnormalities should be corrected before surgery. In animals with experimental intestinal obstruction, administration of crystalloids caused a decrease in plasma oncotic pressure and net loss of fluid into the distended intestinal lumen, whereas colloids transiently increased plasma oncotic pressure and allowed the jejunum to maintain normal absorptive capacity (Allen et al. 1986). Antibiotics effective against gram-negative and gram-positive aerobic and anaerobic bacteria are administered to patients with signs of sepsis or intestinal compromise and can be used prophylactically before surgery. The prognosis depends on the cause of obstruction and severity of clinical abnormalities associated with it. The prognosis ranges from very good for simple foreign bodies to grave for metastatic intestinal neoplasia. If a large portion of the intestine must be removed, the patient may be at risk for developing short-bowel syndrome.

▶ Normal Physiology of the Hepatobiliary System

Bile Formation, Composition, and Flow

Bile is an aqueous solution containing organic and inorganic compounds and electrolytes (Table 16–1) (Pugh and Stone, 1969). Among its unique constituents are bile acids, which are amphipathic organic anions synthesized and conjugated by the liver. The hepatocyte is a polarized secretory epithelial cell with specific transporters localized in the basolateral and canalicular portions of the plasma membrane (Meier 1995). The canaliculus represents a confined space (approximately 1 μm in diameter) formed by a junction between specialized portions of cell membranes from two adjacent hepatocytes. The surfaces defining the canaliculus form a tight junction that functions as an anatomic barrier to solute diffusion. Transport processes in the basolateral hepatocellular and canalicular membranes determine bile acid uptake and biliary excretion. Active transport of osmotically active solutes into the canaliculus provides the driving force for bile flow.

Bile salts are the most concentrated organic solutes in bile and the major determinant of bile secretion. Rate-limiting secretory mechanisms involve bile acid transporters in the canalicular membranes. Bile acids impart unique properties that attenuate the osmotic forces in bile. Formation of bile acid micelles (polymolecular aggregates) protects the intestinal mucosa from highly concentrated solutes and promotes interaction between bile acids and lipids in the intestinal tract, thus facilitating digestion. Almost all bile acids are conjugated (exclusively to taurine in the cat and to taurine or glycine in the dog) and exist as organic anions rather than undissociated acids. Nonabsorbable constituents of bile (e.g., bile acids, phospholipids, cholesterol) are concentrated when water and inorganic electrolytes (e.g., sodium, chloride, bicarbonate) are absorbed from the gallbladder and biliary ducts. Stasis of bile flow or dehydration of the patient can promote a pathologic thickening of bile (inspissated or sticky consistency), whereas choleresis (increased bile flow) produces watery or dilute bile. The bicarbonate concentration of bile exceeds that of plasma and is largely under the influence of secretin. Most of the bicarbonate in bile arises during bile transport through biliary ductules.

Bile formation and flow are driven mainly by osmotic mechanisms. Flow is initiated by bile acid–dependent and –independent mechanisms. In the basal state, equal contributions to flow are derived from canalicular bile salt–dependent and bile salt–independent mechanisms and from ductule processes. In the absence of bile salts, bile flow reaches only 40 to 50% of normal. Transcellular rather than paracellular mechanisms are most important in determining bile composition. Transcellular mechanisms concentrate bile acids and other solutes, whereas paracellular mechanisms permit simple diffusion (water and electrolytes) down electrochemical or osmotic gradients (Fig. 16–9).

There is a direct linear relationship between canalicular bile acid concentrations and bile flow. Non–micelle-forming bile acids (e.g., dehydrocholate) have the greatest effect. Hepatocellular uptake of bile acids is an energy-dependent (ATP-requiring) process linked to sodium transport. This process accounts for approximately 80% of taurocholate uptake but only 50% of unconjugated cholate uptake (Meier 1995). Cytosolic transport of bile acids to canalicular membranes is facilitated by protein carriers. Efflux of bile acids into canaliculi involves several mechanisms including facilitated diffusion dependent on canalicular carrier proteins, an ATP-dependent mechanism, and exocytosis of cytosolic vesicles. Collectively, the transcellular transport of bile acids and micelle formation maintain a marked concentration gradient between bile and blood, permitting biliary concentrations to exceed plasma bile acid concentrations by 100- to 1000-fold.

Bile acid–independent bile flow is mediated by a sodium transport Na^+, K^+-ATPase–linked mechanism, bicarbonate transport (associated with carbonic anhydrase and a canalicular membrane pump), and transport of organic solutes (e.g., glutathione [GSH]). These processes are largely regulated by hormones, including inulin and glucagon.

Bile ducts contribute to bile formation and modification as well as to bile flow. Production of ductular fluid is primarily under the influence of secretin, which regulates spontaneous or basal bile flow. Gastrin (but not pentagastrin) also increases bile duct secretion in dogs, whereas somatostatin decreases ductular bile flow. Increased ductular bile flow results in bile alkalinization and dilution.

TABLE 16–1. Flow and Electrolyte Concentrations of Hepatic Bile

Species	Flow (μL/min/g liver)	Na^+ (mEq/L)	K^+ (mEq/L)	Cl^- (mEq/L)	HCO_3^- (mEq/L)	Taurocholate (mM/L)
Dog	0.19 ($n = 24$)*	171 ($n = 75$)	5.1 ($n = 73$)	66 ($n = 83$)	61 ($n = 83$)	37.2 ($n = 80$)
Cat	0.23 ($n = 5$)	163 ($n = 16$)	4.2 ($n = 16$)	109 ($n = 16$)	24.1 ($n = 16$)	26.1 ($n = 10$)

*n = Number of observations reported.

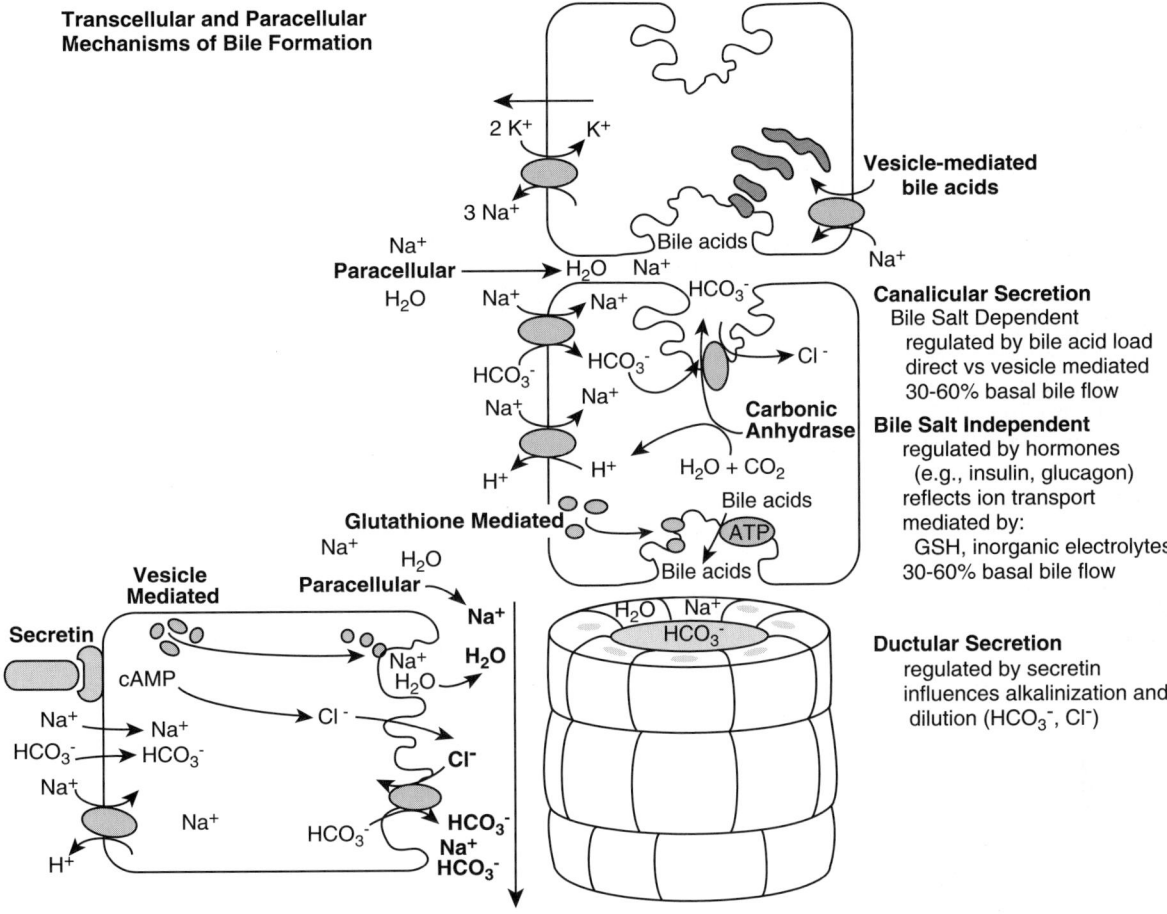

FIGURE 16-9. Transcellular (active pump–dependent) and paracellular (diffusion-dependent) mechanisms of bile formation in the hepatocyte and ductular system. Canalicular secretion depends on both bile salt–dependent and –independent mechanisms. Efflux of bile acids into canaliculi involves facilitated diffusion dependent on canalicular carrier proteins, ATP-dependent mechanisms, and exocytosis of cytosolic vesicles. Bile acid–independent bile flow is mediated by a sodium transport Na+, K+-ATPase linked mechanism, bicarbonate transport (associated with carbonic anhydrase and a canalicular membrane pump), and transport of organic solutes (e.g., glutathione [GSH]). These processes are largely regulated by hormones, including inulin and glucagon. Ductular secretion is largely stimulated by secretin, which initiates spontaneous or "basal" bile flow and bile alkalinization.

Disease states causing bile ductule proliferation also increase bile flow (e.g., cirrhosis, extrahepatic bile duct occlusion, inflammatory disorders). Bile ductules and ducts can also reabsorb bile as shown in cholecystectomized dogs (Erlinger 1987).

Hepatic Functions Influencing Body Fluid Balance and Electrolytes

Considering the broad metabolic responsibilities and interactions of the liver, there are several aspects of hepatic function that influence body fluid and electrolyte balance. Relevant mechanisms include the synthesis of albumin and regulation of intravascular oncotic pressure, direct and indirect effects on hormones influencing water and electrolyte regulation, intrahepatic baroreceptors sensing changes in hepatic perfusion or congestion, and changes in renal tubular electrolyte excretion, water turnover, and glomerular filtration rate (GFR). Although significant metabolic adaptations are initiated by the liver, confusion regarding its influence on water and electrolyte balance exists because of the complexity of the interactions involved and because of the dependence of clinicopathologic markers of renal function and hydration status on hepatic function. Notably, liver synthetic function directly influences serum concentrations of albumin, urea, and creatinine, and hepatic insufficiency directly and indirectly leads to changes in electrolyte balance and water turnover.

Serum Proteins: Albumin and Globulins

ALBUMIN

Albumin accounts for 25% of the proteins synthesized by the liver (Morgan and Peters 1971). Serum albumin concentration reflects the net result of synthesis and secretion from hepatocytes, systemic distribution, and degradation. Being relatively small in size (approximately 66,000 daltons), albumin can be lost from the body or into third spaces by pathologically altered vasculature (e.g., inflammation, vasculitis), gut wall (e.g., lymphangiectasia, severe protein-losing enteropathy), or glomeruli (e.g., glomerulonephritis, amyloidosis) or as a result of hepatic inflammation and sinusoidal hypertension. Impaired or down-regulated albumin synthesis or losses exceeding the synthetic capability of the liver result in hypoalbuminemia of varying severity. The liver has a tremendous reserve capacity for albumin synthesis, and when necessary basal rates of albumin synthesis can more than double (Rothschild et al. 1988).

Despite its importance as an oncotic agent, albumin is not managed as a high-priority protein. Rather, its production fluctuates depending on current physiologic conditions and requirements (Fig. 16–10). The most important variables determining albumin production are nutrition and the interstitial osmotic pressure as sensed by the hepatocyte (Rothschild et al. 1966). The influence of nutrition on albumin production can be dramatic. After a fast or with consumption of a protein-deficient diet, albumin synthesis declines by 50% within 24 h. However, serum albumin concentration reflects this change only after a lag period ranging from days to weeks as a new balance is achieved between exchangeable albumin pools. Feeding excessive calories in a protein-restricted ration augments development of hypoalbuminemia, as does dietary depletion of branched-chain amino acids (Rothschild et al. 1988; Kirsch 1969; Lunn and Austin 1983). Hypoalbuminemia, caused in part by reduced albumin synthesis, can also be a consequence of changes in serum oncotic pressure related to hyperglobulinemia as well as treatment with synthetic colloids (e.g., dextran) (Dich et al. 1973; Rothschild et al. 1965).

After synthesis in the hepatocyte, albumin is released into the space of Disse by exocytosis. It then diffuses into the hepatic sinusoids, where it mingles with the systemic circulation. It is then dispersed into the interstitial space, returning to the systemic circulation through lymphatics and the thoracic duct. In normal animals, 50 to 70% of albumin is located extravascularly, with the highest amounts within interstitial spaces in skin and muscle (Lunn and Austin 1983).

Exactly where albumin catabolism occurs remains controversial, although endothelial cells are believed to be the major site (Yedgar et al. 1983). The half-life of plasma albumin in dogs is estimated to range between 7 and 10 days (Fink et al. 1944; Dixon et al. 1953). No half-life estimate is available for the cat. Although the rate of albumin catabolism is highly variable, the fractional catabolic rate is directly proportional to the plasma albumin concentration and pool size (Hoffenberg 1970). In conditions that cause hypoalbuminemia, the fractional as well as absolute rate of albumin catabolism decreases. The rate of albumin catabolism increases after albumin or synthetic colloid transfusion. Thus, transfusion of albumin or infusions of synthetic colloids may potentiate endogenous hypoalbuminemia by two separate mechanisms. As a consequence of the large space of distribution and numerous mechanisms influencing the synthesis, distribu-

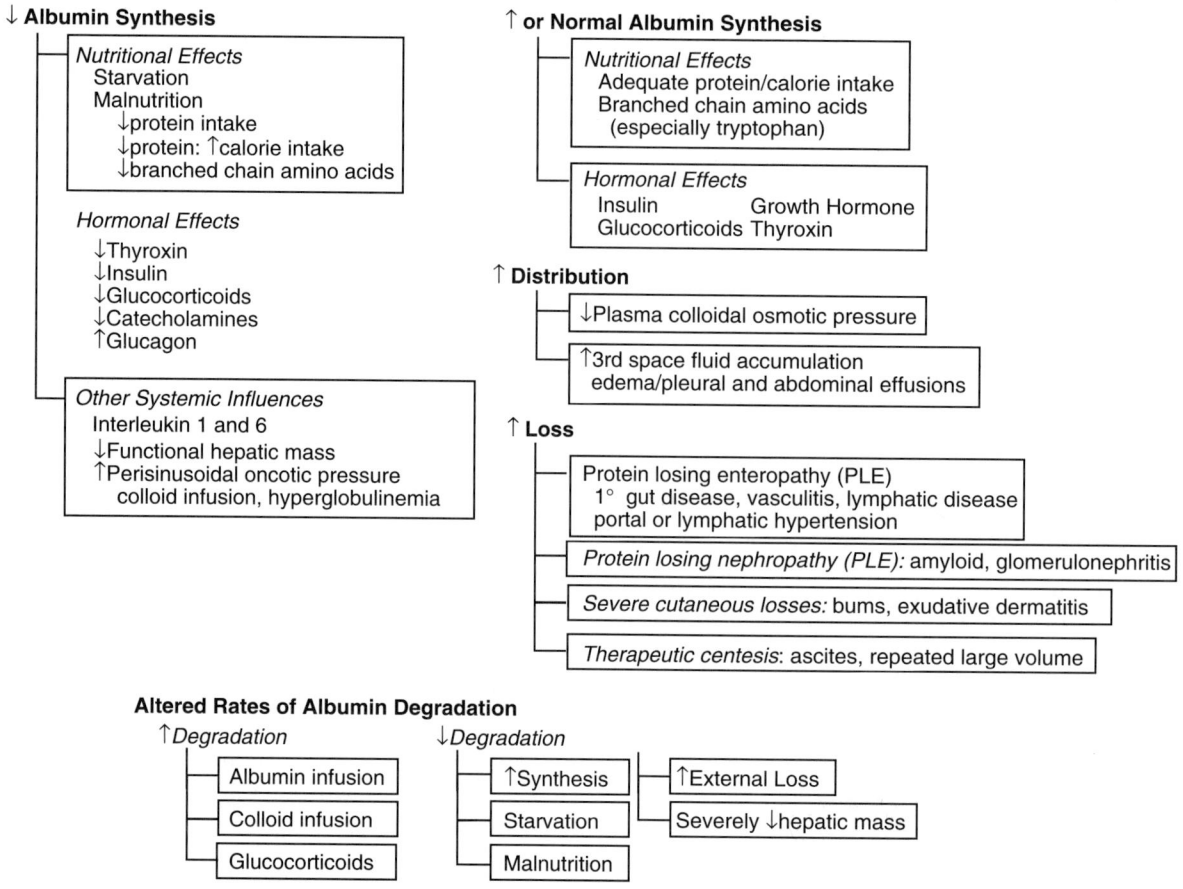

FIGURE 16–10. Factors and conditions influencing albumin synthesis and degradation.

tion, and catabolism of albumin, the serum albumin concentration does not accurately reflect contemporary changes in total body albumin resources or its hepatic synthesis.

GLOBULINS

The plasma globulin concentration reflects a large number of different proteins, some of which are shown in Figure 16–11. The majority of nonimmunoglobulin serum globulins are synthesized and stored in the liver. Many of these globulins function as acute-phase proteins, a group of functionally diverse proteins normally present in very small quantities. The synthesis of acute-phase proteins is rapidly and markedly increased in response to tissue injury or inflammation under the influence of cytokines. These globulins can contribute substantially to an increased total globulin concentration. Nevertheless, determination of the total globulin concentration is not a good measure of liver synthetic function because of the contribution of immunoglobulins to the total globulin concentration.

Hyperglobulinemia is common in animals with acquired hepatic disease. The magnitude of this response may mask hypoalbuminemia if only total serum protein concentration is determined. Along with the acute-phase globulin response, increased globulins reflect systemic immune stimulation secondary to impaired Kupffer cell function, disturbed B- and T-cell function, and development of autoantibodies. In severe hepatic insufficiency, reduced concentration of α-globulins (e.g., haptoglobin, α_1-antitrypsin) and hypoalbuminemia portend a poor prognosis (Sevelius 1995).

Hepatic Nitrogen Metabolism: Detoxification, Excretion, Role in Acid-Base Balance

UREA CYCLE AND GLUTAMINE CYCLE

The liver converts waste nitrogen to an excretable form (Cooper 1996). Nitrogen derived from amino acids can be converted to ammonia directly or indirectly after incorporation into glutamate or aspartate in the liver. Ammonia is subsequently detoxified by conversion to urea (Fig. 16–12). Two mechanisms exist for hepatic nitrogen detoxification. The hepatic urea cycle is best known and involves a linked series of enzymatic reactions conducted in the mitochondria and cytosol of the hepatocyte (see Fig. 16–12). The second mechanism, the glutamine cycle, involves transport of glutamine into mitochondria, where it is converted to ammonia and used as a precursor of carbamoyl phosphate (see Fig. 16–12). The urea cycle is considered a low-affinity system most important during alkalosis, whereas the glutamine cycle is a high-affinity system most important during acidosis. Urea synthesis occurs largely in periportal hepatocytes (zone 1) and glutamine synthesis in the perivenous region (zone 3). Working cooperatively, these systems efficiently cleanse ammonia from portal blood. Approximately 25% of ammonia for urea synthesis is derived directly from portal blood, with the remainder derived from catabolism of proteins, peptides, and amino acids.

Urea synthesis depends on substrate supply, hormonal regulation, nutritional status, and liver cell volume. Regulation of urea cycle enzymes corresponds to the level of dietary nitrogen intake and, possibly, the liver cell volume. The urea cycle is believed by some to play an important role in acid-base homeostasis, as explained by the following reactions (using alanine as an example of an amino acid as a nitrogen source) (Cooper 1996):

$$CH_3CH(CO_2)NH_3 + 3O_2 \rightarrow 2CO_2 + HCO_3^- + NH_4^+ + H_2O$$
(alanine)

Generation of one positive (NH_4^+) and one negative (HCO_3^-) charge has the potential to maintain electroneutrality. However, because physiologic pH is in the range 7.0 to 7.4, only 1% of the ammonia exists as ammonia. The protons represented by the ammonium ions therefore cannot be readily transferred to HCO_3^-; catabolism of large amounts of amino acids or protein can thus

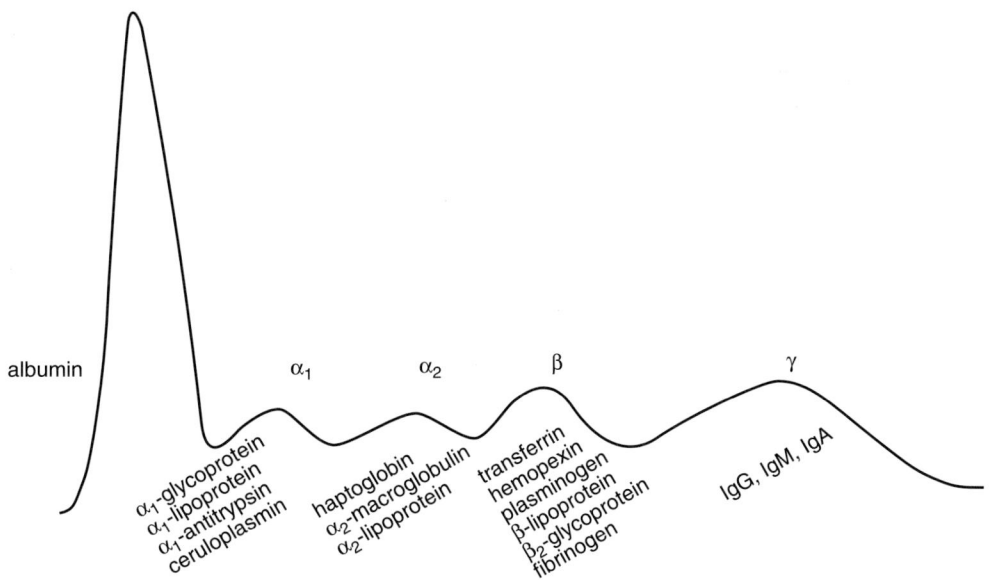

FIGURE 16–11. Diagram showing a cellulose acetate electrophoretogram with representative proteins in their region of mobilization.

generate high bicarbonate concentrations resulting in metabolic alkalosis. Normally, detoxification of ammonia to electroneutral urea prevents changes in systemic pH (Cooper 1996):

$$2NH_4^+ + HCO_3^- \rightarrow NH_2CONH_2 \text{ (urea)} + 2H_2O + H^+$$

$$HCO_3^- + H^+ \rightarrow H_2O + CO_2$$

Net: $2NH_4^+ + 2HCO_3^- \rightarrow NH_2CONH_2 + CO_2 + 3H_2O$

The preceding model is probably an oversimplification. Consumption of a diet composed of a complex mixture of amino acids (anionic, cationic, and sulfate-containing amino acids) results in a net gain of protons that must be excreted or neutralized. Urinary excretion occurs via dihydrogen phosphate (titratable acidity) and renal tubular production of ammonium from glutamine. Traditional concepts of renal tubular acid titration consider ammonium ion formation an important mechanism of acid-base adjustment. Ammonium ions excreted in urine, however, are incapable of titrating acid because they are already protonated (Cooper 1996). An alternative view is that urinary excretion of NH_4^+ represents a mechanism by which the liver is deprived of substrates for urea synthesis, resulting in less bicarbonate neutralization and mitigation of acidosis. According to this hypothesis, the kidneys determine the route of nitrogen disposal whereas the liver plays a more active role in systemic acid-base balance.

DIURETIC IMPAIRMENT OF AMMONIA DETOXIFICATION

Administration of carbonic anhydrase inhibitors (e.g., acetazolamide) and thiazides (e.g., chlorothiazide) can indirectly hasten the development of hyperammonemia in patients with hepatic insufficiency. This adverse effect of diuretic use occurs by inhibition of HCO_3^- generation. Since bicarbonate is necessary for mitochondrial synthesis of carbamoyl phosphate (an essential urea cycle substrate) urea cycle function is impaired (see Fig. 16–12) (Haussinger et al. 1986).

SERUM POTASSIUM CONCENTRATION AND AMMONIAGENESIS

Experimental and clinical observations of potassium depletion and loading suggest that renal ammonia production is intimately linked with potassium homeostasis. Low serum potassium concentrations stimulate and high serum potassium concentrations suppress renal ammoniagenesis (Tannen 1977). A closed-loop regulatory system modulates ammonia production, hydrogen ion homeostasis, and urinary potassium excretion in response to acute and chronic changes in serum potassium concentration.

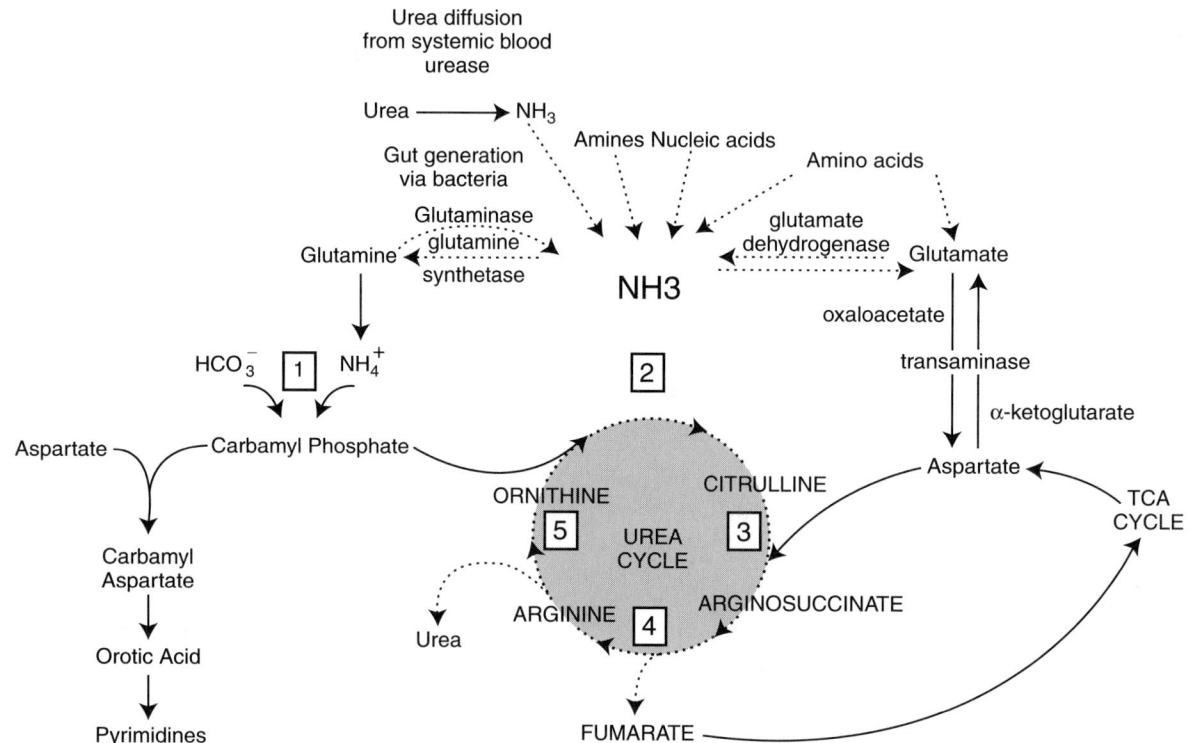

1: Carbamylphosphate Synthetase 1
2: Ornithine Transcarbamylase
3: Argininosuccinate Synthetase
4: Argininosuccinase
5: Arginase

FIGURE 16–12. Diagram showing the biochemical reactions involved with nitrogenous waste production, detoxification, and elimination. See text for explanations.

Pathophysiology of the Hepatobiliary System

Clinical Importance of Hypoalbuminemia

Hypoalbuminemia (serum albumin concentration <1.5 g/dL) alters Starling's forces and favors loss of fluid from the vascular space, hypovolemia, and decreased systemic perfusion pressure. In conjunction with other disturbances in the Starling forces, a transudative effusion and/or edema may develop. The location of third-space fluid accumulation often reflects local causal factors. In hepatic sinusoidal or portal hypertension and sodium retention, as occurs in patients with hepatic fibrosis or cirrhosis, a pure or modified transudate accumulates as ascites in the abdomen.

Many endogenous and exogenous compounds (including drugs) are bound to albumin, and transport of such substances is an important function of albumin. Adverse clinical consequences may arise in hypoalbuminemic patients requiring treatment with highly protein-bound drugs. A larger amount of unbound or "free" drug may increase interactions with receptors and facilitate movement of drug across the blood-brain barrier, potentially resulting in adverse effects.

Hypoalbuminemia is usually accompanied by hypocalcemia (as reflected by measurement of serum total calcium concentration) caused solely by reduced protein-calcium binding. A linear relationship between serum protein and calcium concentrations exists in dogs and can be used to determine the clinical importance of hypocalcemia (Meuten et al. 1982; Bienzle et al. 1993). A consistent relationship between albumin, protein, and calcium concentrations is not apparent in cats (Flanders et al. 1989; Bienzle et al. 1993).

HYPOALBUMINEMIA IN LIVER DISEASE

Although most commonly considered to reflect hepatic synthetic failure, hypoalbuminemia in patients with liver disease is multifactorial. In addition to reduced synthetic capacity, increased distribution into ascites, malnutrition, and a negative acute-phase response may all affect serum albumin concentration. In patients with portal hypertension and ascites, newly synthesized albumin may be released directly into ascitic fluid and may take weeks to reach equilibrium with the exchangeable albumin pool (Rothschild et al. 1969; Zimmon et al. 1969). Some human patients with severe liver disease and hypoalbuminemia maintain normal rates of albumin synthesis. In such patients, water and sodium retention confuses the interpretation of serum protein concentrations. Serum protein concentrations in dogs with hepatic cirrhosis with and without ascites are shown in Figure 16–13.

In inflammatory liver disease, albumin synthesis may be suppressed by inflammatory mediators (e.g., tumor necrosis factor, interleukins) (Baumann and Gauldie 1994; Castell et al. 1990; Koj et al. 1984; Moshage et al. 1987). Suppression of albumin synthesis is usually inversely proportional to the extent of acute-phase reactant (e.g., fibrinogen, haptoglobin, α_1-macroglobulin, antithrombin III, α_1-glycoprotein, α_2-macroglobulin) synthesis and thus has been called a negative acute-phase response. Abnormal polyamine metabolism, caused by altered urea cycle function and methionine metabolism, also can impede albumin synthesis. Inappropriate dietary restriction of protein is the most common correctable cause of hypoalbuminemia in these patients.

Hypoalbuminemia related to hepatic insufficiency is generally not accompanied by a decreased total globulin concentration (see Fig. 16–13). Rather, total globulin concentrations are normal or increased as a result of a disproportionate increase in γ-globulins. Gamma-globulin concentrations increase as a result of increased systemic exposure to gut-derived antigens, microorganisms, and debris normally removed by the hepatic mononuclear phagocytes (Kupffer's cells) and the presence of infectious or immune-mediated processes associated with underlying diseases. Alpha-globulins (particularly haptoglobin), fibrinogen, and antithrombin III concentrations are abnormally low in dogs with end-stage cirrhosis and hepatic synthetic failure (Sevelius and Andersson 1995). The diagnostic utility of these proteins is complicated by the induction of haptoglobin by glucocorticoids and development of coagulopathies that can further deplete fibrinogen and antithrombin III (Harvey and West 1987; Kelly and Summerfield 1987).

The wide range of serum albumin concentrations in normally hydrated cirrhotic dogs with and without ascites demonstrates that hypoalbuminemia is only one factor influencing ascites formation (see Fig. 16–13). In dogs with ascites ($n=52$), the median serum albumin concentration was 2.0 g/dL (range, 1.2–3.2), and in dogs without ascites ($n=50$) the median serum albumin concentration was 2.4 g/dL (range, 0.7–4.2). Median serum globulin concentrations in these dogs were similar, whereas the median plasma fibrinogen concentration was significantly decreased in ascitic dogs (median, 105 mg/dL; range, 30–780 mg/dL) compared with dogs without ascites (median, 165 mg/dL; range, 64–550 mg/dL).

HYPOALBUMINEMIA IN PROTEIN-LOSING ENTEROPATHY

Hypoalbuminemia in patients with severe protein-losing enteropathy (PLE) is related to pathologic changes involving the mucosa, lymphatics, and mesenteric or intestinal vasculature as well as congenital anomalies (William 1996). Usually, mucosal lesions in the stomach and intestines are overt and include erosive or inflammatory changes and vascular or lymphatic congestion. Protein loss occurs via the mucosal vasculature into the enteric lumen or into interstitial spaces and the peritoneal cavity. Intestinal mucosal capillaries have large fenestrations that permit diffusion of macromolecules. It is through these fenestrae that mucosal disease and venous or lymphatic stasis can result in plasma protein loss into the enteric canal. In these circumstances, both albumin and globulins are lost equally, leading to panhypoproteinemia.

Although there is usually histologic evidence of the associated disease process in patients with PLE, proteins can be lost into the stomach or intestines in the absence of morphologic abnormalities. Protein loss in this case occurs as a result of increased permeability at the epithelial tight junctions resulting in intercellular protein leakage (Kaup et al. 1988). The cause of such pathologic

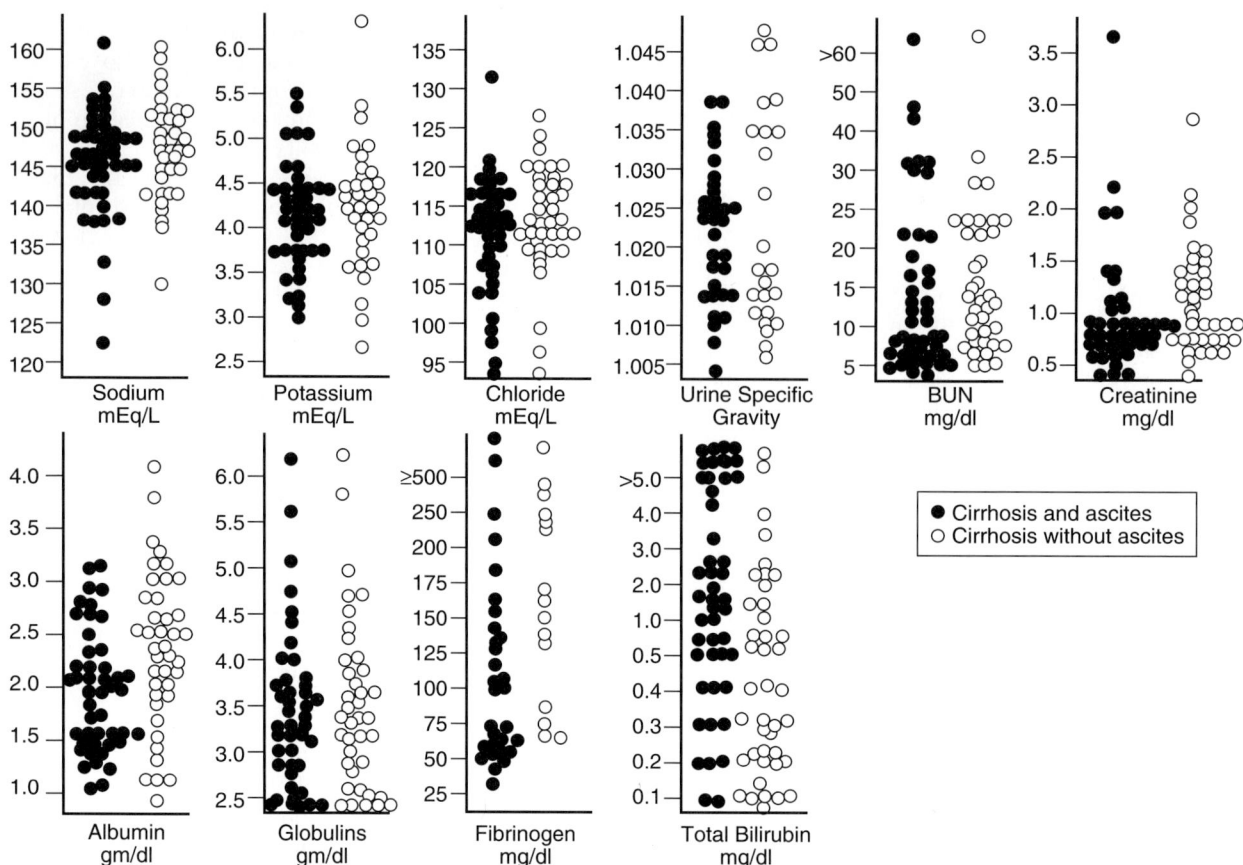

FIGURE 16-13. Scattergram showing the serum electrolytes, BUN, creatinine, total bilirubin, and urine specific gravity in dogs with hepatic cirrhosis. (Data from SA Center, College of Veterinary Medicine, Cornell University, 1998.)

permeability is unclear. Hemorrhage into the enteric canal and degradation of proteins by inflammatory cells in the gut wall and by proteases in epithelial cells also contribute to panhypoproteinemia in PLE. Lymphatic congestion or hypertension causes weeping of protein-rich lymph into the abdominal cavity and enteric canal (Kaup et al. 1988). Lymphatic obstruction also leads to loss of lymphocytes into the intestinal lumen, which is manifested clinically by lymphopenia and, in some cases, immunosuppression.

The most important disorders causing PLE are chronic inflammatory diseases, neoplasia, and circulatory conditions (Williams 1996). Severe panhypoproteinemia suggests underlying hemolymphatic hypertension, enteric mural inflammation, vasculitis, or circulatory disease. Extracorporeal loss of albumin is accompanied by loss of antithrombin III (molecular mass approximately 60,000 daltons) and high-molecular-weight globulins. One exception is the gastrointestinal disorder of the basenji dog in which hyperglobulinemia is maintained (Breitschwerdt et al. 1980).

Most patients with PLE exhibit signs of weight loss and have a history of episodic vomiting and diarrhea. In some, however, there are no clinical signs except abdominal effusion and a tendency for dependent limb edema. Abdominal effusion usually occurs in patients with PLE when serum albumin concentration decreases to 1.0 g/dL, but it may appear at higher albumin concentrations depending on the presence of other conditions favoring portal and lymphatic hypertension and systemic sodium retention. Capillary, or lymphatic hypertension related to local, hepatic, or cardiac causes of circulatory stasis facilitates ascites accumulation at higher serum albumin concentrations than typically occur in PLE patients. Chronic portal hypertension in liver disease, occlusion of the extrahepatic portal venous circulation (caused by stricture, strangulation, or thrombosis), or intestinal or mesenteric vasculitis can lead to enteric protein loss (Sarfeh et al. 1986). Such loss of protein is also thought to contribute to hypoproteinemia associated with cirrhosis and portal hypertension. Similar enteric protein loss is associated with calorie wasting in patients with right-sided congestive heart failure (splanchnic venous and lymphatic congestion) and contributes to cardiac cachexia (Williams 1996).

HYPOALBUMINEMIA IN PANCREATITIS

Hypoalbuminemia may also develop in patients with pancreatitis. In this circumstance, hypoalbuminemia results from vascular or lymphatic leakage in inflamed pancreatic and peripancreatic tissues, adjacent peritonitis, systemic vasculitis caused by release of pancreatic elastases and other enzymes, bleeding tendencies, and protein accumulation in inflammatory abdominal effusion. Usually, these patients do not develop panhypoproteinemia unless large volumes of crystalloid fluids are rapidly infused.

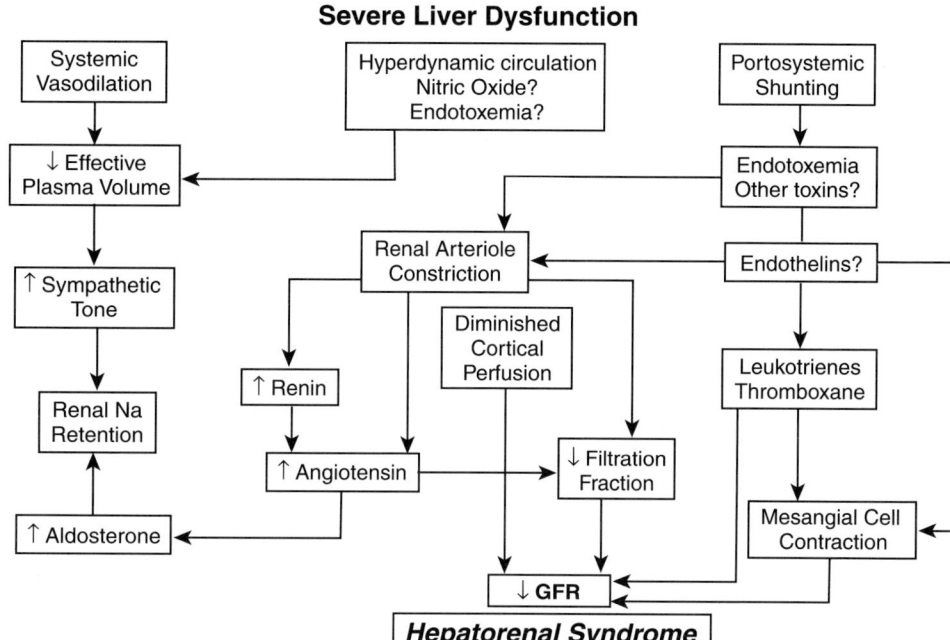

FIGURE 16-14. Pathophysiologic mechanisms of the hepatorenal syndrome as it occurs in human beings.

Water and Sodium Disturbances in Chronic Liver Disease

The most common fluid and electrolyte abnormalities in humans with acquired hepatic insufficiency involve impaired ability to excrete sodium and water and reduced GFR. Sodium retention occurs first, and water retention and impaired GFR are secondary.

THE HEPATORENAL SYNDROME

The *hepatorenal syndrome*, a syndrome of functional renal failure developing in the absence of morphologic renal injury, occurs primarily in human patients with ascites. Presumably, a similar syndrome occurs in veterinary patients. Reduced renal cortical perfusion resulting from increased renal vascular resistance precedes renal failure in this syndrome. The cause of intrarenal vasoconstriction is complex and poorly understood (Fig. 16–14). Factors associated with development of hepatorenal syndrome in humans are listed in Table 16–2. Among the various mechanisms are the renin-angiotensin-aldosterone axis, sympathetic nervous system, atrial natriuretic peptide, nitric oxide, endothelin, prostaglandins, and the renal kallikrein-kinin system. Essential diagnostic criteria for the hepatorenal syndrome in humans include a spontaneously acquired acute decline in GFR, impaired urine sodium excretion (<10 mEq/day), urine osmolality greater than plasma osmolality, and absence of other causes of renal failure.

IMPAIRED RENAL EXCRETION OF SODIUM AND WATER: EXPANSION OF INTRAVASCULAR VOLUME

Cirrhotic humans studied before development of ascites undergo dynamic intravascular volume expansion at least 1 week before overt ascites accumulation. This phase correlates with renal sodium retention (McCullough et al. 1991). A 36% plasma volume expansion occurred in cirrhotic dogs during this active salt-retaining preascitic phase. Two-thirds of the newly acquired volume distributes into the vasodilated splanchnic circulation and one-third into the nonsplanchnic vasculature (Levy 1977a). Formation of ascites is hastened by sodium ingestion or intravenous administration of sodium-containing fluids.

Studies of animals with experimentally induced chronic liver injury have shown a direct relationship between sodium retention and subsequent ascites formation (Levy 1977b; Levy and Allotey 1978; Lopez-Novoa et al. 1980; Jimenez et al. 1985; Gliedman et al. 1970; Unikowsky et al. 1983). Sodium retention occurred before detectable changes in peripheral venous resistance, arterial blood pressure, or cardiac output in dogs with experimentally induced cirrhosis (chronic bile duct occlusion, dimethylnitrosamine). Renal tubular sodium retention also preceded changes in GFR, renal blood flow, filtration fraction, and intrarenal vascular resistance (Levy 1977b). The increase in total body exchangeable sodium correlated more with altered hepatic structure and vasculature

TABLE 16-2. **Factors Associated with Development of the Hepatorenal Syndrome in Humans**

Constant Associations
Ascites
Intravascular volume disturbances

Variable Associations
Gastrointestinal bleeding
Large-volume paracentesis
Overzealous use of diuretics
Progressive jaundice
Sepsis
Nephrotoxic drugs
Nonsteroidal antiinflammatory drugs
Radiographic contrast media

than with mesenteric portal venous hypertension and hypoalbuminemia (Gliedman et al. 1964). Surgical creation of portosystemic shunting in dogs with hepatic cirrhosis abolished portal hypertension and coincidentally the early tendency for renal sodium retention and ascites. In such studies, 20- to 30-pound cirrhotic dogs with shunts were able to maintain neutral sodium balance with intakes as high as 85 mEq/day. Cirrhotic dogs without shunts accumulated sodium at this level of intake (Unikowsky et al. 1983).

ABNORMAL ALDOSTERONE RELEASE AND RESPONSE TO ALDOSTERONE

An inappropriately normal to high aldosterone concentration precedes and accompanies pathologic sodium retention in cirrhosis in both animal models and human patients. Experimentally, both hepatic venous congestion and acute portal hypertension stimulated aldosterone secretion (Better and Schrier 1983). Studies in human cirrhotics and animals have demonstrated an impaired aldosterone "escape phenomenon," a normal physiologic process through which the biologic response to high aldosterone tone is blunted (Better and Schrier 1983). The importance of aldosterone in sodium and water retention in cirrhosis is demonstrated by the efficacy of spironolactone (a specific aldosterone antagonist) in mobilizing ascites and alleviating sodium retention in patients lacking renal dysfunction. This effect can be blunted by administration of metoclopromide, a dopaminergic prokinetic antiemitic known to stimulate aldosterone production (D'Arienzo et al. 1985).

The influence of aldosterone on renal sodium retention is exaggerated in cirrhosis by increased renal sensitivity to the hormone. Clinically, this sensitivity is evidenced by the rapid accumulation of ascites in cirrhotic dogs given glucocorticoids with mineralocorticoid effects.

INTRAHEPATIC BARORECEPTORS

Additional signals encouraging renal sodium and water retention may be derived from the so-called hepatorenal reflex involving hepatic baroreceptors. The importance of sinusoidal hypertension and presumably baroreceptor stimulation in the etiopathogenesis of sodium and water retention has been inferred from several observations (Wong et al. 1995; Somberg et al. 1995). Evidence suggests that physiologic sensors communicating with renal sympathetic efferents modulate renal tubular sodium and water conservation (Kostreva et al. 1980; Levy and Wexler 1987a, b).

PORTOSYSTEMIC SHUNTING

Surgically created portosystemic shunts in normal dogs have been used to clarify the influence of deviated hepatoportal perfusion on sodium and water retention. Ten weeks after end-to-side portocaval shunt construction, plasma volume, systemic blood pressure, and central venous pressures were maintained and there were no changes in GFR, plasma renin activity, or aldosterone concentration (Levy and Wexler 1978). Although some dogs maintained neutral sodium balance after ingestion of 150 mEq sodium per day, others developed ascites (Levy and Wexler 1978). Thus, it appears that portosystemic shunting alone can impair the ability to adapt to increased sodium loads. This finding may explain the observed propensity for ascites formation in some dogs with portosystemic vascular anomalies (PSVAs) after development of mild hypoalbuminemia or after administration of sodium-rich polyionic fluids.

ISOOSMOTIC RENAL SODIUM RETENTION

In most patients with hepatic insufficiency prone to ascites formation, isoosmotic renal sodium retention expands extracellular volume such that total body sodium loading is not reflected in measured plasma concentrations (see Fig. 16–13). However, the important role of sodium in resolution of ascites and edema is evident from the reduction or resolution of ascites after dietary sodium restriction or administration of sodium-wasting diuretics. In humans, the intensity of sodium retention varies among patients, some having high renal sodium excretion and others having urine that is virtually free of sodium. Medical treatment of the latter group is exceedingly difficult. That similar phenomena occur in cirrhotic dogs is indicated by consideration of their diverse urine specific gravities and serum sodium concentrations recorded at the time of initial presentation and the apparent resistance of some of these dogs to sodium-wasting diuretic therapy.

IMPAIRED FREE-WATER EXCRETION AND DILUTIONAL HYPONATREMIA

Some cirrhotic humans (up to 35%) develop impaired free-water excretion causing dilutional hyponatremia (Papper 1958; Papper et al. 1959; Shear et al. 1965, 1966). A similar phenomenon seems comparatively rare in dogs (Fig. 16–13) (Vaamonde 1988; McCullough et al. 1991; Papper and Saxon, 1959; Epstein 1985; Arroyo et al. 1976). Compared with nonascitic cirrhotic dogs, those with ascites have higher median urine specific gravity values but similar BUN, creatinine, and total protein concentrations. As in humans, a normal or increased serum sodium concentration does not predict ascites formation in dogs.

Mechanisms leading to reduced free-water excretion are linked to stimulation of arginine vasopressin (AVP) secretion. The most plausible theories involve the sympathetic nervous system as both a detector and effector mechanism, adjusting extracellular fluid volume and arterial pressure. Activation of the sympathetic nervous system is relatively common in cirrhotic humans. Strategically located sensors detect "fullness" in the systemic circulation, low pressure in atria and pulmonary arteries, and high pressure in carotid arteries, aorta, and juxtaglomerular apparatus. Mechanistically, decreased total body sodium or decreased arterial pressure reduces sympathetic inhibition of AVP secretion, whereas vascular distention causes inhibition of AVP secretion and adjustments in vascular tone (vasoconstriction), cardiac rate, and cardiac contractility. Endothelin may play a modulatory role in the renal AVP response.

Endogenous prostaglandins may also play an important role in regulation of sodium and water balance as well as renal function in patients with cirrhosis. These compounds are normally essential for regulation of renal perfusion and tubular response to AVP. The important regulatory and protective effects of renal prostaglandins become apparent when nonsteroidal antiinflammatory drugs are administered to cirrhotic patients with ascites. These patients experience a profound decrease in renal blood flow and GFR, marked activation of vasoconstrictor systems, and overt sodium and fluid retention.

WATER AND SODIUM DISTURBANCES IN CATS WITH LIVER DISEASE

Cats with hepatic lipidosis (HL) do not develop consistent trends in serum electrolyte concentrations (Fig. 16–15). This is not unexpected as a large number of different conditions causing anorexia and rapid weight loss lead to HL. In a survey of cats with severe HL in which blood and urine samples were collected before fluid therapy was initiated, 14 of 72 had a urine specific gravity less than 1.010, 29 of 114 were hyponatremic, and only 1 was hypernatremic. Cats with chronic cholangitis or cholangiohepatitis also do not develop consistent trends in serum sodium concentrations or urine specific gravity.

Influence of Liver Function on Blood Urea Nitrogen and Serum Creatinine Concentrations

UREA SYNTHESIS

Blood urea nitrogen (BUN) concentration is directly affected by hepatic urea synthesis. Consequently, patients with acquired hepatic insufficiency and those with portosystemic shunting commonly develop subnormal BUN concentrations. This effect is intensified by the common therapeutic maneuver of dietary nitrogen restriction in patients with liver disease. Such extrarenal influences on BUN complicate its clinical utility for assessment of renal function.

CREATININE SYNTHESIS, NEGATIVE NITROGEN BALANCE, LOSS OF LEAN MUSCLE MASS

The liver also plays a major role in the biosynthesis of creatine, an organic nitrogenous compound essential for cell energy metabolism (Fig. 16–16). Creatine is derived from two amino acids; the initial synthetic step is dependent on a rate-limiting enzyme (glycine amidinotransferase) in a wide variety of organs. The next synthetic step occurs primarily in the liver and involves the transfer of a methyl group from S-adenosylmethionine. In hepatic insufficiency, reduced hepatic synthesis of creatine can result in subnormal serum creatinine concentrations. Approximately 98% of creatine is located in muscle tissue, and loss of muscle mass resulting from catabolism or negative nitrogen balance can also result in a subnormal serum creatinine concentration. Studies of humans with hepatic cirrhosis and concurrent renal dysfunction have clearly shown that the serum creatinine concentration in

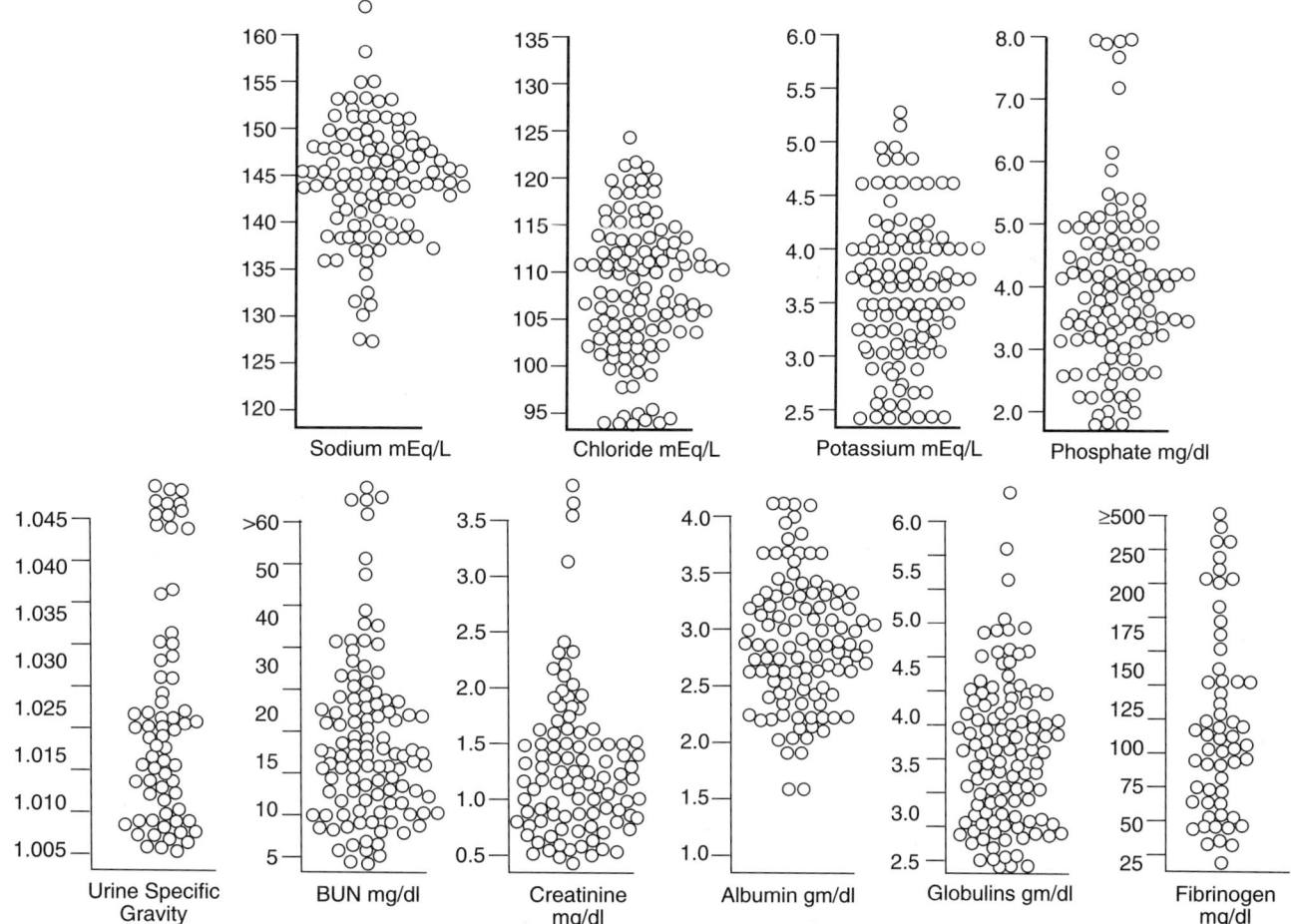

FIGURE 16–15. Scattergram showing serum electrolytes, BUN, creatinine, proteins, and urine specific gravity in cats with hepatic lipidosis. (Data from SA Center, College of Veterinary Medicine, Cornell University, 1998.)

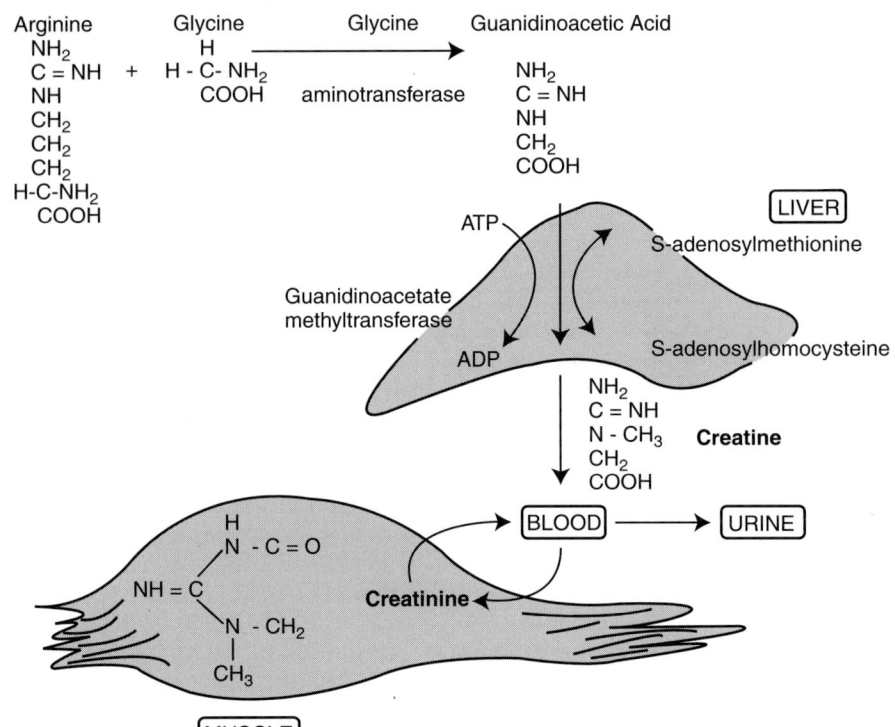

FIGURE 16-16. Diagrammatic representation of hepatic involvement in creatine synthesis. (Adapted from Heymsfield SB, Arteaga C, McManus C, et al.: Measurement of muscle mass in humans: Validity of the 24-hour urinary creatinine method. Am J Clin Nutr 37:478–494, 1983. © American Society for Clinical Nutrition.)

this circumstance fails to reflect impaired GFR (Papdakis and Arieff 1987; Caregaro et al. 1994).

INCREASED WATER TURNOVER AND GLOMERULAR FILTRATION RATE

The influence of hepatic insufficiency on BUN and serum creatinine concentrations is aggravated by increased water turnover and development of supranormal GFR, as shown in dogs with congenital PSVAs (Deppe et al. 1998). Primary polydipsia associated with HE, stimulation of hepatoportal osmoreceptors, and an impaired renal medullary concentration gradient (chronic hypokalemia, low urea synthesis) may each contribute to deranged water balance in these animals (Grauer and Pitts 1987; Tannen 1977; Kozlowski and Krzysztof 1973).

POLYURIA AND POLYDIPSIA

Polydipsia, polyuria, and renal dysfunction may be associated with liver disease in both dogs and cats. Dogs with chronic hepatitis and cats with chronic cholangitis or cholangiohepatitis commonly also have histologic evidence of chronic interstitial nephritis. Some affected dogs concurrently develop glomerulonephritis. Dogs with PSVAs may be presented primarily for polyuria and polydipsia (Grauer and Pitts 1987; Center and Magne 1990). The cause of polydipsia and polyuria in these animals is multifactorial. Mechanisms may include psychogenic polydipsia associated with HE, sensory input detecting diminished hepatoportal blood flow or osmolality, renal medullary washout as a result of subnormal urea concentration, renal tubular dysfunction associated with potassium depletion, or increased concentrations of endogenous steroids (Kozlowski and Krzysztof 1973).

Evaluation of the initial urine concentration before fluid therapy in a group of dogs with PSVAs showed that 47 of 87 had a urine specific gravity below 1.020 and 12 of 87 were hyposthenuric (see Fig. 16–17). Although serum electrolyte concentrations were not significantly associated with urine concentration, subnormal BUN concentration occurred in 58 of 123 dogs and a low normal to subnormal creatinine concentration was found in 83 of 123 dogs. These findings suggest that fluid diuresis contributes to low urine specific gravity in these patients, as supported by the demonstration of a supranormal GFR in dogs with PSVAs in steady-state fluid balance (Deppe et al. 1998). Subnormal BUN concentrations in dogs with PSVAs could impair maintenance of the renal medullary solute gradient necessary for water reabsorption in response to AVP. Low serum creatinine concentration probably reflects reduced muscle mass associated with the young age and small size of affected dogs (many are young small-breed dogs), hepatic insufficiency, and increased water turnover (Heymsfield et al. 1990; Caregaro et al. 1994; Papadakis et al. 1987; Deppe et al. 1998).

Similar mechanisms are likely to be operative in dogs with acquired hepatic insufficiency. Of cirrhotic dogs with ascites (see Fig. 16–13), 15 of 25 with a complete urinalysis had pretreatment urine specific gravity below 1.020. Of these, only 3 of 26 were hyposthenuric. In the same group, 11 of 42 had a low BUN and 21 of 42 had a low or subnormal serum creatinine concentration. In cirrhotic dogs without ascites, 16 of 34 with a complete urinalysis had a specific gravity less than 1.020 and only 1 of 34 was hyposthenuric. In the same group, 20 of 47 dogs had a low BUN concentration and 36 of 47 had a low-normal or subnormal serum creatinine concentration.

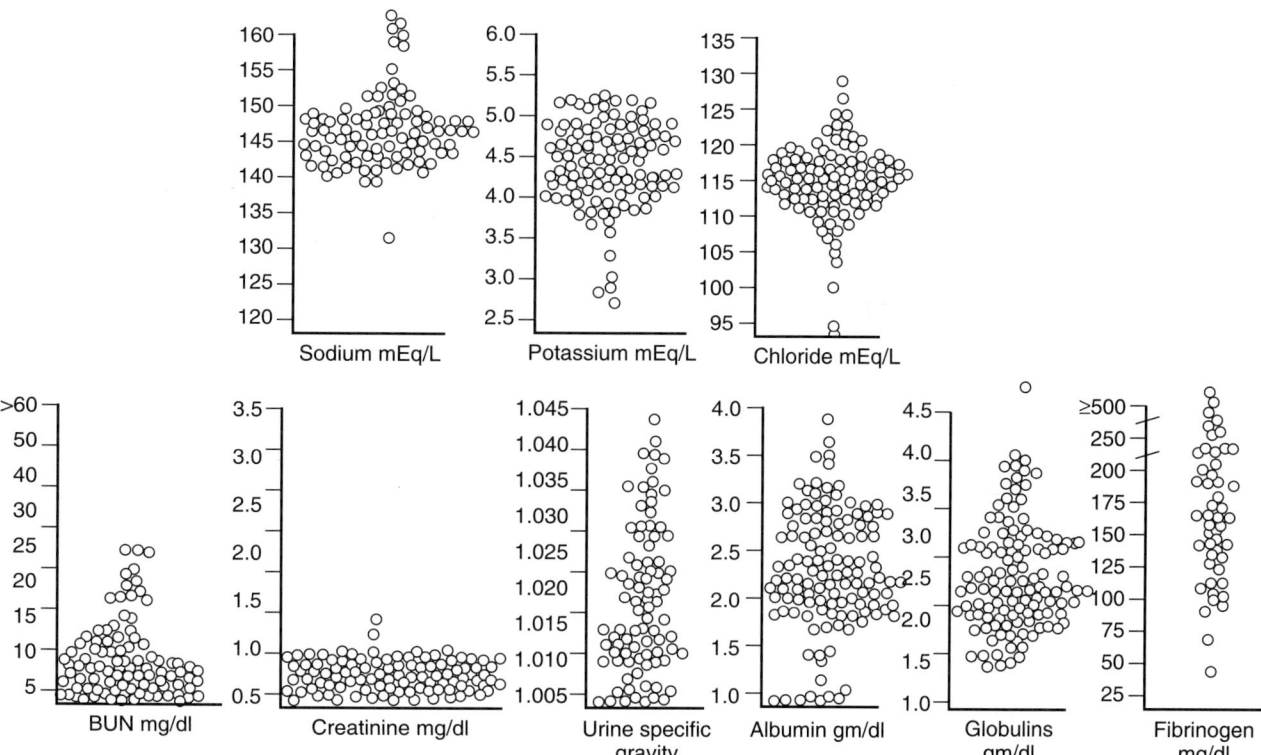

FIGURE 16-17. Scattergram showing serum electrolytes, BUN, creatinine, proteins, and urine specific gravity in dogs with portosystemic venous anomalies. (Data from SA Center, College of Veterinary Medicine, Cornell University, 1998.)

Hypokalemia in Liver Disease

Hypokalemia is a serious electrolyte disturbance associated with hepatic insufficiency (Casey et al. 1965). Contributing factors include deficient caloric intake, vomiting, diarrhea, malassimilation of nutrients, treatment with loop diuretics, and secondary hyperaldosteronism (Tannen 1983). Magnesium deficiency can also complicate hypokalemia by potentiating kaliuresis through its effects on aldosterone (Francisco et al. 1981; Mendelson et al. 1969). Diagnostically, hypokalemia may go unrecognized as a result of the transcellular shift that normally occurs between potassium and hydrogen ions. In order to increase awareness of hypokalemia in cirrhotic humans, it has been suggested that serum potassium concentrations at the lower end of the normal range be considered clinically abnormal (Zavagli 1986). Serum potassium concentrations in dogs with cirrhosis, cats with HL, and dogs with PSVAs are shown in Figures 16–13, 16–15, and 16–17. Frank hypokalemia was present in 32 of 116 cats with HL, in 11 of 48 cirrhotic dogs with ascites, in 10 of 42 cirrhotic dogs without ascites, and in 6 of 113 dogs with PSVAs. Consideration of these data with increased awareness of low-normal values shows that 44 of 116 cats with HL, 34 of 90 cirrhotic dogs (19 of 48 with ascites and 15 of 42 without ascites), and 24 of 104 dogs with PSVAs had subnormal or low-normal serum potassium concentrations. Although the prognosis is significantly worse for cats with HL and hypokalemia, the prognostic significance of hypokalemia has not been evaluated in the other disorders (Center et al. 1993).

It is important to recognize and correct hypokalemia for several reasons. Most important, there is a reciprocal relationship between intra- and extracellular potassium concentrations and renal ammoniagenesis (Tannen 1983; Tannen and Kunin 1976; Good 1987). Infusion of potassium chloride in hypokalemic patients significantly improved central nervous system function in early HE and prolonged survival in cirrhotic humans (Zavagli et al. 1993). Patients given potassium chloride to achieve normokalemia developed a reduction in arterial ammonia concentration and pH, a marked increase in the arterial NH_4^+/NH_3 ratio, a significant decrease in urine pH, and slightly increased 24-h ammoniuria associated with a significantly increased urine NH_4^+/NH_3 ratio. Mechanistically, potassium infused into the hypokalemic patient replaces intracellular hydrogen ions. The displaced cellular hydrogen ions lower blood pH, promoting conversion of ammonia to its less diffusible form (NH_4^+). This small shift in pH is not great enough to stimulate renal ammoniagenesis, although reduced urine pH leads to increased excretion of ammonium ions. This effect may be augmented by increased plasma aldosterone given its ability to increase hydrogen ion delivery into the distal renal tubular fluid (Sebastian et al. 1980).

Hypophosphatemia in Liver Disease

Hypophosphatemia may complicate hepatic insufficiency, respiratory alkalosis, diabetes mellitus, and enteral alimentation in animals (Willard et al. 1987; Adams et al. 1993; Akol et al. 1993; Justin and Hohenhaus 1995). At increased risk are cats with HL associated with diabetes mellitus or pancreatitis, in which symptomatic hypophosphatemia may develop after rapid rehydration, insulin therapy, and refeeding. Serum calcium and phosphorus concentrations in cats with HL are shown in Figure 16–15. Of this group of cats, only 6 of 116 were hypophosphatemic (serum phosphorus concentration ≤ 2.0 mg/dL) at the time of initial presentation. Hypophosphatemia in the patient with liver disease is thought to reflect intracellular shifts of phosphate (Stoff 1982; Forrester and Moreland 1989). Associated complications include hemolytic anemia, weakness (neck ventroflexion in cats), neurologic signs that may be mistaken for those of HE, and impaired phagocyte function (Forrester and Moreland 1989; Craddock et al. 1974; Dawson et al. 1987). Mechanisms of hemolysis involve depletion of red cell energy related to impaired glycolysis and ATP production and diminished ability to maintain reduced glutathione in erythryocytes. Muscle weakness in hypophosphatemia may be severe enough to impair ventilation, leading to ventilatory failure and respiratory acidosis.

Acid-Base Abnormalities in Liver Disease

A variety of acid-base abnormalities may develop in patients with hepatobiliary disease. The most common disturbance in humans with hepatic insufficiency in hepatic coma is respiratory alkalosis, but metabolic acid-base disturbances may also occur (Prytz and Thomsen 1976). Patients with stable cirrhosis and those with portal hypertension attenuated by surgically created portosystemic shunts commonly develop compensated respiratory or metabolic alkalosis. Respiratory akalosis is closely associated with the extent of functional liver impairment rather than the presence of portosystemic shunting and nearly always is compensated (Prytz and Thomsen 1976).

MECHANISM OF RESPIRATORY ALKALOSIS AND METABOLIC ALKALOSIS

Respiratory alkalosis in cirrhosis may be due to reduced arterial oxygen saturation secondary to acquired venoarterial shunting, ventilation-perfusion mismatch (derived from ascites-induced restriction of ventilatory efforts or changes in pulmonary capillaries), a shift to the right in the oxyhemoglobin dissociation curve, direct stimulation of the respiratory center by encephalopathic toxins (e.g., NH_3), or development of central nervous system acidosis (Heinemann et al. 1960). Respiratory alkalosis may also develop as compensation for metabolic acidemia (e.g., lactic acidosis, increased concentrations of free fatty acids, impaired renal tubular acid excretion, or renal hypoperfusion) (Amatuzio and Nesbitt 1950; Record et al. 1975).

MECHANISM OF METABOLIC ALKALOSIS

Metabolic alkalosis in some patients is due to excessive diuretic therapy, repeated vomiting of gastric secretions, or alkali loading arising from transfusion of citrate-anticoagulated blood. Immediately after blood collection, citrate-phosphate-dextran (CPD)–preserved blood has reduced bicarbonate and high citrate concentrations (Emmitt and Narins 1987). During storage, red cell metabolism consumes bicarbonate during glycolysis and lactic acid production. After infusion, citrate-preserved blood products favor development of a metabolic alkalosis because both lactate and citrate can be metabolized to HCO_3^-. The total "potential" bicarbonate concentration in 450 mL of CPD-preserved human blood is approximately 58 mEq/L (the initial 24 mEq/L plasma bicarbonate concentration plus 34 mEq/L citrate) (Emmitt and Narins 1987). Although transfused blood is transiently "acidifying" because of free citric acid, this is quickly counteracted by the metabolism of citrate to CO_2 and water.

Persistent secondary hyperaldosteronism, as occurs in some patients prone to ascites formation, also contributes to metabolic alkalosis. This effect is augmented when administered diuretics increase distal renal tubular delivery of sodium and water. Metabolic alkalosis is also favored by loss of "effective" extracellular volume (Emmitt and Narins, 1987).

Metabolic and respiratory alkalosis are serious complications in patients with liver disease and HE. As shown experimentally in dogs, this acid-base disturbance has the potential to augment central nervous system ammonia uptake and toxicity (Carter et al. 1973).

MECHANISMS OF METABOLIC ACIDOSIS

Metabolic acidosis is more common in patients in the terminal stages of cirrhosis complicated by hypoxia, systemic hypotension, lactic acidosis, and renal dysfunction. Patients who develop lactic acidosis have severely compromised hepatic function and cardiovascular stability.

Blood Gas Abnormalities in Liver Disease

Impaired arterial oxygenation, characterized by an increased alveolar-arterial oxygen gradient ($P_A - PaO_2$ gradient) or overt hypoxemia, is common in humans hospitalized for hepatic cirrhosis (Krowka and Cortese 1985; Agusti et al. 1996). Limited information is available for veterinary patients, but data for a small number of cirrhotic dogs are shown in Figure 16–18. As shown, 12 of 13 cirrhotic dogs had an increased $P_A - PaO_2$ gradient, 7 of 13 were overtly hypoxemic, and 7 of 13 had respiratory alkalosis.

An increased $P_A - PaO_2$ gradient is more sensitive for detection of impaired oxygen exchange than resting P_{O_2}. The $P_A - PaO_2$ gradient considers the $PaCO_2$, which reflects ventilatory effort. Most cirrhotic humans with an increased $P_A - PaO_2$ gradient maintain normal PaO_2 by alveolar hyperventilation, which sustains their respiratory alkalosis. Causes of hypoxia or increased $P_A - PaO_2$ gradient range from impaired ventilation (e.g., limited diaphragmatic and intercostal motion related to tense ascites, ventilatory failure caused by HE or weakness) to less overt conditions creating ventilation-perfusion mismatch and intrapulmonary shunting (vascular dilatation and arteriovenous communications associated with portal hypertension) (Berthelot et al. 1966; Krowka and Cortese 1994).

Ventilation-perfusion mismatch is a common complication in cirrhotic humans. Intrapulmonary vasodilatation results from pathologic accumulation or release of nitric oxide (NO) or other vasoactive substances. These impair the normal hypoxic vasoconstrictor response, which potentiates any factor causing ventilation-perfusion mis-

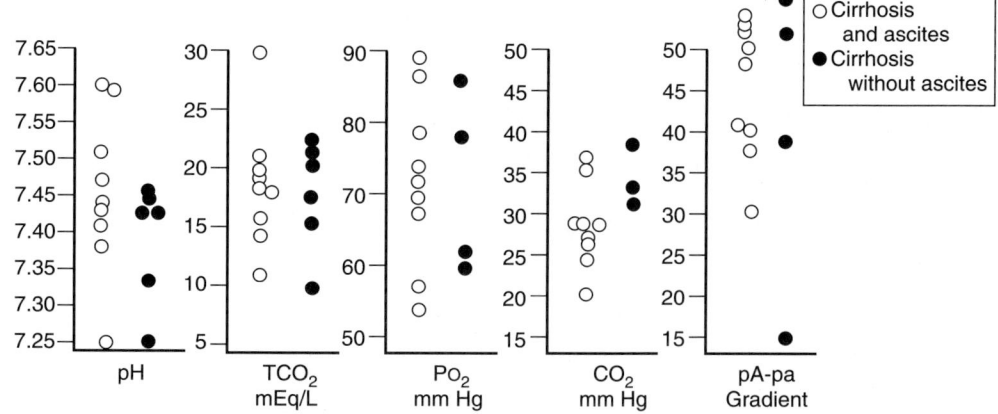

FIGURE 16-18. Diagram showing the arterial blood gases and calculated $P_A-P_{aO_2}$ gradient in dogs with hepatic cirrhosis. (Data from SA Center, College of Veterinary Medicine, Cornell University, 1998.)

match (Rolla et al. 1997; Hedenstierna et al. 1991). Anatomic changes in pulmonary capillaries, documented by radiographic and histologic methods, contribute to the increased $P_A - P_{aO_2}$ gradient in cirrhotic humans. Blood may be shunted through pleural vessels or through diffusely dilated vessels in the intra-alveolar wall. In these patients, sophisticated diagnostic techniques (e.g., contrast echocardiography) are less sensitive than arterial blood gas analysis after 100% oxygen loading for detection of deranged oxygenation ($P_{aO_2} < 400$ mm Hg after 100% O_2 loading indicates the presence of shunting). Although no pharmacologic intervention has alleviated the increased $P_A - P_{aO_2}$ gradient in cirrhotic humans, abnormal gas exchange has resolved after liver transplantation in some (Agusti et al. 1996; Battaglia et al. 1997). This finding suggests that compromised gas exchange is an epiphenomenon of liver failure rather than a result of irreversible anatomic changes in respiratory or vascular structures.

RIGHT SHIFT OF THE OXYHEMOGLOBIN DISSOCIATION CURVE

Gas exchange in some cirrhotics is further compromised by altered hemoglobin-oxygen affinity secondary to increased concentrations of 2,3-diphosphoglycerate (Astrup and Roerth 1973; Rodman et al. 1960). A right shift in the oxyhemoglobin dissociation curve caused by increased 2,3-diphosphoglycerate concentration can be attributed to anemia, hypoxia, alkalosis, or hyperammonemia. Such a right shift impairs release of oxygen at the level of tissues, increasing their vulnerability to hypoxia, free-radical damage, development of acid-base disturbances, and multisystemic organ failure (Burk et al. 1984).

Lactate Metabolism and Lactic Acidosis in Liver Disease

Pyruvate, an intermediate common to several metabolic pathways, is the immediate precursor of lactic acid. Glucose and alanine are the physiologically important pyruvate precursors. Pathologic conditions stimulating conversion of glucose or alanine to pyruvate predispose to lactic acidosis. The enzyme pyruvate dehydrogenase plays an integral role in lactate metabolism, catalyzing the intramitochondrial conversion of pyruvate to acetyl Coenzyme A (acetyl CoA), which enters the Krebs cycle (Fig. 16–19).

Removal of lactic acid normally occurs through three pathways: two depend on hepatic function and the third on renal excretion (Kriesberg 1980). At rest, the liver uses 40 to 60% of endogenously produced lactate by oxidation in the mitochondrial tricarboxylic acid cycle or by conversion of lactate to glucose in the cytosolic Cori cycle (see Fig. 16–19). Each mechanism of lactate metabolism regenerates bicarbonate. Hepatic utilization of lactate depends on substrate uptake, hepatic gluconeogenic capacity, and hepatic blood flow. In the absence of metabolic acidosis or tissue perfusion deficits, hyperlactatemia is usually associated with conditions favoring glycolysis (e.g., high catecholamine concentrations, alkalosis), which increases degradation of pyruvate to lactate (DeGasperi et al. 1997). Respiratory alkalosis, common in cirrhotic patients, is thought to augment lactate production by enhancing phosphofructokinase activity (Frommer 1983). Lactate accumulation is also favored when symptomatic hypoglycemia increases catecholamine release (Fig. 16–19).

Lactic acidosis is a clinical syndrome most commonly associated with tissue hypoxia and hypoperfusion. It is characterized by persistently increased blood lactate concentrations and metabolic acidosis. Because lactate production is a late sign of inadequate oxygen supply, it is neither a sensitive nor an early indicator of impending hepatic insufficiency (Bihari et al. 1985, 1987). Lactic acidemia may also develop in a few conditions without perfusion deficits or hypoxic injury (e.g., diabetes mellitus, renal failure, certain patients with severe hepatic failure, sepsis syndrome) (Frommer 1983; DeGasperi et al. 1997).

Hypoperfusion, hypoxia, and ischemic damage of the liver convert it from a lactate-consuming to a lactate-producing organ (DeGasperi et al. 1997). Intraoperative hypotension, hepatic ischemia, vascular thrombosis, and fulminant hepatic failure can each lead to lactic acidemia. In fulminant hepatic failure, lactic acidemia indicates severe circulatory insufficiency, anaerobic metabolism, and diffuse panlobular parenchymal damage (Bihari et al.

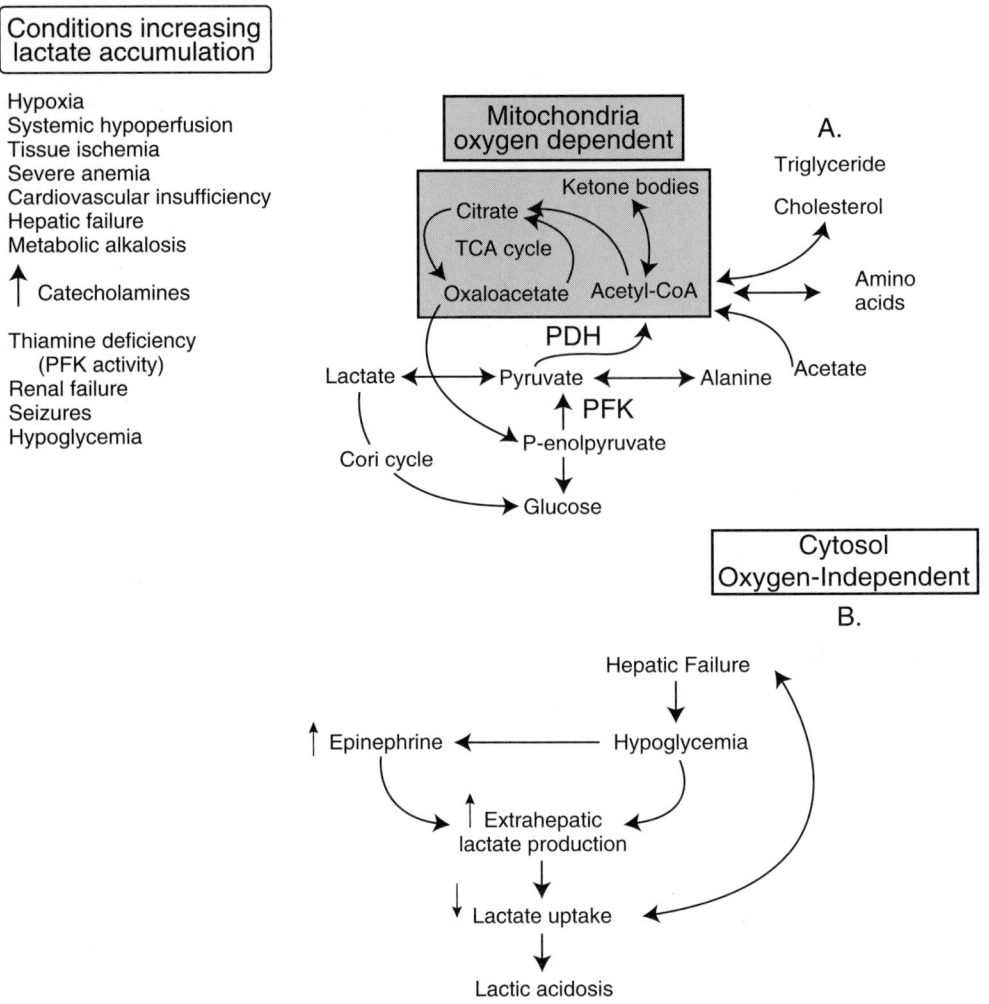

FIGURE 16–19. Metabolic generation and interactions of lactate (A) and the mechanisms leading to lactic acidosis in liver failure (B). PFK = phosphofructokinase; PDH = pyruvate dehydrogenase.

1985). The direct relationship between blood lactate concentration and the severity of hepatic damage permits prognostic use of systemic lactate concentrations in hepatic transplant patients (DeGasperi et al. 1997).

Serum lactate concentrations are measured only rarely in veterinary patients, and the prevalence of lactic acidemia remains unsubstantiated in dogs and cats with most forms of liver disease. However, cats with severe HL have been shown to develop hyperlactatemia (Center et al. 1991). The tendency for affected cats to develop lactate intolerance may be related to impaired mitochondrial function, thiamine deficiency (thiamine is a cofactor for pyruvate dehydrogenase activity), impaired sinusoidal blood flow due to hepatocellular cytosolic expansion with triglyceride, or other underlying disorders causing hypoxia or a predilection for lactic acidosis (e.g., diabetes mellitus, pancreatitis).

Transfusion of stored blood can also be a source of lactic acidosis. Immediately after collection in CPD solution, human blood has reduced bicarbonate concentration, increased $P{CO_2}$ (CO_2 slowly diffuses through the plastic), and a high citrate concentration (Emmitt and Narins 1987). During storage, red cell glycolysis generates lactic acid, which within 14 days reaches a concentration of approximately 12 mEq/L in 450 mL of anticoagulated blood. Comparable studies have not been performed using blood from dogs or cats.

Citrate Metabolism in Liver Disease

Citrate-rich blood products can lead to symptomatic hypercitratemia in patients with hepatic insufficiency. Owing to the chelating capacity of citrate, hypercitratemia can result in ionized hypomagnesemia and hypocalcemia. These electrolyte changes complicate maintenance of normal cardiovascular homeostasis, hemostasis, and other metabolic systems. High citrate loads can also lead to metabolic alkalosis due to hepatic metabolism of citrate to bicarbonate. The CPD solution used as an anticoagulant and preservative for blood components is a mixture of sodium citrate, citric acid, sodium phosphate, and dextrose. A 450-mL unit of blood mixed with 63 mL of CPD solution delivers a final sodium cirate concentration of 34 mEq/L (Emmitt and Narins 1987). Hemorrhagic tendencies aggravated or initiated after transfusion of large amounts of citrate-containing blood or blood products result from ionized hypocalcemia, which impairs appropriate activation of procoagulants.

Cardiovascular Changes in Liver Disease

Humans with cirrhosis and portal hypertension develop dynamic circulatory disturbances. The circulatory system becomes hyperkinetic with increased cardiac output, decreased arterial pressure, and reduced peripheral vascular resistance. These changes lead to peripheral and splanchnic hypotension (Lee 1989). Abnormal myocardial contractility termed cirrhotic cardiomyopathy also contributes to systemic hypoperfusion (Abelmann et al. 1955; Henriksen et al. 1989; Lee et al. 1990). Proposed mechanisms involve neural factors (e.g., false neurotransmitters, alterations in autonomic nervous tone, and adaptations reflecting neuronal damage or impaired end-organ responsiveness), circulating vasodilators, mechanoreceptor-mediated responses, and impaired function of cardiac muscle (Lee et al. 1990; Ma and Lee 1996; Ramond et al. 1986; Laffi et al. 1996). Some studies also have suggested a limited preload reserve impairing cardiac response to hypervolemia because of sodium and water retention (Ingles et al. 1991).

Dogs with experimentally induced cirrhosis and ascites develop a 20% increase in cardiac output that corresponds with reduced peripheral vascular resistance and reduced arterial blood pressure (Levy and Allotey 1978). Similar hyperdynamic adaptations are suspected in clinical patients and probably complicate anesthetic and surgical procedures (Center, unpublished observations).

Changes are most evident in patients with major bile duct occlusion. In these patients, vasodilatory effects and exaggerated vagovagal responses are secondary to biliary tree distention or compression or retention of noxious components of bile (e.g., bile acids, bilirubin).

In humans, primary cardiac disease also can lead to fulminant hepatic failure, reduced hepatic ammonia clearance, and other overt evidence of hepatic insufficiency (Kisloff and Schaffer 1976; Wiesen et al. 1995). This is uncommon in veterinary patients.

Hepatic Encephalopathy

Hepatic encephalopathy is a complex neurophysiologic syndrome involving the central nervous system that implies a critical loss of functional hepatic mass (65–70%) or hepatofugal circulation (portosystemic shunting). The cause of HE is multifactorial. The most highly suspected contributing agents, factors, precipitating conditions, and their mechanisms are summarized in Tables 16–3 and 16–4 and in Figure 16–20 (Center 1996). The onset of clinical signs can be acute or chronic and episodic or progressive. A wide spectrum of clinical signs can develop in dogs and cats. Early or mild subclinical signs are often not recognized (e.g., drowsiness, anorexia, lethargy). Different etiologic mechanisms are thought to underlie acute versus chronic HE on the basis of responses of patients to interventional treatments. Acute HE may be accompanied by cerebral edema, increased intracranial pressure, altered cerebral blood flow, and brain herniation. Cerebral edema develops in 80% of humans with

TABLE 16–3. **Putative Hepatoencephalopathic Toxins and Their Mechanisms**

Ammonia
↓ Microsomal Na^+, K^+-dependent ATPase in brain
↓ ATP availability (ATP consumed in glutamine production)
↑ Excitability (if mild ↑ NH_3)
Disturbed malate-aspartate shuttle
↑ Glycolysis
Brain edema (acute liver failure)
↓ Glutamate, altered glutamate receptors
↑ BBB transport: glutamate, tryptophan, octopamine

Bile Acids
Membranocytolytic effects alter cell or membrane permeability
Blood-brain barrier (BBB) more permeable to other HE toxins
Impaired cellular metabolism due to cytotoxicity

Endogenous Benzodiazepines
Neural inhibition: hyperpolarize neuronal membrane

GABA
Neural inhibition: hyperpolarize neuronal membrane
↑ BBB permeability to GABA in HE
↓ α-Ketoglutarate
Diversion from Krebs cycle for NH_3 detoxification
↓ ATP availability

Aromatic Amino Acids
↓ Neurotransmitter synthesis: ↓ dopa

Altered Neuroreceptors
↑ Production false neurotransmitters

Methionine → Mercaptans (Methanethiol and Dimethydisulfide)
Synergistic with other toxins: NH_3, SCFA
Are gut derived → fetor hepaticus (distinct breath odor in HE)
↓ NH_3 detoxification in brain urea cycle
↓ Microsomal Na^+, K^+-ATPase

Tryptophan
Directly neurotoxic
↑ Serotonin: neuroinhibition

Glutamine
Alters BBB amino acid transport

Short-Chain Fatty Acids
↓ Microsomal Na^+, K^+-ATPase in brain
Uncouple oxidative phosphorylation
Impair oxygen utilization
Displace tryptophan from albumin → ↑ free tryptophan

Phenol (Derived from Phenylalanine and Tyrosine)
Synergistic with other toxins
↓ A multitude of cellular enzymes
Neurotoxic and hepatotoxic

False Neurotransmitters (Tyrosine → Octopamine, Phenylalanine → Phenylethylamine)
Impair norepinephrine action

Abbreviations: BBB = blood-brain barrier; GABA = γ-aminobutyric acid; HE = hepatic encephalopathy; SCFA = short-chain fatty acids.

TABLE 16-4. **Conditions Associated with Development of Hepatic Encephalopathy**

Condition	Mechanism	Condition	Mechanism
Dehydration	Prerenal azotemia	Constipation	↑ Toxin production
	Renal azotemia		↑ Toxin absorption
Azotemia	↑ NH_3	Hemolysis: ↑ RBC breakdown →	↑ Protein
Alkalemia	↑ NH_4 CNS trapping	Blood transfusion:	
Hypokalemia	↑ NH_3 renal formation	↑ RBC breakdown →	↑ Protein: ↑ NH_3
	↑ Alkalemia:	↑ NH_3 content, endotoxins	
	Polyuria and anorexia	GI Hemorrhage	
Hypoglycemia	Neuroglycopenia	RBC digestion →	
Catabolism	Augments NH_3 toxicity	inflammation-	↑ Protein: ↑ NH_3
	↑ Protein turnover: ↑ NH_3	parasitism-	↑ Protein: ↑ NH_3
Infection	↓ Muscle NH_3 detoxication	High dietary protein	↑ Protein: ↑ NH_3
	↑ Protein turnover: ↑ NH_3	(animal, fish, eggs)	
	Urease producers → urea → ↑ NH_3	↑ protein load: ↑ NH_3, aromatic amino acids	
Polydipsia, polyuria	↓ K^+ → alkalosis, ↑ NH_3	↑ many other toxins	
	Inappetence, weakness	Drugs (examples)	
Anorexia	Catabolism	Benzodiazepines	
	↓ K^+, ↓ zinc	Antihistamines	
	Dehydration	Barbiturates	
	Hypoglycemia	Phenothiazines	
		Metronidazole	
		Tetracyclines	
		Methionine	
		Organophosphates	
		Diuretic overdosage	
		Anesthetics	

Abbreviations: CNS = central nervous system; GI = gastrointestinal; RBC = red blood cell.

fulminant hepatic failure and is the most common cause of death. Chronic HE is more often associated with long-standing metabolic derangements influencing neuronal response and brain energy requirements. Thus, chronic HE may be associated with more subtle clinical signs.

Of all the mechanisms of HE investigated, the most compelling and least controversial involve ammonia. Reduced ability to detoxify ammonia in the urea cycle is a consequence of reduced hepatic mass or hepatofugal circulation. Normally, ammonia is derived from the metabolism of amino acids, ingested proteins, and bacterial digestion of nitrogenous substrates (including urea) within the alimentary canal. Increased exposure of the central nervous system to ammonia reflects increased systemic

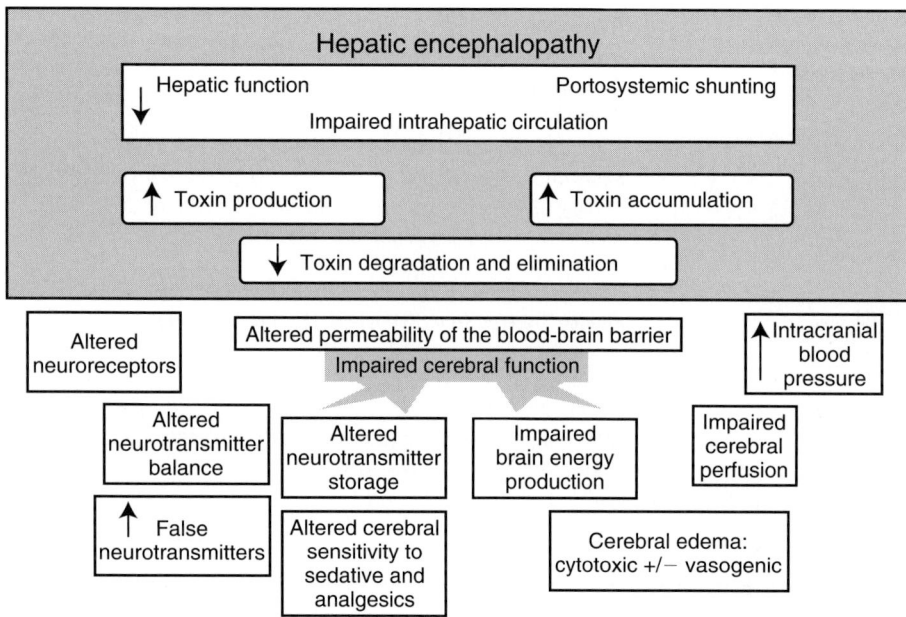

FIGURE 16-20. Pathophysiologic mechanisms of hepatic encephalopathy.

accumulation of ammonia. Nevertheless, hyperammonemia is inconsistently associated with HE. This discordance is attributed by some investigators to entrapment of ammonia in the central nervous system as a result of altered permeability of the blood-brain barrier, known to accompany HE. This phenomenon permits partitioning of ammonia within neural tissues during episodic hyperammonemia.

Neuropathologic consequences of hyperammonemia include early neuroexcitation followed by neuroinhibition, inhibition of cerebral Na^+, K^+-ATPase impairing osmoregulation and maintenance of membrane thresholds, blockade of the γ-aminobutyric acid (GABA) receptor complex, altered amino acid membrane transport, and impairment of cerebral energy production. Hypokalemia and metabolic alkalosis are well known to augment development and persistence of hyperammonemia and HE. Metabolic alkalosis facilitates brain uptake and intracerebral trapping of ammonia as the ammonium ion (NH_4^+) (Zieve 1981; Duffy and Plum 1982). Hypokalemia promotes metabolic alkalosis and HE as a result of increased renal loss of H^+ and tubular ammonia absorption. Severe hypokalemia may also impair urinary concentrating ability, leading to diuresis and dehydration. The resultant prerenal azotemia increases BUN, urea diffusion into the gut, and subsequent enteric ammonia production and uptake into the portal circulation. Weakness and anorexia associated with hypokalemia also favor dehydration, azotemia, and malnutrition, which promote hyperammonemia.

Other concerns important for patients with HE include avoidance of hypoglycemia, constipation, infections, malnutrition, and adverse drug interactions. In some animals, hypoglycemia is an important factor producing encephalopathic signs. Hypoglycemia can directly invoke neurologic and systemic signs (e.g., weakness, lethargy, confusion) as well as production and potentiation of other neurotoxins associated with HE. Constipation is detrimental because many toxins of HE are produced and absorbed in the large intestine. Catabolic conditions and administration of certain drugs may also contribute to HE. Catabolic effects of cachexia, starvation, and glucocorticoid administration increase nitrogenous waste production (ammonia and other toxic metabolites). Antianabolic effects of certain drugs (e.g., tetracyclines) may increase production and release of toxic nitrogenous products. Drugs associated with the GABA receptor (e.g., diazepam, phenobarbital) can directly produce signs of HE or stupor.

TREATMENT OF HEPATIC ENCEPHALOPATHY

MODIFICATION OF ENTERIC SUBSTRATES AND ORGANISMS

Since there are several postulated mechanisms of HE, no single effective treatment is appropriate for all patients in all circumstances. A common approach is directed at correction of hyperammonemia by efforts to reduce enteric and extraintestinal ammonia production and to augment ammonia detoxication (Table 16–5). Orally administered disaccharides fermented in the gut (e.g., lactulose, lactitol, or lactose in the lactase-deficient patient) are commonly used with antimicrobial agents to suppress urease-producing enteric bacteria. Transient repopulation of the gut with beneficial (non–urease-producing) microorganisms (e.g., lactobacilli) may provide short-term benefits. Collectively, these efforts often ameliorate clinical signs of HE. In neurologically impaired patients unable to receive oral medications, cleansing enemas are used to rid the colon of retained toxins and debris and are followed by retention enemas (Table 16–5). Retention enemas contain enteric modulating medications that have effects similar to those described for oral administration.

NUTRITIONAL SUPPORT

Several intravenous nutritional support solutions have been investigated for their influence on HE, correction of hyperammonemia, and reduction of accumulated aromatic amino acids. Solutions rich in branched-chain amino acids and solutions supplemented with urea cycle intermediates, ketoacids, and L-carnitine have been evaluated in animal models (including the dog) and in cirrhotic humans with HE (Center 1996; Salvatore et al. 1964; Zieve et al. 1986; Kircheis et al. 1997; Therrien et al. 1997). Depending on the model and investigative methods, a diversity of results has prevented a general consensus on management strategies. The most interesting and clinically applicable findings involve the parenteral administration of L-carnitine, which has shown promise in the treatment of ammonia toxicity. However, this approach has not yet been applied in clinical patients. Routine total parenteral nutrition solutions have been used safely in dogs and cats with HE by the author, with fluid formula modifications to achieve protein restriction as needed on an individual basis.

In general, nutritional support of the patient suffering from episodic HE is initiated by using a protein-restricted diet as recommended for patients with renal insufficiency. Individual titration is recommended for each patient to establish optimal protein intake.

CEREBRAL EDEMA AND HYPOXIA

Cerebral blood flow varies widely in humans with fulminant hepatic failure. Approximately 67% of these patients develop cerebral lactatemia, thought to reflect their lower cerebral metabolic rate and reduced oxygen availability. Treatment with mannitol and acetylcysteine has improved these abnormalities. Cerebral edema, intracranial hypertension, and cerebral herniation are common causes of death in humans in fulminant hepatic failure or severe HE coma. Brain edema and swelling follow breakdown of the blood-brain barrier (vasogenic edema) and impaired cell osmoregulation (cytotoxic or cellular edema) (Sussman 1996; Center 1996). Poor response to glucocorticoids and better response to mannitol support primary involvement of cytotoxic mechanisms.

Experimentally and clinically in humans, intravenous administration of acetylcysteine reduces cerebral edema in acute hepatic failure. For animals, the acetylcysteine regimen recommended for acetaminophen toxicity is used empirically along with mannitol. Acute hyperventilation should be avoided in patients with HE because it decreases both cerebral blood flow and metabolic rate, increasing the potential for ischemic damage (Wendon et al. 1994). Although cerebral edema complicating liver failure and HE is associated with hypoxia, it is unclear

TABLE 16–5. Methods Used to Modify Enteric Production and Absorption of Toxins

Dietary Modifications
↓ Protein quantity
Altered protein quality: dairy and vegetable preferred
↑ Dietary soluble fiber

Modification of Enteric Microbial Population

Alter enteric pH	Lactose, lactulose, lactitol, fiber
Antimicrobials	
Neomycin	22 mg/kg, PO, q8–12h
Metronidazole	7.5 mg/kg, PO, q8–12h
Amoxicillin	11 mg/kg, q12h
Lactobacilli from live yogurt cultures	
Modify enteric substrates: dietary, nonabsorbable disaccharides fiber	
Lactulose	0.25–0.5 mL/kg, PO, q8–12h
(This is a STARTING dose; start low and gradually work dose up to required amount based on stool consistency)	
Lactitol	0.5–0.75 g/kg, PO, q12h
Lactose	Slightly sweet solution, q12h
Fiber	Metamucil, psyllium
(Each of the above is used to effect, attaining several soft stools per day)	

Direct Elimination of Enteric Microorganisms, Substrates, and Products

Cleansing enemas	5–10 mL/kg, repeat until clear: use warm polyionic fluids as necessary, respect total systemic drug dose
Retention enemas	
Neomycin	15–20 mL 1% solution, q8h
Lactulose	5–15 mg diluted 1:3 with water, q8h
Lactitol	0.5–0.75 g/kg, q12h
Metronidazole	7.5 mg/kg (systemic dose) with water, q12h
Betadine	Dilute 1:10 with water, flush out within 10 min
Dilute vinegar	Dilute 1:10 with water, alters pH, q8–12h
Activated charcoal	Administered and retained in crisis situation

whether hypoxia is causal or develops after brain edema. Impaired brain energy production consistent with HE could lead to reduced membrane Na^+,K^+-ATPase activity, cell swelling, and impaired perfusion (Ede et al. 1987). If an increased $P_A - PaO_2$ gradient is present, affected patients should also be supported with supplemental oxygen.

Abdominal Effusion Related to Liver Disease: Ascites

The pathophysiologic mechanisms underlying ascites formation are complex. No specific clinical characteristics clearly identify patients prone to development of ascites. Serum electrolyte, BUN, creatinine, protein, and total bilirubin concentrations are shown in Figure 16–13 for 109 cirrhotic dogs initially presented with and without ascites (Center SA, unpublished data, 1998).

There are two traditional theories and one unifying theory explaining ascites formation. The *overflow theory* suggests that abnormalities in renal function precipitate hemodynamic changes leading to ascites. Impaired renal sodium excretion and fluid retention lead to an *overflow* of fluid into the systemic vasculature and third-space compartments. In cirrhosis, abdominal effusion accumulates as a result of hepatic sinusoidal, arterial, and portal hypertension. The major discrepancy between this theory and actual hemodynamic changes in cirrhotic humans and dogs is that the arterial vascular compartment remains *relatively* underfilled as a consequence of arterial vasodilatation. Such underfilling persists despite increased plasma volume and cardiac output.

The second traditional theory explaining ascites formation, the *classic underfilling hypothesis*, postulates that reduced oncotic pressure and hepatic sinusoidal hypertension lead to hepatic interstitial edema, increased hepatic lymph flow, and spilling of excess fluid into the peritoneal cavity. Hepatic lymph flow in cirrhosis may be 10 times the normal rate, and lymph formation is thought to exceed lymphatic drainage capacity. Subsequent extravasation of fluid from the hepatic and splanchnic circulation results in systemic hypovolemia detected by intrathoracic and arterial sensors. These signal the need for systemic volume expansion and initiate renal sodium and water retention. The retained fluid cannot adequately expand the vascular compartment because of continued fluid and protein loss into the abdominal cavity, and a self-perpetuating cascade initiates sodium and water retention. Unfortunately, the systemic hemodynamic adaptations in cirrhotic patients with ascites do not coincide with the compensatory responses described by this theory. These patients have peripheral systemic arterial vasodilatation, normal plasma volume, and sodium retention that precede ascites formation (Levy et al. 1977; Lopez-Novoa et al. 1980; Jimenez et al. 1985; Gliedman et al. 1970).

The hypothesis of *peripheral arterial vasodilatation* unifies the two traditional etiopathogenic cascades (Fig. 16–21). This hypothesis proposes that renal adaptations for sodium and water retention are secondary to reduced effective arterial blood volume (Schrier 1988; Better and

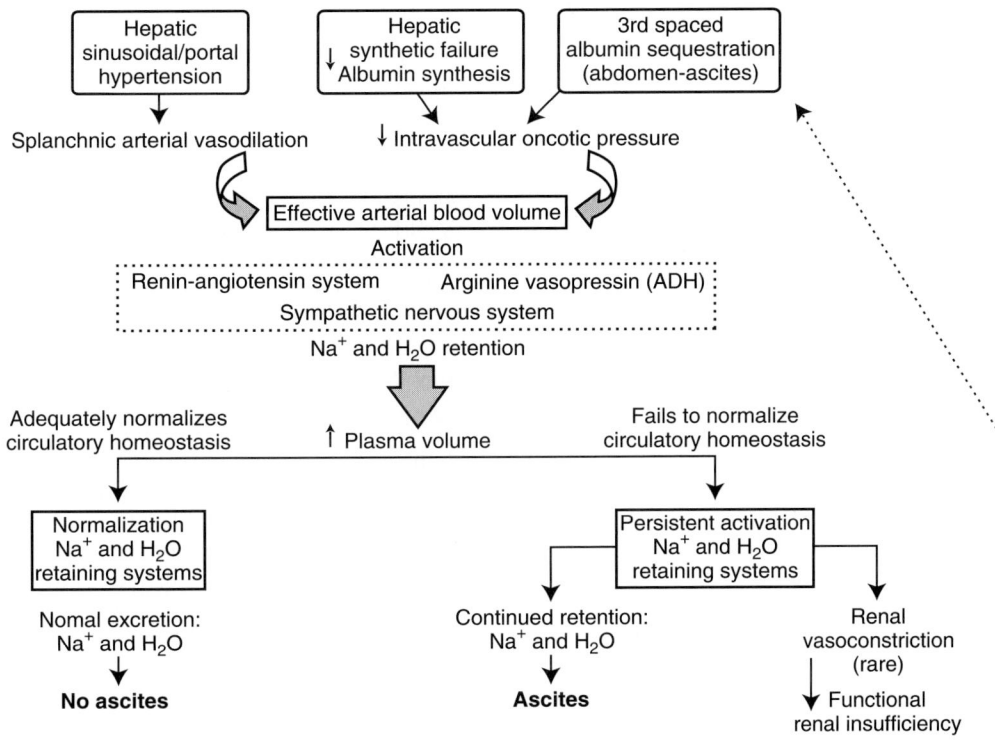

FIGURE 16-21. Pathophysiologic mechanisms according to the unifying theory of ascites formation.

Schrier 1983). *Apparent* arterial vasodilatation or hypovolemia derives from a disproportionate expansion of the arterial vascular compartment and formation of arteriovenous anastomoses. Portal hypertension appears to initiate splanchnic arteriolar vasodilatation. High-pressure baroreceptors, sensing arterial underfilling, stimulate the renin-angiotensin-aldosterone axis and the sympathetic nervous system, causing release of AVP. These mechanisms result in renal sodium and water retention. Functional renal failure, as occurs in the hepatorenal syndrome, can be a severe complication of these responses. Other proposed causes of arterial vasodilatation include increased splanchnic and systemic bile acid concentrations, autonomic nervous system dysfunction, accumulation of false neurotransmitters, exposure to increased concentrations of vasoactive intestinal peptide (VIP), and abnormal liberation of prostaglandins (Better and Schrier 1983; Wong et al. 1997).

ASSESSMENT OF ASCITES

Abdominal effusion should always be biochemically and cytologically evaluated. A sample should be submitted for culture if cytologic evaluation is suggestive of infection. In most dogs with ascites related to liver disease, the fluid is a pure transudate having a total protein concentration less than 2.5 g/dL and specific gravity between 1.010 and 1.015. Cytologically, the fluid is relatively acellular, with only a few mesothelial cells and neutrophils. In the jaundiced patient, the fluid is yellow and a few bilirubin crystals may be observed. Body weight and abdominal girth measurements should be taken as a reference for appraising changes in fluid accumulation. Girth measurements are meaningful only if a consistent method is used. A mark is made on the abdomen with a permanent ink marker and the owner is taught to measure girth circumference with a consistent technique.

▶ Fluid Therapy in Liver Disease
Initial Considerations

Selection of the most appropriate fluid for the patient with hepatobiliary disease must take into consideration the propensity of these patients for third-space fluid accumulation (e.g., edema, ascites), hypoalbuminemia, hyponatremia, hypokalemia, coagulopathies, and hyperlactatemia and whether or not preexisting acid-base disturbances put them at risk for HE. In patients without evidence of synthetic failure or HE, balanced polyionic solutions are appropriate and should be supplemented with KCl as routinely recommended for maintenance needs. Sequential evaluation of hydration and serum electrolyte concentrations is used to guide therapeutic electrolyte adjustments.

Nutritional Considerations

In the patient with severe hepatic dysfunction, critical concerns include the ability to maintain nutritional intake and euglycemia, to avoid azotemia, and to avoid iatrogenic fluid retention (e.g., edema, ascites) as a consequence of hypoalbuminemia. Nutritional support should optimally provide positive nitrogen balance and adequate caloric, vitamin, and micronutrient intake. Protein intake for dogs with HE is initiated at 2.5 g/kg body weight per day, preferably using proteins of vegetable or dairy origin supplemented with soluble and insoluble fiber. Protein intake for cats with HE is initiated at 4.5 g/kg body weight per day with protein having a high biologic value. In cats, it is essential to avoid anorexia and rapid weight loss, which are linked to the development of hepatic lipidosis. Provision of water-soluble vitamin preparations containing B_1 (thiamine) is mandatory. Signs of vitamin B_1 deficiency (Wernicke's encephalopathy) are easily confused with HE and rapidly ameliorated with 50 to 100 mg of thiamine initially administered q12h and then q24h for an initial 3 days and thereafter as part of balanced vitamin supplementation. Vitamin B_{12} is provided in B complex vitamins as a daily supplement for all animals or as specific therapy (1 mg administered by intramuscular injection q7 to q21 days) in animals with subnormal B_{12} concentrations. Low vitamin B_{12} concentrations have been linked to hepatic lipidosis (HL) in some cats and can result from intestinal malabsorption. Nitrogen tolerance is estimated from the patient's response after intake of a normal balanced ration as well as from evidence of hyperammonemia (e.g., measured blood ammonia concentrations, ammonium urate crystalluria, episodic neurobehavioral signs linked to food ingestion). In animals with nitrogen intolerance, dietary modification (protein quantity and quality) and oral treatment with lactulose (0.25 to 1 mL/kg PO q12h or q8h) and metronidazole (7.5 mg/kg PO q12h or q8h) or neomycin (22 mg/kg PO q12h) are recommended. Used together, these drugs synergistically improve nitrogen tolerance (Center 1996). The lactulose dosage must be individually titrated to attain several soft (i.e., pudding-like) stools each day. An excessive dosage of lactulose can result in painful abdominal cramps (as a consequence of drug fermentation), increased peristalsis (overt borborygmus), and diarrhea. Generation of lactic, acetic, and formic acid may rarely lead to metabolic acidosis and dehydration. In humans, hypernatremia has also been an iatrogenic complication of lactulose overdosage (Nelson et al. 1983).

Maintenance of Euglycemia

Patients with hepatic dysfunction may also have insufficient liver and muscle glycogen reserves to maintain glycogenolysis. If hepatic gluconeogenesis is also impaired, these patients are prone to symptomatic hypoglycemia. Animals with portosystemic shunting and those with fulminant hepatic failure are at greatest risk. Neuroglycopenia must be avoided in animals with congenital portosystemic vascular anomalies during surgical and anesthetic procedures, as this can permanently impair their neurologic recovery. In HE, hypoglycemia can intensify neurologic signs by augmenting ammonia-associated brain energy deficits. Intravenous fluids should initially be supplemented with 2.5% dextrose with sequential determinations of blood glucose concentrations guiding precise fluid supplementation with glucose. In patients with symptomatic hypoglycemia, 0.5 to 1 mL/kg of a 50% dextrose solution may be given by rapid intravenous injection. Thereafter, glucose supplementation is sustained by lower concentrations of glucose in a monitored 24-h infusion. The hypertonic nature of glucose-supplemented fluids requires administration into a large central vein. Attention must be given to detection of early signs of phlebitis at the site of fluid administration because these patients have increased susceptibility to endotoxemia and infection. Local and systemic reactions (e.g., fever, pain, regional lymphadenopathy) to phlebitis should be managed by catheter removal, catheter tip culture, and administration of broad-spectrum antimicrobials.

Fluid Therapy in the Patient with Ascites or Edema

When ascites or edema is present before fluid administration or develops after infusion of polyionic solutions, fluid support must be modified to reduce the administered load of sodium. As previously mentioned, ascites can be induced in medium-sized dogs with experimentally induced cirrhosis by ingestion of only 85 mEq of sodium per day. Considering that a 30-lb dog has a maintenance volume requirement of approximately 1 L/day, the sodium content of commonly used polyionic crystalloid solutions promotes ascites formation when maintenance volumes are administered. Selection of commercially available solutions with restricted sodium content or mixing of commercially available solutions to achieve the desired sodium content is necessary for these patients. Slow infusion of both a crystalloid and a colloid is a useful approach for many of these patients because it expands intravascular volume, limits the requirement for crystalloid, and reduces the tendency for third-space fluid sequestration. Crystalloid administration is reduced to 33% of normal maintenance requirements when administered with 20 mL/kg synthetic colloid per day. The potential bleeding complications associated with synthetic colloid use as well as their cost must be carefully considered. See Chapter 23 for more information on colloid therapy.

Treatment of Acid-Base Imbalances in Liver Disease

LACTIC ACIDOSIS

High-anion-gap metabolic acidosis, in the absence of renal failure or administration of unusual drugs, suggests lactic acidemia. In this circumstance, lactate-containing fluids should be avoided. Lactic acidosis in a patient with liver disease suggests the presence of some other complicating condition. At a normal rate of lactate production, abrupt cessation of hepatic lactate metabolism does not result in clinically significant lactate accumulation because of a compensatory increase in lactate extraction by extrahepatic tissues (Woods et al. 1982). Challenging a patient with liver dysfunction by administering lactated Ringer's solution may, however, result in lactate accumulation. Acetated Ringer's solution has therefore been recommended as an alternative alkalinizing solution for patients with serious hepatic dysfunction; each millimole of acetate yields 1 mmol of bicarbonate (Arai et al. 1986; Tanifuji et al. 1983). Similar studies have not been performed in animals, but lactic acidemia has been observed in cats with HL.

METABOLIC ACIDOSIS

If alkalinization is necessary, an $NaHCO_3$ or acetate-containing polyionic solution (e.g., Isolyte) can be used for patients with hepatic insufficiency. Solutions with restricted sodium content should be considered for patients with sodium intolerance (i.e., those with edema or ascites). In general, treatment with alkalinizing solutions or medications should be avoided in patients with signs of HE. Lactate-containing solutions should be avoided in cats with severe hepatic lipidosis. If lactic acidemia is thought to be present, identification and correction of systemic hypoperfusion are warranted. An important potential cause of metabolic acidosis in animals with severe liver disease is renal dysfunction, which may develop as a result of decreased GFR or renal tubular acidosis. Chronic renal disease can coexist with chronic inflammation in other organs, including the liver. Renal tubular acidosis has been recognized in dogs with copper-associated hepatotoxicity or drug-induced fulminant hepatic failure and in cats with HL (Center SA, unpublished observations 1998; Brown et al. 1986).

RESPIRATORY ACIDOSIS

Respiratory acidosis is a grave prognostic finding in patients with liver disease and requires diagnostic investigation. Ventilatory support should be provided if hypoventilation is present, but caution should be exercised to avoid hyperventilation and hypocapnia and the complications of decreased cerebral blood flow and metabolic rate. Calculation of the $P_A - PaO_2$ gradient identifies impaired gas diffusion and ventilation-perfusion mismatch in patients with normal arterial PO_2 values. A $P_A - PaO_2$ gradient above 15 mm Hg warrants consideration of oxygen therapy. Respiratory acidosis and increased $P_A - PaO_2$ gradient portend a grave prognosis in animals with hepatic disease.

RESPIRATORY AND METABOLIC ALKALOSIS

Respiratory alkalosis usually does not cause clinical complications or require intervention. Amelioration of HE often attenuates hyperventilation. If loss of acid-rich gastric juice underlies development of metabolic alkalosis, treatment with an H_2 blocker or acid pump inhibitor (e.g., omeprazole) may allow normalization of systemic pH. In patients with hypokalemia, KCl supplementation of fluids is required for recovery from alkalosis. In the absence of impending ascites or edema, 0.9% NaCl may be administered to replace the chloride deficit. In the presence of ascites or edema, infusion of 0.45% NaCl in 2.5% dextrose is preferable. Induction of a bicarbonate diuresis by administration of the carbonic anhydrase inhibitor acetazolamide can also be effective if conventional therapy fails (Dillingham and Anderson 1987). Rarely, severe metabolic alkalosis may require consideration of acidifying therapy (e.g., infusion of 0.1 N HCl, administration of an HCl precursor such as lysine hydrochloride or arginine monohydrochloride), plasmapheresis, or hemodialysis (Dillingham and Anderson 1987). These methods are rarely used in veterinary medicine. Administration of arginine monohydrochloride, lysine hydrochloride, or hydrochloric acid is considered experimental and would be used only with extreme caution.

A dilute solution of hydrochloric acid can be prepared by dilution of concentrated HCl in distilled water and sterilization using a 0.22-μm filter. The solution is then added to either dextrose or saline to form a 0.1 N solution (100 mEq/L) and administered over 6 to 24 h (Inadomi and Kopple 1987). Diluted HCl is administered only through a large catheter in a central vein. L-Arginine monohydrochloride is commercially available as a 10% solution for intravenous administration (Inadomi and Kopple 1987). L-lysine hydrochloride can be obtained only from a chemical supply house and is suspended to make a 10% solution and then sterilized (Inadomi and Kopple 1987). Metabolism of L-arginine monohydrochloride and L-lysine hydrochloride yields an eqimolar amount of HCl. Many adverse effects have been reported with these solutions, including an adverse reaction to the increased nitrogen load (i.e., induction or aggravation of HE and azotemia) and extracellular movement of potassium with life-threatening hyperkalemia (Bushinsky and Gennari 1978; Inadomi and Kopple 1987).

Colloid Administration in Liver Disease

ALBUMIN

Patients with liver disease, hypoalbuminemia, and third-space fluid accumulation may require administration of albumin or synthetic colloids to facilitate resolution of edema or ascites and expansion of the intravascular compartment. This approach is particularly important when hypovolemia or hypotension occurs during anesthesia and surgery. Selection of the most appropriate colloid for a given situation depends on the required duration of effect, whether or not abnormalities of hemostasis are present, and whether or not other disease processes are aggravating hypoproteinemia. In patients with severe ongoing extracorporeal protein loss (e.g., intestinal loss, urinary loss), administered colloids may have a very short plasma retention time. If hypoalbuminemia is due only to hepatobiliary disease, colloids have a longer plasma retention time.

Plasma administration is ideal for patients with hepatic insufficiency and hypoalbuminemia, and an infusion rate of 10 ml/kg/h is typically used. Using this approach, important coagulation and transport proteins are provided in addition to albumin. Since many patients with liver disease have clinical or subclinical abnormalities of hemostasis, plasma administration may normalize hemostasis. Plasma infusion may also attenuate the tendency for adverse drug interactions involving highly protein-bound medications. Albumin has a much longer retention time than synthetic colloids when extracorporeal protein loss is not a complicating factor (Rudloff and Kirby 1997). The patient's size determines whether plasma administration can reasonably be expected to achieve colloid repletion. Unfortunately, plasma administration can lead to complications associated with hypercitratemia and introduction of endotoxins, pyrogens, or bacteria in contaminated bags (Dillingham and Anderson 1987).

SYNTHETIC COLLOIDS

Dextran and hydroxyethyl starch (HES) are macromolecular colloids developed for use as acute volume expanders. Dextrans are linear polymers of glucose produced by using bacterial enzyme systems. The preferred dextran for oncotic effect is dextran 70, which has an effective half-life of 24 h in normal dogs. HES, a highly branched polymer of glucose (synthetic hydroxyethyl substitute of amylopectin), also has a plasma half-life of 24 h in normal animals (Yacobi et al. 1982). The pharmacokinetics of HES are complex owing to the molecular size and heterogeneity of component polymers. Elimination of HES occurs by glomerular filtration of small polymers, hydrolysis of larger polymers by α-amylase, or reticuloendothelial phagocytosis and metabolism in liver, spleen, and lymph nodes (Mishler 1982). The HES that is retained in reticuloendothelial cells does not appear to have a detrimental effect on organ function in normal dogs, but its effects have not been evaluated in dogs with liver disease or portosystemic shunting (Mishler 1982; Thompson et al. 1970; Parth et al. 1992; Murphy et al. 1965). Although HES expands plasma volume in humans for 12 to 48 h, it increased colloid oncotic pressure for less than 12 h in hypoalbuminemic dogs (Haupt and Rackow 1982; Hulse and Yacobi 1983; Moore and Garvey 1996). When used for oncotic support, synthetic colloids are usually given at a dosage of up to 20 mL/kg/day and can be administered by slow infusion over many hours.

ADVERSE EFFECTS OF SYNTHETIC COLLOIDS IN PATIENTS WITH LIVER DISEASE

Synthetic volume expanders have predictable effects on hemostasis. The risk of bleeding with dextran is related to the dosage and type of dextran used. Hemostatic abnormalities may be related to dilutional effects on one or more coagulation factors, interference with platelet activity, decreased activity of von Willebrand's factor, or increased fibrinolytic activity (Thompson and Gadsden 1965; Lewis et al. 1966; Gollub et al. 1967; Karlson et al. 1967; Garzon et al. 1967; Berqvist 1982; Stump et al. 1985; Symington 1986; Aberg et al. 1977, 1979; Macintyre et al. 1985; Damon et al. 1987; Sanfilippo et al. 1987; Concannon et al. 1992; Dalrymple-Hay et al. 1992). Regardless of cause, hemostatic abnormalities are notable in animals with hepatobiliary disease given dextran 70 (Center SA, unpublished observations). Intraoperative use of dextran 70 in dogs with portosystemic vascular anomalies has resulted in bleeding tendencies in patients assessed presurgically as having normal hemostasis (i.e., normal mucosal bleeding time, prothrombin time, activated partial thromboplastin time, activated coagulation time, and proteins induced by vitamin K absence or antagonism [PIVKA] clotting test). In addition to rapid hemodilution causing a moderate to severe reduction in hematocrit, some patients with liver disease treated with synthetic colloids also have developed transient pulmonary edema.

In normal dogs and humans, the influence of HES on coagulation is dose dependent and negligible when small doses are administered. However, normal dogs do develop a dose-dependent increase in bleeding time after blood replacement with HES. Induced hemostatic abnormalities in humans have involved von Willebrand's factor and factor VIII coagulation activity, and cumulative doses above 30 mL/kg have induced von Willebrand's disease or hemophilia-like syndromes. There are few reports of HES use in veterinary clinical patients and no information regarding its influence on coagulation tests in patients with hepatobiliary disease. Although HES is contraindicated in the presence of severe coagulopathies, its use in dogs with low serum albumin concentration not attributable to liver disease with preexisting coagulation abnormalities resulted in normalization of coagulation in five of seven dogs (Smiley and Garvey 1994).

Acute allergic reactions are possible with use of dextrans and HES. In humans, preformed antibodies reactive with dextran may be induced by certain foods or organisms in the gastrointestinal tract (Morito et al. 1985). Interactions between dextran and antidextran antibodies have been demonstrated in humans with fulminant hepatic failure and acute hepatitis (Morito et al. 1985). Damaged hepatocytes may release dextran-like antigens into the patient's circulation, thus promoting formation of antibodies cross-reactive with dextrans. Dextrans are also adsorbed onto erythrocyte membranes and can cause agglutination or excessive rouleau formation. Induced aggregation can interfere with blood crossmatching often used in patients with liver disease requiring repeated blood transfusions. Adverse effects associated with nonalbumin plasma extenders have been well studied only in healthy dogs. Isovolemic hemodilution with HES and polymerized bovine collagen did not have adverse effects on hepatic histology (Standl et al. 1996). Accumulation of HES in hepatocytes of humans with acute renal failure, however, has been reported (Dienes et al. 1986). Normal dogs receiving hypertonic saline (6%) and dextran 70 at a maximal tolerated dosage (20 mL/kg) developed significant increases in alanine aminotransferase, aspartate aminotransferase, and alkaline phosphatase during the first 72 h (Dubick et al. 1993).

Management of Bleeding Tendencies in Patients with Liver Disease

BLOOD TRANSFUSION AND VITAMIN K_1 ADMINISTRATION

Whole-blood transfusions are indicated for patients with symptomatic anemia or coagulopathy. Anemia usually becomes symptomatic in dogs when the PCV is 18% or less and in cats when the PCV is 15% or less. Cats with liver disease seem predisposed to hemolysis associated with formation of Heinz bodies. Sometimes this occurs after treatment with certain drugs (e.g., vitamin K medications with a propylene glycol diluent), ingestion of onion powder flavoring to enhance food palatability, or development of hypophosphatemia. Coagulation abnormalities in liver disease result from several different deficiencies or abnormalities. The most commonly considered cause of bleeding is factor deficiency derived from hepatic synthetic failure. However, clinical evidence suggests that these patients more often develop a vitamin K–responsive coagulopathy. This observation may be related to intestinal malabsorption (e.g., secondary to abnormal enterohepatic bile acid turnover), insufficient dietary intake, or impaired enteric synthesis of vitamin K secondary to prophylactic antimicrobial therapy. Vitamin K deficiency is avoided or corrected by administration of vitamin K_1 at a dosage of 0.5 to 1.5 mg/kg for two to three treatments at 12-h intervals initially and then once weekly as required. Other conditions that may contribute to bleeding tendencies in patients with liver disease include increased factor consumption or utilization as occurs with extensive gastrointestinal bleeding and disseminated intravascular coagulation. Both dogs and cats with biliary tree obstruction or severe acquired hepatic insufficiency can develop pyloroduodenal ulcers that may lead to lethal gastrointestinal hemorrhage.

If a blood transfusion is required, fresh whole blood is most helpful. Stored blood products can deliver substantial amounts of ammonia, which may exacerbate HE or be a source of infused pyrogen or endotoxin (Schenker et al. 1974). The rate of blood administration depends on the circumstances and urgency imposed by bleeding tendencies. Usually, an infusion rate of 5–10 ml/kg/h is safe and effective.

DDAVP ADMINISTRATION

In addition to blood component therapy, coagulopathies may be ameliorated by administration of 1-deamino-8-D-arginine vasopressin (DDAVP) (0.05 to 0.3 µg/kg diluted in 10 to 20 mL of saline and given IV slowly over 10 minutes or given undiluted SQ) in the perioperative period or during a crisis. Although it is known that DDAVP can mitigate bleeding in humans and animals with hepatobiliary disease, its mechanism of action in this circumstance remains undefined. The benefits in such patients seem too great to be explained on the basis of DDAVP-induced liberation of preformed endothelial von Willebrand's factor. When DDAVP is used, its narrow therapeutic interval (i.e., 4–6 h) of effectiveness and its proposed one-time effect require careful consideration for optimal results. Concern should be given to administration of DDAVP to patients with edema or ascites as DDAVP may augment water accumulation.

HEMORRHAGE CAUSED BY CITRATE LOADING

In very small patients (<10 kg) receiving large quantities of blood or blood components preserved with CPD, acquired hemorrhagic tendency is treated with 0.1 mL/kg of 10% $CaCl_2$ suspended in 10 to 20 mL of 0.9% saline and given over 10 to 20 min (Paula Moon, Section of Anesthesiology, College of Veterinary Medicine, Cornell University, Ithaca, NY, personal communication).

Treatment of Ascites in Liver Disease

Increased abdominal pressure related to tense ascites can increase portal venous pressure. This effect can potentiate gastrointestinal hemorrhage from newly expanded varices, ectatic vessels, or ulcerative lesions, as well as protein loss from the gut. Tense ascites also has negative hemodynamic effects on cardiac output. Studies of patients before and after fluid removal have shown a progressive increase in cardiac output, stroke volume, and ventricular ejection rate during and after therapeutic large-volume paracentesis. Tense ascites can also seriously impair ventilation by restricting diaphragmatic movement and chest expansion.

Management of factors contributing to ascites formation is essential. Treatment must be carefully supervised, as iatrogenic problems related to ascites mobilization (e.g., sodium restriction, paracentesis, diuretic administration) can lead to serious complications (e.g., abnormalities of hydration, electrolytes, and acid-base balance). Optimal treatment requires a polysystemic approach and careful sequential evaluations of the patient.

Before treatment is begun, the patient's weight and abdominal girth are recorded, and serum sodium, potassium, BUN, and creatinine concentrations as well as urine specific gravity are determined to provide baseline information. Dietary sodium restriction and combined use of a loop diuretic (furosemide, 1–2 mg/kg PO q12h) and an aldosterone inhibitor (spironolactone, 1–2 mg/kg PO q12h) are recommended initially. Sodium restriction as proposed for dogs with cardiac or renal disease is instituted. Combined use of furosemide and spironolactone produces a greater diuretic effect and usually is not associated with iatrogenic hypokalemia. If sequential evaluations (every 5 to 7 days) of the patient demonstrate poor ascites mobilization but maintenance of normal serum electrolyte concentrations and adequate renal function and if the owner has consistently fed a sodium-restricted diet, the dosage of each diuretic agent is doubled. If treatment still fails to mobilize ascites after an additional 5 to 7 days, large-volume or total paracentesis is recommended. Alternative treatment with a peritoneovenous shunt prosthesis has been performed in some human patients who do not respond to conventional therapy. Unfortunately, use of peritoneovenous shunting is limited by the frequent occurrence of complications induced by the procedure as well as a high rate of prosthesis obstruction within the first postoperative year (Arroyo et al. 1992). This procedure has rarely been used in animals.

THERAPEUTIC OR TOTAL PARACENTESIS

Therapeutic or large-volume paracentesis usually is quite safe. However, severe consequences (including death) in patients with hepatic cirrhosis have been reported. Characteristic hemodynamic maladaptations in these patients include increased plasma renin activity, increased norepinephrine concentrations, reduced systemic vascular resistance, and an increased hepatic venous pressure gradient (Ruiz-del Arbol et al. 1997). The most common complications of therapeutic abdominocentesis in humans include HE, renal impairment, and hyponatremia (Arroyo et al. 1992). The influence of rapid abdominocentesis on portal pressure and vena caval pressure has been evaluated in humans and dogs. These studies have not disclosed deleterious effects on portal or systemic venous pressure. The effect of large-volume paracentesis on reformation of ascites in cirrhotic dogs treated by sodium restriction or high sodium intake is shown in Figure 16–22 (Levy 1977a). These data explain why sodium restriction is so important in overall management of patients with ascites and must be in place before therapeutic paracentesis is attempted.

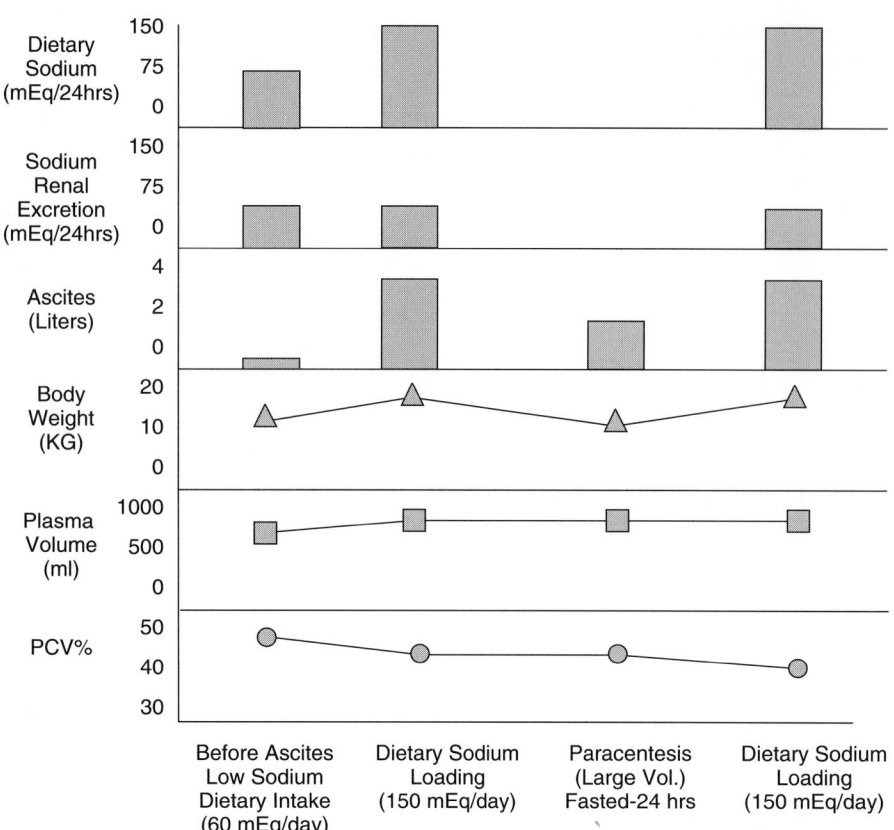

FIGURE 16-22. Experimental data showing the response of cirrhotic dogs to paracentesis and different levels of sodium ingestion. Data derived from five dogs with cirrhosis induced with dimethylnitrosamine (Levy 1977a).

USE OF COLLOIDS IN ASCITES MOBILIZATION

Intravenous colloid administration can facilitate mobilization of ascites in the hypoalbuminemic patient when salt restriction and diuretics are ineffective. In these patients, total paracentesis is coupled with intravenous colloid administration. Without colloids, therapeutic or large-volume paracentesis can lead to contraction of effective circulating blood volume, renal dysfunction, and dilutional hyponatremia.

Total paracentesis coupled with albumin administration is safe and useful for management of intractable ascites. Alternative colloids have been investigated because of the high cost of homologous albumin. In comparative studies, postparacentesis circulatory dysfunction occurred twice as frequently in patients receiving synthetic colloids as in those receiving homologous albumin (Gines et al. 1996). Humans given dextran 70 at 12 h after paracentesis experienced resolution of their hemodynamic abnormalities and became normovolemic (84 ± 14 mL of dextran 70 for each 1000 mL of ascites removed) (Terg et al. 1992). Patients receiving dextran 70 concurrently with paracentesis did not develop significant hemodynamic changes in the first 24 h after paracentesis (Terg et al. 1992). Unfortunately, gastrointestinal bleeding as a complication of dextran infusion precipitated HE in some patients. As a result of the short plasma retention time of dextran 70, some of these patients developed hypovolemia 24 h after paracentesis (Terg et al. 1996). An alternative approach with a more reliable outcome was accomplished by combining smaller volume daily paracentesis with dextran 70 (6 g for each 1000 mL of ascites removed) (Fassio et al. 1992). Compared with diuretic therapy, total paracentesis combined with intravenous dextran 70 resulted in a better outcome and fewer side effects in cirrhotic patients (i.e., there was a high frequency of HE when diuretics alone were used to mobilize ascites) (Sola et al. 1994; Cotrim et al. 1994).

▶ Peritonitis

The peritoneal surface is composed of a single layer of flat mesothelial cells that can exfoliate into the abdomen and transform into activated macrophages. The structure of the peritoneum is supported and maintained by an underlying layer of connective tissue, blood vessels, and lymphatics. In health, the peritoneum functions to protect visceral structures and its large surface area functions to transport water and electrolytes between the peritoneal cavity and circulation. Normally, only minimal quantities of fluid accumulate in the peritoneal cavity (0 to 15 mL depending on the size of the animal). Normal peritoneal fluid is clear; has a pH of 7.4, a specific gravity less than 1.016, and a total protein concentration below 3.0 g/dL; and contains fewer than 3000 nucleated cells per microliter. Noncolloidal solutes (e.g., sodium, potassium, chloride, glucose, urea) are found in the same concentrations as in plasma.

Peritonitis is defined as inflammation of the peritoneal lining as a result of bacterial, traumatic, or chemical injury. When acute and generalized, peritonitis can have serious metabolic consequences and result in altered intestinal motility and function. When inflamed, the peritoneum can sequester large volumes of fluid and electrolytes in the abdominal cavity. The quantity and physicochemical characteristics of the sequestered fluid reflect the underlying pathophysiologic disease mechanisms as well as osmotic solutes, protein exudation, and chemical constituents within the entrapped fluid.

The systemic effects of peritonitis are determined by the nature of the underlying disease process as well as the fluid constituents. Disorders associated with large-volume fluid accumulation (e.g., uroabdomen, pancreatic chemical peritonitis, bile peritonitis, septic peritonitis) can induce systemic hypovolemia, electrolyte derangements, and hypoproteinemia. The most common complications of peritonitis include hypovolemia, hyponatremia, and metabolic acidosis (Fig. 16–23). Fluid and electrolyte disturbances related to peritonitis are commonly complicated by concurrent vomiting of gastric or duodenal fluids and occasionally diarrhea. Without appropriate intervention, even nonseptic peritonitis can lead to systemic dehydration and loss of intravascular oncotic pressure, which can culminate in acute renal failure and death.

Specific Causes of Peritonitis

UROABDOMEN
Peritonitis derived from rupture of the urinary system leads to rapid dehydration, azotemia, hyponatremia, hypochloremia, hyperkalemia, and metabolic acidosis. Determination of fluid creatinine concentration and comparison with serum creatinine concentration discloses a higher creatinine concentration in the abdominal effusion (i.e., ratio of fluid to serum creatinine ≥ 2.0). Comparatively, there is little or no difference between fluid urea nitrogen and BUN concentrations. The relatively larger creatinine molecule delays equilibrium between fluid and blood, whereas the relatively small urea molecule permits rapid diffusion to all compartments.

BILE PERITONITIS
Bile peritonitis is due to rupture of the gallbladder or major biliary ducts. Typically, a large-volume effusion accumulates within 1 week. In some cases, fluid is trapped adjacent to the site of leakage by the omentum. In animals with diffuse bile spillage, dehydration, hyponatremia, hyperbilirubinemia, metabolic acidosis, and sepsis may develop rapidly. Lecithin and bile acids in bile are cytotoxic and cause serosal, peritoneal, and vascular leakiness and inflammation that permit the transmural passage of enteric microbes into the abdominal cavity. Failure to identify the position and structure of the extrahepatic biliary structures on ultrasonographic evaluations supports but does not confirm a diagnosis of biliary tree rupture.

PANCREATIC PERITONITIS
Pancreatitis can result in chemical peritonitis associated with either a localized right quadrant reaction and effusion or diffuse abdominal involvement. Release of activated enzymes damages adjacent visceral structures, serosal surfaces, and microcirculation. Complications include sequestration of plasma proteins and sodium in an exudative effusion, systemic panhypoproteinemia, intravascular volume contraction, ionized hypocalcemia, cardiac ar-

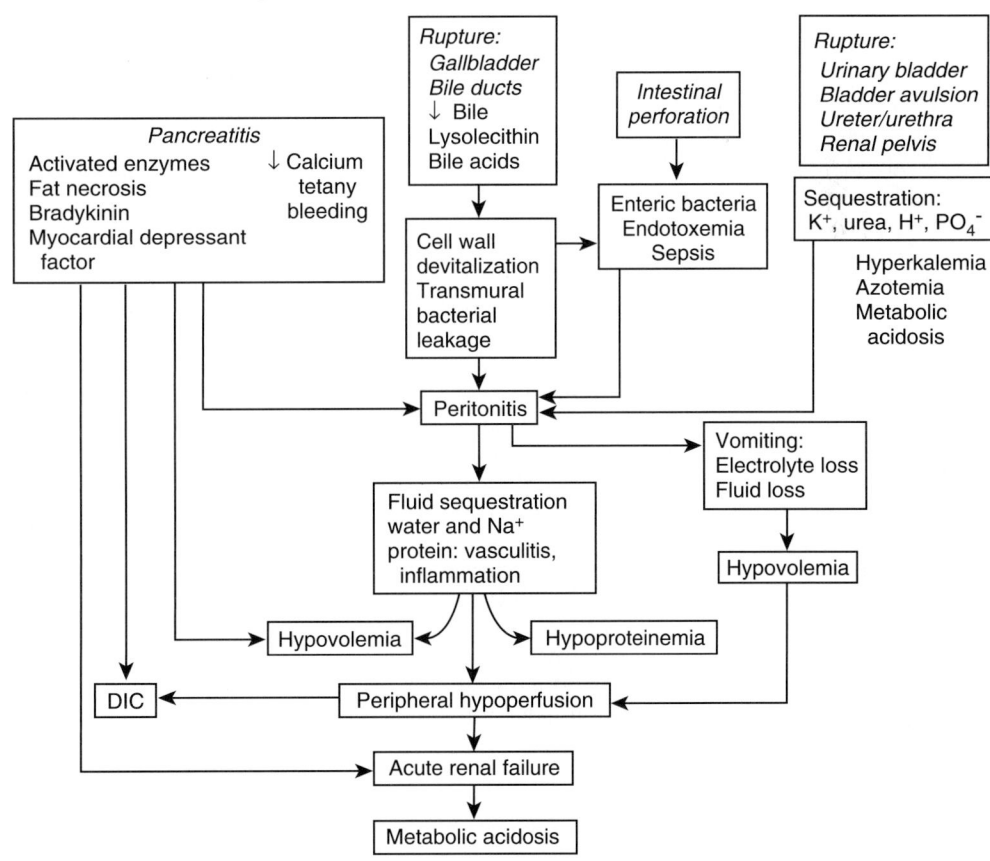

FIGURE 16–23. Pathophysiologic mechanisms and considerations in disorders leading to peritonitis.

rhythmias, pulmonary edema or effusion, biliary tree obstruction, acute hepatic necrosis, acute renal failure, endotoxic shock, and disseminated intravascular coagulation. Determination of pancreatic enzyme activity in the effusion and comparison with serum enzyme activity, cytologic identification of macrophages containing engulfed fat globules, and determination of systemic concentrations of trypsin-like immunoreactive substances (TLI) are helpful diagnostic indicators along with ultrasonographic evaluation of the right cranial abdominal quadrant.

INTESTINAL RUPTURE

Septic peritonitis is commonly associated with endotoxic shock, which may quickly follow viscus perforation. Septic peritonitis causes loss of sodium, water, and proteins into the peritoneal cavity. If it is left untreated, hypovolemia, hyponatremia, acidosis, and acute renal failure develop quickly. Microscopically identifying a mixed bacterial population along with intracytoplasmic organisms within neutrophils and macrophages highly supports a diagnosis of peritonitis caused by bowel rupture.

Treatment of Peritonitis

In all cases of peritonitis, provision of fluids for intravascular volume expansion is critical. In chemical peritonitis associated with uroabdomen or bile peritonitis and in septic peritonitis associated with intestinal rupture, the abdominal cavity should be emptied and lavaged if the patient's status precludes emergency surgery. There is no evidence that abdominal lavage changes the patient's outcome in pancreatitis. If endotoxic shock is suspected, appropriate antimicrobial coverage against enteric opportunists and single-dose glucocorticoid administration for septic shock are appropriate.

Rapid volume expansion may require administration of fluids at shock rates and volume. Fluid administration is best guided by sequential measurements of central venous pressure, systemic blood pressure, and vital signs (e.g., heart rate and rhythm, lung sounds and respiratory rate, body weight). A urinary catheter should be placed to monitor urine production (1–2 ml/kg/h is the minimally acceptable rate). Colloid administration is essential if the serum albumin concentration is below 2.0 g/dL. Plasma should be given to patients with pancreatitis for provision of antiproteases that may attenuate pancreatic enzyme activity. Plasma should also be given to patients manifesting clinical signs or laboratory parameters of disseminated intravascular coagulation. Synthetic colloids may be used for patients with other disorders. Hyponatremia is corrected by infusion of polyionic fluids rich in sodium. Potassium supplementation is essential in nearly all animals with peritonitis with the exception of uroabdomen in which hyperkalemia is present. Severe hyperkalemia in uroabdomen is successfully managed by abdominocentesis followed by abdominal lavage and correction of uroabdomen. In severe cases, treatment with insulin and glucose or administration of calcium gluconate may be required to lower the serum potassium concentration.

REFERENCES

Abelmann WH, Kowalski HJ, and McNeely WF: The hemodynamic response to exercise in patients with Laennec's cirrhosis. *J Clin Invest* 34:690–695, 1955.

Aberg M, Bergentz S, and Hedner U: Effect of dextran and induced thrombocytopenia on the lysability of ex vivo thrombi in dogs. *Acta Chir Scand* 143:91–94, 1977.

Aberg M, Hedner V, and Bergentz S: Effect of dextran on factor VIII and platelet function. *Ann Surg* 189:243–247, 1979.

Adams LG, Hardy RM, Weiss DJ, et al.: Hypophosphatemia and hemolytic anemia associated with diabete mellitus and hepatic lipidosis in cats. *J Vet Intern Med* 7:266–271, 1993.

Agusti AG, Roca J, and Rodriguez-Roisin R: Mechanisms of gas exchange impairment in patients with liver cirrhosis. *Clin Chest Med* 17:49–66, 1996.

Akol KG, Washabau RJ, Saunders HM, et al.: Acute pancreatitis in cats with hepatic lipidosis. *J Vet Intern Med* 7:205–209, 1993.

Allen D, Krietys PR, and Grainger DN: Crystalloids versus colloids: Implications in fluid therapy of dogs with intestinal obstruction. *Am J Vet Res* 47:1751–1755, 1986.

Allen DA, Schertel ER, Muir WW, et al.: Hypertonic saline/dextran resuscitation of dogs with experimentally induced gastric dilation-volvulus shock. *Am J Vet Res* 52:92–96, 1991.

Amatuzio DS and Nesbitt S: A study of pyruvic acid in the blood, spinal fluid and urine of patients with liver disease with and without hepatic coma. *Clin Invest* 29:1486–1490, 1950.

Arai K, Kawamoto M, Yuge O, et al: A comparative study on lactated Ringer and acetated Ringer solution as intraoperative fluid in patients with liver dysfunction. *Masui* 35:793–799, 1986.

Argent BE and Case RM: Pancreatic ducts: Cellular mechanism and control of bicarbonate. In: Johnson LR (ed): *Physiology of the Gastrointestinal Tract*, 3rd ed. New York, Raven Press, p. 1473, 1994.

Arroyo V, Rodes J, Gutierrez-Lizarraga MA, et al.: Prognostic value of spontaneous hyponatremia in cirrhosis with ascites. *Am J Dig Dis* 21:249–256, 1976.

Arroyo V, Gines P, and Planas R: Treatment of ascites in cirrhosis. Diuretics, peritoneovenous shunt, and large-volume paracentesis. *Gastroenterol Clin North Am* 21:237–256, 1992.

Astrup J and Roerth M: Oxygen affinity of hemoglobin and red cell 2,3 diphosphoglycerate in hepatic cirrhosis. *Scand J Clin Lab Invest* 31:311–317, 1973.

August AGN, Roca J, and Rodriguiz-Roisin R: Mechanisms of gas exchange impairment in patients with liver cirrhosis. *Clin Chest Med* 17:49–66, 1996.

Avery ME and Snyder JD: Oral therapy for acute diarrhea: The underused simple solution. *N Engl J Med* 323:891–894, 1990.

Battaglia SE, Pretto JJ, Irving LB, et al.: Resolution of gas exchange abnormalities and intrapulmonary shunting following liver transplantation. *Hepatology* 25:1228–1232, 1997.

Baumann H and Gauldie J: The acute phase response. *Immunol Today* 15:74–80, 1994.

Bergqvist D: Dextrans and haemostasis: A review. *Acta Chir Scand* 31:320–324, 1982.

Berthelot P, Walker JG, Sherlock S, et al.: Arterial changes in the lungs in cirrhosis of the liver and lung spider nevi. *N Engl J Med* 274:291–298, 1966.

Better OS and Schrier RW: Disturbed volume homeostasis in patients with cirrhosis of the liver. *Kidney Int* 23:303–309, 1983.

Bhattacharya SK, Luther RW, Pate JW, et al.: Soft tissue calcium and magnesium content in acute pancreatitis in the dog: Calcium accumulation, a mechanism for hypocalcemia in acute pancreatitis. *J Lab Clin Med* 105:422–427, 1985.

Bhattacharya SK, Crawford AJ, Pate JW, et al.: Mechanism of calcium and magnesium translocation in acute pancreatitis: A temporal correlation between hypocalcemia and membrane-mediated excessive intracellular calcium accumulation in soft tissues. *Magnesium* 7(2):91–102, 1988.

Bienzle D, Jacobs RM, and Lumsden JH: Relationship of serum total calcium to serum albumin in dogs, cats, horses and cattle. *Can Vet J* 34:360–364, 1993.

Bihan D, Gimson AES, Lindridge J, and Williams R: Lactic acidosis in fulminant hepatic failure: Some aspects of pathogenesis and prognosis. *J Hepatol* 1:405–416, 1983.

Bihari D, Gimson AE, Lindridge J, et al: Lactic acidosis in fulminant hepatic failure. Some aspects of pathogenesis and prognosis. *J Hepatol* 1:405–516, 1985.

Bihari D, Gimson AE, Waterson M, et al: Tissue hypoxia during fulminant hepatic failure. *Crit Care Med* 13:1034–1039, 1985.

Bihari D, Smithies M, Gimson A, et al: The effects of vasodilation with prostacyclin on oxygen delivery and uptake in critically ill patients. *N Engl J Med* 317:397–403, 1987.

Binder HJ and Sandle GI: Electrolyte transport in the mammalian colon. In Johnson LR (ed): *Physiology of the Gastrointestinal Tract*, 3rd ed, Vol 2. New York, Raven Press, pp. 2133–2171, 1994.

Breitschwerdt EB, Halliwell WH, Foley CW, et al.: A heritable diarrhetic syndrome in the basenji characterized by malabsorption, protein-losing enteropathy, and hypergammaglobulinemia. *J Am Anim Hosp Assoc* 16:551–560, 1980.

Breitschwerdt EB, Barta O, Waltman C, et al.: Serum proteins in healthy basenjis and basenjis with chronic diarrhea. *Am J Vet Res* 44:326–328, 1983.

Brown SA, Spyridakis LK, and Crowell WA: Distal renal tubular acidosis and hepatic lipidosis in a cat. *J Am Vet Med Assoc* 189:1350–1352, 1986.

Burk RF, Lane JM, and Patel K: Relationship of oxygen and glutathione in protection against carbon tetrachloride induced hepatic microsomal lipid peroxidation and covalent binding in the rat. Rationale for the use of hyperbaric oxygen to treat carbon tetrachloride ingestion. *J Clin Invest* 74:1996–2001, 1984.

Burrows CF: Chronic diarrhea in the dog. *Vet Clin North Am* 13:521, 1983.

Bushinsky DA and Gennari FJ: Life-threatening hyperkalemia induced by arginine. *Ann Intern Med* 89:632–634, 1978.

Butterworth RF, Giguere JF, Michaud J, et al.: Ammonia: Key factor in the pathogenesis of hepatic encephalopathy. *Neurochem Pathol* 6:1–12, 1987.

Butterworth RF, Gaudreau C, Vincelette J, et al.: Thiamine deficiency and Wernicke's encephalopathy in AIDS. *Metab Brain Dis* 6:207–212, 1991.

Caregaro L, Menon F, Angeli P, et al.: Limitations of serum creatinine level and creatine clearance as filtration markers in cirrhosis. *Arch Intern Med* 154:201–205, 1994.

Carter CC, Lifton JF, and Welch MJ: Organ uptake and blood pH and concentration effects of ammonia in dogs determined with ammonia labeled with 10 minute half-lived nitrogen 13. *Neurology* 23:204–213, 1973.

Casey TH, Summerskill WHJ, Bickford RG, et al.: Body and serum potassium in liver disease: II. Relationships to arterial ammonia, blood pH, and hepatic coma. *Gastroenterology* 18:208–215, 1965.

Castell JV, Gomez-Lechon MJ, David M, et al: Acute-phase response of human hepatocytes: regulation of acute-phase protein synthesis by interleukin-6. *Hepatology* 12:1179–1186, 1990.

Center SA: Pathophysiology of liver disease: normal and abnormal function. In Guilford GA, Center SA, Strombeck DR, et al (eds): *Strombeck's Small Animal Gastroenterology*, 3rd ed, Philadelphia,WB Saunders, pp. 553–632, 1996.

Center SA: Unpublished information, College of Veterinary Medicine, Cornell University, 1998.

Center SA and Magne M: Historical, physical examination, and clinicopathologic features of portosystemic vascular anomalies in the dog and cat. *Semin Vet Med Surg (Small Anim)* 5:83–93, 1990.

Center SA, Crawford MA, Guida L, et al.: A retrospective study of cats (n=77) with severe hepatic lipidosis: (1975–1990). *J Vet Intern Med* 7:349–359, 1993.

Center SA, Thompson M, Wood PA, et al: Hepatic ultrastructural and metabolic derangements in cats with severe hepatic lipidosis. Proceedings of the 9th ACVIM Forum, pp. 193–196, 1991.

Chang EB and Rao MC: Intestinal water and electrolyte transport: Mechanisms of physiological and adaptive responses. In Johnson LR (ed): *Physiology of the Gastrointestinal Tract*, 3rd ed. New York, Raven Press, pp. 2027–2081, 1994.

Concannon KT, Haskins S, and Feldman BF: Hemostatic defects associated with two infusion rates of dextran 70 in dogs. *Am J Vet Res* 53:1369–1375, 1992.

Connor H, Woods HF, and Ledinham JG: Comparison of the hepatic uptake and utilization of D($-$) and L($+$) sodium lactate in normal man. *Ann Nutr Metab* 27:481–487, 1983.

Cooke HJ: Role of the "little brain" in the gut in water and electrolyte homeostasis. *FASEB J* 3:127–138, 1989.

Cooke HJ and Reddix RA: Neural regulation of intestinal electrolyte transport. In Johnson LR (ed): *Physiology of the Gastrointestinal tract*, 3rd ed, Vol 2. New York, Raven Press, pp. 2083–2132, 1994.

Cooper AJL: Role of the liver in amino acid metabolism. In Zakim D and Boyer TD (eds): *Hepatology: A Textbook of Liver Disease*, 3rd ed. Philadelphia, WB Saunders Co., pp. 563–604, 1996.

Cornelius LM and Rawlings CA: Arterial blood gas and acid-base values in dogs with various diseases and signs of disease. *JAVMA* 178:992–995, 1981.

Cotrim HP, Garrido V, Parana R, et al.: Paracentesis associated with dextran-70 in the treatment of ascites in patients with chronic liver diseases: A randomized therapeutic study. *Arq Gastroenterol* 31:125–129, 1994.

Craddock PR, Yawata Y, VanSanten L, et al.: Acquired phagocyte dysfunction: A complication of hypophosphatemia of parenteral hyperalimentation. *N Engl J Med* 290:1403–1407, 1974.

Cullen JJ, Caropreso DK, Hemann LL, et al.: Pathophysiology of adynamic ileus. *Dig Dis Sci* 42:731–737, 1997.

Curran PF: Na, Cl, and water transport by rat ileum in vitro. *J Gen Physiol* 43:1137–1148, 1960.

Cuschieri A, Cummings JRG, Meehan SE, et al.: Treatment of acute pancreatitis with fresh frozen plasma. *Br J Surg* 70:710–712, 1983.

Damon L, Adams M, Stricker R, et al.: Intracranial bleeding during treatment with hydroxyethyl starch. *N Engl J Med* 317:964–965, 1987.

D'Arienzo A, Ambrogio G, Di Siervi P, et al.: A randomized comparison of metoclopramide and domperidone on plasma aldosterone concentrations and on spironolactone-induced diuresis in ascitic cirrhotic patients. *Hepatology* 5:854–857, 1985.

Dalrymple-Hay M, Aitchison R, Collins P, et al.: Hydroxyethyl starch induced acquired von Willebrand's disease. *Clin Lab Haematol* 14:209–211, 1992.

Dawson DJ, Babbs C, Warnes TW, et al.: Hypophosphataemia in acute liver failure. *Br Med J* 295:1312–1313, 1987.

DeGasperi A, Mazz E, Corti A, et al: Lactate blood levels in the perioperative period of orthotopic liver transplantation. *Int J Clin Lab Res* 27:123–128, 1997.

Deppe TA, Center SA, Simpson KW, et al: Glomerular filtration rate and renal volume in dogs with congenital portosystemic vascular anomalies before and surgical ligation. *J Vet Intern Med* 13:465–471, 1999.

DiBartola SP: Metabolic acidosis. In DiBartola SP (ed): *Fluid Therapy in Small Animal Practice*. Philadelphia, WB Saunders Co., pp. 216–243, 1992.

DiBartola SP, Johnson SE, Davenport DJ, et al.: Clinicopathologic findings resembling hypoadrenocorticism in dogs with primary gastrointestinal disease. *J Am Vet Med Assoc* 187:60–63, 1985.

Dich J, Hansen SE, and Thieden HID: Effect of albumin concentration and colloid osmotic pressure on albumin synthesis in the perfused rat liver. *Acta Physiol Scand* 89:352–358, 1973.

Dienes HP, Gerharz CD, Wagner R, et al.: Accumulation of hydroxyethyl starch (HES) in the liver of patients with renal failure and portal hypertension. *J Hepatol* 3:223–227, 1986.

Dillingham MA and Anderson RJ: Electrolyte, water, mineral, and acid base disorders in liver disease. In Maxwell MH, Kleeman CR, and Narins RG (eds): *Clinical Disorders of Fluid and Electrolyte Metabolism*, 4th ed. New York, McGraw-Hill Book Company, pp. 879–896, 1987.

Dixon FJ, Maurer PH, and Deichmiller MP: Half-lives of homologous serum albumins in several species. *Soc Exp Bio Med* 83:287–288, 1953.

Dubick MA, Zaucha GM, Korte DW Jr, et al.: Acute and subacute toxicity of 7.5% hypertonic saline–6% dextran-70 (HSD) in dogs. 2. Biochemical and behavioral responses. *J Appl Toxicol* 13:49–55, 1993.

Duffel SJ: Some aspects of pancreatic disease in the cat. *J Small Anim Pract* 16:365–374, 1975.

Duffy TE, Plum F: Hepatic encephalopathy. In Arias I, Popper H, Schachter D, et al (eds): *The Liver: Biology and Pathobiology*. New York, Raven Press, pp. 693–715, 1982.

Ede RJ, Gove CD, Hughes RD, et al: Reduced brain Na^+, K^+-ATPase activity in rats with galactosamine-induced hepatic failure: Relationship to encephalopathy and cerebral oedema. *Clin Sci* 72:365–371, 1987.

Edell ES, Cortese DA, Krowka MJ, et al.: Severe hypoxemia and liver disease. *Am Rev Respir Dis* 140:1631–1635, 1989.

Edmonds CJ: Salts and water. In Smyth DH (ed): *Biomembranes*, Vol 4B, *Intestinal Absorption*. New York, Plenum, pp. 711–759, 1974.

Emmitt M and Narins RG: Mixed acid-base disorders. In Maxwell MH, Kleeman CR, and Narins RG (eds): *Clinical Disorders of Fluid and Electrolyte Metabolism*, 4th ed. New York, McGraw-Hill Book Company, pp. 743–788, 1987.

Epstein M: Derangements of renal water handling in liver disease. *Gastroenterology* 89:1415–1425, 1985.

Erlinger S: Physiology of bile secretion and enterohepatic circulation. In Johnson LR (ed): *Physiology of the Gastrointestinal Tract*, 2nd ed. New York, Raven Press, pp. 1557–1580, 1987.

Farthing MJG: History and rationale of oral rehydration and recent developments in formulating an optimal solution. *Drugs* 36(suppl 4):80–90, 1988.

Fassio E, Terg R, Landeira G, et al.: Paracentesis with dextran 70 vs paracentesis with albumin in cirrhosis with tense ascites. Results of a randomized study. *J Hepatol* 14:310–316, 1992.

Fink RM, Enns R, Kimball CP, et al: Plasma protein metabolism: Observations using heavy nitrogen in lysine. *J Exp Med* 80:455–475, 1944.

Flanders JA, Scarlett JM, Blue JT, et al.: Adjustment of total serum calcium concentration for binding to albumin and protein in cats: 291 cases (1986–1987). *J Am Vet Med Assoc* 194:1609–1611, 1989.

Fordtran JS: Speculations on the pathogenesis of diarrhea. *Fed Proc* 26:1405–1414, 1967.

Forrester SD and Moreland KJ: Hypophosphatemia: Causes and clinical consequences. *J Vet Intern Med* 3:149–159, 1989.

Francisco LL, Sawin LL, and Dibona GF: Mechanism of negative potassium balance in the magnesium-deficient rat. *Proc Soc Exp Biol Med* 168:382–388, 1981.

Frommer JP: Lactic acidosis. *Med Clin North Am* 67:815–829, 1983.

Garzon AA, Cheng C, Lerner B, et al.: Hydroxyethyl starch (HES) and bleeding: An experimental investigation of its effect on hemostasis. *J Trauma* 7:757–766, 1967.

Gines A, Fernandez-Esparrach G, Monescillo A, et al.: Randomized trial comparing albumin, dextran 70, and polygeline in cirrhotic patients with ascites treated by paracentesis. *Gastroenterology* 111:1002–1010, 1996.

Gliedman ML, Girardet RE, Schwartz A, et al.: Hepatic vascular anatomy and manometry in experimental biliary obstruction and ascites. *Surg Gynecol Obstet* 119:749–757, 1964.

Gliedman ML, Carroll HJ, Popowitz L, et al.: An experimental hepatorenal syndrome. *Surg Gynecol Obstet* 131:34–40, 1970.

Gollub S, Schaefer C, and Squitieri A: The bleeding tendency associated with plasma expanders. *Surg Gynecol Obstet* 124:1203–1211, 1967.

Good DW: Effects of potassium on ammonia transport by medullary thick ascending limbs of the rat. *J Clin Invest* 80:1358–1365, 1987.

Grauer GF and Pitts RP: Primary polydipsia in three dogs with portosystemic shunts. *J Am Anim Hosp Assoc* 23:197–200, 1987.

Graves TK, Schall WD, Refsal K, and Nachrenier RF: Basal and ACTH-stimulated plasma aldosterone concentrations are normal or increased in dogs with trichuriasis-associated pseudohypoadrenocorticism. *J Vet Intern Med* 8:287–289, 1994.

Gregory CR, Guiilford WG, Berry CR, et al.: Enteric function in cats after subtotal colectomy for treatment of megacoon. *Vet Surg* 19:216–220, 1990.

Hamer DH and Gorbach SL: Intestinal diarrhea and bacterial food poisoning. In Sleisinger MH: *Gastrointestinal and Liver Disease. Pathophysiology, Diagnosis and Management*, 6th ed, Vol 2. Philadelphia, WB Saunders Co., pp. 1594–1632, 1998.

Happe RP and DeBruijne JJ: Pentagastrin stimulated gastric secretion in the dog (orogastric aspiration technique). *Res Vet Sci* 33:232–239, 1982.

Harper CG and Kril JJ: Neuropathological changes in alcoholics. In Hunt W and Nixon SJ (eds): *Alcohol-Induced Brain Damage*. Research Monograph 22. Washington, DC, National Institutes of Health, pp. 39–70, 1993.

Harvey CJ, Lopez JW, and Hendrick MJ: An uncommon intestinal manifestation of feline infectious peritonitis: 26 cases (1986–1993). *J Am Vet Med Assoc* 209:1117–1120, 1996.

Harvey JW and West CL: Prednisone-induced increases in serum alpha-2-globulin and haptoglobin concentrations in dogs. *Vet Pathol* 24:90–92, 1987.

Haskins SC: Shock. In Kirk RW, Bistner SI, and Ford RB (eds): *Handbook of Veterinary Procedures and Emergency Treatment*, 5th ed. Philadelphia, WB Saunders Co., pp. 33–52, 1990.

Haupt MT and Rackow EC: Colloid osmotic pressure and fluid resuscitation with hetastarch, albumin, and saline solutions. *Crit Care Med* 10:159–162, 1982.

Haussinger D, Kaiser S, Stehle T, et al.: Liver carbonic anhydrase and urea synthesis. The effect of diuretics. *Biochem Pharmacol* 35:3317–3322, 1986.

Heald RD, Jones BD, and Schmidt DA: Blood gas and electrolyte concentrations in canine parvoviral enteritis. *J Am Anim Hosp Assoc* 22:745–748, 1986.

Hedenstierna G, Soderman C, Eriksson L, et al.: Ventilation-perfusion inequality in patients with non-alcoholic liver cirrhosis. *Eur Respir J* 4:711–717, 1991.

Heinemann HO, Emirgil C, and Mijnssen JP: Hyperventilation and arterial hypoxemia in cirrhosis of the liver. *Am J Med* 28:239–246, 1960.

Henriksen HJ, Ring-Larsen H, and Christensen NJ: Autonomic nervous function in liver disease. In Bomzon A and Blendis LM (eds): *Cardiovascular Complications of Liver Disease*. Boca Raton, FL, CRC Press, pp. 63–79, 1989.

Hess RS, Saunders HM, Van Winkle TJ, et al. Clinical, clinicopathologic, radiographic, and ultrasonographic abnormalities in dogs with fatal acute pancreatitis: 70 cases (1986–1995). *J Am Vet Med Assoc* 213:665–670, 1998.

Heymsfield SB, Arteaga C, McManus C, et al.: Measurement of muscle mass in humans: Validity of the 24-hour urinary creatinine method. *Am J Clin Nutr* 37:478–494, 1983.

Heymsfield SB, Waki M, and Reinus J: Are patients with chronic liver disease hypermetabolic? *Hepatology* 11:502–504, 1990.

Hill RC and Van Winkle TJ: Acute necrotizing and acute suppurative pancreatitis in the cat: A retrospective study of 40 cases (1976–1989). *J Vet Intern Med* 7:25–33, 1993.

Hoffenberg R: Control of albumin degradation in vivo and in the perfused liver. In Rothschild MA, Waldmann T (eds): *Plasma Protein Metabolism: Regulation of Synthesis, Distribution and Degradation.* New York, Academic Press, pp. 239–255, 1970.

Horton JW, Dunn CW, Burnweit CA, et al.: Hypertonic saline dextran resuscitation of acute canine bile-induced pancreatitis. *Am J Surg* 158:48–56, 1989.

Hulse J and Yacobi A: Hetastarch: An overview of the colloid and its metabolism. *Drug Intell Clin Pharmacol* 17:334–341, 1983.

Ingles A, Hernandez I, Garcia-Estan J, et al.: Limited cardiac preload reserve in conscious cirrhotic rats. *Am J Physiol* 260: H1912–H1917, 1991.

Inadomi DW and Kopple JD: Fluid and electrolyte disorders in total parenteral nutrition. In Maxwell MH, Kleeman CR, and Narins RG (eds): *Clinical Disorders of Fluid and Electrolyte Metabolism*, 4th ed. New York, McGraw-Hill Book Company, pp. 945–966, 1987.

Izquierdo R, Bermes E Jr, Sandberg L, et al.: Serum calcium metabolism in acute experimental pancreatitis. *Surgery* 98:1031–1037, 1985.

Jacobs RM, Weiser MG, Hall RL, et al.: Clinicopathologic findings of canine parvoviral enteritis. *J Am Anim Hosp Assoc* 16:809–814, 1980.

Jimenez W, Martinez-Pardo A, Arroyo V, et al.: Temporal relationship between hyperaldosteronism, sodium retention and ascites formation in rats with experimental cirrhosis. *Hepatology* 5:245–250, 1985.

Justin RB and Hohenhaus AE: Hypophosphatemia associated with enteral alimentation in cats. *J Vet Intern Med* 9:228–233, 1995.

Karanjia ND, Lutrin FJ, Chang Y-B, et al.: Low dose dopamine protects against hemorrhagic pancreatitis in cats. *J Surg Res* 48:440–443, 1990.

Karlson KE, Garzon AA, Shaftan GW, et al.: Increased blood loss associated with administration of certain plasma expanders: Dextran 75, dextran 40, and hydroxyethyl starch. *Surgery* 62:670–678, 1967.

Kaup FJ, Drommer W, Kersten U, et al.: Ultrastrukturelle untersuchungen bei einem Fall von intestinaler Lymphangiektasie. *Kleintierpraxis* 33:81–86, 1988.

Kelly DA and Summerfield JA: Hemostasis in liver disease. *Semin Liver Dis* 7:182–191, 1987.

Kircheis G, Nilius R, Held C, et al.: Therapeutic efficacy of L-ornithine-L-aspartate infusions in patients with cirrhosis and hepatic encephalopathy: Results of a placebo-controlled, double-blind study. *Hepatology* 25:1351–1360, 1997.

Kirsch RE, Saunders SJ, Frith L, et al: Plasma amino acid regulation of albumin synthesis. *J Nutr* 98:395–403, 1969.

Kisloff B and Schaffer G: Fulminant hepatic failure secondary to congestive heart failure. *Am J Dig Dis* 21:895–900, 1976.

Kitchell BE, Strombeck DR, Cullen J, and Harrold D: Clinical and pathologic changes in experimentally induced acute pancreatitis in cats. *Am J Vet Res* 47:1170–1173, 1986.

Klar E, Herfarth C, and Messmer K: Therapeutic effect of isovolemic hemodilution with dextran 60 on the impairment of pancreatic microcirculation in acute biliary pancreatitis. *Ann Surg* 211:346, 1990.

Koj A, Gauldie J, Regoeczi E, et al: The acute-phase response of cultured rat hepatocytes. *Biochem J* 224:505–514, 1984.

Kostreva DR, Castaner A, and Kampine JP: Reflex effects of hepatic baroreceptors on renal and cardiac sympathetic nerve activity. *Am J Physiol* 238:R390–R394, 1980.

Kozlowski S and Krzysztof D: The role of osmoreception in portal circulation in control of water intake in dogs. *Acta Physiol Pol* 24:325–330, 1973.

Kreisberg RA: Lactate homeostasis and lactic acidosis. *Ann Intern Med* 92:227–237, 1980.

Kreisberg RA: Pathogenesis and management of lactic acidosis. *Annu Rev Med* 35:181–193, 1984.

Krejs GJ: VIPoma syndrome. *Am J Med* 82:37–47, 1987.

Krowka MJ and Cortese DA: Pulmonary aspects of chronic liver disease and liver transplantation. *Mayo Clin Proc* 60:407–418, 1985.

Krowka MJ and Cortese DA: Hepatopulmonary syndrome. Current concepts in diagnostic and therapeutic considerations. *Chest* 105:1528–1537, 1994.

Kruse JA, Zaidi SAJ, and Carlson RW: Significance of blood lactate levels in critically ill patients with liver disease. *Am J Med* 83:77–82, 1987.

Laffi G, Lagi A, Cipriani M, et al.: Impaired cardiovascular autonomic response to passive tilting in cirrhosis with ascites. *Hepatology* 24:1063–1067, 1996.

Lantz GC: The pathophysiology of acute mechanical small bowel obstruction. *Compend Contin Educ Pract Vet* 3:910–917, 1981.

Lebenthal E and Duffey ME: *Textbook of Secretary Diarrhea.* New York, Raven Press, 1990.

Lee SS: Cardiac abnormalities in liver cirrhosis. *West J Med* 151:530–535, 1989.

Lee SS, Marty J, Mantz J, et al.: Densitization of myocardial β-adrenergic receptors in cirrhotic rats. *Hepatology* 12:481–485, 1990.

Levy M: Sodium retention and ascites formation in dogs with experimental portal cirrhosis. *Am J Physiol* 233:F572–F585, 1977a.

Levy M: Sodium retention in dogs with cirrhosis and ascites: Efferent mechanisms. *Am J Physiol* 233:F586–F592, 1977b.

Levy M and Allotey JB: Temporal relationships between urinary salt retention and altered systemic hemodynamics in dogs with experimental cirrhosis. *J Lab Clin Med* 92:560–569, 1978.

Levy M and Wexler MJ: Renal sodium retention and ascites formation in dogs with experimental cirrhosis but without portal hypertension or increased splanchnic vascular capacity. *J Lab Clin Med* 91:520–536, 1978.

Levy M and Wexler MJ: Hepatic denervation alters first-phase urinary sodium excretion in dogs with cirrhosis. *Am J Physiol* 253:F664–F671, 1987a.

Levy M and Wexler MJ: Sodium excretion in dogs with low grade caval constriction: Role of hepatic nerves. *Am J Physiol* 253:F672–F678, 1987b.

Lewis JH, Szeto IL, and Bayer WL: Severe hemodilution with hydroxyethyl starch and dextrans. *Arch Surg* 93:941–950, 1966.

Lifton SJ, King LG, and Zerbe CA: Glucocorticoid deficient hypoadrenocorticism in dogs: 18 cases (1986–1995). *J Am Vet Med Assoc* 209:2076–2081, 1996.

Lloyd KKC and Debas HT: Peripheral regulation of gastric acid secretion. In Johnson LR (ed): *Physiology of the Gastrointestinal Tract*, 3rd ed. New York, Raven Press, pp. 1185–1226, 1994.

Lopez-Novoa JM, Rengel MA, and Hernando L: Dynamics of ascites formation in rats with experimental cirrhosis. *Am J Physiol* 238:F353, 1980.

Lunn PG and Austin S: Excess energy intake promotes the development of hypoalbuminemia in rats fed on low-protein diets. *Br J Nutr* 49:9–16, 1983.

Ma Z and Lee SS: Cirrhotic cardiomyopathy: Getting to the heart of the matter. *Hepatology* 24:451–459, 1996.

Macintyre E, Mackie IJ, Ho D, et al.: The haemostatic effects of hydroxyethyl starch (HES) used as a volume expander. *Intensive Care Med* 11:300–303, 1985.

Macy DW: Feline pancreatitis. In Kirk RW and Bonagura JD (eds): *Current Veterinary Therapy X.* Philadelphia, WB Saunders, pp. 893–896, 1989.

Malik R, Hunt GB, Hinchlifke JM, and Church DB: Severe whipworm infection in the dog. *J Small Anim Pract* 31:185–188, 1990.

McCullough AJ, Mullen KD, and Kalhan SC: Measurements of total body and extracellular water in cirrhotic patients with and without ascites. *Hepatology* 14:1102–1111, 1991.

Meier PJ: Molecular mechanisms of hepatic bile salt transport from sinusoidal blood into bile. *Am J Physiol* 269:G801–G812, 1995.

Melgarejo T, Roheleder J, Williams DA, and Simpson KW: Immunoelectrophoretic characterization of plasma α_1-protease inhibitor in dogs with experimental pancreatitis. *J Vet Intern Med* 10:157, A33, 1996.

Mendelson JH, Ogata M, and Mello NK: Effects of alcohol ingestion and withdrawal on magnesium states of alcoholics: Clinical and experimental findings. *Ann N Y Acad Sci* 162:918–933, 1969.

Metcalf W, Padadopoulos A, Tufaro R, et al.: A clinical physiologic study of hydroxyethyl starch. *Surg Gynecol Obstet* 131:255–267, 1970.

Meuten DJ, Chew DJ, Capen CC, et al.: Relationship of serum total calcium to albumin and total protein in dogs. *J Am Vet Med Assoc* 180:63–67, 1982.

Mishler JM: *Pharmacology of Hydroxyethyl Starch. Use in Therapy and Blood Banking.* Oxford, Oxford University Press, pp. 1–118, 1982.

Mishler JM, Borberg H, Emerson PM, et al.: Hydroxyethyl starch. An agent for hypovolaemic shock treatment II: Urinary excretion in normal volunteers following three consecutive daily infusions. *Br J Clin Pharmacol* 4:591–595, 1977.

Moore LE and Garvey MS: The effect of hetastarch on serum colloid oncotic pressure in hypoalbuminemic dogs. *J Vet Intern Med* 10:300–303, 1996.

Moore R and Carpenter J: Intramural hematoma causing obstruction in three dogs. *J Am Vet Med Assoc* 184:186–188, 1984a.

Moore R and Carpenter J: Intestinal sclerosis with pseudo-obstruction in three dogs. *J Am Vet Med Assoc* 184:830–833, 1984b.

Morgan EH and Peters T: The biosynthesis of rat serum albumin: V. Effect of protein depletion and refeeding on albumin and transferrin synthesis. *J Biol Chem* 246:3500–3507, 1971.

Morito T, Nishimake T, Saito K, et al.: Dextran and antidextran antibodies in the sera of patients with liver diseases. *Int Arch Allergy Appl Immunol* 78:213–217, 1985.

Moseley RH: Fluid and electrolyte disorders and gastrointestinal disease. In Kokko JP and Tannen RL (eds): *Fluid and Electrolytes*. Philadelphia, WB Saunders, p. 675, 1996.

Moshage HJ, Janssen JAM, Franssen JH, et al: Study of the molecular mechanisms of decreased liver synthesis of albumin in inflammation. *J Clin Invest* 79:1635–1641, 1987.

Muir WW: Acid-base and electrolyte disturbances in dogs with gastric dilatation-volvulus. *J Am Vet Med Assoc* 181:229–231, 1982.

Murphy GP, Demaree DE, and Gagnon JA: The renal and systemic effects of hydroxyethyl starch solution infusions. *J Urol* 93:534–539, 1965.

Musch MW, Miller RJ, Field M, et al.: Stimulation of colonic secretion by lipoxygenase metabolites of arachidonic acid. *Science* 217:1255–1256, 1982.

Nelson DC, McGrew WRG, and Hoyumpa AM: Hypernatremia and lactulose therapy. *JAMA* 249:1295–1298, 1983.

Norenberg MD: The astrocyte in liver disease. *Advances in Cellular Neurobiology*. San Diego, CA, Academic Press, pp. 303–352, 1981.

Ohlsson K: Interactions in vitro and in vivo between dog trypsin and dog plasma protease inhibitors. *Scand J Clin Lab Invest* 28:219, 1971.

Ooms L and Degryse A: Pathogenesis and pharmacology of diarrhea. *Vet Res Commun* 10:355–397, 1986.

Owens JM, Drazner FH, and Gilbertson SR: Pancreatic disease in the cat. *J Am Anim Hosp Assoc* 11:83–89, 1975.

Papdakis MA and Arieff AI: Unpredictability of clinical evaluation of renal function in cirrhosis. Prospective study. *Am J Med* 82:945–953, 1987.

Papper S: The role of the kidney in Laennec's cirrhosis of the liver. *Medicine (Baltimore)* 37:299–309, 1958.

Papper S, Belsky JL, and Bleifer KH: Renal failure in Laennec's cirrhosis of the liver I. Description of clinical and laboratory features. *Ann Intern Med* 51:759–765, 1959.

Parth E, Jurecka W, and Szepfalusi Z: Histological and immunohistochemical investigations of hydroxyethyl starch deposits in rat tissues. *Eur Surg Res* 24:13–21, 1992.

Peoples JB: The role of pH in altering serum ionized calcium concentration. *Surgery* 104:370–374, 1988.

Planas R, Gines P, Arroyo V, et al.: Dextran-70 versus albumin as plasma expanders in cirrhotic patients with tense ascites treated with total paracentesis. Results of a randomized study. *Gastroenterology* 99:1736–1744, 1990.

Presig R, Bircher J, and Paumgartner G: Physiologic and pathophysiologic aspects of the hepatic hemodynamics. *Prog Liver Dis* 4:201–216, 1972.

Prytz H and Thomsen AC: Acid-base status in liver cirrhosis. Disturbances in stable, terminal and porta-caval shunted patients. *Scand J Gastroenterol* 11:249–256, 1976.

Pugh P and Stone SL: The ionic composition of bile. *J Physiol (Lond)* 201:50P–51P, 1969.

Ramond MJ, Comay E, and Lebrec D: Alterations in isoprenaline sensitivity in patients with cirrhosis: Evidence of abnormality of the sympathetic nervous activity. *Br J Clin Pharmacol* 21:191–196, 1986.

Rattner DW, Napolitano LM, Corsetti J, et al.: Hypocalcemia in experimental pancreatitis occurs independently of changes in serum nonesterified fatty acid levels. *Int J Pancreatol* 6(4):249–262, 1990.

Record CO, Iles RA, Cohen RD, et al.: Acid-base and metabolic disturbances in fulminant hepatic failure. *Gut* 16:144–149, 1975.

Robinson EP and Hardy RM: Clinical signs, diagnosis and treatment of alkalemia in dogs: 20 cases (1982–1984). *J Am Vet Med Assoc* 192:943–949, 1988.

Rodman T, Sobel M, Close HP, et al.: Arterial oxygen unsaturation and the ventilation-perfusion defect of Laennec's cirrhosis. *N Engl J Med* 263:73–79, 1960.

Rodriguez-Roisin R, Roca J, Agusti AGN, et al.: Gas exchange and pulmonary vascular reactivity in patients with liver cirrhosis. *Am Rev Respir Dis* 135:1085–1092, 1987.

Rolla G, Brussino L, Colagrande P, et al.: Exhaled nitric oxide and oxygenation abnormalities in hepatic cirrhosis. *Hepatology* 26:842–847, 1997.

Romatowski J: Use of oral fluids in acute gastroenteritis in small animals. *Mod Vet Pract* 66:261–263, 1985.

Rose BD: Metabolic alkalosis. In *Clinical Physiology of Acid-Base and Electrolyte Disorders*, 2nd ed. New York, McGraw-Hill, pp. 374–393, 1984.

Rothschild MA, Oratz M, Dessler R, et al: Albumin synthesis in cirrhotic subjects with ascites studied with carbonate.[14] *J Clin Invest* 48:344–350, 1969.

Rothschild MA, Oratz M, and Schreiber SS: Serum albumin. *Hepatology* 8:385–401, 1988.

Rudloff E and Kirby R: The critical need for colloids: selecting the right colloid. *Compend Contin Educ* 19:811–825, 1997.

Ruiz-del Arbol L, Monescillo A, Jimenez W, et al.: Paracentesis-induced circulatory dysfunction: Mechanisms and effect on hepatic hemodynamics in cirrhosis. *Gastroenterology* 113:579–586, 1997.

Ruppin H, Bar-Meir S, Soergel KH, et al.: Absorption of short chain fatty acids by the colon. *Gastroenterology* 78:1500–1507, 1980.

Sacerdoti D, Bolognesi M, Merkel C, et al.: Renal vasoconstriction in cirrhosis evaluated by duplex Doppler ultrasonography. *Hepatology* 17:219–224, 1993.

Sachs G: The gastric H^+/K^+-ATPase. In Johnson LR (ed): *Physiology of the Gastrointestinal Tract*, 3rd ed. New York, Raven Press, p. 1119, 1994.

Sack DA, Chowdhury AMAK, Eusof A, et al.: Oral rehydration of rotavirus diarrhea: A double blind comparison of sucrose with glucose electrolyte solution. *Lancet* 2:280–283, 1978.

Saffer LJ, Dantes DA, and Sobotka H: Utilization of intravenously injected sodium D-lactate as a test of hepatic function. *Arch Intern Med* 62:918–924, 1938.

Salvatore F, Cimino F, d'Ayello-Caracciolo M, et al.: Mechanism of the protection by L-ornithine-L-aspartate mixture and by L-arginine in ammonia intoxication. *Arch Biochem Biophys* 107:499–508, 1964.

Santosham M, Daum RS, Dillman L, et al.: A controlled study of well-nourished children hospitalized in the United States and Panama. *N Engl J Med* 306:1070–1076, 1982.

Sanfilippo MJ, Suberviola PD, and Geimer NF: Development of a von Willebrand–like syndrome after prolonged use of hydroxyethyl starch. *Am J Clin Pathol* 88:653–655, 1987.

Sarfeh IH, Aaronson S, Lombino D, et al: Selective impairment of nutrient absorption from intestines with chronic venous hypertension. *Surgery* 99:266–269, 1986.

Schaer M: A clinicopathologic survey of acute pancreatitis in 30 dogs and 5 cats. *J Am Anim Hosp Assoc* 15:681–687, 1979.

Schenker S, Breen KJ, and Hoyumpa AM: Hepatic encephalopathy: Current status. *Gastroenterology* 66:121–151, 1974.

Schrier RW, Arroyo V, Bernardi M, et al: Peripheral arterial vasodilation hypothesis: A proposal for the initiation of renal sodium and water retention in cirrhosis. *Hepatology* 8:1151–1157, 1988.

Sebastian A, Sutton JM, Hulter HM, et al: Effect of mineralocorticoid replacement therapy on renal acid-base homeostasis in adrenalectomized patients. *Kidney Int* 18:762–763, 1980.

Sellin JH: Intestinal electrolyte absorption and secretion. In Sleisinger MH, Fordtran JS, Feldman M, and Scharschmidt BT (eds): *Gastrointestinal and Liver Disease Pathophysiology, Diagnosis and Management*, 6th ed., Vol 2. Philadelphia, WB Saunders Co., pp. 1451–1471, 1998.

Sevelius E: Chronic liver disease in the dog: A demographic, aetiologic, diagnostic and prognostic study. Thesis, Swedish University of Agricultural Sciences, Department of Pathology, Uppsala, Sweden, 1995.

Sevelius E and Andersson M: Serum protein electrophoresis as a prognostic marker of chronic liver disease in dogs. *Vet Rec* 137:663–667, 1995.

Shear L, Kleinerman J, and Gabuzda GJ: Renal failure in patients with cirrhosis of the liver. I. Clinical and pathologic characteristics. *Am J Med* 39:184–189, 1965.

Shields R: The absorption and secretion of fluid and electrolytes by the obstructed bowel. *Br J Surg* 52:774–779, 1965.

Simon MA, Diez J, and Prieto J: Abnormal sympathetic and renal response to sodium restriction in compensated cirrhosis. *Gastroenterology* 101:1354–1360, 1991.

Simpson KW: Current concepts of the pathogenesis and pathophysiology of acute pancreatitis in the dog and cat. *Compend Contin Educ Pract Vet* 15:247–254, 1993.

Simpson KW: Acute Pancreatitis. In August JR (ed): *Consultations in Feline Internal Medicine III*. Philadelphia, WB Saunders, pp. 91–98, 1997.

Simpson KW and Dykes NL: Diagnosis and treatment of gastrinoma. *Semin Vet Med Surg (Small Anim)* 12:274–281, 1997.

Simpson KW, Alpers DH, DeWille J, et al.: Cellular localization and hormonal regulation of pancreatic intrinsic factor secretion in dogs. *Am J Physiol* 265:G178–188, 1993.

Simpson KW, Shiroma JT, Biller DS, et al.: Ante mortem diagnosis of pancreatitis in four cats. *J Small Anim Pract* 35:93–99, 1994.

Simpson KW, Beechey-Newman N, Lamb CR, et al.: Cholecystokinin-8 induces edematous pancreatitis in dogs which is associated with a short burst of trypsinogen activation. *Dig Dis Sci* 40:2152–2161, 1995.

Sladen GE and Dawson AM: Interrelationships between the absorptions of glucose, sodium and water by the normal human jejunum. *Clin Sci* 36:119–132, 1969.

Sladen GE, Parsons DS, and Dupre J: Effects of bicarbonate on intestinal absorption. *Gut* 9:731, 1968.

Smiley LE and Garvey MS: The use of hetastarch as adjunct therapy in 26 dogs with hypoalbuminemia: A phase two clinical trial. *J Vet Intern Med* 8:195–202, 1994.

Sola R, Vila MC, Andreu M, et al.: Total paracentesis with dextran 40 vs diuretics in the treatment of ascites in cirrhosis: A randomized controlled study. *J Hepatol* 20:282–288, 1994.

Soll AH and Berglindh T: Receptors that regulate gastric acid-secretory function. In Johnson LR (ed): *Physiology of the Gastrointestinal Tract*, 3rd ed. New York, Raven Press, pp. 1139–1169, 1994.

Somberg KA, Lake JR, Romlanovich SJ, et al: Transjugular intrahepatic portosystemic shunts for refractory ascites: Assessment of clinical and hormonal response and renal function. *Hepatology* 21:709–716, 1995.

Standl T, Lipfert B, Reeker W, et al.: Acute effects of complete blood exchanges with ultra-purified hemoglobin solution or hydroxyethyl starch on liver and kidney in the animal model. *Anasthesiol Intensivmed Notfallmed Schmerzther* 31:354–361, 1996.

Stoff JS: Phosphate homeostasis and hypophosphatemia. *Am J Med* 72:489–495; 1982.

Strombeck DR: Small and large intestine: Normal structure and function. In Guilford WG, Center SA, Strombeck DR, et al. (eds): *Strombeck's Small Animal Gastroenterology*, 3rd ed. Philadelphia, WB Saunders, Co., p. 318, 1996.

Stump DC, Strauss RG, Henriksen RA, et al.: Effects of hydroxyethyl starch on blood coagulation, particularly factor VIII. *Transfusion* 25:230–234, 1985.

Sussman NL: Fulminant hepatic failure. In Zakim DL and Boyer TD (eds): *Hepatology: A Textbook of Liver Disease*. Philadelphia, WB Saunders Co., pp. 618–650, 1996.

Symington BE: Hetastarch and bleeding complications. *Ann Intern Med* 105:627–628, 1986.

Tanifuji Y, Kamide M, Shudo Y, et al: Clinical evaluation of acetated ringer as intraoperative fluids for patients with liver cirrhosis. *Masui* 32:1347–1352, 1983.

Tannen RL: Relationship of renal ammonia production and potassium homeostasis. *Kidney Int* 11:453–465, 1977.

Tannen RL: Ammonia and acid base homeostasis. *Med Clin North Am* 67:781–798, 1983.

Tannen RL and Kunin AS: Effect of pH on ammonia production by renal mitochondria. *Am J Physiol* 231:1631–1637, 1976.

Terg R, Berreta J, Abecasis R, et al.: Dextran administration avoids hemodynamic changes following paracentesis in cirrhotic patients. A safe and inexpensive option. *Dig Dis Sci* 37:79–83, 1992.

Terg R, Miguez CD, Castro L, et al.: Pharmacokinetics of dextran-70 in patients with cirrhosis and ascites undergoing therapeutic paracentesis. *J Hepatol* 25:329–333, 1996.

Therrien G, Rose C, Butterworth J, et al.: Protective effect of L-carnitine in ammonia-precipitated encephalopathy in the portacaval shunted rat. *Hepatology* 25:551–556, 1997.

Thillainayagam AV, Hunt JB, and Farthing MJG: Enhancing clinical efficiency of oral rehydration therapy: Is low osmolality the key? *Gastroenterology* 114:197–210, 1998.

Thompson WL and Gadsden RH: Prolonged bleeding times and hypofibrinogenemia in dogs after infusion of hydroxyethyl starch and dextran. *Transfusion* 5:440–446, 1965.

Thompson WL, Fukushima T, Rutherford RB, et al.: Intravascular persistence, tissue storage, and excretion of hydroxyethyl starch. *Surg Gynecol Obstet* 131:965–972, 1970.

Tobias TA and Schertel ER: Shock: Concepts and management. In DiBartola SP (ed): *Fluid Therapy in Small Animal Practice*. Philadelphia, WB Saunders Co., pp. 436–470, 1992.

Twedt DC and Grauer GF: Fluid therapy for gastrointestinal, pancreatic and hepatic disorders. *Vet Clin North Am* 12:463–485, 1982.

Unikowsky B, Wexler MJ, and Levy M: Dogs with experimental

cirrhosis of the liver but without intrahepatic hypertension do not retain sodium or form ascites. *J Clin Invest* 72:1594–1604, 1983.

Vaamonde CA: Renal water handling in liver disease. In Epstein M (ed): *The Kidney in Liver Disease*, 3rd ed, Baltimore, Williams & Wilkins, pp. 31–72, 1988.

Van Slyke KK and Evans EI: The paradox of aciduria in presence of alkalosis caused by hypochloremia. *Ann Surg* 126:545–567, 1947.

Vollmar B, Lang G, Menger MD, et al.: Hypertonic hydroxyethyl starch restores hepatic microvascular perfusion in hemorrhagic shock. *Am J Physiol* 266:H1927–H1934, 1994.

Wall PJ and Record CO: Lactate elimination in man: Effects of lactate concentration and hepatic dysfunction. *Eur J Clin Invest* 9:397–454, 1979.

Washabau RJ and Hall JA: Gastrointestinal motility disorders of dogs and cats. *Eur J Comp Gastroenterol* 2:9–19, 1997.

Wells BT: Use of a gelatin solution in hypovolaemia and toxaemia in small animals. *Vet Rec* 107:85–87, 1980.

Wendon JA, Harrison PM, Keays R, et al: Cerebral blood flow and metabolism in fulminant liver failure. *Hepatology* 19:1407–1413, 1994.

Wiesen S, Reddy KR, Jeffers LJ, et al.: Fulminant hepatic failure secondary to previously unrecognized cardiomyopathy. *Dig Dis* 13:199–204, 1995.

Willard MD, Zerbe CA, Schall WD, et al.: Severe hypophosphatemia associated with diabetes mellitus in six dogs and one cat. *J Am Vet Med Assoc* 190:1007–1010, 1987.

Williams DA: Malabsorption, small intestinal bacterial overgrowth, and protein-losing enteropathy. In Guilford WG, Center SA, Strombeck DR, et al. (eds): *Strombeck's Small Animal Gastroenterology*, 3rd ed. Philadelphia, WB Saunders, pp. 367–380, 1996.

Wilson GP and Burt JK: Intussusception in the dog and cat: A review of 45 cases. *J Am Vet Med Assoc* 164:515–518, 1974.

Wingfield WE, Twedt DC, Moore RW, et al.: Acid-base and electrolyte values in dogs with acute gastric dilatation-volvulus. *J Am Vet Med Assoc* 180:1070–1072, 1982.

Wong F, Girgrah N, and Blendis L: Fluid retention in cirrhosis. Review: the controversy over the pathophysiology of ascites formation in cirrhosis. *J Gastroenterol Hepatol* 12:437–444, 1997.

Wong F, Sniderman K, Liu P, et al: Transjugular intrahepatic portosystemic stent shunt: Effects on hemodynamics and sodium homeostasis in cirrhosis and refractory ascites. *Ann Intern Med* 122:816–822, 1995.

Woods HF, Connor H, and Tucker GT: The role of altered lactate kinetics in the pathogenesis of type B lactic acidosis. *CIBA Found Symp* 87:307–323, 1982.

Yacobi A, Gibson TP, McEntegart CM, et al.: Pharmacokinetics of high molecular weight hydroxyethyl starch in dogs. *Res Commun Chem Pathol Pharmacol* 36:199–204, 1982.

Yedgar S, Carew RE, Pittman RC, et al: Tissue sites of catabolism of albumin in rabbits. *Am J Physiol* 244:E101–E107, 1983

Zavagli G: Anomalie del ricambio del potassia. In Introzzi P (ed): *Trattato Italiano di Medicina Interna*. Part IX, ed 3. Firenze, USES, pp. 1162–1164, 1986.

Zavagli G, Ricci G, Bader G, et al: The importance of the highest normokalemia in the treatment of early hepatic encephalopathy. *Miner Electrolyte Metab* 19(6):362–367, 1993.

Zieve L: The mechanisms of hepatic coma. *Hepatology* 1:360–365, 1981.

Zieve L, Lyftogt C, and Raphael D: Ammonia toxicity: Comparative protective effect of various arginine and ornithine derivatives, aspartate, benzoate, and carbamyl glutamate. *Metab Brain Dis* 1:25–35, 1986.

Zimmon DS, Oratz M, Kessler R, et al: Albumin to ascites: Demonstration of a direct pathway bypassing the systemic circulation. *J Clin Invest* 48:2074–2078, 1969.

CHAPTER 17

Fluid Therapy in Endocrine and Metabolic Disorders

AMY M. GROOTERS

Animals with endocrinopathies or metabolic disorders often develop serious abnormalities of electrolyte and acid-base balance as a complication of their underlying disease. Examples commonly encountered in small animal practice include development of metabolic acidosis and hyperglycemia in patients with diabetic ketoacidosis (DKA), hyponatremia and hyperkalemia in patients with hypoadrenocorticism, and hypotension and coagulopathy in patients with heatstroke. Prompt recognition and treatment of these abnormalities are essential to successful management of patients and require both an understanding of the pathophysiologic mechanisms responsible for their development and familiarity with the advantages and disadvantages of various therapeutic options.

▶ Diabetic Ketoacidosis

Ketoacidosis is a potentially life-threatening complication of diabetes mellitus that is commonly encountered in small animal practice. It is characterized by a complex set of metabolic derangements that stem from relative or absolute insulin deficiency combined with diabetogenic hormone excess. Affected animals are typically presented with signs of multiple organ dysfunction including anorexia, vomiting, lethargy, weakness, tachypnea, and dehydration. Concurrent disorders such as pancreatitis, pneumonia, urinary tract infection, and congestive heart failure often are present. The diagnosis of DKA usually is based on the presence of ketones in the urine of a diabetic animal that is showing signs of systemic illness. Further supportive findings include severe hyperglycemia, dehydration, azotemia, and a high-anion-gap metabolic acidosis. When the diagnosis of DKA has been made, goals of therapy should include correction of hypovolemia, administration of insulin, correction of electrolyte and acid-base imbalances, and treatment of complicating concurrent disorders.

Pathophysiology

Ketoacidosis develops as a result of a shift in the balance between insulin and the counterregulatory hormones (glucagon, cortisol, growth hormone, and catecholamines) that antagonize its actions. The resultant state of relative or absolute insulin deficiency promotes lipolysis, proteolysis, and ketogenesis; stimulates hepatic glucose production; and inhibits glucose utilization, effectively shifting intermediary metabolism in insulin-sensitive tissues from a carbohydrate-metabolizing system to a fat-metabolizing system (Kitabchi and Wall 1995).

LIPOLYSIS AND PROTEOLYSIS

Insulin, through its actions on hormone-sensitive lipase in adipose tissue, is a potent inhibitor of lipolysis (Ganong 1993). Deficiency of insulin therefore permits the breakdown of stored triglycerides into glycerol and free fatty acids, which are presented to the liver as precursors for gluconeogenesis and ketogenesis, respectively. In the absence of insulin, lipolysis is accelerated by catecholamines (which act through β receptors to increase tissue lipase activity) (Ganong 1993) and by growth hormone and cortisol (Feldman and Nelson 1996a). Relative insulin deficiency and counterregulatory hormone excess also promote proteolysis, resulting in increased plasma concentrations of amino acids, which are precursors for hepatic gluconeogenesis (Kitabchi and Wall 1995).

KETOGENESIS AND KETONE UTILIZATION

Enhanced ketone production in DKA results from increased availability of ketoacid precursors (circulating free fatty acids) combined with a shift in hepatic metabolism from fatty acid esterification and triglyceride synthesis to fatty acid oxidation and ketone production. Although both glucagon excess and insulin deficiency have significant effects on hepatic metabolism in DKA, glucagon's role in stimulating ketogenesis is primarily to increase the liver's capacity for fatty acid oxidation, whereas the major contribution of insulin deficiency is to promote mobilization of free fatty acids (McGarry and Foster 1980). Glucagon shifts hepatic metabolism by inhibiting acetyl coenzyme A (CoA) carboxylase (the enzyme that catalyzes conversion of pyruvate to acetyl CoA), which decreases hepatic concentrations of malonyl CoA. Malonyl CoA prevents fatty acid oxidation by blocking the enzyme (carnitine palmitoyltransferase I) that facilitates movement of fatty acids into hepatic mitochondria, where they undergo β-oxidation. Thus, the glucagon-induced decrease in hepatic malonyl CoA stimulates ketogenesis by permitting increased movement of fatty acids into mitochondria for oxidation and ketoacid production (McGarry and Foster 1980; Umpierrez et al. 1996). Peripheral tissue utilization of the ketones produced by this process (mainly β-hydroxybutyrate and acetoacetic acid) is impaired in the presence of insulin deficiency (Sherwin et al. 1976). As a result, they accumulate and eventually overwhelm body buffers, resulting in the high-anion-gap metabolic acidosis that typifies the ketoacidotic state.

GLUCOSE PRODUCTION AND UTILIZATION

Hyperglycemia in DKA results from increased gluconeogenesis, accelerated glycogenolysis, and decreased utilization of glucose by peripheral tissues. Increased gluconeogenesis (the most important factor contributing to hyperglycemia) (Luzi et al. 1988) is caused by glucagon excess and insulin deficiency, which stimulate glucose production by activating phosphoenolpyruvate carboxykinase, the rate-limiting enzyme of gluconeogenesis (Kitabchi and Wall 1995). Proteolysis and lipolysis contribute to increased glucose production by providing additional substrates for gluconeogenesis (amino acids and lactate from muscle and glycerol from fat) (Barrett and DeFronzo 1984). Insulin deficiency and glucagon excess also increase hepatic glucose production by accelerating the breakdown of glycogen stores (glycogenolysis), and glucagon aggravates this effect by inhibiting glycolysis. Decreased utilization of glucose by peripheral tissues (such as muscle) results from insulin deficiency, which is exacerbated by growth hormone and cortisol-induced peripheral insulin antagonism. Catecholamines also impair uptake of glucose by peripheral tissues (Kitabchi and Wall 1995), as do high concentrations of circulating amino acids (Barrett and DeFronzo 1984).

OSMOTIC DIURESIS

Both hyperglycemia and ketonemia contribute to osmotic diuresis in patients with DKA. The resultant volume depletion is compounded by inadequate oral fluid intake and increased losses associated with vomiting. Eventually, volume depletion is severe enough to decrease glomerular filtration, which contributes to the severity of hyperglycemia, and may cause prerenal azotemia. In addition to volume losses, osmotic diuresis results in significant losses of electrolytes, including sodium, potassium, phosphorus, calcium, and magnesium.

Treatment

Therapy for DKA is directed at correction of the metabolic derangements that arise from and contribute to the ketoacidotic state. Goals of treatment include improving tissue perfusion by replacing fluid deficits and expanding circulatory volume, correcting acid-base and electrolyte imbalances, decreasing serum glucose concentrations, eliminating serum ketoacids, identifying and treating concurrent disorders, and preventing complications of therapy. These goals are met through appropriate fluid and insulin administration, electrolyte supplementation, careful monitoring of the patient, and ancillary therapy for complicating disorders.

Fluid Therapy

Replacement of volume and electrolyte deficits is essential for successful management of DKA; therefore, fluid administration should be the first priority in treating the ketoacidotic patient. Fluid therapy is critical not only for restoring vascular volume and tissue perfusion but also for preserving circulatory volume when insulin-induced resolution of hyperglycemia causes plasma osmolality to drop. Fluid administration helps to resolve hyperglycemia by diluting glucose in the extracellular space, by increasing peripheral insulin delivery and glucose utilization (Rosenbloom and Hanas 1996; Diehl and Wheeler 1992), and by improving renal perfusion, thereby increasing urinary excretion of glucose (Kitabchi and Wall 1995; Waldhausl et al. 1979; Owen et al. 1981). Fluid therapy alone can significantly lower blood glucose concentrations, as evidenced by decreases of up to 80% over 12 to 24 h in hyperglycemic hyperosmolar human patients receiving intravenous fluids without insulin (Ennis et al. 1994). Fluid administration also reduces concentrations of counterregulatory hormones (Waldhausl et al. 1979; DeFronzo et al. 1994), which may improve cellular sensitivity to subsequent insulin administration. On the other hand, fluid therapy alone does not appear to reduce the severity of metabolic acidosis or decrease serum ketone concentrations in ketoacidotic patients (Waldhausl et al. 1979; Owen et al. 1981; Lebovitz 1995; Sacks et al. 1979; Foster and McGarry 1983).

FLUID THERAPY BEFORE INSULIN ADMINISTRATION

Because of the beneficial effects of fluid therapy in DKA, some physicians advocate rehydration for several hours before insulin administration (Kitabchi and Wall 1995; Gonzalez-Campoy and Robertson 1996). This recommendation is supported by the fact that fluid therapy has been used alone for up to 17 h without clinical deterioration in people with DKA (Waldhausl et al. 1979). Although the clinical effects of rehydration without insulin therapy have not been evaluated in small animals, data for human patients suggest that fluid administration for 1 to 2 h before insulin therapy may be beneficial in ketoacidotic dogs and cats. Two clear indications for initiating fluid therapy before insulin administration are severe hyperglycemia associated with hypotension (Barrett and DeFronzo 1984) and the presence of significant hypokalemia (serum potassium concentration < 2.5–3.0 mEq/L) at the time of presentation (Umpierrez et al. 1996; DeFronzo et al. 1994). Administration of insulin to patients with severe hyperglycemia causes a shift of glucose and water from the extracellular to the intracellular space, resulting in a sudden decrease in intravascular volume that could exacerbate any preexistent hypotension and precipitate vascular collapse (DeFronzo et al. 1994; Nichols and Crenshaw 1995). Similarly, insulin therapy can worsen hypokalemia by causing an intracellular shift of potassium; therefore, in patients with significant hypokalemia at the time of presentation, parenteral potassium supplementation should begin before insulin administration (Umpierrez et al. 1996; DeFronzo et al. 1994).

CHOICE OF FLUID TYPE

Although ketoacidotic patients are more deficient in free water than electrolytes, isotonic fluids should be administered initially because of their ability to expand circulatory volume and enhance renal perfusion (Kitabchi and Wall 1995; Umpierrez et al. 1996; Lebovitz 1995; Macintire 1995). The initial fluid of choice is 0.9% saline, which aids in replacing both sodium and volume deficits. In patients presented with signs of hypovolemic shock, colloids are preferred for initial fluid therapy (Umpierrez et al. 1996; Diehl and Wheeler 1992; Hillman 1987).

Despite severe hyperglycemia and sometimes azotemia, most DKA patients are not severely hyperosmolar because of their concurrent sodium deficits. However, when the occasional ketoacidotic patient with severe hyperosmolality (measured or calculated* serum osmolality > 350 mOsm/kg) is encountered, some clinicians recommend initial administration of hypotonic fluids, such as 0.45% saline (Feldman and Nelson 1996a; Nichols and Crenshaw 1995). Complications associated with initial administration of hypotonic fluids result from a rapid drop in extracellular fluid osmolality, which facilitates movement of free water into the intracellular space, potentially leading to cerebral edema (Hammond and Wallis 1992; Harris et al. 1991; Rosenbloom 1990). There is evidence that chronic hyperosmolality associated with hyperglycemia results in accumulation of intracellular solutes called idiogenic osmoles or osmolytes, which serve to maintain cerebral intracellular volume in the presence of high serum osmolality (Harris et al. 1990; Harris et al. 1993). Because intracellular concentrations of osmolytes cannot change quickly, a rapid decrease in serum osmolality produces an osmotic gradient that favors movement of water into cerebral cells. Although cerebral edema does not develop during the treatment of ketoacidotic dogs and cats as often as it does in juvenile human patients, care must still be taken not to decrease serum osmolality too rapidly.

A second disadvantage of the initial use of hypotonic fluid in DKA is the fact that water cannot be retained in the vascular space in the presence of decreasing extracellular osmolality. Therefore, hypotonic fluids are less effective than isotonic fluids for restoring circulatory volume and tissue perfusion. For these reasons (and because serum hyperosmolality typically resolves fairly rapidly as blood glucose concentration decreases in response to isotonic fluid and insulin therapy), the author rarely uses hypotonic fluids in the initial treatment of ketoacidosis.

After restoration of intravascular volume with an isotonic solution, fluid therapy may be switched to hypotonic (0.45%) saline, which more closely matches the water and sodium content of fluid lost through osmotic diuresis (Kitabchi and Wall 1995; Umpierrez et al. 1996). Once serum glucose concentration has fallen below 250 mg/dL,

---

*Serum osmolality can be calculated as osmolality (mOsm/kg) = $2(Na + K) + (glucose/18) + (BUN/2.8)$, where BUN is blood urea nitrogen.

enough 50% dextrose should be added to the fluids to make a 2.5 to 5% dextrose solution. This provides a carbohydrate substrate and allows continued insulin administration (which is necessary to resolve the ketosis) without the development of hypoglycemia.

RATE AND VOLUME OF FLUID ADMINISTRATION

In most ketoacidotic patients, an attempt should be made to replace the hydration deficit over the first 24 h while also supplying maintenance fluid needs and matching ongoing losses. More conservative rates should be used for animals with evidence of cardiac disease. Patients showing signs of shock (prolonged capillary refill time, pale mucous membranes, weak pulses) should initially receive colloid solutions (if available) or more rapid infusions of normal saline. If evidence of circulatory failure is not present, there does not appear to be any benefit from rapid fluid infusion. In fact, one study in human patients indicated that slower rates of fluid administration were more effective than rapid rates in correcting the metabolic derangements associated with DKA (Adrogue et al. 1989). Once the hydration deficit has been replaced, the rate of fluid administration should be based on maintenance requirements, ongoing gastrointestinal or urinary losses, degree of azotemia, and serial evaluation of the patient's clinical condition and body weight.

Insulin Therapy

Administration of insulin is necessary for resolving ketosis as well as for decreasing blood glucose concentration. Serum insulin concentrations of 15 to 30 μU/mL inhibit release of free fatty acids from tissues, decrease glycogenolysis, and enhance peripheral ketone utilization (Chiasson et al. 1976). Insulin concentrations of 50 to 100 μU/mL are required to inhibit hepatic gluconeogenesis (Barrett and DeFronzo 1984), whereas concentrations of 100 to 200 μU/mL are required for stimulation of peripheral glucose utilization (Barrett and DeFronzo 1984; Christensen and Orskov 1968). Therefore, any serum concentration of insulin that decreases blood glucose concentration will also effectively inhibit lipolysis and ketogenesis and stimulate ketone uptake. In patients with DKA, ketone metabolism is optimized at insulin concentrations that cause maximal inhibition of ketogenesis and glycogenolysis without marked stimulation of peripheral glucose utilization (Macintire 1993). The effectiveness of insulin therapy in DKA is dependent in large part on adequate restoration of circulatory volume and tissue perfusion by appropriate fluid administration.

Before the early 1970s, high doses of insulin were recommended for treatment of DKA in people because insulin resistance associated with counterregulatory hormone excess was presumed to be present. However, studies of human patients published since that time have demonstrated that low-dose insulin therapy (producing plasma insulin concentrations of approximately 100 μU/mL) is as effective as high-dose therapy for resolving the metabolic alterations associated with DKA but is associated with a much lower frequency of complications, such as hypoglycemia and hypokalemia (Luzi et al. 1988; Alberti et al. 1973; Kitabchi et al. 1976; Burghen et al. 1980).

Only rapidly acting insulin with a short duration of action (regular crystalline insulin) should be used in the treatment of DKA. Regular insulin can be administered to ketoacidotic dogs and cats either as a continuous intravenous infusion or as intermittent intramuscular injections. Because of its effectiveness, safety, and convenience, the low-dose intramuscular protocol is recommended for the majority of small animal patients (Feldman and Nelson 1996a; Diehl and Wheeler 1992). Either technique used in combination with appropriate fluid therapy typically resolves severe hyperglycemia within 12 h. Care must be taken not to decrease blood glucose concentrations too quickly because rapid shifts in plasma osmolality can result in loss of vascular volume or development of cerebral edema. Ketosis takes significantly longer than hyperglycemia to resolve (usually 2–3 days); therefore, it is essential to continue regular insulin therapy beyond resolution of hyperglycemia.

CONTINUOUS INTRAVENOUS INSULIN ADMINISTRATION
Intravenous (IV) infusion is the method of choice for administration of insulin to human DKA patients (Kitabchi and Wall 1995; Umpierrez et al. 1996) and has been shown to be safe and effective for treating dogs and cats (Macintire 1993). Its major drawbacks are the need for an infusion pump, placement of two IV lines per patient, and the fact that frequent monitoring of blood glucose concentration is necessary to prevent hypoglycemia (Diehl and Wheeler 1992; Macintire 1995). To prepare the infusion, regular insulin (2.2 U/kg for dogs; 1.1 U/kg for cats) is added to 250 mL of 0.9% NaCl and administered at a rate of 10 mL/h in a line separate from the IV fluids (Macintire 1993). Because insulin binds to plastic tubing, the first 50 mL should be run through the IV line and then discarded (Peterson et al. 1976). Blood glucose should be assessed every 1 to 2 h and the rate of insulin infusion adjusted as needed to ensure that blood glucose concentrations do not decline more quickly than 100 mg/dL/h. This protocol has been shown to produce plasma insulin concentrations of 100 to 200 μU/mL in dogs and gradually decrease blood glucose concentrations to 250 mg/dL or less within 12 h in the majority of affected dogs (Macintire 1993). When blood glucose falls below 250 mg/dL, enough 50% dextrose should be added to the IV fluids to make a 2.5 to 5% dextrose solution. The insulin infusion can be continued as before until ketonemia is resolved, with blood glucose concentration assessed every 2 to 4 h and the infusion rate adjusted as needed to maintain blood glucose concentrations between 75 and 300 mg/dL. Alternatively, the IV infusion can be discontinued, and regular insulin can be administered subcutaneously at a dosage of 0.5 U/kg every 6 to 8 h (Feldman and Nelson 1996a).

LOW-DOSE INTRAMUSCULAR INSULIN ADMINISTRATION
Intermittent low-dose intramuscular (IM) administration is an effective and reliable alternative to continuous IV infusion that provides practitioners with a more practical and convenient technique for insulin administration (Feldman and Nelson 1996a; Sacks et al. 1979; Chastain and Nichols 1981; Wheeler 1988), and is the author's preferred method of treatment. Low-dose IM administration has been shown to produce serum insulin concentrations of approximately 100 μU/mL in dogs (Feldman and Nelson 1996a) and in people (Kitabchi et al. 1976, 1979). With this protocol, regular insulin is administered initially at a dosage of 0.25 U/kg IM. Blood glucose concentration is reevaluated every 1 to 2 h, and repeated doses of regular insulin at 0.1 to 0.2 U/kg IM are administered every 1 to 2 h as needed to decrease blood glucose concentrations slowly. A drop in blood glucose concentration of 50 to 100 mg/dL every hour is optimal; the goal should be to lower blood glucose to a concentration of 250 mg/dL or less over 6 to 10 h. When the blood glucose concentration reaches 250 mg/dL, two changes in therapy should be made: (1) regular insulin therapy should be switched to 0.5 U/kg given subcutaneously every 6 to 8 h, and (2) enough 50% dextrose should be added to the IV fluids to make a 5% dextrose solution. Subcutaneous regular insulin therapy is continued (with dosage adjustments made to maintain blood glucose concentrations between 75 and 300 mg/dL) until ketosis has resolved.

SWITCHING TO MAINTENANCE INSULIN THERAPY
Regular insulin administration (by either the intermittent IM or continuous IV method) should be maintained until serum and urine ketones have cleared, concurrent disorders (such as pancreatitis) have resolved, the patient is eating and drinking without vomiting, and IV fluids can be discontinued (usually 2–4 days). At that time, insulin therapy should be switched to a longer acting maintenance insulin (such as NPH, Lente or Ultralente) administered once or twice daily.

Potassium Supplementation

In most ketoacidotic patients, total body stores of potassium are deficient because of kaliuresis associated with osmotic diuresis as well as decreased intake and increased gastrointestinal losses of potassium (Nardone et al. 1978). Therefore, hypokalemia is a common pretreatment finding in ketoacidotic patients (Bruskiewicz et al. 1997; Crenshaw and Peterson 1996; Ling et al. 1977). However, serum potassium concentration may be normal or even high at the time of initial presentation because of a shift of potassium from the intracellular to the extracellular compartment (Diehl and Wheeler 1992; Nichols and Crenshaw 1995). This extracellular shift classically has been attributed to the metabolic acidosis associated with DKA, which was thought to cause an exchange of potassium ions for hydrogen ions that were moving into cells (Foster and McGarry 1983; Kreisberg 1978). However, later evidence demonstrated that insulin deficiency, hyperglycemia, and decreased urinary potassium excretion associated with poor renal perfusion are equally important factors contributing to the maintenance of normal or high serum potassium concentrations in DKA patients (Adrogue et al. 1986).

Treatment for DKA typically is associated with a rapid decrease in serum potassium concentration caused by an insulin-mediated shift of potassium back into the intracellular compartment, as well as by resolution of metabolic acidosis, dilution of potassium in the extracellular space, and increased kaliuresis associated with improved renal perfusion (Kitabchi and Wall 1995; Nichols and Crenshaw 1995). For this reason, potassium supplementation usually is required during treatment of DKA, even in patients that are not initially hypokalemic.

Guidelines for parenteral potassium supplementation during treatment of ketoacidosis are listed in Table 17–1. Whenever possible, supplementation should be based on serial measurement of serum potassium concentration. If serum potassium concentration is not known, 30 to 40 mEq/L of potassium chloride should be added to the IV fluids. To avoid potential adverse cardiac effects, IV potassium should not be given at a rate of more than 0.5 mEq/kg/h. In animals that are oliguric, potassium supplementation should be withheld until renal perfusion and urine output have improved.

Phosphorus Supplementation

Phosphorus wasting in patients with DKA occurs as a result of osmotic diuresis, impaired phosphate reabsorption in the proximal tubule associated with insulin deficiency (DeFronzo et al. 1976), and acidosis-induced inhibition of renal tubular phosphate reabsorption (DeFronzo et al. 1994; Knochel 1977). Despite chronic phosphorus depletion, however, serum phosphorus concentrations often are normal or only mildly decreased at the time of initial presentation because insulin deficiency and hypertonicity cause a shift of phosphate from the intracellular to the extracellular space (Nichols and Crenshaw 1995; Crenshaw and Peterson 1996; Kebler et al. 1985). In addition, in animals with concurrent chronic renal disease or prerenal azotemia, hyperphosphatemia initially may be present (Bruskiewicz et al. 1997).

Correction of insulin deficiency, dehydration, and hypertonicity during treatment of DKA decreases serum phosphorus concentration and may result in the development of severe hypophosphatemia (<1.5 mg/dL) within the first 12 to 24 h of therapy (Kebler et al. 1985; Willard et al. 1987). Potential consequences of severe hypophosphatemia include hemolytic anemia, decreased erythrocyte 2,3-diphosphoglycerate concentration resulting in decreased tissue oxygenation, muscle weakness, rhabdomyolysis, seizures, and stupor (Knochel 1977; Willard et al. 1987; Adams et al. 1993; Forrester and Moreland 1989). Fortunately, although the development of hypophosphatemia during treatment for DKA is common, clinical consequences of hypophosphatemia are observed infrequently and usually are limited to the development of hemolytic anemia (Nichols and Crenshaw 1995; Bruskiewicz et al. 1997; Schaer 1977).

Phosphate supplementation should be considered if hypophosphatemia is associated with hemolysis or if serum phosphorus concentration falls below 1.0 to 1.5 mg/dL (Hardy and Adams 1989). The recommended initial phosphate dosage is 0.01 to 0.03 mmol/kg/h for 6 to 24 h as needed to increase serum phosphorus concentration above 2.0 to 2.5 mg/dL (Hardy and Adams 1989). However, higher doses (0.03–0.12 mmol/kg/h for 6 to 24 h) may be required for correction of severe hypophosphatemia in some patients with DKA (Nichols and Crenshaw 1995). Phosphate should be added to calcium-free IV fluids and can be administered as either the potassium or sodium salt. Potassium phosphate solutions provide 3.0 mmol of phosphate and 4.4 mEq of potassium per milliliter. Sodium phosphate solutions provide 3.0 mmol of phosphate and 4.0 mEq of sodium per milliliter. Serum phosphorus concentration should be reevaluated every 6 to 8 h during parenteral phosphate supplementation. Phosphate supplementation is contraindicated for patients with hypercalcemia, hyperphosphatemia, or oliguria. Potential complications of parenteral phosphate supplementation include hyperphosphatemia, hypocalcemia, soft tissue mineralization, hypotension, and renal failure (Knochel 1977; Forrester and Moreland 1988).

Routine phosphate supplementation aimed at preventing the development of hypophosphatemia in patients with DKA has been advocated by some authors who suggest that 50% of the required amount of potassium be administered as potassium chloride and 50% as potassium phosphate (Feldman and Nelson 1996a; Bruskiewicz et al. 1997). However, the effectiveness of such supplementation for decreasing mortality, preventing consequences of hypophosphatemia, or improving the clinical course of DKA has not yet been demonstrated (Becker et al. 1983; Keller and Berger 1980; Fisher and Kitabchi 1983). In fact, hemolytic anemia associated with hypophosphatemia may develop despite routine potassium phosphate supplementation (Bruskiewicz et al. 1997). In addition, significant hypocalcemia has been associated with parenteral phosphate administration in both veterinary and human patients with DKA (Adams et al. 1993; Fisher and Kitabchi 1983; Winter et al. 1979). Because the potassium deficit in DKA patients greatly exceeds the phosphorus deficit, it is not surprising that routine supplementation of potassium phosphate based on the potassium deficit may result in hyperphosphatemia and hypocalcemia (Adams et al. 1993).

Bicarbonate Administration

For the majority of animals with DKA, fluid administration (which increases urinary excretion of ketoacids) and insulin therapy (which enhances ketone utilization and inhibits ketone production) are all that are necessary to correct the metabolic acidosis. However, in animals with severe metabolic acidosis (blood pH < 7.2, serum bicarbonate concentration < 10 mEq/L), the deleterious effects of acidemia may prompt the clinician to consider further therapy. Administration of bicarbonate to these

TABLE 17–1. **Guidelines for Potassium Supplementation in Patients with Diabetic Ketoacidosis**

Initial Serum Potassium Concentration (mEq/L)	Addition of KCl to Fluids
>5.5	Wait 2 h, then add 20 mEq/L
4.0–5.0	Add 20–40 mEq/L
3.0–4.0	Add 40–60 mEq/L
<3.0	Add 60–80 mEq/L

patients is controversial (DeFronzo et al. 1994; Nichols and Crenshaw 1995). This is due in part to the fact that clinical and biochemical benefits of bicarbonate therapy in ketoacidotic patients have not been convincingly demonstrated. Studies of people have found no difference in the rate of change of blood pH or plasma bicarbonate concentration or in the time required to recover from ketoacidosis between patients treated with and without bicarbonate (Lever and Jaspan 1983), even when the initial acidosis was severe (Morris et al. 1986).

In addition, bicarbonate administration may be associated with a number of potentially harmful effects. As part of a negative feedback system that helps to maintain acid-base homeostasis by allowing blood pH to regulate ketoacid production, acidemia inhibits ketogenesis and free fatty acid availability (Hood and Tannen 1989, 1994). Therefore, correction of the acidemia by administration of bicarbonate results in an increase in ketone production and may delay resolution of ketonemia (Okuda et al. 1996; Hale et al. 1984).

Administration of bicarbonate also has the potential to exacerbate electrolyte disturbances associated with DKA. Because correction of acidosis promotes movement of potassium into cells (Adrogue and Madias 1981), significant hypokalemia may be more likely to develop in patients that receive bicarbonate. Bicarbonate administration also can decrease ionized serum calcium concentrations (Chew et al. 1989) and may exacerbate preexistent hypocalcemia (Bruskiewicz et al. 1997). In addition, overzealous bicarbonate therapy may result in later development of metabolic alkalosis as plasma ketones are metabolized and may aggravate preexistent hyperosmolality.

Acidemia causes a shift of the oxygen-hemoglobin curve to the right, and it has been suggested that rapid correction of acidosis with bicarbonate (which shifts the curve back to the left) might impair tissue oxygen delivery. However, a clinically significant effect of bicarbonate administration on tissue oxygen delivery in ketoacidotic patients has been difficult to demonstrate (Munk et al. 1974). Another concern about bicarbonate therapy has been the potential development of paradoxical central nervous system (CNS) acidosis (Posner and Plum 1967). Administration of bicarbonate increases blood pH, which decreases the ventilatory drive, causing a rise in P_{CO_2}. Because the blood-brain barrier is more permeable to CO_2 than to bicarbonate, the additional CO_2 diffuses into the CNS more rapidly than the exogenously administered bicarbonate. Although this could theoretically decrease the pH in the CNS, serial measurement of cerebrospinal fluid pH in human patients with DKA has failed to demonstrate such an effect (Morris et al. 1986). In addition, there is evidence that the medullary drive for hyperventilation persists for 18 h or more after correction of metabolic acidosis (Kreisberg 1978).

For all these reasons, bicarbonate therapy should be considered only when acidemia is severe (blood pH less than 7.10–7.15, plasma bicarbonate concentration < 8 mEq/L). When it is administered, bicarbonate should be given at a dose of 0.2 × body weight (kg) × (desired plasma bicarbonate concentration − patient's plasma bicarbonate concentration) over 2 to 6 h. Blood gases should be monitored serially after bicarbonate administration; the goal of therapy should be to increase blood pH to 7.2 or plasma bicarbonate concentration to 10 to 12 mEq/L.

▶ Hyperosmolar Diabetic Coma

Hyperglycemic hyperosmolar nonketotic diabetic coma is a rare complication of diabetes mellitus that is characterized by severe hyperglycemia and hyperosmolality, severe dehydration, absence of significant ketosis, and variable degrees of CNS depression (Feldman and Nelson 1996a; Wheeler 1988). It often is associated with renal dysfunction, which worsens the prognosis for recovery (Feldman and Nelson 1996a).

Pathophysiology

Like diabetic ketoacidosis, hyperglycemic hyperosmolar nonketotic diabetes (HHND) develops in response to a state of relative insulin deficiency that results in increased hepatic glucose production and decreased peripheral glucose utilization. Unlike the situation in DKA, however, ketosis is minimal or absent. This probably occurs because endogenous insulin concentrations in patients with HHND are adequate to prevent lipolysis but inadequate to inhibit hepatic glucose production or to stimulate peripheral glucose utilization (Chupin et al. 1981; Lorber 1995). Other potential reasons for the lack of ketosis in HHND include lower concentrations of counterregulatory hormones and free fatty acids (Gerich et al. 1971; Lindsey et al. 1974; Gordon and Kabadi 1976) and hyperosmolality-induced suppression of lipolysis (Turpin et al. 1979).

The magnitude of hyperglycemia typically is more severe (600 to 1600 mg/dL) in HHND than in DKA (Feldman and Nelson 1996a). This often is related to impaired renal function in patients with HHND, which may be the result of preexisting primary renal disease or may develop as a result of severe volume depletion associated with prolonged osmotic diuresis (Wheeler 1988). In addition, the lack of ketosis may contribute to the severity of hyperglycemia because, unlike patients with DKA that are presented for signs of systemic illness associated with ketosis, patients with HHND may not be presented to the veterinarian until signs associated with severe hyperosmolality occur (Feldman and Nelson 1996a).

Neurologic signs in patients with HHND may result from the effects of initial hyperosmolality (which causes a shift of water from the intracellular to the extracellular space) or from the development of cerebral edema associated with rapid correction of hyperosmolality during treatment. These signs can range from mild depression to coma and are proportional to the severity of hyperosmolality (Wheeler 1988).

Treatment

Goals of therapy for HHND are similar to those for DKA and include expansion of circulatory volume, resolution of hyperglycemia and hyperosmolality, correction of electrolyte imbalances, and identification and treatment of concurrent disorders. Additional considerations that are more often applicable in treating HHND include avoiding a rapid decrease in plasma osmolality (which may precipitate cerebral edema), maintaining adequate blood pressure in the presence of hypovolemia as plasma osmolality drops, monitoring urine output, and treating renal failure.

Fluid therapy aimed at restoring circulatory volume is essential in treating HHND. If azotemia or signs of hypotension are present, isotonic fluids (0.9% NaCl) should be given initially to expand vascular volume and improve renal perfusion (Lorber 1995). When circulatory function is adequate, hypotonic fluids (0.45% NaCl) should be administered, with the goal of replacing approximately half of the patient's estimated volume deficit over the first 24 h in addition to meeting maintenance fluid requirements. Potassium and phosphorus supplementation should be based on measurement of serum electrolyte concentrations, especially in animals with renal dysfunction.

Insulin-induced movement of glucose and water from the extracellular to the intracellular space in patients with severe hyperglycemia can cause a sudden decrease in intravascular volume, which may precipitate vascular collapse in animals with preexistent hypovolemia (DeFronzo et al. 1994; Nichols and Crenshaw 1995). Therefore, insulin therapy should be withheld in HHND until circulatory volume has been reestablished by administering intravenous fluids for several hours (Macintire 1995; Wheeler 1988). Protocols for insulin administration in HHND are the same as those for DKA and should be adjusted as needed to prevent rapid correction of hyperglycemia.

▶ Acute Adrenocortical Insufficiency

Hypoadrenocorticism is an endocrinopathy that most often develops in young to middle-aged female dogs and is characterized by chronic, intermittent, nonspecific signs of illness. Animals may be presented to the veterinarian during the chronic phase of the disease because of lethargy, anorexia, vomiting, diarrhea, weight loss, weakness, trembling, or polyuria and polydipsia (Kintzer and Peterson 1997; Melian and Peterson 1996). However, in some animals the subtle signs of hypoadrenocorticism go unnoticed until precipitation of an acute hypovolemic crisis, which often is referred to as an addisonian crisis. When this occurs, patients are presented with signs of hypovolemic shock and severe weakness. Successful management of this potentially life-threatening crisis is dependent on rapid administration of intravenous fluids to correct hypovolemia, recognition and treatment of electrolyte and acid-base derangements (especially hyperkalemia), and parenteral administration of glucocorticoids.

Pathophysiology

Adrenocortical insufficiency is characterized by inadequate secretion of glucocorticoids and mineralocorticoids by the adrenal cortex. Aldosterone, the principal mineralocorticoid secreted by the adrenal cortex, promotes renal reabsorption of sodium and water and renal excretion of potassium and hydrogen ions. Cortisol and corticosterone, the principal adrenocortical glucocorticoids, stimulate appetite, help to maintain normal blood glucose concentration and normal blood pressure, promote free-water loss through the kidneys, protect against shock, and help the animal respond to stress. Insufficient secretion of these hormones in dogs with hypoadrenocorticism thus may lead to hypovolemia, hypotension, hyponatremia, hyperkalemia, metabolic acidosis, hypoglycemia, and shock.

Addison's disease (primary hypoadrenocorticism) results from destruction of the adrenal cortices. Secondary hypoadrenocorticism results from insufficient secretion of adrenocorticotropic hormone (ACTH) from the pituitary gland and in small animals usually is caused by excessive or prolonged administration of exogenous glucocorticoids. In most cases of primary adrenocortical insufficiency, both glucocorticoid (cortisol) production and mineralocorticoid (aldosterone) production are inadequate. However, in secondary hypoadrenocorticism only glucocorticoids are deficient. The most common cause of hypoadrenocorticism in small animal patients is idiopathic atrophy of the adrenal cortices, which is probably the result of an immune-mediated process.

Clinical Signs and Laboratory Abnormalities

Animals with acute adrenocortical insufficiency typically are presented with signs of lethargy, hypovolemia (e.g., pale mucous membranes, weak femoral pulses, prolonged capillary refill time), and profound weakness. Bradycardia (caused by the effects of hyperkalemia on the heart) is present in approximately one-third of dogs in addisonian crisis (Hardy 1995; Feldman and Nelson 1996b). Because hypovolemia from other causes usually is associated with tachycardia, the presence of bradycardia in an animal with shock should alert the clinician to the possibility of hypoadrenocorticism. Evidence of severe gastrointestinal hemorrhage (hematemesis, melena) occasionally is present (Medinger et al. 1993).

Classical clinicopathologic abnormalities associated with acute adrenocortical insufficiency include hyponatremia, hyperkalemia, azotemia, and mild to moderate normal-anion-gap metabolic acidosis. Although hyponatremia and hyperkalemia are present in most dogs with acute adrenocortical insufficiency, not all affected dogs demonstrate these classic electrolyte changes (Lifton et al. 1996; Sadek and Schaer 1996). When hypoadrenal dogs without hyponatremia and hyperkalemia are presented in a state of collapse, their clinical signs often are related to significant hypoglycemia or severe gastrointestinal hemorrhage (Lifton et al. 1996).

Although the azotemia associated with hypoadrenocorticism typically is prerenal in origin, urinary concentrating ability often is impaired as a result of chronic hyponatremia and loss of the renal medullary concentration gradient (Feldman and Nelson 1996b; Tyler et al. 1987). As a result, urine specific gravity usually is less than 1.030. Hypercalcemia and hypoglycemia each are present in approximately 30% of dogs with acute adrenocortical insufficiency (Melian and Peterson 1996; Feldman and Nelson 1996b; Peterson and Feinman 1982;

Peterson et al. 1996). Hematologic abnormalities include mild nonregenerative anemia or polycythemia (related to hemoconcentration) and lack of a stress leukogram (Peterson et al. 1996).

Diagnosis

The ACTH stimulation test is the test of choice for the diagnosis of hypoadrenocorticism. In animals with suspected acute adrenocortical insufficiency, the ACTH stimulation test should be started as soon as fluid therapy has been initiated. All dogs with primary hypoadrenocorticism have a subnormal response to ACTH. Plasma cortisol concentrations are measured before and 2 h after IM administration of 2.2 U/kg (40 U maximum) of ACTH gel (Acthar gel HP; Rhone-Poulenc-Rorer). Alternatively, 0.25 mg of synthetic ACTH (cosyntropin, Cortrosyn; Organon) is given intravenously with baseline and 1-h cortisol sampling. Normal dogs have resting cortisol concentrations of 1 to 5 µg/dL and stimulate to a range of 6 to 20 µg/dL. Plasma cortisol concentrations fail to increase after ACTH stimulation in dogs with primary hypoadrenocorticism; in fact, many have pre- and post-ACTH cortisol concentrations below the normal resting range (<1 µg/dL). Dogs with secondary hypoadrenocorticism typically show a slight, but still subnormal, response to ACTH stimulation.

It often is necessary to administer glucocorticoid therapy to a dog in a hypoadrenal crisis before the ACTH stimulation test can be completed. Because prednisone and prednisolone interfere with the radioimmunoassay of cortisol, they should not be administered before or during adrenal function testing. If glucocorticoid therapy is necessary before the post-ACTH cortisol sample has been drawn, dexamethasone should be chosen because it does not interfere with the cortisol assay.

Treatment

Goals of therapy for acute adrenocortical insufficiency include restoration of normal circulatory volume; correction of hyponatremia, hyperkalemia, and metabolic acidosis; replacement of glucocorticoids; and recognition and treatment of the detrimental effects of hyperkalemia on the heart. Because acute adrenocortical insufficiency is a medical emergency, it is essential to initiate therapy immediately for any animal with clinical signs suggestive of acute hypoadrenocorticism; confirmation of the diagnosis can be pursued once steps have been taken to restore adequate circulatory volume and resolve life-threatening hyperkalemia.

Fluid Therapy

Because shock and circulatory collapse are the most common causes of death in patients with acute adrenocortical insufficiency, rapid infusion of large volumes of isotonic fluid should be the first priority. Normal saline (0.9% NaCl) is the fluid of choice. Lactated Ringer's solution (despite its 4 mEq/L potassium concentration) can be administered if normal saline is not available. If hypoglycemia is present, 50% dextrose should be added to the fluids to make a 5% solution. Ideally, this solution should be administered through a central vein.

Fluids should be administered through an indwelling intravenous catheter at a rate of 40 to 80 mL/kg/h over the first 1 to 2 h. After that time the rate should be decreased to two to three times normal maintenance fluid requirements and adjusted on the basis of an ongoing assessment of the animal's volume status and urine production. After normal circulatory volume has been restored, maintenance fluid therapy should be continued until the animal is eating and drinking. Although the azotemia associated with hypoadrenocorticism usually resolves with fluid therapy, primary renal damage may occur as a result of prolonged renal hypoperfusion; thus urine production should be monitored and appropriate therapy (e.g., dopamine infusion) instituted if oliguria does not resolve with initial volume restoration.

Glucocorticoid Replacement

Parenteral glucocorticoids should be administered after fluid therapy has been initiated. Rapidly acting glucocorticoid formulations include hydrocortisone sodium succinate (Solu-Cortef, Upjohn; 2–4 mg/kg IV), dexamethasone sodium phosphate (Azium-SP, Schering; 1–2 mg/kg IV), dexamethasone (Azium, Schering; 0.5–1 mg/kg IV slowly), and prednisolone sodium succinate (Solu-Delta-Cortef, Upjohn; 15–20 mg/kg IV). Dexamethasone often is the initial choice because it does not interfere with the cortisol radioimmunoassay and thus can be given immediately before or during the ACTH stimulation test. High-dose glucocorticoid administration may need to be repeated in 6 h. As the dog improves, the glucocorticoid dose is reduced to maintenance (prednisone, 0.2 mg/kg/day) over 3 to 5 days. Oral glucocorticoid therapy should be initiated when vomiting resolves.

Mineralocorticoid Replacement

Rapidly acting parenteral mineralocorticoid formulations are no longer available. However, volume expansion with normal saline usually is sufficient for correction of the hypovolemia, hyponatremia, and hyperkalemia associated with mineralocorticoid deficiency. Maintenance mineralocorticoid therapy with desoxycorticosterone pivalate (Percorten-V, Novartis; 2.2 mg/kg IM q25d) can be initiated during initial therapy for acute adrenocortical insufficiency and may provide some mineralocorticoid activity within the first 24 h of therapy (Feldman and Nelson 1996b).

Management of Hyperkalemia

Rapid volume expansion alone is sufficient for correction of hyperkalemia in the majority of patients with acute adrenocortical insufficiency. However, if serum potassium concentration is greater than 7.5 mEq/L (or if atrial standstill or severe bradyarrhythmias are present), more aggressive therapy should be considered (see Chapter 5). Options include intravenous administration of glucose (with or without insulin), sodium bicarbonate, or 10% calcium gluconate. Glucose acts by driving potassium into the intracellular compartment and is administered as a bolus of 10% dextrose (4–10 mL/kg) given IV over 30 to 60 min with saline (Feldman and Nelson 1996b). Regular insulin, which also acts to drive potassium into cells, is administered subcutaneously or intramuscularly at a dosage of 0.1 to 0.2 U/kg, followed by at least 2 g of dextrose (20 mL of 10% dextrose) for every unit of insulin given.

Because correction of acidosis promotes movement of potassium into cells (Adrogue and Madias 1981), bicarbonate therapy may be indicated if life-threatening hyperkalemia is associated with significant metabolic acidosis (see later). Finally, when hyperkalemia is deemed immediately life threatening, intravenous administration of 10% calcium gluconate (2–10 mL given slowly over 10–20 min while monitoring the electrocardiogram) can be used to protect myocardial cells temporarily while other measures are taken to lower serum potassium concentration (DiBartola and de Morais 1992). This is rarely necessary in animals with hypoadrenocorticism.

Correction of Metabolic Acidosis

The metabolic acidosis associated with hypoadrenocorticism typically is mild to moderate and usually can be corrected by fluid therapy alone. However, if severe metabolic acidosis is present (pH < 7.1; bicarbonate < 10 mEq/L), administration of sodium bicarbonate (given at a dose of 0.2 × body weight [kg] × [desired plasma bicarbonate concentration − patient's plasma bicarbonate concentration] over 2 to 6 h) is indicated. Sodium bicarbonate should not be added to calcium-containing fluids (such as lactated Ringer's solution) because precipitation can occur. Blood gases should be monitored serially after bicarbonate administration; the goal of therapy should be to raise the blood pH to 7.2 or the plasma bicarbonate concentration to 12 mEq/L.

▶ Hypoglycemia

A number of differential diagnoses must be considered when hypoglycemia is encountered in the small animal patient (Table 17–2). Mild to moderate hypoglycemia in an otherwise stable patient usually is treated by managing or resolving the underlying cause of the hypoglycemia and providing multiple feedings or oral glucose supplementation. However, patients that are presented to the veterinarian in an acute hypoglycemic crisis associated with neurologic signs require parenteral glucose supplementation. After hypoglycemia has been identified in such a patient, initial therapy should consist of an intravenous bolus of 50% dextrose given slowly to effect (usually 2–15 mL). Neurologic signs associated with hypoglycemia should respond to dextrose administration within 1 to 2 min. The initial dextrose bolus should be followed with a continuous intravenous infusion of 5% dextrose, which may need to be continued for several days, depending on the underlying cause of the hypoglycemia. If a balanced electrolyte solution is indicated, dextrose can be added to either normal saline or lactated Ringer's solution at 100 mL of 50% dextrose per liter to make a 5% dextrose solution. Because of its hypertonicity, this solution should

TABLE 17–2. Causes of Hypoglycemia in Small Animal Patients

1. Excess insulin
   - Islet cell tumors (insulinoma)
   - Iatrogenic insulin overdose
2. Hepatic disease
   - End-stage liver disease
   - Portosystemic shunt
   - Glycogen storage disease
3. Extrapancreatic tumors that produce insulin-like substances
   - Leiomyoma and leiomyosarcoma (gastrointestinal, splenic)
   - Hepatoma, hepatic carcinoma
   - Hemangiosarcoma
4. Endocrine disorders
   - Hypoadrenocorticism
   - Growth hormone deficiency
5. Juvenile-onset hypoglycemia
   - Idiopathic hypoglycemia of toy breed puppies
   - Glycogen storage diseases
6. Sepsis
7. Hunting dog hypoglycemia
8. Pregnancy-associated hypoglycemia
9. Polycythemia
10. Artifactual—sample handled incorrectly

be administered through a catheter in a central vein if possible.

▶ Heatstroke

Heatstroke is an often fatal condition of extreme hyperthermia that occurs when the heat-dissipating mechanisms of the body are overcome by an acute increase in heat-producing factors, such as environmental conditions or exercise (Holloway 1992). The resultant effects of thermic injury on the body are widespread, and multiple organ failure often ensues. Successful therapy is dependent on early recognition, rapid intervention, careful monitoring, and aggressive management of potentially life-threatening complications, such as cardiac arrhythmias, acute renal failure, and disseminated intravascular coagulation.

Pathophysiology

Direct thermal injury associated with heatstroke affects nearly every system of the body. Effects on the cardiovascular system are characterized by decreased systemic vascular resistance, hypovolemia, and myocardial ischemia, hemorrhage, and necrosis, which often result in the development of tachyarrhythmias. Early in the course of heatstroke, cardiac output is increased (as a result of peripheral vasodilatation) and blood flow is preferentially distributed away from splanchnic vascular beds in order to maintain blood pressure. However, as the disorder progresses, cardiac output decreases, hypovolemia worsens, and compensatory distribution of blood flow fails, resulting in hypotension and cardiovascular collapse (Holloway 1992).

Thermal damage to megakaryocytes, consumption of platelets and clotting factors, decreased production of clotting factors secondary to hepatic damage, and widespread endothelial damage leading to disseminated intravascular coagulation all contribute to the development of severe coagulopathies in animals with heatstroke (Holloway 1992; Ruslander 1992). In the gastrointestinal tract, extensive epithelial damage and poor tissue perfusion lead to profuse gastrointestinal bleeding and disruption of the mucosal barrier, which predisposes the animal to development of gram-negative bacteremia and sepsis (Holloway 1992). Direct thermal injury and prolonged splanchnic hypoperfusion contribute to hepatic injury in animals with heatstroke and may cause severe hepatic dysfunction (Holloway 1992).

Acute renal failure is a common complication of heatstroke (Krum and Osborne 1977) and results from renal hypoperfusion, direct thermal injury to renal tubular cells, and thrombosis associated with disseminated intravascular coagulation (Schrier et al. 1970). Deleterious effects on the central nervous system include neuronal injury and death; cerebral edema, hemorrhage, or infarction; and hypothalamic damage and dysfunction (Ruslander 1992). This hypothalamic damage may predispose affected animals to subsequent episodes of hyperthermia. Acid-base abnormalities associated with heatstroke include metabolic acidosis (related to tissue hypoperfusion and lactic acid production) and respiratory alkalosis (related to excess panting).

Treatment

The goals of therapy for heatstroke are to lower core body temperature, to provide aggressive cardiovascular support, and to manage secondary complications as they arise. Cooling the patient is the first priority and, if possible, should be initiated by the owners before transporting the pet to the veterinary hospital. The animal should be removed from the hot environment and soaked with cool water. Ice-water baths are contraindicated because they promote cutaneous vasoconstriction, which impairs heat loss (Holloway 1992). Circulation of air over the patient with the use of fans increases evaporative cooling. When core body temperature reaches 39°C (102°F), cooling should be discontinued to avoid development of hypothermia.

Isotonic fluids (normal saline or lactated Ringer's solution) should be administered in volumes up to 90 mL/kg (dog) or 70 mL/kg (cat) in the first 1 to 2 h to restore circulatory volume and treat cardiovascular shock. The amount and rate of fluid administration should be based on the degree of hypovolemia and hypoperfusion, as assessed by monitoring capillary refill time, femoral pulse quality, central venous pressure, urine output, and severity of gastrointestinal hemorrhage. Blood products (fresh frozen plasma or fresh whole blood) should be administered to patients with signs of disseminated intravascular coagulation. Packed red blood cells or fresh whole blood may be needed for treatment of anemia resulting from gastrointestinal hemorrhage, especially if it is associated with coagulopathy. Glucocorticoids have not been shown to be beneficial in the routine treatment of heatstroke but may be indicated if the patient shows signs of cerebral edema (Holloway 1992; Ruslander 1992). Nonsteroidal antiinflammatory agents are contraindicated in the treatment of heatstroke because they have the potential to exacerbate gastrointestinal and renal damage (Holloway 1992; Ruslander 1992) and are not effective in lowering body temperature in heatstroke patients.

Intravenous fluid therapy support and close monitoring should be continued for several days after initial emergency management because many of the complications of heatstroke do not develop until 48 to 72 h after the initial hyperthermic insult. These include acute renal failure, severe thrombocytopenia, cardiac arrhythmias, seizures, hepatic failure, and sepsis.

REFERENCES

Adams LG, Hardy RM, Weiss DJ, et al.: Hypophosphatemia and hemolytic anemia associated with diabetes mellitus and hepatic lipidosis in cats. *J Vet Intern Med* 7:266–721, 1993.

Adrogue HJ, and Madias NE: Changes in plasma potassium concentration during acute acid-base disturbances. *Am J Med* 71:456–467, 1981.

Adrogue HJ, Lederer ED, Suki WN, et al.: Determinants of plasma potassium levels in diabetic ketoacidosis. *Medicine (Baltimore)* 65:163–172, 1986.

Adrogue HJ, Barrero J, and Eknoyan G: Salutary effects of modest fluid replacement in the treatment of adults with diabetic ketoacidosis. Use in patients without extreme volume deficit. *JAMA* 262:2108–2113, 1989.

Alberti KG, Hockaday TD, and Turner RC: Small doses of intramuscular insulin in the treatment of diabetic "coma." *Lancet* 2:515–522, 1973.

Barrett EJ and DeFronzo RA: Diabetic ketoacidosis: Diagnosis and treatment. *Hosp Pract (Off Ed)* 19:89–95, 99–104, 1984.

Becker DJ, Brown DR, Steranka BH, et al.: Phosphate replacement during treatment of diabetic ketosis. Effects on calcium and phosphorus homeostasis. *Am J Dis Child* 137:241–246, 1983.

Bruskiewicz KA, Nelson RW, Feldman EC, et al.: Diabetic ketosis and ketoacidosis in cats: 42 cases (1980–1995). *J Am Vet Med Assoc* 211:188–192, 1997.

Burghen GA, Etteldorf JN, Fisher JN, et al.: Comparison of high-dose and low-dose insulin by continuous intravenous infusion in the treatment of diabetic ketoacidosis in children. *Diabetes Care* 3:15–20, 1980.

Chastain CB and Nichols CE: Low-dose intramuscular insulin therapy for diabetic ketoacidosis in dogs. *J Am Vet Med Assoc* 178:561–564, 1981.

Chew DJ, Leonard M, and Muir WD: Effect of sodium bicarbonate infusions on ionized calcium and total calcium concentrations in serum of clinically normal cats. *Am J Vet Res* 50:145–150, 1989.

Chiasson JL, Liljenquist JE, Finger FE, et al.: Differential sensitivity of glycogenolysis and gluconeogenesis to insulin infusions in dogs. *Diabetes* 25:283–291, 1976.

Christensen NJ and Orskov H: The relationship between endogenous serum insulin concentration and glucose uptake in the forearm muscles of nondiabetics. *J Clin Invest* 47:1262–1268, 1968.

Chupin M, Charbonnel B, and Chupin F: C-peptide blood levels in keto-acidosis and in hyperosmolar non-ketotic diabetic coma. *Acta Diabetol Lat* 18:123–128, 1981.

Crenshaw KL and Peterson ME: Pretreatment clinical and laboratory evaluation of cats with diabetes mellitus: 104 cases (1992–1994). *J Am Vet Med Assoc* 209:943–949, 1996.

DeFronzo RA, Goldberg M, and Agus ZS: The effects of glucose and insulin on renal electrolyte transport. *J Clin Invest* 58:83–90, 1976.

DeFronzo RA, Matsuda M, and Barrett EJ: Diabetic ketoacidosis:

A combined metabolic-nephrologic approach to therapy. *Diabetes Rev* 2:209–238, 1994.

DiBartola SP and deMorais HSA: Disorders of potassium: Hypokalemia and hyperkalemia. In DiBartola SP (ed): *Fluid Therapy in Small Animal Practice*, 1st ed. Philadelphia, WB Saunders, pp. 89–115, 1992.

Diehl KJ and Wheeler SL: Pathogenesis and management of diabetic ketoacidosis. In Kirk RW and Bonagura JD (eds): *Current Veterinary Therapy XI*. Philadelphia, WB Saunders, pp. 359–363, 1992.

Ennis ED, Stahl EJVB, and Kreisberg RA: The hyperosmolar hyperglycemic syndrome. *Diabetes Rev* 2:115–126, 1994.

Feldman EC and Nelson RW: Diabetic ketoacidosis. In Feldman EC and Nelson RW (eds): *Canine and Feline Endocrinology and Reproduction*, 2nd ed. Philadelphia, WB Saunders, pp. 392–421, 1996a.

Feldman EC and Nelson RW: Hypoadrenocorticism. In Feldman EC and Nelson RW (eds): *Canine and Feline Endocrinology and Reproduction*, 2nd ed. Philadelphia, WB Saunders, pp. 266–306, 1996b.

Fisher JN, and Kitabchi AE: A randomized study of phosphate therapy in the treatment of diabetic ketoacidosis. *J Clin Endocrinol Metab* 57:177–180, 1983.

Forrester SD and Moreland KJ: Hypophosphatemia. Causes and clinical consequences. *J Vet Intern Med* 3:149–159, 1989.

Foster DW and McGarry JD: The metabolic derangements and treatment of diabetic ketoacidosis. *N Engl J Med* 309:159–169, 1983.

Ganong WF: Energy balance, metabolism, and nutrition. *Review of Medical Physiology*, 16th ed. Norwalk, CT, Appleton & Lange, p. 278, 1993.

Gerich JE, Martin MM, and Recant L: Clinical and metabolic characteristics of hyperosmolar nonketotic coma. *Diabetes* 20:228–238, 1971.

Gonzalez-Campoy JM and Robertson RP: Diabetic ketoacidosis and hyperosmolar nonketotic state: Gaining control over extreme hyperglycemic complications. *Postgrad Med* 99:143–152, 1996.

Gordon EE and Kabadi UM: The hyperglycemic hyperosmolar syndrome. *Am J Med Sci* 271:252–268, 1976.

Hale PJ, Crase J, and Nattrass M: Metabolic effects of bicarbonate in the treatment of diabetic ketoacidosis. *Br Med J (Clin Res Ed)* 289:1035–1038, 1984.

Hammond P and Wallis S: Cerebral oedema in diabetic ketoacidosis (editorial). *BMJ* 305:203–204, 1992.

Hardy RM: Hypoadrenal gland disease. In Ettinger SJ and Feldman EC (eds): *Textbook of Veterinary Internal Medicine*, 4 ed. Philadelphia, WB Saunders, pp. 1579–1592, 1995.

Hardy RM and Adams LG: Hypophosphatemia. In Kirk RW and Bonagura JD (eds): *Current Veterinary Therapy X*. Philadelphia, WB Saunders, pp. 43–47, 1989.

Harris GD, Fiordalisi I, Harris WL, et al.: Minimizing the risk of brain herniation during treatment of diabetic ketoacidemia: A retrospective and prospective study [published erratum appears in *J Pediatr* 118:166–167, 1991]. *J Pediatr* 117:22–31, 1990.

Harris GD, Lohr JW, Fiordalisi I, et al.: Brain osmoregulation during extreme and moderate dehydration in a rat model of severe DKA. *Life Sci* 53:185–191, 1993.

Hillman K: Fluid resuscitation in diabetic emergencies—A reappraisal. *Intensive Care Med* 13:4–8, 1987.

Holloway SA: Heatstroke in dogs. *Compend Contin Educ Pract Vet* 14:1598–1604, 1992.

Hood VL and Tannen RL: Regulation of acid production in ketoacidosis and lactic acidosis. *Diabetes Metab Rev* 5:393–409, 1989.

Hood VL and Tannen RL: Maintenance of acid-base homeostasis during ketoacidosis and lactic acidosis. *Diabetes Rev* 2:177–194, 1994.

Kebler R, McDonald FD, and Cadnapaphornchai P: Dynamic changes in serum phosphorus levels in diabetic ketoacidosis. *Am J Med* 79:571–576, 1985.

Keller U and Berger W: Prevention of hypophosphatemia by phosphate infusion during treatment of diabetic ketoacidosis and hyperosmolar coma. *Diabetes* 29:87–95, 1980.

Kintzer PP and Peterson ME: Primary and secondary canine hypoadrenocorticism. *Vet Clin North Am Small Anim Pract* 27:349–357, 1997.

Kitabchi AE and Wall BM: Diabetic ketoacidosis. *Med Clin North Am* 79:9–37, 1995.

Kitabchi AE, Ayyagari V, and Guerra SM: The efficacy of low-dose versus conventional therapy of insulin for treatment of diabetic ketoacidosis. *Ann Intern Med* 84:633–638, 1976.

Kitabchi AE, Young R, Sacks H, et al.: Diabetic ketoacidosis: reappraisal of therapeutic approach. *Annu Rev Med* 30:339–357, 1979.

Knochel JP: The pathophysiology and clinical characteristics of severe hypophosphatemia. *Arch Intern Med* 137:203–220, 1977.

Kreisberg RA: Diabetic ketoacidosis: New concepts and trends in pathogenesis and treatment. *Ann Intern Med* 88:681–695, 1978.

Krum SH and Osborne CA: Heatstroke in the dog: a polysystemic disorder. *J Am Vet Med Assoc* 170:531–535, 1977.

Lebovitz HE: Diabetic ketoacidosis. *Lancet* 345:767–772, 1995.

Lever E and Jaspan JB: Sodium bicarbonate therapy in severe diabetic ketoacidosis. *Am J Med* 75:263–268, 1983.

Lifton SJ, King LG, and Zerbe CA: Glucocorticoid deficient hypoadrenocorticism in dogs: 18 cases (1986–1995). *J Am Vet Med Assoc* 209:2076–2081, 1996.

Lindsey CA, Faloona GR, and Unger RH: Plasma glucagon in nonketotic hyperosmolar coma. *JAMA* 229:1771–1773, 1974.

Ling GV, Lowenstine LJ, Pulley LT, et al.: Diabetes mellitus in dogs: A review of initial evaluation, immediate and long-term management, and outcome. *J Am Vet Med Assoc* 170:521–530, 1977.

Lorber D: Nonketotic hypertonicity in diabetes mellitus. *Med Clin North Am* 79:39–52, 1995.

Luzi L, Barrett EJ, Groop LC, et al.: Metabolic effects of low-dose insulin therapy on glucose metabolism in diabetic ketoacidosis. *Diabetes* 37:1470–1477, 1988.

Macintire DK: Treatment of diabetic ketoacidosis in dogs by continuous low-dose intravenous infusion of insulin. *J Am Vet Med Assoc* 202:1266–1272, 1993.

Macintire DK: Emergency therapy of diabetic crises: Insulin overdose, diabetic ketoacidosis, and hyperosmolar coma. *Vet Clin North Am Small Anim Pract* 25:639–650, 1995.

McGarry JD and Foster DW: Regulation of hepatic fatty acid oxidation and ketone body production. *Annu Rev Biochem* 49:395–420, 1980.

Medinger TL, Williams DA, and Bruyette DS: Severe gastrointestinal tract hemorrhage in three dogs with hypoadrenocorticism. *J Am Vet Med Assoc* 202:1869–1872, 1993.

Melian C and Peterson ME: Diagnosis and treatment of naturally occurring hypoadrenocorticism in 42 dogs. *J Small Anim Pract* 37:268–275, 1996.

Morris LR, Murphy MB, and Kitabchi AE: Bicarbonate therapy in severe diabetic ketoacidosis. *Ann Intern Med* 105:836–840, 1986.

Munk P, Freedman MH, Levison H, et al.: Effect of bicarbonate on oxygen transport in juvenile diabetic ketoacidosis. *J Pediatr* 84:510–514, 1974.

Nardone DA, McDonald WJ, and Girard DE: Mechanisms in hypokalemia: Clinical correlation. *Medicine (Baltimore)* 57:435–446, 1978.

Nichols R and Crenshaw KL: Complications and concurrent disease associated with diabetic ketoacidosis and other severe forms of diabetes mellitus. In Bonagura JD (ed): *Current Veterinary Therapy XII*. Philadelphia, WB Saunders, pp. 384–387, 1995.

Okuda Y, Adrogue HJ, Field JB, et al.: Counterproductive effects of sodium bicarbonate in diabetic ketoacidosis. *J Clin Endocrinol Metab* 81:314–320, 1996.

Owen OE, Licht JH, and Sapir DG: Renal function and effects of partial rehydration during diabetic ketoacidosis. *Diabetes* 30:510–518, 1981.

Peterson L, Caldwell J, and Hoffman J: Insulin adsorbance to polyvinylchloride surfaces with implications for constant-infusion therapy. *Diabetes* 25:72–74, 1976.

Peterson ME and Feinman JM: Hypercalcemia associated with hypoadrenocorticism in sixteen dogs. *J Am Vet Med Assoc* 181:802–804, 1982.

Peterson ME, Kintzer PP, and Kass PH: Pretreatment clinical and laboratory findings in dogs with hypoadrenocorticism: 225 cases (1979–1993). *J Am Vet Med Assoc* 208:85–91, 1996.

Posner JB and Plum F: Spinal-fluid pH and neurologic symptoms in systemic acidosis. *N Engl J Med* 277:605–613, 1967.

Rosenbloom AL: Intracerebral crises during treatment of diabetic ketoacidosis. *Diabetes Care* 13:22–33, 1990.

Rosenbloom AL and Hanas R: Diabetic ketoacidosis (DKA): Treatment guidelines. *Clin Pediatr (Phila)* 35:261–266, 1996.

Ruslander D: Heat stroke. In Kirk RW and Bonagural JD (eds): *Current Veterinary Therapy XI*. Philadelphia, WB Saunders, pp. 143–146, 1992.

Sacks HS, Shahshahani M, Kitabchi AE, et al.: Similar responsiveness of diabetic ketoacidosis to low-dose insulin by intramuscular injection and albumin-free infusion. *Ann Intern Med* 90:36–42, 1979.

Sadek D and Schaer M: Atypical Addison's disease in the dog: A retrospective survey of 14 cases. *J Am Anim Hosp Assoc* 32:159–163, 1996.

Schaer M: A clinical survey of thirty cats with diabetes mellitus. *J Am Anim Hosp Assoc* 13:23–27, 1977.

Schrier RW, Hano J, Keller HI, et al.: Renal, metabolic, and circulatory responses to heat and exercise. Studies in military recruits during summer training, with implications for acute renal failure. *Ann Intern Med* 73:213–223, 1970.

Sherwin RS, Hendler RG, and Felig P: Effect of diabetes mellitus and insulin on the turnover and metabolic response to ketones in man. *Diabetes* 25:776–784, 1976.

Turpin BP, Duckworth WC, and Solomon SS: Simulated hyperglycemic hyperosmolar syndrome. Impaired insulin and epinephrine effects upon lipolysis in the isolated rat fat cell. *J Clin Invest* 63:403–409, 1979.

Tyler RD, Qualls CW Jr, Heald RD, et al.: Renal concentrating ability in dehydrated hyponatremic dogs. *J Am Vet Med Assoc* 191:1095–1100, 1987.

Umpierrez GE, Khajavi M, and Kitabchi AE: Review: Diabetic ketoacidosis and hyperglycemic hyperosmolar nonketotic syndrome. *Am J Med Sci* 311:225–233, 1996.

Waldhausl W, Kleinberger G, Korn A, et al.: Severe hyperglycemia: Effects of rehydration on endocrine derangements and blood glucose concentration. *Diabetes* 28:577–584, 1979.

Wheeler SL: Emergency management of the diabetic patient. *Semin Vet Med Surg (Small Anim)* 3:265–273, 1988.

Willard MD, Zerbe CA, Schall WD, et al.: Severe hypophosphatemia associated with diabetes mellitus in six dogs and one cat. *J Am Vet Med Assoc* 190:1007–1010, 1987.

Winter RJ, Harris CJ, Phillips LS, et al.: Diabetic ketoacidosis. Induction of hypocalcemia and hypomagnesemia by phosphate therapy. *Am J Med* 67:897–900,

CHAPTER 18

Fluid and Diuretic Therapy in Heart Failure

JOHN D. BONAGURA   LINDA B. LEHMKUHL   HELIO AUTRAN DE MORAIS

Congestive heart failure (CHF) is a clinical syndrome characterized by cardiac dysfunction, abnormal hemodynamics, neurohormonal activation, release of cytokines, and renal retention of sodium and water. Heart failure is triggered by a cardiac or vascular lesion that impairs cardiac output. Although the underlying disorders and resultant clinical presentations vary, the compensations activated in response to reduced cardiac output are largely stereotypic. These compensations support arterial blood pressure (ABP) but, when chronically activated, also yield a maladaptive state that causes substantial morbidity and mortality.

Advanced CHF, as well as the therapy of this syndrome, often is associated with alterations in renal function and a variety of fluid, electrolyte, and serum biochemical abnormalities. Some of these disturbances are mild and seemingly well tolerated, but others, such as hyponatremia and acute renal failure, indicate severe circulatory dysfunction and a need for urgent therapy (Kaloyanides 1980). There are circumstances in which cardiac patients actually require fluid therapy to maintain optimal ventricular filling and prevent deterioration of renal function. It is more common, however, for fluid therapy to aggravate fluid accumulation in a previously compensated cardiac patient. Safe restoration of fluid and electrolyte balance in the patient with circulatory failure is challenging. To orchestrate such treatment, the clinician must appreciate the pathophysiology of heart failure and the compensatory changes that develop. This chapter addresses some of the clinically relevant pathophysiologic and therapeutic aspects of heart failure.

Much of our understanding of hemodynamics, renal function, and neurohumoral activity in circulatory failure stems from experimental studies performed in dogs (Paradiso et al. 1995; Francis and McDonald 1995). Studies of fluid therapy in spontaneous CHF in dogs and cats, however, are largely unavailable. Accordingly, the recommendations offered here represent our interpretation of relevant animal studies as well as personal experience with the treatment of dogs and cats in CHF.

▶ The Normal Circulation

The central circulation is regulated largely by a need to maintain plasma volume, mean ABP, and tissue perfusion. Of prime importance is the maintenance of normal effective plasma volume and ABP in the central circulation (Rose 1994; Schrier and Abraham 1999). These two variables depend on cardiac output, systemic vascular impedance, and renal regulation of sodium and water excretion. The reflexes that control the circulation have evolved so that blood pressure and plasma volume are maintained within a narrow range even in the presence of sudden physiologic stresses, such as exercise, hypotension, or hemorrhage. Blood pressure and plasma volume are monitored by different mechanoreceptors and osmoreceptors located in the arteries, veins, heart, kidney, and central nervous system. Ultimately, two factors—cardiac output and systemic vascular resistance (more precisely, vascular impedance)—determine ABP (Fig. 18–1). A change in either one of these two variables causes a parallel change in blood pressure. Numerous physiologic variables can affect cardiac output and vascular impedance (Table 18–1), and many of these factors are perturbed in CHF. Of particular relevance in this chapter are determinants of plasma volume in health and disease (Table 18–2). Plasma volume is a major contributor to venous pressure and cardiac filling. The serum sodium concentration, as described more fully in Chapter 3, plays a central role in determining plasma volume. Renal tubular activity, vascular dynamics, hormones, and other vasoactive factors regulate sodium balance. Abnormalities of sodium excretion are pivotal to the development of CHF.

Attention also must be directed to the microcirculation and factors controlling fluid movement across capillaries. Tissue perfusion is crucial for organ functions such as the formation of urine, muscle contraction, and exchange of oxygen and carbon dioxide. Assuming the maintenance of adequate mean ABP, vascular resistance largely governs tissue perfusion across the arterial side of the microcirculation. Vascular resistance for any regional circulation is the sum of structural, autonomic, hormonal, and local vasoactive factors (see Table 18–1). Conversely,

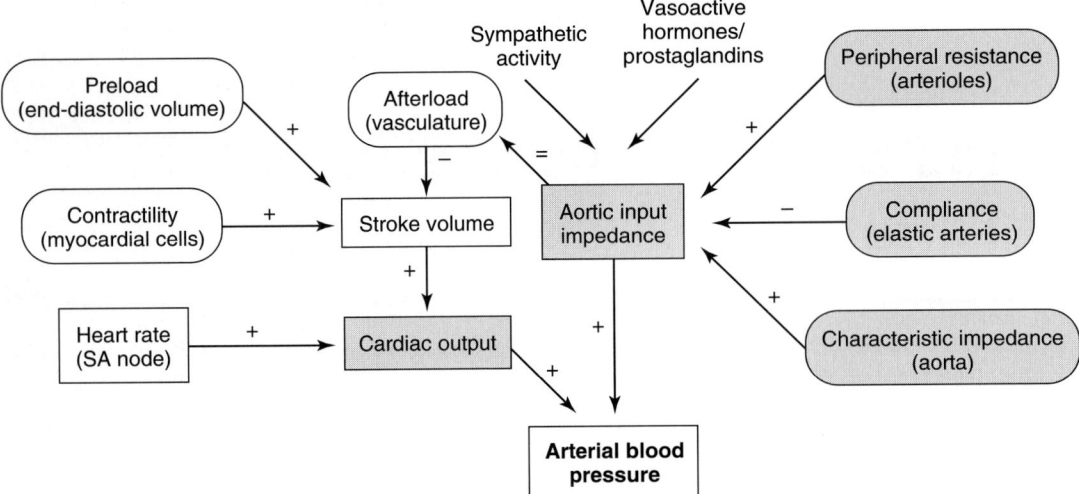

FIGURE 18–1. Control of arterial blood pressure. Arterial blood pressure is a function of the cardiac output and the arterial impedance. Contractility, preload, and afterload determine the stroke volume, which, multiplied by the heart rate, yields the cardiac output. Changes in arterioles, elastic arteries, and the aorta all influence the aortic input impedance (afterload). (+) = increases in the parameter increase aortic input impedance, stroke volume, cardiac output, or arterial blood pressure; (−) = increases in the parameter decrease aortic input impedance or stroke volume. (Modified from de Morais HSA: Pathophysiology of heart failure and clinical evaluation of heart function. In Ettinger SJ and Feldman EC [eds]: *Textbook of Veterinary Internal Medicine,* 5th ed. Philadelphia, WB Saunders Co., 2000.)

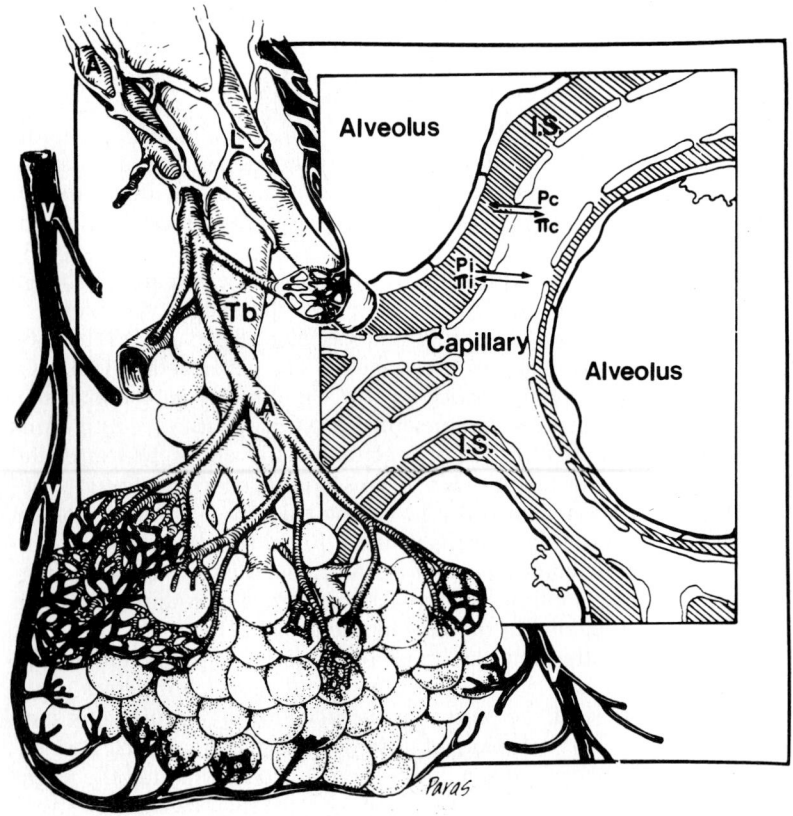

FIGURE 18–2. Microcirculation of the respiratory unit. The arteriole branches into the capillary plexus surrounding alveoli. Starling's forces controlling fluid movement into or out of the capillary or interstitial space (IS) are indicated. Capillary hydrostatic pressure in the lung must generally exceed 20 to 25 mm Hg before edema develops. Chronically, even higher hydrostatic pressures can be tolerated before edema develops. This is explained by the increased lymphatic drainage of the interstitium that develops in chronic edematous states. P_c = capillary hydrostatic pressure, which forces fluid into the interstitium; π_c = capillary colloid osmotic pressure due principally to albumin, which causes fluid to be retained within the capillary; P_i = interstitial hydrostatic pressure, which is negative in the lung; π_i = interstitial colloid osmotic pressure, which is controlled by pulmonary lymphatics and maintains the interstitium relatively free of albumin; A = arteriole; V = venule; L = lymphatic vessel; Tb = terminal bronchiole. (From Ware WW and Bonagura JD: Pulmonary edema. In Fox PR [ed]: *Canine and Feline Cardiology.* Philadelphia, WB Saunders Co., p. 252, 1999. Medical illustration by Felicia Paras.)

TABLE 18-1. **Factors Controlling Arterial Blood Pressure**

Variables Affecting Cardiac Output
Venous pressure and venous return
    Plasma volume
    Renal regulation of sodium and water
    Serum albumin
    Venous tone
        Sympathetic activity
        Local factors (e.g., kinins)
Ventricular diastolic function
    Venous pressure and venous return
    Myocardial relaxation
    Ventricular chamber compliance
    Pericardial restraint
    Ventricular filling
Ventricular systolic function
    Myocardial contractility
    Preload (ventricular end-diastolic volume)
    Afterload (arterial impedance)
    Valvular function
Electrical activity of the heart
    Heart rate
    Cardiac rhythm and conduction

Variables Affecting Systemic Vascular Impedance
Vasoconstriction
    Sympathetic nervous system
    Angiotensin II
    Arginine vasopressin (ADH)
    Endothelin
    Some prostaglandins
Vasodilatation
    Atrial natriuretic peptide (ANP)
    Brain natriuretic peptide (BNP, ventricular origin)
    Some prostaglandins (e.g., prostacyclin)
    Endothelium-derived relaxation factor (nitric oxide)
Aortic dynamic compliance

Arterial and Cardiac Baroreceptor (Mechanoreceptor) Reflexes

---

plasma volume and venous pressure exert the greatest effect at the venous end of the capillary. The interplay of hydrostatic pressures, oncotic pressures, capillary permeability, and lymphatic function determines whether the interstitium and serous body cavities accumulate or remain free of excess solute and water (Kaloyanides 1980; Starling 1894; Taylor 1982). The effect of these so-called Starling forces on fluid dynamics is summarized in Figure 18–2.

▶ The Circulation in Heart Failure

Heart failure is characterized clinically by hemodynamic abnormalities triggered by cardiac dysfunction (Kinugawa and Thames 1995). The causes of heart failure include numerous structural and functional disorders of the cardiac valves, myocardium, pericardium, and blood vessels, as well as sustained cardiac arrhythmias (Table 18–3). In response to impaired cardiac output, potent homeostatic mechanisms are activated that preserve perfusion of the brain and heart but at the expense of less vital regional circulations. Preservation of blood pressure mandates dramatic alterations in neural, hormonal, renal, and cardiovascular function and structure. These adaptations (summarized in Table 18–4) include activation of the sympathetic nervous system (Francis 1985; Ware et al. 1990), neurohormonal activation (Packer 1985; Francis and McDonald 1995), increased systemic vascular resistance (Francis et al. 1984, 1985) and impedance (Eaton et al. 1993), reduction of autonomic reflex activity (Zucker et al. 1979; Kinugawa and Thames 1995), and cardiac dilatation and hypertrophy (Katz 1990; Gaasch and Freeman 1995). Heart failure also alters renal function (Zucker et al. 1979; Paradiso et al. 1995) and enhances reabsorption of sodium and water (Watkins et al. 1976; Cannon 1977). In combination, these potent control systems are capable of maintaining normal ABP in all but the most severe cases of cardiac failure.

Hemodynamic abnormalities in the central circulation and microcirculation in CHF (Table 18–5) can be traced to both decreased cardiac performance and renal retention of sodium and water (Schrier 1988; Rose 1994; Paradiso et al. 1995). Decreased cardiac output, valvular insufficiency, or diminished ventricular compliance increases ventricular end-diastolic pressure, which is transmitted

TABLE 18-2. **Factors Regulating Plasma Volume in Heart Failure**

Controlled Variables
Arterial blood pressure (arterial and ventricular mechanoreceptors)
Plasma osmolality (central nervous system)
Serum sodium concentration (juxtaglomerular apparatus)
Renal perfusion pressure (kidney)
Atrial volume and pressure (left atrium)

Effectors Modifying Renal Glomerular and Tubular Function
Norepinephrine (sympathetic activity)
Renin-angiotensin
Arginine vasopressin (ADH)
Aldosterone
Renal blood flow (and distribution)
Natriuretic peptides (ANP, BNP)

Plasma Protein (Albumin)

Drug Therapy
Diuretics
    Loop diuretics (furosemide, bumetanide, torsemide)
    Thiazide diuretics (hydrochlorothiazide)
    Potassium-sparing diuretics (triamterene, amiloride)
    Spironolactone (blocks renal effects of aldosterone)
    Carbonic anhydrase inhibitors (acetazolamide)
Angiotensin-converting enzyme inhibitors (captopril, enalapril, benazepril, lisinopril)
Digitalis glycosides and other cardiotonic drugs
Vasodilator drugs (hydralazine, nitrates, angiotensin-converting enzyme inhibitors)

Fluid Balance
Fluid therapy (volume and type)
Dietary sodium intake
Voluntary water intake
Gastrointestinal function

TABLE 18-3. Causes of Heart Failure

Valvular Heart Disease
Congenital malformations
    Aortic stenosis
    Mitral valve malformation
    Pulmonic stenosis
    Tricuspid valve malformation
Acquired diseases
    Degenerative, myxomatous atrioventricular valvular disease
    Ruptured chordae tendineae
    Bacterial endocarditis

Myocardial Diseases
Malformations: defects of the atrial and ventricular septum
Dilated cardiomyopathy
Hypertrophic cardiomyopathy
Restrictive cardiomyopathy (endomyocardial fibrosis)
Undefined feline cardiomyopathies
Atrial muscle degeneration
Right ventricular cardiomyopathy
Myocarditis
Secondary myocardial diseases (hyperthyroidism, acromegaly, hypertension)

Pericardial Diseases
Idiopathic pericardial hemorrhage/pericarditis
Cardiac neoplasia leading to pericardial effusion
Infectious

Vascular Diseases
Malformation: patent ductus arteriosus
Arteriovenous fistula
Heartworm disease

High-Output States
Anemia
Thyrotoxicosis

Cardiac Arrhythmia
Chronic bradyarrhythmia
Chronic tachyarrhythmia

TABLE 18-4. Neurohormonal, Renal, and Cardiovascular Activities in Congestive Heart Failure

Autonomic
Heightened sympathetic nervous system activity
    Increased heart rate
    Augmentation of myocardial contractility
    Vasoconstriction
    Release of renin
Blunting of arterial blood pressure reflexes

Hormonal or Autocrine
Vasoconstricting or sodium-retaining systems
    Activation of the renin-angiotensin-aldosterone system
    Release of arginine vasopressin (antidiuretic hormone)
    Release of vasoactive prostaglandins and local vasoconstricting factors
        Endothelin-1
        Thromboxane
        Neuropeptide Y
Vasodilating or natriuretic systems
    Release of natriuretic peptides (impaired responsiveness of end organ)
    Increased basal nitric oxide (reduced release after receptor stimulation)
    Increased release of prostaglandins (E_2, I_2)
    Decrease in kallikreins
    Increased dopamine
    Decreased calcitonin gene-related peptide
Increased release of tumor necrosis factor and other cytokines

Renal
Efferent arteriolar constriction (via angiotensin II)
Increased filtration fraction (ratio of glomerular filtration rate to renal plasma flow)
Redistribution of renal blood flow
Increased sodium and water reabsorption

Cardiovascular
Cardiac adaptations
    Ventricular dilatation
    Ventricular hypertrophy
    Tissue changes (e.g., fibrosis, hypertrophy, altered collagen matrix)
    Intrinsic changes in cardiac isoenzymes
    Down-regulation of cardiac beta receptors
Vascular adaptations
    Vasoconstriction
    Increased systemic vascular resistance and arterial impedance
    Redistribution of blood flow
    Vascular remodeling

TABLE 18-5. Hemodynamic Consequences of Congestive Heart Failure

Reduced cardiac output
Increased systemic vascular resistance and arterial impedance
Increased pulmonary vascular resistance
Increased plasma volume
Increased ventricular end-diastolic pressure
Increased venous pressure
    Systemic (central) venous pressure
    Pulmonary venous pressure
Increased capillary hydrostatic pressure
    Edema
    Serous cavity effusions

---

back to the venous and capillary beds ("backward" failure). Higher venous and capillary pressures are augmented by renal fluid retention and expansion of the plasma volume. Renal sodium and water retention as a consequence of reduced cardiac output often is described in the medical literature as "forward" heart failure (Rose 1994). Forward failure, in this regard, does not refer to clinical signs of low cardiac output but instead describes the renal responses triggered by low cardiac output. Forward failure is a critical factor in the development of edema and effusions in right-sided and biventricular heart failure. These concepts and some of the factors responsible for increased venous and capillary pressures are shown in Figure 18-3. The important role of the kidney in the pathogenesis of edema and effusions is discussed later in this chapter.

Venous hypertension and increased end-diastolic pressure enhance cardiac filling and allow the ventricle to generate a greater contractile response. As shown in Figure 18-4, ventricular stroke volume is directly related to ventricular filling pressure (Swan et al. 1970; Franciosa et al. 1983). High venous pressure also maintains cardiac filling when ventricular compliance is decreased, as in

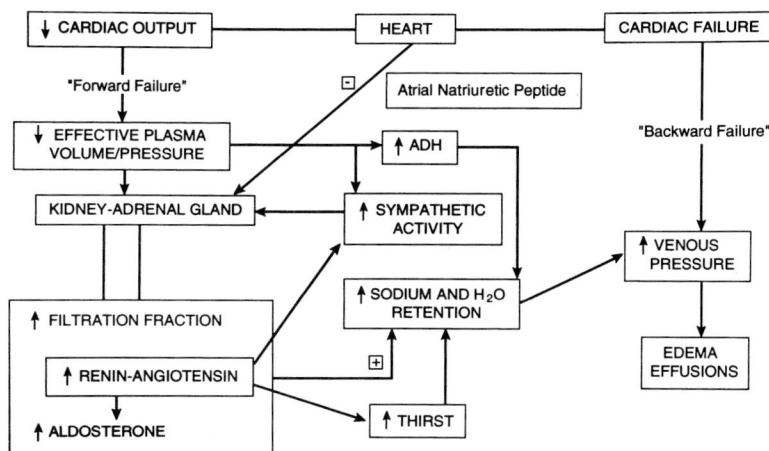

FIGURE 18–3. Prominent mechanisms responsible for fluid accumulation in heart failure. The development of pulmonary edema, subcutaneous edema, or the transudative effusions in body cavities can be explained by the combined effects of abnormally high venous pressure and renal retention of sodium and water. Ventricular systolic or diastolic failure increases venous pressure behind the failing ventricle ("backward" failure). This may be the predominant mechanism of edema formation in acute left-sided heart failure. In contrast, chronic heart failure, especially when right-sided or biventricular in nature, is characterized by avid sodium retention. Although atrial distention causes the release of atrial natriuretic peptide (ANP), the effects of sympathetic activity, angiotensin II, aldosterone, vasopressin (ADH), and local vasoconstrictor factors dominate, leading to vasoconstriction in systemic vessels and increased sodium and water reabsorption in the renal tubules. This is a simplified view as other local and systemic factors can be involved. (Modified from Bonagura JD: Fluid management of the cardiac patient. *Vet Clin North Am Small Anim Pract* 12:503, 1982.)

hypertrophic cardiomyopathy, pericardial disease, or gross ventricular dilatation (Gaasch and Freeman 1995) (see Fig. 18–4, lower panel). The clinical relevance of this relationship becomes obvious when the edematous patient is treated with diuretics and venous pressures, ventricular filling, and cardiac output decline, causing systemic hypotension or prerenal azotemia.

The term *congestive heart failure* implies a situation of increased venous and capillary hydrostatic pressures, increased transudation of fluid across capillary walls, and net accumulation of fluid in the interstitial compartment (i.e., edema) or serous body cavities (i.e., effusion). A safety margin normally prevents this accumulation of fluid, and venous pressures must increase substantially (usually to two or three times above the normal upper limit) before edema develops (Guyton and Lindsey 1959; Taylor 1982; Weaver and Carrico 1984; Staub 1984). Development of pulmonary edema in the dog usually requires left atrial pressure to rise acutely above 20 mm Hg (Guyton and Lindsey 1959). Substantial increases in lymphatic drainage permit much higher pressure to be tolerated chronically (Cannon 1977; Dumont et al. 1963). In addition to increased venous pressures, hypoalbuminemia can contribute to edema formation (Guyton and Lindsey 1959; Wiener-Kronish et al. 1987). As a consequence of variable lymphatic drainage and other factors such as capillary permeability and compartment compliance, edema is not uniformly distributed in the tissues (Weaver and Carrico 1984). This nonuniform distribution is evident clinically inasmuch as acute cardiogenic pulmonary edema in the dog is most prominent in perihilar and in right-sided lung lobes.

The edema of CHF develops predominantly in the capillary beds drained by the failing side of the heart. This finding is pertinent because CHF is classified clinically as left sided, right sided, or biventricular. Increased pulmonary venous and capillary hydrostatic pressures cause pulmonary edema (see Fig. 18–2), the cardinal finding of left-sided CHF. Right-sided CHF causes increased systemic venous pressures and leads to jugular venous distention or pulsation, hepatic congestion, ascites, or (infrequently in small animals) subcutaneous edema. Increased systemic venous pressure even may contribute to pulmonary edema formation (Miller et al. 1978). Pleural effusions develop as a result of left-sided, right-sided, or, most often, biventricular failure. This finding can be explained by the dual venous drainage of the pleural surfaces (i.e., parietal drainage is systemic whereas visceral drainage is pulmonary). Although veterinary textbooks usually attribute pleural effusion to isolated right-sided CHF, this is not common in human patients. Pleural effusion correlates better with pulmonary capillary wedge pressure than with right atrial pressure (Wiener-Kronish et al. 1987). Similarly, pleural effusions in small animals most often indicate biventricular CHF. Although pleural effusion does occur in some dogs and cats with predominantly right-sided cardiac disease (e.g., pulmonic stenosis, tricuspid malformation), ascites is more common. Clinically significant pleural effusions are rare in animals with isolated right ventricular failure caused by heartworm-induced pulmonary hypertension (Calvert and Rawlings 1988; Thrall and Calvert 1983). Conversely, pleural effusions are common when end-stage CHF develops in dogs with severe mitral regurgitation, pulmonary hypertension, and secondary right ventricular dysfunction or in cats with severe cardiomyopathy.

The relative contribution of renal sodium retention in CHF probably depends on the type and acuteness of

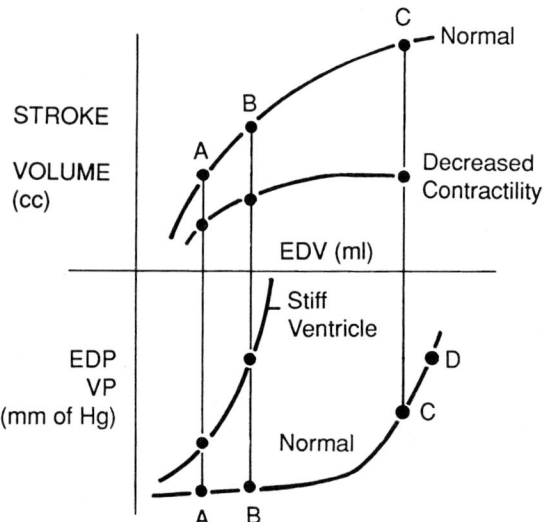

FIGURE 18-4. Ventricular function curves in heart failure. Ventricular function curves demonstrate the potential relationships between venous pressure (a determinant of ventricular filling and end-diastolic volume), ventricular compliance or distensibility (which determines the venous and atrial pressures required to fill the ventricle), and stroke volume (determined by ventricular end-diastolic volume, ventricular afterload, and myocardial contractility). The top of the graph demonstrates ventricular systolic function and the lower curves demonstrate ventricular filling dynamics.

Top: When inotropic ("contractile") state and afterload are held constant, the ventricular stroke volume depends on cardiac filling (preload), although this relationship is depressed in patients with myocardial failure. Patients treated with excessive dosages of diuretics may develop inadequate ventricular filling, leading to decreased stroke volume and cardiac output and causing prerenal azotemia. Reduction of diuretic dosage or fluid therapy is generally required to reestablish cardiac output.

Bottom: Ventricular distensibility—the tangent of any point on the diastolic pressure-volume curve—depends on the amount of ventricular hypertrophy, myocardial fibrosis, and the volume of the ventricle. Animals with stiff ventricles resulting from ventricular hypertrophy or myocardial fibrosis require high ventricular filling pressures and are poorly tolerant of fluid infusions. Note that increased cardiac filling can progress only at disproportionately higher venous pressures, a situation that predisposes to pulmonary edema. Recognize that even dilated ventricles can develop diastolic dysfunction (lower right). Once the grossly dilated ventricle reaches a certain point, distensibility decreases. Compare the slope at the extreme right of this diastolic filling curve with that of the smaller, hypertrophied ventricle. The benefit of diuretic therapy in this setting can be appreciated, as even small reductions in plasma volume and preload may permit the ventricle to fill at substantially lower venous pressures.

heart failure. The development of ascites, pleural effusion, or subcutaneous edema in right-sided or biventricular cardiac failure is accompanied by avid renal sodium retention (see next section). Dramatic weight loss, often exceeding 5 kg in large-breed dogs, may be observed after successful diuresis. This degree of weight loss after diuretic therapy is quite uncommon in isolated left-sided failure. Thus, successful therapy of right-sided CHF depends in the short term on initiation of a brisk diuresis. Long-term management hinges on improving cardiac function, reducing neurohormonal activation, and overcoming the potent sodium-retaining effects of forward cardiac failure.

In contrast to right-sided or biventricular CHF, severe left-sided heart failure can develop without substantial sodium retention or weight gain (Hollander and Judson 1956). Two common examples in veterinary medicine can be cited. The first example is rupture of a mitral chorda tendinea in an older dog with previously stable mitral regurgitation. The sudden increase in mitral regurgitant volume increases mean left atrial and pulmonary capillary pressures, leading to peracute pulmonary edema. The second example is a cat with hypertrophic cardiomyopathy and a noncompliant left ventricle (see Fig. 18–4, lower left curve). It is not uncommon for severe pulmonary edema to follow a bout of protracted tachycardia (e.g., stress). Development of pulmonary edema in these situations can be explained by acute deterioration of left ventricular systolic or diastolic performance that rapidly increases left atrial and pulmonary venous pressures. Although diuresis is an important treatment in this situation, short-term success may hinge on therapy that reduces mitral regurgitant fraction (i.e., afterload reduction) or improves diastolic ventricular function.

Another issue of relevance to CHF and fluid therapy of the cardiac patient is the relative size of the vascular compartments. The vascular compliance of the pulmonary circulation is much smaller than that of the systemic circulation, and sudden expansion of the plasma volume usually increases pulmonary venous pressure more than systemic venous pressure. This is particularly true in the patient with left-sided heart disease and explains why some dogs and cats develop pulmonary edema after intravenous administration of a so-called maintenance volume of crystalloid solution. Furthermore, central venous pressure (CVP) cannot be used to gauge the effect of intravenous fluid therapy on left-sided cardiac filling pressures, especially in the setting of isolated left-sided CHF (Rose 1994). Owing to differences in vascular compliance and cardiac function, left-sided filling pressures may increase much more rapidly than CVP.

▶ Renal Function in Heart Failure

Remarkably, the kidney often is able to maintain glomerular filtration in the setting of decreased blood pressure or cardiac output. Decreases in renal perfusion are countered by dilatation of the afferent arteriole mediated by the release of prostaglandin E_2, and constriction of the efferent arteriole primarily by angiotensin II. Efferent arteriolar constriction also is augmented by arginine vasopressin (antidiuretic hormone, ADH), norepinephrine, and atrial and brain natriuretic peptides (ANP and BNP) (Paradiso et al. 1995). These microvascular responses increase glomerular filtration pressure, increase filtration fraction, and maintain glomerular filtration in the setting of reduced renal blood flow (Packer et al. 1986a; Ritz and Nowack 1990; Suki 1989) (also see Chapter 2).

The renal response to decreased cardiac output is central to the pathogenesis of edema and effusions in heart failure. Studies of induced right-sided heart failure in dogs have demonstrated avid retention of administered salt loads (Barger et al. 1961). Numerous mechanisms have been identified for persistent sodium retention in CHF (see Fig. 18–3). These alterations include redistribution of renal blood flow (Barger et al. 1961; Priebe et al. 1980), enhanced tubular sodium reabsorption (Auld et al. 1971; Levy 1972; Millard et al. 1972), release of prostaglandins (Oliver et al. 1981; Dzau et al. 1984; Dzau and Swartz 1987), greater renal sympathetic nerve activity (Higgins et al. 1972; Osborn et al. 1983; Cohn et al. 1984; Levine et al. 1982; Schrier et al. 1971; Thomas and Marks 1978), increased renal interstitial pressure (Migdal et al. 1977; Granger 1986), and increased hormonal activity. The last includes increases in vasopressin (ADH) (Cannon 1977; Riegger et al. 1982), angiotensin II, and aldosterone (Freeman et al. 1979; Levens 1990; Riegger et al. 1984; Cohn and Levine 1982; Creager et al. 1981; Dzau et al. 1981; Gottlieb and Weir 1990; Hall et al. 1977; Hirsch et al. 1990; Ichikawa et al. 1984; Keane and Shapiro 1990; Kubo 1990; Packer et al. 1986a, 1986b; Ritz and Nowack 1990; Suki 1989) (see Table 18–4). Presumably, these mechanisms also operate in animals with spontaneous heart failure (Reinhardt et al. 1977).

Particular emphasis has been placed on the increased concentrations of renin, angiotensin II, and aldosterone found in patients with CHF (Packer 1985). There are numerous triggers for the release of renin in the cardiac patient. One mechanism is the stimulation of renal β-adrenergic receptors by sympathetic efferent traffic activated in response to hypotension. Renin also is released in response to reduced renal blood flow related to heart failure or volume depletion caused by diuretic therapy of CHF. Severe sodium restriction, especially in dogs with signs of heart disease but without overt CHF, can lead to renin release (Pedersen 1996). Clinically, the effects of angiotensin II and aldosterone can be mitigated in part by drugs that inhibit formation of angiotensin II (angiotensin-converting enzyme [ACE] inhibitors such as enalapril) or drugs that block the AT-1 receptor of angiotensin II such as losartan and candesartan (Table 18–6).

Other factors promote renal fluid retention in CHF. Changes in intrarenal blood flow can lead to redistribution of flow to the salt-conserving juxtamedullary nephrons (Levy 1972; Lifschitz and Schrier 1973; Cannon 1977). Increased filtration fraction maintains glomerular filtration rate but predisposes to renal tubular reabsorption of water (see Chapter 2). Arginine vasopressin (ADH) also plays a role. In CHF, increases in plasma ADH concentration probably represent nonosmotic release in response to low ABP (Paradiso et al. 1995). Increased thirst (mediated by angiotensin II), when combined with increases in ADH, can contribute to free-water retention and hyponatremia (Mettauer et al. 1986; Dzau and Hollenberg 1984; Packer et al. 1984). Endothelin is released from endothelial cells in CHF. This hormone reduces renal blood flow, glomerular filtration rate, and urinary sodium excretion (Paradiso et al. 1995; Margulies et al. 1990). The sequence in which these mechanisms are activated varies with the type and severity of heart failure (Rose 1994; Francis and McDonald 1995). It is clear, however, that with deterioration in cardiac function sodium- and water-retaining mechanisms are exacerbated and further expansion of the plasma volume occurs. Blunting the renal response generally requires appropriate medical treatment of CHF, progressive restriction of dietary sodium, and administration of diuretics.

In CHF, the vasoconstrictive and sodium-retaining mechanisms overwhelm local and systemic vasodilator and natriuretic systems. Distention of the atria, for example, signals the release of ANP, which normally causes diuresis and vasodilatation. Although an increased circulating concentration of ANP can be measured in dogs with experimentally induced CHF, it also has been shown that the renal response to this hormone is blunted or antagonized (Riegger et al. 1988; Cogan 1990; Molina et al. 1988). If dogs or people with CHF are treated with pharmacologic doses of ANP, however, or if the degradation of ANP is reduced by administration of a neutral endopeptidase inhibitor, diuresis may follow (Molina et al. 1988; O'Connor et al. 1998).

▶ Cardiovascular Drugs and Renal Function

Effects of Diuretics on Renal Function

Diuretics used in management of CHF prevent reabsorption of solute and water, leading to increased urine flow. Diuretics are essential to both the short- and long-term management of CHF. The clinical pharmacology of these drugs and effects on renal function (Table 18–7) are relevant to understanding their effectiveness and limitations.

All of the commonly used diuretics, except spironolactone, are delivered by renal blood flow and secreted in the proximal tubule. Circulatory failure, reduced renal blood flow, or primary renal failure may reduce the renal delivery of a diuretic. In the case of renal failure, endogenous organic acids can compete with furosemide for transport across the proximal nephron. Once secreted into the filtrate, a diuretic inhibits salt and water transport via a specific mechanism and at relatively specific sites along the nephron (Rose 1991; Jackson 1996; Opie et al. 1995).

Figure 18–5 demonstrates the general sites of action of the commonly used diuretics. The importance of understanding these details can be illustrated by two examples. First, the potency of a diuretic depends on the ability of cells distal to the site of diuretic action to reabsorb sodium and water. Initially in CHF, loop diuretics, which act on the thick portion of Henle's loop, are highly effective. However, in severe chronic CHF the more distal tubular cells can increase their reabsorption of sodium and water and overcome the effects of the diuretic (Rose 1994). This problem can be counteracted with additional treatment such as the combination of hydrochlorothiazide and spironolactone, which acts on the distal nephron. This type of sequential nephron blockade can induce a marked diuresis in some dogs. A second example pertains to the adverse effects of diuretics. Loop diuretics increase the delivery of sodium to cells of the late distal convoluted tubules and collecting ducts. At those sites, sodium is reabsorbed in exchange for potassium (under the influence of aldosterone) or hydrogen ions that are secreted (Jackson 1996). These ion exchange mechanisms have the potential to cause hypokalemia or metabolic alkalosis, especially with high doses or chronic therapy.

TABLE 18-6. **Effects of Cardiovascular Drugs on Renal Function**

Pharmacologic Class	Examples	Mechanism of Action	Effects on Renal Function
Angiotensin-converting enzyme inhibitors	Captopril, benazepril, enalapril, lisinopril, ramipril	Inhibit converting enzyme, preventing conversion of AT-1 to AT-2; also reduce degradation of vasodilator kinins	Reduce the activity of the renin-angiotensin-aldosterone system; can reduce intraglomerular filtration pressure by blocking angiotensin II–mediated vasoconstriction of the efferent arteriole
Angiotensin receptor blockers	Losartan, candesartan	Block AT-1 receptors of angiotensin II	As described for angiotensin-converting enzyme inhibitors; may also affect tissue renin-angiotensin-aldosterone systems
Catecholamines	Dobutamine, dopamine	Stimulate beta and alpha receptors to increase cardiac output and blood pressure; low doses of dopamine stimulate dopaminergic receptors in renal arterioles	Increase renal perfusion pressure; dilate renal blood vessels (dopamine)
Digitalis glycosides	Digoxin	Sensitize baroreceptors	Reduce sympathetic nerve activity; may reduce activation of the renin-angiotensin system
Diuretics*	Loop diuretics (furosemide) Thiazide diuretics Potassium-sparing diuretics (amiloride, spironolactone)	Prevent reabsorption of electrolytes and water at various sites along the renal tubules Furosemide (administered IV) can release atrial natriuretic peptide and prostaglandins	Increase urine volume and urinary electrolyte loss; high dose can precipitate volume depletion and acute renal failure; IV furosemide may cause dilation of renal arterioles
Neutral endopeptidase inhibitors	Sinorphan, ecadotril	Prevent degradation of atrial natriuretic peptide	Renal vasodilatation, increase urinary loss of sodium and water
Vasodilators	Hydralazine, sodium nitroprusside, prazosin	Dilate systemic arterioles by diverse mechanisms (e.g., generation of nitric oxide; α-adrenergic blockade)	May increase renal perfusion; if hypotension develops renal blood flow can decrease

*Also see Table 18–7.

The carbonic anhydrase inhibitors, such as acetazolamide, act on the proximal tubule by inhibiting bicarbonate reabsorption. These diuretics are limited in effectiveness because they induce metabolic acidosis and the loop of Henle and distal nephron can reabsorb much of the increased salt and water that is delivered to these segments. Carbonic anhydrase inhibitors are rarely if ever used in CHF.

Furosemide, ethacrynic acid, bumetanide, and torsemide exert their effects on the ascending limb of Henle's loop. These so-called loop diuretics block the Na^+-K^+-$2Cl^-$ cotransporter (symport) and prevent the active transport across the tubular lumen of two chloride ions, one sodium ion, and a potassium ion. Loop diuretics are potent with a good dose response ("high ceiling"). This is related to the high capacity for reabsorbing filtrate at this site (normally about 25% of the filtrate is reabsorbed at this site). Loop diuretics impair urinary dilution because dilution of the filtrate is a normal function of this segment. Urinary concentration also is impaired because blocking the Na^+-K^+-$2Cl^-$ carrier impedes development of a hypertonic renal interstitium. After administration of a loop diuretic, there are substantial losses of chloride, sodium, water, and other electrolytes (including potassium, magnesium, and calcium) in the urine. Intravenous administration of furosemide may cause release of vasodilator prostaglandins that increase renal blood flow (Bourland et al. 1977; Patak et al. 1979; Nomura et al. 1981; Packer et al. 1987).

The thiazide and thiazide-like diuretics act on the cortical distal convoluted tubule by competing with the luminal Na-Cl cotransporter and preventing movement of NaCl into the distal tubular cells. This effect impairs the ability to dilute urine (and excrete solute-free water) but does not necessarily affect urine concentration, which is a medullary function. Accordingly, in hyponatremia, when there is impaired free-water clearance, the thiazide diuretics are relatively contraindicated (Kaloyanides 1980; Rose 1991). The overall potency of thiazide diuretics is limited, in part because about 90% of the filtrate already has been reabsorbed before the distal nephron has been reached.

The late distal tubules and collecting ducts are sites of sodium reabsorption, aldosterone-controlled secretion of potassium ions, ADH-mediated water reabsorption, and urine concentration. Diuretics acting at these sites (e.g., spironolactone, amiloride, triamterene) initiate diuresis by preventing movement of sodium through luminal channels, either by directly blocking the channels (amiloride, triamterene) or by antagonizing the effect of aldosterone (spironolactone). These drugs also exert a potassium-sparing effect and often are classified by that description. They act very distally in the nephron, and their quantitative potential to inhibit sodium reabsorption

TABLE 18–7. Diuretics

Diuretic Class	Examples	Primary Site of Action	Mechanisms of Action	Adverse Effects in Dogs and Cats
Carbonic anhydrase inhibitors	Acetazolamide	Proximal tubules	Inhibit membrane and cytoplasmic carbonic anhydrase	Metabolic acidosis
Loop diuretics	Furosemide Bumetanide Torsemide Ethacrynic acid	Thick ascending loop of Henle	Block Na^+-K^+-$2Cl^-$ cotransporter (symport)	Volume depletion, azotemia, hypokalemia, hypomagnesemia, hyponatremia, ototoxicity
Thiazides Thiazide-like diuretics	Hydrochlorothiazide Chlorthalidone Metolazone	Distal convoluted tubules	Block the Na^+-Cl^- cotransporter (symport)	As described for loop diuretics Potential for hyponatremia Ventricular arrhythmias (from hypokalemia)
Potassium-sparing diuretics Aldosterone antagonists	Triamterene Amiloride Spironolactone	Late distal tubules Collecting ducts	Inhibit renal epithelial sodium channels (triamterene, amiloride) Inhibit mineralocorticoid receptors (spironolactone)	Hyperkalemia

is low, resulting in a weak diuretic effect. The diuretic effect of spironolactone depends on prevailing aldosterone concentrations (which are low in animals prescribed appropriate doses of ACE inhibitors). The main value of these drugs is for maintenance of normal serum potassium concentration or antagonism of aldosterone-induced cardiac injury (Sun and Weber 1998; Weber 1999).

There are a number of clinically relevant issues regarding the dosage and administration of diuretics (Dirks et al. 1966; Seely and Dirks 1977; Suki et al. 1965; Rose 1991). Many of the commonly used diuretics are organic anions at physiologic pH and are highly bound to serum proteins. To be effective, the diuretic must be delivered to the urinary space by glomerular filtration or active secretion in the proximal renal tubule. Active secretion is the more important mechanism because the drug is concentrated in tubular fluid. Reduced renal perfusion associated with heart failure, as well as primary renal disease, may limit the effectiveness of a diuretic unless a high dosage is employed and the drug is sufficiently

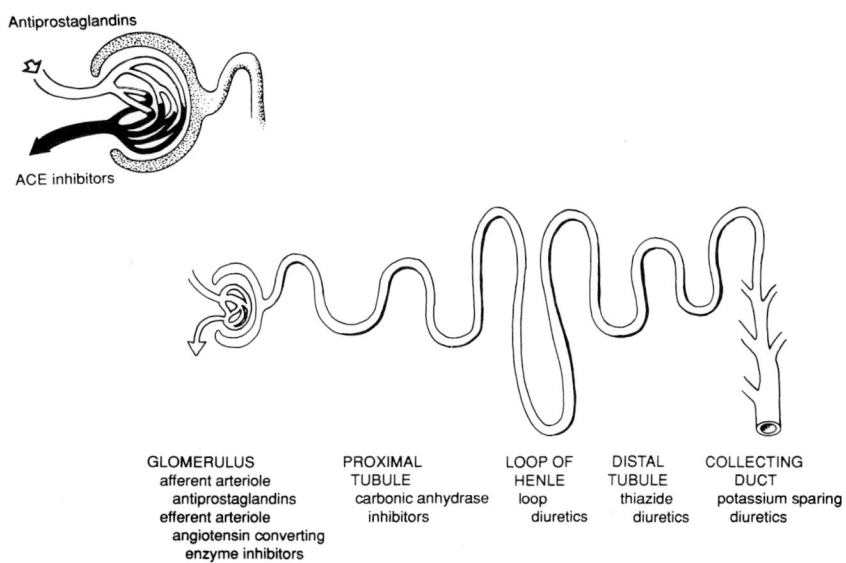

FIGURE 18–5. Renal effects of diuretics and angiotensin-converting enzyme (ACE) inhibitors in heart failure. This schematic drawing of the nephron indicates potential sites of action of various diuretic and vasodilator drugs. Acetazolamide, a carbonic anhydrase inhibitor, acts principally on the proximal tubules. Drugs acting on this segment are rarely if ever used in the management of congestive heart failure. Furosemide, bumetanide, torsemide, and ethacrynic acid act principally by impairing chloride transport in the loop of Henle, whereas the thiazides, spironolactone, triamterene, and amiloride act on more distal segments of the nephron. ACE inhibitors, such as enalapril, may interrupt the effects of angiotensin at a number of sites in the nephron. Of importance in heart failure is drug-induced vasodilatation in the efferent arteriole that can lower intraglomerular pressure, decrease filtration fraction, and precipitate acute renal failure.

concentrated in renal tubular fluid. The concern about renal perfusion is one rationale for initial high-dose, intravenous administration of furosemide in patients with severe CHF. Gastrointestinal absorption of diuretics such as furosemide may be impaired in CHF, especially with right-sided failure and intestinal edema. Temporarily switching from oral to parenteral administration of furosemide can have a dramatic diuretic benefit in some patients. Pain, administration of opiates (which stimulate ADH release), high sodium intake, and acute worsening of heart failure all represent clinical situations in which diuretics may fail and the dosage requirement for successful diuresis may be substantially higher.

Diuretic therapy triggers neurohormonal responses (Francis and McDonald 1995) and diuretic monotherapy is no longer considered appropriate for management of CHF. Diuretic-induced volume depletion leads to renal retention of salt and water. This effect is mediated by decreased tubular flow rate, salt retention in segments of the nephron unaffected by the diuretic used, increased sympathetic activity, and activation of the renin-angiotensin-aldosterone system (Rose 1994). Consequently, most patients with moderate CHF should be treated with an ACE inhibitor and a diuretic. If diuretic monotherapy is prescribed, administration of the drug three times daily may become necessary, and even at this frequency the diuretic may become less effective ("braking" effect).

The dosage of diuretics used must be effective but should be carefully controlled to prevent the common complications of dehydration, azotemia, and electrolyte imbalance (see later). The initial dosage of furosemide chosen for a patient with life-threatening pulmonary edema often is high (2–5 mg/kg, IV q1–3h) to ensure diuresis. Symptomatic improvement, brisk diuresis, and decline in pulmonary capillary wedge pressure often develop within 1 to 2 h of administration of furosemide, but a lag period (24–48 h) may be noted between obvious clinical improvement and clearing of radiographic pulmonary densities. After initial therapy, a lower daily dosage of furosemide is chosen (2–4 mg/kg q12h in dogs and 1 mg/kg q12–24h in cats), but adjustments may be required during the first week of therapy. Owing to the potential for overzealous diuresis and iatrogenic renal failure and electrolyte disturbances, the clinician should evaluate serum biochemistry every 24 to 48 h until the patient is eating and drinking satisfactorily. After a stable diuretic course of 2 to 3 weeks, most dogs maintain relatively normal renal function and serum potassium concentration unless a decompensating factor (e.g., vomiting, anorexia) intervenes. This is especially true when ACE inhibitors are prescribed concurrently because they reduce aldosterone concentration and decrease potassium loss. Thus, stable serum creatinine and potassium concentrations over two or three reevaluation periods are likely to be maintained for some time (Rose 1994). The overall dosage of diuretics should be limited by using combination therapy for CHF, including progressive sodium restriction, ACE inhibitors, and digoxin if there are no contraindications (Parmley 1985; Keene and Rush 1989). Cats receiving furosemide are more prone to develop mild to moderate azotemia and hypokalemia than are dogs, even at dosages that are 50% lower than daily dosages used for dogs.

Effects of Other Cardiovascular Drugs on Renal Function

Angiotensin II is one of the factors responsible for efferent arteriolar vasoconstriction and increased filtration fraction in CHF. The ACE inhibitors, such as enalapril, may antagonize efferent arteriolar constriction sufficiently in some patients to cause an abrupt fall in glomerular perfusion pressure. This effect is especially likely in volume-depleted patients. The result is acute renal failure, with serum creatinine concentration often exceeding 5 mg/dL. Renal failure in this setting generally can be reversed by reducing diuretic dosage, lowering the dosage of the ACE inhibitor, and providing judicious fluid therapy (see later in this chapter). After volume repletion, the dosage of the ACE inhibitor gradually is increased over 2 to 4 weeks, and the drug combination is adjusted while monitoring body weight, clinical signs of CHF, ABP, and serum creatinine concentration.

Normal autonomic responses to changes in blood pressure are blunted in CHF (Higgins et al. 1972). This allows sympathetic activity to dominate in experimental models of cardiac failure. Sympathetic nerve activity can increase renin release and affect renal blood flow (Paradiso et al. 1995). Digitalis glycosides such as digoxin appear to exert a neurotropic effect and restore baroreceptor sensitivity and parasympathetic tone, and this effect is independent of the inotropic action of the drug (Thames 1979; Kinugawa and Thames 1995). By this or some other effect, digoxin also can blunt the renin-angiotensin-aldosterone system in CHF.

Aspirin and other antiprostaglandin drugs may be deleterious in CHF patients, preventing prostaglandin-in-

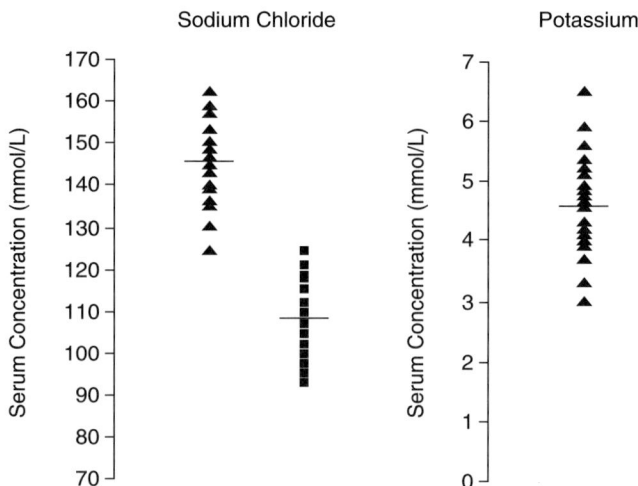

FIGURE 18–6. Serum sodium, chloride, and potassium concentrations of 39 dogs with CHF at the time of admission to the hospital. The individual values are plotted for each dog (some values overlap). The mean value is shown as a horizontal line. Median values (not shown) are sodium, 148 mEq/L; chloride, 109 mEq/L; potassium, 4.6 mEq/L.

duced dilatation of the afferent arteriole and antagonizing the effects of furosemide. The renal effects of other cardiac drugs are summarized in Table 18–6.

▶ Serum Biochemical Abnormalities in Congestive Heart Failure

The majority of serum biochemical abnormalities in heart failure can be attributed to alterations in renal function, changes in dietary intake of water and electrolytes, diuretic and other drug therapy, and drug toxicosis. Most alterations are mild, and two surveys of serum biochemical concentrations of patients at our hospitals have failed to demonstrate severe changes in the majority of cardiac patients (Figs. 18–6 and 18–7) (Bonagura and Ware 1986; Bonagura and Lehmkuhl 1992). Nevertheless, some animals with CHF develop substantial disorders of fluid and electrolyte balance that may require fluid therapy and adjustment of cardiac medications.

Sodium

Serum sodium concentration usually is normal in heart failure (see Fig. 18–6), but total body sodium and total body water are likely to be increased. Severe right-sided or biventricular CHF can be associated with hyponatremia. Salt wasting secondary to concurrent diuretic use may contribute to hyponatremia, but it is uncommon for low serum sodium concentration in an edematous patient to be caused solely by salt depletion. Multiple factors are probably involved (Mettauer et al. 1986; Dzau and Hollenberg 1984; Packer et al. 1984; Fichman et al. 1971; Friedman et al. 1989). One likely cause of hyponatremia in CHF is dilution resulting from markedly reduced renal free-water clearance (see Chapter 3). This effect probably is mediated by the nonosmotic release of arginine vasopressin (ADH) and indicates insufficient cardiac output. Continued release of ADH and polydipsia are important factors to be considered in the pathogenesis of hyponatremia in the patient with CHF. In one study of dogs with CHF, dogs with severe heart failure caused by dilated cardiomyopathy were more likely to develop hyponatremia (Ware et al. 1990). Activation of the renin-angiotensin-aldosterone system is predictable in the setting of severe CHF, and glomerular filtration pressure may depend largely on efferent arteriolar constriction mediated in part by angiotensin II (Packer et al. 1986a; Ritz and Nowack 1990). Consequently, ACE inhibitors must be used very carefully in such patients. Such treatment, however, often is effective in improving CHF and, despite a reduction in serum aldosterone concentration, increasing serum sodium concentration (see section on therapy of fluid and electrolyte imbalances).

Potassium

Serum potassium concentration may be normal, increased, or decreased in patients with heart failure (see Fig. 18–6). Mild *hyperkalemia* may be observed in acute low-output heart failure because of an abrupt reduction in glomerular filtration rate. Overzealous administration of potassium salts and potassium supplementation in the presence of potassium-sparing diuretics, beta blockers, or ACE inhibitors are causes of iatrogenic hyperkalemia. Profound hyperkalemia can occur in cats with CHF and concurrent aortic thromboembolism. This probably is related to multiple factors, such as muscle necrosis, reperfusion of infarcted tissues (Pion and Kittleson 1989), metabolic acidosis, and renal failure with inadequate urinary excretion of potassium. Management of life-threatening hyperkalemia may be required as discussed in Chapter 5.

Hypokalemia is particularly injurious because it predisposes to digitalis intoxication and muscular weakness and may induce cardiac arrhythmias. Hypokalemia in the cat has been linked to abnormal taurine metabolism and taurine deficiency–associated myocardial failure (Dow et al. 1992). Numerous factors predispose to hypokalemia in the cardiac patient (Rose 1994). Anorexia resulting from chronic disease or digitalis intoxication can lead to inadequate potassium intake. Cardiac cachexia and tissue wasting also lead to increased potassium loss. The renin-angiotensin-aldosterone system may be important because potassium excretion is enhanced by aldosterone. Fortunately, aldosterone concentrations are readily reduced by administration of an ACE inhibitor. Reduced renal perfusion may influence potassium handling because inadequate delivery of sodium to the distal tubule causes potassium to be secreted with organic acids (Kaloyanides 1980; Rose 1991). Kaliuresis of variable magnitude occurs with diuretic therapy unless a potassium-sparing diuretic, such as spironolactone or triamterene, or an ACE inhibitor is prescribed. We have observed hypokalemia even when potassium-sparing diuretics have been administered. Cats

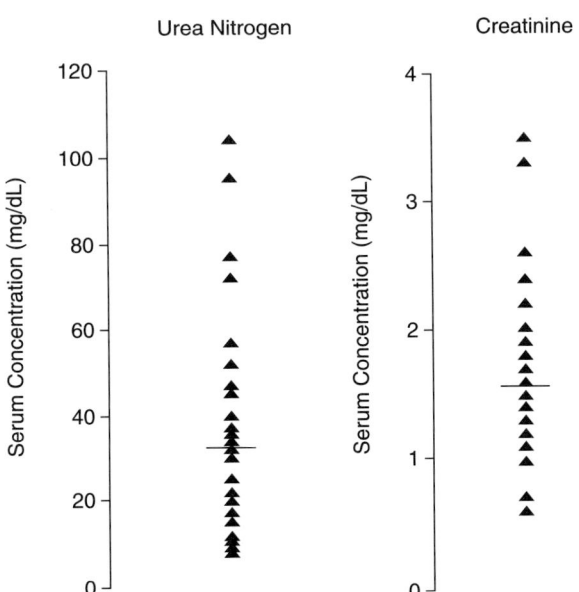

FIGURE 18–7. Serum (blood) urea nitrogen (BUN) and serum creatinine concentrations of 39 dogs with CHF at the time of admission to the hospital. The individual values are plotted for each dog (some values overlap). The mean value is shown as a horizontal line. Median values (not shown) are BUN, 25 mg/dL; creatinine, 1.4 mg/dL.

seem particularly prone to diuretic-induced hypokalemia. The potent loop diuretics, such as furosemide, also promote kaliuresis by accelerating delivery of sodium to the distal nephron, leading to an overall increase in the rate of sodium-potassium exchange (Kaloyanides 1980; Rose 1991; Cobb and Michell 1992). Combination diuretic therapy is especially likely to lead to hypokalemia, even in the presence of ACE inhibitors or spironolactone. Lastly, metabolic alkalosis is a frequent complication of volume contraction, vomiting, or diuretic-induced chloriuresis (Rose 1991, 1994). Alkalosis increases the concentration of potassium in the renal tubular cell and promotes its secretion into the tubular fluid.

Other Electrolytes

Serum chloride concentration usually is normal in heart failure (see Fig. 18–6). It is common, however, for an animal to develop mild hypochloremia after diuretic therapy. Mild hypochloremia is the most commonly observed diuretic-induced electrolyte disturbance in our practice. This observation probably is due to the inhibitory effect of furosemide and other loop diuretics on chloride transport and may be associated with a small but commensurate increase in serum bicarbonate concentration as estimated by the total CO_2. Serum calcium and phosphorus concentrations are normal in CHF unless renal failure or another unrelated disorder is present. *Hypomagnesemia* has received little attention in veterinary medicine, but it is common in human patients undergoing diuresis induced by loop diuretics (Decarli et al. 1986; Swales 1982; Ryan 1987). The potential importance of magnesium is emphasized by the association of hypomagnesemia with cardiac arrhythmias and the use of magnesium infusions to treat digitalis-induced cardiac arrhythmias in human patients. Serum magnesium concentration in dogs with CHF did not decrease significantly after furosemide therapy in one study of dogs (Edwards 1991) but was 20% lower than that of a control population in another study of dogs (Cobb and Michell 1992). Digitalis also has been shown to increase urinary magnesium excretion.

Acid-Base Disturbances

Blood pH in heart failure is the product of competing factors that alter acid-base balance. Complex acid-base disorders are common because of disturbances in tissue oxygenation and in pulmonary and renal function. As a result, simple determination of total CO_2 without direct measurement of blood pH and calculation of bicarbonate may lead to erroneous conclusions (see Chapters 9–12). In our experience, respiratory alkalosis and metabolic acidosis are the most commonly encountered acid-base disorders in acute heart failure. Mild metabolic alkalosis is not uncommon in patients receiving chronic diuretic therapy.

Metabolic acidosis may be caused by a stagnant circulation with hypoxia and lactic acidemia (Fulop et al. 1973), by prerenal azotemia, or by tissue ischemia as may occur with aortic thromboembolism. In uncomplicated cases, the venous pH and bicarbonate concentrations are mildly decreased and arteriovenous oxygen difference is increased. In severe CHF, with avid vasoconstriction, mixed venous PO_2 often is lower than 30 mm Hg. *Respiratory acidosis* is a less common but more serious complication and indicates the presence of severe respiratory failure, pulmonary edema, compression atelectasis (from pleural effusion), or respiratory muscle fatigue. Respiratory acidosis is characterized by the development of arterial hypoxemia and hypercapnia and a decrease in blood pH unless a mixed disorder is present (see Chapter 12). *Metabolic alkalosis,* with increased bicarbonate concentration and blood pH, is common and often is a complication of diuretic therapy with resultant volume contraction (contraction alkalosis) and renal loss of chloride and potassium (Kaloyanides 1980; Rose 1991). Vomiting, a common complication of digitalis intoxication, also leads to chloride loss and metabolic alkalosis. *Respiratory alkalosis* with a low PCO_2 may be detected in some patients because animals with moderate pulmonary edema tend to hyperventilate.

Serum Proteins

Serum protein concentration frequently is decreased in severe heart failure, especially in dogs with right-sided or biventricular failure. In a survey of dogs with CHF and atrial fibrillation, about one-fourth had low serum protein concentrations (Bonagura and Ware 1986). Concurrent disorders (e.g., liver disease, renal disease, gastrointestinal disease) also may influence serum protein concentration.

The mechanisms responsible for decreased serum protein concentration in CHF are undetermined. Possible explanations include lymphatic loss of protein through a congested intestine, decreased hepatic synthesis, cardiac cachexia, and enhanced endothelial permeability caused by increased capillary pressure and hypoxia. Ascitic fluid is higher in protein concentration than is a transudate collecting in the pleural space because the hepatic sinusoid is more leaky than other capillary beds. Consequently, considerable protein can pool in the peritoneal cavity of a cardiac patient with ascites, and the protein concentration in ascitic fluid can exceed 3.5 g/dL. Repeated abdominal paracentesis also can contribute to total body depletion of protein. Plasma volume contraction after diuretic therapy usually increases serum protein concentration, but total serum protein concentration may remain subnormal or in the low-normal range. Hypoproteinemia in dogs with CHF caused by heartworm disease may be related to glomerular injury and renal protein loss. Dramatic proteinuria has been observed in heartworm-infected dogs with concurrent renal amyloidosis.

There are a number of clinical consequences of hypoproteinemia in CHF. Effective plasma volume is decreased further when moderate to severe hypoalbuminemia develops. As demonstrated in experimental studies of dogs with left atrial hypertension, edema is more likely to occur at lower venous pressures when there is hypoalbuminemia (Guyton and Lindsey 1959). Marked protein loss through the gut may indicate a need for additional nutritional support. Hypoalbuminemia also predisposes to metabolic alkalosis (see Chapter 10). Infusions of plasma may be required in the patient with severe hypoalbuminemia and may promote a substantial diuresis.

TABLE 18–8. Causes of Azotemia in Heart Failure

Renal Disease
Preexisting renal disease
Renal thromboembolism (feline cardiomyopathy, bacterial endocarditis)
Heartworm disease (glomerulonephritis, amyloidosis)

Inadequate Renal Blood Flow
Dehydration
    Anorexia and hypodipsia
    Vomiting
    Water restriction (by the client or veterinarian)
Severe heart failure (low cardiac output, hypotension)

Drug Related
Volume contraction resulting from diuretics
Angiotensin-converting enzyme inhibitors (hypotension, efferent arteriolar vasodilatation)
Vasodilator therapy (hypotension)
Digitalis intoxication (secondary to anorexia or vomiting)

Renal Function Tests

The blood urea nitrogen (BUN) and serum creatinine concentrations may increase in CHF, indicating reduced glomerular filtration. There are several reasons for development of azotemia in heart failure, but the most common are preexisting renal disease, reduced cardiac output, and iatrogenic problems (i.e., overzealous use of diuretics and ACE inhibitors). Common causes of azotemia in dogs or cats with CHF are listed in (Table 18–8).

Approximately 25% of dogs with CHF are azotemic at the time of admission (Bonagura and Ware 1986) (also see Fig. 18–7). The magnitude of azotemia generally is mild to moderate. Renal function should be assessed both before and after initiation of therapy. Azotemia is common in patients with dilated cardiomyopathy and cardiogenic shock and may improve only after aggressive therapy with inotropic agents and reestablishment of hydration (see section on therapy of fluid and electrolyte imbalances). The development of azotemia in a patient with previously normal renal function suggests overzealous diuresis, an adverse reaction to an ACE inhibitor, inappropriate water restriction, or a worsening of heart failure. Return of serum creatinine concentration to normal after intravenous or subcutaneous administration of a crystalloid solution or after reduction of drug dosage indicates a prerenal or drug-induced cause of azotemia. Acute renal failure that responds promptly to intravenous administration of a crystalloid solution has been observed in some dogs treated with ACE inhibitors (see earlier).

▶ Therapy of Heart Failure

Overall management of fluid balance in the cardiac patient requires effective treatment of CHF and control of edema. The initial goals of heart failure therapy include increasing arterial PO_2, reducing oxygen demand, and decreasing venous pressure and the tendency to edema formation. Additional aims include maintaining cardiac output, ABP, and tissue perfusion. In-hospital therapy is needed for animals with moderate to severe CHF. Eventually, a long-term home treatment plan is prescribed.

Hospital Therapy

The first goals are attained with supplemental oxygen therapy and sedation as needed to reduce distress or air hunger. Dogs can be sedated with morphine (initial dosage of 0.05–0.1 mg/kg IM), but one must recognize that vomiting after morphine injection occasionally precipitates cardiac arrest. An alternative sedative protocol for dogs uses a mixture of acepromazine (0.025 mg/kg) with either buprenorphine (0.005 mg/kg IM) or butorphanol (0.2 mg/kg IM). Stress in cats can be alleviated with an acepromazine-butorphanol combination (0.1 mg/kg acepromazine and 0.25 mg/kg butorphanol IM). In the presence of a moderate to large pleural effusion, thoracocentesis is performed to decrease pulmonary atelectasis. Tense ascites, sufficient to impair ventilation, is reduced by abdominocentesis. About one-third of the total ascitic volume is drained. The high protein content of hepatic lymph and the dynamic equilibrium between the third-space and plasma compartments argue against complete drainage of the peritoneal space (Rose 1994). Pulmonary edema sufficient to cause respiratory failure and respiratory muscle fatigue is an indication for artificial ventilation. Diuresis with furosemide (initial dosage of 2–5 mg/kg IV) and venodilator therapy (e.g., nitroglycerin ointment or sodium nitroprusside) act in concert to reduce venous and capillary hydrostatic pressures.

Cardiac output and tissue perfusion are increased by unloading the left ventricle by administering arteriolar dilators and providing inotropic support if needed. The need for arteriolar dilators depends on the cause and severity of CHF, and vasodilator therapy constitutes a more aggressive approach with the risk of inducing systemic hypotension. Vasodilators such as hydralazine (1–2 mg/kg PO q12h), enalapril (0.5 mg/kg PO q24h or q12h), and sodium nitroprusside (1–5 μg/kg/min by constant-rate infusion) are useful in specific situations (Bonagura and Rush, in press). Inotropic support with dobutamine (2.5–10 μg/kg/min) or dopamine (2–10 μg/kg/min) is particularly helpful in animals with dilated cardiomyopathy, whereas dogs with mitral regurgitation or cats with hypertrophic cardiomyopathy rarely need inotropic support in the hospital setting. These treatments are titrated to achieve a systolic ABP of 90 to 120 mm Hg.

Home Therapy

Chronic therapy of CHF often involves treatment with an ACE inhibitor. A fundamental feature of CHF is dominance of vasoconstrictive–sodium-retaining mechanisms over competing vasodilator-natriuretic systems (Francis and McDonald 1995). Chronic activation of the sympathetic nervous system and the renin-angiotensin-aldosterone system also can injure the myocardium, blood vessels, and other tissues (Hirsch et al. 1995; Sun and Weber 1998). Several studies, including clinical trials in veterinary medicine, have emphasized the beneficial effect of pharmacologic blockade of these systems on both morbidity and mortality in CHF (Riegger et al. 1984; Creager and Cusco 1995; Shimoyama et al. 1995; IMPROVE Study Group 1995; COVE Study Group 1995). Two prospective North American studies of dogs in CHF have demonstrated the efficacy of enalapril at 0.5 mg/kg PO q24h or q12h (IMPROVE Study Group 1995; COVE Study Group 1995). A European study of benazepril use in dogs with CHF yielded similar results at dosages of 0.5 mg/kg q24h or q12h. Alternatively, lisinopril (0.25–0.5 mg/kg q24h or q12h) can be prescribed. Cats with chronic CHF also can benefit from ACE inhibition. Although the initial dosage is low (0.25–0.5 mg/kg q48h PO), higher dosages are tolerated by some cats (0.25–0.5 mg/kg q12h PO).

Thus, the typical home therapy of CHF in dogs includes an ACE inhibitor as described before, furosemide (2–4 mg/kg PO q24h to q8h), and often digoxin (0.005–0.01 mg/kg PO q12h). When CHF is complicated by atrial fibrillation, treatments may be needed in addition to digoxin. For example, treatment with either diltiazem (0.25–1.0 mg/kg q8h PO) or propranolol (0.1–0.6 mg/kg q8h PO) allows better control of ventricular rate response in atrial fibrillation. These negative inotropic drugs, however, must be used carefully in CHF. They should be initiated at a low dosage and gradually increased to the desired effect. Other dietary measures may be considered. The addition of omega-3 fatty acids found in fish oil may inhibit cytokines and reduce cardiac cachexia (Freeman et al. 1998). Typical dosages are 30 to 40 mg/kg PO daily for eicosapentaenoic acid (EPA) and 20 to 25 mg/kg PO daily for docosahexaenoic acid (DHA). Nutriceuticals, such as taurine or L-carnitine, may be indicated for some patients (Kittleson et al. 1997).

Increasingly, emphasis is being placed on treatments that reduce the deleterious effects of neurohormones on cardiac and vascular tissues. Similar to the angiotensin-converting enzyme inhibitors, β-adrenergic blockers improve left ventricular ejection fraction and inhibit myocardial remodeling and fibrosis in humans and in animal models of myocardial failure (Bristow 1997). Careful dose titration is critical, as the negative inotropic effects can worsen CHF. Another advance has been renewed interest in blocking tissue renin-angiotensin-aldosterone systems by administration of the aldosterone antagonist spironolactone (Weber 1999). This therapy has produced substantial benefits in human patients with CHF. Although these treatments require more study in animals, they seem particularly relevant for dogs with dilated cardiomyopathy.

Home management of the cat with progressive CHF or recurrent pulmonary edema or pleural effusion secondary to cardiomyopathy often includes furosemide (1–2 mg/kg PO q24h or q12h) and enalapril. Digoxin (one-fourth of a 0.125-mg tablet q48h) also is prescribed for dilated or restrictive cardiomyopathy. Diltiazem (30 mg of a sustained-release product, initially q24h) often is recommended for long-term management of feline hypertrophic cardiomyopathy. Specific treatment plans for hospital and home management of CHF in dogs and cats can be found elsewhere (Bonagura and Rush, in press; Bonagura and Lehmkuhl 1999).

Refractory Edema and Effusions

Some patients become refractory to diuretic therapy and continue to develop edema or effusions (Rose 1991). Three commonly encountered examples of this problem are (1) progressive ascites and pleural effusion in dogs with biventricular heart failure, (2) progressive pleural effusion in cats with cardiomyopathy, and (3) recurrent pulmonary edema in dogs with left-sided heart failure. Successful therapy of some of these patients may be attained by skillful use of cardiac medications (O'Connor et al. 1998) and by addressing the following points:

- Ensure medication compliance and educate the client about medications, dosages, and methods of administration.
- Consistently enforce a low-sodium diet.
- Enforce rest.
- Optimize current medication dosages, especially the daily dosage of an ACE inhibitor.
- Adjust the dosage or route of administration of furosemide.
- Consider using combination diuretic therapy.
- Improve left-sided heart function.
- Identify and treat extracardiac complications such as hyperthyroidism, anemia, and hypertension.

The first three points are straightforward but by no means easy to achieve. With progressive CHF, the sodium intake should be progressively limited unless the patient is hyponatremic. Periods of enforced rest are useful in mobilizing edema and decreasing cardiac work. Rest alone can lead to considerable diuresis in patients with right-sided CHF. The remaining guidelines require some explanation.

Current medication dosages should be optimal for the stage of CHF. The effect of an ACE inhibitor in CHF may be dose dependent (Van Veldhuisen et al. 1998). Frequently, veterinarians prescribe ACE inhibitors but do not always maximize the dosage for fear of precipitating hypotension or renal failure. For both enalapril and benazepril, the daily dosage should be increased to at least 0.5 mg/kg PO q12h. If ABP is satisfactory (i.e., systolic pressure > 90 mm Hg), even higher dosages (0.75 mg/kg q12h) may be considered. In addition, in dogs with predominately left-sided CHF, a second vasodilator can be prescribed (see later). Unless there is a contraindication to digitalization (e.g., complex ventricular ectopia, atrioventricular block, sinus node disease, moderate to severe renal failure), digoxin should be prescribed. The dosage should yield a trough serum digoxin concentration of 0.8 to 1.2 ng/mL, but trough concentrations as high as 2 ng/mL may be acceptable.

Modifying the daily or individual diuretic dosage may be necessary, especially in dogs with chronic renal failure, in dogs that develop severe polydipsia, and in those with apparent intestinal malabsorption of furosemide. Low dosages of furosemide (i.e., 1–2 mg/kg q12h or q24h), in combination with an ACE inhibitor, are quite effective in patients with mild heart failure. Patients with renal failure or low cardiac output, however, may require higher dosages to deliver sufficient active drug to the renal tubules (Gerlag and van Meijel 1988). In the case of furosemide, gradually increasing the dosage and frequency from 2 mg/kg q12h to 6 mg/kg q8h may be sufficient to cause maximal inhibition of chloride and sodium reabsorption. Once this "ceiling" effect is achieved, no further diuresis develops with that individual dosage (Rose 1991). This is especially true with the loop diuretics (e.g., furosemide, bumetanide), which typically have a short duration of action (see previous section on diuretics). Furosemide may be poorly absorbed by a congested intestine (Vasko et al. 1985), and the clinician may wish to consider subcutaneous administration of furosemide in patients with refractory ascites and pleural effusion. Frequently, the same daily dosage, given subcutaneously instead of orally, leads to substantial diuresis. We have taught clients to administer furosemide subcutaneously to their animals, and such therapy can be beneficial when used chronically. One approach involves replacement of one oral dose of furosemide by an identical dose, administered subcutaneously, on Monday, Wednesday, and Friday. If the dog responds favorably, the frequency is reduced to twice weekly.

Combination diuretic therapy represents another option for the patient with refractory edema or effusion (Rose 1991; Heinemann 1978; Oster et al. 1983). The combination of two or three agents acting on different segments of the nephron may be more effective than the use of a single drug. Most clinicians begin therapy with furosemide, and addition of a thiazide or spironolactone, drugs that act on the distal cortical segments, may overcome the compensatory increase in distal salt and water retention that occurs with chronic furosemide therapy. One approach is to administer furosemide PO q8h and a hydrochlorothiazide-spironolactone (or hydrochlorothiazide-triamterene) combination tablet in place of one of the furosemide doses. The patient is evaluated clinically and by serum biochemistry after 5 days. If serum biochemistry is acceptable but congestion persists, the hydrochlorothiazide-spironolactone combination can be given twice daily. The patient then is reexamined in 7 days. This combination therapy has a potassium-sparing effect, but profound hyponatremia and hypokalemia occur occasionally. This combination diuretic treatment can be recommended for dogs with progressive ascites or pleural effusion unless there is significant hyponatremia (i.e., <130 mEq/L). Thiazide diuretics are avoided in dogs or cats with hyponatremia. Angiotensin-converting enzyme inhibitors (Kluger et al. 1982; Dzau and Hollenberg 1984; Rouse et al. 1987) and other treatments that improve cardiac function are preferred (Keene and Rush 1989; Loeb et al. 1977). These treatments are discussed in the next section.

Refractory pulmonary edema in dogs caused by mitral valve disease or cardiomyopathy should be managed by ensuring optimal digitalization, maximal dosages of an ACE inhibitor, and effective diuretic therapy with furosemide. When this approach fails, a second vasodilator can be prescribed to unload the left ventricle and reduce the mitral regurgitant fraction. Many dogs tolerate the combination of hydralazine (0.5–1 mg/kg PO q12h) or amlodipine (0.05–0.1 mg/kg PO q24h) with an ACE inhibitor. Treatment should be initiated in the hospital with frequent monitoring of ABP. Systolic pressure should be titrated to 85 to 90 mm Hg. When the dog is released from the hospital, the client is advised to report any clinical signs of hypotension. Potent inotropic-vasodilator drugs (inodilators), such as milrinone and pimobendan, also have been efficacious in some dogs with refractory CHF, but these drugs are not widely available. Cats with recurrent pulmonary edema caused by hypertrophic cardiomyopathy often respond when enalapril is added to therapy with furosemide and the calcium channel blocker diltiazem.

▶ Therapy of Fluid and Electrolyte Imbalances in Congestive Heart Failure

Indications

The cardiac patient, in contrast to many other sick animals, is not an ideal candidate for parenteral fluid therapy. Volume expansion poses substantial risks in terms of increasing venous pressures, sodium retention, and edema. In managing cardiac patients, we prefer to offer water (of low sodium content) ad libitum, provide a sodium-restricted but palatable diet, treat CHF medically, and allow the patient's kidneys to correct any fluid and electrolyte disturbances. This approach may lack technical sophistication, but it often works well in the clinical setting. Dogs are especially resilient to the complications of diuretic therapy provided their intake of water and food is adequate. In fact, it is common to observe a dog or cat begin drinking shortly after receiving successful therapy for life-threatening pulmonary edema or pleural effusion.

Unfortunately, some patients with heart failure do develop problems that require fluid and electrolyte supplementation. Indications for fluid therapy in the patient with CHF include persistent anorexia, dehydration, renal failure, moderate to severe hypokalemia, digitalis intoxication, drug-induced hypotension, gastroenteritis, anemia, and serious metabolic (e.g., diabetes mellitus), neoplastic, or infectious diseases. Another indication is the need for intravenous infusion to deliver drugs such as dobutamine, sodium nitroprusside, or lidocaine. When animals with heart disease undergo general anesthesia, a catheter should be placed and intravenous fluids administered. Ventricular filling in pericardial disease requires higher than normal venous pressures, and this abnormality may demand volume expansion with parenteral fluid therapy.

Thus, a number of situations may necessitate fluid therapy in the cardiac patient. What fluid should be infused? The following recommendations are based on our clinical experience and theoretical considerations for fluid, electrolyte, and diuretic therapy in patients with CHF. Controlled, prospective evaluations of such therapy in dogs and cats are unavailable. The following discussion considers basic principles of therapy; selection of fluids, additives, and rates of administration; monitoring of the patient (including Swan-Ganz catheterization); and our approach to some specific problems related to fluid therapy in the cardiac patient.

Parenteral Solutions

FLUID VOLUME

The daily fluid volume is guided by the current state of edema, estimated maintenance needs (40–60 mL/kg/day), hydration status, body weight, oral fluid intake, estimated urine output, total serum protein concentration, serum sodium concentration, serum creatinine concentration, and, when available, central venous and pulmonary capillary wedge pressures. It is prudent to consider a minimal fluid infusion initially (e.g., no more than 30–40 mL/kg/day) and to assess the effect of fluid therapy on the patient. The daily volume should be infused slowly and distributed evenly over 24 h to reduce the risk of pulmonary edema and pleural effusion. The choice of fluid depends largely on concerns about sodium retention (see later). The intravenous route of administration is preferred, but either 0.45% NaCl in 2.5% dextrose or lactated Ringer's solution can be given subcutaneously if necessary. When the patient can drink, fluid therapy is tapered, low-sodium fresh water is supplied ad libitum, and dietary sodium intake is regulated while ensuring a palatable diet.

The CHF patient continues to retain sodium, and diuretics must be given concurrently to prevent untoward retention of sodium derived from the diet or crystalloid therapy. Although it may seem paradoxical to administer diuretics to a patient receiving fluid therapy, these drugs are important adjuncts to the overall fluid and electrolyte management in treatment of the edematous cardiac patient (Kaloyanides 1980; Hamlin et al. 1965; Rose 1991). Diuretic therapy also promotes redistribution of extracellular water from edematous sites to the venous system. Furosemide and the thiazides also act initially to increase glomerular filtration rate (possibly by releasing vasodilating prostaglandins). After diuresis and contraction of the plasma volume, however, cardiac filling and glomerular filtration rate decrease unless the patient drinks adequately or receives supplemental fluid therapy. A fine balance is required, and the clinician must learn to control the risk of edema while preventing an increase in BUN or serum creatinine concentration.

SODIUM

Dogs with cardiac failure do not respond normally to a sodium load, and after saline infusion, marked retention of sodium and water can occur (Barger et al. 1961). Healthy dogs can maintain normal serum sodium concentration with a diet containing sodium at only 0.5 mEq/kg/day (11.5 mg/kg/day) (Michell 1989; Morris et al. 1976). This amount is equivalent to approximately 175 mg of sodium or 435 mg of sodium chloride per day for a 15-kg dog. A 14.75-oz can of Canine Prescription Diet H/d (Hill's) contains 108 mg sodium (20 mg sodium per 100 kcal; 538 kcal per can), and a 12.5-oz can of CV-Formula (Purina) contains 130 mg sodium (20 mg/100 kcal; 571 kcal/can). A 2.5-oz jar of chicken baby food contains approximately 40 to 60 mg sodium. A number of over-the-counter dog foods also are relatively restricted in sodium (e.g., Cycle Senior, Alpo Senior). The extent of dietary sodium restriction required in animals with CHF has not been determined, but it seems prudent to limit daily sodium intake to less than 12 mg/kg/day in dogs with advanced cardiac failure. The average sodium content of Feline Prescription Diet H/d (Hill's) is 354 mg per 14.25-oz can (70 mg/100 kcal; 506 kcal/can), and a 5.5-oz can of CV-Formula (Purina) contains 112 mg sodium (50 mg/100 kcal; 223 kcal/can). Dietary sodium requirements for cats in CHF are not available.

The clinician also must be mindful of the sodium content of crystalloid solutions. Normal saline solution (0.9% NaCl) contains 154 mEq of sodium per liter. Therefore, 500 mL of 0.45% NaCl in 2.5% dextrose contains 37.5 mEq (862 mg) of sodium, an amount that conceivably represents the minimal daily requirement for a normal 75-kg dog. If severe metabolic acidosis is present (pH < 7.1–7.2), and sodium bicarbonate must be added to the fluid, an additional sodium load is imposed (see Chapter 10). There are 23 mg of sodium per milliequivalent of sodium bicarbonate, and this sodium load must be considered when calculating daily sodium intake.

On the basis of these concepts, either 5% dextrose or 0.45% NaCl in 2.5% dextrose, supplemented with potassium chloride, is recommended when routine fluid therapy is required for rehydration, maintenance of hydration, or drug infusions in patients with CHF. Unfortunately, therapy with 5% dextrose or 0.45% NaCl in 2.5% dextrose is sometimes associated with inadequate free-water excretion, weight gain, hyponatremia, and hypokalemia. These electrolyte disturbances are similar to those observed when some dogs and cats with severe CHF are treated with diuretics and given free access to water. Development of hyponatremia in this clinical setting is especially common in cats. Because of the potential for hyponatremia, some clinicians prefer to administer small volumes of a balanced crystalloid, such as lactated Ringer's solution, that contains sodium chloride in concentrations closer to those of normal extracellular fluid. The short-term use (<12 h) of such sodium-replete fluids usually is well tolerated, provided the volume is small and the rate of infusion slow (e.g., 2.5–5 mL/kg/h). Therapy of hyponatremia is discussed later and in Chapter 3.

POTASSIUM SUPPLEMENTATION

Potassium (as the chloride salt) is administered routinely to cardiac patients receiving fluid therapy. Administration of glucose-containing, salt-poor solutions, especially during diuretic therapy of anorexic patients, tends to lower serum potassium concentration. Typical intravenous potassium dosages of 0.5–2.0 mEq/kg/day are given using accepted guidelines for intravenous administration of potassium (see Chapter 5). For hypokalemic animals, higher dosages of potassium chloride are used up to a rate not to exceed 0.5 mEq/kg/h intravenously. Oliguria, hyperkalemia, and concurrent administration of potassium-sparing diuretics, beta blockers, or ACE inhibitors are relative contraindications for parenteral potassium therapy, unless serum potassium concentration is known to be low. When providing the patient with oral potassium chloride supplementation, the clinician should consider that there is 1 mEq of potassium in each 89 mg of potassium chloride salt (or in 234 mg of potassium gluconate).

BLOOD PRODUCTS

Moderate to severe anemia increases the demand for cardiac output and can precipitate CHF. In most cases, the packed cell volume must fall below 22% or it must drop rapidly for cardiac complications to occur. Although anemia alone can cause high-output heart failure, the development of pulmonary edema or pleural effusion is even more common in the setting of a preexisting heart disease such as cardiomyopathy or chronic valvular heart disease. Anemic patients often receive fluid therapy to maintain blood pressure and organ perfusion, and this poses another risk for the dog or cat with underlying cardiac dysfunction. Similarly, the hemoglobin solution Oxyglobin expands plasma volume and can cause CHF in susceptible patients. Management of these animals involves medical therapy of CHF, treatment of the underlying cause of anemia, and often a slow infusion of packed cells to reduce the demand for cardiac output.

Managing Electrolyte Disorders in CHF

Electrolyte disturbances, notably hypokalemia, hypochloremia, and metabolic alkalosis, are common complications of diuretic therapy. Digitalis intoxication with anorexia and vomiting can have similar effects. Mild reductions in serum chloride concentration are of limited concern but hypokalemia should be avoided in cardiac patients because it predisposes to cardiac arrhythmias, digitalis intoxication, muscle weakness (and necrosis), and renal fibrosis and may decrease serum taurine concentration in cats (Dow et al. 1992). Fortunately, most dogs do not develop marked hypokalemia during the initial hospital therapy of CHF (Bonagura and Lehmkuhl 1992). With the widespread use of ACE inhibitors (which spare potassium loss), hypokalemia also is relatively uncommon during chronic management of CHF, except in the settings of digitalis intoxication, vomiting, or prolonged anorexia or when combination diuretic therapy is prescribed. Cats are more prone to hypokalemia. Even a 1-day course of parenteral furosemide can lower serum potassium concentration in cats. Hypokalemia is common with chronic furosemide administration in cats unless prevented by an ACE inhibitor or potassium supplementation.

Hypokalemia can be prevented in the hospital setting by encouraging food intake and supplementing parenteral fluids with KCl (see earlier). Routine oral potassium supplementation is needed only when diuretics are administered chronically, but neither an ACE inhibitor nor potassium-sparing diuretic is part of the treatment plan. In such cases, a KCl "salt substitute" can be sprinkled on the food, or the client can administer a prescription formulation of potassium gluconate or potassium chloride daily. As a rule, potassium supplementation should not be given with an ACE inhibitor because hyperkalemia may develop. Use of oral potassium supplements and the hospital management of severe hypokalemia are described in detail in Chapter 5.

Serum sodium concentration generally is normal in cardiac patients, and the finding of hyponatremia is a serious sign. Low serum sodium concentration in the setting of excess extracellular fluid volume suggests decreased effective arterial blood volume with impaired renal water excretion related to persistent release of ADH. Diuretics also may contribute to hyponatremia (and hypochloremia) by causing hypokalemia, inducing plasma volume depletion and release of ADH, and impairing function in the diluting segments of the nephron (Kaloyanides 1980; Fichman et al. 1971; Friedman et al. 1989). Thiazide diuretics are especially likely to cause hyponatremia because they favor excretion of relatively concentrated urine. These abnormalities are exacerbated by increased water intake associated with polydipsia, which can be prominent in dogs with CHF, or by infusion of a sodium-poor crystalloid. The general causes of and approach to hyponatremia are described in Chapter 3.

Therapy of hyponatremia in CHF is difficult. Mild hyponatremia (130–145 mEq/L in dogs) simply is an indication to adjust cardiac therapy. Moderate hyponatremia (<130 mEq/L), especially when associated with prerenal azotemia, is an indication for cage rest, mild water restriction, frequent determination of body weight and serum biochemistry, and vigorous therapy of CHF. Furosemide is continued because studies in human patients suggest that furosemide may promote the formation of more dilute urine, thereby increasing free-water clearance, whereas thiazides do not (Rose 1991). Thiazide diuretics should be discontinued. If the patient is receiving fluids, either lactated Ringer's solution or 0.9% NaCl, supplemented with KCl, should be used initially at conservative infusion rates (e.g., 20–30 mL/kg per 24 h). Infusion for 48 to 72 h of a catecholamine (dobutamine or dopamine) or an inodilator such as amrinone or pimobendan (if available) should be considered to increase cardiac output. Gradually increasing the dosage of ACE inhibitor up to the maximal dosage tolerated (at least 0.5 mg/kg of enalapril or benazepril q12h) is important to antagonize the renin-angiotensin-aldosterone system (Dzau and Hollenberg 1984; Packer et al. 1984). Despite the theoretical concern that an ACE inhibitor would reduce serum sodium concentration, clinical experience in this setting is just the opposite. Severe hyponatremia (<120 mEq/L) requires water restriction and cautious infusion of 0.9% saline to prevent the neurologic consequences of hyponatremia (see Chapter 3). Mannitol may increase delivery of filtrate to the distal diluting segments of the nephron and increase free-water clearance. With few exceptions, patients with CHF and severe hyponatremia have been unresponsive to therapy. Therapy with ADH analogues that block the effects of this hormone on the distal nephron may become available in the future (Schrier and Abraham 1999).

Monitoring of Patients

Cardiac patients require careful monitoring of clinical, hematologic, cardiac, and hemodynamic variables. It is important to tabulate and establish the trend of important clinical signs: body temperature, respiratory rate and depth, breath sounds, heart rate, heart rhythm, mucous membrane color and refill time, pulse strength, attitude, noninvasively determined arterial blood pressure, and pulse oximetry if available (Table 18–9). Frequent determination of such simple variables as water and food intake, estimated urine output, body weight, infused fluid

TABLE 18-9. Evaluation of the Cardiac Patient

Inspection and Examination
Body weight
Estimated hydration
Jugular venous pressure
Arterial blood pressure (indirect or direct)
Body temperature
Pulse rate and quality
Respiratory rate
Pattern of ventilation
Cardiac auscultation
Pulmonary auscultation and percussion
Level of consciousness
Muscle strength
Mucous membrane color and capillary refill time
Evaluation for ascites (measurement of girth)

Laboratory Evaluation
Blood urea nitrogen and serum creatinine
Serum electrolytes (sodium, potassium, chloride)
Blood gas tensions (Po_2, Pco_2)
Blood pH and bicarbonate

Chest Radiograph
Evaluation of heart size
Pulmonary vascularity
Pulmonary infiltrates or edema
Pleural effusion

Electrocardiogram
Heart rate and rhythm
ST segment (myocardial perfusion or ischemia)
T wave

Determination or Calculation of:
Intravenous fluid requirements
Oral water intake
Urinary output
Total daily sodium intake (intravenous and dietary)
Total daily potassium intake (intravenous and dietary)
Total daily caloric intake
Environmental temperature and humidity

Hemodynamic Measurements
Central venous pressure (right-sided filling pressures)
Pulmonary capillary wedge pressure (left-sided filling pressures)
Cardiac output

Current Therapy
Diuretic drugs
Crystalloid and additives
Cardiotonic agents, including digitalis
Vasodilators and angiotensin-converting enzyme inhibitors
Additional measures: paracentesis, oxygen, antiarrhythmic drugs, bronchodilator, omega-3 fatty acids

---

volume, and diuretic dosage provides the clinician with useful information about fluid dynamics and the need for fluid therapy. Serial determination of serum creatinine, sodium, and potassium concentrations is useful for adjusting fluid, diuretic, and cardiac therapy. Physical and radiographic signs of fluid accumulation may indicate a need to reduce fluid volume and increase diuretic dosage or consider additional treatments, such as vasodilator drugs. More accurate hemodynamic information can be obtained using a percutaneously placed pulmonary arterial catheter, as described in the following section. The effect of fluid therapy on central and pulmonary venous pressures is a prime concern in patients with heart failure and can be a major determinant of the rate of fluid administration. Insufficient venous pressure reduces cardiac output whereas very high pressures promote formation of edema. In heart failure, an optimal venous pressure is necessary to maintain cardiac output, but pulmonary venous pressures above 20 mm Hg and central venous pressures (CVPs) above 10 to 12 cm H_2O may be associated with formation of edema.

The CVP is simple to measure using an indwelling jugular venous catheter, and its determination quantifies and indicates the directional changes of right heart filling pressures. Inspection and estimation of jugular venous pressure provide similar qualitative information. A CVP line is quite useful in guiding fluid management of seriously ill patients without heart disease, but CVP is *not* an accurate reflection of pulmonary venous pressure in CHF. The ability of the left and right ventricles to accept and pump blood may be quite different in CHF. Accordingly, the effects of a volume infusion on the left ventricle and pulmonary circulation may not be accurately gauged by measuring the filling pressures of the right ventricle (Swan et al. 1970; Forrester et al. 1976; Franciosa et al. 1983). It is quite common to observe animals with high pulmonary venous pressure but relatively low CVP. This is especially true after diuretic therapy. Even in animals with right-sided CHF, ascites may continue to develop despite a relatively low CVP, possibly as a result of avid sodium retention, hypoproteinemia, or the development of cardiac cirrhosis and portal hypertension secondary to chronic hepatic congestion.

In order to obtain measurements of pulmonary venous and left-sided cardiac filling pressures, a catheter must be advanced into a lobar pulmonary artery under fluoroscopic or pressure-monitored guidance (Fig. 18–8). Special end-hole, balloon-tipped catheters (Swan-Ganz) can be used to occlude pulmonary arterial flow temporarily, permitting measurement of the damped left atrial pressure waveform, which is transmitted through the valveless pulmonary venous and capillary beds (Swan et al. 1970; Forrester et al. 1976; Franciosa et al. 1983; Keene and Rush 1989). The mean value of such a determination is called the *pulmonary capillary wedge pressure* and is equivalent to the mean left ventricular filling pressure (but not equivalent to the end-diastolic pressure in some patients) (Fig. 18–9). Pulmonary edema generally is associated with pulmonary capillary wedge pressures above 20 to 25 mm Hg. These values are guidelines, and even higher values may not be associated with edema in chronic left-sided heart failure. The clinician can measure the pressure filling the left ventricle and estimate the tendency to form pulmonary edema by determining whether low (<7 mm Hg), optimal (12–18 mm Hg), or high (>20 mm Hg) venous pressures are present in the cardiac patient (Franciosa et al. 1983) (see Figs. 18–9 and 18–10). The rate of fluid administration, diuretic dosage, and cardiac therapy are guided by these measurements. Marked reductions in pulmonary capillary wedge pressure

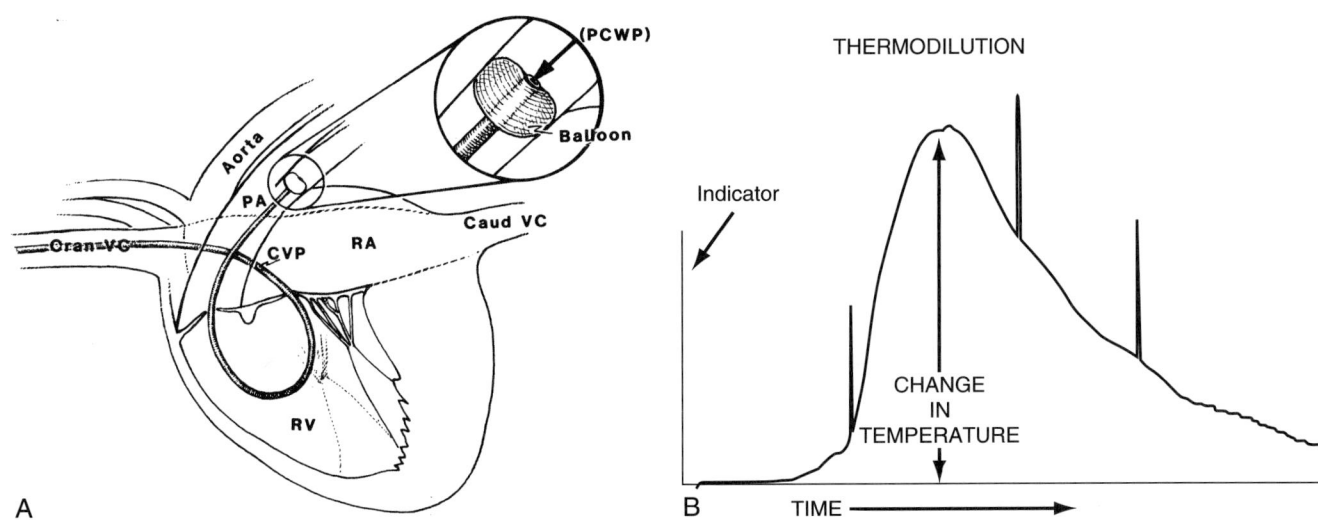

FIGURE 18–8. Swan-Ganz pulmonary catheterization. *(A)* Determination of central venous pressure and pulmonary capillary wedge pressure. Determination of right and left ventricular filling pressures (left lateral view). A balloon-tipped, flow-directed catheter (Swan-Ganz) is inserted into the jugular vein and passed through the cranial vena cava (Cran VC), right atrium (RA), right ventricle (RV), and pulmonary artery (PA). Two independent catheter lumina permit pressure determinations in both the right atrium and the pulmonary artery. The proximal lumen in the RA measures the central venous pressure (CVP), and the distal tip measures the PA pressure. When the balloon is inflated, blood flow is temporarily occluded and the pulmonary capillary wedge pressure (PCWP) is measured (inset). Caud VC = caudal vena cava. *(B)* Cardiac output curve of a 21-kg dog in heart failure. The curve was obtained using a Swan-Ganz catheter equipped with a distal thermistor tip for measuring blood temperature. The recording demonstrates the change in blood temperature that developed after 3 mL of iced 5% dextrose was injected into the right atrial port of the catheter. Cardiac output is inversely related to the area under the curve. The calculated cardiac output in this case was 2.3 L/min. (*A* from Bonagura JD: Fluid management of the cardiac patient. *Vet Clin North Am Small Anim Pract* 12:509, 1982.)

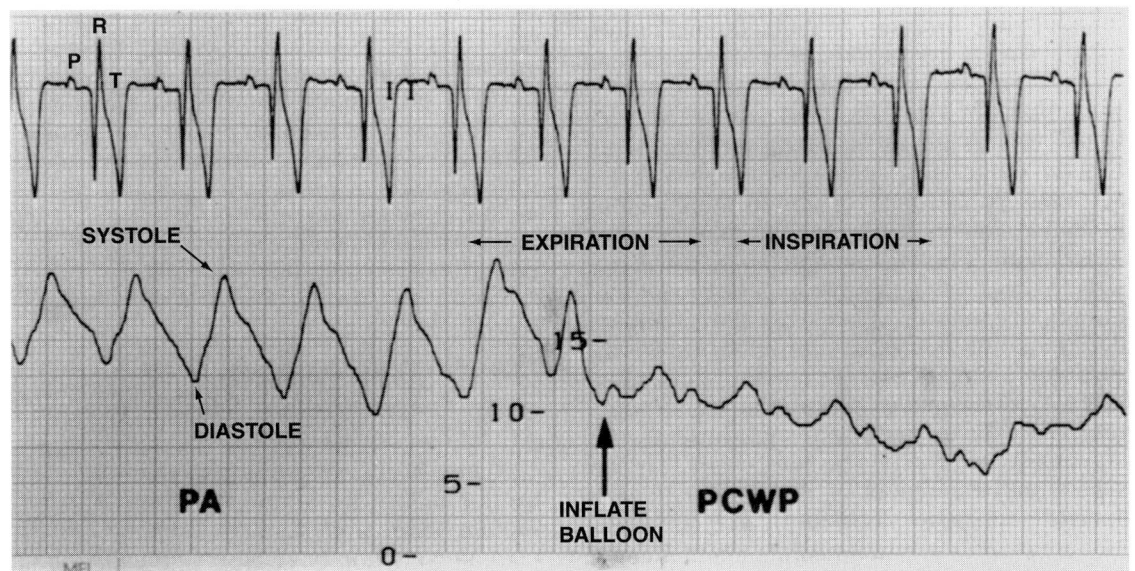

FIGURE 18–9. Pressure tracing recorded from the pulmonary artery of a dog undergoing diuretic treatment of congestive heart failure. The pulmonary artery pulsatile pressure and occlusion (wedge) pressure are indicated. Balloon inflation is complete at the arrow. Notice that the pulmonary artery diastolic pressure is closely related to the wedge pressure. The pulmonary artery diastolic pressure is often used to track changes in the wedge pressure (provided there is no pulmonary vascular disease). Variations in the pressure recording baseline are related to ventilation. Measurements are generally made during expiration to avoid the "dips" associated with negative intrapulmonary pressures.

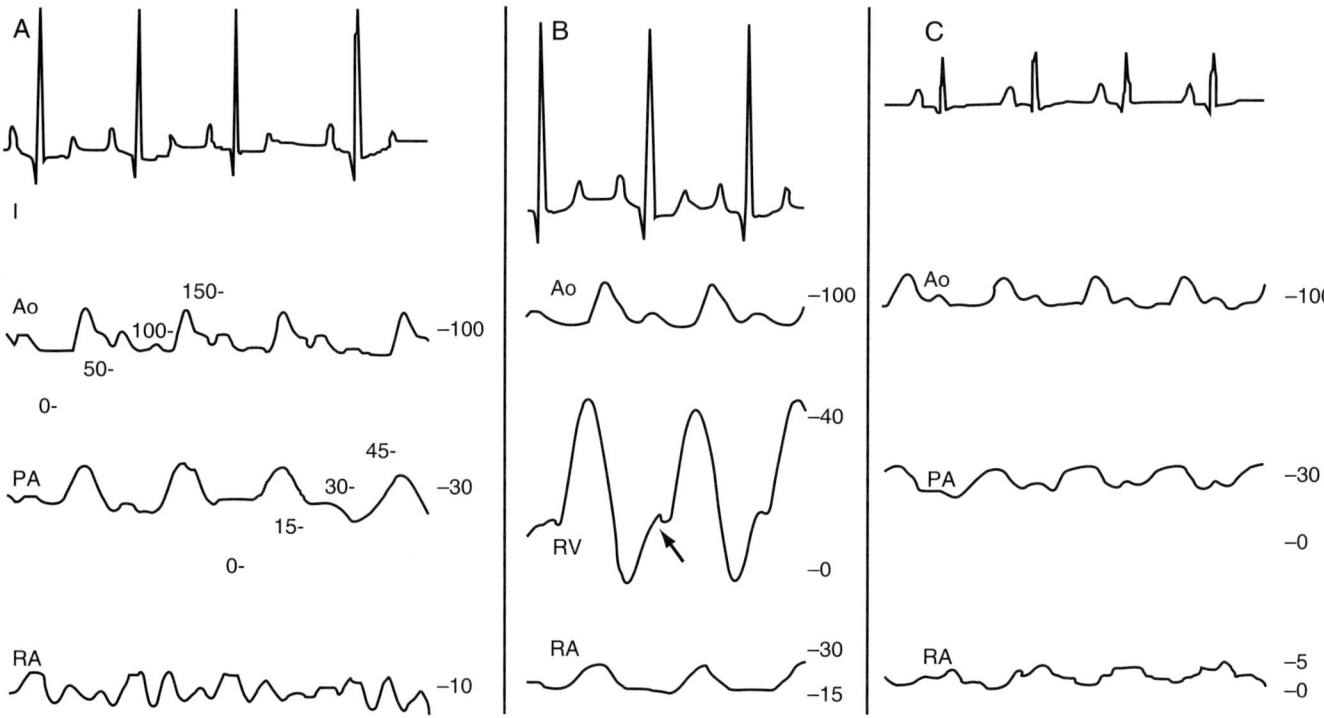

FIGURE 18-10. *(A)* Electrocardiogram and pressure recordings from a standing dog with dilated cardiomyopathy and biventricular cardiac dysfunction. There is pulmonary hypertension secondary to abnormally high wedge pressure (not shown) and left-sided cardiac dysfunction. The pulmonary artery pressures are approximately 39/23 (systolic/diastolic) mm Hg. The right atrial pressure (central venous pressure) is also abnormally high, with a mean value of approximately 9 mm Hg. Scales indicate mm Hg for the adjacent curves. Ao = pressure in the descending aorta; PA = pressure in the pulmonary artery; RA = pressure in the right atrium. *(B)* ECG and pressure recordings from a standing dog with dilated cardiomyopathy and mitral and tricuspid regurgitation during infusion of 0.9% saline solution. Volume expansion has led to a marked increase in the right atrial pressure (mean, 16 mm Hg). The right ventricular pressure (RV) tracing also indicates an increase in the end-diastolic ventricular pressure (arrow). Pulmonary hypertension from left-sided heart failure accounts for the increase in systolic RV pressure (42 mm Hg, normal is < 25 mm Hg). Scales on the right indicate mm Hg for the preceding curves. *(C)* ECG and pressure recordings from a standing dog with mitral regurgitation and mild left-sided heart failure. Pulmonary hypertension secondary to abnormally high wedge pressure (not shown) and left-sided cardiac dysfunction are present. The pulmonary artery pressures are approximately 34/25 (systolic/diastolic) mm Hg. The wedge pressure in this case was approximately 23 mm Hg. Despite the high left-sided filling pressures, note that right atrial pressure is normal, with a mean (central venous pressure) value of approximately 3 mm Hg. Scales on the right indicate mm Hg for the preceding curves.

can be observed in some patients after administration of furosemide, hydralazine, or sodium nitroprusside.

Cardiac output also can be measured when the catheter is equipped with a thermistor near the catheter tip and a cardiac output computer is available (see Fig. 18–8B). With this information, four potential *hemodynamic subsets* may be encountered (Forrester et al. 1976):

- Normal cardiac output and normal pulmonary capillary wedge pressure (the normal situation)
- Normal cardiac output with high pulmonary capillary wedge pressure predisposing to edema (left-sided CHF with volume expansion)
- Low cardiac output and low pulmonary capillary wedge pressure (volume depletion, as with excessive diuresis)
- Low cardiac output and high pulmonary capillary wedge pressure (severe left-sided heart failure; cardiogenic shock)

The CVP also can be measured through dual-port Swan-Ganz catheters (see Fig. 18–8A). In biventricular CHF both the wedge pressure and CVP are abnormally high (see Figs. 18–9 and 18–10). With excessive diuresis of the patient, both pressures are reduced. A relatively common situation after diuresis in primary left-sided heart failure is persistently high wedge pressure with relatively low (<5 mm Hg) CVP. This situation can lead to reduced right-sided filling and prerenal azotemia. Reducing the diuretic dosage improves cardiac output but may exacerbate pulmonary edema.

REFERENCES

Auld RB, Alexander EA, and Levinsky NG: Proximal tubular function in dogs with thoracic caval constriction. *J Clin Invest* 50:2150–2158, 1971.

Barger AC, Yates FE, and Rudolph AM: Renal hemodynamics and sodium excretion in dogs with graded valvular damage, and in congestive failure. *Am J Physiol* 200:601–608, 1961.

Bonagura JD and Lehmkuhl LB: Fluid therapy in heart failure. In Dibartola SJ (ed): *Fluid Therapy in Small Animal Practice*, 1st ed. Philadelphia, WB Saunders Co., pp. 529–553, 1992.

Bonagura JD and Lehmkuhl LB: Cardiomyopathy. In Birchard SJ and Sherding RG (eds): *Saunders Manual of Small Animal Practice*, 2nd ed. Philadelphia, WB Saunders Co., in press.

Bonagura JD and Rush J: Heart failure. In Birchard SJ and Sherding RG (eds): *Saunders Manual of Small Animal Practice*, 2nd ed. Philadelphia, WB Saunders Co., in press.

Bonagura JD and Ware WA: Atrial fibrillation in the dog: Clinical findings in 81 cases. *J Am Anim Hosp Assoc* 22:111–120, 1986.

Bourland WA, Day DK, and Williams HE: The role of the kidney in the early nondiuretic action of furosemide to reduce elevated left atrial pressure in the hypervolemic dog. *J Pharmacol Exp Ther* 202:221–229, 1977.

Braunwald E: Pathophysiology of heart failure. In Braunwald E (ed): *Heart Disease: A Textbook of Cardiovascular Medicine*. Philadelphia, WB Saunders Co., pp. 426–448, 1988.

Bristow MR: Mechanism of action of beta-blocking agents in heart failure. *Am J Cardiol* 80:26L–40L, 1997.

Calvert CA and Rawlings CA: Canine heartworm disease. In Fox PR (ed): *Canine and Feline Cardiology*. New York, Churchill Livingstone, pp. 519–549, 1988.

Cannon PJ: The kidney in heart failure. *N Engl J Med* 296:26–32, 1977.

Cobb M and Michell AR: Plasma electrolyte concentrations in dogs receiving diuretic therapy for cardiac failure. *J Small Anim Pract* 33:526–529, 1992.

Cogan MG: Atrial natriuretic peptide. *Kidney Int* 37:1148:1160, 1990.

Cohn JN and Levine TB: Angiotensin-converting enzyme inhibition in congestive heart failure: The concept. *Am J Cardiol* 49:1480–1483, 1982.

Cohn JN, Levine TB, Olivar MT, et al.: Plasma norepinephrine as a guide to prognosis in patients with chronic congestive heart failure. *N Engl J Med* 311:819–823, 1984.

Co-operative Veterinary Enalapril (COVE) Study Group: Controlled clinical evaluation of enalapril in dogs with heart failure—Results of the Cooperative Veterinary Enalapril Study Group. *J Vet Intern Med* 9:243–252, 1995.

Creager MA and Cusco JA: Treatment of congestive heart failure with angiotensin-converting enzyme inhibitors. In McCall D and Rahimtoola SH (eds): *Heart Failure*. New York, Chapman & Hall, pp. 316–344, 1995.

Creager MA, Halperin JL, Bernard DB, et al.: Acute regional circulatory and renal hemodynamic effects of converting-enzyme inhibition in patients with congestive heart failure. *Circulation* 64:483–489, 1981.

Decarli C, Spouse G, and Larosa JL: Serum magnesium levels in symptomatic atrial fibrillation and their relation to rhythm control by intravenous digoxin. *Am J Cardiol* 57:956–959, 1986.

Dirks JH, Cirksena WJ, and Berliner RW: Micropuncture study of the effect of various diuretics on sodium reabsorption by the proximal tubules of the dog. *J Clin Invest* 45:1875–1885, 1966.

Dow SJ, Fettman MJ, Smith KR, et al.: Taurine depletion and cardiovascular disease in adult cats fed a potassium-depleted acidified diet. *Am J Vet Res* 53:402–405, 1992.

Dumont AE, Clauss RH, Reed GE, et al.: Lymph drainage in patients with congestive heart failure: Comparison with findings in hepatic cirrhosis. *N Engl J Med* 269:949–952, 1963.

Dzau VJ and Hollenberg NK: Renal response to captopril in severe heart failure: Role of furosemide in natriuresis and reversal of hyponatremia. *Ann Intern Med* 100:777–781, 1984.

Dzau VJ and Swartz SL: Dissociation of the prostaglandin and renin-angiotensin systems during captopril therapy for chronic congestive heart failure secondary to coronary artery disease. *Am J Cardiol* 60:1101–1105, 1987.

Dzau VJ, Colucci WS, Hollenberg NK, et al.: Relation of the renin-angiotensin-aldosterone system to clinical state in congestive heart failure. *Circulation* 63:645–651, 1981.

Dzau VJ, Packer M, Lilly LS, et al.: Prostaglandins in severe congestive heart failure: Relation to activation of the renin-angiotensin system and hyponatremia. *N Engl J Med* 310:347–352, 1984.

Eaton GE, Cody RJ, and Brinkley PF: Increase in aortic impedance precedes peripheral vasoconstriction at the early stage of ventricular failure in the paced canine model. *Circulation* 88:2714–2721, 1993.

Edwards JN: Magnesium and congestive heart failure. *Proceedings, American College of Veterinary Internal Medicine*. New Orleans, pp. 679–680, 1991.

Fichman MP, Vorherr H, Kleeman CR, et al.: Diuretic-induced hyponatremia. *Ann Intern Med* 75:853–863, 1971

Forrester JS, Diamond G, Chatterjee K, et al.: Medical therapy of acute myocardial infarction by application of hemodynamic subsets. *N Engl J Med* 295:1404–1413, 1976.

Franciosa JA, Dunkman WB, Wilen M, et al.: "Optimal" left ventricular filling pressure during nitroprusside infusion for congestive heart failure. *Am J Med* 74:457–464, 1983.

Francis GS: Neurohumoral mechanisms involved in congestive heart failure. *Am J Cardiol* 55:15A–21A, 1985.

Francis GS: Neuroendocrine activity in congestive heart failure. *Am J Cardiol* 66:33D–39D, 1990.

Francis GS and McDonald KM: Neurohumoral mechanisms in heart failure. In McCall D and Rahimtoola SH (eds): *Heart Failure*. New York, Chapman & Hall, pp. 90–116, 1995.

Francis GS, Goldsmith SR, Levine TB, et al.: The neurohumoral axis in congestive heart failure. *Ann Intern Med* 101:370–377, 1984.

Francis GS, Siegel RM, Goldsmith SR, et al.: Acute vasoconstrictor response to intravenous furosemide in patients with chronic congestive heart failure. Activation of the neurohumoral axis. *Ann Intern Med* 103:1–6, 1985.

Freeman LM, Rush JE, Kehayias JJ, et al.: Nutritional alterations and the effect of fish oil supplementation in dogs with heart failure. *J Vet Intern Med* 12:440–448, 1998.

Freeman RH, Davis JD, Williams GM, et al.: Effects of the oral angiotensin converting enzyme inhibitor, SQ 14225 in a model of low cardiac output in dogs. *Circ Res* 45:540–545, 1979.

Friedman E, Shadel M, Halkin H, et al.: Thiazide-induced hyponatremia. *Ann Intern Med* 110:24–30, 1989.

Fulop M, Horowitz M, Aberman A, et al.: Lactic acidosis in pulmonary edema due to left ventricular failure. *Ann Intern Med* 79:180–186, 1973.

Gaasch WH and Freeman GL: Functional properties of normal and failing hearts. In McCall D and Rahimtoola SH (eds): *Heart Failure*. New York, Chapman & Hall, pp. 14–29, 1995.

Gerlag PGG and vanMeijel JJM: High-dose furosemide in the treatment of refractory congestive heart failure. *Arch Intern Med* 148:286–291, 1988.

Gottlieb SS and Weir MR: Renal effects of angiotensin-converting enzyme inhibition in congestive heart failure. *Am J Cardiol* 66:14D–21D, 1990.

Granger JP: Regulation of sodium excretion by renal interstitial hydrostatic pressure. *Fed Proc* 45:2892–2896, 1986.

Guyton AC and Lindsey AW: Effect of elevated left atrial pressure and decreased plasma protein concentration on the development of pulmonary edema. *Circ Res* 7:649–657, 1959.

Hall JE, Guyton AC, Jackson TE, et al.: Control of glomerular filtration rate by the renin-angiotensin system. *Am J Physiol* 233:F366–F372, 1977.

Hamlin RL, Smith RC, Powere TE, et al.: Efficacy of various diuretics in normal dogs. *J Am Vet Med Assoc* 146:1417–1420, 1965.

Heinemann HO: Right-sided heart failure and the use of diuretics. *Am J Med* 64:367–369, 1978.

Higgins CB, Vatner SF, Eckberg DL, et al.: Alterations in the baroreceptor reflex in conscious dogs with heart failure. *J Clin Invest* 51715–724, 1972.

Hirsch AT, Pinto YM, Schunkert H, et al.: Potential role of the tissue renin-angiotensin system in the pathophysiology of congestive heart failure. *Am J Cardiol* 66:22D–32D, 1990.

Hirsch AT, Muellerleile M, and Dzau VJ: Cardiovascular tissue angiotensin systems: Activation and actions in heart failure. In McCall D and Rahimtoola SH (eds): *Heart Failure*. New York, Chapman & Hall, pp. 117–134, 1995.

Hollander W and Judson WE: The relationship of cardiovascular and renal hemodynamic function to sodium excretion in patients with severe heart disease but without edema. *J Clin Invest* 35:970–979, 1956.

Ichikawa I, Pfeffer JM, Pfeffer MA, et al.: Role of angiotensin II in the altered renal function of congestive heart failure. *Circ Res* 55:669–675, 1984.

IMPROVE Study Group: Acute and short-term hemodynamic, echocardiographic, and clinical effects of enalapril maleate in dogs with naturally acquired heart failure: Results of the Invasive Multicenter Prospective Veterinary Evaluation of Enalapril study. *J Vet Intern Med* 9:234–242, 1995.

Jackson EK: Diuretics. In Hardman JG, Limbird LE, Molinoff PB, et al.: *Goodman & Gilman's The Pharmacological Basis of Therapeutics*, 9th ed. New York, McGraw-Hill, pp. 685–714, 1996.

Kaloyanides GJ: Pathogenesis and treatment of edema with special reference to the use of diuretics. In Maxwell MH and Kleeman CR (eds): *Clinical Disorders of Fluid and Electrolyte Metabolism*. New York, McGraw-Hill, pp. 647–701, 1980.

Katz AM: Cardiomyopathy of overload: A major determinant of prognosis in congestive heart failure. *N Engl J Med* 322:100–110, 1990.

Keane WR and Shapiro BE: Renal protective effects of angiotensin-converting enzyme inhibition. *Am J Cardiol* 65:491–531, 1990.

Keene BW and Rush JE: Therapy of heart failure. In Ettinger SJ (ed.): *Textbook of Veterinary Internal Medicine*, 3rd ed. Philadelphia, WB Saunders Co., pp. 939–975, 1989.

Kinugawa T and Thames MC: Baroreflexes in heart failure. In McCall D and Rahimtoola SH (eds): *Heart Failure*. New York, Chapman & Hall, pp. 30–45, 1995.

Kittleson M, Keene B, Pion PD, et al.: Results of the Multicenter Spaniel Trial (MUST): Taurine and carnitine responsive dilated cardiomyopathy in American cocker spaniels with decreased plasma taurine concentration. *J Vet Intern Med* 11:204–211, 1997.

Kluger J, Cody RJ, and Laragh JH: The contribution of sympathetic tone and the renin-angiotensin system to severe chronic congestive heart failure: Response to specific inhibitors (prazosin and captopril). *Am J Cardiol* 49:1667–1674, 1982.

Kubo SH: Neurohormonal activation and the response to converting enzyme inhibitors in congestive heart failure. *Circulation* 81(suppl III):107–114, 1990.

Levens NR: Control of renal function by intrarenal angiotensin II in the dog. *J Cardiovasc Pharmacol* 16(suppl 4):565–569, 1990.

Levine TB, Francis GS, Goldsmith SR, et al.: Activity of the sympathetic nervous system and renin-angiotensin system assessed by plasma hormone levels and their relation to hemodynamic abnormalities in congestive heart failure. *Am J Cardiol* 49:1659–1666, 1982.

Levy M: Effects of acute volume expansion and altered hemodynamics on renal tubular function in chronic caval dogs. *J Clin Invest* 51:922–938, 1972.

Lifschitz MD and Schrier RW: Alterations in cardiac output with chronic constriction of thoracic inferior vena cava. *Am J Physiol* 225:1364–1370, 1973.

Loeb HS, Bredakis J, and Gunnar RM: Superiority of dobutamine over dopamine for augmentation of cardiac output in patients with chronic low output cardiac failure. *Circulation* 55:375–381, 1977.

Margulies KG, Hilderbrand FL, Lerman A, et al.: Increased endothelin in experimental heart failure. *Circulation* 82:2226–2232, 1990.

Mettauer B, Rouleau J-L, Bichet D, et al.: Sodium and water excretion abnormalities in congestive heart failure. *Ann Intern Med* 105:161–167, 1986.

Michell AR: Physiological aspects of the requirement for sodium in mammals. *Nutr Res Rev* 2:149–160, 1989.

Migdal S, Alexander EA, and Levinsky NG: Evidence that decreased cardiac output is not the stimulus to sodium retention during acute constriction of the vena cava. *J Lab Clin Med* 89:809–816, 1977.

Millard RW, Higgins CB, Franklin D, et al.: Regulation of the renal circulation during severe exercise in normal dogs and dogs with experimental heart failure. *Circ Res* 31:881–888, 1972.

Miller WC, Simi WW, and Rice DL: Contribution of systemic venous hypertension to the development of pulmonary edema in dogs. *Circ Res* 43:598–600, 1978.

Molina CR, Fowler MB, McCrory S, et al.: Hemodynamic, renal, and endocrine effects of atrial natriuretic peptide infusion in severe heart failure. *J Am Coll Cardiol* 12:175–186, 1988.

Morris ML, Patton RL, and Teeter SM: Low sodium diet in heart disease: How low is low? *Vet Med Small Anim Clin* 9:1225–1227, 1976.

Nomura A, Yasuda H, Minami M, et al.: Effect of furosemide in congestive heart failure. *Clin Pharmacol Ther* 30:177–182, 1981.

O'Connor CM, Gattis WA, and Swedberg K: Current and novel pharmacologic approaches in advanced heart failure. *Am Heart J* 135:S249–S263, 1998.

Oliver JA, Sciacca RR, Pinto J, et al.: Participation of the prostaglandins in the control of renal blood flow during acute reduction of cardiac output in the dog. *J Clin Invest* 67:229–237, 1981.

Opie LH, Kaplan NM, and Poole-Wilson PA: Diuretics. In Opie LH (ed): *Drugs for the Heart*, 4th ed. Philadelphia, WB Saunders Co., pp. 83–103, 1995.

Osborn JL, Holdaas H, Thames MD, et al.: Renal adrenoreceptor mediation of antinatriuretic and renin secretion responses to low frequency renal nerve stimulation in the dog. *Circ Res* 53:298–305, 1983

Oster JR, Epstein M, and Smoller S: Combination therapy with thiazide-type and loop diuretic agents for resistant sodium retention. *Ann Intern Med* 99:405–406, 1983.

Packer M: Neurohumoral interactions and adaptations in congestive heart failure. *Am J Cardiol* 55:1A–10A, 1985.

Packer M, Medina N, and Yshak M: Correction of dilutional hyponatremia in severe chronic heart failure by converting-enzyme inhibition. *Ann Intern Med* 100:782–789, 1984.

Packer M, Lee WH, and Kessler PD: Preservation of glomerular filtration rate in human heart failure by activation of the renin-angiotensin system. *Circulation* 74:766–774, 1986a.

Packer M, Lee WH, Medina N, et al.: Influence of renal function on the hemodynamic and clinical responses to long-term captopril therapy in severe chronic heart failure. *Ann Intern Med* 104:147–154, 1986b.

Packer M, Lee WH, Medina N, et al.: Functional renal insufficiency during long-term therapy with captopril and enalapril in severe chronic heart failure. *Ann Intern Med* 106:346–354, 1987.

Paradiso G, Bakris GL, and Stein JH: The kidney and heart failure. In McCall D and Rahimtoola SH (eds): *Heart Failure*. New York, Chapman & Hall, pp. 135–158, 1995.

Parmley WW: Pathophysiology of congestive heart failure. *Am J Cardiol* 55:9A–14A, 1985.

Patak RV, Fadem SZ, Rosenblatt SG, et al.: Diuretic-induced changes in renal blood flow and prostaglandin E excretion in the dog. *Am J Physiol* 236:F494–F500, 1979.

Pedersen HD: Effects of mild mitral-valve insufficiency, sodium-intake, and place of blood-sampling on the renin-angiotensin system in dogs. *Acta Vet Scand* 37:109–118, 1996.

Pion PD and Kittleson MD: Therapy for feline aortic thromboembolism. In Kirk RW: *Current Veterinary Therapy X*. Philadelphia, WB Saunders Co., pp. 295–301, 1989.

Priebe H, Heimann JC, and Hedley-Whyte J: Effects of renal and hepatic venous congestion on renal function in the presence of low and normal cardiac output in dogs. *Circ Res* 47:883–890, 1980.

Reinhardt HW, Kaczmarczy KG, Eisele R, et al.: Left atrial pressure and sodium balance in conscious dogs on a low sodium intake. *Pflugers Arch* 370:59–66, 1977.

Riegger GA, Liebau G, and Kochsiek K: Antidiuretic hormone in congestive heart failure. *Am J Med* 72:49–52, 1982.

Riegger GA, Liebau G, Holzschuh M, et al.: Role of the renin-angiotensin system in the development of congestive heart failure in the dog as assessed by chronic converting-enzyme blockade. *Am J Cardiol* 53:614–618, 1984.

Riegger GA, Elsner D, Kroner EP, et al.: Atrial natriuretic peptide in congestive heart failure in the dog: Plasma levels, cyclic guanidine monophosphate, ultrastructure of atrial myoendocrine cells, and hemodynamic, hormonal, and renal effects. *Circulation* 77:398–406, 1988.

Ritz E and Nowack R: Detrimental and beneficial effects of converting enzyme inhibitors on the kidney. *J Cardiol Pharmacol* 16(suppl 4):570–575, 1990.

Rose BD: Diuretics. *Kidney Int* 39:336–352, 1991.

Rose BD: *Clinical Physiology of Acid-Base and Electrolyte Disorders*, 4th ed. New York, McGraw-Hill, 1994.

Roudebush P, Allen TA, Kuehn NF, et al.: The effect of combined therapy with captopril, furosemide, and a sodium-restricted diet on serum electrolyte concentrations and renal function in normal dogs and dogs with congestive heart failure. *J Vet Intern Med* 8:337–342, 1994.

Rouse D, Dalmeida W, Williamson FC, et al.: Captopril inhibits the hydro-osmotic effect of ADH in the cortical collecting tubule. *Kidney Int* 32:845–850, 1987.

Ryan MP: Diuretics and potassium/magnesium depletion: Directions for treatment. *Am J Med* 82(suppl 3A):38–47, 1987.

Schrier RW: Pathogenesis of sodium and water retention in high output and low output cardiac failure, nephrotic syndrome, cirrhosis and pregnancy. *N Engl J Med* 319:1065–1072; 1127–1134, 1988.

Schrier RW and Abraham WT: Hormones and hemodynamics in heart failure. *N Engl J Med* 341:577–585, 1999.

Schrier RW, Humphreys MH, and Ufferman RC: Role of cardiac output and the autonomic nervous system in the antinatriuretic response to acute constriction of the thoracic superior vena cava. *Circ Res* 29:490–498, 1971.

Seely JF and Dirks JH: Site of action of diuretic drugs. *Kidney Int* 11:1–8, 1977.

Shimoyama H, Sabbah HN, Rosman H, et al.: Effects of long-term therapy with enalapril on severity of functional mitral regurgitation in dogs with moderate heart failure. *J Am Coll Cardiol* 25:768–772, 1995

Skorecki KL and Brenner BM: Body fluid homeostasis in congestive heart failure and cirrhosis with ascites. *Am J Med* 72:323–338, 1982.

Starling EH: The influence of mechanized factors on lymph production. *J Physiol* (Lond) 10:14–155, 1894.

Staub NC: Pathophysiology of pulmonary edema. In Staub NC and Taylor AE (eds): *Edema*. New York, Raven Press, pp. 719–746, 1984.

Suki WN: Renal hemodynamic consequences of angiotensin-converting enzyme inhibition in congestive heart failure. *Arch Intern Med* 149:669–673, 1989.

Suki WN, Rector FC Jr, and Seldin DW: The site of action of furosemide and other sulfonamide diuretics in the dog. *J Clin Invest* 44:1458–1469, 1965.

Sun Y and Weber KT: Cardiac remodelling by fibrous tissue—Role of local factors and circulating hormones. *Ann Med* 30(suppl1):S3–S8, 1998.

Swales JD: Magnesium deficiency and diuretics. *Br Med J* 285:1377–1378, 1982.

Swan HJC, Ganz W, Forrester J, et al.: Catheterization of the heart in man with use of a flow-directed balloon-tipped catheter. *N Engl J Med* 283:447–451, 1970.

Taylor AE: Capillary fluid filtration: Starling forces and lymph flow. *Circ Res* 49:557–575, 1982.

Thames MD: Acetylstrophanthidin-induced reflex inhibition of canine renal sympathetic nerve activity mediated by cardiac receptors with vagal afferents. *Circ Res* 44:8–15, 1979.

Thomas JA and Marks BH: Plasma norepinephrine in congestive heart failure. *Am J Cardiol* 41:233–243, 1978.

Thrall DE and Calvert CA: Radiographic evaluation of canine heartworm disease coexisting with right heart failure. *Vet Radiol* 24:124–126, 1983.

Van Veldhuisen DJ, Genth-Zoth S, Brouwer J, et al.: High- versus low-dose ACE inhibition in chronic heart failure: A double-blind, placebo-controlled study of imidapril. *J Am Coll Cardiol* 32:1811–1818, 1998.

Vasko MR, Brown-Cartwright D, Knochel JP, et al.: Furosemide absorption altered in decompensated congestive heart failure. *Ann Intern Med* 102:314–318, 1985.

Ware WA, Lund DD, Subieta AR, et al.: Sympathetic activation in dogs with congestive heart failure caused by chronic mitral valve disease and dilated cardiomyopathy. *J Am Vet Med Assoc* 197:1475–1481, 1990.

Watkins L Jr, Burton JA, Haber E, et al.: The renin-angiotensin-aldosterone system in congestive failure in conscious dogs. *J Clin Invest* 57:1606–1617, 1976.

Weaver LJ and Carrico CJ: Congestive heart failure and edema. In Staub NC and Taylor AE (eds): *Edema*. New York, Raven Press, pp. 543–562, 1984.

Weber KT: Aldosterone and spironolactone in heart failure [editorial]. *N Engl J Med* 341:709–717, 1999.

Wiener-Kronish JP, Goldstein R, Matthay RA, et al.: Lack of association of pleural effusion with chronic pulmonary arterial and right atrial hypertension. *Chest* 92:967–970, 1987.

Zucker IH, Share L, and Gilmore JP: Renal effects of left atrial distension in dogs with chronic congestive heart failure. *Am J Physiol* 236:H554–H560, 1979.

CHAPTER 19

Fluid Therapy During Intrinsic Renal Failure

DENNIS J. CHEW

Normal renal function, including maintenance of extracellular fluid volume and osmolality, normal electrolyte concentrations, and acid-base balance, is essential for stability of the internal milieu. Excretion of metabolic waste products, biosynthesis of hormones, and degradation of reabsorbed peptides are additional essential renal functions. The amount of water and electrolytes presented to and processed by the kidneys on a daily basis is enormous. Consequently, it is not surprising that failure of normal renal function is associated with failure to regulate the volume and composition of the extracellular fluid. An overview of normal renal function is presented in Chapter 2.

Intrinsic (primary) renal failure is present whenever functional and histopathologic lesions in the kidneys result in accumulation of nitrogenous waste products (e.g., urea, creatinine) in the blood. Loss of at least 75% of renal excretory function (reversible or irreversible) must occur before blood urea nitrogen (BUN) or serum creatinine concentrations become increased (i.e., before azotemia is detected). Serum phosphorus concentration becomes increased with further loss (85% or more) of excretory renal function.

Intrinsic renal failure may be divided into failure with acute or chronic causes (Polzin et al. 1989; Chew and DiBartola 1989). A specific diagnosis is important in establishing a prognosis and making adjustments in therapy but is not necessary for the initial treatment of the patient with intrinsic (primary) renal failure. The approach to fluid therapy in the patient with renal failure is similar regardless of the specific histologic diagnosis.

Intrinsic renal failure occurs in both dogs and cats with similar frequency, but chronic renal failure (CRF) may occur with greater frequency in older cats than in older dogs (Lulich et al. 1992). A survey found renal disease to be more prevalent in cats than dogs receiving care at veterinary clinics (Lund et al. 1999). Chronic renal failure is much more common than acute renal failure (ARF) in both species. Acute renal failure was diagnosed in approximately 30% of dogs with renal disease in one series (Vaden et al. 1997) but in only 5% in another study (Behrend et al. 1996). Isolated ischemic events accounted for 33% of the cases in dogs, followed by 22% in which no underlying cause could be found, 21% with isolated exposure to a nephrotoxicant, 18% with multiple disorders, and 5% with isolated miscellaneous disorders (e.g., leptospirosis, pyelonephritis, renal lymphoma) (Vaden et al. 1997). In a series of dogs with hospital-acquired ARF, 72% had been exposed recently to a nephrotoxicant and 14% had undergone anesthesia within the previous 2 weeks; chronic heart disease, neoplasia, and fever were conditions commonly associated with ARF (Behrend et al. 1996).

Both CRF and ARF may be subdivided into oliguric or nonoliguric forms (Table 19–1). Chronic renal failure is usually characterized by polyuria, but affected animals may be transiently oliguric when dehydrated and permanent oliguria develops during terminal decompensation. Patients with ARF can be either oliguric or nonoliguric. Animals with ARF are often clinically more ill, on the basis of history, clinical signs, and laboratory evaluation, than those with compensated CRF. Decompensated CRF patients, however, may be as sick as those with ARF. "Acute-on-chronic" renal failure is a common situation in which acute prerenal azotemia caused by vomiting, anorexia, and hypodipsia aggravates preexisting azotemia. The CRF patient also is at greater risk for developing acute tubular necrosis resulting from ischemia caused by dehydration. Thirty-five percent of dogs with hospital-acquired renal failure had preexisting renal disease (Behrend et al. 1996). Severe anemia may necessitate blood transfusion in both CRF patients and those with ARF. Hypoproteinemia arising from chronic glomerular disease may require plasma transfusion, but this aspect of therapy

TABLE 19–1. **Renal Failure Syndromes Requiring Fluid Therapy**

Common	Uncommon
Polyuric chronic renal failure	Oliguric chronic renal failure
Oligoanuric acute renal failure	Nephrotic syndrome
Nonoliguric acute renal failure	

TABLE 19-2. Uremic Signs and Problems That May Require Fluid Therapy Support

Gastrointestinal
  Anorexia
  Vomiting
  Diarrhea
  Hypodipsia
Altered urine production
  Polydipsia
  Polyuria
  Oliguria
  Anuria
Blood
  Anemia
    Lack of production
    Blood loss
    Decreased red cell life span
  Hypoproteinemia
    Blood loss
    Increased glomerular permeability

is not addressed in this chapter. See Table 19–2 for a list of the clinical abnormalities that may require fluid therapy in patients with renal failure.

Parenteral fluid therapy is the most important consideration in the initial treatment of uremic patients with severe clinical signs and laboratory abnormalities (those referred to as in a uremic "crisis"). Fluid therapy goals include extracellular fluid volume expansion, correction of serious electrolyte and acid-base disturbances, reduction of the magnitude of azotemia, and provision of red blood cells when needed. Nutritional support during early stabilization has not received much emphasis but is probably important. Fluid therapy must be integrated with other treatments in the uremic patient. In oliguric intrinsic renal failure, the patient must be monitored for retention of water and electrolytes, whereas losses of water and electrolytes must be replaced in patients with polyuric intrinsic renal failure.

▶ General Principles and Goals

Rarely is the exact nature of the underlying disease process responsible for intrinsic renal failure known at the time therapy must be instituted. Consequently, treatment and further diagnostic testing must be carried out simultaneously. Table 19–3 presents an overview of the goals of fluid therapy in the patient with renal failure, and Table 19–4 presents a recommended diagnostic and therapeutic approach.

The primary aim of therapy during severe uremia is to correct alterations in the patient's internal milieu. Ideally, this allows the patient to live long enough to allow repair of renal damage during acute injury and hypertrophy of remnant viable nephrons during chronic injury, resulting in improved renal function and ability to sustain life without extensive medical support. Existing renal lesions are not directly amenable to therapy. Adequate extracellular fluid volume must be maintained to maximize renal perfusion and assist in excretory function. Fluid therapy during uremic crises usually is successful at least until a definitive diagnosis and prognosis can be made.

Intravenous fluid therapy also offers the clinician an avenue for intensive diuresis of the patient with renal failure so that azotemia is reduced. A combination of fluid administration for rehydration, maintenance, and mild volume expansion and diuretic administration can be used in an attempt to increase glomerular filtration rate (GFR), renal blood flow (RBF), and renal tubular fluid flow rate in animals with apparent primary (intrinsic) renal failure. Blood urea nitrogen, serum creatinine, and serum phosphorus concentrations decrease if this therapy successfully increases GFR. Blood urea nitrogen concentration can decrease without a change in GFR because increased renal tubular fluid flow rate reduces passive tubular reabsorption of urea, but creatinine is not affected by changes in tubular flow rate (Finco and Duncan 1976; Finco

TABLE 19-3. General Goals of Parenteral Fluid Therapy for Uremic Patients

Survival
  Temporary
    Awaiting a specific diagnosis
    Formulating a prognosis
    Awaiting results of a renal biopsy
    Awaiting implementation of dialysis
  Long-standing
    Recompensation in CRF
    Reclamation of renal function and histology in ARF
Reduction in magnitude of azotemia
  Improvement in renal function or resolution of renal lesions
  Maximization of endogenous renal excretory function
    Correct prerenal component
    Increase GFR
    Increase tubular flow rate (with or without an increase in GFR)
    Preferential decrease in BUN versus serum creatinine
Improved quality of life

TABLE 19-4. Initial Diagnostic and Therapeutic Sequence for the Uremic Patient

Obtain baseline data (before any treatment)
  Body weight, skin turgor, vital signs
  PCV and total protein, urinalysis
  BUN, serum creatinine, serum phosphorus
  Sodium, potassium, chloride
  Total CO_2 or blood gases
Rule out prerenal and postrenal azotemia immediately
Start fluid treatments
Fluid challenge response
Rule out other potentially reversible causes for decreased GFR
  Urinary tract infection
  Hypercalcemia
  Hypokalemia and potassium depletion
  Leptospirosis
Determine the cause of the intrinsic renal failure
  Complete urinalysis
    Urine specific gravity before fluids
    Urine dipstrip
    Fresh urine sediment
  Urine protein-to-creatinine ratio
  Urine culture
  Renal imaging
    Radiography
    Ultrasonography
    Excretory urography
  Renal biopsy
Repeat baseline data during fluid treatments

1997). For these reasons, BUN concentration often decreases out of proportion to serum creatinine concentration when diuresis ensues.

Initial therapy for uremic animals is directed toward correction of all potential prerenal factors that may be contributing to the azotemia. The intravenous route is used for fluid administration to ensure rapid access to the circulation and to maximize renal perfusion. The volume of fluid administered must be chosen and monitored carefully because animals that remain oligoanuric may become overhydrated by excessive fluid infusion, whereas it may be difficult to administer sufficient fluid volume to correct dehydration in animals with severe polyuria. Overhydration also may occur in animals without oliguria if their ability to excrete a water load is severely impaired.

The most life-threatening fluid, electrolyte, and acid-base disturbances should be corrected first while searching for the potential causes of intrinsic renal failure. Drugs capable of causing ARF (e.g., aminoglycosides) should be discontinued. Hypovolemia usually is corrected over a period of 4 to 6 h to enhance renal perfusion rapidly. Loss of renal autoregulatory function may prevent kidneys damaged by ischemia, nephrotoxins, or chronic disease from protecting themselves against ongoing or future episodes of reduced renal perfusion. Further renal injury is sustained in these instances if renal hypotension develops or persists. Fluid therapy regimens for treatment of uremic patients have not been standardized in veterinary medicine, and what follows is largely based on empirical experience.

▶ Initial Stabilization

Route of Fluid Administration

The oral and subcutaneous routes of fluid administration are not satisfactory for the initial phase of treatment of severely uremic patients. The azotemic patient may be vomiting and have unreliable gastrointestinal absorption of water and electrolytes. Subcutaneous absorption of fluid also may be unreliable, especially if moderate or severe dehydration is present. Also, it is difficult to administer large volumes of fluid by the subcutaneous route. Consequently, the intravenous route is essential during the initial treatment of uremic patients with substantial dehydration, severe ongoing fluid losses (e.g., vomiting, diarrhea, polyuria), or serious disturbances of electrolyte and acid-base balance.

Placement of a sterile indwelling jugular venous catheter is preferred for the initial management of severe uremia so that central venous pressure (CVP) can be monitored during aggressive fluid administration. Fluid administration should be discontinued temporarily or markedly curtailed if CVP exceeds 13 cm H_2O or if it increases acutely by 2 cm H_2O or more during any 10-min period. A fluid challenge with 20 mL/kg administered over 10 min can be used to assess the likelihood of subsequent volume overload. The CVP should not increase more than 2 cm H_2O if cardiovascular function is normal (Chew 1991). If available, measurement of pulmonary capillary wedge pressure can provide an earlier warning about impending volume overload.

Rehydration

Fluid needs for rehydration can be calculated (estimated percentage of dehydration × body weight in kilograms = liters required) or administered as two to three times maintenance fluid needs (i.e., 80–180 mL/kg/day). Hypovolemic shock, if present, should be treated with fluids administered at a rate of 90 mL/kg/h with or without CVP monitoring until cardiovascular status has been stabilized. Further fluids are administered to match sensible (urinary volume), insensible (respiratory and gastrointestinal losses of approximately 20 mL/kg/day), and contemporary (an estimated volume from vomiting and diarrhea) fluid losses. Urine output is variable in patients with intrinsic renal failure, and it is advisable to place an indwelling urinary catheter to monitor urine output and facilitate fluid therapy for the initial 24 to 48 h. Alternatively, urine can be collected in a metabolic cage. For cats, the weight of the litter pan can be sequentially determined. Visualization of urinations and serial palpation of bladder filling during fluid therapy are the least reliable methods for determining urine production.

Urine Output

RECOGNITION OF OLIGURIA

Prompt recognition of oliguria is important because it dictates the volume of fluid that can be safely administered. Oliguria at presentation may be due to hypovolemia (due to hypodipsia, anorexia, vomiting, and diarrhea), severe intrarenal damage, or both. Although not present initially, oliguria occasionally has developed later during treatment of patients with ARF and CRF. Development of oliguria at any point during the course of treatment mandates meticulous attention to further fluid infusion to avoid overhydration.

Oliguria has been defined variably as less than 0.27 mL/kg/h (English 1974), less than 0.48 mL/kg/h (DiBartola et al. 1980; Polzin et al. 1989), and less than 1.0 to 2.0 mL/kg/h (Haskins 1979). Normal dogs and cats produce a minimal urine volume of approximately 1.0 mL/kg/h if not under the stress of acute study (Bentinck-Smith and French 1989; Hamlin and Rasjian 1964; Smith et al. 1964), whereas dogs suddenly caged without food produced approximately half this volume (DiBartola et al. 1980). Liberal criteria should be used to document oliguria in uremic patients. Urine production of less than 1.0 mL/kg/h (24 mL/kg/day) is considered absolute oliguria, whereas urine production of 1.0 to 2.0 mL/kg/h during IV fluid infusion is considered relative oliguria. Healthy kidneys are expected to produce a brisk diuresis (urine output ranging from 2.0 to 5.0 mL/kg/h) after IV administration of fluids for correction of dehydration and expansion of the extracellular fluid volume (Ross 1989). A prompt and brisk diuresis during IV fluid infusion suggests that initial oliguria was probably physiologic (prerenal) in nature.

Anuria (0 mL/kg/h in 18%) and oliguria (0.1–1.0 mL/kg/h in 43%) were documented in over 60% of 44 dogs with ARF whose urine output was measured. Normal urine output (1–2 mL/kg/h in 25%) and polyuria (>2 mL/kg/h in 14%) were found in the remaining dogs (Vaden et al. 1997). Dogs that were oliguric (<0.25 mL/kg/h) at the time of diagnosis of hospital-acquired ARF and that remained oliguric after at least 6 h of fluid therapy were 20 times more likely to die or be euthanized than were dogs with greater urine production (Behrend et al. 1996).

"INS AND OUTS"

Direct measurement of urine output allows the clinician to match fluid therapy to the needs of the dehydrated animal with either severe oliguria or diuresis. When this approach is not used, there is a tendency to overestimate the fluid requirement in an oliguric animal (resulting in overhydration) and to underestimate the fluid requirement in an animal undergoing extensive diuresis (resulting in failure to correct dehydration). Using this technique, the day is divided into six 4-h intervals. Other intervals (e.g., every hour, every 6 h, every 8 h) may be chosen on the basis of the animal's condition. The fluid requirement for this interval is determined using both insensible (20 mL/kg divided by 6 for a 4-h interval) and measured sensible (urine volume) losses over the same period. The measured volume of sensible (urinary) losses from the previous 4-h period is given back to the patient in the next 4-h period along with the calculated insensible requirement. Previously calculated dehydration needs are replaced first, and then the "ins and outs" method just described is carried out. This close attention to fluid volume is of benefit in the initial treatment of critically ill animals, especially when cardiovascular and renal status is uncertain.

Fluid Quality

Normal saline (0.9% NaCl) often is the initial fluid of choice for intravascular rehydration because it contains abundant sodium (154 mEq/L) and is devoid of potassium. The type of fluid chosen for correction of dehydration should be based on the patient's serum sodium concentration (see later). When rehydration has been accomplished, hypotonic fluids (0.45% NaCl in 2.5% dextrose; 5% dextrose) may be used for maintenance needs in order to prevent the development of hypernatremia. Hypernatremia commonly develops in patients with primary renal failure that receive fluids high in sodium relative to sodium maintenance needs (e.g., lactated Ringer's solution, 0.9% NaCl) for several days. Hypotonic fluids (e.g., 0.45% NaCl in 2.5% dextrose) should be considered for maintenance after initial rehydration of these patients in order to avoid development of hypernatremia.

Potassium supplementation of fluids must be monitored carefully by measurement of serum potassium concentration. Serum potassium concentration is affected by urine output, renal excretory function, metabolic acidosis, oral intake, and rate of parenteral fluid administration (see Chapter 5). In general, potassium supplementation is not recommended during the initial hours of stabilization until renal excretory function has been maximized and the serum potassium concentration measured, especially if the patient is oliguric. Supplementation of fluids with potassium often is needed during polyuric renal failure, but the magnitude of potassium supplementation should be less than that used in patients with normal renal function. Rather than the usual 20 to 30 mEq/L of KCl per liter of fluids, 10 to 20 mEq/L may be more appropriate in patients with renal failure.

Metabolic Abnormalities

Dogs and cats with compensated CRF generally have normal serum sodium, potassium, and chloride concentrations. Electrolyte and acid-base disorders commonly develop, however, in patients with decompensated CRF and ARF with severe reductions in GFR (Behrend et al. 1996; Brown et al. 1985; DiBartola et al. 1987; Thrall et al. 1984; Vaden et al. 1997). Hyperkalemia, hypokalemia, hypernatremia, hyponatremia, hyperphosphatemia, hypocalcemia, and metabolic acidosis are the abnormalities most likely to be encountered. Depending on the severity of these metabolic abnormalities, specific treatment may be required.

SODIUM

Serum sodium concentration often is normal in dehydrated uremic patients as a consequence of isonatremic fluid loss (e.g., polyuria, diarrhea). Some patients, however, have hypernatremia when losses of free water have been greater than sodium losses. Hypernatremia commonly develops after uremic patients are treated for several days with replacement solutions containing large amounts of sodium. Hypernatremia also may develop after several doses of sodium bicarbonate administered for treatment of metabolic acidosis. Less commonly, patients with renal failure have dehydration and hyponatremia because of continued water consumption and dilution of extracellular fluid sodium concentration after isonatremic sodium losses. In addition, the hypercatabolic state results in increased endogenous water production that can contribute to overhydration and hyponatremia if the additional water cannot be excreted by the kidneys (Feld et al. 1990).

Isotonic isonatremic fluid solutions (Normosol, lactated Ringer's solution, or 0.9% NaCl) are indicated for the initial correction of dehydration in patients with normal serum sodium concentrations. After hypovolemic shock has been corrected with isotonic fluids, hypotonic solutions (0.45% NaCl or 5% dextrose in water) are indicated for patients with initially high serum sodium concentrations. Usually, isotonic solutions are administered to patients with hyponatremia in an effort to provide sodium and water with the expectation that the excess water will be excreted by the kidneys and the serum sodium concentration returned to normal. Rarely, hypertonic sodium chloride solutions (3% NaCl) may be needed for treatment of severe and symptomatic hyponatremia (see Chapter 3).

CHLORIDE

Serum chloride concentration usually parallels serum sodium concentration during free-water loss. Proportionally more chloride may be lost during vomiting of gastric fluid, and in some uremic patients hypochloremia may develop. The fluid of choice in this instance is 0.9% NaCl (see Chapter 4).

POTASSIUM

HYPERKALEMIA

Life-threatening hyperkalemia is most likely to be encountered in severely oliguric patients, especially when metabolic acidosis is severe. Mild to moderate hyperkalemia can develop in patients with poor renal function receiving IV fluids supplemented with potassium salts. Hyperkalemia usually is not a problem in CRF unless severe oliguria or metabolic acidosis develops. Hyperkalemia was uncommon in dogs with intrinsic ARF in one study. Serum potassium concentration was less than 5.0 mEq/L in 75% of affected dogs despite the presence of oligoanuria in over 60% of the dogs (Vaden et al. 1997). Severe hyperkalemia is more likely in azotemic dogs and cats with urethral obstruction, uroabdomen, or hypoadrenocorticism. Mean serum potassium concentration was 6.26 mEq/L in a series of male cats with urethral obstruction and serum potassium concentration was above the reference range in over 50% of affected cats (Drobatz and Hughes 1997). Serial or continuous electrocardiographic (ECG) monitoring is recommended in these instances because severe hyperkalemia can lead to life-threatening cardiac arrhythmias. The electrocardiogram can be useful in detecting the deleterious physiologic effects of hyperkalemia (see Chapter 5).

Hyperkalemia can be managed temporarily by volume expansion with 0.9% NaCl and sodium bicarbonate infusion (1–4 mEq/kg, IV). Any ECG changes compatible with hyperkalemia should be managed to stabilize the cardiac rhythm. These measures are discussed in Chapter 5 and include sodium bicarbonate infusion, infusion of hypertonic glucose solutions, and administration of calcium gluconate. Glucose infusion may be preferred over sodium bicarbonate when total calcium or ionized calcium concentrations are precariously low because an infusion of alkali may further lower ionized and total calcium concentrations. Glucose infusions also are preferred over bicarbonate if seizures already are a problem or if metabolic alkalosis exists. Calcium gluconate directly counteracts the effect of potassium on the heart but does not lower serum potassium concentration. Calcium salts may have an additional benefit in patients with hypocalcemia but also may have the disadvantage of promoting soft tissue mineralization if hyperphosphatemia is present.

The electrocardiogram should revert to normal within minutes of these treatments, but they provide only temporary relief from the effects of hyperkalemia. Maximizing renal excretory function and maintaining blood pH and bicarbonate within the normal range help lower serum potassium concentration more permanently. Chronic hyperkalemia may be treated with an ion exchange resin (sodium polystyrene sulfonate) or may require dialysis. The treatment of hyperkalemia is discussed in detail in Chapter 5, peritoneal dialysis is discussed in Chapter 25, and hemodialysis is discussed in Chapter 26.

HYPOKALEMIA

Hypokalemia is most likely to occur at presentation in patients with polyuric renal failure, especially when anorexia is present. Hypokalemia is much more common than hyperkalemia in animals with CRF, and it occurs more commonly in cats than in dogs. Hypokalemia also may develop later after rehydration with potassium-deficient fluids, during periods of spontaneous diuresis, and during periods of intensive therapeutic diuresis.

Hypokalemia apparently can be either a consequence of or cause of CRF, especially in cats (Buffington et al. 1991; DiBartola et al. 1987; Dow 1988; Dow et al. 1987, 1989; Fettman 1989). Chronic hypokalemia can cause functional renal lesions (e.g., defective urinary concentrating ability, decreased GFR), structural renal lesions, and CRF. Chronic metabolic acidosis and potassium depletion in cats apparently can result in CRF, but the exact mechanisms remain unknown. The fractional urinary excretion of potassium may be high at a time when serum potassium concentration is low in cats with primary renal failure. The same phenomenon occasionally has been observed in dogs with CRF. Cats with marked potassium depletion and hypokalemia may demonstrate truncal weakness manifested by ventroflexion of the head and inability to move.

Potassium should be added cautiously to daily fluids (see Table 5–4 in Chapter 5) in animals with primary renal failure. Serum potassium concentration should be measured serially to ensure that hyperkalemia does not develop, because excretion of an acute potassium load is delayed in patients with renal failure (see Chapter 5). Severe hypokalemia usually is defined as a potassium concentration of 2.5 mEq/L or less and often is associated with clinical signs. Serum potassium concentrations of 2.0 mEq/L or less are life threatening (see Chapter 5).

It has been recommended that, if possible, IV fluids be avoided during the initial treatment of cats with primary renal failure and severe hypokalemia. This recommendation was based on the observation of paradoxical further lowering of serum potassium concentration or failure of serum potassium concentration to increase after potassium supplementation of IV fluids in cats with chronic potassium depletion (Dow 1988; Dow et al. 1987, 1989). This may be a result of extracellular fluid volume expansion and has been observed despite maximal rates of potassium supplementation with fluids containing up to 80 mEq/L potassium. Instead of supplementing IV fluids with potassium, oral supplementation with potassium gluconate is recommended for the correction of severe hypokalemia during the first 12 to 24 h. After this time, aggressive fluid therapy with potassium supplementation can be instituted. An initial daily dosage of 5 to 10 mEq of potassium gluconate (Kaon elixir 20 mEq/15 mL, diluted one to one with water) divided b.i.d. to t.i.d. is recommended until serum potassium concentration approaches the normal range (Dow et al. 1987, 1989). Afterward, 3 to 8 mEq/day is given orally for maintenance of serum potassium concentration and this dosage is tapered to 2 to 4 mEq/day for chronic maintenance (Dow et al. 1987, 1989). Alternatively, subcutaneous fluids containing up to 35 mEq/L potassium chloride can be given at the time of initial oral supplementation. In this case, volume expansion and concomitant diuresis are not as great as those observed with IV fluids, resulting in less dilution of extracellular fluid potassium concentration and less renal excretion of the administered potassium. Correction of severe hypokalemia using the regimen just described has been remarkably successful within 24 h in the author's experience.

Potassium depletion and hypokalemia at concentrations of 2.0 mEq/L or less may result in paralysis of respiratory muscles and require ventilatory support. In these instances, infusion of IV fluids containing 80 to 150 mEq/L potassium may be justified at the maximal rate of 0.5 mEq/kg/h. Dopamine infusion at 0.5 µg/kg/min has been suggested as another possible acute rescue measure for severe hypokalemia, as this may allow translocation of intracellular potassium to extracellular fluid (Dow 1988; Dow et al. 1987, 1989). The action of dopamine on adrenal cortical receptors also selectively inhibits angiotensin II–induced aldosterone secretion (Carcoana and Hines 1996), which could be helpful in minimizing kaliuresis.

PHOSPHORUS

HYPERPHOSPHATEMIA

Hyperphosphatemia is a frequent finding in patients with ARF and CRF and it may be severe (>10 mg/dL). Hyperphosphatemia may be excessively severe compared with the increase in BUN or serum creatinine concentrations in patients with ARF. Acute hyperphosphatemia in the absence of primary renal injury is not deleterious to renal excretory function or renal histology but may be of consequence in the development of further primary renal injury during both acute and chronic intrinsic renal failure. During ARF, hyperphosphatemia may contribute to worsening of histologic lesions and excretory function through a number of proposed mechanisms, including renal mineralization, direct nephrotoxicity, and renal vasoconstriction (Zager 1982).

Hyperphosphatemia also can adversely influence the progression of CRF in dogs and cats and contribute to the development of hypocalcemia during CRF and ARF. At present, it is not known whether rigorous control of serum phosphorus concentration during the uremic crises of patients with ARF or CRF will improve recovery of renal excretory function or enhance healing of renal lesions. Despite this, it seems clinically prudent to make an effort to reduce serum phosphorus concentration to some degree, preferably to within the normal range. Less severe hyperphosphatemia was associated with improved survival in a group of dogs with hospital-acquired ARF (Behrend et al. 1996).

There is no specific fluid therapy designed to counteract increased serum phosphorus concentration. Therapeutic efforts to increase GFR, however, also tend to decrease serum phosphorus concentration. If the patient is not vomiting, intestinal phosphorus-binding agents (e.g., aluminum hydroxide, calcium carbonate, calcium acetate) should be administered in an attempt to maintain serum phosphorus concentration below 6.0 mg/dL. Phosphorus binders are much more effective when given with meals but may lower serum phosphorus concentration in anorexic patients, presumably by binding phosphorus in gastrointestinal secretions (Schiller et al. 1989). See Chapter 7 for more information on the use of phosphate binders.

HYPOPHOSPHATEMIA

Hypophosphatemia is an unlikely occurrence in patients with primary renal failure. Rarely, excessive treatment with intestinal phosphorus binders and intensive diuresis results in transient hypophosphatemia.

CALCIUM

Approximately 50 to 75% of dogs with CRF had normal serum calcium concentrations in one report (Chew and Nagode 1990), depending on whether the serum total or ionized calcium concentration was measured (see Chapter 6). Similarly, 10 to 40% of these patients had hypocalcemia, and 6 to 14% were hypercalcemic. Approximately 75% of cats with CRF had normal serum total calcium concentrations, whereas 15% had hypocalcemia and 12% had hypercalcemia (DiBartola et al. 1987). Mean serum calcium concentration was normal in dogs with ARF, but 25% of affected dogs had concentrations less than the reference range (Vaden et al. 1997).

Serum total calcium concentration can markedly underestimate the severity of ionized hypocalcemia, especially in azotemic patients. Seventy-five percent of cats with urethral obstruction and azotemia had low ionized calcium concentrations, but serum total calcium concentrations were simultaneously low in only 27% of patients. Low total calcium concentrations predicted low ionized calcium concentrations in these cats, but normal total calcium concentrations did not accurately predict low ionized calcium concentrations (Drobatz and Hughes 1997).

Symptomatic hypocalcemia (i.e., tremors, seizures, muscular weakness, muscular rigidity) is not common in patients with renal failure but may require IV administration of calcium salts when it does occur (see Chapter 6). Administered calcium, however, may interact with an increased serum phosphorus concentration, resulting in metastatic mineralization of various soft tissues, including the heart and kidneys. Hypocalcemia has been attributed to mass law interactions between calcium and phosphorus when serum phosphorus has been very high and also to deficits of calcitriol (reduced intestinal absorption of calcium and increased skeletal resistance to parathyroid hormone). Measures to decrease serum phosphorus concentration may increase serum calcium concentration through more favorable mass law ionic interactions between phosphorus and calcium. Symptomatic hypocalcemia appears to be more common in dogs with ethylene glycol poisoning and ARF, but it also can be seen after $NaHCO_3$ therapy and reductions in serum ionized calcium concentration.

Hypercalcemia occasionally is encountered in dogs and cats with CRF (Chew and Nagode 1990; DiBartola et al. 1987; Finco and Rowland 1978). Hypercalcemia in these instances usually is mild, but some dogs with renal failure have been observed to have serum total calcium concentrations of approximately 14 mg/dL (Ross 1989). In most instances, dogs with CRF and hypercalcemia have an associated ionized calcium concentration that either is normal or low (Chew and Nagode 1990; Nachreiner and Refsal 1990; Refsal et al. 1998). Accordingly, these patients do not require specific therapy for hypercalcemia. When serum ionized calcium concentration is increased, specific therapy to lower the ionized calcium concentration is warranted (see Chapter 6).

MAGNESIUM

Serum magnesium concentration may be increased in patients with severe renal failure (Chew and Nagode 1990). Ionized and total magnesium concentrations occasionally are increased in dogs and cats with renal failure (Summers et al. 1999). Total serum magnesium concentrations were increased in 11 of 14 cats with urethral obstruction (Drobatz and Hughes 1997). Magnesium-containing drugs, such as antacids, should be avoided because any absorbed magnesium may not be readily excreted by the kidneys and could exacerbate hypermagnesemia. Hypomagnesemia has been associated with peritoneal dialysis with dialysate that did not contain magnesium (Crisp et al. 1989) (see Chapter 8).

METABOLIC ACIDOSIS

Metabolic acidosis is commonly associated with severe reductions in renal mass and GFR. In CRF, there is a progressive inability to excrete hydrogen ions because total urinary ammonia excretion declines with the reduction in renal mass. Increased serum phosphorus concentration also contributes to the degree of metabolic acidosis in both ARF and CRF (see Chapter 9). The degree of metabolic acidosis often is well compensated in patients with stable CRF owing to renal tubular adaptation and respiratory hyperventilation. Patients with decompensated CRF or ARF, however, often have severe metabolic acidosis. Ethylene glycol poisoning frequently is associated with severe metabolic acidosis in the early phases after ingestion and metabolism to organic acids (Grauer et al. 1984; Thrall et al. 1984).

Metabolic acidosis may be severe (blood pH < 7.2) and require treatment. In the absence of blood gas analysis, a total CO_2 concentration lower than 15 mEq/L on a routine serum biochemistry panel in a patient with primary renal failure usually indicates the presence of metabolic acidosis severe enough to require alkali supplementation. More aggressive correction of metabolic acidosis is indicated if hyperkalemia also is present. To correct metabolic acidosis, sodium bicarbonate is added to calcium-free maintenance fluids at a dosage of 1 to 5 mEq/kg, depending on the severity of the acidosis. Alternatively, the bicarbonate deficit of the extracellular space can be calculated from blood gas data using the formula 0.3 × body weight (kg) × base deficit = mEq of bicarbonate to be given over several hours, or one-fourth to one-half given as a slow bolus with the remainder given in maintenance fluids.

This method requires use of serial blood gas analysis and adjustment of therapy on the basis of the results. Hypernatremia, hyperosmolality, metabolic alkalosis, lowering of serum ionized calcium concentration with resultant seizures, and paradoxical cerebrospinal fluid acidosis are all potential problems during alkali therapy (Chew et al. 1989) (see Chapter 10).

Intensive Diuresis

The goal of intensive diuresis is to increase the turnover of body water, electrolyte, and metabolic waste products. It is hoped that diuresis will result in loss of some substances that have accumulated in the uremic environment and have caused many of the clinical signs of uremia. Any increases of GFR, RBF, and urine flow rate may be independent of one another. In certain instances, GFR actually increases during diuresis, but in other cases an increase in urine production is not accompanied by increased GFR. An increase in urine volume should not be equated with improved renal excretory function. In some cases, it is not possible to increase urine flow.

Most studies in humans have failed to show any benefit of mannitol or furosemide either prophylactically or as treatment for established nephrotoxic or ischemic ARF (Conger 1995; Shilliday and Allison 1994; Thadhani et al. 1996). The use of diuretics is justified to increase urine output and thus facilitate fluid therapy, but no data suggest that diuretics improve clinical outcome. The ability of diuretics to alter favorably the course of a uremic crisis is not established in veterinary medicine, but most clinicians administer them anyway. Success with these agents includes decreased magnitude of azotemia and conversion from oligoanuria to increased urine flow. Diuretics are most commonly used in states of oliguria, usually those associated with ARF. Osmotic diuretics and furosemide have been used to augment urinary flow in animals with polyuric CRF, but their superiority over rehydration and mild extracellular fluid volume expansion has not been established. The use of diuretics in patients with polyuric renal failure sometimes is not advocated on the grounds that urine production may become excessive and result in dehydration. Theoretically, however, these patients could benefit from diuretics that cause vasodilatation, increased GFR, increased RBF, and natriuresis, but this has not been studied. In all instances, rehydration should be completed before administration of diuretics (Chew 1990; Chonko and Grantham 1987; Kirby 1989; Levinsky et al. 1983).

Conversion from Oliguria to Nonoliguria

Oliguria and persistence of azotemia during initial fluid therapy may result from inadequate correction of renal perfusion or intrarenal vasoconstriction or be a result of the underlying renal damage. To distinguish among these possibilities, a fluid "push" often is advocated to ensure that clinically nondetectable dehydration or hypovolemia is not the cause of the oliguria. Extracellular fluid volume expansion may override some forms of intrarenal vasoconstriction. A fluid volume of approximately 3 to 5% (30–50 mL/kg) of the animal's body weight has been recommended after the correction of apparent dehydration (Finco 1977). The rationale for this additional fluid load is that dehydration of 3 to 5% of body weight may be clinically undetectable, and renal function may improve when additional fluid is administered. Slight overhydration is preferable to ongoing dehydration and possible further renal damage (Polzin et al. 1989). If oliguria persists after this maneuver, it is likely to be pathologic. This fluid administration must be closely monitored because an animal with severely diseased kidneys may not be able to tolerate this volume expansion, and overhydration may result. Performing a fluid push with CVP monitoring may be safer, but even this approach does not guarantee avoidance of overhydration.

The use of diuretics to convert oliguria to nonoliguria should be considered after rehydration has been accomplished (Chew 1990; Chonko and Grantham 1987; Kirby 1989; Levinsky et al. 1983). Rehydration allows greater delivery of the diuretic to the kidney, and beneficial effects are more likely to occur. If diuresis is initiated before rehydration, dehydration could result in additional renal injury. It is easier to manage patients that are nonoliguric because hyperkalemia and overhydration are less likely to occur and the severity of nitrogenous waste product retention may be less. It is not certain whether conversion from oliguria to nonoliguria after diuretic administration changes the natural course of the disease or merely identifies animals with less severe underlying renal lesions (Levinsky et al. 1983). Animals that remain oliguric despite diuretic administration have a poor prognosis because of the relative impracticality of dialysis.

Dextrose, mannitol, furosemide, and dopamine (or combinations of these) are the diuretics most often employed in attempts to convert oliguria to nonoliguria. Administration of diuretics to normal animals can increase GFR, RBF, tubular fluid flow rate, and osmolar clearance. Decreased release of renin and inhibition of tubuloglomerular feedback are features of some diuretics that are theoretically attractive in the treatment of ARF (Chonko and Grantham 1987; Levinsky et al. 1983). Reduced transport of sodium by damaged tubules after use of diuretics has the potential advantage of limiting further injury in acute but sublethally injured tubular cells, particularly those located in areas of relative hypoxia (outer medulla and the pars recta and thick ascending limb of the loop of Henle) (Brezis et al. 1991; Schrier et al. 1987).

The phase of ARF during which diuretics are given dramatically influences their ability to improve renal function. In some experimental models, diuretics given prophylactically can preserve renal excretory function, but the extent of tubular necrosis may not be limited. In experimental animals and some clinical trials in humans, diuretics were most effective when given prophylactically, somewhat effective if given during the induction phase, and least effective when given during the maintenance phase of ARF. Mannitol or furosemide given prophylactically to human patients with CRF who were about to undergo radiocontrast agent infusion provided less renoprotection than observed in those who received 0.45% sodium chloride infusion alone (Solomon et al. 1994). Radiocontrast-induced vasoconstriction was overcome in human patients by the infusion of mannitol or atrial natriuetic peptide but both infusion groups experienced a similar extent of ARF (Kurnik et al. 1990).

Although diuretic administration may not result in immediate improvement of renal excretory function, conversion from oliguria to nonoliguria represents some measure of success. In the author's experience, oliguric animals in the maintenance phase of ARF usually can be converted to nonoliguria by administration of diuretics, with the notable exception of patients with oligoanuria caused by ethylene glycol poisoning (Thrall et al. 1984). Usually, conversion to nonoliguria occurs without a detectable increase in GFR and is characterized by an increase in urine volume without reduction of the magnitude of azotemia. Increased tubular flow rate has the potential to relieve obstruction of tubular lumina and, secondarily, to improve GFR. It is important that adequate IV fluid administration be maintained to prevent dehydration and additional renal injury in patients that experience a marked increase in urine volume after diuretic administration.

During attempts to initiate diuresis, careful attention must be given to body weight, urine output, and changes in BUN or serum creatinine concentration. After the hydrated body weight of the patient has been established as a baseline, attempts should be made to maintain body weight while administering diuretics. Progressive weight loss during attempts to maintain diuresis indicates dehydration, whereas progressive weight gain indicates overhydration.

Meticulous attention to fluid therapy is required after diuresis has been established by administration of diuretics or spontaneous renal repair because there is a tendency toward dehydration, hyponatremia, and hypokalemia that may persist for weeks.

HYPERTONIC DEXTROSE

Osmotic diuresis using 20% dextrose in water has been used at a total daily dosage of approximately 22 to 66 mL/kg. Solutions containing 2.5 or 5% dextrose do not provide sufficient dextrose to initiate diuresis. To create hyperglycemia, a 20% dextrose solution is administered at a rate of 2 to 10 mL/min for the first 10 to 15 min. This is followed by administration at a rate of 1 to 5 mL/min. Alternatively, the dextrose dosage can be calculated as 0.5 to 1.0 g/kg infused over 15 to 20 min (Ross 1989).

The development of glucosuria indicates that sufficient hyperglycemia has been achieved to saturate renal tubular transport of glucose. Urine output should approach 1 to 4 mL/min if this procedure has been successful in initiating diuresis. After this dose has been given, a polyionic solution (e.g., lactated Ringer's solution) is administered IV to prevent dehydration and electrolyte depletion. This treatment is repeated two to three times daily as needed. If adequate urine volume is not produced, further attempts at osmotic diuresis using hypertonic dextrose are not warranted.

Some authors have stated that hypertonic dextrose may be as effective as mannitol in promoting diuresis and that dextrose has the additional advantage of being less expensive and easily detected in the urine. An additional advantage of hypertonic dextrose solutions is that it may be possible to combine increased urine flow rate with provision of some calories. The salutary effects of dextrose solutions on renal function and urinary flow rate, however, have not been rigorously compared with those of other diuretics. It is the author's opinion that other diuretics are more potent in conversion of oliguria to nonoliguria.

MANNITOL

Mannitol may be used as an alternative to dextrose in promoting osmotic diuresis. No controlled studies support the use of mannitol prophylactically or during established ARF in human patients (Conger 1995). Mannitol administration results in extracellular fluid volume expansion, which favors increased GFR and reduced tubular sodium reabsorption, but the beneficial effects of mannitol are not simply the result of volume expansion, because the same effect is not observed after volume expansion with 0.9% NaCl (Levinsky et al. 1983). After filtration, mannitol exerts a hyperosmotic effect along the entire nephron and also inhibits renin release (Levinsky et al. 1983), which may be important in forms of ARF that are dependent on the renin-angiotensin-aldosterone system. Mannitol may induce release of atrial natriuetic peptide which may contribute to its salutary effects on renal function (see later) (Kurnik et al. 1990). After renal ischemia, mannitol attenuates a deleterious rise in intramitochondrial calcium concentration and also acts as a free-radical scavenger (Shilliday and Allison 1994).

Mannitol may be superior to dextrose in promoting diuresis in animals with ARF when cellular swelling is important in the maintenance of oliguria or reduced GFR. Dextrose equilibrates with intracellular and extracellular fluid spaces, but mannitol remains within the extracellular space and consequently may be more effective in reversing cellular swelling. Mannitol also may be superior to furosemide in the treatment of ARF in patients that are not yet overhydrated.

Mannitol may be infused at an initial dosage of 0.25 to 0.50 g/kg body weight given intravenously over 3 to 5 min to initiate diuresis. Mannitol is available for injection as a 25% solution. Diuresis is expected within 20 to 30 min after infusion. The concerns about dextrose also apply to mannitol, but there is no practical way to monitor the appearance of mannitol in the urine. If a beneficial effect is seen (increased urine flow rate or reduction in the magnitude of azotemia), intermittent bolus injections or constant infusion as a 5 to 10% solution may be necessary to maintain this salutary effect. To maintain diuresis, a 5 to 10% mannitol solution may be administered IV at 2 to 5 mL/min. Mannitol may be diluted in lactated Ringer's solution to provide fluid needs. The total daily dosage of mannitol should not exceed 2 g/kg (Osborne et al. 1972), because high-dose mannitol therapy has been reported to cause ARF in some human patients (Brezis et al. 1991) and has been associated with nervous system toxicity in functionally anephric dogs (Silber and Thompson 1972).

If a beneficial effect (urine production 1 to 3 mL/min) (Osborne et al. 1972) is not seen within an hour, mannitol infusion is discontinued because additional doses may not be excreted and may result in severe hyperosmolality, hyponatremia, hypervolemia, pulmonary edema, and congestive heart failure. Animals that are already overhydrated should not be given mannitol.

FUROSEMIDE

Furosemide (Lasix) may be given as the initial therapy, after mannitol has failed to have a salutary effect, or in combination with dopamine (see later). Furosemide may promote diuresis when dextrose and mannitol have failed to do so. This loop diuretic acts by inhibiting the reabsorption of chloride in the thick ascending limb of the loop of Henle after secretion by the proximal tubule. A small amount of the administered dose is filtered (Chonko and Grantham 1987). It also may impair tubuloglomerular feedback (Brezis et al. 1991).

A dosage of 2 to 4 mg/kg is administered IV, and this dosage may be doubled or even tripled if no beneficial effect is seen within 30 to 60 min. When successful, diuresis may last as long as 2 h, and furosemide may be given every 8 h to maintain diuresis.

Furosemide can result in permanent or reversible ototoxicity and deafness in human patients, usually when given at high dosages or to patients with renal failure (Weiner and Mudge 1985). Hearing impairment in dogs and cats receiving furosemide for primary renal failure has not been investigated. High dosages (e.g., 50 mg/kg) of furosemide administered to normal dogs may cause hypotension, apathy, and staggering, and a dosage of 10 mg/kg administered to normal cats caused apathy and anorexia (Polzin et al. 1989). Furosemide potentiates the severity and rapidity of tubular injury in some types of experimental ARF, including aminoglycoside nephrotoxicity, but the mechanism of such injury is unclear (Adelman et al. 1979; Levinsky et al. 1983). On the basis of these studies, furosemide should not be given to patients as treatment for ARF caused by aminoglycosides. Furosemide exacerbated renal injury in these dogs when given at the same time as the nephrotoxin, but furosemide has not been studied as a treatment for ARF caused by aminoglycoside administration in hydrated dogs. In one study of hospital-acquired ARF, all three dogs that received a combination of gentamicin and furosemide therapy did not survive (Behrend et al. 1996).

DOPAMINE AND OTHER DOPAMINERGIC AGENTS

Dopamine is a catecholamine capable of interacting with two subtypes of dopamine receptors (DA-1 and DA-2), as well as with α- and β-adrenergic receptors (Brooks et al. 1990b; Smith et al. 1990). Interaction with adrenergic receptors can limit its usefulness, however, because of the tachycardia and increased systemic and renal vascular resistance that follow vasoconstriction at higher dosages.

Dopamine receptors have been identified at both vascular and tubular sites. Dopamine receptors that regulate renal vasodilatation have been demonstrated in the kidney of the dog, rat, and rabbit but not in the feline kidney (Clark et al. 1991b). Proximal renal tubules of rats, rabbits, and human beings contain specific dopamine receptors that inhibit sodium and water reabsorption when stimulated, but detailed characteristics of these receptors are not yet available (Clark et al. 1991b).

Postsynaptic DA-1 receptors cause vasodilatation of renal, mesenteric, coronary, and cerebral vascular beds (Goldberg and Rajfer 1985). The second type of dopamine receptor (DA-2) is located on postganglionic sympathetic nerve endings and ganglia, and activation of these receptors inhibits the release of norepinephrine. These receptors also are located in the emetic center of the brain (Goldberg and Rajfer 1985).

The first type of dopamine receptor has not been identified in glomeruli but is found in nonglomerular renal vessels (Hammond and Cutler 1989). Stimulation of DA-1 receptors results in direct vasodilatation, whereas DA-2 receptor activation indirectly results in vasodilatation by inhibiting release of norepinephrine from postganglionic sympathetic nerve endings with subsequent reduction of tonic sympathetic vasoconstriction (Aronson et al. 1990; Frederickson et al. 1985; Hammond and Cutler 1989; Smith et al. 1990). Stimulation of DA-2 receptors also can result in nausea and vomiting (Smith et al. 1990). These receptors have been identified in the glomeruli and tubules of the rat kidney (Frederickson et al. 1985). The first type of receptor also has been identified in the juxtaglomerular cells of the rat kidney, and when stimulated it increases renin secretion (Lokhandwala and Hegde 1990), but inhibition of renin release has been noted by others (Denton et al. 1996).

After dopamine administration, RBF usually is increased to a greater degree than is GFR (Frederickson et al. 1985; Hammond and Cutler 1989). When they occur, increases in GFR may be a consequence of increased cardiac output rather than a direct renal effect. In some species, however, GFR is highly dependent on RBF, and increased RBF could contribute to increased GFR. Increased RBF and decreased renal vascular resistance occurred in a dose-dependent manner in anesthetized dogs receiving dopamine at rates of 1 to 48 µg/kg/min (Hahn et al. 1982). In dogs, the effects of dopamine on RBF and electrolyte excretion are mediated by activation of DA-1 receptors, and these effects are abolished by administration of the DA-1 specific receptor antagonist SCH 23390 (Frederickson et al. 1985). Renal vasodilatation mediated via DA-2 vascular receptor activation is considered important by some investigators (Hammond and Cutler 1989). Dopamine causes natriuresis largely by inhibition of Na^+,K^+-adenosinetriphosphatase in the proximal tubule, medullary thick ascending limb of Henle's loop, and cortical collecting duct via DA-1 and DA-2 receptor interaction. The effect of dopamine to limit oxygen consumption in high-risk tubules could limit tubular injury and accelerate renal repair in ARF. Free-water excretion also is enhanced because dopamine inhibits the central release of antidiuretic hormone (ADH) and antagonizes the action of ADH at the collecting tubule (Denton et al. 1996).

The renal response to dopamine infusion varies by species, dosage, and degree of renal impairment. Pronounced differences in the response to dopamine exist between dogs and cats. "Renal-dose" dopamine (0.2–2.0 µg/kg/min) activates both dopamine DA-1 and DA-2 receptors, whereas β-adrenergic receptors are activated at higher dosages (2–5 µg/kg/min) and α-adrenergic receptors become increasingly activated at even higher dosages (>5 µg/kg/min) (Carcoana and Hines 1996; Harper and Savage 1997). An ideal dosage of dopamine for beneficial renal effects is one at which dopaminergic and β-adrenergic effects exceed vasoconstrive α-adrenergic effects (<5 µg/kg/min) (Carcoana and Hines 1996). The beneficial renal effects of dopamine are more likely in patients with less severe azotemia (i.e., in patients earlier in the acute renal disease process) at the time dopamine infusion is started (Conger 1995; Lindner et al. 1979). Increased RBF, increased urine volume, decreased urine osmolality, and increased urinary fractional excretions of electrolytes typically occur during dopamine infusion in dogs (Frederickson et al. 1985; Hahn et al. 1982). In dogs, GFR is either increased or unchanged during dopamine infusion (Frederickson et al. 1985). Low-dose dopamine infusion (<10 µg/kg/min) increases RBF largely as a consequence of efferent arteriolar dilatation (Hammond and Cutler 1989). High-dose dopamine infusion (≥10 µg/kg/min) predominantly activates α-adrenergic receptors. Renal α-adrenergic receptor activation results in renal vasoconstriction. Renal α-adrenergic receptors are located on renal tubular cells and produce antidiuretic and antinatriuretic effects when stimulated (Hammond and Cutler 1989). Activation of β-adrenergic receptors in the kidney may enhance renin release (Hammond and Cutler 1989).

Fenoldopam, a specific DA-1 receptor agonist, is more specific and potent than dopamine in causing renal vasodilatation in dogs (Brooks and DePalma 1993; Clark et al. 1991a; Hahn et al. 1982). Fenoldopam and derivatives that maintain increased RBF are well absorbed from the intestinal tract of the dog (Brooks et al. 1990a). Fenoldopam maintained or increased RBF despite systemic arterial hypotension in anesthetized dogs in one study (Aronson et al. 1990). Increased systemic arterial pressure and tachycardia do not occur with fenoldopam, because, unlike dopamine, it does not stimulate adrenergic receptors. Renal perfusion is maintained at higher dosages of fenoldopam despite induction of systemic hypotension. Fenoldopam stimulated release of renin in anesthetized dogs, an effect that opposes fenoldopam's inhibition of tubular function and its vasodepressor actions (Clark et al. 1991a). Oral and IV fenoldopam given to a small number of dogs with spontaneous chronic renal insufficiency increased RBF nearly 100% over baseline, whereas GFR as estimated by creatinine clearance increased by 25 to 50% (Brooks et al. 1990b). Fenoldopam ameliorated cyclosporine-induced nephrotoxicity in rats (Brooks et al. 1990c) and provided renal protection during subacute amphotericin nephrotoxicity in dogs. Some enhanced recovery of renal function was seen during acute amphotericin nephrotoxicity (Nichols et al. 1992). Fenoldopam increased renal reserve for RBF but not for GFR in dogs in which amino acids were simultaneously infused (Brooks and DePalma 1993).

YM435 is a new potent and selective dopamine DA-1 receptor agonist with no α- or β-adrenoreceptor agonist activity. Infusion of YM435 in anesthetized dogs caused RBF to increase more than 10 times as much as with dopamine infusion. Renal blood flow also was slightly increased over that achieved with fenoldopam infusion (Yatsu et al. 1997c). YM435 can overcome renal vasoconstriction of afferent and efferent arterioles induced by angiotensin II and endothelin in rats (Takenaka et al. 1993) and angiotensin II or norepinephrine in dogs (Yatsu et al. 1997b). Increased RBF, GFR, urinary flow rate, and urinary sodium excretion followed infusion of YM435 in anesthetized dogs in a dose-dependent manner without effect on heart rate (Yatsu et al. 1997a) YM435 reversed angiotensin II–induced decreases in RBF, GFR, and urine flow rate in the same study of dogs and prevented decreases induced by renal nerve stimulation or platelet-activating factor. Infusion of YM435 reversed decreases in GFR, urinary flow rate, and urinary sodium excretion that occurred after 1 h of renal ischemia in experimental dogs but not when the infusion was stopped. Beneficial effects were not observed during infusion of 0.9% saline (Yatsu et al. 1998).

In the normal cat, diuresis occurs during dopamine infusion but increases in GFR and RBF are not observed. The cat apparently does not have specific dopamine receptors in its renal vasculature or tubules (Clark et al. 1991b; Wasserman et al. 1980). Fenoldopam does not cause any renal effects in anesthetized cats (Clark et al. 1991b), suggesting that dopamine receptors either do not exist or are present in low numbers in the kidneys of this species. Despite this, diuresis and natriuresis ensue during dopamine infusion in cats. This effect is probably due to stimulation of α-adrenergic receptors that increase blood pressure and decrease sodium reabsorption in the late distal tubule and collecting tubule (Clark et al. 1991b). This diuretic response can be abolished by nonselective α-adrenergic antagonists but not by selective dopamine receptor antagonists (Clark et al. 1991b). "Pressure diuresis" may partially explain the diuresis during dopamine infusion at dosages of approximately 10 μg/kg/min because systemic arterial blood pressure is increased at this dosage in cats (Clark et al. 1991b).

The so-called renal-dose dopamine (a dosage below the vasopressor dosage, often 2–5 μg/kg/min) has surprisingly little documentation to support its use in clinical patients in either human (Denton et al. 1996; Shilliday and Allison 1994; Thadhani et al. 1996) or veterinary medicine. Efficacy studies of dopamine in clinically uremic dogs or cats with or without oliguria are not available. On the basis of results for experimental dogs and cats and clinical trials in human patients, dopamine infusion for the conversion of oliguria to nonoliguria seems reasonable. In oliguric human patients, dopamine infusion can result in diuresis and natriuresis after high-dose furosemide therapy has failed to establish diuresis (Hammond and Cutler 1989). Low-dose dopamine infusion (4 μg/kg/min) attenuated the adverse effects of ibuprofen on RBF in a canine model of endotoxic shock and counteracted the vasoconstrictive effects of systemically administered norepinephrine (Fink et al. 1985).

The potentially beneficial effects of dopaminergic compounds have been studied in human patients with CRF. In these patients, dopamine infusion increased GFR and RBF (Hammond and Cutler 1989). In another study of human patients with advanced CRF, GFR did not increase, but RBF, urine flow, and sodium excretion were increased after dopamine infusion (Hammond and Cutler 1989). Oral ibopamine has been given to human patients with CRF in an attempt to retard progressive deterioration of excretory renal function, and increased creatinine clearance, diuresis, and natriuresis were observed (Casagrande et al. 1989).

In human patients, there is marked individual variation in the rate of dopamine infusion required to achieve activation of various receptors. Consequently, patients must be carefully monitored in order to achieve the desired effect (Goldberg and Rajfer 1985). Variation in the response to dopamine may be due to differences in the number or sensitivity of dopamine receptors among different species and among individuals in a given species (Trim et al. 1989). The side effects of dopamine may be severe and counterproductive to renal excretory function.

Therefore, dopamine must be infused accurately at a low dosage, usually 1 to 5 μg/kg/min. Such precise infusion is best achieved with an infusion pump. A large vein should be chosen for infusion of dopamine to avoid vasoconstriction that may be associated with a relatively high concentration of dopamine locally. Otherwise, ischemia and necrosis can occur, and extravasation of dopamine-containing fluids warrants the same concern (Hosgood 1990).

Dopamine should not be administered in fluids containing sodium bicarbonate or in other alkaline fluids, because the drug is inactivated in an alkaline environment (Brezis et al. 1991; Hammond and Cutler 1989). Metoclopramide is a DA-2 receptor antagonist (Smith et al. 1990). Consequently, intermittent injection or constant infusion of metoclopramide (Reglan) to control vomiting should be avoided or discontinued during dopamine infusion.

Dopamine hydrochloride (Intropin) is available as single-dose vials of 200, 400, or 800 mg. The vial containing 200 mg per 5 mL vial is most appropriate for small animal patients and provides 40 mg/mL. Dopamine must always be diluted before administration. It can be added safely to most commercially available saline or dextrose-containing solutions and is stable in fluids at room temperature for at least 24 h.

Dopamine can be diluted by adding 0.75 mL of Intropin (30 mg) to 500 mL of 0.9% NaCl or lactated Ringer's solution. This results in a dopamine concentration of 60 μg/mL. A separate IV line is recommended for infusion of dopamine to ensure accuracy of dose administration. Alternatively, two IV lines can be connected by a Y-piece administration set to one IV catheter. Dopamine is administered via one IV line, and the other IV line is used to administer fluids for maintenance and rehydration. First, the total number of micrograms per minute to be infused is calculated, and then the number of drops per minute required to achieve this dose is calculated. An infusion pump is set at this number of drops per minute. In the absence of an infusion pump, an administration set that delivers 60 drops/mL (pediatric drip chamber) is used. Each drop contains 1 μg of dopamine. For example, to infuse dopamine at 2 μg/kg/min to a 10-kg dog, 20 μg/min is required. This can be accomplished using a 60 drop/mL drip chamber at 20 drops/min or 1 drop per 3 s. Alternatively, 50 mg (1.25 mL of a 40 mg/mL solution) of dopamine may be added to 500 mL of fluids, resulting in a dopamine concentration of 100 μg/mL, and the drip rate is adjusted accordingly (Cornelius 1983).

Electrocardiographic monitoring is recommended during dopamine infusion to ensure rapid detection of arrhythmias. The resting heart rate should be determined and recorded after hydration but before starting the dopamine infusion. The heart rate should be determined every 15 min for the first hour and hourly thereafter if no problems have been encountered. A sudden increase in heart rate (>180/min in dogs or >200/min in cats) indicates the need to reduce the rate of dopamine infusion. Emergence of a serious cardiac arrhythmia (e.g., ventricular tachycardia) during dopamine infusion may preclude further administration of the drug. Promptly discontinuing dopamine infusion usually results in cessation of cardiac arrhythmias. Animals with underlying cardiac disease may be more susceptible to arrhythmias during dopamine infusion, but this usually is not a problem at the low dosage of dopamine employed for renal effects. Serial blood pressure measurements may be helpful in detection of adrenergic receptor activation when higher dosages of dopamine (≥ 5 μg/kg/min) are employed in attempts to convert oliguria to nonoliguria. The infusion rate should be decreased if systemic arterial blood pressure continuously increases during dopamine infusion.

It is the author's impression that oliguric renal failure that has failed to respond to mannitol or furosemide may be converted to nonoliguria after combined infusion of dopamine and furosemide. Experimental studies in dogs showed this combination to be superior to either dopamine or furosemide alone in maintaining GFR, RBF, osmolar clearance, and urine flow during a model of nephrotoxic ARF (Lindner et al. 1979). A synergistic effect of dopamine in combination with furosemide has been found for the conversion of oliguria to nonoliguria in human patients with ARF. A salutary response necessitates prior volume repletion and institution of combination therapy diuretics within 24 h of the onset of oliguria (Hammond and Cutler 1989). Dopamine-induced renal vasodilatation may increase the delivery of furosemide to its site of action in the ascending limb of Henle's loop (Schwartz and Gewertz 1988).

Most of the author's experience with combined use of dopamine and furosemide has been in dogs, but this regimen has been used safely in cats. Dopamine is continuously infused at a rate of 2 to 5 μg/kg/min in combination with furosemide at 1 mg/kg/h given by IV bolus injections. If no improvement occurs within 6 h, additional efforts to convert oliguria to nonoliguria with dopamine are unlikely to be successful, and the infusion should be discontinued. This combination regimen often is selected by clinicians as a last resort, but it may be more beneficially employed in the initial management of oliguric ARF. As noted earlier, decreased BUN and serum creatinine concentrations do not necessarily accompany an increase in urine production.

Studies of the more potent and specific dopaminergic renal vasodilators and natriuretics should be undertaken in the future to determine their ability to alter the course of uremic crises in dogs and cats. It may prove valuable to study higher dosages of dopamine after α- and β-adrenergic blockade. Felodipine is a calcium channel blocker with renal vasodilatory and natriuretic properties that also warrants further study in the treatment of uremic crises (DiBona 1985; Pettersson et al. 1987). Recovery of GFR is more rapid in human patients with intrinsic ARF when they are treated with the calcium channel blocking agent verapamil or gallopamil (Conger 1995).

Atrial natriuretic peptide (ANP) causes diuresis, natriuresis, increased GFR, and maintenance of RBF during periods of increased vasoconstriction (Kurnik et al. 1990). Atrial natriuretic peptide promotes both vasodilatation of the afferent arteriole and vasoconstriction of the efferent arteriole, an effect that selectively increases GFR independently of RBF (Humes 1995). Atrial natriuretic peptide also may provide renoprotection independently of its hemodynamic effects in that renal tubular cell exfoliation, necrosis, and cast formation are reduced and ATP regeneration is enhanced. Atrial natriuretic peptide exerts beneficial effects immediately after ischemia and also during established postischemic ARF in which sustained increases in GFR and tubular function may occur (Humes 1995; Shilliday and Allison 1994). Atrial natriuretic peptide prevented radiocontrast-induced renal vasoconstriction in a study of dogs and proved beneficial in models of ischemic and nephrotoxic ARF (Kurnik et al. 1990). Results from a multicenter study of human patients with ARF suggest that atrial natriuretic peptide may be beneficial in patients with oliguria (Kurnik et al. 1990). Clinical trials in human patients with established acute tubular necrosis are being conducted (Humes 1995). Atrial natriuretic peptide was most beneficial when started earlier in the course of ARF in human patients (Conger 1995). High doses of atrial natriuretic peptide cause peripheral vasodilatation that can result in systemic hypotension as a limiting factor. A combination of atrial natriuretic peptide and dopamine may provide the beneficial effects of atrial natriuretic peptide without the hypotension (Shilliday and Allison 1994).

Failure to Convert Oliguria to Nonoliguria

When oliguria persists, it is imperative to curtail drastically the daily volume of IV fluids administered in order to avoid overhydration. Fluids should not be discontinued unless the animal is already obviously overhydrated (i.e., inappropriate weight gain, subcutaneous edema, pulmonary edema, distended jugular veins). Fluid administration should be adjusted in patients with persistent oliguria to replace insensible losses (respiratory and normal gastrointestinal losses are approximately 20 mL/kg/day) and contemporary fluid losses from vomiting or diarrhea (this volume must be estimated).

Providing insensible fluid needs may allow the animal to survive long enough for spontaneous diuresis to occur. Dialysis may be required to maintain life if the animal is severely uremic, has severe hyperkalemia and metabolic acidosis, or is markedly overhydrated. Peritoneal dialysis is discussed in Chapter 25 and hemodialysis is discussed in Chapter 26. Therapeutic phlebotomy may be a lifesaving maneuver in a critically overhydrated patient. Acute removal of approximately 25% of the patient's blood volume (approximately 20 mL/kg) may be useful in this setting.

Blood

Transfusion with whole blood or packed red cells is indicated if the packed cell volume (PCV) is less than 20% and may be of benefit in some patients with PCV values of 20 to 25% (see Chapter 21). Packed red blood cells are preferable in overhydrated patients. Transfusion with whole blood is satisfactory if overhydration is not present or if total plasma protein concentration is less than 5.0 g/dL.

Severe anemia may be apparent at presentation in animals with advanced CRF or may develop later in those with ARF. Anemia often becomes apparent only after correction of intravascular dehydration or may develop suddenly after gastrointestinal blood loss in both ARF and CRF patients. Anemia usually is not apparent in the early phases of ARF, but it frequently becomes apparent during a protracted maintenance phase, especially when the magnitude of azotemia is severe.

Blood loss through gastrointestinal ulceration can be severe yet may go undetected until melena is observed later. Blood loss may be aggravated by poor platelet function and capillary fragility in uremia at a time when replacement with new red blood cells (reticulocytes and nucleated red blood cells) is inefficient because of reduced renal erythropoietin production by the diseased kidneys. Shortened red blood cell life span and suppression of bone marrow as a consequence of uremia also may contribute to anemia (Chew and DiBartola 1989; Polzin et al. 1989). Lastly, repeated blood sampling for diagnostic testing and ongoing crystalloid fluid therapy contribute to the observed anemia. Concomitant management of gastrointestinal ulcers with H-2 receptor blocking drugs (e.g., cimetidine, ranitidine, famotidine, nizatidine) and sucralfate and a reduction in the magnitude of azotemia aid in reduction of blood loss.

Nutritional Aspects of Management

Treatment of human patients with ARF with parenteral alimentation solutions containing amino acids and glucose resulted in a more rapid decrease in serum creatinine concentration and lower mortality (Conger 1995). Primary renal failure is a catabolic state (Brezis et al. 1991; Polzin et al. 1989) in which breakdown of body proteins potentiates the observed increases in BUN, serum phosphorus, serum potassium, and hydrogen ion concentrations. Most animals with severe uremia are anorexic and consequently suffer protein-calorie malnutrition, which may become life threatening. Spontaneous intake of nutrients is unlikely in animals that remain severely azotemic (BUN > 100 mg/dL) during initial medical management of a uremic crisis. Some animals resume nutrient intake after medical therapy has reduced the severity of gastrointestinal ulceration, central stimuli for vomiting have been blunted, and the magnitude of azotemia has been reduced. Animals undergoing successful dialysis often eat on their own.

Some form of nutritional support usually is prescribed for anorexic uremic animals with decompensated CRF or protracted ARF. The aim of nutritional therapy is to promote anabolism and reduce endogenous protein catabolism, which serves as a source of nitrogenous solutes, phosphorus, potassium, and hydrogen ions. Force-feeding can be attempted but often is not successful in providing enough nutritional support. Nutrient intake should consist of a reduced quantity of high-quality protein. Sufficient nonprotein calories must be supplied to prevent the dietary protein source from being catabolized for energy.

Some sparing of body protein can be accomplished by hypertonic glucose infusion, particularly when administered in conjunction with amino acids during total parenteral nutrition (Brezis et al. 1991; Chew and DiBartola 1989; Polzin et al. 1989). The BUN is reduced in these instances as a consequence of reduced catabolism and enhanced anabolism, and this may improve the animal's quality of life. In addition, provision of nutrients during renal healing may facilitate the recovery process, but the proper nutrient composition in this setting is not known. Care must be taken to prevent overhydration when administering hypertonic alimentation solutions to patients with oliguria. Infusion of 20 to 25% dextrose to supply caloric needs and of a balanced amino acid solution at 0.3 g/kg/day via a jugular catheter has been recommended for parenteral nutritional support (Finco and Barsanti 1983). Standard glucose supplementation of IV fluids at 2.5 or 5% dextrose does not provide sufficient nonprotein calories to prevent catabolism of endogenous proteins. Total parenteral nutrition is discussed in Chapter 22.

Enteral alimentation using nasogastric tube feedings can be attempted after initial reduction of azotemia by fluid therapy and medical management of the gastrointestinal manifestations of uremia using H-2 receptor blocking drugs, metoclopramide, and sucralfate. Nasogastric tube feedings are relatively easy to maintain and are well tolerated by cats and most dogs. In the absence of more specific information regarding nutritional requirements during uremic episodes in dogs or cats, commercially available liquid diets for human and veterinary patients have been used for nasogastric tube feedings at the Ohio State University Veterinary Teaching Hospital. Some severely azotemic animals are able to tolerate nasogastric tube feedings quite well. Pulse feedings four to six times per day through the nasogastric tube are often tolerated without vomiting. Continuous pump infusion of liquid nutrition is frequently tolerated when previous pulse feedings resulted in vomiting. Pureed veterinary foods designed to reduce waste retention during renal failure do not flow through small-diameter nasogastric tubes well but can be administered readily through a gastrostomy tube. If long-term nutritional support is necessary during support of renal healing, placement of a gastrostomy tube facilitates this therapy.

▶ Monitoring the Effects of Fluid Therapy

Frequent monitoring of the patient in uremic crisis is essential, especially during the first 3 days, when these patients are likely to be most unstable and rapid changes are most likely.

Serial body weight measurements using the same scale facilitate proper fluid therapy during initial management. Weight gain sufficient to account for rehydration should occur during the initial 24 h of IV fluid therapy. Failure to gain weight during attempts at rehydration indicates that an inadequate volume of fluid has been administered, possibly because of underestimation of ongoing losses through vomiting or diarrhea. Precise body weight should be determined three to four times during the first 24 h of hospitalization to ensure that rehydration is being accomplished. Mild progressive weight loss should occur thereafter in the absence of caloric intake. Failure to lose some weight during this period can be a clue that inappropriate fluid retention has occurred. It is easy to overlook gradual fluid accumulation that ultimately may lead to clinical signs related to overhydration. Anticipated daily weight loss for anorexic animals has been estimated as 0.1 to 0.3 kg body weight per 1000 kcal of daily caloric need (Finco 1977) or 0.5 to 1.0% of body weight per day (English 1974). Body weight should be determined twice daily for the duration of hospitalization to ensure that a sudden inappropriate increase in body weight does not occur. On the other hand, sudden excessive loss of body weight may indicate episodes of unappreciated fluid loss and dehydration that could threaten ongoing renal healing.

Measurement of urine output via an indwelling urethral catheter facilitates fluid therapy decisions in conjunction with serial body weight as described previously. Animals that have questionable urine output after the administration of fluids for rehydration should have a urinary catheter placed at this time. The hour-to-hour decision-making process during fluid challenges and diuretic treatments is facilitated by precise quantitative information about urine output.

Packed cell volume and total plasma protein (TPP) concentration should be determined twice daily for the first 48 h and daily thereafter while the patient is receiving parenteral fluids. This can be helpful in documenting intravascular rehydration (decreasing PCV and TPP), overhydration (progressively decreasing PCV and TPP), dehydration (increasing PCV and TPP), or blood loss (decreasing PCV and TPP). The amount of blood withdrawn for each PCV and TPP determination should be minimized by using a 25-gauge needle and filling the microhematocrit tube directly from the hub of the needle when a drop of blood first appears.

Serial physical examination is focused on evaluation of hydration, because overhydration can result in death of the animal and dehydration can lead to further renal injury. The subcutaneous tissues may feel gelatinous ("slippery") during overhydration before the development of overt peripheral edema. Increased lung sounds and respiratory rate may indicate early overhydration as well as pneumonia or compensatory hyperventilation in response to metabolic acidosis. Jugular venous distention suggests hypervolemia or overt congestive heart failure. Ongoing hemorrhage (e.g., gastrointestinal blood loss) should be suspected when mucous membranes suddenly become pale.

Serial measurements of serum biochemistry are necessary to determine whether the animal's azotemia is responding to treatment. Frequent serum biochemical evaluation is indicated for patients with progressive or rapid changes in BUN and creatinine concentrations, those with persistent oliguria, and those that suddenly develop polyuria. Patients with severe electrolyte or acid-base disturbances should be followed more frequently than those with relatively stable biochemistry. Adjustment of the dosage of oral phosphorus-binding agents is based on serial measurement of serum phosphorus concentra-

Chest radiographs, urine culture, and blood culture should be considered for patients that develop fever, cough, or leukocytosis with a left shift during hospitalization. Intravenous catheter sites should be inspected. The intravenous catheter should be removed and its tip cultured when catheter sepsis is suspected. Maintenance of IV catheters is discussed further in Chapter 14.

Renal biopsy should be performed if it is not clear whether the intrinsic renal disease is chronic or acute. The finding of acute lesions on renal biopsy may justify further expense and effort, whereas severe chronic lesions associated with nonresponsive uremia may warrant euthanasia.

Outcome During Fluid Treatments of Uremic Crises

Ideally, fluid therapy provides sufficient time for adequate renal healing, improved renal excretory function, and at least partial resolution of azotemia and the clinical signs of uremia. The magnitude of residual azotemia and loss of other renal functions (e.g., concentrating ability, acidifying ability) after the withdrawal of aggressive fluid therapy determine whether an animal can eventually be treated without administration of parenteral fluids.

Fluid therapy may not be sufficient for patients with renal failure and advanced irreversible loss of excretory function. In these cases, the serum concentrations of urea nitrogen, creatinine, phosphorus, and other unmeasured uremic solutes do not decrease sufficiently to allow adaptation to the uremic environment. The nature of the underlying renal disease, the extent of systemic uremic signs, and the presence of concomitant abnormalities in other organ systems interact to determine whether survival is possible. Many animals with severe uremia are euthanized because of severe clinical signs that do not improve rapidly during initial treatment. Electrolyte imbalances, acid-base disturbances, uremic solute retention, hormonal dysfunction, hematologic abnormalities, and malnutrition can be extensive and difficult to manage effectively.

In the absence of dialysis, persistence of oliguria or development of oliguria during fluid and diuretic treatment of dogs with ARF is associated with a poor prognosis (Behrend et al. 1996; Brown et al. 1985; Vaden et al. 1997). Nonoliguric renal failure was common in one study of aminoglycoside nephrotoxicity (Brown et al. 1985), but 50% of affected patients were oliguric in a later report (Behrend et al. 1996). The prognosis is worse for dogs with oliguric forms of aminoglycoside nephrotoxity, but the absence of oliguria does not guarantee survival. The prognosis is grave for dogs or cats that develop anuric ARF, a situation most likely to develop in ethylene glycol intoxication (Grauer et al. 1984; Kersting and Nielsen 1966; Nunamaker et al. 1971; Rowland 1987; Thrall et al. 1984). Anuric ARF also may be encountered in cats after ingestion of Easter or day lilies (Hall 1999). Dogs and cats with severe oliguric ARF have been shown to survive with return of renal function and urine production after several months of hemodialysis (Cowgill 1995; Cowgill and Langston 1996; Langston et al. 1997).

Many animals with acute decompensation of CRF can be successfully treated if a substantial proportion of their azotemia is prerenal in nature. In these cases, the goal is to return the animal to its previous level of azotemia by careful rehydration.

The outlook is not so good for animals with intrinsic ARF. In a series of dogs with intrinsic ARF, more than 50% died or were euthanized, whereas 24% survived with CRF and 19% returned to normal as evaluated by serum creatinine concentration (Vaden et al. 1997). Similarly, of a series of dogs with hospital-acquired ARF, 38% survived, 24% died, and 38% were euthanized (Behrend et al. 1996). In dogs with ARF, severe azotemia (serum creatinine concentration > 10 mg/dL), hypocalcemia (< 8.6 mg/dL), anemia (PCV < 33%), proteinuria, ethylene glycol ingestion, and disseminated intravascular coagulation were associated with failure to survive, but advanced age was not a factor (Vaden et al. 1997). Odds ratios for failure to survive were lowest for dogs with presenting serum creatinine concentrations of 1.8 to 5.0 mg/dL, intermediate for those serum creatinine concentrations of 5.1 to 10.0, and very high for dogs with serum creatinine concentrations in excess of 10.0 mg/dL. Dogs that did not survive hospital-acquired ARF in another study had higher serum phosphorus and anion gap concentrations than dogs that survived. In the same study, dogs that were older than 7 years or had oliguria at presentation also were at increased risk for failure to survive. Unlike the findings in the other study, however, magnitude of azotemia at the time of diagnosis did not predict survival despite the fact that mean serum creatinine and BUN concentrations were lower in survivors. Maximal BUN and serum creatinine concentrations also failed to predict survival in this study (Behrend et al. 1996). When intrinsic ARF in dogs is due to leptospirosis, aggressive fluid therapy and administration of antibiotics often lead to resolution of nephritis and survival (Brown et al. 1996; Harkin and Gartrell 1996; Rentko et al. 1992). In the unusual circumstance in which hospital-acquired ARF follows use of nafcillin, the prognosis for recovery of normal renal function is fair. Four of seven dogs regained normal renal function, two had persistent isosthenuria with normal BUN and creatinine concentrations, and one was euthanized because of failure to respond to treatment (Pascoe et al. 1996).

Prognosis for survival and recovery of adequate renal function after episodes of intrinsic ARF require clinical consideration and integration of the cause of renal failure, severity of histopathologic renal injury, severity of laboratory abnormalities, other organ system dysfunctions, response time after initial therapy, adequacy of response to therapy, and access to dialysis. In the future, targeted therapy to augment renal hemodynamics with atrial natriuretic peptide, assisted recovery of denuded tubular basement membranes with growth factors, and resolution of intratubular obstruction with disintegrins and fluid therapy may improve prognosis for recovery from intrinsic ARF (Humes 1995; Thadhani et al. 1996).

How long should one wait for the return of adequate renal function? There is no well-defined period in patients with renal failure over which the magnitude of azotemia substantially diminishes as renal lesions heal and renal function improves, if this occurs at all. Consequently, the duration of treatment is determined individually for each patient. Fluid therapy is continued as long as the BUN, serum creatinine, and serum phosphorus concentrations are progressively decreasing to a level tolerated by the patient.

Long-term supportive care may be required for animals in which the magnitude of severe azotemia either does not decrease or actually increases during initial aggressive fluid therapy. Some animals tolerate severe azotemia during acute or chronic renal failure better than others. In these patients, meticulous attention to fluid therapy is indicated for 2 to 4 weeks during ARF, for 5 to 7 days during uncomplicated decompensated CRF, and for 2 to 4 weeks during acute-on-chronic renal failure. This usually provides adequate time for the diseased kidneys to undergo healing of acute lesions or recompensation in chronic renal disease. The time required for renal compensation and improved clinical condition is quite variable and depends on the extent of renal injury.

In the absence of dialysis, euthanasia should be considered for animals with severe azotemia and clinical signs of uremia if clinical and laboratory improvement is not seen after 5 to 7 days of intensive treatment. Dialysis may substantially lessen the patient's discomfort by reducing the magnitude of azotemia. Early and aggressive hemodialysis has been shown to improve the prognosis for survival of ARF in dogs and cats (see Chapter 26). Animals that remain severely oliguric, develop progressive oliguria, or develop overhydration during aggressive fluid therapy probably should be euthanized if dialysis is not an option. Likewise, euthanasia should be considered for animals with intractable hyperkalemia or severe metabolic acidosis.

Bacterial infections are important complications during the management of uremic crises and may result in death. Uremic patients have diminished host defenses at a time when indwelling urinary catheterization is necessary to monitor urine output and placement of an intravenous catheter is required to administer fluids. Urinary tract infection is a common cause of bacterial sepsis in dogs (Calvert and Dow 1990). Recumbency may favor the development of pneumonia in the septic animal and increases the risk of aspiration pneumonia after episodes of vomiting.

Severe encephalopathy and uremic pneumonitis may be manifestations of advanced renal failure that are not readily treated. Blood loss into the gastrointestinal tract can be severe. Gastrointestinal ulcers that contribute to hemorrhage, diarrhea, and vomiting may continue to develop despite conventional medical management of uremia. Malnutrition can become severe when nutrient intake is absent or poor and when catabolism is increased. Such malnutrition results in severe loss of lean body mass.

Tapering Parenteral Fluid Therapy

If oliguria persists despite attempts at intensive diuresis, the volume of administered fluid is immediately reduced until diuresis ensues. Replacement of insensible fluid losses is continued at approximately 20 mL/kg/day, and contemporary losses from vomiting or diarrhea are replaced.

In nonoliguric patients, the volume of fluid administered is reduced gradually after BUN and serum creatinine concentrations have decreased substantially. Alternatively, fluids are tapered if BUN and serum creatinine concentrations remain increased but are stable for three consecutive days after an initial reduction in the magnitude of azotemia and improved clinical status. It has been the author's experience that animals with BUN concentrations above 100 mg/dL and serum creatinine concentrations above 8 mg/dL after aggressive fluid therapy are not likely to be managed adequately with fluids, and certainly not when fluid therapy is withdrawn.

Patients with polyuric renal failure have an obligatory diuresis, and successful tapering of IV fluids depends on increased spontaneous fluid intake by the animal (drinking and eating) and reduced fluid losses through vomiting or diarrhea. Fluid therapy should not be abruptly discontinued during the treatment of uremic patients in order to avoid development of dehydration and a subsequent sudden increase in the magnitude of azotemia. In general, parenteral fluid volume is reduced by approximately 25% daily for each of two to three consecutive days before discontinuing fluid therapy. It is important to monitor the patient closely during this time to ensure that the animal remains well hydrated (as determined by skin turgor and stable body weight) and that the magnitude of azotemia either stabilizes or decreases. A substantial increase in BUN and serum creatinine concentrations in conjunction with deterioration of the animal's clinical condition necessitates resumption of fluid therapy. During more rapid tapering of IV fluids, it is advisable to provide supplemental fluids subcutaneously.

Some animals with worsening azotemia after initial tapering of fluid volume can successfully undergo a later reduction of fluid volume after an additional few days of full fluid support. At that time, the tapering of fluid therapy should be more gradual. Some uremic patients develop a worsening degree of azotemia after each tapering of IV fluids and cannot be successfully treated. In some instances, chronic fluid loading by the subcutaneous route (administered by the owners at home) can alleviate the degree of azotemia to an extent that the animal remains functional.

REFERENCES

Adelman AD, Spangler WL, Beasom F, et al: Furosemide enhancement of experimental gentamicin nephrotoxicity. *J Infect Dis* 140:342–352, 1979.

Aronson S, Goldberg LI, Roth S, et al: Preservation of renal blood flow during hypotension induced with fenoldopam in dogs. *Can J Anaesth* 37:380–384, 1990.

Behrend EN, Grauer GF, Mani I, et al: Hospital-acquired acute renal failure in dogs: 29 cases (1983–1992). *J Am Vet Med Assoc* 208:537–541, 1996.

Bentinck-Smith J and French TW: A roster of normal values for dogs and cats. In Kirk RW (ed): *Current Veterinary Therapy X.* Philadelphia, WB Saunders Co., pp 1335–1345, 1989.

Brezis M, Rosen S, and Epstein FH: Acute renal failure. In Brenner BM and Rector FC (eds): *The Kidney.* Philadelphia, WB Saunders Co., pp 993–1061, 1991.

Brooks DP, and DePalma D: The dopamine DA-1 receptor agonist fenoldopam enhances amino-acid–induced hyperemia in dogs. *Pharmacology* 47:43–49, 1993.

Brooks DP, DePalma PD, Cyronak MJ, et al: Identification of fenoldopam prodrugs with prolonged renal vasodilator activity. *J Pharmacol Exp Ther* 254:1084–1089, 1990a.

Brooks DP, Goldstein R, Koster PF, et al: Effect of fenoldopam in dogs with spontaneous renal insufficiency. *Eur J Pharmacol* 184:195–199, 1990b.

Brooks DP, Drutz DJ, and Ruffolo RR Jr: Prevention and complete reversal of cyclosporine A–induced renal vasoconstriction and nephrotoxicity in the rat by fenoldopam. *J Pharmacol Exp Ther* 254:375–379, 1990c.

Brown CA, Roberts AW, Miller MA, et al.: *Leptospira interrogans* serovar *grippotyphosa* infection in dogs. *J Am Vet Med Assoc* 209:1265–1267, 1996.

Brown SA, Barsanti JA, and Crowell WA: Gentamicin-associated acute renal failure. *J Am Vet Med Assoc* 186:686–690, 1985.

Buffington CA, DiBartola SP, and Chew DJ: Effect of low potassium commercial nonpurified diet on renal function of adult cats. *J Nutr* 121:S91–S92, 1991.

Calvert CA and Dow SW: Cardiovascular infections. In Greene CE (ed): *Infectious Diseases of the Dog and Cat,* 2nd ed. Philadelphia, WB Saunders Co., pp 97–113, 1990.

Carcoana OV and Hines RL: Is renal dose dopamine protective or therapeutic? Yes. *Crit Care Clin* 12:677–685, 1996.

Casagrande C, Merlo L, Ferrini R, et al.: Cardiovascular and renal action of dopaminergic prodrugs. *J Cardiovasc Pharmacol* 14(suppl 8):540–559, 1989.

Chew DJ: Acute intrinsic renal failure. 14th Kal Kan Symposium, Columbus, OH, pp 69–92, 1991.

Chew DJ, and DiBartola SP: Diagnosis and pathophysiology of renal disease. In Ettinger SJ (ed): *Textbook of Veterinary Internal Medicine,* 3rd ed, Vol 2. Philadelphia, WB Saunders Co., pp 1893–1961, 1989.

Chew DJ, Leonard M, Muir W: Effect of sodium bicarbonate infusions on ionized calcium and total calcium concentrations in serum of clinically normal cats. *Am J Vet Res* 50:145–150, 1989.

Chew DJ, and Nagode LN: Renal secondary hyperparathyroidism. Fourth Annual Meeting of the Society for Comparative Endocrinology, Washington, DC, pp 17–26, 1990.

Chonko AM and Grantham JJ: Treatment of edema states. In Maxwell MH, Kleeman CR, and Narins RG (eds): *Clinical Disorders of Fluid and Electrolyte Metabolism,* 4th ed. New York, McGraw-Hill, pp 429–460, 1987.

Clark KL, Hilditch A, Robertson MJ, and Drew GM: Effects of dopamine DA1-receptor blockade and angiotensin converting enzyme inhibition on the renal actions of fenoldopam in the anaesthetized dog. *J Hypertens* 9:1143–1150, 1991a.

Clark KL, Robertson MJ, and Drew GM: Do renal tubular dopamine receptors mediate dopamine-induced diuresis in the anesthetized cat? *J Cardiovasc Pharmacol* 17:267–276, 1991b.

Conger JD: Interventions in clinical acute renal failure: What are the data? *Am J Kidney Dis* 26:565–576, 1995.

Cornelius LM: Fluid therapy in the uremic patient. In Kirk RW (ed): *Current Veterinary Therapy VIII.* Philadelphia, WB Saunders Co., pp 989–994, 1983.

Cowgill LD: Application of peritoneal and hemodialysis in the management of renal failure. In Osborne CA and Finco DR (eds): *Canine and Feline Nephrology and Urology.* Baltimore, Williams & Wilkins, pp. 335–367, 1995.

Cowgill LD, and Langston CE: Role of hemodialysis in the management of dogs and cats with renal failure. *Vet Clin North Am Small Anim Pract* 26:1347–1378, 1996.

Crisp MS, Chew DJ, DiBartola SP, and Birchard SJ: Peritoneal dialysis in dogs and cats: 27 cases (1976–1987). *J Am Vet Med Assoc* 195:1262–1266, 1989.

Denton MD, Chertow GM, and Brady HR: "Renal-dose" dopamine for the treatment of acute renal failure: Scientific rationale, experimental studies and clinical trials. *Kidney Int* 50:4–14, 1996.

DiBartola SP, Chew DJ, and Jacobs G: Quantitative urinalysis including 24 hour protein excretion in the dog. *J Am Anim Hosp Assoc* 16:537–546, 1980.

DiBartola SP, Rutgers HC, Zack PM, and Tarr MJ: Clinicopathologic findings associated with chronic renal disease in cats: 74 cases (1973–1984). *J Am Vet Med Assoc* 190:1196–1202, 1987.

DiBona GF: Effects of felodipine on renal function in animals. *Drugs* 29(suppl 2):168–175, 1985.

Dow SW: Studies of potassium depletion in cats. 12th Annual Kal Kan Symposium, Columbus, OH, pp 61–64, 1989.

Dow SW, Fettman MJ, Curtis CR, and LeCouteur RA: Hypokalemia in cats: 186 cases (1984–1987). *J Am Vet Med Assoc* 194:1604–1608, 1989.

Dow SW, LeCouteur RA, Fettman MJ, and Spurgeon TL: Potassium depletion in cats: Hypokalemic polymyopathy. *J Am Vet Med Assoc* 191:1563–1568, 1987.

Drobatz KJ and Hughes D: Concentration of ionized calcium in plasma from cats with urethral obstruction. *J Am Vet Med Assoc* 211:1392–1395, 1997.

English PB: Acute renal failure in the dog and cat. *Aust Vet J* 50:384–392, 1974.

Feld LG, Cachero S, and Springate JE: Fluid needs in acute renal failure. *Pediatr Clin North Am* 37:337–350, 1990.

Fettman MJ: Feline kaliopenic polymyopathy/nephropathy syndrome. *Vet Clin North Am Small Anim Pract* 19:415–432, 1989.

Finco DR: Fluid Therapy. In Kirk RW (ed): *Current Veterinary Therapy VI*. Philadelphia, WB Saunders Co., pp 3–12, 1977.

Finco DR: Kidney function. In Kaneko JJ, Harvey JW, and Burss ML (eds): *Clinical Biochemistry of Domestic Animals*, 5th ed. San Diego, Academic Press, pp 441–484, 1997.

Finco DR and Barsanti JA: Parenteral nutrition during a uremic crisis. In Kirk RW (ed): *Current Veterinary Therapy VIII*. Philadelphia, WB Saunders Co., pp 994–996, 1983.

Finco DR and Duncan JR: Evaluation of blood urea nitrogen and serum creatinine concentrations as indicators of renal dysfunction: A study of 111 cases and review of related literature. *J Am Vet Med Assoc* 168:593–601, 1976.

Finco DR and Rowland GN: Hypercalcemia secondary to chronic renal failure in the dog: A report of four cases. *J Am Vet Med Assoc* 173:990–994, 1978.

Fink M, Nelson R, and Roethal R: Low-dose dopamine preserves renal blood flow in endotoxin shocked dogs treated with ibuprofen. *J Surg Res* 38:582–591, 1985.

Fredrickson ED, Bradley T, and Goldberg L: Blockade of renal effects of dopamine in the dog by the DA1 antagonist SCH 23390. *Am J Physiol* 249:F236–F240, 1985.

Goldberg LI and Rajfer SI: Dopamine receptors: Applications in clinical cardiology. *Circulation* 72:245–248, 1985.

Grauer GF, Thrall MA, Henre BA, et al: Early clinicopathologic findings in dogs ingesting ethylene glycol. *Am J Vet Res* 45:2299–2303, 1984.

Hahn RA, Wardell JR, Sarau HM, and Ridley PT: Characterization of the peripheral and central effects of SK&F 82526, a novel dopamine receptor agonist. *J Pharmacol Exp Ther* 223:305–313, 1982.

Hall JO: Nephrotoxicity of Easter lily (*Lilium longiflorum*) when ingested by cats. *J Am Vet Med Assoc*, in press.

Hamlin RL and Rasjian RJ: Water intake and output and quantity of feces in healthy cats. *Vet Med* 59:746–747, 1964.

Hammond PG and Cutler RE: Dopamine, dopaminergic agents, and the kidney. Part 1: Pharmacology, vascular and tubular effects. *Dial Transplant* 18:36–37, 1989.

Harkin KR and Gartrell CL: Canine leptospirosis in New Jersey and Michigan: 17 cases (1990–1995). *J Am Anim Hosp Assoc* 32:495–501, 1996.

Harper L and Savage CO: The use of dopamine in acute renal failure (letter). *Clin Nephrol* 47:347–349, 1997.

Haskins SC: Anesthetic management of the end-stage renal failure patient. *Calif Vet* 33:13–15, 1979.

Hosgood G: Pharmacologic features and physiologic effects of dopamine. *J Am Vet Med Assoc* 197:1209–1211, 1990.

Humes HD: Acute renal failure: Prevailing challenges and prospects for the future. *Kidney Int Suppl* 50:S26–S32, 1995.

Kersting EJ, and Nielsen SW: Experimental ethylene glycol poisoning in the dog. *Am J Vet Res* 27:574–582, 1966.

Kirby R: Acute renal failure as a complication in the critically ill animal. *Vet Clin North Am Small Anim Pract* 19:1189–1208, 1989.

Kurnik BR, Weisberg LS, Cuttler IM, and Kurnik PB: Effects of atrial natriuretic peptide versus mannitol on renal blood flow during radiocontrast infusion in chronic renal failure. *J Lab Clin Med* 116:27–36, 1990.

Langston CE, Cowgill LD, and Spano JA: Applications and outcome of hemodialysis in cats: A review of 29 cases. *J Vet Intern Med* 11:348–355, 1997.

Levinsky NG, Bernard DB, and Johnston PA: Mannitol and loop diuretics in acute renal failure. In Brenner BM and Lazarus JM (eds): *Acute Renal Failure*. Philadelphia, WB Saunders Co., pp 712–722, 1983.

Lindner A, Cutler RE, and Goodman WG: Synergism of dopamine plus furosemide in preventing acute renal failure in the dog. *Kidney Int* 16:158–166, 1979.

Lokhandwala MF and Hegde SS: Cardiovascular dopamine receptors: Role of renal dopamine and dopamine receptors in sodium excretion. *Pharmacol Toxicol* 66:237–243, 1990.

Lulich JP, Osborne CA, O'Brien TD, et al. Feline renal failure: Questions, answers, questions. *Compend Cont Ed Pract Vet* 14:127–151, 1992.

Lund EM, Armstrong PJ, Kirk CA, et al: Health status and population characteristics of dogs and cats examined at private veterinary practices in the United States. *J Am Vet Med Assoc* 214:1336–1341, 1999.

Nachreiner RF and Refsal KR: The use of parathormone, ionized calcium and 25-hydroxyvitamin D assays to diagnose calcium disorders in dogs. *8th Annual Forum, American College of Veterinary Internal Medicine,* Washington, DC, pp 251–254, 1990.

Nichols AJ, Koster PF, Brooks DP, and Ruffolo RR Jr: Effect of fenoldopam on the acute and subacute nephrotoxicity produced by amphotericin B in the dog. *J Pharmacol Exp Ther* 260:269–274, 1992.

Nunamaker DM, Medway W, and Berg P: Treatment of ethylene glycol poisoning in the dog. *J Am Vet Med Assoc* 159:310–314, 1971.

Osborne CA, Low DG, and Finco DR: Fluid therapy in renal failure. In Osborne CA, Low DG, and Finco DR (eds): *Canine and Feline Urology*. Philadelphia, WB Saunders Co., pp 291–309, 1972.

Pacoe PJ, Ilkiw JE, Kass PH, and Cowgill LD: Case-control study of the association between intraoperative administration of nafcillin and acute postoperative development of azotemia. *J Am Vet Med Assoc* 208:1043–1047, 1996.

Pettersson K, Noble MIM, Bjorkman J-A, et al: The positive inotropic effect of felodipine in isovolumically beating dog heart. *J Cardiovasc Pharmacol* 10(suppl 1):S112–S118, 1987.

Polzin D, Osborn C, and O'Brien T: Diseases of the kidneys and ureters. In Ettinger SJ (ed): *Textbook of Veterinary Internal Medicine*, 3rd ed, Vol 2. Philadelphia, WB Saunders Co., pp 1962–2046, 1989.

Refsal KR, Nachreiner RF, and Graham PA: Laboratory assessment of hypercalcemia. *16th Annual American College of Veterinary Internal Medicine Forum,* San Diego, pp 646–647, 1998.

Rentko VT, Clark N, Ross LA, and Schelling SH: Canine leptospirosis. A retrospective study of 17 cases. *J Vet Intern Med* 6:235–244, 1992.

Ross LA: Fluid therapy for acute and chronic renal failure. *Vet Clin North Am Small Anim Pract* 19:343–359, 1989.

Rowland J: Incidence of ethylene glycol intoxication in dogs and cats seen at Colorado State University Veterinary Teaching Hospital. *Vet Hum Toxicol* 29:41–44, 1987.

Schiller LR, Santa Ana CA, Sheikh MS, et al: Effect of the time of administration of calcium acetate on phosphorus binding. *N Engl J Med* 320:1110–1113, 1989.

Schrier RW, Arnold PE, van Putten VJ, et al: Cellular calcium in ischemic acute renal failure. *Kidney Int* 32:313, 1987.

Schwartz LB, and Gewertz BL: The renal response to low dose dopamine. *J Surg Res* 45:574–588, 1988.

Shilliday I and Allison ME: Diuretics in acute renal failure. *Ren Fail* 16:3–17, 1994.

Silber SJ and Thompson N: Mannitol induced central nervous system toxicity in renal failure. *Invest Urol* 9:310, 1972.

Smith GW, Farmer JB, Ince F, et al: FPL 63012AR: A potent D1-receptor agonist. *Br J Pharmacol* 100:295–300, 1990.

Smith RC, Haschen T, Hamlin RL, and Smith CR: Water and electrolyte intake and output and quantity of feces in the healthy dog. *Vet Med* 59:743–746, 1964.

Solomon R, Werner C, Mann D, et al: Effects of saline, mannitol, and furosemide to prevent acute decreases in renal function induced by radiocontrast agents. *N Engl J Med* 331:1416–1420, 1994.

Summers A, Chew DJ, and Buffington CAT: Serum ionized magnesium and calcium concentrations in a population of sick dogs and cats. *Compend Cont Ed Pract Vet Suppl,* in press.

Takenaka T, Forster H, and Epstein M: Characterization of the renal microvascular actions of a new dopaminergic (DA1) agonist, YM435. *J Pharmacol Exp Ther* 264:1154–1159, 1993.

Thadhani R, Pascual M, and Bonventre JV: Acute renal failure. *N Engl J Med* 334:1448–1460, 1996.

Thrall MA, Grauer GF, and Mero KN: Clinicopathologic findings in dogs and cats with ethylene glycol intoxication. *J Am Vet Med Assoc* 184:37–41, 1984.

Trim CM, Moore JN, and Clark ES: Renal effects of dopamine infusion in conscious horses. *Equine Vet J Suppl* 7:124–128, 1989.

Vaden SL, Levin J, and Breitschwerdt EB: A retrospective case-control of acute renal failure in 99 dogs. *J Vet Intern Med* 11:58–64, 1997.

Wasserman K, Huss R, and Kullman R: Dopamine-induced diuresis in the cat without changes in renal hemodynamics. *Arch Pharm* 312:77–83, 1980.

Weiner IM and Mudge GH: Diuretics and other agents employed in the mobilization of edema fluid. In Gilman AG, Goodman LS, Rall TW, and Murad F (eds): *The Pharmacologic Basis of Therapeutics.* New York, Macmillan Publishing, pp 887–907, 1985.

Yatsu T, Arai Y, Takizawa K, et al: Renal effect of YM435, a new dopamine D1 receptor agonist, in anesthetized dogs. *Eur J Pharmacol* 322:45–53, 1997a.

Yatsu T, Takizawa K, Kasia-Nakagawa C, et al: Hemodynamic characterization of YM435, a novel dopamine DA1 receptor agonist, in anesthetized dogs. *J Cardiovasc Pharmacol* 29:382–388, 1997b.

Yatsu T, Uchida W, Inagaki O, et al: Dopamine DA1 receptor agonist activity of YM435 in the canine renal vasculature. *Gen Pharmacol* 29:229–232, 1997c.

Yatsu T, Arai Y, Takizawa K, et al: Effect of YM435, a dopamine DA1 receptor agonist, in a canine model of ischemic acute renal failure. *Gen Pharmacol* 31:803–807, 1998.

Zager RA: Hyperphosphatemia: A factor that provokes severe experimental acute renal failure. *J Lab Clin Med* 100:230–239, 1982.

CHAPTER 20

Shock Syndromes in Veterinary Medicine

PATHOPHYSIOLOGY, CLINICAL RECOGNITION, AND TREATMENT

THOMAS K. DAY

Shock is a complex series of physiologic events that result from a variety of causes and clinical diseases in veterinary medicine. Veterinary patients can be presented in shock, develop shock during the diagnosis and treatment of a wide variety of medical and surgical diseases, or develop shock in the postoperative period. The most challenging medical and surgical diseases have shock as a component or possible sequela of the disease process. In human medicine, the postoperative period is one in which shock occurs more commonly. All of the shock syndromes in veterinary medicine can result in high morbidity and mortality if not recognized and treated immediately. Advances in our knowledge of the pathophysiology of shock and shock syndromes combined with advances in noninvasive and invasive monitoring techniques have resulted in the ability to anticipate, recognize, and treat shock syndromes more effectively. This chapter provides the current philosophy on the pathophysiology, recognition, monitoring techniques, and treatment regimens of shock.

▶ Definition of Shock

A true understanding of the shock syndromes must begin with the definition of shock. Shock is not defined by tachycardia, hypotension, circulatory collapse, stupor, coma, pale mucous membranes, or dehydration. These clinical signs may be associated with shock and are easily recognized, but they are common to many other conditions. The underlying problem or inciting event of all causes of shock is a decrease in effective blood flow and oxygen delivery to tissues that does not meet the demand of the tissues (Muir 1990). The decrease in blood flow can occur by many mechanisms, either cardiac or vascular in nature, as described by the traditional categorization of shock. Poor tissue perfusion initiates a complex series of events that eventually result in altered cellular metabolism, cellular death, organ failure, and ultimately the death of the animal. Simply stated, shock can be defined as an imbalance between oxygen delivery and oxygen consumption, such that the delivery of oxygen does not meet the needs of the tissues.

▶ Pathophysiology

The delivery of oxygen to the tissues must meet the oxygen consumption demands of the tissues. In the normal animal, oxygen consumption by the tissues is relatively constant. Clinical syndromes that can result in increased tissue oxygen consumption include status epilepticus, tremorogenic toxins (e.g., strychnine, mold), heatstroke, and malignant hyperthermia. A systematic, formula-oriented description of oxygen delivery variables may be beneficial in understanding all of the possible mechanisms by which oxygen delivery can be altered to produce shock (Table 20–1). The delivery of oxygen is dependent on cardiac output and the content of oxygen in arterial blood. Cardiac output is the product of heart rate and stroke volume, which consists of preload, afterload, myocardial contractility, and myocardial synchrony (cardiac rhythm). The content of oxygen in arterial blood consists of the amount of hemoglobin and the saturation of the existing hemoglobin with oxygen. Alteration of any of the determinants of oxygen delivery can result in inadequate oxygen in the tissues.

One variable that was not mentioned in the definition of shock that we commonly measure during anesthesia and critical care is blood pressure. Blood pressure is the product of cardiac output and systemic vascular resistance. By definition, it is the lateral force that the blood exerts on the blood vessel wall at any given portion of the vascular system. Blood pressure is not synonymous with blood flow and cannot be mistaken as cardiac output (cardiac output actually is a determinant of blood pressure). Therefore, blood pressure is not a primary determinant of oxygen delivery but may be only a sign that cardiac output (which is a determinant of oxygen delivery) may be inadequate.

TABLE 20-1. **Oxygen Delivery Variables, Equations, and Normal Values**

Term and Abbreviation	Formula	Normal Value
Oxygen delivery (DO_2)	$DO_2 = CO \times CaO_2$	500–800 mL/min/m²
O_2 content in arterial blood (CaO_2)	$CaO_2 = (Hb \times 1.34 \times SaO_2) + (PaO_2 \times 0.003)$	16–22 mL O_2/dL
O_2 content in mixed venous blood (CvO_2)	$CvO_2 = (Hb \times 1.34 \times SvO_2) + (PvO_2 \times 0.003)$	12–17 mL O_2/dL
Arterial-venous O_2 content difference (oxygen extraction)	$Ca\text{-}vO_2 = CaO_2 - CvO_2$	3–5 mL O_2/dL
Oxygen consumption (VO_2)	$VO_2 = (CaO_2 - CvO_2) \times CO$	100–150 mL/min/m²
Cardiac output (CO)	$CO = MAP/SVR$	150–200 mL/kg/min

Abbreviations: SaO_2 = saturation of oxygen in arterial blood; SvO_2 = saturation of oxygen in venous blood; MAP = mean arterial blood pressure; SVR = systemic vascular resistance.

The nature of shock is such that the primary initiating event is poor tissue perfusion. A decrease in arterial blood pressure, regardless of the cause (decreased cardiac output or decreased systemic vascular resistance), initiates a neurohormonal response intended to increase intravascular volume and cardiac output (Fig. 20–1) (Guyton 1991). Specialized stretch receptors located in the aorta and carotid arteries detect a decrease in cardiac output. A neural signal transmitted to the vasomotor center of the medulla oblongata results in release of the inhibition of the sympathetic center and depresses the parasympathetic center. The adrenal medulla plays a large role in the neurohormonal response by releasing epinephrine and norepinephrine. The overall result is an increase in heart rate, contractility, and vasoconstriction (arterial and venous).

Other extrinsic responses to a decrease in cardiac output include aldosterone release from the adrenal medulla, which acts to retain sodium and water. The renin-angiotensin-aldosterone feedback reinforces an increase in systemic vascular tone. The pituitary releases adrenocorticotropic hormone (ACTH) and vasopressin (antidiuretic hormone, ADH). The combination of catecholamine stimulation and ACTH release increases circulating cortisol, which mobilizes substrates necessary for energy production. The renal tubules are affected by ADH and further retain water to increase intravascular volume.

The main goal of the neural and neurohormonal response to shock is to sustain or reestablish intravascular volume and blood flow to tissues. Blood flow to organs is controlled by both intrinsic and extrinsic factors. Autoregulation is a process that regulates normal blood flow in states of mild hypoperfusion. This is especially true with the cerebral and coronary vasculature. In the early stages of shock (see later), blood flow is maintained to the brain and heart at the expense of other organs including the intestinal tract, liver, and kidney.

The vasoconstriction that occurs in major arteries and veins as a result of the neurohormonal response to shock also occurs at the capillary level. Both precapillary and postcapillary vessels constrict. Precapillary constriction results in decreased perfusion to tissues. As shock progresses and oxygen supply decreases, anaerobic metabolism ensues. The combination of decreased oxygen supply and anaerobic metabolism alters the reaction of the terminal vessels in response to continual sympathetic stimulation. In this situation, the precapillary vessels dilate while the postcapillary vessels remain constricted. The results are increased blood flow to the capillary system and "pooling" in the venules. This volume shift is in addition to hypovolemia in the macrocirculation. In addition to the macrocirculation effects, the increased hydrostatic filtration pressure in the capillaries causes fluid loss in the tissues. The changes in the microcirculation have been termed *circulus vitiosus* of shock (Fig. 20–2) (Neugebauer et al. 1994). The changes at the capillary level also are responsible for what is termed maldistribution of blood flow.

Shock also interferes with other regulatory systems that influence normal homeostasis. Endorphins, enkephalins, neuropeptides, and cytokines are mediators that regulate normal homeostasis. The cytokines have received a great deal of attention, especially in relation to septic shock syndromes (Purvis and Kirby 1994; Kirby 1995). The cytokines are released in response to local tissue damage (see later) and include substances such as interleukin-1, tumor necrosis factor, interleukin-6, platelet-activating factor, and nitric oxide. In fact, more than 150 locally produced mediators have been implicated in shock (Neugebauer et al. 1994). The mononuclear phagocytes are the most critical cells in initiating the release of cytokines.

A prerequisite for developing adequate therapy, especially in systemic inflammatory response syndrome (SIRS) and septic shock, is exact knowledge of the physiology and pathophysiology of the cytokines and other mediators. Mediator release occurs at variable times throughout the shock process. Many of the mediators may have positive roles, whereas others may contribute to the hemodynamic, pulmonary, and circulatory effects of shock. Unfortunately, the current role of a single "shock" toxin is not clear and is quite dependent on the state of shock progression and the experimental conditions studied. Therefore, no single therapeutic intervention has been discovered that can terminate the shock process.

▶ Clinical Stages of Shock

Three clinical stages of shock have been described to elucidate the progression of the shock process: compensatory stage, early decompensatory stage, and decompensatory (terminal) stage (Table 20–2) (Rudloff and Kirby 1994). As described before, the initiating event is an acute decrease in tissue perfusion. When the normal compensatory neurohormonal response to restore blood volume and maintain the metabolic needs of the tissues is unsuccessful in restoring perfusion, shock ensues. As cardiac output decreases and autoregulation is lost, there is a rapid progression from compensatory to early decompensatory to decompensatory (terminal) shock.

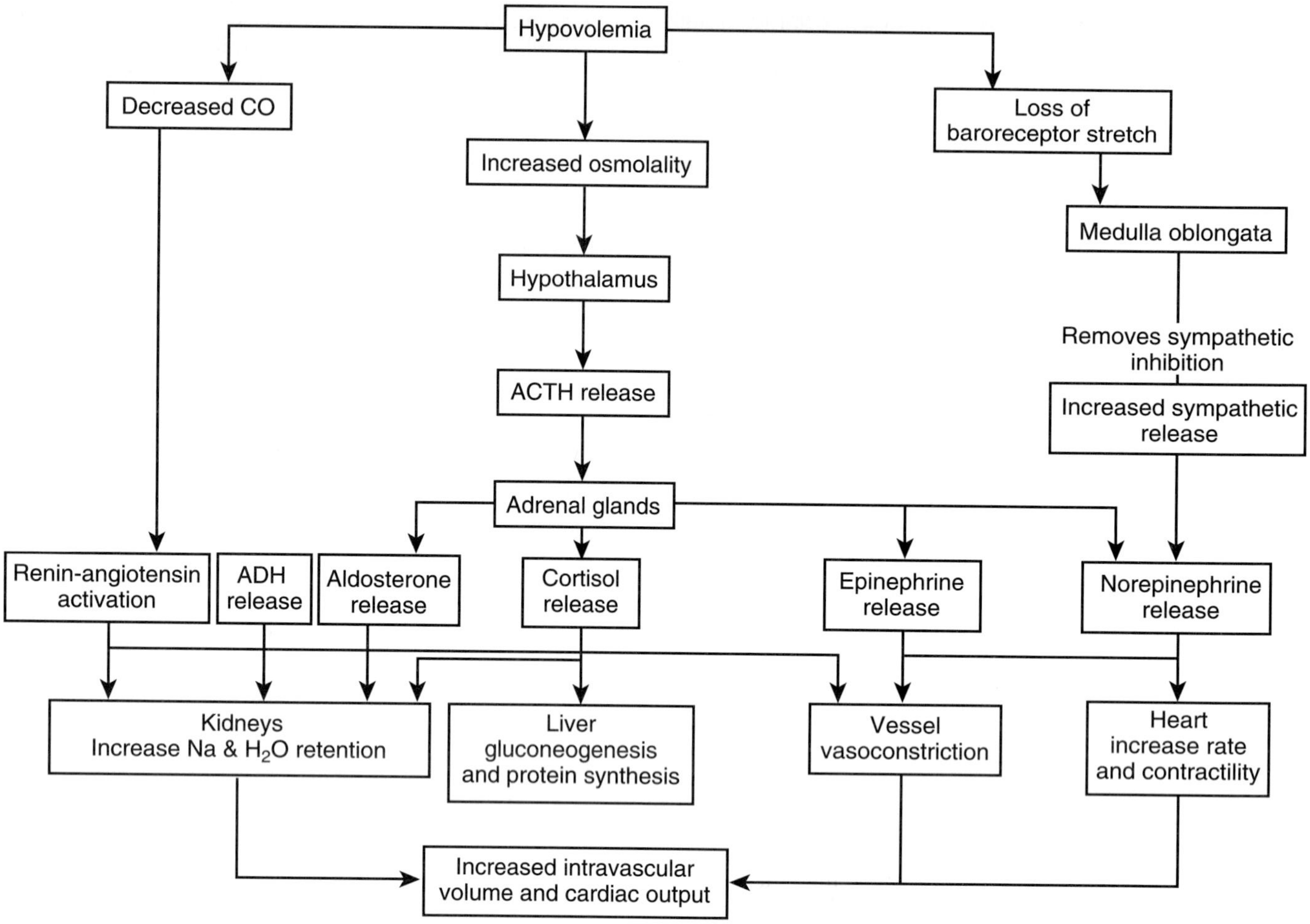

FIGURE 20–1. Neurohormonal responses to a decrease in intravascular volume.

Compensatory Stage

The compensatory stage of shock occurs as a result of baroreceptor-mediated release of catecholamines. Systemic vascular resistance (arteries and veins), heart rate, and contractility increase to produce an increase in cardiac output. The neurohormonal response described earlier also aids in increasing venous return via water retention, in addition to movement of interstitial fluid to the intravascular space. These compensatory mechanisms require a large amount of energy, resulting in a hypermetabolic state at the cellular level. The increased metabolic state produced in the compensatory stage of shock requires an above-normal amount of oxygen to be delivered. Additional substrates required to produce energy are provided by the actions of glucagon, ACTH, cortisol, and growth hormone. The compensatory stage of shock can maintain adequate cardiac output during mild to moderate acute loss of intravascular volume. The hypermetabolic state cannot be maintained indefinitely. As intravascular volume remains inadequate, systemic vascular resistance begins to decrease, cardiac dysfunction occurs, and decompensation begins.

Early Decompensatory Stage

The early decompensatory stage of shock is marked by redistribution of blood flow to preferred organs (heart

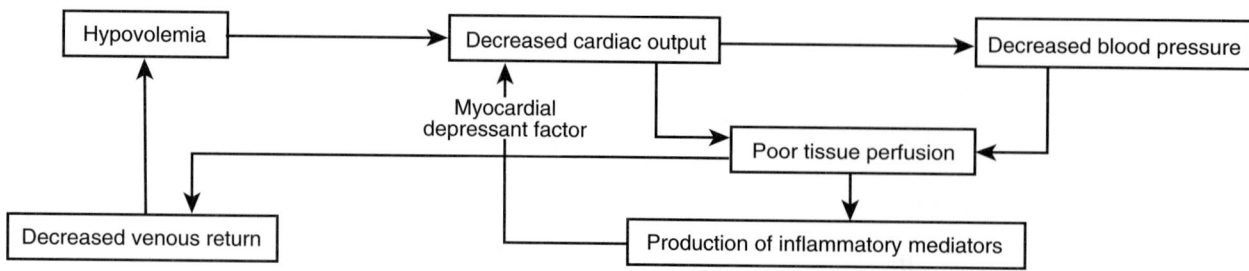

FIGURE 20–2. Circulatory events that lead to the vicious circle (circulus vitiosus) of shock.

SHOCK SYNDROMES IN VETERINARY MEDICINE

TABLE 20-2. Clinical Stages and Signs of Shock

Clinical Stage of Shock	Characteristics	Clinical Signs
Compensatory stage	Increases in CO, HR, and SVR Neurohormonal response Hypermetabolic, hyperdynamic state	Mild increases in HR, RR Normal mentation and blood pressure "Brick" red MM, CRT < 1 s
Early decompensatory stage	Redistribution of blood flow to heart and brain Consumption of oxygen dependent upon oxygen delivery Development of lactic acidosis	Tachycardia, tachypnea, pale MM, poor CRT, weak pulse, poor mentation, usually hypothermic, hypotension
Decompensatory (terminal) stage	Autoregulatory escape, sympathetic center lost, chronotropic and inotropic response lost	Low heart rate in spite of low CO, absent CRT, severe hypotension

Abbreviations: CO = cardiac output; HR = heart rate; SVR = systemic vascular resistance; RR = respiratory rate; CRT = capillary refill time; MM = mucous membranes.

and brain) with further decreases in oxygen delivery to all other organs. Oxygen consumption in tissues becomes dependent on oxygen delivery, and anaerobic metabolism, lactic acidosis, and tissue hypoxia result. As lactic acidosis progresses, cellular integrity is lost, resulting in accumulation of arachidonic acid. Arachidonic acid accumulation is the primary stimulus for production of prostaglandins, leukotrienes and other chemical mediators that incite SIRS (see later discussion).

Organ response to the redistribution of blood flow during early decompensatory shock varies. Intestinal integrity may be compromised, resulting in microulceration. Normal intestinal flora can translocate to the bloodstream through the compromised mucosa. The pancreas responds to hypoxia by releasing myocardial depressant factor, which decreases myocardial contractility, predisposes the heart to cardiac arrhythmias, and depresses the reticuloendothelial system. Vasoconstriction of the pulmonary vasculature results in microvascular shunting and impairment of oxygen transport. Blood is shunted from the cortical to juxtamedullary nephrons, and constriction of the afferent glomerular arterioles can reduce renal blood flow enough to produce oliguria and induce tubular necrosis.

Decompensatory (Terminal) Stage

Prolonged tissue hypoxia can result in a phenomenon termed autoregulatory escape. The local responses override the sympathetic-mediated vasoconstriction and massive vasodilatation occurs in all organs, including the heart and brain. Complete circulatory collapse is the end point of autoregulatory escape. The sympathetic center of the brain no longer functions and the chronotropic and inotropic response is lost. This is the final event in all types of shock and is termed decompensatory (terminal) shock.

▶ Clinical Signs of Shock

Compensatory Stage

The clinical signs of compensatory shock are commonly overlooked by veterinarians. The hyperdynamic cardiovascular system can easily be mistaken to be normal. Although heart rate and respiratory rate are usually increased (in some cases heart rate is only mildly increased), mucous membranes are injected (bright pink to reddish in color), capillary refill is more rapid than normal (usually less than 1 s), mentation is normal, blood pressure is normal to increased, and pulse pressure is normal to increased (bounding pulses). Adequate volume resuscitation (fluid therapy, discussed later) is immediately warranted to remove the stimulus for the hypermetabolic state and prevent the decompensatory stage of shock. Injected mucous membranes may not be as consistent a clinical entity in cats as in dogs.

Early Decompensatory Stage

Clinical signs of the early decompensatory stage of shock are most commonly observed. Tachycardia, normal to decreased pulse pressure, hypotension, pale mucous membranes, prolonged capillary refill time, mental depression, and decreased body temperature are all signs of early decompensatory shock. Aggressive fluid resuscitation is required to stop the pathologic process, reduce morbidity (e.g., sepsis, renal failure), and prevent mortality. Cats may not necessarily show signs of tachycardia as do dogs. Cats that have all the signs of shock except tachycardia should be considered in a state of shock and treated appropriately.

Decompensatory (Terminal) Stage

Clinical signs of decompensatory (terminal) shock include low heart rate despite low cardiac output and severe hypotension, pale or cyanotic mucous membranes, absent capillary refill, weak or absent pulses, decreased heart sounds, low body temperature, no urine production, and stupor or coma. Cardiopulmonary arrest is imminent without very aggressive resuscitation and organ support. The decompensatory stage of shock commonly is not responsive to aggressive fluid resuscitation.

▶ Classification of Shock Syndromes

Historically, shock has been classified into various categories and etiologies. The traditional categorization of the types of shock is based on (1) alteration of the variables that determine oxygen delivery and (2) associated clinical signs and laboratory findings (Shoemaker 1995). Heart failure (cardiogenic shock) results in a decrease in myocardial contractility and decreased oxygen delivery. Massive losses of intravascular volume (hypovolemic or hemorrhagic shock) result in a decrease in oxygen delivery. Septic shock and, to some extent, traumatic shock result in a maldistribution of blood flow to the tissues at the level of the capillary circulation, at times in the presence of normal cardiac output. The traditional categorization of shock also includes anaphylactic shock.

A more functional classification of shock also has been developed and is based on the hemodynamic defects involved and not necessarily the specific etiology (Muir 1990). The functional categories of shock include hypovolemic, cardiogenic, vasogenic (distributive), and obstructive. Hypovolemic shock can occur by loss of intravascular volume of any etiology including dehydration, blood loss, and "third-space" loss of fluids in the intestinal tract. Cardiogenic shock can occur as a result of any cardiovascular abnormality. Sepsis, endotoxemia, anaphylaxis, and neurogenic injury, including trauma, all can be described as manifesting a vasogenic mechanism of shock. Obstructive shock actually is a form of cardiogenic shock and includes cardiac tamponade, pulmonary thromboembolism, caval syndrome, and intracardiac tumors. Shock in the gastric dilatation-volvulus (GDV) syndrome also can be classified as obstructive.

Shock also has been categorized on the basis of normal or abnormal circulatory mechanisms (Tobias et al. 1992). The emphasis of this classification is on the dynamics of precapillary and postcapillary vascular changes that occur and the resultant redistribution and pooling of blood. The traditional and functional categories of shock have been used as examples with this classification of shock.

The traditional categorization of shock is simplistic and easy to understand, yet it is seriously misleading (Shoemaker 1995). There is a tendency to approach a one-dimensional, easy to understand diagnosis of shock with a simplistic, one-dimensional approach to therapy. Unfortunately, shock is complex; it does not begin with a common pathophysiologic event and does not necessarily end with survival after a simple universal initial treatment. Each etiology of shock sets in motion a complex series of events that include neural and hormonal responses as well as numerous inflammatory cascades.

Another example of the complex nature of the classifications of shock is use of the term distributive shock. The term distributive has been used to describe various types of high-flow shock under the assumption that blood flow is not normally distributed to tissue beds. Used in this context, "distributive shock" is a theoretical designation of a type of shock syndrome that is not defined by criteria that can be easily measured in a clinical setting. Maldistribution of blood flow has been documented in people in clinically accessible microscopic vascular beds (e.g., sclera, liver, nail bed). Direct observations have documented the phenomenon of maldistribution of blood flow, but such measurements are not necessarily representative of all areas and are not quantitative measures of the extent of maldistribution throughout the body. Therefore, maldistribution of blood flow is a physiologic concept that may be relevant to all shock states (Shoemaker 1995). Clinically measurable, quantitative criteria are required for distributive shock to qualify as a specific type of shock.

The various classifications of shock syndromes in veterinary and human medicine have been created in an attempt to simplify a complex series of physiologic events. Unfortunately, laboratory research and clinical experiences have not supported any one classification of the shock syndromes as being the easiest to understand or teach. The purpose of this chapter is not to create yet another classification scheme of shock but to describe the common presentations of shock syndromes in a manner that is simpler to understand. It is important to remember that the three clinical stages of shock presented previously occur in any shock syndrome, regardless of the classification, and should be viewed as the "tip of the iceberg" with respect to therapeutic intervention. The presentation of the patient should rank as the first and most important aspect of the shock syndromes, and valuable time should not be wasted deciding which classification scheme best describes the patient. Granted, the clinical presentation and treatment of a patient in cardiogenic shock are notably different from those of a patient with hemorrhagic shock and from those of a patient meeting the criteria for SIRS. This chapter emphasizes the concepts that (1) there are important initial decisions based on physical examination that determine the clinical stage of shock, (2) initial therapy is based on the clinical stage of the specific shock syndrome, and (3) the classification of the etiology of shock, response to initial therapy, and laboratory and other diagnostic evaluations all determine further therapeutic interventions. The following description of the common shock syndromes is meant not to oversimplify the complex nature of shock but to present a logical, clinical approach to shock therapy.

Shock syndromes of greatest importance in veterinary medicine can best be described as a combination of both traditional and functional classifications and include hypovolemic (including hemorrhagic and anaphylactic) shock, SIRS (septic shock), traumatic (surgical, postoperative, blunt trauma) shock, and cardiogenic shock (including obstructive).

Hypovolemic Shock

Hypovolemia can be either absolute or relative in nature and is a common presentation of shock. Hemorrhagic shock is considered an absolute cause of hypovolemia because an actual loss of intravascular blood volume has occurred. Common clinical presentations include hemoperitoneum secondary to hemorrhage from splenic or hepatic neoplasia, coagulopathies (anticoagulant rodenticide toxicity, thrombocytopathies), gastrointestinal hemorrhage, epistaxis, and traumatic lacerations of arteries or other major blood vessels (Crystal and Cotter 1992). Nonhemorrhagic shock is associated with relative hypovolemia as there is no direct loss of blood from the intravascular space. The primary physiologic event is either loss of plasma volume or pooling of blood in venous capacitance vessels. Examples of loss of plasma volume include severe dehydration and third-space loss (e.g., peritoneum, intestinal tract). Anaphylactic shock occurs as a result of immunoglobulin E–mediated release of vasoactive substances that produces massive vasodilatation and pooling of as much as 60 to 80% of the circulating blood volume (Mueller and Noxon 1990).

Systemic Inflammatory Response Syndrome and Septic Shock

Systemic inflammatory response syndrome reflects the body's defense against circulating bacterial toxins (Kirby

1995; Purvis and Kirby 1994; Shoemaker et al. 1993a, 1993b). Various terms have been used to describe the systemic changes that occur when bacteria invade the bloodstream, including the sepsis syndrome. Physical examination findings and diagnostic parameters are used to help determine whether a patient fulfills the criteria of SIRS (Table 20–3). The presence of bacteria, bacterial toxins, or inflammatory mediators in a patient with the cardiovascular criteria that determine a state of shock separates septic shock from all other forms of shock. Both medical diseases and surgical procedures can result in SIRS.

Gram-negative and gram-positive bacteria that invade the circulation can liberate toxins or toxinlike substances that stimulate a cellular response and mediator release. Mononuclear cells, phagocytes, neutrophils, vascular endothelium, and platelets are the target cells for the lipid A portion of the endotoxin molecule (gram-negative bacteria) and peptidoglycans (gram-positive bacteria). Cytokines that initiate a variety of events leading to shock are liberated from the target cells (see later discussion). Examples of the cytokines are tumor necrosis factor, interleukins, platelet-activating factor, and nitric oxide.

The primary effects of the cytokines on the cardiovascular system are vasodilatation, increased vascular permeability that can result in loss of intravascular volume, and myocardial dysfunction. Three types of shock can occur as a result of SIRS: (1) hypovolemia secondary to increased vascular permeability, (2) maldistribution of blood flow caused by cytokine-induced vasodilatation, and (3) cardiogenic shock caused by decreased cardiac performance secondary to circulating myocardial depressant factor (Shoemaker et al. 1993a, 1993b). Clinically, high-output and low-output states of septic shock have been observed. In the high-output state, mild vasodilatation produced by the effects of cytokines on the vasculature results in an increase in cardiac output. Mucous membranes are bright red, capillary refill time is shortened, core body temperature is usually increased, and peripheral pulses are bounding. In the low-output state, peripheral vasodilatation overwhelms the cardiovascular system and, combined with poor ventricular performance in the latter stages of sepsis, cardiac output decreases. Mucous membranes are pale, capillary refill time is prolonged, core body temperature is decreased, pulses are weak, and blood pressure is low.

The clinical diagnosis of SIRS implies that some primary insult has resulted in the secondary response of SIRS and septic shock. Identification and treatment of the primary insult are vital to successful management. After inflammatory mediators have been released from mononuclear cells, therapy primarily is supportive. As of yet, no single "silver bullet" therapy has been developed to antagonize the effects of cytokines. Failure to initiate therapy immediately or ineffective therapeutic intervention can result in severe organ damage and the development of multiple organ dysfunction syndrome (MODS). A common cause of death in septic shock is MODS.

The most important point to remember is that vasodilatation and increased vascular permeability dominate the cardiovascular effects of SIRS and septic shock and aggressive, appropriate fluid therapy and cardiovascular support are crucial in successful treatment. The combination of cardiovascular effects results in a maldistribution of blood flow to tissues, at times in the presence of normal or increased cardiac output. Common clinical examples of SIRS include pancreatitis, heatstroke, pyometra, septic peritonitis, GDV, snake envenomation, neoplasia, and multiple trauma.

Traumatic Shock

Traumatic shock is a common occurrence in veterinary medicine. Traumatic shock can occur as a result of accidental blunt trauma or in the postoperative period after extensive soft tissue and orthopedic surgery. The two mechanisms of shock that occur are hypovolemia and maldistribution of blood flow at the capillary level secondary to neurogenic mechanisms or pain-induced vasoconstriction. The surgical operation can be viewed as controlled trauma that allows us to know the time and type of inciting event that may produce shock (Bishop et al. 1993). Acute blood loss is an obvious cause of hypovolemia that can induce shock. Tissue damage and ischemia also can set in motion the series of events that constitute SIRS. Adequate and aggressive monitoring of the patient allows immediate intervention. Shock after accidental trauma is similar to surgical shock, but wider variations in the patterns of shock occur with accidental trauma because of marked differences in the extent and location of injuries and delays in therapeutic intervention.

Pain and Shock

Pain can result in cardiovascular changes that resemble shock or can potentiate the shock process. Many patients, after either blunt trauma or extensive surgery (soft tissue or orthopedic), have pain as a primary cause of the physiologic changes that can result in shock. Vasoconstriction secondary to pain can produce a decrease in blood flow and oxygen delivery that can be severe enough to decrease oxygen delivery.

Cardiogenic Shock

Cardiogenic shock can be associated with cardiac disease of any cause, acquired or congenital. Cardiogenic shock is an uncommon presentation during the postoperative period, but when it occurs in this setting it is very serious. Most patients with postoperative cardiogenic shock have undetected underlying cardiovascular disease, but animals

TABLE 20–3. Criteria for Systemic Inflammatory Response Syndrome*

Rectal temperature	>103.5°F, <100°F
Heart rate	>160 beats per minute (dog)
	>250 beats per minute (cat)
Respiratory rate	>20 breaths per minute
Paco$_2$	<32 mm Hg
White blood cell count	>12,000, <1000, or >10% bands

*A patient is considered to have SIRS if two or more of the criteria are fulfilled.

with compensated heart failure secondary to mitral valve insufficiency may be at greater risk for developing postoperative cardiogenic shock.

The clinical signs of cardiogenic shock are similar to those of other types of shock with notable exceptions. Respiratory distress and exercise intolerance or collapse are prominent features, and bilateral crackles related to pulmonary edema may be heard on thoracic auscultation. Cardiac murmurs also are prominent. Jugular distention may be prominent (jugular veins are collapsed in other types of shock) and mucous membranes may have a greater tendency to become cyanotic. Arrhythmias also are common at presentation in patients with cardiogenic shock and can be a primary cause of decreased cardiac output and decreased oxygen delivery.

Obstructive shock has been classified as a form of cardiogenic shock. Decreased ventricular filling results in decreased cardiac output and decreased oxygen delivery. Examples of obstructive shock include pericardial tamponade secondary to pericardial effusion, caval syndrome of heartworm disease, pulmonary thromboembolism, and intracardiac neoplasia. The dilated stomach in patients with GDV can decrease ventricular filling as a result of obstruction of the caudal vena cava and can be a source of shock.

▶ Treatment

The most successful approach to therapy of shock syndromes commences with anticipation of events that could lead to states of inadequate perfusion. Under most circumstances, however, the clinician cannot anticipate events that will lead to a state of shock except in the postoperative period. Early recognition and intervention also are important in the successful treatment of shock. A quotation from Shoemaker and Kram (1991) provides an effective philosophy of shock therapy: "The single most important factor in successful resuscitation from shock is time. . . . rapid expeditious therapy in early stages may lead to good results, but adequate therapy that is delayed may be ineffective." Advances in fluid types and monitoring techniques, although not a substitute for delays in providing therapy, have increased the likelihood of successful initial therapy.

Standard ABCs of Resuscitation

The standard ABCs of resuscitation (*airway, breathing, bleeding, circulation*) should be the initial therapy for all shock patients. A patent airway should be established and maintained at all times. Abnormal breathing patterns should be recognized. Supplemental oxygen should be delivered at a high flow rate (5 L/min) by face mask or by the "blow by" technique if the animal resists a face mask. In most intraoperative and postoperative patients, an endotracheal tube is in place. If not, be certain that the patient is able to breathe adequately and provide supplemental oxygen.

The standard ABCs can be expanded to the postoperative patient and include anesthetic drugs. All anesthetic drugs that may have deleterious effects on the cardiovascular system should be antagonized or eliminated. All alpha$_2$ agonists should be antagonized because their expected cardiovascular responses include decreased cardiac output.

Controversy exists on whether or not to antagonize the opioid agonists. Bradycardia is not typically a side effect of opioids during shock. In most instances, the sympathetic response overrides the parasympathomimetic effects of opioid agonists. Analgesia is an important component in the treatment of the shock syndromes, and consequently most opioids should not be antagonized. The most important reason to antagonize an opioid would be respiratory depression. Opioid agonists are most likely to produce deleterious respiratory depression. Therefore, the opioid agonist-antagonists are in greater favor as analgesics during shock.

The phenothiazines cannot be antagonized, but knowledge of their use aids in therapy. The benzodiazepines have minimal effects on the cardiovascular system and do not require antagonists. The inhalation anesthetics are eliminated primarily by respiration. Both halothane and isoflurane can have deleterious effects on the cardiovascular system, including decreased cardiac output (halothane) and decreased systemic vascular resistance (isoflurane). Isoflurane also is a potent respiratory depressant.

Circulatory support begins by control of internal and external bleeding. The primary method of circulatory support is fluid therapy in all of the shock syndromes, with the exception of cardiogenic shock (Table 20–4).

TABLE 20–4. Fluid Choices for Patients in Shock

Fluid Type	Dosage	Indications for Use
Crystalloids (lactated Ringer's solution, 0.9% NaCl, Normosol, Plasma-Lyte)	90 mL/kg as fast as possible (dog) 55 mL/kg as fast as possible (cat)	Acute volume resuscitation, interstitial fluid replacement (dehydration)
Hypertonic solutions (7% NaCl, 23.4% NaCl)	4 mL/kg over 5 min for a 7% solution; see Table 20–5 for dilution of 23.4% NaCl with colloid	Acute volume resuscitation in normally hydrated animals
Colloids		
Whole blood	22 mL/kg/h maximum	>30% loss of blood
Plasma	10–20 mL/kg	Loss of oncotic pressure, secondary hemostatic disorders
Packed red blood cells	Based on PCV	Hemolytic anemia, oxygen-carrying source
Hemoglobin-based oxygen carriers (Oxyglobin)	15–30 mL/kg	Hemolytic anemia, acute loss of intravascular volume
Hetastarch, pentastarch	10–20 mL/kg initial bolus (dog) 20 mL/kg/day infusion	Acute volume resuscitation, source of oncotic pressure

Volume Resuscitation

Vascular access must be obtained to begin adequate volume resuscitation. Fluids placed in the subcutaneous tissue or peritoneal cavity are not considered adequate for shock therapy. The neurohormonal response to low cardiac output results in peripheral vasoconstriction and poor absorption of fluids administered subcutaneously or intraperitoneally. In addition, as described subsequently, crystalloid fluids require administration as rapidly as possible to expand the intravascular space effectively.

The central veins (e.g., jugular vein) allow larger volumes of crystalloids to be administered faster, although jugular vein catheterization requires more time. Catheterization of a peripheral vein should be completed before placing a catheter in the jugular vein, and the decision to place an indwelling catheter in the jugular vein should be made on the basis of the initial response to fluid therapy and the underlying cause of shock. Peripheral venous catheterization is simpler and a patent catheter can be obtained in a fraction of the time required for jugular venous catheterization. Appropriate peripheral veins readily available include the cephalic and lateral saphenous veins in dogs and the cephalic and medial saphenous veins in cats. A clinical syndrome in which placing a catheter in the lateral saphenous vein is contraindicated is GDV in dogs. The dilated stomach prevents an adequate volume of fluids from reaching the heart. More than one peripheral vein may be necessary to administer adequate volumes of fluids in very large dogs or to administer two or more different types of fluids. Venous cutdown procedures may become necessary in patients with no visible veins as a result of severe hypotension and poor peripheral circulation.

The type of catheter that is used also can be an important factor in the speed of fluid administration. A large-gauge, short, over-the-needle catheter placed in a peripheral vein allows administration of larger volumes of fluid more rapidly than a smaller gauge, long, through-the-needle catheter placed in a central (e.g., jugular) vein.

The intraosseous route of administration may be of value in patients weighing less than 2 kg, especially puppies and kittens. Intraosseous placement of large-gauge needles in the trochanteric fossa, tibial crest, iliac wing, or proximal humerus can allow rapid administration of any type of fluid (see Chapter 14).

CRYSTALLOIDS

Isotonic crystalloid fluids historically have been the most commonly recommended type of initial fluid therapy for the shock patient, but the basis for the popularity of crystalloids is unclear (Marino 1998b). Two experiments were performed in the 1960s that may have popularized crystalloid fluid therapy for animals and people with hemorrhagic shock (Moore 1965; Shores et al. 1964). One experiment showed that the physiologic response to mild hemorrhage is a shift of fluid from the interstitial space to the intravascular space (Moore 1965). The second experiment provided information that survival was improved in an animal model of hemorrhagic shock when crystalloids were administered simultaneously with reinfusion of the blood that was removed (Shores et al. 1964).

The conclusions from these two experiments, which have endured over the years, are that an interstitial fluid deficit is a major consequence of hemorrhage and that crystalloid fluid replacement is important for survival. Changes in interstitial fluid occur only when blood loss is less than 15% of total blood volume. When blood volume loss exceeds 15%, intravascular volume must be supported by a fluid type that will not move into the interstitial space.

Crystalloids effectively replenish the interstitial space. Dehydration is defined as loss of water in the extravascular tissue (interstitial and intracellular). Tonicity of the interstitial compartment increases as fluid is lost, which promotes movement of fluid out of the intravascular space. Severe dehydration can result in poor tissue perfusion but the terms dehydration and perfusion should not be used simultaneously. Crystalloids contribute to effective fluid resuscitation when used with colloids when dehydration also is present.

Another consequence of large volumes of crystalloid fluids is decreased intravascular oncotic pressure caused by dilution of impermeable protein anions (Marino 1998b). Decreased oncotic pressure impairs maintenance of intravascular volume and promotes extravasation of fluids into the interstitial space.

Approximately 75 to 85% of isotonic crystalloids move to the interstitial space within the first hour after intravenous administration (Griffel and Kaufman 1992). For example, if an animal loses 300 mL of intravascular volume, approximately 1200 mL of isotonic crystalloid must be administered. Therefore, crystalloid fluids do not maintain intravascular volume or tissue perfusion for extended periods and should not be considered the sole source of intravascular fluid support for shock patients. Massive crystalloid administration can actually produce body compositional changes similar to those of the late stages of shock: expanded total body water and interstitial water with contracted plasma volume and intracellular fluid (Shoemaker 1995). Increased interstitial water and excessive total body water do not correlate with corrected intravascular deficits. Hypovolemia can occur in the presence of interstitial edema. Increased amounts of interstitial fluid do not play a role in circulatory function and actually may impair oxygen transport by impairing diffusion of oxygen from the intravascular space to the cells.

Examples of isotonic crystalloids include lactated Ringer's solution, physiologic saline, Plasma-Lyte A, and Normosol-R. Hyperchloremic metabolic acidosis has been reported after administration of large doses of physiologic saline. Normosol-R contains acetate as a buffer and can cause hypotension during rapid infusion. The rate of administration of isotonic crystalloids in dogs and cats historically has been stated to be 90 mL/kg/h and 55 mL/kg/h, respectively. However, because of the rapid extravasation of crystalloids to the interstitial space, the recommended rate of administration to dogs and cats has been revised to 90 and 55 mL/kg, respectively, *as rapidly as possible*. The entire shock dose should be administered within 10 to 15 min. Administration can be hastened by utilizing pressurized fluid infusion systems; large-gauge, short catheters; and multiple catheters. This rate of administration is effective for the treatment of compensatory shock, which may be the only clinical stage of shock that responds to volume expansion before extravasation to the interstitial space and does not require further aggressive intravascular support.

Most normal, healthy animals can tolerate the additional interstitial volume for short periods of time. Most of the interstitial fluid is either returned to the intravascular space via lymphatics or excreted by the kidneys. Although crystalloids historically have been recommended for initial fluid therapy in shock (except for cardiogenic shock), the veterinarian should consider the clinical stage of shock and the possible detrimental effects of large volumes of crystalloid solutions.

During the postoperative period, most anesthetized patients have received large volumes of crystalloid fluids, effectively diluting intravascular proteins and the interstitial space and predisposing the patient to interstitial edema. Therefore, crystalloid solutions are contraindicated and other types of intravascular volume support (e.g., colloids, hypertonic fluids) are more beneficial if inadequate perfusion states develop in the postoperative period.

The patient with SIRS also benefits from other types of intravascular volume expansion in addition to crystalloids, because an important component of SIRS is increased capillary membrane permeability. The goal with SIRS patients is to maintain intravascular volume with colloids and attempt to avoid interstitial edema (especially in the lung and the brain) that may occur with very large doses of crystalloids.

COLLOIDS

Colloid oncotic pressure (COP) is important in maintaining fluid balance between the intravascular and interstitial compartments (Concannon 1993; Kirby and Rudloff 1997). The primary source of oncotic pressure within the intravascular compartment is albumin (69,000 daltons), and normal COP in an animal with 7.3 g/dL protein is approximately 28 mm Hg. Synthetic colloids were produced with molecular weights similar to that of albumin. Body composition changes in shock and the pathophysiology of SIRS can create disturbances in COP and fluid balance that require appropriate use of colloids.

Colloid solutions are divided into biologic (e.g., whole blood, albumin, plasma) and synthetic (hetastarch, pentastarch, dextrans, gelatins, hemoglobin-based oxygen carriers, HBOCs) (see Chapters 15 and 23). Biologic colloids are indicated in specific conditions but rarely are used alone in shock therapy. Most biologic colloids are used in addition to other types of fluid therapy (e.g., crystalloids, hypertonic solutions, synthetic colloids). Whole-blood transfusions may be warranted as a primary fluid choice during hemorrhagic shock, but caution must be taken to avoid potential complications including transfusion reaction, hemolysis of red blood cells, citrate toxicity, and hypocalcemia. The recommended rate of whole-blood transfusion has been reported not to exceed 22 mL/kg/h, but some clinical situations require administration as fast as possible (Crystal and Cotter 1992). Whole blood is not a practical primary source of intravascular volume support because of lack of readily available blood donors and the large volumes required for larger dogs.

Hemorrhagic shock secondary to traumatic hemoperitoneum can be treated by the technique of autotransfusion in addition to synthetic colloid and crystalloid fluid therapy (Marino 1998a; Brooks 1992; Crowe and Devey 1994). In most instances, autotransfusion of blood from the peritoneal cavity does not supply active platelets or clotting factors. Potential complications include dyspnea, respiratory insufficiency, and disseminated intravascular coagulation secondary to red blood cell fragments or other microaggregates. The number of microaggregates can be minimized by administering blood collected from the peritoneal space through a commercial blood filter. Blood that has been in the peritoneal cavity for several days or hemorrhage as a result of suspected splenic or hepatic neoplasia should not be used for autotransfusion.

The primary oncotic activity of plasma (75%) is produced by albumin. The COP of albumin is nearly identical to that of plasma (25 mm Hg) (Kirby and Rudloff 1997). Intuitively, albumin could be considered the ideal colloid solution. However, it is incorrect to assume that albumin distributes only to the intravascular space. Albumin distributes throughout the extracellular space, and the amount of time it spends in the intravascular space is longer than that of a crystalloid but shorter than that of hetastarch. The plasma half-life of albumin is 16 h and more than 90% of infused albumin remains in the intravascular space.

Rarely is there a need for plasma transfusion as the sole fluid therapy for shock in veterinary patients, with the rare exception of severe burn injury in which there is massive loss of protein and hypovolemia. Albumin is packaged as either a 5% or 25% solution. A 5% solution can be administered at 10 to 20 mL/kg as rapidly as necessary during shock (Rudloff and Kirby 1994). Many institutions and clinics may be severely limited in their in-house supply of fresh, frozen, or fresh frozen plasma.

Packed red blood cells (PRBCs) have been considered colloids, but the red blood cell itself does not exert COP. Red blood cells alone cannot expand intravascular volume, but administration of PRBCs increases the oxygen-carrying capacity of the existing intravascular volume. There are valid clinical situations in which PRBCs are indicated for shock patients to increase the oxygen-carrying capacity of the blood (see later), but PRBCs should not be considered a type of fluid for volume expansion.

Synthetic colloids are high-molecular-weight substances that remain in the vascular space. Hydroxyethyl starch (hetastarch) is the most commonly used synthetic colloid (Kirby and Rudloff 1997; Marino 1998b). The use of dextran 70 has decreased because of complications, whereas hetastarch administration has few known clinical complications. Pentastarch is a low-molecular-weight derivative of hetastarch that currently is not approved for use in the United States. A gelatin-based colloid fluid (VetaPlasma) also is available for use in dogs and cats.

The primary purpose of colloid solutions is to provide volume expansion and oncotic pressure by remaining in the intravascular space and attracting sodium and water from the interstitial space. Colloids are used primarily as initial therapy for early decompensatory and decompensatory (terminal) shock and are valuable in the treatment of shock in the postoperative period when large amounts of crystalloids have been administered, saturating the interstitial space. Colloid solutions are the primary method of initial and continued volume expansion in patients with SIRS (Kirby and Rudloff 1997). Colloids replace intravascular deficits only, and crystalloids also should be administered to replace interstitial deficits that may be present or that may be created by administration of colloids and hypertonic solutions.

The molecular weight of each colloid determines its oncotic pressure (Concannon 1993). A colloid solution has a wide range of molecule sizes. Two terms are used to measure the size of colloid molecules: weight average molecular weight (M_w) and number average molecular weight (M_n). The M_w is determined by light scattering and is not as accurate a measure of the size of the colloid as M_n, which is the arithmetic mean of the range of molecular weights in the solution. The M_w is larger than the M_n, and as the molecular weight distribution of the colloid becomes narrower, M_w approaches and eventually equals M_n. Albumin (69,000 daltons) is used as a reference to compare oncotic activity.

Dextran 70 is synthesized from sucrose by the bacterium *Leuconostoc mesenteroides* and is processed to a clinically useful size. The M_w of dextran 70 is approximately 70,000 (hence the name dextran 70) and 80% of the molecules have molecular weights between 20,000 and 200,000 daltons. The size of dextran 70 is similar to that of albumin, and it would appear that dextran 70 is the ideal colloid solution. However, the M_n of dextran 70 may be as low as 39,000. Administration of dextran 70 results in an 80 to 100% expansion of plasma volume. Its plasma half-life is approximately 25.5 h with a 24-h duration of clinical effect. Coagulopathy is the main side effect and is dose related. The bleeding tendencies have been attributed to coating of platelets, precipitation and dilution of clotting factors, increased thrombolysis and decreases in von Willebrand's factor and factor VIII activity. Dextran 70 should not be administered to animals with coagulation disorders or thrombocytopenia. Administration of dextran 70 at 20 mL/kg over 20 to 30 min to dogs resulted in decreased von Willebrand's factor antigen concentration and factor VIII activity, and buccal mucosal bleeding time and partial thromboplastin time were increased. Dextrans are adsorbed onto the red blood cell membranes and can interfere with crossmatching of future blood products for transfusion. Although spontaneous bleeding has not been reported in dogs, I have observed a marked decrease in effective coagulation of blood from incision and catheter sites. Consequently, I do not recommend dextran 70 for surgical patients or patients for which invasive monitoring will be used. The dosage of dextran should not exceed 20 mL/kg/day as a combination of bolus and constant-rate infusion. This dosage has been exceeded without apparent adverse effects.

Hydroxyethyl starch (hetastarch) is produced by a chemical modification of amylopectin, which is a complex carbohydrate molecule similar to glycogen. Hetastarch also has a wide range of M_w in solution (M_w = 480,000), but 80% of the molecules have molecular weights between 30,000 and 2,000,000 daltons. The M_n of hetastarch is 69,000. Administration of hetastarch at 20 mL/kg results in a 70 to 200% (average 141%) increase in plasma volume because of a COP of 30 mm Hg, which exceeds the COP of plasma (25 mm Hg). The plasma half-life of hetastarch is 25.5 h and the duration of volume expansion is 12 to 48 h, with longer retention time related to higher doses. Hetastarch prolongs partial thromboplastin time, but clinical bleeding has not been reported in human or veterinary patients. Hetastarch does not interfere with platelet function, but hetastarch administration over several days can result in interference with crossmatching.

The dosage of hetastarch used clinically is 10 to 20 mL/kg in the dog and 10 to 15 mL/kg in the cat (Rudloff and Kirby 1994). This initial dosage is administered as a rapid bolus in dogs and over 10 to 15 min in cats, because rapid administration has been reported to cause nausea in cats. This initial dosage has been exceeded without adverse effects. A constant-rate infusion of 20 mL/kg/day can be administered after the initial bolus if the animal's disease process and cardiovascular status require continued colloid therapy. Hetastarch has been a useful, lifesaving colloid solution, especially in patients with SIRS.

Pentastarch is an analogue of hetastarch and has a lower M_w than hetastarch (264,000 versus 450,000). Pentastarch originally was used for leukophoresis in people and currently is being investigated as a colloidal plasma expander (Rainey and Road 1994). Pentastarch has clinical qualities similar to those of hetastarch with fewer potential side effects. The COP of pentastarch is approximately 40 mm Hg, which should result in volume expansion 1.5 times greater than that with plasma.

A gelatin (oxypolygelatin) colloidal plasma expander (VetaPlasma) currently is available on the veterinary market. Information about this product is limited, but the M_w is approximately 30,000 to 35,000 and there is an approximately 65 to 75% increase in plasma volume after removal of 50% of blood volume and administration of an equal volume of oxypolygelatin solution. Duration of clinical effect was 2 to 4 h and an increase in partial thromboplastin time occurred, but there was no report of clinical bleeding. The small molecular size and limited time of effective plasma expansion are unlikely to be of great benefit, but gelatin colloids may be more effective than crystalloid solutions.

The metabolism of synthetic colloids depends primarily on the size of the molecule. Dextran molecules smaller than 20,000 daltons and hetastarch molecules smaller than 72,000 daltons are rapidly excreted via renal glomerular filtration. Hetastarch is hydrolyzed in the plasma by α-amylase, resulting in hyperamylasemia. The larger molecules of dextran and hetastarch are degraded by the reticuloendothelial system. Other molecules are absorbed into the interstitial space and recirculated through the lymphatic system.

HBOCs have been studied as a replacement for whole blood or packed red blood cells (PRBCs) and as an ideal fluid for resuscitation during shock. The two acellular oxygen carriers that have been evaluated are hemoglobin solutions (stroma-free hemoglobin, pyridoxylated hemoglobin, polymerized hemoglobin) and perfluorocarbon emulsions. HBOCs must effectively transport oxygen and support circulatory hemodynamics. The most useful features of HBOCs include lack of a need to do crossmatching, ready availability, stability at room temperature, long storage time, prolonged residence and activity in the vascular space, and effective oxygen transport without supplemental oxygen.

The HBOC Oxyglobin, which is a polymerized hemoglobin of bovine origin, has been released to the veterinary market. Oxyglobin is a universally compatible fluid that immediately enhances oxygen-carrying capacity by providing a hemoglobin source to plasma. In addition to oxygen-carrying capacity, Oxyglobin exerts a colloid effect in blood, potentially making it the ideal fluid for resuscitation. Its shelf life is approximately 2 years at room temperature and supplemental oxygen is not required for the positive effects on oxygen-carrying capacity. Compared with whole blood, Oxyglobin has a higher P_{50} (partial pressure of O_2 at which hemoglobin is 50% saturated), which allows oxygen to be delivered to the tissues more readily. The oxygen affinity of Oxyglobin is dependent on chloride and not 2,3-diphosphoglycerate, as in red blood cells. The half-life of Oxyglobin is dose dependent and generally is 24 h at clinically useful dosages. The COP of Oxyglobin is approximately 28 mm Hg.

The most common adverse effects of Oxyglobin administration are transient and include discoloration of mucous membranes, sclera, and urine; mild gastrointestinal effects (vomiting, diarrhea); and an increase in central venous pressure (CVP). The increase in CVP actually may be an advantage of Oxyglobin for shock patients.

The primary use of Oxyglobin for most veterinary patients is for anemia, whether it is due to hemolysis, blood loss, or ineffective erythropoiesis. There also is great interest in the use of Oxyglobin for patients with hypovolemic or hemorrhagic shock and especially SIRS, because of the colloidal effects of Oxyglobin in addition to its ability to increase oxygen delivery. Oxyglobin will probably play a crucial role in the management of shock syndromes in veterinary medicine in the near future (see Chapters 15 and 21).

CRYSTALLOIDS OR COLLOIDS?

Neither crystalloids nor colloids administered alone have resulted in an increase in survival in human patients with hypovolemic shock (Bisonni et al. 1993; Shoemaker and Kram 1991). Colloids provide superior intravascular volume support, based on physiology and clinical experience. An interesting analogy, called the "hole in the bucket," has been presented in the medical literature to help resolve the argument over whether crystalloids or colloids should be used for intravascular volume expansion (Marino 1998b). Imagine that the goal of therapy is to expand intravascular volume by filling a bucket. The volume of crystalloid required to expand intravascular volume (i.e., fill the bucket) is approximately three times the volume of colloid required. Assuming that the bucket filled with colloid is full, it will be necessary to punch holes in the bucket filled with crystalloid to allow excess fluid to escape and prevent overflow. The question is, if the goal is to fill the bucket with fluid, do you want to punch holes in the bucket and make the bucket more difficult to fill? It would certainly be more efficient to fill the bucket without having to punch holes in it to deliver a volume of crystalloid equivalent to the volume of colloid.

HYPERTONIC SOLUTIONS

Hypertonic crystalloid solutions (7% and 23.4% NaCl) became popular in veterinary medicine in the 1980s and were described as small-volume resuscitation (Schertel 1992) (see Chapter 24). A single bolus of 7% NaCl (4 mL/kg) provides plasma volume expansion comparable to that of colloids at one-fourth the volume. The primary mechanism of action is provision of an immediate ionic attraction to allow movement of water from the interstitial space to the intravascular space. Hypertonic saline also has been reported to increase myocardial contractility and dilate precapillary blood vessels that may play a role in the maldistribution of blood flow.

The duration of effects is similar to that of isotonic crystalloids and additional intravascular support with colloids is required to maintain effective volume expansion. A convenient method for administering hypertonic saline with a colloid is to dilute 23.4% NaCl with 6% hetastarch (preferred) or 6% dextran 70 to make a 7.5% solution and infuse at a dosage of 4 mL/kg. The rate of administration of all hypertonic saline solutions should not exceed 1 mL/kg/min, and therefore solutions should be administered over a 5-min period in dogs and cats.

Complications of hypertonic saline administration may occur when solutions are infused too rapidly and include bradycardia, hypotension, bronchoconstriction, and rapid, shallow breathing. The mechanism of the cardiopulmonary effects may involve a reflex mediated by the vagus nerve and the lungs, but atropine does not blunt the response (Schertel et al. 1985). Slow administration is highly recommended and does not induce this reflex. Cellular dehydration is another potential complication of administering hypertonic solutions, an effect that is more likely when multiple doses are used or when hypertonic saline is used for patients that are dehydrated. Hypernatremia can occur when more than two doses are administered in close succession. Serum sodium concentration should be monitored if more than two doses are required.

Hypertonic solutions, either alone or in combination with colloids, are useful alternatives for fluid resuscitation in the postoperative patient that has required intravascular volume support and received large volumes of crystalloid fluids. Hypertonic saline and colloids do not place more burden on an already saturated interstitial space and may be beneficial in partially correcting some interstitial edema states. Hypertonic solutions are contraindicated for patients with hypernatremia and severely dehydrated patients.

COMBINATION FLUID THERAPY

Combinations of fluids are the most effective method of fluid therapy, especially for early decompensatory shock, decompensatory (terminal) shock states, and shock secondary to dehydration and third-space loss of fluids. Isotonic and hypertonic crystalloid fluids can be combined with hetastarch to produce effective intravascular volume expansion at lower total volumes than for isotonic crystalloid solutions alone in patients with compensatory shock. Isotonic crystalloids may not be as effective in early decompensatory shock and SIRS and are not effective in decompensatory (terminal) shock. Hetastarch lowers the total amount of isotonic crystalloids required by 40 to

TABLE 20–5. Quick Reference for the Combination of 23.4% NaCl and 6% Hetastarch (4 mL/kg)*

Weight (lb)	Weight (kg)	mL 23.4% NaCl	mL Hetastarch
2	1	1.3	2.7
5	2	2.6	5.4
10	4.5	6	12
15	7	9	18
20	9	12	24
25	11	15	30
30	14	19	38
35	16	21	42
40	18	24	48
45	20.5	27	54
50	23	31	62
55	25	33	66
60	27	36	72
65	29.5	39	78
70	32	43	86
75	34	45	90
80	36	48	96
85	38.5	51	102
90	41	55	110
95	43	57	114
100	45.5	61	122
125	57	76	152
150	68	91	182

*Administer no faster than 1 mL/kg/min.

60%, which can be useful for volume resuscitation in very large dogs. A combination of 23.4% NaCl and hetastarch (Table 20–5) followed by smaller volumes of crystalloids is useful. Intravascular volume expansion is rapid and sustained, and the dose of crystalloids required to maintain the interstitial space is reduced. Another important reason to administer crystalloids in most types of shock is that both hypertonic solutions and colloids can produce a state of relative dehydration in the interstitial space.

In summary, if the goal of immediate fluid resuscitation is to expand the intravascular space, colloids should be used. If the goal of immediate fluid resuscitation is to expand the entire extracellular space, crystalloids should be used. If the goal is to expand both the intravascular and extracellular spaces, both colloids with or without hypertonic solutions and crystalloids should be used.

CARDIOGENIC SHOCK

Adequate volume resuscitation is the single most important treatment for all types of shock with the notable exception of cardiogenic shock. Fluid redistribution from the lungs to the circulation, inotropic support, and antiarrhythmic therapy are the primary goals of therapy in cardiogenic shock. An animal that has received therapy to reduce or redistribute intravascular volume may actually become dehydrated and volume depleted. Fluid therapy is warranted for these patients and appropriate monitoring should determine both the type and rate of fluid therapy in patients treated for cardiogenic shock. Current investigations have provided evidence that low dosages and slow administration of colloids may provide the necessary volume to maximize cardiac output in some patients with heart failure.

▶ Ancillary Supportive Therapy

Other treatment regimens should be employed after volume replacement, especially when the patient is not responsive to initial therapy. Shock should be treated on the basis of knowledge of pathophysiology and not necessarily initial clinical observations (Shoemaker 1995). In most instances, for example, if the animal is hypotensive, vasopressors should not be administered immediately. Likewise, diuretics should not be administered immediately to treat oliguria in the shock patient. Further treatment should be based on monitoring the effectiveness of initial fluid therapy (see later).

Support of the Cardiovascular System

Evidence of poor perfusion (e.g., hypotension, increased CVP, oliguria) after initial resuscitation with appropriate fluid therapy is an indication for use of drugs to support cardiac output and blood pressure. Clinicians can anticipate the probable need for continued pharmacologic cardiovascular support from the cause of shock. Animals that have evidence of prolonged shock, decompensatory shock, and SIRS are likely to require drugs that act on the cardiovascular system to support blood flow and blood pressure. The primary class of drugs useful in these situations is the inotropes. Inotropes require adequate intravascular volume to be effective and are ineffective in states of uncorrected hypovolemia. Examples of inotropes that can be used in patients with continued evidence of poor output despite adequate volume expansion include the sympathomimetic agents dobutamine and dopamine.

Dobutamine is a synthetic sympathomimetic agent that exerts effects on the β_1-adrenoceptors of the myocardium to increase the force of contraction. Dobutamine exerts weak effects on β_2-adrenoceptors located on blood vessels to produce mild vasodilatation. The combination of mild arterial vasodilatation and increased force of myocardial contraction results in increased cardiac output without a dramatic increase in arterial blood pressure. The dosage range of dobutamine is wide (2–15 μg/kg/min), but most clinicians begin with continuous-rate infusion of 2 to 5 μg/kg/min and increase the dosage as needed on the basis of hemodynamic monitoring. Adequate intravascular volume is required for dobutamine to exert positive inotropic effects (Klein 1977). The most common side effect of dobutamine infusion is development of ventricular arrhythmias. The dobutamine infusion should be temporarily discontinued if ventricular arrhythmias occur and can be safely restarted at a lower infusion rate upon cessation of the arrhythmias. Dobutamine has minimal effects on the heart rate.

Dopamine is a precursor of norepinephrine and exerts dose-dependent effects. Low infusion rates (1–5 μg/kg/min) stimulate dopaminergic receptors in renal, coronary, and cerebral arteries, resulting in arterial dilatation. Somewhat higher infusion rates (5–10 μg/kg/min) produce a sympathomimetic effect by stimulating β_1-adrenergic receptors in the sinus node and myocardium, resulting in a positive chronotropic and inotropic effect. Cardiac output is increased as a result of increased heart rate and force of myocardial contraction. Blood pressure is increased to a greater extent than occurs with dobutamine. High infusion rates (>10 μg/kg/min) stimulate α_1-adrenergic receptors located on arterial blood vessels and result in vasoconstriction and increased blood pressure. The most common side effect of dopamine is development of ventricular arrhythmias. Heart rate should increase with a moderate infusion rate of dopamine.

Vasopressors such as epinephrine (0.1–0.3 μg/kg/min) can be used during life-threatening states of hypotension that are refractory to initial fluid resuscitation. The goal of vasopressors is to raise blood pressure sufficiently to maintain blood flow to the heart and brain. Use of vasopressors should be considered temporary, as vasoconstriction occurs in other tissues and decreases blood flow and organ function. The most common side effects of epinephrine are ventricular arrhythmias, including ventricular fibrillation. Other vasopressors that can be administered include the α_1-adrenoceptor agonist methoxamine (0.05–0.2 mg/kg IV), norepinephrine (0.01–0.4 μg/kg/min), and dopamine in a high-dose infusion (>10 μg/kg/min).

Antiarrhythmic Therapy

Any type of arrhythmia can occur during shock, but ventricular arrhythmias (e.g., ventricular premature complexes, paroxysmal ventricular tachycardia, ventricular tachycardia) are most common. Arrhythmias that occur during shock before initial volume resuscitation are most likely the result of inadequate myocardial perfusion and may respond to volume expansion alone. Cardiogenic shock is a notable exception because arrhythmias may be the primary cause of decreased cardiac output and corresponding shock. Other causes of ventricular arrhythmias, depending on the cause of shock, include trauma, electrolyte imbalances, SIRS, hypoxemia, anemia, pain, and underlying cardiac disease.

The decision to treat ventricular arrhythmias should be based on several factors beyond the number of premature ventricular complexes (PVCs) that occur during 1 min. There is little debate that isolated PVCs rarely require antiarrhythmic therapy and that rapid ventricular tachycardia (>200 PVCs per minute) almost always requires treatment. There is, however, considerable debate on whether or not to administer antiarrhythmic drugs in many other clinical settings, especially considering the arrhythmogenic effects of many agents.

The least supported reason to administer antiarrhythmic therapy is the number of PVCs that occur in 1 min. Many guidelines state that when more than 20 PVCs occur per minute, antiarrhythmic therapy should be instituted. However, if the patient's blood pressure is not affected and there is no evidence of a serious arrhythmia (e.g., R-on-T phenomenon), there is little reason to administer drugs. Ventricular premature complexes that occur in the following patterns should be treated: bigeminy, trigeminy, paroxysmal and sustained ventricular tachycardia, and multiform PVCs. Ventricular arrhythmias that affect hemodynamics (blood flow and blood pressure) should always be treated. Close coupling of the QRS and T wave (R-on-T phenomenon) should always be treated, as this presentation predisposes to ventricular tachycardia and ventricular fibrillation.

Antiarrhythmic drugs are indicated for arrhythmias that persist after initial fluid resuscitation, administration of analgesic agents (see later), and correction of electrolyte disturbances. Intravenous bolus and continuous-rate infusions are the preferred methods of administration. The antiarrhythmic agents most commonly used during shock include lidocaine and procainamide.

Lidocaine usually is considered the first choice for ventricular arrhythmias. It is administered as an intravenous bolus (2 mg/kg) followed by a continuous-rate infusion (40–80 μg/kg/min) if needed. Lidocaine has a very short half-life and a very large volume of distribution and usually warrants continuous-rate infusion to maintain adequate plasma concentrations. Common side effects include vomiting and seizures. Hypotension can occur at very large doses.

Procainamide may be administered intravenously (3–6 mg/kg) as a bolus followed by a continuous-rate infusion (10–40 μg/kg/min) if lidocaine is ineffective. Procainamide depresses contractility to a greater degree than lidocaine, but both agents are considered proarrhythmic in nature.

Ventricular arrhythmias that do not respond to initial administration of antiarrhythmic drugs should be considered refractory arrhythmias. A logical approach should be used to determine the reason for ineffective antiarrhythmic therapy. Electrolytes should be evaluated because potassium is required for lidocaine and procainamide to be effective. Intravascular volume should be adequate as determined by monitoring cardiovascular variables such as CVP. Appropriate analgesia should be administered and adequate oxygenation of arterial blood should be maintained based on blood gas analysis. Serum magnesium concentration should be determined if refractory ventricular arrhythmias are present after all the preceding variables have been determined to be adequate. This is especially true in patients that may have chronic underlying disease.

Antiarrhythmic therapy should be discontinued slowly to determine whether additional therapy is warranted. There is no firm guideline on the rate at which lidocaine or procainamide infusions should be decreased. Patients without underlying cardiac disease should have complete resolution of ventricular arrhythmias.

Analgesia

Pain and the physiologic response to pain can be detrimental to the shock patient. The primary physiologic effects of pain are manifested by the cardiovascular system and include increased heart rate, vasoconstriction, and arrhythmias. Vasoconstriction secondary to unrelieved pain, inadequate intravascular volume, and poor myocardial function can dramatically lower cardiac output. Adequate and safe analgesia should be provided for almost all patients with signs of shock. This approach is especially true for trauma patients and those with SIRS.

Opioid analgesics are preferred for patients in shock (Table 20–6). The opioid agonist-antagonist butorphanol (0.2–0.6 mg/kg IV) is a safe and effective analgesic agent.

SHOCK SYNDROMES IN VETERINARY MEDICINE

TABLE 20-6. Useful Intravenous or Intramuscular Analgesics for Dogs and Cats in Shock

Agent	Dose and Route	Approximate Duration	Comments
Butorphanol	0.2–0.6 mg/kg, IV or IM	2–4 h	Rarely causes bradycardia, minimal respiratory depression
Buprenorphine	0.01–0.1 mg/kg, IV or IM	2–6 h	Rarely causes bradycardia, minimal respiratory depression
Oxymorphone	0.05–0.1 mg/kg, IV or IM	2–4 h	Dose-dependent bradycardia and respiratory depression
Morphine	0.1–0.2 mg/kg/h infusion (dogs only)	Continuous	Minimal respiratory and cardiovascular (heart rate) depression

Butorphanol produces little effect on cardiovascular and pulmonary function. The approximate duration of action ranges from 2 to 4 h. Other alternatives include the opioid agonist buprenorphine (0.01–0.1 mg/kg IV). Oxymorphone can suppress pulmonary function in a dose-dependent manner. Buprenorphine has little effect on the cardiopulmonary system.

A viable alternative for continuous analgesia is a constant-rate intravenous infusion of morphine (0.1–0.2 mg/kg/h). Although morphine can decrease heart rate and impair pulmonary function at higher doses, administration as an intravenous infusion at the recommended dosage has little effect on cardiopulmonary function. Morphine is relatively inexpensive and, when used appropriately, provides adequate analgesia and produces few side effects.

The duration of analgesic therapy should be determined by the initiating cause of pain. An animal that has sustained a fracture should have analgesia administered continuously or on a predetermined schedule until the fracture can be repaired. An animal with SIRS secondary to peritonitis also should have continuous administration of analgesia. Analgesic agents can be decreased and discontinued when the clinician is confident that the patient is no longer showing signs of pain.

Antibiotic Therapy

The decision to administer antibiotics should be based on several factors including the stage of shock and the underlying problem. Antibiotics are not indicated for patients in the compensatory stage of shock unless there is obvious evidence of external trauma. However, antibiotics should be administered to patients in decompensatory shock or with evidence of external trauma. Cultures of blood, urine, peritoneal or pleural fluid, and any discharges should be submitted whenever possible before antibiotic administration.

Bacterial translocation from the intestinal tract to the bloodstream may occur during the decompensatory stages of shock and during reperfusion injury. Broad-spectrum antibiotics such as first-generation cephalosporins (e.g., cefazolin, 20 mg/kg IV) are indicated during initial fluid resuscitation. Continuation of antibiotics should be determined by monitoring the patient.

Patients with septic shock secondary to SIRS require intravenous administration of broad-spectrum bactericidal antibiotics. Blood for cultures can be collected before administration of antibiotics, but delay in therapy and marginal yield of organisms in blood cultures may deter collection of blood for culture. First-generation cephalosporins are economical, efficacious, and often the first choice of antibiotics. When adequate perfusion is established or the animal does not seem to respond to initial antimicrobial therapy, an aminoglycoside (e.g., amikacin, 5 mg/kg IV) can be administered while closely monitoring urine output. The aminoglycosides provide additional coverage for gram-negative organisms. Surgical removal of a septic focus, if present, is indicated.

Controversy on Glucocorticoid Use in Shock Syndromes

Glucocorticoid administration as an initial therapy has been advocated for most shock patients and in the past 50 years was suggested for all shock patients (Tobias and Schertel 1992). Clinicians must use a common sense approach to the administration of any therapy for the treatment of shock, including corticosteroids, and not utilize these agents reflexly.

The primary benefit and strongest argument for the use of glucocorticoids is their strong antiinflammatory effect (Rudloff and Kirby 1994). Of particular interest is the prevention of cytokine production by macrophages. Potent components of SIRS, such as tumor necrosis factor, interleukin-1, interleukin-6, and platelet-activating factor are inhibited by glucocorticoids. Glucocorticoids inhibit cyclooxygenase and lipoxygenase activity stimulated by cytokines and inhibit production of eicosanoids (prostaglandins, thromboxanes, leukotrienes). The earlier glucocorticoids are administered in the inflammatory response, the better the inhibition of cytokines and eicosanoids. In addition to their potent antiinflammatory effect, glucocorticoids reduce reperfusion injury. The effects of reperfusion injury are best prevented if glucocorticoids are present at the time of reperfusion of tissues. This effect is difficult to achieve in the clinical setting. The two most commonly administered glucocorticoids are dexamethasone sodium phosphate (1 mg/kg IV) and prednisolone sodium succinate (10–20 mg/kg IV).

Glucocorticoids relax arterioles and venules and can improve microcirculation. Although this is a positive cardiovascular effect, glucocorticoid administration is not recommended in the presence of hypovolemia without adequate fluid resuscitation because relaxation of peripheral vessels can produce hypotension. Sudden death has been reported in people after rapid administration of glucocorticoids.

The potential deleterious effects of glucocorticoids are numerous and include the previously described effects on the cardiovascular system. Gastrointestinal effects include development of ulcers that are attributed to antiprostaglandin activity and subsequent decrease in mucosal blood flow. There is an argument against the use of glucocorticoids in advanced stages of shock when the integrity of the intestinal mucosa may be compromised, resulting in microulceration. Glucocorticoids impair the cellular immune response and can predispose to bacterial infection. The beneficial effects of glucocorticoids have been reported by some investigators as being useful only with the concurrent administration of antibiotics to counteract suppression of the immune system (Neugebauer et al. 1994).

Because of the negative effects of glucocorticoids on the cellular immune response, glucocorticoids generally are contraindicated in patients that have signs of SIRS or are considered to be in septic shock (Neugebauer et al. 1994; Rudloff and Kirby 1994; Shoemaker et al. 1993a). There is some evidence that glucocorticoids can have beneficial effects in septic shock if administered before or shortly after shock ensues by reducing products created by the inflammatory cascade (Neugebauer et al. 1994). Administration before shock, however, is impossible in nonhospitalized patients. Two large, multicenter, clinical trials in people provided evidence that glucocorticoids have negative effects on patients in septic shock (Bone et al. 1987; Veterans Administration 1987). These two studies have resulted in the recommendation not to administer glucocorticoids to patients in septic shock. My opinion is that corticosteroids are not indicated in patients in shock.

Bicarbonate Therapy

Recommendations on the use of sodium bicarbonate in patients with shock have changed in the literature. Bicarbonate is no longer routinely recommended for shock patients (Neugebauer et al. 1994; Shoemaker 1995). Animals in shock usually have metabolic acidosis because of decreased tissue perfusion and it has previously been recommended that the acidosis be treated with sodium bicarbonate. Metabolic acidosis related to poor tissue perfusion, however, should be treated by increasing tissue perfusion. In most instances, improving tissue perfusion reverses metabolic acidosis. Animals with underlying disease that may predispose to metabolic acidosis (e.g., bicarbonate loss related to diarrhea or renal disease) usually require additional intervention.

The degree of metabolic acidosis in shock depends on the severity and duration of poor tissue perfusion. Mild metabolic acidosis (pH 7.2–7.4) has few metabolic consequences. Animals with compensatory or early decompensatory shock of short duration usually have mild metabolic acidosis. Animals with prolonged early decompensatory shock or decompensatory (terminal) shock may have severe metabolic acidosis (pH < 7.2) Severe metabolic acidosis (pH < 7.2) decreases cardiac performance and can predispose the heart to ventricular arrhythmias. Acute metabolic acidosis can also result in a transient hyperkalemia related to transcellular shifting of potassium from the intracellular to extracellular space.

Current recommendations for administration of bicarbonate begin with documentation of metabolic acidosis by blood gas analysis (DiBartola 1992). Prophylactic administration of sodium bicarbonate is no longer recommended. Bicarbonate should be administered only when the pH is 7.1 to 7.2 and administered only in amounts necessary to increase the pH to 7.2. An 8.4% sodium bicarbonate solution is high in sodium and can result in volume overload, decreased serum ionized calcium concentration, "overshoot" metabolic alkalosis, paradoxical central nervous system acidosis, and hypokalemia caused by a transcellular shift of potassium from the extracellular to intracellular space. Current recommended dosages range from 0.25 to 1.0 mEq/kg IV administered as a bolus over 10 to 15 min. Repeated blood gas analysis determines the effect of the initial dose.

Blood Products

Some clinical situations require administration of blood or blood products. Hemorrhagic shock from excessive blood loss usually requires administration of whole blood (preferred), PRBCs, or an HBOC (Oxyglobin). The extent of acute blood loss cannot be determined reliably by monitoring the packed cell volume (PCV) alone, as the PCV is likely not to decrease for several hours after acute blood loss. Monitoring clinical signs or quantitating the amount of blood loss should facilitate the decision to administer blood or blood products. In most instances, crystalloid, colloid, or hypertonic fluid therapy should be instituted first because whole blood or blood products may not be immediately available. In addition, external or internal blood loss must be controlled for administration of blood or blood products to be effective.

The amount of blood administered usually is based on a mathematical formula, but such formulas are based on the animal's current PCV and the desired increase in PCV. As mentioned previously, however, the PCV may not change acutely although the animal's vital signs may indicate the need for blood. The amount of blood to administer can be estimated without using the PCV as a guide. Most animals can tolerate a 10 to 15% loss of blood acutely without requiring blood transfusion. Acute blood loss of more than 20% usually requires blood transfusion in addition to initial fluid therapy. Most animals that lose more than 50% of their blood acutely do not survive for an extended period of time. Therefore, estimating an approximate percentage blood loss and multiplying by blood volume (90 mL/kg in dogs or 70 mL/kg in cats) can provide an initial volume of blood to administer. One should be cautious when using this approach to calculate the volume of blood to be transfused, because it represents a very crude estimate. The animal should be monitored closely for its response to blood administration and for potential complications, including volume overload, transfusion reactions, and metabolic acidosis or hypocalcemia secondary to massive doses of anticoagulant (anticoagulant citrate dextrose solutions).

HBOCs (e.g., Oxyglobin) have been developed to provide a readily available source of oxygen-carrying fluid.

Advantages include no transfusion reactions, ready availability off the shelf at room temperature, and colloidal effects. The effects can last more than 24 h, depending on the dose administered. Internal or external hemorrhage must be controlled for this approach to be effective. The colloidal effects associated with Oxyglobin in addition to its oxygen-carrying capability make it an attractive fluid for maximum volume resuscitation and oxygen delivery. For example, synthetic colloids (hetastarch) provide colloidal effects and support cardiac output but do not have oxygen-carrying capacity.

▶ Monitoring

Many variables can be monitored in the shock patient, including physical findings (e.g., mucous membrane color, capillary refill time, pulse rate and quality, heart rate, respiratory rate), arterial blood pressure (by invasive or noninvasive means), PCV, urine output, CVP, cardiac output, and blood gases (arterial and venous). Which of these is the most important variable to monitor? Which variable gives the clinician the most valuable information? The answers to these questions depend on the pathophysiology of shock in the patient in question. Oxygen transport variables (e.g., cardiac output, content of oxygen in arterial and venous blood, oxygen consumption, and oxygen delivery) provide the most important and most accurate information. Unfortunately, most veterinary practices do not have the capability to monitor oxygen transport variables. Many of the easily measured variables may be normal, and the animal still can progress to end-stage organ failure and death. Therefore, the information that can be obtained by the clinician must be used carefully to make decisions about further therapeutic intervention.

Another common question is how often to monitor the patient in shock. The answer depends upon the clinical status of the patient. The most critically ill patients require continuous, even minute-by-minute monitoring, whereas more stable patients require less frequent monitoring. Clinical judgment must be used to determine the interval of monitoring.

Physical Parameters

Physical parameters are important and simple to monitor for trends that may be early indications of deterioration or improvement in cardiovascular status. The interpretation of these parameters is subjective and final decisions should be confirmed with more objective monitoring techniques. Peripheral pulse rate and rhythm; respiratory rate, rhythm, and effort; mucous membrane color; and capillary refill time provide subjective information on the status of the cardiopulmonary system. Other physical parameters that are important include the animal's mentation, character of peripheral pulses, and assessment of the jugular veins.

Packed Cell Volume and Total Plasma Proteins

Measurements of PCV and total plasma proteins provide essential information. The PCV provides information on the oxygen-carrying potential of the blood as hemoglobin is the major contributor to the content of oxygen in arterial blood. Acute changes in blood volume may not be reflected in the PCV (see earlier). The PCV should be maintained between 25 and 35% in all critically ill animals. Blood or blood products should be considered when the PCV falls below 20% acutely and the animal is showing signs of decreased oxygen delivery (e.g., tachypnea, exercise intolerance, decreased mentation). Many patients with a chronic decrease in PCV may not require blood products until the PCV falls below 15%.

Measurement of total plasma proteins provides information on many variables. The color of the plasma can identify hemolysis or icterus. The refractometer reading of the total plasma proteins can provide subjective information on the COP. Evaluation of the COP is essential for maintenance of intravascular volume. Proteins are large molecules that are maintained within the intravascular space. The presence of these large, nondiffusible molecules creates a force that draws water into the vascular space. A decreased concentration of proteins related to blood loss or extravasation from the intravascular space because of defects in the endothelium (as in SIRS) results in decreased COP. A decrease in COP can cause loss of intravascular water to the interstitial space and predispose to interstitial edema. The total plasma protein concentration should remain above 3.5 g/dL to maintain adequate COP. Colloid therapy should be strongly considered when the total plasma protein concentration falls below 3.5 g/dL. Colloid oncotic pressure can be measured directly with an oncometer. The COP of plasma is normal patients is approximately 25 mm Hg and values of 18 to 20 mm Hg are found in critically ill patients (Aldrich and Haskins 1995).

Central Venous Pressure

The CVP can provide valuable information regarding right ventricular function and intravascular volume status and is relatively easy to monitor in most veterinary practices. Monitoring of CVP involves placement of an indwelling jugular catheter with the tip of the catheter in the thoracic cranial vena cava. If the animal has appropriate right-sided heart function, CVP provides information on filling pressures of the heart (preload). The CVP should range between 10 and 15 cm H_2O in the shock patient, although normal CVP values range from 0 to 2 cm H_2O. Other determinants of CVP must also be considered when interpreting values, including intrathoracic pressure and venous distensibility.

Should all animals in shock have CVP monitored? The answer to this question depends on the primary presenting problem. For example, an animal that presents in shock secondary to pancreatitis and SIRS should have CVP monitored as soon as possible. On the other hand, the dog that presents after blunt trauma with no indication of internal bleeding probably does not require CVP monitoring. In the latter situation, most clinicians would rather administer the initial fluid resuscitation, monitor the animal closely, and, if there are signs of continued shock, place a jugular catheter for CVP monitoring and locate the source of continued intravascular volume deficiency.

Appropriate fluid resuscitation should result in an increase in CVP. However, the nature of crystalloid therapy is such that intravascular volume expansion is temporary because of normal movement of the crystalloid into the interstitial space. A general rule is that if the CVP increases to an acceptable value after initial fluid resuscitation with crystalloids but then falls below 3 cm H_2O and physical parameters also deteriorate, further therapy is warranted. A rapid decrease in CVP also may indicate acute blood loss.

Arterial Blood Pressure

Arterial blood pressure is defined as the force that is exerted by the blood on the arterial wall. Arterial blood pressure is not cardiac output, and it should not be assumed that adequate blood pressure is synonymous with adequate cardiac output. In fact, cardiac output is a determinant of mean arterial blood pressure (mean arterial pressure = cardiac output × systemic vascular resistance). If systemic vascular resistance is increased secondary to vasoconstriction, the result is increased blood pressure. However, cardiac output actually can decrease during hypertension. An animal in pain can have hypertension yet have a lower than normal cardiac output. The animal with poor myocardial performance because of SIRS and vasoconstriction caused by pain or hypothermia can have very poor cardiac output. Therefore, blood pressure monitoring should be used in addition to other monitoring techniques to provide the most accurate assessment of cardiovascular status.

Arterial blood pressure can be measured by direct or indirect methods. Direct measurement of arterial blood pressure requires a catheter placed in a peripheral artery (usually dorsal pedal or femoral), a pressure transducer, and a monitor. Accurate measurement of systolic, diastolic, and mean arterial pressures can be obtained with proper positioning of the transducer (level of the heart) and adequate calibration of equipment. The arterial waveform also can be monitored for early deterioration of the cardiovascular system (i.e., flattening of the waveform). Placement of an arterial catheter is a challenge, especially in patients weighing less than 10 kg, and the equipment is expensive, which may deter many clinicians from measuring arterial blood pressure directly.

Indirect measurement of arterial blood pressure is most feasible for the practicing veterinarian. The most important factor to remember with indirect methods is that the values obtained are not necessarily accurate, especially in smaller animals (<10 kg). However, the trend of values obtained is extremely important and should be considered more than the actual values.

The two available methods of indirect arterial blood pressure monitoring are oscillometric and Doppler ultrasonic. The oscillometric method (Dinamap) involves placement of an appropriate-sized blood pressure cuff over a peripheral artery. The mechanism of blood pressure measurement is to determine the oscillation of the artery at systolic and mean arterial pressures and convert this measurement to a numerical blood pressure. The diastolic pressure is the pressure at which the maximum oscillation has decreased by 80%. Therefore, diastolic pressure measurements are least accurate. The most common artery used is the dorsal pedal artery, although the coccygeal and metacarpal arteries have been used with less success. The area over the artery should be clipped and the animal should be placed in lateral recumbency to ensure that the limb is near the level of the heart. Appropriate cuff size is critical to obtain adequate readings. The width of the cuff should be approximately 40% of the circumference of the limb. A cuff that is too large results in falsely decreased values, and a cuff that is too small results in falsely increased values. The oscillometric method provides systolic, diastolic, and mean arterial pressures as well as heart rate. The primary disadvantages of the oscillometric method include the cost of the equipment and inaccurate or unobtainable values in animals weighing 5 to 10 kg.

The Doppler ultrasonic method uses the Doppler effect to detect movement of red blood cells past a crystal that emits Doppler waves. Each pulse of blood is converted to a sound that can easily be heard. The crystal is placed over the metacarpal artery with an appropriate-sized cuff placed proximal to the crystal. A sphygmomanometer is attached to the cuff and inflated until no sound is detected. The pressure is slowly reduced until the first audible pulse is detected. Only systolic blood pressure is measured on a reliable basis, although diastolic pressure can also be obtained. The first audible pulse is the systolic blood pressure as indicated on the sphygmomanometer. The pressure continues to be slowly removed from the cuff until the audible signal changes tone. The change in tone occurs at the diastolic blood pressure. Advantages of the Doppler method include detection of an audible pulse, reasonable cost, and reliable use in very small patients.

Oxygen Transport Variables

Oxygen transport variables (e.g., cardiac output, content of oxygen in arterial and venous blood, oxygen consumption, and oxygen delivery) provide the most valuable information on cardiovascular function, but the cost of instrumentation and need to place specialized catheters tend to limit the use of these parameters.

CARDIAC OUTPUT

Cardiac output is defined as the total output of blood from the heart and is synonymous with blood flow. Cardiac output measurement requires thermodilution catheters to be placed in the pulmonary artery and a cardiac output computer. Although the cost of Doppler ultrasound equipment is high, the technique to determine blood flow with an ultrasound probe is less difficult than placement of a thermodilution catheter. However, I have conducted experimental trials that indicate Doppler ultrasound may not be a reliable method to determine cardiac output in patients in shock.

URINE OUTPUT

Urine output can be used as an indirect measurement of renal blood flow and therefore as an indirect measurement of cardiac output. If urine production decreases below 1 mL/kg/h in an animal without previously detected renal disease, low cardiac output should be suspected. Urine production is relatively easy to monitor by placement of a urethral catheter and hourly recording of urine production.

OXYGEN CONTENT

Determination of oxygen content variables requires arterial and mixed venous blood gas determinations. Most of the variables in Table 20–1 are calculated. The assessment of adequate cardiopulmonary function ultimately is determined by oxygen delivery variables.

Blood Gas Analysis

Arterial and venous blood gas analysis can provide valuable information about cardiopulmonary function. The production of portable "point of care" blood gas analyzers has greatly increased the clinician's ability to monitor blood gases. Laboratory blood gas analyzers cost $10,000 to $30,000 or more, whereas portable blood gas analyzers can be purchased for approximately $5000. One disadvantage of blood gas analysis (arterial or venous) is that the results obtained represent a single moment in time. The status of the patient may be changing minute by minute, which may limit the value of intermittent blood gas analysis. Also, the partial pressure of oxygen reflects the amount of oxygen dissolved in plasma. Saturation of hemoglobin with oxygen is much more important because oxygen is delivered by hemoglobin in the red blood cell. The saturation of hemoglobin can be determined from the oxyhemoglobin dissociation curve.

Arterial blood gas analysis provides information about gas exchange in the lung and arterial acid-base balance. Arterial blood samples are collected from the femoral or dorsal pedal artery in a heparinized syringe. The partial pressure of oxygen in arterial blood (PaO_2) is correlated with oxygen exchange in the lung. Acid-base balance is discussed in Chapters 9 to 12.

A true mixed venous blood gas sample must be obtained from the pulmonary artery, which requires placement of specialized catheter. The partial pressure of oxygen in mixed venous blood (PvO_2) represents information about perfusion of tissues on a global basis. Normal PvO_2 values range from 35 to 45 mm Hg. Values below 30 mm Hg indicate poor perfusion of the peripheral tissues. If a thermodilution catheter is not placed in the pulmonary artery to collect blood for PvO_2 determination, a jugular catheter placed to monitor CVP can be used to collect a venous blood sample that may approximate a true mixed venous sample. The blood gas variable that can predict survival in human patients is PvO_2 (see later).

Pulse Oximetry

Pulse oximetry allows continuous monitoring of the saturation of hemoglobin with oxygen (SaO_2). The PaO_2 provides information about oxygen dissolved in plasma, whereas SaO_2 provides information about the ability of the red blood cell to carry oxygen. To be of value, pulse oximetry requires pulsatile flow of blood to the periphery. Many patients in shock have decreased blood flow to the periphery, which limits the effectiveness of pulse oximetry. In addition, the device is applied to the tongue for the most accurate readings, a technique that is difficult in the conscious patient. Other areas where the probe may be placed include the ear, axilla, vulva, and prepuce. A rectal probe may be of value in the conscious patient.

▶ Predictors of Outcome

Normal cardiovascular and pulmonary parameters do not correlate with survival. Many critically ill human patients with normal values die. The goal of volume resuscitation and other therapy for shock is to maintain supranormal cardiovascular parameters (Tuchschmidt et al 1992). Most of the oxygen transport variables should be 50 to 60% above normal values. If these variables cannot be monitored, CVP, urine output, and blood pressure should all exceed normal values by 50% or more while normal heart rate and rhythm and oxygenation are maintained.

As already mentioned, PvO_2 indicates perfusion of peripheral tissues. In human patients, PvO_2 values between 28 and 35 mm Hg represent poor perfusion requiring immediate treatment. Most human patients with PvO_2 below 28 mm Hg do not survive (Snyder 1982). Other negative predictors of outcome include advanced age, irreversible primary disease, and thrombocytopenia.

▶ Other Concerns

The following aspects of fluid resuscitation are beyond the scope of this chapter but are of great importance when treating patients with severe shock and shock secondary to trauma. They are mentioned briefly here.

Resuscitation-Induced Hemorrhage and Hypotensive Resuscitation

The hypotensive patient with uncontrolled internal hemorrhage is a challenge. Fluid resuscitation should begin before surgical intervention, but aggressive fluid resuscitation may increase blood pressure and cardiac output sufficiently to exacerbate hemorrhage (Crowe and Devey 1994). Hypotensive resuscitation is defined as fluid therapy administered at rates and volumes below current recommendations with an end point below normal or supranormal values of blood pressure (Marino 1998a). The optimal end point of this type of resuscitation has not been determined. Blood pressures higher than presentation but lower than normal have been suggested. More clinical information on hypotensive resuscitation is necessary before precise recommendations can be made. I administer a colloid (hetastarch) as a 5 ml/kg IV bolus or crystalloids (e.g., lactated Ringer's, 0.9% NaCl) as a 50 ml/kg IV bolus as resuscitation for uncontrolled internal hemorrhage in preparation for surgical exploration.

Postresuscitation Injury

Most clinicians have witnessed deterioration of patients that seemingly have been resuscitated successfully from advanced stages of shock. The gastrointestinal tract and brain seem to be most susceptible to injury after successful fluid resuscitation, but multiple organ failure also can occur. Two processes have been implicated in injury after successful resuscitation: the no-reflow phenomenon and reperfusion injury (Marino 1998a).

NO-REFLOW PHENOMENON
Perfusion can be decreased even after seemingly adequate fluid resuscitation. Several mechanisms have been proposed to explain this phenomenon, including calcium-induced vasoconstriction, leukocyte plugging of the microvasculature, and vascular compromise caused by edema of surrounding tissues. Lack of flow to the brain can result in cerebral edema. Lack of flow to the intestinal tract can result in translocation of intestinal pathogens and lead to postresuscitation septicemia, SIRS, and septic shock. The occurrence and severity of the no-reflow phenomenon seem to be related to the duration of poor perfusion during shock. At present there is no therapy that can prevent the no-reflow phenomenon.

REPERFUSION INJURY
The phenomenon of reperfusion injury has been well established and can occur in any organ after adequate resuscitation. Toxic oxygen metabolites are known to be produced by a cascade of events that result in the production of superoxide and hydroxyl radicals. As with the no-reflow phenomenon, reperfusion injury can occur in any organ, but its effects on the brain are most detrimental to the survival of the patient. Antioxidants, corticosteroids, calcium channel blockers, free-radical scavengers and iron chelators have been studied as potential treatments but no single approach has been determined to be most effective. The most effective therapy is likely to be one that can be administered before resuscitation, which is nearly impossible in the clinical setting.

Fluid Therapy for Shock with Concurrent Head Trauma and Pulmonary Contusions

Patients in shock with concurrent head trauma and pulmonary contusions present special challenges to fluid therapy. Head trauma patients with cerebral edema are probably not able to handle large volumes of crystalloid fluids because most of the crystalloid extravasates to the interstitium within 1 h of administration. Many patients with head trauma deteriorate soon after crystalloid administration. Hypertonic saline and synthetic colloids, either alone or in combination, are the fluids of choice for patients with head trauma (see Table 20–5). Crystalloid therapy should be administered cautiously.

Fluid therapy in patients with pulmonary contusions is controversial (Hackner 1995). In this clinical setting, the alveolar-capillary membranes have sustained damage and the alveoli have been flooded with blood. Administration of large volumes of crystalloids potentially may worsen the clinical signs associated with pulmonary contusions. That this outcome necessarily occurs, however, has not been determined in laboratory or clinical studies. Clinically, the current recommendation is similar to that for patients with cerebral edema. Consequently, hypertonic solutions and colloids, or a combination of the two, are the treatment of choice, with judicious administration of crystalloids.

Clinical Examples of Fluid Therapy for the Three Stages of Shock

COMPENSATORY SHOCK
A 2-year-old male mixed-breed dog weighing 20 kg is presented after being hit by a car 20 min earlier. The dog walks into the clinic and seems normal. Physical examination shows hydration, normal; heart rate, 150/min; respiratory rate, 90/min; mucous membranes, bright red; capillary refill time, <1 s; strong femoral pulses; normal blood pressure. The dog is in compensatory shock and requires fluid therapy. An 18-gauge catheter is placed in a cephalic vein. Fluid options include 1.8 L of lactated Ringer's solution or 80 mL of 7% NaCl plus 500 mL of lactated Ringer's solution. Physical parameters after therapy include heart rate, 80/min; respiratory rate, 30/min; mucous membranes, pink; capillary refill time, 2 s. The dog is observed for 12 h for other injuries and released.

EARLY DECOMPENSATORY SHOCK
A 5-year-old female mixed-breed dog weighing 25 kg is presented after being hit by a car 2 to 4 h earlier. The dog also has a luxation of the coxofemoral joint. The dog is in lateral recumbency with a decreased level of consciousness. Physical examination shows hydration, normal; heart rate, 180/min; respiratory rate, 90/min; mucous membranes, pale; capillary refill time, difficult to elicit; weak femoral pulses; hypotension (70 mm Hg systolic blood pressure); and mild abdominal distention. Abdominocentesis shows hemoabdomen. This dog is in early decompensatory shock (hemorrhagic and traumatic) and requires aggressive fluid therapy and monitoring. An oxygen mask is placed and oxygen delivered at 5 L/min. An 18-gauge catheter is placed in the cephalic vein and therapy begins as another catheter is being placed in the jugular vein. External pressure is applied to the legs and caudal abdomen. Fluid options include 125 mL of 7% NaCl alone or with 1 L of lactated Ringer's solution, 500 mL of 6% of hetastarch, or 125 mL of 7% NaCl plus 500 mL of 6% hetastarch. Central venous pressure, arterial blood pressure (Doppler), and physical parameters are monitored continuously for several hours until the dog is stable. Analgesia is administered in the form of a parenteral opioid (butorphanol or oxymorphone). The coxofemoral luxation should not be addressed until the animal is adequately stabilized. Two hours later, the abdominal hemorrhage is not progressing, arterial blood pressure now is 150 mm Hg, mucous membranes are pink, capillary refill time is 2 s, and CVP has remained between 8 and 12 cm H_2O. The external pressure is slowly removed and blood pressure remains steady.

DECOMPENSATORY (TERMINAL) SHOCK AND SIRS
A 10-year-old 10-kg male schnauzer is presented after 24 h of intractable vomiting and diarrhea. The dog had eaten garbage 2 days previously. The dog is in lateral recumbency with severe abdominal pain and with a decreased level of consciousness. Physical examination shows hydration, 10% dehydrated; heart rate, 70/min; respiratory rate, 60/min; mucous membrane, pale; capillary refill time, cannot be elicited; rectal temperature, 37°C; no palpable femoral pulses; barely audible heart

sounds; severe hypotension (50 mm Hg systolic blood pressure). The dog is in decompensatory (terminal) shock and requires aggressive fluid therapy and cardiovascular support. An oxygen mask is placed and oxygen delivered at 5 L/min. Twenty-gauge catheters are placed in both cephalic veins and therapy begins as a catheter is being placed in the jugular vein. Fluid therapy includes 1 L of lactated Ringers solution as fast as can be administered via one cephalic catheter and then at twice maintenance rate and 200 mL of 6% hetastarch via the other cephalic catheter. Antibiotics, analgesia (morphine infusion), and heparin (minidose) are administered. The CVP is monitored by means of the jugular catheter and arterial blood pressure is continuously monitored or repeatedly assessed. The dog does not produce urine after initial fluid therapy, blood pressure decreases, and CVP increases. The dog may be in cardiac failure or unresponsive to fluid therapy because of decreased oncotic pressure secondary to SIRS and increased vascular permeability. Venous blood gas analysis shows a PvO_2 of 30 mm Hg. Fluid therapy is continued, 6% hetastarch (50 mL) is repeated, another hetastarch infusion (20 mL/kg/day) is begun for oncotic support, and dobutamine infusion (5 μg/kg/min) is started. One hour later, the dog begins to show a response: urine production is 3 mL/kg/h, CVP decreases, blood pressure increases, and the dog begins to respond to verbal commands.

REFERENCES

Aldrich J and Haskins SC: Monitoring the critically ill patient. In Bonagura JD (ed): *Current Veterinary Therapy XII*. Philadelphia, WB Saunders Co., p. 98, 1995.

Bishop MH, Shoemaker WC, Appel PL, et al: Influence of time and optimal circulatory resuscitation in high-risk trauma. *Crit Care Med* 21:56, 1993.

Bisonni RS, Holtgrave DR, Lawler F, et al: Colloids versus crystalloids in fluid resuscitation: An analysis of randomized controlled trials. *J Fam Pract* 32:387–390, 1991.

Bone RC, Fisher CJ Jr, Clemmer TP, et al: A controlled clinical trial of high-dose methylprednisolone in the treatment of severe sepsis and septic shock. *N Engl J Med* 317:653–658, 1987.

Brooks M: Transfusion medicine. In Murtaugh RJ and Kaplan PM (eds): *Veterinary Emergency and Critical Care Medicine*. St. Louis, Mosby Year Book, p. 543, 1992.

Concannon KT: Colloid oncotic pressure and the clinical use of colloidal solutions. *J Vet Emerg Crit Care* 3:49–62, 1993.

Crowe DT and Devey JJ: Assessment and management of the hemorrhaging patient. *Vet Clin North Am Small Anim Pract* 24:1095–1122, 1994.

Crystal MA and Cotter SM: Acute hemorrhage: A hematologic emergency in dogs. *Compend Contin Educ* 14:1, 1992.

DiBartola SP: Metabolic acidosis. In DiBartola SP (ed): *Fluid Therapy in Small Animal Practice*. Philadelphia, WB Saunders Co., p. 216, 1992.

Griffel MI and Kaufman BS: Pharmacology of colloids and crystalloids. *Crit Care Clin* 8:235–254, 1992.

Guyton AC: Transport of oxygen and carbon dioxide in the blood and body fluids. In Guyton AC (ed): *Textbook of Medical Physiology*, 8th ed. Philadelphia, WB Saunders Co., p. 433, 1991.

Hackner SG: Emergency management of traumatic pulmonary contusions. *Compend Contin Educ* 17:677–686, 1995.

Kirby R: Septic shock. In Bonagura JD (ed): *Current Veterinary Therapy XII*. WB Saunders Co., p. 139, 1995.

Kirby R and Rudloff E: The critical need for colloids: Maintaining fluid balance. *Compend Contin Educ* 19:705–719, 1997.

Klein LW: Cardiovascular therapeutics. In Parillo JE (ed): *Current Therapy in Critical Care Medicine*, 3rd ed. St. Louis, CV Mosby, p. 72, 1977.

Lutz H: Animal experiments on the effect of colloidal plasma substitutes in hemorrhagic shock in the dog. *Bibl Haematol* 33:232–247, 1969.

Marino PL: Hemorrhage and hypovolemia. In Marino PL (ed): *The ICU Book*, 2nd ed. Baltimore, Williams & Wilkins, p. 207, 1998a.

Marino PL: Colloid and crystalloid resuscitation. In Marino PL (ed): *The ICU Book*, 2nd ed. Baltimore, Williams & Wilkins, p. 228, 1998b.

Moore FD: The effects of hemorrhage on body composition. *N Engl J Med* 273:567–577, 1965.

Mueller DL and Noxon JO: Anaphylaxis: Pathophysiology and treatment. *Compend Contin Educ* 12:2, 1990.

Muir WW: Overview of shock. Proceedings of the 14th Annual Kal Kan Symposium. Emergency/Critical Care, p. 7, 1990.

Neugebauer E, Lechleuthner A, Rixen D, et al: Pharmacotherapy of shock. In Chernow B (ed): *The Pharmacologic Approach to the Critically Ill Patient*, 3rd ed. Baltimore, Williams & Wilkins, p. 1104, 1994.

Purvis D and Kirby R: Systemic inflammatory response syndrome: Septic shock. *Vet Clin North Am Small Anim Pract* 24:1225–1247, 1994.

Rainey TG and Read CA: Pharmacology of colloids and crystalloids. In Chernow B (ed): *The Pharmacologic Approach to the Critically Ill Patient*, 3rd ed. Baltimore, Williams & Wilkins, p. 272, 1994.

Rudloff E and Kirby R: Hypovolemic shock and resuscitation. *Vet Clin North Am Small Anim Pract* 24:1015–1039, 1994.

Schertel ER: Hypertonic fluid therapy. In DiBartola SP (ed): *Fluid Therapy in Small Animal Practice*. Philadelphia, WB Saunders Co., p. 471, 1992.

Schertel ER, Schneider DA, Zissimos AG, et al: Cardiopulmonary reflexes induced by osmolality changes in the airways and pulmonary vasculature. *Fed Proc* 44:835, 1985.

Shoemaker WC: Diagnosis and treatment of shock syndromes. In Shoemaker WC, Ayers S, Grenvick A, et al. (eds): *Textbook of Critical Care*, 3rd ed. Philadelphia, WB Saunders Co., pp. 85–101, 1995.

Shoemaker WC and Kram HB: Comparison of the effects of crystalloids and colloids on hemodynamic oxygen transport, mortality and morbidity. In Simmon RS and Udeko AJ (eds): *Debates in General Surgery*. Chicago, Year Book Medical Publishers, 1991.

Shoemaker WC, Appel PL, Kram HB, et al: Temporal hemodynamics and oxygen transport patterns in medical patients with sepsis and septic shock. *Chest* 104:1529, 1993a.

Shoemaker WC, Appel PL, Kram HB, et al: Sequence of physiologic patterns in surgical septic shock. *Crit Care Med* 21:1876, 1993b.

Shores T, Carrico J, and Lightfoot S: Fluid therapy in hemorrhagic shock. *Arch Surg* 88:688–693, 1964.

Snyder JV and Carroll GC: Tissue oxygenation: A physiological approach to a clinical problem. *Curr Probl Surg* 19:650–719, 1982.

Tobias TA and Schertel ER: Shock. In DiBartola SP (ed): *Fluid Therapy in Small Animal Practice*. Philadelphia, WB Saunders Co., p. 436, 1992.

Tuchshmidt J, Fried J, Astiz M, et al: Supranormal oxygen delivery improves mortality in septic shock patients. *Chest* 102:216–220, 1992.

Veterans Administration Systemic Sepsis Cooperative Group: Effect of high-dose glucocorticoid therapy on mortality in patients with clinical signs of systemic sepsis. *N Engl J Med* 317:659–665, 1987.

Ware WA: Shock. In Murtaugh RJ and Kaplan PM (eds): *Veterinary Emergency and Critical Care Medicine*. St. Louis, Mosby Year Book, p. 163, 1992.

Special Therapy

SECTION 5

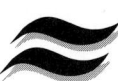

CHAPTER 21

Blood Transfusions and Blood Substitutes

ANN E. HOHENHAUS   VIRGINIA RENTKO

At first glance, a chapter describing blood transfusion and blood substitutes may seem out of place in a textbook on fluid therapy, but there are many similarities between fluids, such as lactated Ringer's solution, and blood. Like crystalloid and colloid solutions, blood products are not used to treat disease; they are supportive therapies given to correct deficiencies in the patient until the underlying disease process can be treated. For example, a red blood cell transfusion is given to replace red blood cells lost because of a traumatic laceration. The transfusion of red blood cells increases the oxygen-carrying capacity of the blood, allowing surgical repair of the laceration; it is not the primary treatment for hemorrhage.

Both blood transfusions and fluid therapy must be carefully assessed before inclusion in a treatment plan. Both can cause volume overload and electrolyte disturbances and can transmit infection if the solution becomes contaminated with a pathogenic microbe (Yaphe et al. 1993; Killen et al. 1971; Freeman et al. 1994). Before using either crystalloid solutions or blood products, the veterinarian should assess the risk-to-benefit ratio for the recipient. Despite the potential negative effects of transfusion, most veterinarians view it as lifesaving therapy that allows the transfusion recipient to receive other necessary treatments such as surgery, chemotherapy, or medical care (Howard et al. 1992).

The three major differences between crystalloid and colloid solutions and blood products are their immunogenicity, availability, and cost. The immunogenicity of blood products stems from the proteins and cellular material in the blood. Because crystalloid solutions lack proteins and cellular material, they are not considered immunogenic; however, certain colloid solutions such as hydroxyethyl starch have been reported to cause acute anaphylaxis in rare instances in human beings (Ring and Messmer 1977). The mechanism of this reaction is unknown.

Crystalloid and colloid solutions are readily available because they can be manufactured according to market demand. Blood products can be produced only by a living animal, and production is limited to the donor's physiologic capability to produce blood. Availability of blood for transfusion is further limited by the small number of commercial canine and feline blood banks that provide a convenient source of blood for the veterinary practitioner (Table 21–1). Furthermore, blood products require a more regulated storage environment and have a significantly shorter shelf life than crystalloid or colloid solutions, making blood a less convenient product to stock and use in a veterinary hospital.

The actual costs associated with canine blood transfusions are not known, but veterinarians estimate the cost of a transfusion of 500 mL of whole blood to range from $25 to more than $300 (Howard et al. 1992). The cost of 500 mL of lactated Ringer's solution is less than a dollar.

Despite the fact that the first documented transfusion was given to a dog in 1665 by Richard Lower at Oxford University, veterinary transfusion medicine scientifically and technologically lags behind its counterpart in human medicine (Lower 1989). Information in this chapter is based on animal studies whenever possible. When none is available, currently accepted guidelines in human medicine are applied to the veterinary patient. The purpose of this chapter is to provide the reader with:

1. A basic understanding of the theory of blood component therapy
2. Information on the technical aspects of obtaining blood for transfusion
3. Suggestions for the administration and monitoring of transfusions
4. A description of a recently approved blood substitute for use in dogs

▶ Basics of Blood Components

The best way to preserve and store blood for transfusion is to separate whole blood into its component parts. Appropriate use of blood components not only conserves the products but also allows the most specific and safe product to be used for each animal. When blood components are used instead of whole blood for transfusion, two dogs can benefit from 1 unit of whole blood. For example, a plasma transfusion can counteract the anticoagulant effects of rodenticide intoxication in one dog

TABLE 21-1.	Veterinary Blood Banks
Animal Blood Bank PO Box 1118 Dixon, CA 95620 800 243-5759	Hemopet 938 Stanford Street Santa Monica, CA 90403 310 828-4804
"Buddies for Life" Canine Blood Bank 1940 South Telegraph Road Bloomfield Hills, MI 48302-0245 248 334-6877	Midwest Animal Blood Services 120 East Main Street Stockbridge, MI 49285 517 851-8244
Eastern Veterinary Blood Bank 2138-B Generals Highway Annapolis, MD 21401 800 949-3822	Penn Animal Blood Bank Veterinary Hospital of the University of Pennsylvania 3850 Spruce Street Philadelphia, PA 19104 215 573-PABB

while blood cells from the same donor can provide enhanced oxygen-carrying capacity for a second, anemic dog. Component transfusions also have been used in cats, although preparation of components is more difficult because of the small volume of blood collected from donor cats (Henson et al. 1994; Schneider 1995).

Veterinarians must become familiar with the use of blood components, because blood components are the predominant products available through commercial blood banks. Component therapy requires planning to acquire and coordinate the equipment and donors for successful blood collection. Preparation of blood components from whole blood requires that the blood from the donor be collected into the anticoagulant-containing bag of a multibag plastic blood collection system. The whole blood then is separated into packed red blood cells and plasma by differential centrifugation and the plasma transferred into one or more of the satellite bags via the sterile tubing linking the bags. The bags are separated, and packed red blood cells are stored in a refrigerator while plasma is frozen. Blood collected into glass bottles is not amenable to centrifugation and cannot be processed into components. In addition, storage of blood in a glass bottle results in lower concentrations of 2,3-diphosphoglycerate and ATP than storage of blood in plastic bags (Eisenbrandt and Smith 1973a). Most general practitioners do not have access to the type of centrifuge required for proper separation of blood into components. It is possible to acquire a used centrifuge or request the local blood bank to process the blood collected by the veterinarian. However, production of components is not feasible for most veterinarians. The technical aspects of component production are not included in this chapter but can be found elsewhere (Schneider 1995; Mooney 1992).

The most commonly used blood products and their indications and suggested dosages are described below. The dosage of a blood product depends on the physical state of the patient and the response of the patient to the treatment; in essence, the treatment is "to effect." Too much blood has been transfused if the patient becomes polycythemic or develops volume overload. No maximal dose has been defined.

Whole Blood

Whole blood is the blood collected from the donor plus the anticoagulant. No standards have been established for the volume of blood that constitutes 1 unit. When a human blood collection system is used for dogs, 450 ± 45 mL of blood plus 63 mL of anticoagulant is collected and often is designated as 1 unit. Whole blood contains red blood cells, clotting factors, proteins, and platelets and is the product most commonly transfused into dogs and cats (Howard et al. 1992). As a starting point, the dosage for whole blood is 10 to 22 mL/kg.

Packed Red Blood Cells

Packed red blood cells are the cells and a small amount of plasma and anticoagulant that remains after the plasma is removed from 1 unit of whole blood. If 450 mL of blood is collected, the volume of packed red blood cells obtained is approximately 200 mL. Because the plasma has been removed, the total volume transfused is less than 1 unit of whole blood but has the same oxygen-carrying capacity as 1 unit of whole blood. Packed red blood cells are used only to treat anemia because they do not contain significant numbers of platelets or clotting factors. The initial dosage of packed red blood cells is 6 to 10 mL/kg.

Fresh Frozen Plasma

Fresh frozen plasma is the plasma obtained from 1 unit of whole blood plus the anticoagulant. It contains all clotting factors, which, if frozen at −30°C, maintain activity for 1 year. The albumin is preserved at that temperature for 5 years. When stored at −30°C, the plastic storage bag becomes brittle and if not carefully handled can crack, rendering the plasma unusable. For this reason, plasma is stored in special boxes to protect the plastic bag and must be handled carefully before transfusion (Fig. 21–1). Fresh frozen plasma can be used to treat a congenital deficiency of clotting factors such as von Willebrand's disease or hemophilia A and B. Acquired coagulopathies such as rodenticide intoxication, liver disease coagulopathy, and disseminated intravascular coagulation resulting in hemorrhage are treated with fresh frozen plasma. Fresh frozen plasma should not be used as a source of albumin, for volume expansion, or for nutritional support (National Institutes of Health 1985). Calculations suggest that plasma would need to be given at a dosage of 45 mL/kg to increase the albumin concentration by 1 g/dL, making plasma treatment for hypoalbuminemia cost prohibitive (Wardrop 1997). Plasma should be given to effect, which, in the case of coagulopathies, is until active bleeding ceases (Kristensen 1995). For the treatment of coagulation disorders, 6 to 10 mL/kg is the recommended starting dosage. Multiple doses may be required to control bleeding because of the short half-life of clotting factors.

Cryoprecipitate

Cryoprecipitate is prepared from fresh frozen plasma by thawing the plasma at 0 to 6°C. A white precipitate forms

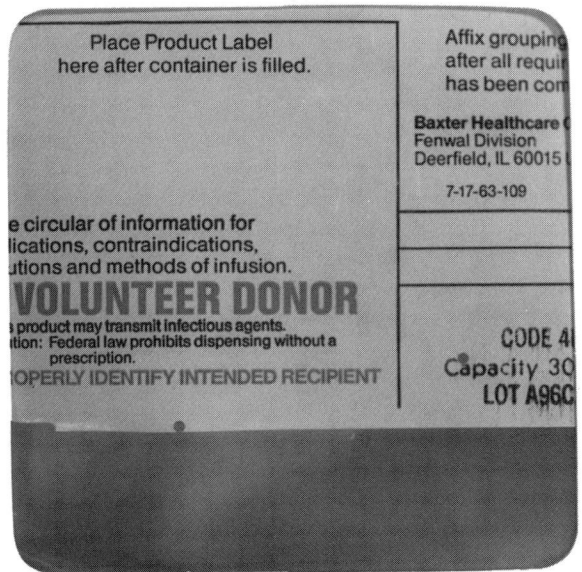

FIGURE 21-1. A typical box for protecting fresh frozen plasma stored in plastic bags. (Courtesy of Baxter Healthcare, Deerfield, IL.)

and the plasma is removed after centrifugation and saved as cryo-poor plasma. The remaining cryoprecipitate is considered 1 unit of cryoprecipitate and is a concentrated source of von Willebrand's factor, fibrinogen, and factors XIII and VIII (antihemophilia factor). It is useful in the treatment of deficiencies of these clotting factors and is handled in the same manner as fresh frozen plasma. Cryoprecipitate may be the blood product of choice for the treatment of von Willebrand's disease, because the larger, more hemostatically active von Willebrand's multimers are concentrated into a smaller volume than in fresh frozen plasma (Ching et al. 1994). The dosage is 1 unit per 10 kg body weight (Meyers et al. 1992).

Platelet-Rich Plasma and Platelet Concentrate

Platelet-containing components are prepared from fresh whole blood by centrifugation at a slower rate than is used for production of packed red blood cells and plasma (Mooney 1992). The platelets are suspended in plasma to facilitate transfusion. Storage and shipping of platelets are impractical because they require a temperature of 20 to 24°C, special plastic bags, and continuous agitation (Allyson et al. 1997). Transfused platelets have been shown to be rapidly destroyed in human patients with immune-mediated thrombocytopenia and, because immune-mediated thrombocytopenia is a common cause of profound thrombocytopenia in dogs, most cases of thrombocytopenia-mediated hemorrhage are not amenable to successful platelet transfusion. If a platelet transfusion is given, the dosage is the platelets collected from 1 unit of whole blood per 10 kg body weight.

▶ Sources of Blood and Blood Products for Transfusion

The most convenient source of blood for a veterinary clinic is a commercial blood bank. Currently, there are only a few commercial veterinary blood banks in the United States, and they cannot adequately supply all of the small animal practices in the country with blood (see Table 21-1). Moreover, only one of the blood banks is currently supplying cat blood (Midwest Blood Services). Veterinary school blood donor programs may serve as an additional source of blood for the practitioner (Howard et al. 1992). Most small animal practitioners borrow a donor from an employee or maintain a blood donor on the premises (Howard et al. 1992). Borrowing a donor from either an employee or a client is a frequently used, if less convenient, option and is less expensive than maintaining an in-hospital donor.

Maintaining donors on the premises is advantageous because they are readily available for donation and their health status and disease exposure can be controlled, but the expense associated with feeding, housing, and caring for a blood donor is significant (Hohenhaus 1992). At Tufts University, the cost of annual housing and maintenance for a blood donor cat for 1 year was estimated as between $1200 and $1500 (Bucheler and Cotter 1993). In addition, the donor occupies space that could be used for client-owned animals, an important consideration for a clinic with limited cage space. Some institutions have instituted outpatient blood donor programs (Bucheler and Cotter 1992). Donors are recruited from clients or employees. Collecting blood from stray animals may be unsafe, because infectious disease exposure and vaccination status are unknown, and this practice may be considered unethical.

▶ Blood Donor Selection

Identification of donor dogs and cats before blood is needed is essential to allow blood type to be determined and health status of the donor to be assessed before blood collection, thus ensuring the safety of the blood being transfused.

Dogs

More than 40 years ago, the best blood donor was believed to be a large, quiet dog so that anesthesia would not be necessary during blood collection (Majilton and Kelley 1951). This belief has not changed. A canine blood donor should be big enough to donate 450 mL (1 unit) of blood safely in one donation. Donating that volume of blood allows collection into commercially manufactured blood collection bags designed to facilitate sterile processing of components. Dogs weighing ≥27 kg have donated 1 unit of blood for 2 years at 3-week intervals (Potkay and Zinn 1969). Dogs selected as donors also should have an easily accessible jugular vein to facilitate venipuncture.

Greyhounds have been promoted as ideal blood donors because of their gentle disposition, high hematocrits, and lean body type, which simplifies blood collection (Green 1982). Many greyhounds are euthanized because of poor racing performance, and these dogs are available from racetracks, breeders, and rescue organizations (Giger 1993).

Veterinarians choosing greyhounds as blood donors should be aware of certain breed idiosyncrasies that affect the management of a greyhound donor. The greyhound idiosyncrasies most important in transfusion medicine are the high red blood cell count, packed cell volume, and hemoglobin concentration and low white blood cell and platelet counts compared with those of mixed-breed dogs (Porter and Canaday 1971; Sullivan et al. 1994). A syndrome of multifocal skin ulceration often accompanied by limb edema or acute renal failure has been reported in young adult greyhounds, and we have seen the skin ulceration form of this disease in greyhound blood donors (Carpenter et al. 1988). This syndrome is known as cutaneous and renal glomerular vasculopathy of greyhounds and has been called "Alabama rot" at the racetrack (Cowan et al. 1997). No infectious agents were identified in a group of 18 dogs with cutaneous and renal glomerular vasculopathy, and dogs developing azotemia had a poorer prognosis than those without azotemia. Because the etiology of this disease is unknown, donation should be postponed during an episode of vasculopathy. Greyhounds in Florida have a seroprevalence of babesiosis of 46% (Taboada et al. 1992). Because the origin of greyhounds obtained as blood donors cannot always be determined, all greyhounds being considered as donors should have serologic testing for *Babesia* performed and dogs with positive titers should be excluded as donors.

Although 13 canine blood groups or blood type systems have been described, only 8 groups are recognized as international standards, and typing sera are available for only 6 types (Table 21–2). Red blood cells can be negative or positive for a given blood type, except for the DEA 1 system, which has three subtypes, dog erythrocyte antigen (DEA) 1.1, 1.2, and 1.3. Canine red blood cells can be negative for all three subtypes (a DEA 1–negative blood type) or positive for any one of the three subtypes. Naturally occurring alloantibodies that cause serologic incompatibility without prior sensitization by transfusion do not appear to cause transfusion incompatibility in the dog.

The blood type of the ideal canine blood donor currently is in dispute. Among the six blood groups for which typing sera are available, a transfusion reaction has been attributed to antibody against DEA 1.1 induced by a DEA 1.1–positive transfusion in a DEA 1.1–negative recipient (Giger et al. 1995). In theory, red blood cells expressing

TABLE 21–2. **Blood Types in Dogs and Cats for Which Typing Antisera Currently Exist**

Dogs	
Dog erythrocyte antigen (DEA)	1.1, 1.2
	3
	4
	5
	7
Cats	
Type	A
	B
	AB

DEA 1.2 can sensitize a DEA 1.2–negative transfusion recipient, resulting in an acute hemolytic transfusion reaction if a second transfusion of DEA 1.2–positive blood is given. In a laboratory setting, antibodies against DEA 1.2 have been reported to cause transfusion reactions, but clinical reports of hemolytic transfusion reactions mediated by anti–DEA 1.2 antibodies are lacking. Approximately 45% of dog red blood cells are positive for DEA 7. Dog erythrocyte antigen 7 is believed to be structurally related to an antigen found in common bacteria. A naturally occurring antibody against DEA 7 has been described in 20 to 50% of DEA 7–negative dogs, and may result in accelerated removal of DEA 7–positive cells from a DEA-negative donor with anti–DEA 7 antibodies (Smith 1991). On the basis of this information, the recommendation has been made to select donors that are negative for DEA 1.1, 1.2, and 7. Others suggest that the donor dog also have red blood cells positive for DEA 4 to be designated a universal donor (Hale 1995). The importance of DEA 3 and 5 in blood donor selection remains to be determined.

One other feature that should be considered before selecting a dog as a blood donor is the dog's plasma von Willebrand factor concentration. Von Willebrand's disease is the most common inherited coagulopathy in dogs and has been reported in many breeds of dogs and in dogs of mixed breeding as well. Because of the high frequency of this disease in the canine population, a canine blood donor is likely to be used to transfuse a dog with von Willebrand's disease–induced hemorrhage, and a donor with a normal concentration of von Willebrand's factor is essential to provide that deficient coagulation factor.

Cats

The physical requirements for a feline blood donor are similar to those for a canine donor. The ideal feline donor is a large cat, more than 5 kg in body weight, with a pleasant disposition. Easily accessible jugular veins facilitate collection of blood, and choosing a shorthaired cat decreases the clipping required before phlebotomy. We prefer to avoid brachycephalic cats as donors because they seem to require greater skill in venipuncture.

It is essential to determine the blood type of potential donors. Only one feline blood group system has been identified with three blood types: A, B, and AB (Auer and Bell 1981). Unlike dogs, cats have naturally occurring alloantibodies against type A or type B cells (Giger and Bucheler 1991). Cats of blood type B have strong hemagglutinating antibodies of the immunoglobulin M (IgM) type against type A cells, and cats of blood type A have weak hemolysin and hemagglutinating antibodies of the IgM and IgG types against type B cells. The clinical significance of these alloantibodies is threefold. First and most important, a cat may have a transfusion reaction without sensitization from a previous transfusion; second, type A kittens born to a type B queen are at risk for neonatal isoerythrolysis (Casal et al. 1996); and third, the antibodies are useful in determining the blood type of a cat.

Donors of both type A and type B blood must be available so that compatible transfusions can be provided. Incompatible transfusions result in shortened red blood cell survival in the transfusion recipient and, potentially, death; therefore, the serologic compatibility between recipient and donor must be determined before every transfusion in cats (Giger and Bucheler 1991). Donors of type A blood are easy to find, because over 99% of the domestic cats in the United States are type A (Auer and Bell 1981). The prevalence of domestic cats with type B blood varies geographically. In the United States, the western states have the highest percentage of type B cats, 4 to 6% (Giger et al. 1991b). Australia has the highest reported percentage of type B cats in their domestic cat population, 73%. In Europe, the frequency of blood type B in domestic cats varies from 0% in Finland to 14.9% in France (Giger et al. 1993). Some purebred cats have a higher frequency of type B individuals in their population (Giger et al. 1991a). The British shorthair and the Devon rex have been reported to have the highest proportion of type B individuals, approximately 50%. The Siamese, Oriental shorthair, Burmese, Tonkinese, American shorthair, and Norwegian forest cat breeds have not been reported to have any members with type B blood. Blood type AB is extremely rare, occurring in 0.14% of cats in the United States and Canada (Griot-Wenk et al. 1996). Fortunately, a type AB donor is not required for successful transfusion of a type AB cat. Blood from a type A cat is adequate.

▶ Blood Donor Health Maintenance

A safe blood supply begins with healthy blood donors. All blood donors should undergo a complete physical examination, complete and differential blood count, biochemical profile, and fecal examination yearly. Recommended vaccinations for canine donors include distemper, hepatitis, parainfluenza, parvovirus, and rabies. In addition to rabies vaccinations, feline donors need vaccinations against rhinotracheitis, calicivirus, and panleukopenia. Because the ideal feline blood donor lives in a closed environment and is not exposed to other cats, the authors believe vaccinations against feline leukemia virus (FeLV) and feline infectious peritonitis (FIP) vaccines are unnecessary in donor cats.

▶ Blood Donor Screening

Screening blood donors for infectious diseases transmitted via blood transfusion is an integral part of maintaining a safe blood supply. Infectious disease screening of canine blood donors varies within the various geographic regions of the United States. All donor dogs should be tested annually for heartworms and treated with heartworm preventative on the schedule recommended for pet dogs in the region. *Babesia canis* and *Haemobartonella canis* have been reportedly transmitted to a dog by blood transfusion (Freeman et al. 1994; Lester et al. 1995). Donor dogs should have negative *B. canis* titers, but splenectomy of donor dogs to facilitate identification of *B. canis* and *H. canis* carriers is controversial. Serologic testing for *Brucella canis* may be useful in eliminating dogs with brucellosis, especially dogs with unknown breeding history. Dirofilariasis, ehrlichiosis, and trypanosomiasis can be transmitted via transfusion; consequently, donors should have negative titers to these infectious agents. Transfusion-transmitted borreliosis has not been documented in humans but could theoretically occur. Dogs should not donate if they are ill or have a fever, vomiting, or diarrhea. Using donors with these signs has resulted in *Yersinia enterocolitica* contamination of units of human blood (Galloway and Jones 1986).

Outdoor cats should not be used as blood donors, because most infectious diseases potentially transmitted to cats via transfusion can be prevented by confining cats indoors. Potential donor cats should be screened for FeLV, feline immunodeficiency virus (FIV), and certain other feline infectious agents. Because FeLV infection can take up to 3 months to become patent, cats being considered as donors should be screened monthly for FeLV for three consecutive months. Testing for FIV antibodies can be performed simultaneously. *Bartonella henselae* has been transmitted to cats via infected blood (Kordick and Breitschwerdt 1997). Cats with positive cultures for *B. henselae* should not be used as blood donors. Because fleas are the vector of *B. henselae*, flea control is essential in donor cats. Cats that are infected with *Haemobartonella felis* also should be eliminated from the donor pool. Screening of donor cats for feline infectious peritonitis (FIP) is problematic, because there is no reliable test to differentiate the FIP virus from the enteric coronavirus.

▶ Equipment and Supplies for Collection of Blood

Skin Preparation

Strict aseptic technique must be used during the collection process to prevent contamination of blood. Solutions and equipment used for the collection process should be single-use products whenever possible to prevent inadvertent contamination of blood (Hohenhaus et al. 1997). After clipping the hair over the venipuncture site, the skin is scrubbed. The ideal skin preparation regimen for animals is yet to be determined, but in human blood donors a 30-s, 70% isopropyl scrub followed by a 2% iodine tincture resulted in better skin surface disinfection than alcohol followed by chlorhexidine or green soap (Goldman et al. 1997). Venipuncture is accomplished without touching the scrubbed area.

Anticoagulant Solutions

Several different solutions are available to anticoagulate and preserve blood for transfusion (Table 21–3). Anticoagulants provide no nutrients to preserve red cell metabolism during storage. Anticoagulant-preservative solutions have been designed to provide nutrients to maintain red blood cell function during storage. The most common anticoagulant solution for preservation of canine red blood cells is citrate phosphate dextrose adenine (CPDA-1), because it is the solution found in commercially prepared, multiple-bag systems. It can be withdrawn from the injection port via syringe and used in the storage of feline red blood cells collected in a syringe. Maximal storage time for feline blood has yet to be determined but may be as long as 35 days (Buchler and Cotter 1994). Acid/citrate/dextrose or anticoagulant/citrate/dextrose (ACD) formula B can be used to store either canine or feline blood (Eisenbrandt and Smith 1973; Marion and Smith 1983). Additive solutions are added to packed red blood cells after the plasma is removed. Additive solutions that have been evaluated in dogs are Adsol (Fenwal Laboratories, Baxter Health Care Corporation, Deerfield, IL) and Nutricel (Miles Pharmaceutical Division, West Haven, CT) (Wardrop et al. 1994, 1997b). Storage times for canine red blood cells with these solutions are approximately 5 weeks. Additive solutions have not been evaluated using feline blood.

Collection of Blood from Dogs

Dogs that have not donated blood before may require sedation, whereas dogs that have donated one or more times often do not. If sedation is necessary, we prefer butorphanol (0.1 mg/kg, IV, 10 to 15 min before the donation). This calms the donor but does not induce lateral recumbency. Some prefer to collect blood from dogs in lateral recumbency, especially if the femoral artery is used (Schneider 1995). The choice is strictly a matter of personal preference and skill. Acepromazine is not recommended for sedation because it causes hypotension and platelet dysfunction.

The flow of blood into the bag can occur via gravity or by suction. Blood collected by suction does not have a greater rate of hemolysis than that collected by gravity flow and it can be collected more rapidly (Eibert and Lewis 1997). Suction collection of blood is facilitated by a device (Vacuum Chamber) manufactured by the Animal Blood Bank (Dixon, CA). This device requires an external vacuum source during collection of blood.

Collection of Blood from Cats

It is unusual to find a feline blood donor that does not require sedation during blood donation. We prefer a combination of ketamine (10 mg) and diazepam (0.5 mg) administered IV for cats. Other protocols using midazolam and isoflurane have been described (Schneider 1995). If the sedative agent is to be given IV, a peripheral vein (cephalic or medial saphenous) should be used to preserve the jugular veins for blood collection.

No system is available commercially that is adequate for the collection of blood from cats because of the small volume of blood that can safely be withdrawn from a cat. Typically, anticoagulant is placed in one or two large syringes (25–60 mL), depending on the volume of blood to be collected (see Table 21–3). A large (19-gauge) butterfly needle is used for jugular venipuncture so that if a second syringe of blood is to be collected, the full syringe can be removed and the second syringe connected without a second venipuncture. By the definition of the American Association of Blood Banks, this is an "open" system, and blood collected in this manner should not be transfused more than 24 h after collection (Walker 1993). A closed system has been described for the collection of blood from cats (Price 1991). A commercially available vacuum system can be used for collecting blood from cats, but some authors find this system less satisfactory than the syringe method (Schneider 1995; Kaufman 1992).

▶ Administration of Blood and Plasma

Careful attention should be paid to the unit of blood before transfusion. The most common reason for an acute hemolytic transfusion reaction in human patients is clerical error—the wrong unit of blood is released from the blood bank or a unit of blood is given to a patient who was not intended to receive a transfusion (Szama 1990). In veterinary medicine, it is crucial to confirm that the blood comes from the correct species in addition to being typed and matched to the patient requiring a transfusion. Also, red blood cells in the bag should be examined for a normal red color and consistency. Bacterially contaminated blood often appears brown because of the forma-

TABLE 21–3. Anticoagulants and Preservatives for Blood

Canine Blood		
Anticoagulant	Ratio with blood	Storage time at 0–6°C
Heparin	625 U/50 mL blood	For immediate transfusion
3.8% sodium citrate	1 mL/9 mL blood	For immediate transfusion
Anticoagulant-preservative	Ratio with blood	Storage time at 0–6°C
CPDA-1	1 mL/7 mL blood	20 days
ACD "B"	1 mL/7–9 mL blood	21 days
Additive solutions	100 mL/250 mL packed red blood cells	37–42 days
Feline Blood		
Anticoagulant	Ratio with blood	Storage time at 0–6°C
Heparin	625 U/50 mL blood	For immediate transfusion
3.8% sodium citrate	1 mL/9 mL blood	For immediate transfusion
Anticoagulant-preservative	Ratio with blood	Storage time at 0–6°C
ACD "B"	1 mL/7–9 mL blood	30 days
Additive solutions		Not evaluated

tion of methemoglobin, deoxygenation, and hemolysis (Hohenhaus et al. 1997).

Blood and plasma can be administered via several routes. Most commonly, blood is given intravenously. The diameter of the catheter used for transfusion is important in determining the rate of blood flow, because blood flows more slowly through a small catheter; however, small-diameter catheters have not been associated with increased risk of hemolysis during transfusion (Walker 1993).

The intraosseous route can be used successfully for administration of blood and plasma (Otto et al. 1989). In normal dogs, 93 to 98% of red blood cells administered through an intraosseous catheter are found in the peripheral circulation within 5 min (Clark and Woodley 1959). This rapid and simple method is especially useful for animals with vascular collapse and extremely young puppies and kittens. Special intraosseous catheters are available, but a spinal needle, bone marrow aspiration needle, over-the-needle catheter, and even an ordinary hypodermic needle can be used. Sites for the placement of the intraosseous catheter include the trochanteric fossa of the femur, the medial tibia, and the iliac crest. Blood flows rapidly through an intraosseous catheter, and rate of administration should be monitored closely. Plasma can be administered intraperitoneally in emergency situations, but red blood cells are slowly and poorly absorbed via this route, and it is not recommended for red blood cell transfusions.

A blood transfusion administration set should be used for any transfusion of blood or component, because the incorporated filter removes blood clots and debris that could cause embolism. The filter typically used in veterinary medicine is 170 μm in size. For small-volume transfusions, an 18-μm filter that can be attached to intravenous tubing is useful. A blood administration set does not remove air from stored blood, and although glass bottles are convenient blood collection systems because they do not require an extrinsic vacuum source, the risk of air embolism is increased when blood is collected into glass bottles.

The American Association of Blood Banks is explicit in stating that no medications may be added to blood or component (Walker 1993). In addition, no fluid should be added to blood except 0.9% sodium chloride when it is necessary to decrease the viscosity of packed red blood cells. Fluids containing calcium such as lactated Ringer's solution may overcome the anticoagulant properties of citrate, resulting in coagulation of the blood. Solutions such as 5% dextrose in water are hypotonic and may induce hemolysis.

The recommended rate of transfusion of red blood cells depends on the status of the recipient. In massive hemorrhage, the transfusion should be given as rapidly as possible. In a normovolemic, stable transfusion recipient, some clinicians recommend a rate of 0.25 mL/kg for the first 30 min, after which the rate is increased if no reaction is seen (Turnwald and Pichler 1985). In patients with heart disease, a rate of 4 mL/kg/h should not be exceeded (Green 1982). Plasma can be given more rapidly (4–6 mL/min) (Killingworth 1984). Whatever the rate chosen, it should be rapid enough to complete the transfusion within 4 h of initiation because of the risk of bacterial growth in blood maintained at room temperature for a prolonged period.

Control of delivery rate can be accomplished by use of infusion pumps to deliver a preset volume over a specific period of time. The use of infusion pumps must be limited to devices approved for use with blood, because some infusion pumps can result in hemolysis of red blood cells as a result of excessive pressure. Blood can be pumped at a rate of 50, 100, or 200 mL/h using the IVAC 530 pump without significant hemolysis (Stiles and Raffe 1991).

Because blood and plasma are stored in a refrigerator or freezer, warming of blood before transfusion has been recommended to prevent hypothermia in the transfusion recipient. Warming of blood is probably necessary only if a large volume of blood is to be given or the recipient is a neonate. For adult animals receiving a single unit of blood, the blood can be administered directly from the refrigerator. Warming blood has the potential for excessive heating, causing red blood cell membrane damage and hemolysis or bacterial growth if contamination is present. Blood warming devices that employ dry heat, radiowaves, microwaves, or electromagnetic energy are available, but cost often is prohibitive. Refrigerated human blood can be warmed quickly by mixing it with warm (45–60°C) 0.9% saline in a 1:1 ratio without damage to red blood cells (Iserson and Huestis 1991). This method has not been tested for dogs or cats. Once blood is warmed to 37°C, it deteriorates rapidly and, if not used, should be discarded. Fresh frozen plasma must be thawed before transfusion. A method for thawing canine fresh frozen plasma in a microwave oven has been described, but we have found this unsatisfactory because of uneven heating by household microwave ovens (Hurst et al. 1987). Plasma can be thawed at room temperature; if the thawing time needs to be shortened, the plasma can be placed into a plastic bag and thawed in a 37°C water bath. The plastic bag is necessary to prevent contamination of the infusion ports in the water bath. Plasma should be used within 4 h of thawing.

Because blood does not contain any antibacterial agents, it must be refrigerated until used. If the clinical status of the animal requires that the transfusion be given more slowly, the blood can be split into smaller units with a transfer bag. One portion is transfused while the other is returned to the refrigerator until the first half of the transfusion is completed. In patients with cardiac disease that are at risk for volume overload, the risk can be minimized by use of packed red blood cells, which require infusion of a smaller volume than whole blood. Diuretics can be administered before transfusion to decrease intravascular volume in cardiac patients.

Transfusion recipients should be monitored during transfusion to allow early detection of a transfusion reaction. Rectal temperature, heart rate, and respiratory rate should be recorded every 10 min during the first 30 min and every 30 min thereafter. The patient should be monitored for vomiting, diarrhea, urticaria, and hemoglobinuria or hemoglobinemia. Changes in vital signs or clinical status may indicate a transfusion reaction. Patients developing volume overload become tachypneic or dyspneic and tachycardic. In patients receiving large transfusions (≥ one blood volume in 24 h) of stored blood, serum potassium and calcium concentrations should be monitored frequently to detect hyperkalemia or hypocalcemia.

▶ Transfusion Reactions

Definition

A transfusion reaction consists of the range of immunologic and metabolic changes that occur during or after administration of a blood product. Four classes of transfusion reactions have been described (Table 21–4). Acute transfusion reactions occur during or within a few hours after a transfusion, and delayed transfusion reactions occur after the completion of the transfusion. The delay may be months to years. The classic transfusion reaction, or the acute hemolytic transfusion reaction caused by transfusion of incompatible red blood cells, is an example of an acute immunologic transfusion reaction. The three other classes of transfusion reactions are acute nonimmunologic, delayed immunologic, and delayed nonimmunologic. Reports describing transfusion reactions in dogs and cats are limited. (Freeman et al. 1994; Henson et al. 1994; Wardrop 1997; Giger et al. 1991; Lester et al. 1995; Giger and Akol 1990; Auer and Bell 1982; Yuile et al. 1948; Wardrop et al. 1997a; Giger et al. 1995).

Acute Immunologic Transfusion Reactions

Acute immunologic transfusion reactions occur because antibodies that elicit an immune response are present in the plasma of either the donor or recipient. The sequelae of an acute immunologic transfusion reaction are rapid, often irreversible, and sometimes fatal. Current theories of the pathogenesis of acute hemolytic transfusion reaction in humans propose that hemolysis induces the release of cytokines such as tumor necrosis factor, interleukin-1, -6, and -8, complement, endothelium-derived relaxing factor (nitric oxide), and endothelin, which result in the clinical syndrome of disseminated intravascular coagulation, shock, and acute renal failure (Capon and Goldfinder 1995). The pathophysiology of acute hemolytic transfusion reaction in dogs and cats must differ in some manner from that described in human beings, because acute renal failure is not reported to be a feature in dogs and cats (Giger et al. 1995; Giger and Akol 1990; Auer and Bell 1982; Yuile et al. 1948).

The best example of an acute hemolytic transfusion reaction in veterinary medicine occurs when type A red blood cells are administered to a type B cat. In the recipient cat, naturally occurring alloantibodies and complement bind to the transfused red blood cells and cause hemolysis. Clinical signs described in cats having an acute hemolytic transfusion reaction include fever, vomiting, lethargy, and icterus (Auer and Bell 1982). Laboratory testing often identifies a positive Coombs' test, rapidly declining packed cell volume, and rising serum bilirubin concentration.

Dogs having an acute hemolytic transfusion reaction show clinical signs similar but not identical to those observed in cats. Most affected dogs exhibit fever, restlessness, salivation, incontinence, and vomiting. Some dogs develop shock, and an occasional dog experiences acute death. Plasma and urine hemoglobin concentrations increase within minutes of transfusion. Incompatible cells are reported to be cleared from the circulation in less than 2 h. Dogs of blood type DEA 1.1–negative that have previously been sensitized by a transfusion of DEA 1.1–positive cells are at greatest risk for an acute hemolytic transfusion reaction (Giger et al. 1995).

Other acute immunologic transfusion reactions reported in dogs and cats include nonhemolytic fever and urticaria (Henson et al. 1994; Wardrop 1997; Callan et al. 1996). In human beings, nonhemolytic fever is due to antibodies to donor white blood cells and urticaria occurs as a result of antibodies to donor plasma proteins. Urticaria is the most common reaction to plasma transfusion (Wardrop 1997).

Delayed Immunologic Transfusion Reactions

Delayed immunologic transfusion reactions are classified as delayed hemolysis, transfusion-induced immunosuppression, posttransfusion purpura, and graft-versus-host disease. These reactions are not preventable by crossmatching or blood typing. Delayed hemolytic transfusion reactions invariably occur in persons who have been previously sensitized to allogeneic red blood cell antigens by transfusion or pregnancy. Even though compatible blood is given to a patient, the recipient may develop antibodies against any one of the hundreds of red blood cell antigens present on the transfused cells. An amnestic response to the antigens on the transfused red blood cells results in a delayed hemolytic transfusion reaction that occurs 7 to 10 days after a transfusion and is a well-described complication of red cell transfusion in humans. It has not been reported in dogs, but there is no reason it could not occur. Fever is the most common sign of a delayed hemolytic transfusion reaction in humans. Icterus also may be noticed 4 to 7 days after a transfusion.

Posttransfusion purpura has been described (Wardrop et al. 1997a) in a dog with hemophilia A that had previously received a transfusion. Five to 8 days after subsequent transfusions, thrombocytopenia and petechiation were evident. Blood collected during a thrombocytopenic

TABLE 21–4. **Classification of Transfusion Reactions**

Acute immunologic	Delayed immunologic
Acute hemolytic reaction	Delayed hemolytic
Febile nonhemolytic reaction	Posttransfusion purpura
Urticaria	Delayed nonimmunologic
Acute nonimmunologic	Infectious disease transmission
Hypocalcemia	FeLV, FIP, FIV
Embolism (air or clotted blood)	*Babesia, Haemobartonella*
Endotoxic shock	
Hyperkalemia	
Circulatory overload	
Bacterial contamination of blood	

episode was positive for platelet-bound IgG, indicating an immune mechanism for platelet destruction.

Acute Nonimmunologic Transfusion Reactions

Typically, acute nonimmunologic transfusion reactions are caused by physical changes of the red blood cells during collection, storage, or administration or by contamination of the blood product by infectious agents. Embolism is caused by the formation of clots and other debris during collection and storage of blood. Also, during storage, the ATP content of red blood cells falls and some cells undergo hemolysis, resulting in leakage of potassium out of the cells into the storage medium. A large transfusion of stored blood can result in hyperkalemia, but this is rare unless the patient has renal failure or preexisting hyperkalemia. Also, in instances of massive transfusion, ionized hypocalcemia can result from citrate used as an anticoagulant complexing with calcium, which leads to myocardial dysfunction and potential cardiac arrest as well as tetany (Killen et al. 1971).

One consequence of collecting blood in glass bottles is a greater likelihood of venous air embolism, which causes sudden-onset pulmonary vascular obstruction, a precordial murmur, hypotension, and death caused by respiratory failure. Dogs and cats with chronic severe anemia or compromised cardiac and pulmonary function are at greater risk for circulatory overload and pulmonary edema than those without cardiopulmonary disease.

Transfusion of blood contaminated by bacteria, microfilaria, spirochetes, or protozoa from an inadequately screened blood donor results in transmission of the infectious agent and, eventually, clinical signs of the disease in the recipient. Endotoxic shock results from transfusion of blood that is heavily contaminated with endotoxin-producing bacteria. Clinical signs in cats transfused with blood contaminated by bacteria have been reported to include collapse, vomiting, diarrhea, and acute death, although most cats exhibited no abnormalities when receiving bacterially contaminated blood (Hohenhaus et al. 1997). Shock developed in one dog that received a transfusion contaminated by *Babesia canis* (Freeman et al. 1994).

Physical damage to red blood cells, such as by freezing or overheating during storage or warming, causes hemolysis of red blood cells. The patient exhibits hemoglobinuria and hemoglobinemia without evidence of other signs of an acute hemolytic transfusion reaction, such as fever, vomiting, or collapse.

Delayed Nonimmunologic Transfusion Reactions

In human beings, human immunodeficiency virus, hepatitis virus, and cytomegalovirus infections are documented as late effects of transfusion. The transmission of infection to a recipient cat from a donor cat infected with FeLV, FIV, or FIP would be a veterinary example of a delayed nonimmunologic transfusion reaction.

Evaluation of a Patient with a Suspected Transfusion Reaction

Therapeutic management of transfusion reactions varies depending on the classification of the reaction. Treatment for a delayed transfusion reaction consists of treating the acquired infection appropriately. It is important to recognize the late effects of transfusion and not mistake them for another disease process. Because of the life-threatening nature of acute hemolytic transfusion reactions, immediate intervention is critical.

In all animals suspected of having some form of acute transfusion reaction, the transfusion should be stopped and samples of the patient's blood and urine obtained for baseline evaluation of biochemical, hematologic, and coagulation values. The unit of blood should be inspected to ensure it is from the appropriate species and is the intended unit based on the crossmatch or blood type. The urine can be visually inspected to determine the presence or absence of hemoglobin. A Gram stain and bacterial culture of both blood remaining in the bag and a sample of the recipient's blood should be done. The rectal temperature of the recipient should be compared with the pretransfusion value. A transfusion-associated fever is defined as an increase in 1°F over the pretransfusion temperature (Walker 1993). The cardiovascular system should be monitored via electrocardiogram and blood pressure measurement. Immediate evaluation of ionized calcium and serum potassium concentrations would be useful, but certain electrocardiographic changes suggest hypocalcemia (long QT interval with a normal heart rate) or hyperkalemia (decreased height of P waves, loss of P waves, or widening of the QRS complex with large T waves) if rapid measurement of serum electrolyte concentrations cannot be performed.

Venous access and blood pressure should be maintained via an infusion of a crystalloid solution such as lactated Ringer's solution or 0.9% sodium chloride. Intravenous administration of short-acting glucocorticoids may suppress some of the mediators of acute hemolytic transfusion reactions and lessen the clinical progression, but their efficacy in transfusion reactions has not been evaluated in veterinary patients. When the evaluation of a patient with a suspected transfusion reaction suggests that an acute hemolytic transfusion reaction is occurring, the blood typing and crossmatching must be repeated to determine whether a laboratory error is responsible for the reaction. When fever occurs without evidence of hemolysis and the Gram stain is negative for bacterial contamination, the transfusion may be restarted.

Drug Therapy for Transfusion Reactions
(Table 21–5)

Nonhemolytic, febrile transfusion reactions do not require treatment, but antipyretics may be used if the patient is uncomfortable. Transfusion of bacterially contaminated units of blood can cause shock, which is managed with volume expansion and pressor agents as well as empirical antibiotic administration based on the results of the Gram stain. If urticaria resulting from plasma administration is diagnosed, it should be treated with

TABLE 21–5. Drug Dosages and Route of Administration for Use in Transfusion Reactions

Short-acting glucocorticoids
    Methylprednisolone succinate, 30 mg/kg IV once
    Dexamethasone sodium phosphate, 4–6 mg/kg IV once
Diphenhydramine, 2 mg/kg IV as required
Regular insulin, 0.5 U/kg IV given with 50% dextrose 2 g per unit of insulin as required
Calcium gluconate (10% solution)
    50–150 mg/kg IV over 20–30 min; discontinue if bradycardia occurs
    Repeat if hypocalcemia persists
Calcium chloride (10% solution)
    50–150 mg/kg IV, over 20–30 min; discontinue if bradycardia occurs
    Repeat if hypocalcemia persists
Furosemide, 2–4 mg/kg IV
Nitroglycerin paste (2%), ¼ to 1 in. applied to skin
    Monitor blood pressure, may cause hypotension
Aspirin, 10 mg/kg PO once

short-acting glucocorticoids and antihistamines. The plasma transfusion then may be restarted at a slower rate and the recipient observed carefully. Hyperkalemia in a transfusion recipient is treated similarly to hyperkalemia in any patient (see Chapter 5). The transfusion should be discontinued and normal saline administered because it does not contain potassium and facilitates renal excretion of potassium. Intravenous administration of insulin, followed by administration of 50% dextrose and frequent monitoring of blood glucose and potassium concentrations until serum potassium concentration normalizes, may be sufficient. Routine, empirical administration of calcium to transfusion recipients cannot be recommended because of the risk of hypercalcemia and increased myocardial irritability, but animals with ionized hypocalcemia secondary to massive transfusion should be treated with calcium gluconate or calcium chloride to effect (Cote et al. 1987). Dogs and cats that develop volume overload with transfusion are treated with oxygen supplementation, diuretics, and vasodilators. Improvement should be seen within 1 to 2 h.

Prevention Strategies

A special effort is not necessary to prevent transfusion reactions. Simply by following the transfusion medicine guidelines discussed here with reference to donor selection, blood typing, blood storage, and administration, most transfusion reactions can be prevented. Crossmatching is a specific procedure designed to minimize acute transfusion reactions. It can be performed in most veterinary clinics.

CROSSMATCHING

Crossmatching detects antibodies in the plasma of the recipient or donor that may cause an acute hemolytic transfusion reaction. A transfusion reaction may still occur despite a compatible crossmatch. Crossmatching does not prevent sensitization to red blood cell antigens, which may result in a hemolytic reaction during future transfusions, because it detects only antibodies that are currently present in the donor or recipient. Because of the infrequent occurrence of preformed alloantibodies in dogs, it has been proposed that a crossmatch is not necessary before a first transfusion in a dog. If the dog needs a second transfusion more than 4 to 5 days after the first transfusion, a crossmatch is clearly indicated at that time.

A special situation with reference to blood typing and crossmatching exists in cats. When blood typing is unavailable, crossmatching prevents an A-B mismatch transfusion in a cat. In cats, an incompatible crossmatch with a known type A donor strongly suggests that the potential recipient is a type B cat because of the preformed alloantibodies that exist in all type B cats before any transfusion.

CROSSMATCH PROCEDURE

Performing crossmatching is an intimidating but actually quite simple procedure once all the equipment is assembled (Table 21–6). Multiple descriptions of the procedure have been published, all of which describe the same basic procedure with minor variations (Bucheler and Cotter 1992; Giger 1992; Smith 1991). Not all protocols recommend the use of phosphate-buffered saline, others have an additional step at the end using species-specific Coombs' reagent to increase test sensitivity, and some recommend that tubes be incubated at 4, 37, and 42°C. Following is our protocol:

1. Obtain EDTA-anticoagulated blood from the recipient and the potential donor or the crossmatch tubing segments of blood from the units being considered for transfusion.
2. Centrifuge both donor and recipient blood for 5 min at $1000 \times g$.
3. Using pipettes, remove the plasma and save in separate labeled tubes.
4. Wash the red blood cells by adding phosphate-buffered saline to the red cells to fill the tube. Resuspend the red cells in the saline by tapping the bottom of the tube with a finger.
5. Centrifuge the red cells and saline for 5 min at $1000 \times g$. Pipette off saline, and discard.
6. Repeat steps 4 and 5 twice.
7. After the third washing of the red cells in saline, resuspend the red cells to a 3 to 5% solution. It will appear bright cherry red in color.
8. For each potential donor, mix 2 drops of recipient plasma and 1 drop of donor red cell suspension for the major crossmatch. Mix gently.
9. For each potential donor, mix 2 drops of donor plasma and 1 drop of recipient red cell suspension for the minor crossmatch. Mix gently.

TABLE 21–6. Equipment for Performing Crossmatching

1 mL of EDTA blood from the recipient
1 mL of EDTA blood from the potential donor(s)
Tabletop centrifuge
3 mL test tubes (sterility not required)
0.9% saline or phosphate-buffered saline
Disposable pipettes
Test tube rack

TABLE 21–7. **Crossmatch Incompatibility**

0	No agglutination
Trace	Microscopic agglutination
1+	Many small agglutinates admixed with free cells
2+	Large agglutinates mixed with smaller clumps
3+	Many large agglutinates
4+	Single agglutinate, no free cells

10. For the recipient control, mix 2 drops of recipient plasma and 1 drop of recipient red cell suspension. Mix gently.
11. Incubate the tubes at room temperature for 15 min.
12. Centrifuge the tubes for 15 s at $1000 \times g$.
13. Observe the plasma for hemolysis.
14. Resuspend the centrifuged cells by shaking gently.
15. Observe the red blood cells for agglutination.

INTERPRETATION

Hemolysis or agglutination in a crossmatch indicates transfusion incompatibility. The degree of agglutination is graded 0 to 4+ (Table 21–7 and Fig. 21–2). Units of blood that are incompatible should not be used. If all available units are incompatible, the least reactive unit should be chosen. When the recipient control shows hemolysis or agglutination, the crossmatch cannot be interpreted. This is common in patients with hemolytic anemia.

BLOOD TYPE

Blood type is important in preventing A-B mismatch transfusions in cats and preventing sensitization caused by giving DEA 1.1–positive blood to a DEA 1.1–negative dog. Blood typing of both dogs and cats can be performed by a reference laboratory, but this is not convenient in emergency situations. Commercially available blood typing cards for feline types A, B, and AB and canine type DEA 1.1 are available from DMS Laboratories (2 Darts Mill Road, Flemington, NJ) (Fig. 21–3). The typing kit contains all necessary equipment and reagents to determine these blood types in approximately 3 min. We have found that sick cats are often typed as AB when the cards are used but when retested in a reference laboratory are actually type A.

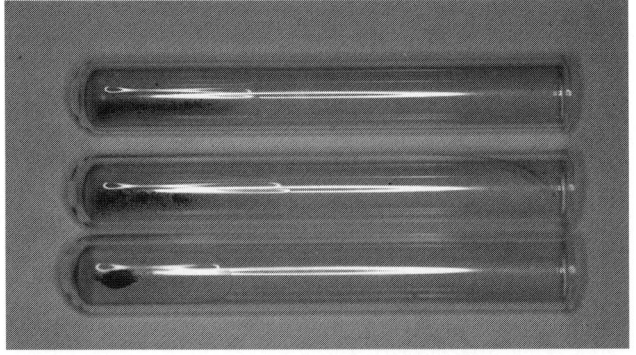

FIGURE 21–2. Three tubes demonstrating increasing degrees of crossmatch incompatibility. From top to bottom the tubes are graded 1+, 2+, and 4+.

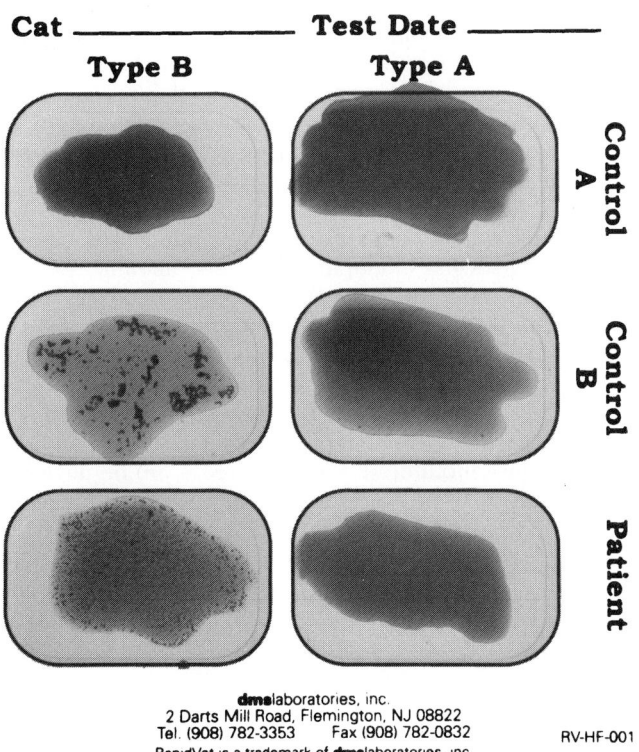

FIGURE 21–3. A feline blood typing card. The patient is blood type B. (Courtesy of DMS Laboratories, Inc., Flemington, NJ.)

▶ Veterinary Hemoglobin-Based Oxygen-Carrying Fluid (Blood Substitute)

Previously, a red blood cell transfusion was the only therapy available to increase the oxygen-carrying capacity of blood. Now, another option is available. A hemoglobin-based oxygen-carrying fluid, Oxyglobin (Biopure Corp., Cambridge, MA), has been approved by the Food and Drug Administration for use in the dog. Oxyglobin (hemoglobin glutamer-200 [bovine]) is ultrapurified, polymerized hemoglobin of bovine origin (13 g/dL) in a modified Ringer's lactate solution with a physiologic pH (7.8). The hemoglobin polymers range in molecular mass from 65 to 500 kd, with an average of 200 kd. The viscosity is low compared with that of blood (1.3 and 3.5 centipoise, respectively) and the solution is isosmotic (300 mOsm/kg) with blood. The concentration of methemoglobin, the inactive form of hemoglobin, is ≤10%. Oxyglobin can be stored at room temperature or refrigerated (2–30°C) for up to 2 years. Its intravascular half-life is dose dependent (30 to 40 h at a dosage of 30 mL/kg), as measured in healthy dogs. More than 90% of the administered dose is expected to be eliminated from the body by 5 to 7 days after infusion. The oxygen half-saturation pressure (P-50) of Oxyglobin is greater than that of canine blood (38 and 30 mm Hg, respectively). This increase in P-50 facilitates offloading of oxygen from the hemoglobin. The hemoglobin is packaged in the deoxygenated state in an overwrap that is impermeable to oxygen.

Complications of severe anemia result from poor oxygenation of tissues. Restoration of adequate tissue oxygenation typically is achieved by administering a blood transfusion. Improvement in the clinical signs of anemia results from a corresponding increase in hemoglobin concentration, which, in turn, increases the arterial oxygen content of the blood. The increased oxygen content of the blood supplied by Oxyglobin also relieves the clinical signs of anemia.

Oxyglobin has been tested in a multicenter clinical trial in dogs with moderate to severe anemia (packed cell volume 6–23%). Sixty-four dogs in need of blood transfusion were studied, including those with anemia related to blood loss ($n = 25$), hemolysis ($n = 30$), or ineffective erythropoiesis ($n = 9$) (Rentko et al. 1996). Thirty dogs were randomized to the Oxyglobin group and 34 dogs to an untreated control group. Dogs in both groups were monitored for a decrease in hemoglobin concentration or a deterioration in physical condition, at which time they received additional oxygen-carrying support. If additional oxygen-carrying support was needed, Oxyglobin-treated dogs received packed red blood cells ($n = 1$) and untreated control dogs received Oxyglobin ($n = 19$). Treatment success was defined as lack of need for additional oxygen-carrying support for 24 h. The success rate in treated dogs (95%) was significantly greater than that in control dogs (32%). This difference between treated and control dogs was significant, regardless of the cause of anemia. To date, no clinical data regarding the use of Oxyglobin in cats have been reported.

The use of Oxyglobin as an oxygen-carrying solution eliminates some of the pretransfusion testing required with red blood cell transfusions. No reconstitution or preparation of Oxyglobin is necessary before infusion. Blood typing and crossmatching are not necessary because the red blood cell membrane, which is the major cause of transfusion incompatibility, has been removed during the manufacturing process. Repeated dosing of Oxyglobin has not been evaluated clinically. Laboratory studies of repeated use are ongoing.

Treatment with Oxyglobin results in some temporary changes in physical findings. After treatment, a transient discoloration (yellow, brown, or red) of the mucous membranes, sclera, urine, and sometimes skin occurs. At the recommended dosage of 30 mL/kg, the potential exists for overexpansion of the vascular volume, particularly in normovolemic animals. Rates of administration >10 mL/kg/h in anemic, clinically ill dogs sometimes resulted in increased central venous pressure, with or without pulmonary edema or other respiratory signs of circulatory overload. In the clinical trial, vomiting occurred in 35% of the dogs that received Oxyglobin. Diarrhea, fever, and death also were seen in approximately 15% of Oxyglobin-treated dogs; however, the association with Oxyglobin or the underlying disease could not be determined. These findings were most common in dogs with immune-mediated hemolyic anemia that received Oxyglobin.

The presence of Oxyglobin in serum may cause artifactual changes in the results of serum chemistry tests. Interference by Oxyglobin depends on the analyzers and reagents used, but is not typical of hemolysis (Moreira et al. 1997; Cullas et al. 1997). Blood samples for analysis should be collected before infusion. A list of valid chemistry tests by analyzer is included in the product labeling. Results of any clinical chemistry test performed with serum containing Oxyglobin should be interpreted with consideration of the validity of the test. In general, all tests using colorimetric techniques are invalid, but other methodologies also show some interference. No interference is seen with hematologic or coagulation parameters except when optical methods are used for measuring prothrombin time and activated partial thromboplastin time. Dipstick measurements (pH, glucose, ketones, protein) of urine are inaccurate when gross discoloration of the urine is present. The urine sediment is not affected.

This oxygen-carrying fluid has been tested widely in the laboratory in a variety of species. Experimental models include hemorrhagic shock in dogs and cats, tumor oxygenation in rats, and surgical blood loss in dogs (Harringer et al. 1992; Walton 1996; Teicher et al. 1993; Standl et al. 1996). The clinical applications of Oxyglobin are now being evaluated.

REFERENCES

Allyson K, Abrams-Ogg ACG, and Johnstone IB: Room temperature storage and cryopreservation of canine platelet concentrates. *Am J Vet Res* 58:1338–1347, 1997.

Auer L and Bell K: The AB blood group system in cats. *Anim Blood Groups Biochem Genet* 12:287–297, 1981.

Auer L and Bell K: Blood transfusion reactions in the cat. *J Am Vet Med Assoc* 180:729–730, 1982.

Bucheler J and Cotter SM: Outpatient blood donor program. In Hohenhaus A (ed): *Problems in Veterinary Medicine*. Philadelphia, JB Lippincott, pp. 572–582, 1992.

Bucheler J and Cotter SM: Setting up a feline blood donor program. *Vet Med* 88:838–845, 1993.

Bucheler J and Cotter SM: Storage of feline and canine whole blood in CPDA-1 and determination of the posttransfusion viability. *J Vet Intern Med* 8:172, 1994.

Callan MB, Oakley DA, Shofer FS, et al.: Canine red blood cell transfusion practice. *J Am Anim Hosp Assoc* 32:303–311, 1996.

Callas DD, Clark TL, Moriera PL, et al.: In vitro effects of a novel hemoglobin-based oxygen carrier on the routine chemistry, therapeutic drug, coagulation, hematology, and blood bank assays. *Clin Chem* 43:1744, 1997.

Capon SM and Goldfinder D: Acute hemolytic transfusion reaction, a paradigm of the systemic inflammatory response: New insights into pathophysiology and treatment. *Transfusion* 35:513–520, 1995.

Carpenter JL, Andelman NC, Moore FM, et al.: Idiopathic cutaneous and renal glomerular vasculopathy of greyhounds. *Vet Pathol* 25:401–407, 1988.

Casal ML, Jezyk PF, and Giger U: Transfer of colostral antibodies from queens to their kittens. *Am J Vet Res* 57:1653–1658, 1996.

Ching YNLH, Meyers KM, Brassard JA, et al.: Effect of cryoprecipitate and plasma on plasma von Willebrand factor multimeters and bleeding time in Doberman pinschers with type-I von Willebrand's disease. *Am J Vet Res* 55:102–110, 1994.

Clark CH and Woodley CH: The absorption of red blood cells after parenteral injection at various sites. *Am J Vet Res* 10:1062–1066, 1959.

Cote CJ, Drop LJ, Daniels, et al.: Calcium chloride versus calcium gluconate: Comparison of ionization and cardiovascular effects in children and dogs. *Anesthesiology* 66:465–470, 1987.

Cowan LA, Mertzke DM, Fenwick BW, et al.: Clinical and clinicopathologic abnormalities in greyhounds with cutaneous and renal glomerular vasculopathy. *J Am Vet Med Assoc* 210:789–793, 1997.

Eibert M and Lewis DC: Post transfusion viability of stored canine red blood cells after vacuum facilitated collection. *J Vet Intern Med* 11:143, 1997.

Eisenbrandt DL and Smith JE: Evaluation of preservatives and containers for storage of canine blood. *J Am Vet Med Assoc* 163:988–990, 1973a.

Eisenbrandt DL and Smith JE: Use of biochemical measures to estimate viability of red blood cells in canine blood stored in acid citrate dextrose solution with and without added ascorbic acid. *J Am Vet Med Assoc* 163:984–987, 1973b.

Freeman MJ, Kirby BM, Panciera DL, et al.: Hypotensive shock syndrome associated with acute *Babesia canis* infection in a dog. *J Am Vet Med Assoc* 204:94–96, 1994.

Galloway SJ and Jones PD: Transfusion acquired *Yersinia enterocolitica*. *Aust N Z J Med* 16:248–250, 1986.

Giger U: Feline transfusion medicine. *Probl Vet Med* 4:600, 1992.

Giger U: Where to get blood donors? (letter) *J Am Vet Med Assoc* 202:705–706, 1993.

Giger U and Akol KG: Acute hemolytic transfusion reaction in an Abyssinian cat with blood type B. *J Vet Intern Med* 4:315–316, 1990.

Giger U and Bucheler J: Transfusion of type-A and type-B blood to cats. *J Am Vet Med Assoc* 198:411–418, 1991.

Giger U, Bucheler J, and Patterson DF: Frequency and inheritance of A and B blood types in feline breeds of the United States. *J Hered* 82:15–20, 1991a.

Giger U, Griot-Wenk M, Bucheler J, et al.: Geographical variation of the feline blood type frequencies in the United States. *Feline Pract* 19:22–27, 1991b.

Giger U, Gorman NT, Hubler M, et al.: Frequencies of feline A and B blood types in Europe. *Anim Genet* 23(suppl 1):17–18, 1993.

Giger U, Gelens CJ, Callan MB, et al.: An acute hemolytic transfusion reaction caused by dog erythrocyte antigen 1.1 incompatibility in a previously sensitized dog. *J Am Vet Med Assoc* 206:1358–1362, 1995.

Goldman M, Roy G, Frechette N, et al.: Evaluation of donor skin disinfection methods. *Transfusion* 37:309–312, 1997.

Green CE: Blood transfusion therapy: An updated overview. *Proceedings of the American Animal Hospital Association*, pp. 187–189, 1982.

Griot-Wenk ME, Callan MB, Chisholm-Chait A, et al.: Blood type AB in the feline AB blood group system. *Am J Vet Res* 57:1438–1442, 1996.

Hale AS: Canine blood groups and their importance in veterinary transfusion medicine. *Vet Clin North Am Small Anim Pract* 25:1323–1332, 1995.

Harringer W, Hodakowski GT, Svizzero T, et al.: Acute effects of massive transfusion of bovine hemoglobin blood substitute in a canine model of hemorrhagic shock. *Eur J Cardiothorac Surg* 6:649, 1992.

Henson MS, Kristensen AT, Armstrong PJ, et al.: Feline blood component therapy: Retrospective study of 246 transfusions. *J Vet Int Med* 8:169, 1994.

Hohenhaus A: Management of the inpatient canine blood donor. *Probl Vet Med* 4:565, 1992.

Hohenhaus AE, Drusin LM, and Garvey MS: *Serratia marcescens* contamination of feline whole blood in a hospital blood bank. *J Am Vet Med Assoc* 210:794–798, 1997.

Howard A, Callan B, Sweeny M, et al.: Transfusion practices and costs in dogs. *J Am Vet Med Assoc* 210:1697–1701, 1992.

Hurst TS, Turrentine MA, and Johnson GS: Evaluation of microwave-thawed canine plasma for transfusion. *J Am Vet Med Assoc* 190:863–865, 1987.

Iserson KV and Huestis DW: Blood warming: Current applications and techniques. *Transfusion* 31:558–571, 1991.

Kaufman PM: Management of the feline blood donor. *Probl Vet Med* 4:555, 1992.

Killen DA, Grogan EL, Gower RE, et al.: Response of canine plasma-ionized calcium and magnesium to the rapid infusion of acid-citrate-dextrose (ACD) solution. *Surgery* 70:736–741, 1971.

Killingsworth C: Use of blood and blood components for feline and canine patients. *J Am Vet Med Assoc* 185:1452–1455, 1984.

Kordick DI and Breitschwerdt EB: Relapsing bacteremia after blood transmission of *Bartonella henselae* to cats. *Am J Vet Res* 58:492–497, 1997.

Kristensen AT: General principles of small animal blood component administration. *Vet Clin North Am Small Anim Pract* 25:1277–1290, 1995.

Lester SJ, Hume JB, and Phipps B: *Haemobartonella canis* infection following splenectomy and transfusion. *Can Vet J* 36:444–445, 1995.

Lower R: [A treatise on the heart on the movement and colour of the blood and on the passage of the chyle into the blood.] In Franklin KJ (ed): Special Edition, the Classics of Medicine Library. Birmingham, AL, Gryphon Editions, p. xvi, 1989.

Majilton EA and Kelley LL: The blood and plasma bank. *Vet Med* 46:226–232, 1951.

Marion RS and Smith JE: Posttransfusion viability of feline erythrocytes stored in acid citrate dextrose solution. *J Am Vet Med Assoc* 183:1459–1460, 1983.

Meyers KM, Wardrop KJ, and Meinkoth J: Canine von Willebrand's disease; pathobiology, diagnosis and short-term treatment. *Compend Contin Educ* 14:13–22, 1992.

Mooney SC: Preparation of blood components. *Probl Vet Med* 4:594, 1992.

Moreira PL, Lansden CC, Clark TL, et al.: Effect of Hemopure® on the performance of Ektachem and Hitachi clinical analyzers. *Clin Chem* 43:1790, 1997.

National Institutes of Health Consensus conference: Fresh-frozen plasma: Indications and risks. *JAMA* 253:551–553, 1985.

Otto CM, Kaufman GM, and Crowe DT: Intraosseous infusion of fluids and therapeutics. *Compend Contin Educ* 11:421–430, 1989.

Porter JA and Canaday WR: Hematologic values in mongrel and greyhound dogs being screened for research use. *J Am Vet Med Assoc* 159:1603–1606, 1971.

Potkay S and Zinn RD: Effects of collection interval, body weight, and season on the hemograms of canine blood donors. *Lab Anim Care* 19:192–197, 1969.

Price LS: A method for collecting and storing feline whole blood. *Vet Tech* 7:561–563, 1991.

Rentko VT, Wohl J, Murtaugh R, et al.: A clinical trial of a hemoglobin based oxygen carrier (HBOC) fluid in the treatment of anemia in dogs. *J Vet Intern Med* 10:177, 1996.

Ring J and Messmer K: Incidence and severity of anaphylactoid reactions to colloid volume substitutes. *Lancet* 1:466–468, 1977.

Schneider A: Blood components: Collection, processing and storage. *Vet Clin North Am Small Anim Pract* 25:1245–1261, 1995.

Smith CA: Transfusion medicine: The challenge of practical use. *J Am Vet Med Assoc* 198:474–452, 1991.

Smith JE: Erythrocytes. *Adv Vet Sci Comp Med* 36:9–55, 1991.

Standl T, Horn P, Wilhelm S, et al.: Bovine hemoglobin is more potent than autologous red blood cells in restoring muscular tissue oxygenation after profound isovolaemic hemodilution in dogs. *Can J Anaesth* 43:714, 1996.

Stiles J and Raffe MR: Hemolysis of canine fresh and stored blood associated with peristaltic pump infusion. *Vet Emerg Crit Care* 1:50–53, 1991.

Sullivan PS, Evans HL, and McDonald TP: Platelet concentration and hemoglobin function in greyhounds. *J Am Vet Med Assoc* 205:838–841, 1994.

Szama K: Reports of 355 transfusion associated deaths: 1976–1985. *Transfusion* 30:583–590, 1990.

Taboada J, Harvey JW, Levy MG, et al.: Seroprevalence of babesiosis in greyhounds in Florida. *J Am Vet Med Assoc* 200:47–50, 1992.

Teicher BA, Schwartz GN, Sotomayor EA, et al.: Oxygenation of tumors by a hemoglobin solution. *J Cancer Res Clin Oncol* 120:85, 1993.

Turnwald GH and Pichler ME: Blood transfusion in dogs and cats. Part II. Administration, adverse effects and component therapy. *Compend Contin Educ* 7:115–126, 1985.

Walker RH (ed): *Technical Manual*, 11th ed. Bethesda, MD, American Association of Blood Banks, 1993.

Walton RS: Polymerized hemoglobin versus hydroxyethyl starch in an experimental model of feline hemorrhagic shock. Proceedings of Fifth IVECC Symposium, 1996.

Wardrop KJ: Canine plasma therapy. *Vet Forum* 14:36–40, 1997.

Wardrop KJ, Owen TJ, and Meyers KM: Evaluation of an additive solution for preservation of canine red blood cells. *J Vet Intern Med* 8:253–257, 1994.

Wardrop KJ, Lewis D, Marks S, et al.: Posttransfusion purpura in a dog with hemophilia A. *J Vet Intern Med* 11:261–263, 1997a.

Wardrop KJ, Tucker RL, and Munai K: Evaluation of canine red blood cells stored in a saline, adenine and glucose solution for 35 days. *J Vet Intern Med* 11:5–8, 1997b.

Yaphe W, Giovengo S, and Moise NS: Severe cardiomegaly secondary to anemia in a kitten. *J Am Vet Med Assoc* 202:961–964, 1993.

Yuile CL, VanZandt TF, Ervin DM, et al.: Hemolytic reactions produced in dogs by transfusion of incompatible dog blood and plasma. *Blood* 4:1232–1239, 1948.

CHAPTER 22

Parenteral Nutrition

REBECCA L. REMILLARD

▶ Clinical Importance

At any age, patients with inadequate nutrient intake become malnourished. Malnutrition is an imbalanced intake of calories and/or nitrogen to support tissue metabolism, and it undermines proper medical or surgical therapeutic management of the animal. Malnutrition is far more common in veterinary patients than currently is recognized. Hospitalized veterinary patients are more commonly protein and calorie deficient because of a decreased total dietary intake. Patients resting in a cage have been mistakenly assumed to require little or no nutrition when, in fact, their needs are significant. The major consequences of malnutrition in all patients are decreased immunocompetence, decreased tissue synthesis and repair, and altered intermediary drug metabolism.

Immunocompetence

The relationship between nutrition and immunity is reciprocal. A malnourished animal is more susceptible to infections and a septic patient is more likely to be anorectic, which results in malnutrition. Nutrient imbalances decrease immune function, which increases the risk of disease, and conversely, certain diseases alter some nutrient requirements (Semba et al. 1997; Burkholder and Swecker 1990; Fischer and Glory 1984). Malnutrition causes impaired cell-mediated responses, secretory immunoglobulin A production, phagocytosis, complement function, antibody affinity, and cytokine production (Chandra 1981, 1988, 1991, 1992b; Shikora et al. 1994; Redmond et al. 1991). Protein-calorie deficiencies limit amino acid and nucleotide substrates for cell proliferation and result in reduced circulating numbers of T lymphocytes and helper and suppressor cells (Kahan 1981; Kulkarni et al. 1986; Ortiz and Betancourt 1984; Chandra and Kumari 1994). Single-nutrient deficiencies of zinc, iron, vitamin B_6, vitamin A, copper, and selenium also impair immune function (Chandra 1992a; Meydani 1990; Grimble 1990). Immunoglobulins and circulating antibodies are maintained at relatively low concentrations during malnutrition but are highly responsive to refeeding. Numbers of T4 helper cells and T8 cytotoxic suppressor cells in malnourished people quickly return to normal with feeding (Kahan 1981; Chandra 1983; Chandra et al. 1982). Postoperatively fed beagles had serum globulin concentrations twofold greater than dogs not fed postoperatively (Moss 1978). In summary, the immune system is dependent upon and responsive to nutritional intake.

Tissue Synthesis and Repair

Tissue synthesis and wound healing are functions of both local and whole-body nutrition (Crane 1989). Locally, amino acids and carbohydrates are needed for collagen and ground substance synthesis. Fibroblasts require energy to synthesize RNA, DNA, and ATP for protein synthesis. Migration of fibroblasts and epithelial and endothelial cells also requires energy. At distant sites, the liver has energy and protein needs specifically for fibronectin, complement, and glucose synthesis. The bone marrow requires nutrients for platelet, leukocyte, and red cell production. Transportation of these components and oxygen to wound sites demands the muscular activities of respiration and cardiac work. The normal continuous cycle of protein turnover (synthesis and degradation) in the body is altered with tissue trauma and during healing. In a rat model, the rates of protein synthesis and degradation were increased after trauma (Stein et al. 1976). Other protein turnover studies have measured a 91% increase in protein synthesis with a 10% increase in protein degradation in perioperatively fed people (Kien et al. 1978). However, perioperatively fasted people had only a 50% increase in protein synthesis with a 79% increase in protein degradation (Birkham et al. 1980). Therefore, proper nutrition for local tissue synthesis and wound healing is dependent on adequate whole-body nutrition.

Intermediary Drug Metabolism

All nutrients are essential for the maintenance of normal cellular structure and function (Parke 1991). Cellular activities are dependent on and regulated by the actions of peptides, lipids, vitamins, and minerals as the substrates, enzymes, coenzymes, and cofactors of intermediary metabolism. Nutrient deprivation alters the normal metabolic synergy responsible for ion gradients, membrane potentials, production of high-energy phosphate compounds, and antioxidant defenses. Nutritional support containing little or no lipid decreases hepatic cytochrome P-450 concentration and activity, which significantly decreases specific drug clearances (Knodell 1990; Raftogianis et al. 1995). Protein-calorie deficiency may result in (1) decreased hepatic biotransformation of some antibiotics, (2) decreased serum proteins that bind and transport drugs throughout the body, and (3) decreased renal blood flow, which decreases the rate of drug elimination and increases the possibility of drug toxicity (Walter-Sack and Klotz 1996). Therefore, protein-calorie malnutrition may alter the normal or expected metabolism of some drugs, which may in turn alter their therapeutic effect even when given at recommended dosages (Albrecht et al. 1986; Varma 1981; Anderson 1988; Krishnaswamy 1990). Patients receiving calories and protein are expected to have more normal drug distribution, metabolism, and elimination than animals deprived of nutritional support.

In veterinary patients, malnutrition is associated with increased morbidity and mortality. Diseased and debilitated patients require adequate calories and protein daily to maintain optimal immune function, tissue synthesis and repair, and normal metabolic reactions. The American College of Veterinary Nutrition has recommended that nutrition problem solving include assessment of the patient, the current food, and the feeding method used. Assessment of these three aspects of cases identifies patients in need of nutritional support in order to avoid or reduce protein-calorie deficiencies and the associated complications. A hospital feeding plan then can be developed to better meet the nutritional needs of the patient.

▶ Assessment of the Patient

The goal of assessment is to establish the animal's nutrient needs with respect to its disease condition. Although inadequate nutrient intake is known to complicate many disorders, anorexia traditionally has been viewed as a secondary problem that will improve when the primary disease problem has been resolved (i.e., "they'll eat when they feel better"). It is better to be proactive and recognize the value of administering calories and protein to our patients (i.e., "they'll feel better when they eat").

Diseased or debilitated patients, whether hospitalized or not, require frequent assessment regardless of their age or life stage. Nutritional assessment involves the evaluation of a number of parameters taken together to determine whether a patient is suffering from protein-calorie malnutrition and which specific nutritional interventions are necessary. A veterinary nutritional assessment protocol should include history, physical examination with special attention to specific risk factors, body condition score, and laboratory tests (Buffington 1994). Weight and diet history, physical examination, and body condition are relatively easy parameters to collect, but key laboratory or immunologic tests that correlate well with nutritional status have not been identified. To date, few clinical studies have been performed in veterinary patients to determine which parameters are applicable and how accurate they are in determining nutritional status and outcome (Michel 1993).

History

Reviewing the animal's medical history helps to determine the current nutritional status of the patient. The signalment defines the patient on the basis of species, breed, age, gender, reproductive status, activity level, and environment. Medical histories should reveal previous medical, surgical, and drug therapies to help understand the patient's appetite and ability to assimilate nutrients. Food intake, dietary, and weight histories help identify patients that are malnourished.

It is important to note the physiologic status of the patient. Noting the gender, reproductive status, age, and activity level of a patient aids in the nutritional evaluation. Reproductive status (intact vs. neutered) is known to alter metabolic rate and energy needs in animals (Root et al. 1996; Flynn et al. 1996). The metabolic processes of growth, gestation, and lactation do not necessarily cease when the animal becomes acutely ill. It may take days of poor energy intake before the hormonal stimuli for growth, gestation, or lactation are down-regulated.

Animals fed homemade, table food, vegetarian, or single-item diets are at greater risk of having subclinical nutritional imbalances. Diets designed, formulated, or prepared by owners rarely are nutritionally complete, balanced, or consistent. These patients not only may have protein-calorie malnutrition but also are more likely to have several vitamin and mineral imbalances, such as calcium and trace mineral deficiencies or subclinical vitamin A or D toxicity.

Patients with a 3-day or longer history of nausea, vomiting, or diarrhea are at increased risk of malnutrition because these findings indicate that nutritional intake has been suboptimal for some time before presentation. Nutrient intake may be voluntarily decreased with nausea, and nutrient digestion and absorption may have been compromised with vomiting or diarrhea.

Physical Examination

All patients should receive a complete physical examination including an accurate determination of body weight and an estimate of body condition. Weight changes must be viewed as a proportion or percentage of "normal, usual, or optimal" weight within a certain time period as opposed to absolute changes in units (i.e., pounds or grams lost). Weight loss of more than 10% over 7 days is clinically significant and warrants further assessment. It is more difficult to determine accurately a 450-g weight change in a 4.5-kg cat than a 4.5-kg change in a 45-kg dog; consequently, cats should be weighed on a scale with increased sensitivity between 0 and 15 kg. As a point of reference, a weight gain or loss of 10 to 15% over several days is most likely a hydration problem and should be corrected first with other medical therapies or fluid management. Pets on designated weight loss programs typically lose 1 to 2% of their body weight per week (Laflamme 1993).

Body condition estimation is a more subjective evaluation of the patient's tissue composition relative to weight (i.e., fat, muscle, and bone) (Thatcher et al. 1998). A body condition score adds valuable information to the breed and body weight data. Fat stores are an indication of previous energy intake (i.e., decreased fat stores indicate low energy intake and vice versa). The presence of muscle wasting implies that protein intake has been insufficient because body muscle mass has been the source of net protein synthesis. Survival rates in people have been directly correlated with available muscle mass. Loss of more than 25 to 30% of body protein compromises the immune system and muscle strength, and death results from infection, pulmonary failure, or both (Matthews and Fong 1993). Several days of preoperative nutritional support in such a patient are advisable if surgery may be safely postponed. There is evidence that only 2 to 3 days of positive energy and protein intake are required to up-regulate hepatic and muscle anabolic enzymes (Zeiderman et al. 1989; Wernerman et al. 1986). In one study of human patients, there was 77% agreement between three independent clinicians' nutritional assessment of the same 64 patients, and clinical judgment of nutritional risk correlated well ($R^2 = 0.73$) with objective data such as weight loss history, serum albumin, transferrin, and cholesterol (Lupo et al. 1993). The clinical assessment of poor body weight and condition has merit and adds significantly to overall assessment of the patient's risk.

Laboratory Data and Other Clinical Information

Laboratory data for a malnourished or dehydrated patient are too difficult to assess as a single data set. Laboratory and other diagnostic tests should be viewed in the context of the patient's history, physical examination findings, and all subsequent laboratory data.

Changes in laboratory test results related to malnutrition are indistinguishable from those related to disease processes, but results should be reviewed with malnutrition in mind. In normally hydrated patients, red blood cell number and size, hemoglobin content, urea nitrogen, potassium, albumin, total protein concentration, and white blood cell count can add to the nutritional assessment of the patient. Red blood cells, hemoglobin, albumin, and total protein have moderate half-lives of 1 to 8 weeks and are an indication of the energy and protein status of the animal over the preceding weeks to months. Dogs fed a protein-deficient diet (4%) with adequate calorie intake (fat 19%) had lower than normal serum albumin and total protein concentrations but normal globulin concentration after 4 weeks (Davenport et al. 1994). Several studies in people have demonstrated that a low serum albumin concentration correlates with complications, but the sensitivity of serum albumin concentration as a single variable is very low (Anderson et al. 1984).

Serum potassium and urea nitrogen concentrations also may be decreased in anorectic animals because these are largely affected by diet on a day-to-day basis. Urea nitrogen, however, tends to increase in end-stage starvation because, with depleted fat stores, muscle is metabolized for energy. Serum creatine kinase concentration also has been evaluated as a marker of feline malnutrition in anorexia and refeeding (Fascetti et al. 1997). Creatine kinase concentration, however, may be abnormal in many disease states (Kitagawa et al. 1991; Antonas 1994).

Risk Factors

Several additional factors increase the patient's risk for malnutrition while hospitalized.

ANOREXIA AND CACHEXIA

Anorexia may be partial or complete. If an animal is consuming no food for a period of time beyond that considered normal for the patient, the anorexia is complete. If the animal consumes some food but less than that considered a normal daily intake for the patient, anorexia is partial. In general, an animal not eating for more than 48 h or consuming less than 50% of normal intake for more than 3 days should be considered cause for concern and noted to have a form of anorexia. Cats and dogs with a history of complete anorexia for three or more days, or any animal with a history of partial anorexia for several weeks, should be considered malnourished.

Cachexia is a state of general illness and malnutrition with profound organ disability. It has been recognized in people that cachexia or low body condition scores are associated with increased risk of complications (Windsor 1993). Loss of peripheral (skeletal) and central (visceral) proteins may have adverse anatomic and functional consequences in animals. These effects include anemia, reduced heart muscle mass and function, decreased pulmonary mechanical function, and a diminished respiratory drive as well as altered intestinal morphology and mildly impaired absorptive abilities (Gran 1983; Biden and Taylor 1983; Heymsfield et al. 1988). Dogs and cats with long-standing cancer, cardiac disease, or renal disease can present in a cachectic state with or without metabolic accommodation.

Metabolic accommodation now is recognized in people and probably exists in the dog and cat as well. Accommodation occurs when energy equilibrium has been reestablished at a constant but lower food intake and lean tissue wasting has been arrested just before becoming fatal. Accommodation in people is successful when (1) total lean tissue depletion is less than that considered critical, (2) weight is low but stable, and (3) serum albumin concentration and total peripheral white blood cell count are normal with intact delayed cutaneous hypersensitivity (Bistrian 1984; Hoffer 1994). This condition of accommodation in people, with the exception of intact delayed cutaneous hypersensitivity, accurately describes some chronically ill animals (i.e., those with chronic renal, hepatic, or cardiac insufficiency). Geriatric chronically ill, cachectic cats and dogs may be maintained at a less than optimal body weight and condition for some time, even though important organ function deficits are apparent. Metabolic rate has been down-regulated and protein turnover has been altered to establish a fragile homeostasis. This homeostasis can be maintained in some pets for weeks to months until a new stress supervenes. These animals often do not survive additional stresses such as trauma, surgery, infection, and tumors as might a similarly afflicted healthy animal. These patients should be considered malnourished.

DAYS OF FOOD DEPRIVATION

During food deprivation, under the influence of endocrine changes, energy is drawn from endogenous stores. Animals utilize different proportions of stored body carbohydrate, fat, and protein to maintain blood glucose concentration throughout the course of starvation in order to maintain vital functions for as long as possible. The adaption from the fed to the starved state is one in which fuel usage by the animal shifts from using primarily a mixture of fuels to using fatty acids as the primary fuel. Carbohydrate and fat metabolism is profoundly altered during the first week of starvation. An understanding of these metabolic changes, primarily in the liver, during simple starvation is essential to understanding the underlying metabolic alterations during anorexia, illness, and cachexia.

As blood glucose concentration falls below 120 mg/dL in mammalian liver cells, glucokinase becomes less active, and the liver becomes a net exporter of glucose in order to maintain blood glucose concentrations. Omnivores, such as the dog, maintain blood glucose concentrations during the first 2 days of food deprivation through glycogenolysis. Glycogenolysis begins within 4 to 5 h of fasting and the liver exports glucose in order to maintain normal blood glucose concentration. The blood glucose concentration is maintained by glycogenolysis for only another 12 to 28 h, and gluconeogenesis using fat and protein stores must maintain it thereafter (Cahill and Owen 1967). In carnivores, such as the cat, blood glucose concentration is maintained by gluconeogenesis from fat and protein stores beginning interprandially because hepatic glycogen stores are minimal. Hepatic glycogen storage in carnivores is relatively small compared with that in omnivores, in part because of lower glycogen synthase and glucokinase activities.

Gluconeogenesis by the liver and kidney using glycerol, lactate, and gluconeogenic amino acids is initiated by glucagon but later maintained by glucocorticoids. Adipose tissue supplies glycerol for glucose production and fatty acids for energy, and muscle catabolism releases gluconeogenic amino acids, lactic acid, and pyruvate to the liver for glucose production (Welbern and Moldawer 1984). By the third day of food deprivation in all mammals, there is a reduction in metabolic rate to slow fat and muscle catabolism in an effort to survive long-term starvation. Animals receiving less than their daily energy requirement, regardless of the circumstances (i.e., food deprivation or anorexia), decrease their metabolic rate by increasing the concentration of reverse triiodothyronine, thereby decreasing the demand for energy (Vagenakis et al. 1975).

Simultaneously with these changes in gluconeogenesis in the first few days of food deprivation, the liver releases ketone bodies from fatty acids as an alternative fuel for non–glucose-dependent tissues. Ketone bodies are essential for maintaining an energy supply to all tissues because fatty acids are water insoluble and must be carried in blood bound to albumin. Once converted to ketone bodies, fatty acids are water soluble, do not require albumin, and can provide a lipid fuel to cells at a much higher blood and interstitial fluid concentration. The rise in blood ketone concentrations causes an enzymatic change in peripheral tissues to promote ketone use and decrease glucose demand, which also conserves body protein and effectively spares glucose for nonadaptive tissues. Ketosis in food deprivation is an appropriate physiologic response to provide a readily diffusible lipid fuel for muscles, kidney, peripheral nerves, and brain during periods of starvation, and their production can be maintained until adipose tissue is depleted.

By day 5 of food deprivation in all mammals, endocrine changes have mandated a metabolic shift to oxidizing endogenous fatty acids and ketone body utilization. In simple starvation, blood glucose concentration remains low; therefore insulin decreases, which allows lipolysis. In the disease state, catecholamines and corticosteroids dominate, which also stimulates lipolysis. Therefore, fat from adipose tissue becomes the main fuel for the body in states of starvation and anorexia (Owen et al. 1969). Muscles begin using ketone bodies for energy to spare glucose. Skeletal muscles also catabolize branched amino acids, exporting the nitrogen as alanine and to a lesser extent as glutamine, thereby providing nitrogen for hepatic synthesis of essential proteins and carbons for hepatic and renal glucose synthesis (Felig et al. 1969). Essential amino acids, however, are reserved for protein synthesis and incorporated into citric acid cycle intermediates and are not burned for energy if at all possible. Fatty acid oxidation somewhat spares oxidation of amino acids for energy, which helps maintain muscle protein stores throughout starvation until the end stages (Fulks et al. 1975). Overall, blood glucose concentration is maintained throughout starvation within the low to normal range for nonadaptive tissues (e.g., erythrocytes, central nervous system, renal medullary cells).

As described, animals utilize different proportions of stored body carbohydrate, fat, and protein to maintain blood glucose concentration and other vital functions at different times during the first week of food deprivation. In adaptation from the fed to the starved state, fuel usage by the animal shifts from primarily using a mixture of fuels to primarily using fat as the fuel. A patient's dietary history indicates the number of "no-food" days. Matching the number of no-food days with this pattern of hepatic fuel utilization is important in selecting the first refeeding formula. The refeeding formula should contain a complete balance of nutrients but should have a carbohydrate, fat, and protein profile that the liver can immediately utilize to minimize the metabolic complications of refeeding.

Nutrients of Concern

Identifying only the nutrients that are important in the management of specific diseases or conditions greatly simplifies clinical nutrition by directing the clinician's attention to adjusting only the few key nutrients rather than all 43 nutrients for the cat or 36 nutrients for the dog.

ENERGY

Diseased patients have metabolic rates and energy requirements that are less than those of a comparable normal healthy individual under maintenance conditions. In protein-calorie malnutrition without disease or injury, decreased triiodothyronine concentration progressively decreases the metabolic rate in an effort to conserve bodily functions until appropriate calorie intake resumes. Triiodothyronine concentrations decrease within 24 h of fasting or caloric restriction and may be 40 to 50% below fed concentrations within 3 days. However, with an ongoing disease process or traumatic injury, the neuroendocrine response to stress increases metabolic rate above that observed in simple starvation. The metabolic rate of an anorectic, sick, or traumatized patient is therefore greater than that of an animal in simple uncomplicated starvation but less than that of an animal in the normal healthy state (Remillard and Armstrong 1998). Knowing the patient's approximate caloric requirement is important because administering nutrition in excess of metabolic need causes metabolic complications. Overfeeding patients is possible and commonly occurs with parenteral nutritional support. Excessive carbohydrate has been associated with hyperglycemia, hypercapnia, fatty liver, increased ventilatory drive, and failure to wean from a ventilator (Deitel et al. 1983; Pilbeam et al. 1983). Excessive fat administration has been associated with hyperlipidemia, hypoxia, increased rate of infection, and a higher postoperative mortality rate (Chang and Silvis 1974; Lowry and Brennan 1979; Hirai et al. 1979).

In human hospitals, the trend has been to feed patients less than previously prescribed. The current recommendation is to feed hospitalized patients at approximately 80% of their energy requirement during illness, which probably is the resting energy requirement (RER) for most patients (Tallado-Rodriguez and Christian 1988). Respiration calorimetry measurements of more than 3000 human patients with a wide variety of diseases, specifically excluding hyperthyroidism, demonstrated that 90% of the patients were within ±15% of their RER (Boothby and Sandiford 1924). Nutritional support teams in major hospitals currently begin feeding patients at or near their RERs and then adjust intake accordingly on the basis of regular nutritional assessments (McMahon 1993; Forse 1995). The majority of hospitalized critically ill people receive energy intakes between 25 and 35 kcal/kg/day (DeBiasse and Wilmore 1994; Woolfson 1983).

Diseased and debilitated veterinary patients presumably are similar to critically ill people and have metabolic rates and energy requirements near their RER. There have been a few preliminary respiration calorimetry measurements in ill dogs with specific disease conditions (Ogilvie et al. 1996a, 1996b; Walton et al. 1996). It is now suggested that hospitalized veterinary patients be fed at their calculated RER, realizing that their actual energy requirement is likely to change over the time course of the disease process and recovery. The daily RER is 30 kcal/kg for adult dogs, 40 kcal/kg for cats, and 50 kcal/kg for either species under 2.3 kg. Feeding patients at the RER is a rational and safe starting estimate that decreases the probability of metabolic complications. Regular nutritional assessment of veterinary patients is highly recommended in order to make adjustments to these initial feeding rates.

Some diseased patients apparently have energy requirements greater than RER as determined by bedside indirect respiration calorimetry in people (Mann et al. 1985). For example, people with head and brain injury have been found to have energy requirements 40% above (1.4 ×) resting values (Ott et al. 1990). Brain injury apparently increases oxygen consumption and acute-phase protein synthesis, which in turn increases the patients' caloric and protein requirements above RER. Severely burned patients also may have energy and protein requirements above RER, depending on the extent of skin damage and surface area exposed (Wilmore et al. 1974). The body loses heat, moisture, and proteins from these areas of skin damage. Similar increases in energy needs probably occur in dogs and cats. In these cases, it is advisable to begin feeding at RER and then increase intake over several days as tolerated by the patient. Slightly underfeeding the patient is preferable to overfeeding.

The veterinary patient's actual metabolic rate can only be approximated in a clinical setting. The energy requirement of these patients initially should be assumed to be the RER. Nutrient intake then can be increased relative to the degree of trauma, disease, or complications as indicated by patient's response and laboratory data over the next few days. The majority of veterinary patients respond positively to initial feedings at RER and metabolic complications with feeding rarely occur.

PROTEIN

Protein in the body is not static but is always in a flux between synthesis and breakdown. Protein synthesis requires that amino acids be present within cells at the correct time and ratio so that proteins may be constructed successfully. Protein degradation involves the release of amino acids, and if an amino acid is deaminated, the carbon skeleton (glucose or fat) is oxidized for energy and the amino group enters the hepatic urea cycle and ultimately is excreted in the urine. Under most circumstances, about 15% of the RER comes from the oxidation of amino acids (Woolfson 1983; Kinney 1988). Hence, proteins contribute very little, compared with fats and carbohydrates, toward meeting the total energy need. Calculating and adjusting for protein calories is of minor consequence when feeding at RER and need not be done. The most conservative and simplest method is to provide the entire caloric need with fat and carbohydrate, meet the protein requirement entirely with amino acids, and not try to estimate what fraction of the protein will be catabolized for energy.

Protein administration should be in balance with calories delivered. Sufficient calories must be available from fat or glucose before amino acids are used for tissue synthesis and repair (Mallet 1984; Porta and Hartroft 1970; Truswell et al. 1969). Excessive protein feeding requires energy expenditure to rid the body of excess nitrogen, which may not be handled well by the liver and kidneys. Feeding excess protein can result in azotemia or hyperammonemia and accompanying clinical signs of encephalopathy. Conversely, insufficient protein intake has been linked to low serum albumin concentration, poor immune response, poor healing, and increased risk of dehiscence and muscle wasting. The most efficient use of protein occurs when 1 to 6 g of protein per 100 kcal of RER is administered. Protein delivered per 100 kcal of energy is not the same as per kilogram body weight.

Administering 1 to 6 g of protein on a body weight basis delivers more (~40%) than on an energy basis and has, in a few intolerant animals, resulted in encephalopathic signs.

In formulating nutritional support, it is prudent first to provide for the total caloric need with fat and carbohydrate and then meet the protein requirement. It is important to remember that if sufficient calories are supplied to the patient as either fat or carbohydrate, protein may not be burned for energy and more likely will be used for protein synthesis. A starting average of 2 to 4 g protein per 100 kcal RER can be used for most patients in which the ability to handle protein waste products is not in question and in which there are no known protein losses. Protein intake then may be adjusted on the basis of the patient's needs and ability to handle these initial protein recommendations. Patients with falling serum albumin concentration may require 5 to 6 g/100 kcal RER, whereas patients with azotemia may tolerate only 1 to 2 g per 100 kcal RER.

B VITAMINS

These water-soluble vitamins are coenzymes that are vital to optimal hepatic metabolism of energy substrates. Folic acid, thiamine, riboflavin, niacin, pantothenic acid, pyridoxine, and B_{12} are essential for hepatic metabolism of glucose, fat, and protein. They are essential coenzymes for the Krebs cycle, ATP production, and red blood cell metabolism. They are required in small amounts compared with other nutrients but are required daily and are not optional for tissue energy metabolism to operate efficiently. All patients that are not eating but are receiving fluids should have B vitamins added to their fluids. These vitamins are easily and inexpensively replaced and should be included in all forms of nutritional support.

FAT-SOLUBLE VITAMINS AND MINERALS

Fat-soluble vitamins A, D, E, and K rarely are needed by hospitalized patients except in specific disease conditions. Most patients have adipose and hepatic stores of the fat-soluble vitamins sufficient to meet metabolic needs for months to years. Macrominerals such as calcium, phosphorus, magnesium, sodium, and potassium rarely are needed by patients over and above amounts required to correct and maintain serum electrolyte concentrations. Whole-body stores of these minerals often are not the problem; rather, abnormal distribution between intra- and extracellular fluid compartments is the problem, and this imbalance should be corrected or nearly corrected before nutritional support is begun. Zinc, copper, manganese, chromium, and selenium are vital cofactors for optimal hepatic and peripheral metabolism of energy substrates, and these trace minerals should be included in all forms of nutritional support.

▶ Assessment of Food and Feeding Method

Ideally, all critically ill patients should consume at least enough of a complete and balanced food to meet their RER daily. Patients' requirements for all other nutrients need not be calculated when a diet contains nonenergy nutrients properly balanced with the caloric density of the product. When the patient consumes the proper amount of a balanced diet, all other nutrient needs have been met, unless there are particularly high losses (e.g., protein, electrolytes). Hospitalized patients eating single-item foods such as meat, baby food, or treats do not have complete and balanced nutrient intakes.

Daily reviews of critically ill patients should include an assessment of actual food intake. In many cases, feeding orders of critically ill patients are written by the attending clinician, and they should be clear and complete. In a multicenter study of 276 dogs with an average 4-day hospital stay, 20% of nearly 900 written feeding orders were clear, complete, and accurate (Remillard et al. 1997). Properly written hospital feeding orders identify a specific food product with the amount, frequency, and route of intake specified, if not by mouth.

Recording the intake of critically ill patients is essential to determine whether nutritional support is necessary. In addition to having complete feeding orders, the medical record should contain the time of day and amount actually offered to the patient. Consumption can be simply recorded as some percentage of the food offered (0, 50, or 100%). If feeding orders are properly written and consumption is recorded, after 24 h of hospitalization it will be apparent whether or not the patient is consuming sufficient food to meet its RER and whether additional nutritional support is required. In the previous study of 276 hospitalized dogs, a positive energy intake (>95% RER) was achieved on only 27% of 821 dog-days recorded whereas a negative energy intake (<95% RER) was observed on the majority of the dog-days (Remillard et al. 1997). When food intake is determined to be less than the patient's RER or the food consumed is not a complete and balanced product for three or more days, nutritional support is needed.

▶ Determine a Parenteral Nutrition Plan

Devising a feeding plan for critically ill patients requires complete knowledge of the case and often must be individually tailored because of the unique circumstances of each case. Nutritional plans require an understanding of the patient's metabolic state relative to changes in metabolism as anorexia or NPO (nothing by mouth) orders continue. The patient with a preexisting condition (e.g., renal, cardiac, or hepatic compromise) requiring specific nutritional modifications must be understood and these special needs incorporated in the new nutritional plan. Prior knowledge that a patient requires other medical and surgical procedures also should be taken into account when formulating a nutritional plan. Lastly, nutritional plans also should take into consideration the clinician's long-term treatment plan and owner's expectations.

Selection of Patients

Any patient with a suspected or documented food intake less than its calculated daily RER for more than 3 days is a candidate for nutritional support. There are only two routes by which nutrients can be supplied to the body, enteral and parenteral. Enteral feeding can provide adequate nutrition simply and cost effectively whether done orally or by feeding tube. Enteral feeding usually is the method of choice because using the gastrointestinal tract is less expensive, stimulates the immune system, and avoids most metabolic complications except diarrhea. Nutrients must be administered parenterally, however, when the small intestine is not functioning adequately to meet the patient's RER and nitrogen requirements. These two methods of nutritional support are not mutually exclusive, and parenterally supplementing calories and protein above what the patient consumes voluntarily to meet the RER is possible in most veterinary practices. Therefore, overall medical assessment of the patient with particular attention to gastrointestinal tract function is essential in deciding how nutritional support should be provided.

Parenteral nutrition (PN) is a valuable asset in meeting a patient's daily resting energy and protein requirements. Proper selection of patients, however, is important to the successful use of PN. Patients with concurrent small-intestinal conditions known or suspected to impair absorption and not expected to be resolved within the next 3 days are good candidates for PN. Depending on the size of the patient, it is not cost effective to administer PN as the only nutritional support for less than a 3-day course. There is a substantial initial cost to compounding (~$50), but many bags can be made at one time. When this cost is spread over 3 or more days, the procedure becomes cost effective. Hence, proper selection of patients mandates that the patient is expected to be hospitalized for several more days because instituting PN for only 1 or 2 days is of questionable cost benefit. When PN is provided in conjunction (e.g., peripheral infusion of 20% lipids) with enteral intake, however, a course of less than 3 days may be cost effective and nutritionally beneficial.

Parenteral nutritional support should not be initiated until the patient is hemodynamically stable with major electrolyte and acid-base abnormalities, severe tachycardia, hypotension, and volume deficits corrected or nearly normal (Table 22–1). Nutritional support should not be initiated until the patient is hemodynamically stable because administering enteral or parenteral nutrition may further compromise unstable patients. Electrolyte and acid-base abnormalities and blood glucose concentration also should be corrected before instituting nutritional support. Severe tachycardia, hypotension, and volume deficits must be corrected before starting nutritional support (Minard and Kudsk 1994). A practical goal is to begin nutritional assessment and support within 24 h of determining that RER intake is inadequate (Burkholder 1995; Devey et al. 1995).

Several examples of patients for which PN is appropriate have been published, but only careful consideration of the preceding criteria can ensure that veterinary patients benefit from PN (Remillard and Thatcher 1989; Lippert and Buffington 1992). Parenteral nutritional support is valuable for patients with inflammatory bowel (small and large) disease, parvovirus gastroenteritis or other causes of impaired gastrointestinal motility, peritonitis, pancreatitis, intestinal lymphoma, or short-bowel syndrome. Patients that are recumbent because of neurologic conditions and have questionable swallowing reflexes with risk of aspiration during oral or tube feedings also may benefit from PN. Parenteral administration of nutrition has been used initially in cats with hepatic lipidosis; in animals with facial fractures, megaesophagus, or pneumonia; and in other patients with high anesthetic risk (e.g., lung lobe torsion or contusions, diaphragmatic hernia). Parenteral nutrition can be administered to most patients until they are more stable and can tolerate placement of feeding tubes. Septic or anemic patients or those with severe upper respiratory infections have persistently poor appetites and may benefit from PN supplementing their low enteral intake of food. Patients with a poor appetite and large heat or protein losses (e.g., continuous-suction chest or abdominal drains, large areas of skin loss because of burn or degloving injury) also benefit from PN because of their less than adequate oral intake. Parenteral nutrition can be used to augment poor enteral intake that does not meet the patient's RER. Administering only intravenous lipids to supplement oral intake of food is successful in meeting the patient's daily RER.

The goal of PN support is to deliver all or part of the patient's RER, but the logistics of this support must be determined on a case-by-case basis. General guidelines are discussed to help establish a protocol, but the need for attentiveness, initiative, and ingenuity in meeting the patient's nutritional needs should never be underestimated because no two cases are alike.

Nomenclature

It is not necessary for PN in veterinary medicine to be *total* parenteral nutrition (TPN). Only human patients fed for many months to years require TPN (i.e., meeting daily total caloric, essential amino and fatty acid, fat- and water-soluble vitamin, and macro-, micro- and ultratrace element requirements). In veterinary medicine, PN attempts to meet the patient's estimated RER, most (but not all) essential amino and fatty acid, some water-soluble vitamin, and selected macro- and micro-element requirements. There are several valid reasons why TPN is not attempted in veterinary medicine. First, the time frame over which PN is administered to animals is relatively short (3–14 days) compared with that used in people, in whom long-term feeding is for 10 days and longer. The shorter time frame of nutritional support allows omission of nutrients normally stored in the body (e.g., fat-soluble vitamins). Until there is a demand by owners for a longer

TABLE 22–1. Criteria of Patients for Total Nutrient Admixture Administration

Hemodynamically stable with major electrolyte and acid-base abnormalities, severe tachycardia, hypotension, and volume deficits corrected or nearly within normal limits

Food intake less than calculated daily resting energy requirement for more than 3 days

Concurrent small-intestinal condition that is known or suspected to be impaired

Expected to be hospitalized for at least the next 3 days

period of support (weeks to months), PN in animals will consist of only the most essential and immediately needed nutrients (e.g., electrolytes, calories, amino acids, B vitamins). Second, adding all available nutrients to a PN solution would require multiple single-nutrient additions of specially prepared products (e.g., glutamine). These are cost prohibitive and difficult to justify on a short-term basis. Third, as more nutrient compounds are added to the solution, the risk of incompatibility increases and the possibility of an insoluble precipitate forming is greater. This risk is of less concern on a short-term basis. Therefore, PN in veterinary medicine currently consists only of essential nutrients, because TPN is limited by precise nutritional knowledge, cost, and pharmacokinetic principles.

Parenteral Products

Compounding PN solutions is not feasible for most veterinary practices, but PN can be administered to patients in most practices. Individual PN solutions of dextrose, lipid and amino acids, vitamins, and microminerals can be combined into a "three-in-one" or total nutrient admixture (TNA). Total nutrient admixture refers to one bag containing a mixture of parenteral solutions to meet a particular patient's fluid, RER, amino acid, electrolyte, and B vitamin needs for a 24-h period. This is a convenient method requiring only one bag, an administration set, and an infusion pump.

ENERGY SOLUTIONS

A TNA solution should supply an energy source sufficient to meet, but not exceed, the patient's daily RER. Many of the metabolic complications of PN may be due to administering energy in excess of the patient's expenditure (Veterans Affairs 1991; Lippert et al. 1993; Hirai et al. 1979; Lowry and Brennan 1979; Chang and Silvis 1974). This "hyperalimentation" actually exceeds the patient's ability to use the exogenous energy sources and produces the adverse metabolic effects commonly associated with PN. In people, the recommendations are to feed at RER instead of RER times some disease factor (McMahon 1993; Forse 1995; DeBiasse and Wilmore 1994). Multiplying RER by a disease factor is no longer recommended for veterinary patients. Dog and cat maintenance energy requirements are also now thought to be lower than previously published (Thatcher et al. 1998).

Energy routinely is provided to veterinary patients receiving PN as dextrose and lipid. Both dextrose and lipid are strongly recommended in a TNA as sources of energy. Several companies provide dextrose and lipid products of various strengths and attributes. Dextrose solutions, usually derived from hydrolyzed cornstarch, range from 2.5 to 70% glucose. These solutions have an osmolality range (between 126 and 3530 mOsm/L) that is directly proportional to their glucose concentration (American Hospital 1997). Dextrose solutions are maintained within the pH range 3.5 to 5.5 and have been autoclaved to prolong shelf life at room temperature. Lipid (10, 20, or 30%) products were reintroduced in the 1970s and contain emulsified fat particles (0.5 μm size) of either soybean oil or safflower oil and glycerin. These solutions contain both linoleic and linolenic acids. Lipid emulsions are maintained within the pH range 6.0 to 8.9 and have an osmolality range of 260 to 310 mOsm/L (American Hospital 1997). Most TNA solutions formulated for veterinary patients have 50% dextrose (2525 mOsm/L) and 20% lipid (260 mOsm/L).

DEXTROSE-TO-LIPID RATIO

It is generally thought that the optimal calorie source is a mixture of glucose and fat, but the precise ratio is not known (Stein 1986). The primary reason for a mixed fuel source is to decrease the possibility of fat deposition in the liver in the event that any one metabolic pathway that handles either fat or dextrose becomes overloaded. The initial recommendation has been that fat not constitute more than 60% of the calorie intake.[*] The potential negative effects of a high-fat infusion were centered around the potential for thrombosis and atherosclerosis and the overall unknown effect of synthetic chylomicrons on blood vessels when administered to people for longer than 10 days. All adverse effects reported in people with fat administration have occurred during infusion at rates providing lipid energy in excess of energy expenditure (Klein and Miles 1994; Mashima 1979; Meguid et al. 1984; Adamkin et al. 1984). Other than the potential problem of thrombosis, there appears to be little substantiation to date of why lipid could not provide more than 60% of the veterinary patient's RER.

When PN is begun, most patients have not consumed daily RER for at least 3 days and often much longer. The proportion of dextrose to lipid in the PN solution should mirror the current metabolic fuel utilization by the liver. Fewer metabolic complications arise if the dextrose-to-lipid ratio in the PN solution is well tolerated by the liver. By the fifth day of anorexia, patients should receive the majority (60–90%) of their calculated RER as lipid because the liver is utilizing glycerol and fatty acids from endogenous fat for gluconeogenesis (Nordenstrom et al. 1983). There is much evidence to suggest that there is a demand for a substantial proportion of calories as fat in the starving and diseased state. For example, a shift in the preferred fuel from glucose to endogenous fat has been identified in septic animals. In acutely septic rats, those given fat-free parenteral glucose had extensive mobilization of endogenous fat, whereas nonseptic rats had no mobilization of endogenous fat when given a fat-free high-glucose solution (Stein 1986). Fat is well oxidized in septic people. In fact, as the severity of sepsis increased, the amount of fat oxidized increased and the capacity to oxidize glucose decreased (Stoner et al. 1983). People with pancreatitis have an altered metabolism characterized by a decreased capacity to oxidize glucose, a peripheral resistance to insulin, and consequently hyperglycemia (Helton 1993). Giving high doses of glucose at a time when the animal's natural response is to minimize glucose utilization does not result in optimal use of administered glucose. This is the most likely cause of the hyperglycemia commonly reported as a complication of PN in people and veterinary patients (Veterans Affairs 1991). Second,

---

[*]Prescribing information for Intralipid intravenous fat emulsion. Cutter Laboratories, Berkeley, CA, 1981.

hyperglycemia impairs immune function, and the high blood glucose concentrations in people receiving PN have been associated with a higher infection rate than observed in enterally fed patients (McMahon 1997). The higher rate of infection associated with PN administration is more likely to be related to overfeeding of dextrose and the subsequent hyperglycemia, which depresses immune function.

High-fat TNA solutions (60–90%) have been used for more than 500 animals receiving PN over a 5-year period (Remillard RL, unpublished data, 1993–1998) and there have been no unusual metabolic or hematologic complications associated with these infusions. In fact, when central venous access is limited and the animal requires fluid therapy at or below maintenance, administering a lipid emulsion IV and delivering 100% of the RER as fat not only is possible but also has been well tolerated. Most patients receiving high-fat PN solutions that do not exceed RER do not develop hyperglycemia on the basis of regular urine glucose checks, as was common in previous reports (Lippert et al. 1993). Hyperglycemia actually is better controlled in patients with diabetes mellitus, pancreatitis, and septicemia because a TNA providing 80% of the calories as fat contains only 1 to 2% dextrose. Intravenous infusion of a lipid emulsion does, however, routinely cause an increase in plasma triglyceride concentration. The consequences in veterinary patients, if any, of persistent hypertriglyceridemia for several days is unknown. This effect should not be considered true hyperlipidemia because most patients clear the lipid particles within 30 min of stopping the infusion. The plasma half-life of dietary chylomicrons after IV infusion of soybean or safflower oil emulsions in dogs ranged from 7 to 16 min (Edgren and Meng 1962; Kesterson 1978). It is important that the TNA infusion pump be stopped 30 min before blood sampling because lipemia associated with PN administration interferes with some serum biochemistry tests. Often, the plasma lipid profiles of dogs and cats with preexisting hyperlipidemia have not been clearly defined. The lipids in TNA solutions are composed of chylomicrons containing triglycerides, and this knowledge may be useful in treating animals with hyperlipidemia that receive PN.

Administering a PN solution to adults and infants for weeks to years has been reported to cause steatosis, intrahepatic cholestasis, periportal inflammation, and cirrhosis. Fatty infiltration of the liver is the earliest and most common abnormality noted (Carpentier et al. 1993). This undesirable relationship between long-term parenteral feeding and hepatic histopathology has been recognized in people and other species and is thought to be multifactorial (Freund 1991; Nussbaum and Fischer 1991). These complications are not specific to PN, dextrose, or lipid emulsions. A balanced formulation of dextrose and lipid is now encouraged for patients with hepatic disease because replacing a portion of the glucose with lipid ameliorates some hepatic histopathology (Nussbaum et al. 1992). At this time, it is unusual for veterinary patients to receive PN for more than 2 weeks, and the hepatic complications associated with prolonged PN administration are unlikely to be observed. Lipid infusions have been reported to cause coagulopathies and thrombocytopenia in people and animals when administered in high doses at rapid rates. Slow continuous infusions of lipids, however, have had little or no perceived effect on platelet number or aggregation, bleeding time, and immune function in a clinical setting.

PROTEIN SOLUTIONS

Patients must receive a source of nitrogen and essential amino acids, and such solutions are available containing 3.5 to 15% amino acids. These solutions are maintained within the pH range 5.3 to 6.5, have an osmolality range of 300 to 1400 mOsm/L, and also may contain electrolytes and/or dextrose at various concentrations (American Hospital 1997). The most commonly used product in veterinary medicine is an 8.5% amino acid and electrolyte solution (1160 mOsm/L). Most amino acid solutions contain all of the essential amino acids for dogs and cats except taurine. Some specialized pediatric amino acid products do, however, contain taurine. Protein should be provided at a ratio of 1 to 6 g protein per 100 kcal of energy. Adult dogs do well with 2 to 3 g of protein, whereas adult cats require 3 to 4 g of protein per 100 kcal. In animals with renal or hepatic insufficiency, lower ratios (1–2 g per 100 kcal RER) are recommended. When there are increased protein needs (e.g., albumin losses, chest tube drain), higher ratios of protein to energy are recommended (5–6 g per 100 kcal RER). When protein is provided at these ratios to energy, patients rarely develop azotemia related to PN administration.

ELECTROLYTE SOLUTIONS

The electrolyte abnormalities that occur during administration of PN involve the major intracellular solutes, potassium and phosphorus. Potassium and phosphorus are translocated intracellularly when energy solutions are administered (Forrester and Moreland 1989). Potassium moves into cells along with glucose in response to insulin and during correction of acidosis. A TNA formulated from an 8.5% amino acid solution with electrolytes and lactated Ringer's solution contains approximately 12 mEq K^+/L, which usually is not adequate to maintain normal serum potassium concentration. Potassium can be added to the PN solution using a 2 mEq/mL KCl solution. If the patient is normokalemic when PN is initiated, a solution containing 30 mEq K^+/L most often maintains normokalemia. If the patient is hypokalemic when PN is started, a solution containing 40 to 80 mEq K^+/L is required. If the patient is hyperkalemic when PN is initiated, no potassium supplementation is recommended, but daily monitoring of serum potassium concentration is advised.

Phosphorus moves into cells with refeeding because of increased production of high-energy phosphate compounds (Hardy and Adams 1989). Animals receiving PN rarely become hypophosphatemic. Phosphorus from lipids (15 mmol/L) and amino acid plus electrolyte (30 mmol/L) usually provide an adequate concentration of phosphorus in the TNA (5–10 mmol/L). If warranted, phosphorus can be added to the PN solution using a 3 mmol/mL sodium or potassium phosphate solution. For hyperphosphatemic animals, the quantity of amino acids administered must be lowered to achieve a lower phosphorus concentration in the TNA.

VITAMIN SOLUTIONS

Few veterinary patients require fat-soluble vitamins during PN unless there is a history of prolonged weight loss, inappetence, and decreased fat absorption. For animals with long-term fat malabsorption, fat-soluble vitamin supplementation is warranted, and it is much simpler and more cost effective to administer 1 mL of a combined vitamin A, D, and E product* intramuscularly one time. This dose supplies fat-soluble vitamins for approximately 3 months.

Water-soluble vitamins, however, must be supplied daily with the TNA. Most veterinary vitamin B products do not contain all 11 B-complex vitamins but rather contain a few selected ones. Some B vitamins are not compatible in the same solution (e.g., folic acid and riboflavin are incompatible). Considering the recommendations of the American Association of Feed Control Officials (AAFCO) for dogs and cats, and given the vitamin concentrations available in commonly used products,† the recommended dose of 1 mL of B vitamins per 100 kcal exceeds the daily minimum allowance of dogs and cats by 5- to 100-fold, depending on the B vitamin in question. There should be little concern about overdosage because B vitamins are water soluble. Some clinicians administer the antioxidant vitamin C to ill dogs and cats (especially those with chronic liver disease) as a precautionary measure but there is no documented need or recommended dose to date. The vitamin C recommendation for people receiving TNA is 200 to 225 mg/day (Demetroiu and Jones 1993).

Some B vitamins are light labile. Preparations of B vitamins are maintained in a light-resistant bottle between 15 and 30°C. Riboflavin, perhaps the most light-labile B vitamin, undergoes a 50% decrease in activity after 8 h under indoor fluorescent lighting (Smith et al. 1988). Given the AAFCO recommended dose of riboflavin and the concentration of riboflavin in the TNA at 1 mL of B vitamins per 100 kcal RER, the patient would receive the daily recommended amount of riboflavin within the first 2 h of TNA therapy. Hence, covering the IV fluid bag to protect B vitamins probably is not necessary. Second, the addition of lipid increases the opacity of the final solution, reduces light penetration, and precludes the need to protect the PN solution from light (Smith et al. 1988). In summary, adding B vitamins is a low-cost but effective means of optimizing energy metabolism at the tissue level.

MICROMINERAL SOLUTIONS

When possible, zinc, copper, manganese, chromium, and selenium should be added to the PN solution directly. A four- to five-trace-element combination solution is available in multiple-dose vials at a reasonable cost (Jeejeebhoy 1981). On the basis of the AAFCO daily trace mineral recommendations for the healthy dog and cat and given the mineral concentration available in commonly used products,* copper appears to be the limiting trace element. The recommended dosage therefore is 1 mL of trace element solution per 100 kcal daily.

DRUG ADDITIONS

Although it is most convenient to administer drugs intravenously with the TNA, extreme caution must be used before any medications are added. Drug and TNA solution compatibility studies are ongoing and there are published lists of drugs known to be compatible and safe (Dickerson et al. 1993). The drugs of most interest to veterinarians that can be incorporated into a three-in-one mixture are listed in Table 22-2. The *Handbook on Injectable Drugs* is updated and published every 2 years and can be consulted for more current information on drug compatibility with PN solutions (Trissel 1996). Once a drug has been added to the day's TNA solution, a decision to discontinue that medication can be costly because a new bag of TNA solution must be compounded. Use of a second peripheral catheter or a double-lumen central catheter therefore may be preferable to adding drugs to PN solutions.

Compounding

TNA formulations are designed specifically for one patient on the basis of current body weight, daily fluid requirement, approximate protein need, and ability to handle glucose as opposed to lipid. The TNA solution should be formulated first to meet the patient's RER and protein needs. Second, the total fluid volume is adjusted using a conventional crystalloid solution to meet the patient's daily fluid requirement. Finally, electrolytes are adjusted as needed (usually only potassium is required) and water-soluble vitamins and trace minerals are added (Table 22-3).

There are several methods by which a veterinarian may compound or obtain a premixed TNA for a particular patient. Some human hospitals mix PN solutions in their own pharmacies, and most formulate PN solutions for veterinarians. The veterinarian, however, must provide the prescription (see Table 23-3) and the final cost is much greater than that with any other method of com-

TABLE 22-2. Drugs Compatible with Total Nutrient Admixture Parenteral Nutrition Solutions

Aminophylline	Diphenhydramine	Lidocaine
Ampicillin	Dopamine	Metoclopramide
Cefazolin	Erythromycin	Penicillin G
Chloramphenicol	Furosemide	Phytonadione
Cimetidine	Gentamicin	Ranitidine
Clindamycin	Heparin	Ticarcillin
Digoxin	Insulin (regular)	

From Dickerson RN, Brown RO, and White KG: Parenteral nutrition solutions. In Rombeau JL and Caldwell MD (eds): Parenteral Nutrition, 2nd ed. Philadelphia, WB Saunders Co., pp. 310–333, 1993.

---

*Vital E-A + D containing 100 KIU of A, 10 KIU of D, and 300 IU of α-tocopherol per mL. Schering-Plough Animal Health Corp., Kenilworth, NJ.

†B-vitamin complex containing 50 mg thiamine, 2 mg riboflavin, 100 mg niacin, 2 mg pyridoxine, 10 mg pantothenic acid, 0.4 ppm B_{12} per mL. Butler Co., Columbus, OH.

*MTE-4 containing 1 mg zinc, 0.1 mg manganese, 0.4 mg copper, 4 μg chromium. Fujisawa USA, Deerfield, IL.

TABLE 22-3. **Standard Total Nutrient Admixture Formulation—Calculation Worksheet**

	Cat Example
Patient Data Needed	
1. Current body weight in kg = _____	4.1 kg
2. Calculate RER as kcal/day = _____	200 kcal/day
3. Expected fluid rate in mL/kg/day = _____	70 mL/kg
4. Calories from fat as % = _____	80%
5. Protein/calorie ratio as g/100 kcal RER = _____	4 g/100 kcal
6. Potassium concentration as mEq/L = _____	30 mEq/L
Parenteral Solution Formula	
Determine volume of fat and dextrose needed daily:	
Fat	
Calculate RER calories from fat = _____	$200 \times 0.80 = 160$ kcal
Calculate volume of 20% (2 kcal/mL) lipid needed = _____	160 kcal/2 kcal/mL = 80 mL/day
Dextrose	
Calculate RER calories from dextrose = _____	$200 - 160 = 40$ kcal
Calculate volume of 50% (1.7 kcal/mL) dextrose needed = _____	40 kcal/1.7 kcal/mL = 24 mL/day
Determine volume of amino acid solution needed daily:	
Calculate grams of protein needed = _____	4 g/100 kcal × RER = 8 g protein/day
Calculate volume of 8.5% amino acid needed = _____	8 g/0.085 g/mL = 94 mL/day
Determine volume of B vitamins and trace minerals needed daily:	
Calculate B vitamins needed = _____	1 mL/100 kcal × RER = 2 mL/day
Calculate trace minerals needed = _____	1 mL/100 kcal × RER = 2 mL/day
PN total volume = mL lipid + mL dextrose + mL amino acid + mL B vitamins + mL trace minerals	
$\quad$ = 80 + 24 + 94 + 2 + 2 = 202 mL	
Determine volume of lactated Ringer's solution (LRS) needed to meet daily fluid requirement:	
Daily fluid volume requested = _____	70 mL/kg × 4.1 kg = 287 mL/day
LRS required is daily total − PN total = _____	287 − 202 = 85 mL
Determine potassium supplementation:	
K^+ from LRS (4 mEq/L) = _____	0.085 L × 4 mEq/L = 0.4 mEq
K^+ from amino acid solution (60 mEq/L) = _____	0.094 L × 60 mEq/L = 5.6 mEq
Total K^+ mEq in TNA solution = _____	0.4 mEq + 5.6 mEq = 6 mEq
Desired final K^+ concentration in TNA = _____	30 mEq/L × 0.287 L = 8.6 mEq
Additional KCl mEq required = _____	8.6 mEq − 6 mEq = 2.6 mEq
KCl mL (2 mEq/mL) required = _____	2.6 mEq/2 mEq/mL = 1.3 mL
Summary	
Daily TNA prescription:	
$\quad$ 20% lipid $\quad$ _____	= 80 mL
$\quad$ 50% dextrose $\quad$ _____	= 24 mL
$\quad$ 8.5% amino acid with electrolytes $\quad$ _____	= 94 mL
$\quad$ B vitamins $\quad$ _____	= 2 mL
$\quad$ Trace minerals $\quad$ _____	= 2 mL
$\quad$ KCl $\quad$ _____	= 1.3 mL
$\quad$ LRS $\quad$ _____	= 85 mL
	Total = 288 mL
Calculated mOsm/L:	
$\quad$ 20% lipid × 260 mOsm/L	0.080 L × 260 = 20.8
$\quad$ 50% dextrose × 2525 mOsm/L	0.024 L × 2525 = 60.6
$\quad$ 8.5% amino acid with electrolytes × 1160 mOsm/L	0.094 L × 1160 = 109
$\quad$ LRS × 300 mOsm/L	0.085 L × 300 = 25.5
	0.288 L = 215.9 particles
$\quad$ Total mOsm/L = 215.9 particle/0.288 total volume = 750 mOsm/L	

pounding. Some veterinary schools, large referral hospitals, and private veterinary practices maintain parenteral solution compounders, supplies, and equipment not only for their own use but also to formulate and sell bags of TNA directly to practitioners. This is the safest, most convenient and economical method of obtaining a TNA solution for the occasional patient that requires PN in most practices.

TNA or all-in-one bags can be compounded by one of three methods, each of which has been previously described (Remillard and Thatcher 1989). Briefly, the least desirable method is to use a syringe to transfer each nutrient solution (dextrose, amino acid, lipid) into a sterile empty fluid bag. This method is the most time consuming and has the highest risk of contamination because of the multiple injections required. The second method uses a closed-circuit fluid system in which the all-in-one bag comes with a preattached three-lead transfer set. Each lead, with a vented filter spike, is inserted directly into the individual nutrient solutions (dextrose, amino acid, lipid) and transferred directly into the all-in-one bag by gravity flow. This method is faster and safer than the syringe method, but transfer of exact quantities (±50 mL) is not possible. This method may be economical when the number of patients requiring PN is relatively low (two or three per month). Both the syringe and gravity feed methods usually leave partially unused bottles of dextrose, fat, and amino acids.

The third method, used by most human hospitals and large referral veterinary hospitals, requires a high-speed closed-circuit fluid compounder that pumps three or four nutrient solutions (dextrose, amino acid, lipid, fluid) directly into one bag within 60 s. Each nutrient solution is accurately transferred to within 1 mL and the system has a mean error of less than 2% (Fig. 22–1). The setup can be used for any number of bags over a 24-h period, after which the setup should be discarded. Multiple bags of TNA for several patients can be made efficiently at one time using partial bottles of dextrose, fat, and amino acids. Making bags of TNA with a compounder is safe, fast, accurate, efficient, and can be done routinely by a veterinary technician (McClendon 1981). I have used a computerized compounder to formulate over 1500 TNA bags over a 5-year period, and there have been no suspected or confirmed instances of mixing errors or microbial contamination during formulation (Remillard RL, unpublished data, 1993–1998).

The diverse composition of the TNA solution increases the risk of physicochemical incompatibilities (Driscoll et al. 1995). All-in-one or TNA solutions, however, can be stored by refrigeration for 7 to 14 days. The integrity of the lipid emulsion usually is the limiting factor. In a TNA, fat particles can aggregate and the larger particles migrate to the surface of the solution, creating a "whiter" band at the top of the TNA solution. This process is called creaming and can easily be reversed by gentle mixing. It is of no danger to the patient. When the negative surface charge of the emulsion is neutralized, however, destabilization of the emulsion progresses irreversibly to coalescence (Driscoll et al. 1986). The process of coalescence is irreversible because of the presence of two immiscible phases of oil and water and is associated with a dark yellow color, either in a line across the top portion of the TNA or as large yellow globules throughout the TNA solution. The addition of B vitamins to the TNA solution gives it a uniform light yellow color, and this appearance should not be confused with coalescence. No bags with evidence of coalescence should be administered to a patient because the larger particles may cause fat embolism in pulmonary capillaries (Leveen et al. 1961; Atik 1978).

Adding divalent cations (e.g., calcium, magnesium) to the TNA solution is not advisable because the positive charge can destabilize the negatively charged surface of the fat particle, break the emulsion, and cause coalescence. The addition of components that decrease the final pH of the solution to 5.0 or less also causes the emulsion to break. Individual dextrose solutions are maintained at pH 5.0 to minimize microbial growth, whereas amino acid solutions are buffered to pH 6.0. When mixing a TNA solution, it is important to add the lipid last or when there is a large volume of a higher pH fluid already in the PN bag.

Administration

TNA solutions can be delivered to the patient by a central, peripheral, intraosseous, or intraperitoneal catheter. TNA solutions with an osmolality less than 600 mOsm/L may be administered via peripheral vein, whereas solutions with an osmolality greater than 600 mOsm/L should be administered into a central vein to decrease the risk of thrombophlebitis. Ideally, the catheter should be dedicated to PN administration and should not be used for blood sampling, medication or blood product administration, or central venous pressure monitoring. When venous access is limited, however, the PN catheter may be used for blood sampling and administering medications when adequately flushed before and after the interruption in PN administration. Excellent aseptic catheter handling

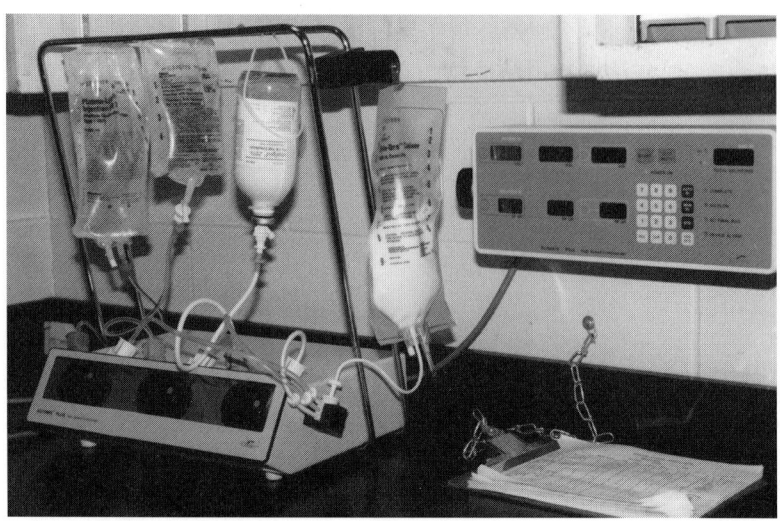

FIGURE 22–1. Photograph of a three-station TNA compounder.

techniques, as with any other fluid therapy, should be used during these line interruptions.

PERIPHERAL VEIN INFUSION

There is increased interest in human medicine in administering PN via a peripheral vein because of the increased risk and additional expense associated with central venous catheters and as a result of newer catheter materials that decrease the incidence of peripheral vein thrombophlebitis (Payne-James and Khawaja 1993; Everitt and McMahon 1994; Kohlhardt et al. 1994; Matsusue et al. 1995; Daly et al. 1985; Isaacs et al. 1977; Maden et al. 1992). Phlebitis is the principal complication occurring within the first 72 h of PN in 26 to 48% of patients (Bayer-Berger et al. 1989). The incidence of phlebitis is significantly increased when TNAs that contain amino acids, potassium, or antibiotics and have an osmolality greater than 600 mOsm/L are used (Gazitua et al. 1979). There are no published clinical reports of administering TNA solutions by peripheral vein to dogs or cats. However, PN solutions without heparin and with osmolality of 600 mOsm/L or less, when administered to veterinary patients using a peripheral catheter have resulted in thrombophlebitis in approximately 15% of cases within 24 to 48 h (Remillard RL, unpublished data using 2.5-cm Vialon catheters, May 1997). Administering fat calories by peripheral vein to dogs and cats is easily accomplished without complications using an isomolar 20% lipid solution piggybacked with standard fluid therapy in sufficient daily volumes to meet RER (Remillard RL, unpublished data using 2.5-cm Vialon catheters, May 1997).

Peripherally inserted central lines can be used in dogs and cats for administering TNA solutions. Cats are smaller than most dogs but have higher protein requirements and sometimes have restrictive fluid allowances. Therefore, the final osmolality of the PN solutions used in cats can be 600 to 800 mOsm/L, and such a solution ideally should be administered into a large vein. Placing a 10- to 20-cm polyurethane* or silicone† catheter into the femoral or saphenous vein and advancing it into the caudal vena cava is possible in the cat. Placing a similar but longer polyurethane or silicone catheter in the lateral saphenous vein and advancing to the caudal vena cava is possible in small dogs. TNA solutions >600 mOsm/L have been administered successfully using peripherally inserted central lines in both dogs and cats.

CENTRAL VEIN INFUSION

A single- or multiple-lumen polyurethane or silicone elastomer catheter may be placed percutaneously or by a cutdown procedure in the external jugular vein of most dogs and cats. The tip of the catheter should be located in the cranial vena cava or right atrium of the heart. Catheters made of silicone elastomer and polyurethane are softer and less irritating and therefore have fewer mechanical and septic complications, and they are less thrombogenic (but more expensive) than the polytetrafluoroethylene (Teflon) catheters commonly used in veterinary patients for fluid administration. For long-term applications (>3 days), silicone and polyurethane are acceptable catheter materials. These central catheters are changed as dictated by individual patients' problems and not at predetermined time intervals. Although initially expensive to place, these catheters may remain in place and be used throughout an entire hospital stay, which may lower overall catheter costs.

Multiple-lumen catheters allow multipurpose venous access for administering incompatible fluid and drug therapies or different fluids at different rates. Although use in veterinary patients has not been adequately evaluated, their use for PN administration has been associated with an increase in septic complications in people (McCarthy et al. 1987). No known or suspected cases of sepsis have been encountered in dogs receiving PN via dual-lumen jugular catheters (Armstrong JP, unpublished data).

OTHER ROUTES OF INFUSION

Intraosseous infusion of electrolytes, amino acids, dextrose, and vitamins has been successfully performed in dogs (Otto et al. 1989). There are no known literature citations referring to intraosseous infusion of lipid. However, successful intraperitoneal infusion of a TNA solution (850 mOsm/L) for longer than 20 days was reported in 19 normal dogs and in 12 normal dogs that had undergone intestinal resection (Moran et al. 1989; Garcia-Gamito et al. 1991). A 10% lipid solution intraperitoneally infused into 2- to 3-month-old beagles was absorbed from the peritoneal cavity over a 4-h period (Klein et al. 1983). These routes may be considered when venous access is not available.

Catheter Complications

The most clinically significant problem during TNA administration involves the catheter. The most common problem seen with a TNA catheter is thrombophlebitis. Infection is much less common.

THROMBOPHLEBITIS

Thrombophlebitis is a response of the intima of the vein to the unique combination of the chemical composition of the infusate, the nature of the catheter material, and the mechanical features of catheter placement, including the ratio of catheter to vessel size. Intravenous catheters reduce blood flow and can induce thrombophlebitis within 72 h, regardless of infusate. Therefore, it often is recommended that Teflon catheters be changed every 3 days. The catheter material is thought to be the single most important factor in the severity of infusion thrombophlebitis (Gaukroger et al. 1988; McKee et al. 1989). Catheter material contributes to thrombosis through three characteristics: roughness, stiffness, and predilection for platelet adhesion (Linder et al. 1984). Teflon° intravenous catheters have been routinely used in veterinary medicine as short peripheral catheters because they are easy to insert, inexpensive, and have caused relatively

---

*L-Cath (16 and 18 gauge), Luther Medical Products, Santa Ana, CA. Central venous (20 to 16 gauge) catheters, Cook Veterinary Products, Bloomington, IL.

†Silicone (20 to 16 gauge) catheters (50 to 60 cm) can be cut to appropriate lengths. Cook Critical Care, Bloomington, IL.

°Jelco (24 gauge, 5 cm). Critikon, Tampa, FL.

low rates of phlebitis (Hershey et al. 1984). Vialon* (a polyetherurethane hydromer) has become available, and catheters made of this material are easier to insert, have lower infiltration rates, and are less thrombogenic than Teflon catheters (McKee et al. 1989; Myles et al. 1981). Several studies comparing peripheral Teflon, Silastic (silicone), and polyurethane catheters and PN administration have been completed (Kohlhardt et al. 1992; Reynolds et al. 1995; Linder et al. 1984). In summary, it appears that catheter materials placed in order of increasing thrombogenicity would be Vialon (lowest), polyurethane, silicone, and Teflon (highest) (Borow and Crowley 1985; di Costanzo et al. 1988).

In people, the incidence of thrombophlebitis also can be reduced by adding low-dose heparin (0.5–1 U/mL) or hydrocortisone (10 mg/L) to the TNA solution (Imperial et al. 1983; Roongpisuthipong et al. 1994; Alpan et al. 1984). This dose of heparin has not affected normal hemostasis in people but has prolonged catheter patency by reducing phlebitis at the catheter tip. A low incidence of thrombophlebitis has been reported in dogs and cats with 1 U of sodium heparin per milliliter of TNA, a dose that does not affect coagulation function in animals with normal hemostasis. There have been no comparative veterinary studies, however, on whether heparin or hydrocortisone reduces phlebitis in peripheral catheters.

INFECTION

Infectious complications with intravenous infusions have been recognized for more than 40 years and now are primarily associated with substandard catheter care. Most catheter-related episodes of septicemia are due to microbial invasion at the catheter wound, either during or after insertion (Bozzetti 1985; Maki et al. 1977). Hospitals that use solutions containing iodine to disinfect the skin and that emphasize catheter site asepsis have significantly lower rates of positive catheter cultures and septicemia (Maki et al. 1973). Catheter placement for PN administration must be carried out meticulously. The catheter bandage and administration sets should be changed at least every other day if not daily. At the time of bandage change, the venipuncture site is cleaned with a solution containing iodine and examined for redness, edema, or swelling. A topical antibiotic ointment that has antifungal and antibacterial properties should be applied at the catheter-skin junction.

Also, hematogenous seeding of the catheter tip thrombi can occur from other sources, such as urinary tract infections, abscesses, pneumonia, or intestinal bacterial translocation. In a prospective study of 200 consecutive patients receiving PN, 75% of the catheters removed in association with septicemia were determined, retrospectively, not to have been the cause of the infection (Ryan et al. 1974). Other infectious sites were subsequently identified in most patients.

Infusion of contaminated fluid is a third, but unlikely, source of infection when the TNA has been compounded in a closed-circuit fluid system. It has been commonly stated that TNA solutions favor microbial growth. However, current TNA solutions with crystalline amino acids do not favor microbial growth as previously thought. Previous statements and cautions were based on the use of a dextrose and protein hydrolysate solution, which is no longer available (Herruzo-Bareara et al. 1984). The protein hydrolysate products contained peptides or ammonia that bacteria used for growth. The crystalline amino acid products currently used in TNA do not contain peptides or ammonia. They are hypertonic and acidic and therefore exhibit antibacterial effects (Goldmann et al. 1972; Wilkinson et al. 1973). There is conflicting evidence concerning whether bacteria grow slowly or not at all in TNA solutions (Scheckelhoff et al. 1986; Rowe et al. 1987). Fungi can proliferate in admixtures, but refrigeration at 4°C suppresses all microbial growth. Lipid emulsions alone, on the other hand, do support growth of gram-positive and gram-negative bacteria and fungal organisms if contaminated. The Centers for Disease Control recommended that lipid emulsions be discarded after 12 h except in TNA systems, which can hang for 24 h (Simmons et al. 1982). The TNA solution can be maintained for several days in the refrigerator but should be administered at room temperature. It is prudent not to extend the delivery of any one bag more than 24 to 36 h. In summary, as with any other type of fluid therapy, infections can be attributed either to lack of aseptic technique at the catheter insertion site or to contamination that occurred during manipulation of administration lines. Septicemia resulting from contaminated fluids occurs far less often than catheter-related sources of infection when TNAs are compounded and administered properly.

Combination of Enteral and Parenteral Nutrition

There has been renewed interest in human medicine in the use of tube feeding and its advantages over PN (Adams et al. 1986; Moore and Jones 1986). There is increasing evidence that prolonged fasting (>3 days) is associated with enterocyte deterioration and decreased gastrointestinal immunity (Alverdy et al. 1985). A possible source of infection with parenteral administration is translocation of enteric bacteria because of a compromised intestinal mucosal barrier. A combination of enteral and parenteral administration has been suggested because infusion of small quantities of a liquid diet has been beneficial in preventing intestinal mucosal deterioration (Remillard et al. 1998a, 1998b; Andrassey et al. 1979, 1985). In addition, intestinal adaptations after disease and intestinal hypertrophy after surgery require the presence of intraluminal nutrients, and food intake has been shown to promote intestinal hyperplasia and brush border enzyme activity (Hermann-Zaidius 1986). Therefore, some enteral feeding is recommended for patients receiving parenteral nutritional support, if possible. Both feeding the small bowel and feeding the patient are important.

▶ Monitoring

Regular reassessment is a critical step in successful nutritional management of a critically ill patient regardless of whether the enteral or parenteral route, or a combination, is used. While the patient is in the hospital, a review of

---

*Insyte (24–18 gauge, 5 cm). Becton-Dickinson, Sandy, UT.

the patient's food intake or successful administration of nutritional support should be done at least daily. Body weight should be recorded daily, but body condition score is unlikely to change during the course of a hospital stay. Laboratory assessments specifically for patients receiving PN are not necessary beyond what is routinely done for critically ill patients.

Changes in serum electrolyte and glucose concentrations are the most common alterations seen with TNA administration. The most common features of refeeding syndrome are hypokalemia and hypophosphatemia. There can be significant electrolyte shifts from the extracellular to the intracellular compartment as energy and amino acids are reintroduced. Regular urine glucose checks are adequate for monitoring hyperglycemia. Determination of blood glucose concentration need be done only when the urine becomes positive for glucose. Although other parameters are used to assess the nutritional status of patients, most parameters do not change with nutritional support during the course of hospitalization. Laboratory parameters such as albumin and total protein concentrations, red blood cell count, and hemoglobin concentration are unlikely to change in less than 2 weeks. Many patients do, however, show subjective improvement in attitude and posture within 24 to 48 h of administering PN.

REFERENCES

Adamkin DH, Gelke KN, and Andrews BF: Fat emulsions and hypertriglyceridemia. *JPEN* 8:563–567, 1984.

Adams S, Dellinger EP, Wurtz MJ, et al.: Enteral versus parenteral nutritional support following laparotomy for trauma: A randomized prospective trial. *J Trauma* 26:882–891, 1986.

Albrecht R, Pelissier MA, Miladi N, et al.: Protein restriction and metabolism on xenobiotics. *Ann Nutr Metab* 30:73–80, 1986.

Alpan G, Eyal F, Springer C, et al.: Heparinization of alimentation solutions administered through peripheral veins in premature infants: A controlled study. *Pediatrics* 74:375–378, 1984.

Alverdy J, Chi HS, and Sheldon GF: The effect of parenteral nutrition on gastrointestinal immunity. *Ann Surg* 202:681–684, 1985.

American Hospital Formulary Service: Drug Information 1997. American Society of Health System Pharmacists, 1997.

Anderson CF, Moxness K, Meister J, et al.: The sensitivity and specificity of nutrition-related variables in relationship to the duration of hospital stay and the rate of complications. *Mayo Clin Proc* 59:477–483, 1984.

Anderson KE: Influences of diet and nutrition on clinical pharmacokinetics. *Clin Pharmacokinet* 14:325–346, 1988.

Andrassey RJ, Mahour GH, Harrison MR, et al.: The role and safety of early postoperative feeding in the pediatric surgical patient. *J Pediatr Surg* 14:381–385, 1979.

Andrassy RJ, Dubois T, Page CP, et al.: Early postoperative nutritional enhancement utilizing enteral branched-chain amino acids by way of a needle catheter jejunostomy. *Am J Surg* 150:730–734, 1985.

Antonas KN: Nutrition status and the laboratory (letter). *Nutrition* 10:88–89, 1994.

Atik M: Hemodynamic changes following infusion of intravenous fat emulsions. *Int J Pharm* 1:141–150, 1978.

Bayer-Berger M, Chiolero R, and Freeman J: Incidence of phlebitis in peripheral parenteral nutrition: Effect of the different nutrient solutions. *Clin Nutr* 8:181–186, 1989.

Biden TJ and Taylor KW: Effects of ketone bodies on insulin release and islet-cell metabolism in the rat. *Biochem J* 212:371–377, 1983.

Birkham RH, Long CL, Fitkins D, et al.: Effects of major skeletal trauma on whole body protein turnover in man measured by L-[^{14}C]-leucine. *Surgery* 88:294–300, 1980.

Bistrian BR: Nutritional assessment of the hospitalized patient: A practical approach. In Wright RA and Heymsfield S (eds): *Nutritional Assessment*. Boston, Blackwell Scientific, pp. 183–205, 1984.

Boothby WM and Sandiford I: Basal metabolism. *Physiol Rev* 4:69–161, 1924.

Borow M and Crowley JG: Evaluation of central venous catheter thrombogenicity. *Acta Anaesthesiol Scand Suppl* 81:59–64, 1985.

Bozzetti F: Central venous catheter sepsis. *Drug Gynecol Obstet* 161:293–301, 1985.

Buffington CA: Nutritional support of critically ill patients, why bother? *Proceedings of IVECCS*, San Antonio, pp. 323–326, 1994.

Burkholder WJ: Metabolic rates and nutrient requirements of sick dogs and cats. *J Am Vet Med Assoc* 206:614–618, 1995.

Burkholder WJ and Swecker WS: Nutritional influences on immunity. *Semin Vet Med Surg (Small Anim)* 5(3):154–166, 1990.

Cahill GF and Owen OE: Starvation and survival. *Trans Am Clin Climatol Assoc* 79:13–20, 1967.

Carpentier YA, Gossum AV, Dubois DY, et al.: Lipid metabolism in parenteral nutrition. In Rombeau JL, Caldwell MD: *Clinical Nutrition: Parenteral Nutrition*, 2nd ed. Philadelphia, WB Saunders Co., pp. 35–74, 1993.

Chandra RK: Immunodeficiency in undernutrition and overnutrition. *Nutr Rev* 39:225–231, 1981.

Chandra RK: Numerical and functional deficiency in T helper cells in protein-energy malnutrition. *Clin Exp Immunol* 51:126–132, 1983.

Chandra RK: Nutritional regulation of immunity: An introduction. In Chandra RK (ed): *Nutrition and Immunology*. New York, Alan R Liss, pp. 1–8, 1988.

Chandra RK: Immunocompetence is a sensitive and functional barometer of nutritional status. *Acta Paediatr Scand Suppl* 374:129–132, 1991.

Chandra RK: Nutrition and immunoregulation. Significance for host resistance to tumors and infectious diseases in humans and rodents. *J Nutr* 122:754–757, 1992a.

Chandra RK: Protein-energy malnutrition and immunological responses. *J Nutr* 122:597–600, 1992b.

Chandra RK and Kumari S: Nutrition and immunity: An overview. *J Nutr* 124:1433s–1435s, 1994.

Chandra RK, Gupta S, and Singh H: Inducer and suppressor T cell subsets in protein-energy malnutrition. Analysis by monoclonal antibodies. *Nutr Res* 2:223–232, 1982.

Chang S and Silvis SE: Fatty liver produced by hyperalimentation of rats. *Am J Gastroenterol* 62:410–418, 1974.

Crane SW: Nutritional aspects of wound healing. *Semin Vet Med Surg* 4:263–267, 1989.

Daly JM, Masser E, Hansen L, et al.: Peripheral vein infusion of dextrose/amino acid solutions +/- 20% fat emulsion. *JPEN* 9:296–299, 1985.

Davenport DJ, Mostardi RA, Richardson DC, et al.: Protein-deficient diet alters serum alkaline phosphatase, bile acids, proteins and urea nitrogen in dogs. *J Nutr* 124:2677s–2679s, 1994.

DeBiasse MA and Wilmore DW: What is optimal nutritional support? *New Horiz* 2(2):122–130, 1994.

Deitel M, Williams VP, and Rice TW: Nutrition and the patient requiring mechanical ventilatory support. *J Am Coll Nutr* 2:25–32, 1983.

Demetroiu AA and Jones LK: Vitamins. In Rombeau JL and Caldwell MD (eds): *Clinical Nutrition; Parenteral Nutrition*, 2nd ed. Philadelphia, WB Saunders Co., pp. 184–202, 1993.

Devey JJ, Crowe DT, Kirby R, et al.: Postsurgical nutritional support (letter). *J Am Vet Med Assoc* 206:1673–1675, 1995.

Dickerson RN, Brown RO, and White KG: Parenteral nutrition

solutions. In Rombeau JL and Caldwell MD (eds): *Clinical Nutrition: Parenteral Nutrition*, 2nd ed. Philadelphia, WB Saunders Co., pp. 310–333, 1993.

di Costanzo J, Sastre B, Choux R, et al.: Mechanism of thrombogenesis during total parenteral nutrition: Role of catheter composition. *JPEN* 12:190–194, 1988.

Driscoll DF, Baptista RJ, Bistrian BR, et al.: Practical considerations regarding the use of total nutrient admixtures. *Am J Hosp Pharm* 43:416–419, 1986.

Driscoll DF, Bhargava HN, Li L, et al.: Physicochemical stability of total nutrient admixtures. *Am J Health Syst Pharm* 52:623–634, 1995.

Edgren B and Meng HC: The removal of dietary chylomicrons and artificial fat emulsions from the circulation of rats and dogs. *Acta Physiol Scand* 56:237–243, 1962.

Everitt NJ and McMahon MJ: Peripheral intravenous nutrition. *Nutrition* 10(1):49–57, 1994.

Fascetti AJ, Mauldin GE, and Mauldin GN: Correlation between serum creatine kinase activities and anorexia in cats. *J Vet Intern Med* 11:9–13, 1997.

Felig P, Owen OE, Wahren J, et al.: Amino acid metabolism during prolonged starvation. *J Clin Invest* 48:584–594, 1969.

Fischer JE and Glory ME: Protein depletion and immunity in the hospitalized patient. In Wrought RA and Heymsfield S (eds): *Nutritional Assessment*. Boston, Blackwell Scientific, pp. 111–129, 1984.

Flynn MF, Hardie EM and Armstrong PJ: Effect of ovariohysterectomy on maintenance energy requirements in cats. *J Am Vet Med Assoc* 209:1572–1581, 1996.

Forrester SD and Moreland KJ: Hypophosphatemia: Causes and clinical consequences. *J Vet Intern Med* 3:149–159, 1989.

Forse RA: Nutrition in critical care. In *Malnutrition in the Hospitalized Patient*. Boston, New England Deaconess Hospital and Harvard Medical School, May 5, 1995.

Freund HR: Abnormalities of liver function and hepatic damage associated with total parenteral nutrition. *Nutrition* 7(1):1–6, 1991.

Fulks RM, Li F, and Goldberg A: Effects of insulin, glucose and amino acids on protein turnover in rat diaphragm. *J Biol Chem* 250:290–298, 1975.

Garcia-Gamito FJ, Moran JM, Mehedero G, et al.: Long term peritoneal nutrition in dogs, both normal and after intestinal resection. *Int Surg* 76:235–240, 1991.

Gaukroger PB, Roberts JG, and Manners TA: Infusion thrombophlebitis: A prospective comparison of 645 Vialon and Teflon cannulae in anaesthetic and postoperative use. *Anaesth Intensive Care* 16:265–271, 1988.

Gazitua R, Wilson K, Bistrian BR, et al.: Factors determining peripheral vein tolerance to amino acid infusions. *Arch Surg* 114:897–900, 1979.

Goldmann DA, Martin WT, and Worthington JW: Growth of bacteria and fungi in total parenteral nutrition solutions. *Am J Surg* 126:314–318, 1971.

Grant JP: Clinical impact of protein malnutrition on organ mass and function. In Blackburn GL, Grant JP, and Young VR (eds): *Amino Acids: Metabolism and Medical Applications*. Boston, John Wright, pp. 347–358, 1983.

Grimble RF: Nutrition and cytokine action. *Nutr Res Rev* 3:193–210, 1990.

Hardy RM and Adams LG: Hypophosphatemia. In Kirk RW: *Current Veterinary Therapy X: Small Animal Practice*. Philadelphia, WB Saunders Co., pp. 43–47, 1989.

Helton WS: Intravenous nutrition in patients with acute pancreatitis. In Rombeau JL and Caldwell MD (eds): *Clinical Nutrition; Parenteral Nutrition*, 2nd ed. Philadelphia, WB Saunders Co., pp. 442–461, 1993.

Hermann-Zaidius MG: Malabsorption in adults: Etiology, evaluation and management. *J Am Diet Assoc* 86:1171–1178, 1986.

Herruzo-Bareara R, Garcia-Caballero J, Vera-Cortes L, et al.: Growth of microorganisms in parenteral nutrition solutions. *Am J Hosp Pharm* 41:1178–1180, 1984.

Hershey DO, Tomford JW, McLaren CE, et al.: The natural history of intravenous catheter associated phlebitis. *Arch Intern Med* 144:1373–1375, 1984.

Heymsfield SB, Hoff RD, Gray TF, et al.: Heart diseases. In Kinney JM, Jeejeebhoy KN, Hill GL, et al. (eds): *Nutrition and Metabolism in Patient Care*. Philadelphia, WB Saunders Co., pp. 477–509, 1988.

Hirai Y, Sanda Y, Fujiwara T, et al.: High calorie infusion-induced hepatic impairments in infants. *JPEN* 3:146–150, 1979.

Hoffer LJ: Starvation. In Shils ME, Olson JA, and Shike M (eds): *Modern Nutrition in Health and Disease*, 8th ed, Vol 2. Lea & Febiger, Philadelphia, pp. 927–949, 1994.

Imperial J, Bistrian BR, Bothe A, et al.: Limitation of central vein thrombosis in total parenteral nutrition by continuous infusion of low-dose heparin. *J Am Coll Nutr* 2:63–73, 1983.

Isaacs JW, Millikan WJ, Stackhouse J, et al.: Parenteral nutrition of adults with a 900 milliosmolar solution via peripheral veins. *Am J Clin Nutr* 30:552–559, 1977.

Jeejeebhoy KN: Trace element requirements in parenteral nutrition. Report of the Second Ross Conference on Medical Research. Nutritional assessment—Present status, future directions and prospects. Columbus, OH, pp. 76–77, 1981.

Kahan BD: Nutrition and host defense mechanisms. *Surg Clin North Am* 61:557–570, 1981.

Kesterson J: Acute intravenous clearance study of 10% and 20% safflower oil emulsions and 10% and 20% Intralipid in dogs. Chicago, Abbott Laboratories, Study T77–527, 1978.

Kien Cl, Young VR, Rohrbaugh DK, et al.: Increased rates of whole body protein synthesis and breakdown in children recovering from burns. *Ann Surg* 187:383–391, 1978.

Kinney JM: Energy metabolism: Heat, fuel and life. In Kinney JM (ed): *Nutrition and Metabolism in Patient Care*. Philadelphia, WB Saunders Co., pp. 3–34, 1988.

Kitagawa H, Kano M, Sasaki Y, et al.: Serum creatine kinase in dogs with dirofilariasis. *J Vet Med Sci* 53:569–575, 1991.

Klein MD, Coran AG, Drongowski RA, et al.: The quantitative transperitoneal absorption of a fat emulsion: Implications for intraperitoneal nutrition. *J Ped Surg* 18:724–731, 1983.

Klein S and Miles JM: Metabolic effects of long-chain and medium chain triglyceride emulsions in humans (editorial). *JPEN* 18:396, 1994.

Knodell RG: Effects of formula composition on hepatic an intestinal drug metabolism during enteral nutrition. *JPEN* 14:34–38, 1990.

Kohlhardt SR, Smith RC, Wright CR, et al.: Fine-bore peripheral catheters verses central venous catheters for delivery of intravenous nutrition. *Nutr* 8:412–417, 1992.

Kohlhardt SR, Smith RC, and Wright CR: Peripheral versus central intravenous nutrition: Comparison of two delivery systems. *Br J Surg* 81:66–70, 1994.

Krishnaswamy K: Drug metabolism and pharmacokinetics in malnourished children. *Clin Pharmacokinet* 17(suppl):68–88, 1989.

Kulkarni AD, Fanslow WC, Drath DB, et al.: Influence of dietary nucleotide restriction on bacterial sepsis and phagocytic cell function in mice. *Arch Surg* 121:169–172, 1986.

Laflamme DP: Body condition scoring and weight maintenance. *Proceedings of the North American Veterinary Conference*, Vol 7, pp. 290–291, 1993.

Leveen HH, Giordano P, and Spletzer J: The mechanism of removal of intravenous fat. Its relationship to toxicity. *Arch Surg* 83:311–321, 1961.

Linder LE, Curelaru I, Gustavsson B, et al.: Material thrombogenicity in central venous catheterization: A comparison between soft antebrachial catheters of silicone elastomer and polyurethane. *JPEN* 8:399–406, 1984.

Lippert AC and Buffington CA: Parenteral nutrition. In DiBartola

SP (ed): *Fluid Therapy in Small Animal Practice*. Philadelphia, WB Saunders Co., pp. 384–418, 1992.

Lippert AC, Fulton RB, and Parr A: A retrospective study of the use of total parenteral nutrition in dogs and cats. *J Vet Intern Med* 7:52–64, 1993.

Lowry SF and Brennan MF: Abnormal liver function during parenteral nutrition: Relation to infusion excess. *J Surg Res* 26:300–307, 1979.

Lupo L, Pannarale O, Altomare D, et al.: Reliability of clinical judgement in evaluation of the nutritional status of surgical patients. *Br J Surg* 80:1553–1556, 1993.

Maden M, Alexander DJ, and McMahon MJ: Influence of catheter type on occurrence of thrombophlebitis during peripheral intravenous nutrition. *Lancet* 339:101–103, 1992.

Maki DG, Goldmann DA, and Rhame FS: Infection control in intravenous therapy. *Ann Intern Med* 79:867–887, 1973.

Maki DG, Weise CE, and Sarafin HW: A semiquantitative culture method for identifying intravenous catheter-related infection. *J Med* 296:1305–1309, 1977.

Mallet JO: Calculating parenteral feedings: A programmed instruction. *J Am Diet Assoc* 84:1312–1320, 1984.

Mann S, Westenskow DR, and Houtchens BA: Measured and predicted caloric expenditure in the acutely ill. *Crit Care Med* 13:173–177, 1985.

Mashima Y: Effect of calorie overload on puppy livers during parenteral nutrition. *JPEN* 3:139–145, 1979.

Matsusue S, Nishimura S, Koizumi S, et al.: Preventive effect of simultaneously infused lipid emulsions against thrombophlebitis during postoperative peripheral parenteral nutrition. *Surg Today* 25:667–671, 1995.

Matthews DE and Fong Y: Amino acid and protein metabolism. In Rombeau JL and Caldwell MD (eds): *Clinical Nutrition; Parenteral Nutrition*, 2nd ed. Philadelphia, WB Saunders Co., pp. 75–112, 1993.

McCarthy MC, Shives JK, Robinson RJ, et al.: Prospective evaluation of single and triple lumen catheters in total parenteral nutrition. *JPEN* 11:259–262, 1987.

McClendon RR: Clinical evaluation of the IV formulator for fabricating TPN solutions. *Am J Intraven Ther Clin Nutr* 8:17–20, 1981.

McKee JM, Shell JA, Warren TA, et al.: Complications of intravenous therapy: A randomized prospective study—Vialon vs. Teflon. *J Intraven Nurs* 12:288–295, 1989.

McMahon MM: Nutritional assessment of the hospitalized patient. In *Hyperalimentation: A Practical Approach*. Boston, New England Deaconess Hospital and Harvard Medical School, September 15, 1993.

McMahon MM: Management of hyperglycemia in hospitalized patients receiving parenteral nutrition. *Nutr Clin Pract* 12:35–38, 1997.

Meguid MM, Akahoshi MP, Jeffers S, et al.: Amelioration of metabolic complications of conventional total parenteral nutrition. *Arch Surg* 119:1294–1298, 1984.

Meydani SN: Dietary modulation of cytokine production and biological functions. *Nutr Rev* 48:361–369, 1990.

Michel K: Prognostic value of clinical nutritional assessment in canine patients. *J Vet Emerg Crit Care* 3(2):96–104, 1993.

Minard G and Kudsk KA: Is early feeding beneficial? How early is early? *New Horiz* 2(2):156–163, 1994.

Moore EE and Jones TN: Benefits of immediate jejunostomy feeding after major abdominal trauma—A prospective randomized study. *J Trauma* 26:874–881, 1986.

Moran JM, Limon M, Mehedero G, et al.: Long term peritoneal nutrition in dogs: Metabolic and histopathological results. *Nutrition* 5(2):89–93, 1989.

Moss G: Immediately postoperative full nutrition and sepsis resistance: Immune globulin synthesis (abstract). *JPEN* 1:36, 1978.

Myles PS, Buckland MR, and Burnett WJ: Single verses double occlusive dressing technique to minimize infusion thrombophlebitis: Vialon and Teflon cannulae reassessed. *Anaesth Intensive Care* 19:525–529, 1991.

Nordenstrom J, Askanazi J, Elwyn DH, et al.: Nitrogen balance during total parenteral nutrition. *Ann Surg* 197:27–33, 1983.

Nussbaum MS and Fischer JE: Pathogenesis of hepatic steatosis during total parenteral nutrition. *Surg Annu* 23:1–11, 1991.

Nussbaum MS, Li S, Bower RH, et al.: Lipid addictions to total parenteral nutrition prevents hepatic steatosis in rats by lowering the portal venous insulin/glucagon ratio. *JPEN* 16:106–109, 1992.

Ogilvie GK, Salman MD, Kesel ML, et al.: Effect of anesthesia and surgery on energy expenditure determined by indirect calorimetry in dogs with malignant and nonmalignant conditions. *Am J Vet Res* 57:1321–1326, 1996a.

Ogilvie GK, Walters LM, Salman MD, et al.: Resting energy expenditure in dogs with nonhematopoietic malignancies before and after excision of tumors. *Am J Vet Res* 57:1463–1467, 1996b.

Ortiz R and Betancourt M: Cell proliferation in bone marrow cells of severely malnourished animals. *J Nutr* 114:472–476, 1984.

Ott L, Young B, Phillips R, et al.: Brain injury and nutrition. *Nutr Clin Pract* 5:68–73, 1990.

Otto CM, Kaufman GM, and Crowe DT: Intraosseous infusion of fluids and therapeutics. *Compend Contin Educ* 11:421–430, 1989.

Owen OE, Felig P, Morgan AP, et al.: Liver and kidney metabolism during prolong starvation. *J Clin Invest* 48:574–583, 1969.

Parke DV: Nutritional requirements for detoxication of environmental chemicals. *Food Addit Contam* 8:381–396, 1991.

Payne-James JJ and Khawaja HT: First choice for total parenteral nutrition: The peripheral route. *JPEN* 17:468–478, 1993.

Pilbeam SP, Head A, Grossman GD, et al.: Undernutrition and the respiratory system: Part 1. *Respir Ther* 65–69, 1983.

Pilbeam SP, Head A, Grossman GD, et al.: Undernutrition and the respiratory system: Part 2. *Respir Ther* 72–78, 1983.

Porta EA and Hartroft WS: Protein deficiency and liver injury. *Am J Nutr* 23:447–461, 1970.

Raftogianis RB, Franklin MR, and Galinsky RE: The depression of hepatic drug conjugation reactions in rats after lipid-free total parenteral nutrition administered via the portal vein. *JPEN* 19:303–309, 1995.

Redmond HP, Leon P, Lieberman MD, et al.: Impaired macrophage function in severe protein-energy malnutrition. *Arch Surg* 126:192–196, 1991.

Remillard RL, Armstrong PJ, Davenport DL: Assisted feeding in hospitalized patients: Enteral and parenteral nutrition. In Hand M, Thatcher CD, and Remillard RL (eds): *Small Animal Clinical Nutrition*, 4th ed. Mark Morris Institute, Topeka, KS, 1999, in press.

Remillard RL and Thatcher CD: Parenteral nutritional support in the small animal patient. *Vet Clin North Am Small Anim Pract* 19:1287–1306, 1989.

Remillard RL, Darden D, Michel K, et al.: Caloric intake of hospitalized canine patient (abstract). Purina Nutrition Forum, St Louis, June 1997.

Remillard RL, Dudgeon DL, and Yardley J: Atrophied small intestinal responses of piglets to oral feedings of milk. *J Nutr* 128:2727S–2729S, 1998a.

Remillard RL, Guerino F, Dudgeon DL, et al.: Intravenous glutamine or limited enteral feedings in piglets: Amelioration of small intestinal disuse atrophy. *J Nutr* 128:2723S–2726S, 1998b.

Reynolds JV, Walsh K, Ruigrok J, et al.: Randomized comparison of silicone verses Teflon cannulas for peripheral intravenous nutrition. *Ann R Coll Surg Engl* 75:447–449, 1995.

Roongpisuthipong C, Puchaiwatananon O, Songchitsomboon S, et al.: Hydrocortisone, heparin and peripheral intravenous infusion. *Nutrition* 10:211–213, 1994.

Root M, Johnston SD, and Olson PN: The effect of prepuberal and postpuberal gonadectomy on heat production measured by indirect calorimetry in male and female domestic cats. *Am J Vet Res* 57:371–374, 1996.

Rowe CE, Fukuyama TT, and Martinoff JT: Growth of microorganisms in total nutrient admixtures. *Drug Intell Clin Pharm* 21:633–638, 1987.

Ryan JA, Abel RM, Abbott WM, et al.: Catheter complications in total parenteral nutrition: A prospective study of 200 consecutive patients. *N Engl J Med* 290:757–761, 1974.

Schecekelhoff DJ, Mirtallo MJ, Ayers LW, et al.: Growth of bacteria and fungi in total nutrient admixtures. *Am J Hosp Pharm* 43:73–77, 1986.

Semba RD, Meydani SN, Kramer TR, et al.: Micronutrient influences on immune response. Conference on Nutrition and Immunity as part of the International conference series on Nutrition and Health Promotion. International Life Sciences Institute, Atlanta, May 5–7, pp. 9–18, 1997.

Shikora SA, Blackburn GL, and Forse RA: Nutrition and immunology: Clinician's approach. In Forse RA (ed): *Diet, Nutrition and Immunity.* Boca Raton, FL, CRC Press, pp. 9–21, 1994.

Simmons BP, Hotton TM, Wong ES, et al.: CDC guidelines for prevention of intravascular infections. *Infect Control* 3:52–67, 1982.

Smith JL, Canhan JE, and Wells PA: Effect of phototherapy light, sodium bisulfite, and pH on vitamin stability in total parenteral nutrition admixtures. *JPEN* 12:394–402, 1988.

Stein TP: Protein metabolism and parenteral nutrition. In Rombeau JL and Caldwell MD (eds): *Clinical Nutrition: Parenteral Nutrition,* 1st ed. Philadelphia, WB Saunders Co., pp. 100–134, 1986.

Stein TP, Oram-Smith JC, Wallace HW, et al.: The effect of trauma on protein synthesis. *J Surg Res* 21:201–203, 1976.

Stoner HB, Little RA, Frayn KN, et al.: The effect of sepsis on the oxidation of carbohydrate and fat. *Br J Surg* 70:32–35, 1983.

Tallado-Rodriquez J, and Christou NV: Clinical assessment of hose defense. *Surg Infect* 13:353–369, 1988.

Thatcher CD, Hand M, and Remillard RL: Small animal clinical nutrition: An iterative process. In Hand M, Thatcher CD, and Remillard RL (eds): *Small Animal Clinical Nutrition,* 4th ed. Topeka, KS, 1999.

Trissel LA: *Handbook on Injectable Drugs,* 9th ed. Bethesda, MD, American Society of Hospital Pharmacies, 1996.

Truswell AS, Hanson JDL, Watson CE, et al.: Relation of serum lipids and lipoproteins to fatty liver in kwashiorkor. *Am J Nutr* 22:568–576, 1969.

Vagenakis AG, Burger A, Portnay GI, et al.: Diversion of peripheral thyroxine metabolism from activating to inactivating pathways during complete fasting. *J Clin Endocrinol Metab* 41:191–194, 1975.

Varma DR: Protein deficiency and drug interactions. *Drug Dev Res* 1:183–198, 1981.

The Veterans Affairs Total Parenteral Nutrition Cooperative Study Group: Perioperative total parenteral nutrition in surgical patients. *N Engl J Med* 325:525–532, 1991.

Walter-Sack I and Klotz U: Influence of diet and nutritional status on drug metabolism. *Clin Pharmacokinet* 31:47–64, 1996.

Walton RS, Wingfield WE, Oglivie GK, et al.: Energy expenditure in 104 postoperative and traumatically injured dogs with indirect calorimetry. *J Vet Emerg Crit Care* 6(2):71–79, 1996.

Welborn MB and Moldawer LL: Glucose metabolism. In Rombeau JL and Rolandelli RH (eds): *Clinical Nutrition Enteral and Tube Feeding,* 3rd ed. Philadelphia, WB Saunders Co., pp. 61–80, 1984.

Wernerman J, von der Decken A, and Vinnars E: Polyribosome concentration in human skeletal muscle after starvation and parenteral or enteral refeeding. *Metabolism* 35:447–451, 1986.

Wilkinson WR, Flores LL, and Pagones JN: Growth of microorganisms in parenteral nutritional fluids. *Drug Intell Clin Pharm* 7:226–231, 1973.

Wilmore DW, Long JM, Mason AD, et al.: Catecholamines: Mediator of the hypermetabolic response to thermal injury. *Ann Surg* 180:653–666, 1974.

Windsor JA: Underweight patients and the risks of major surgery. *World J Surg* 17:165–172, 1993.

Woolfson AMJ: Amino acids—Their role as an energy source. *Proc Nutr Soc* 42:489–495, 1983.

Zeiderman MR, King RFGJ, Young GA, et al.: Metabolic changes in human liver associated with pre-operative intravenous nutrition. *Clin Sci* 77:343–349, 1989.

CHAPTER 23

Fluid Therapy with Macromolecular Plasma Volume Expanders

DEZ HUGHES

> *Those who fill our professional ranks are habitually conservative. This salutary mental attitude expresses itself peculiarly in our communal relations; namely, when a new idea appears which is more or less subversive to old notions and practices, he who originates the idea must strike sledge hammer blows in order to secure even a momentary attention. This must then be followed by a long, patient, propaganda and advertising until in the grand finale, the public, indifferent at first, is aroused, proceeds to discuss, and finally accepts the iconoclastic proposal as a long-accepted fact of its own invention and asks wonderingly, "Why such a bother? What after all is new about this? We knew it long ago!"*
>
> Howard A. Kelly. Electrosurgery in gynaecology. Ann Surg 93:323, 1931.

In the late nineteenth century, Ernest Starling proposed the concept that fluid exchange across vessels was governed by the balance between hydrostatic and osmotic pressure gradients between the intravascular and interstitial fluid compartments (Starling 1896). A hydrostatic pressure gradient in excess of the osmotic gradient at the arterial end of the capillary bed results in a net transudation of fluid into the interstitium. At the venous end of the capillary bed, plasma proteins (which cannot pass out of the blood vessels) exert an osmotic force in excess of the hydrostatic gradient, resulting in a net fluid flux into vessels. More than a century of research has confirmed that Starling's hypothesis provides the foundation for microvascular fluid exchange; however, it also has revealed that the anatomy and physiology of the microvasculature, interstitium, and lymphatic system are much more complex. Consequently, a much deeper understanding of transvascular fluid dynamics is necessary for a logical and rational approach to intravenous therapy with fluids containing macromolecules. This chapter assumes the reader is familiar with the information given in Chapter 1 explaining the fluid compartments of the body and the mechanisms of water and solute flow among compartments. Although this chapter discusses the anatomy, physiology, and biophysics of transvascular fluid dynamics in some depth, comprehensive reviews and texts are available on the subject for a more complete discussion of solute and solvent exchange among the microvasculature, interstitium, and lymphatics (Staub and Taylor 1984; Aukland and Reed 1993; Rippe and Haraldsson 1994). The main aim of this chapter is to address the complexities and controversies of colloid therapy while avoiding the bias apparent in many articles dealing with the crystalloid-colloid controversy. A deeper appreciation of the relevant issues should ensure a more rational approach to deciding whether or not colloid therapy is appropriate. For additional information, the reader is referred to several reviews of colloid fluid therapy available in the veterinary (Concannon 1993; Rudloff and Kirby 1997, 1998a, 1998b; Matthews 1998; Kirby and Rudloff 1997; Smiley 1992) and human medical literature (Falk et al. 1989; Mishler 1984; Roberts and Bratton 1998).

▶ The Microvascular Barrier

In simple terms, the microvascular barrier is a capillary wall that is impermeable to protein. In addition to the endothelial cell and capillary basement membrane, a luminal surface layer (the glycocalyx) and the interstitial matrix contribute to the selective permeability of the microvascular barrier (Aukland and Reed 1993; Rippe and Haraldsson 1994; Wissig and Charonis 1984). The glycocalyx coats the luminal aspect of the endothelial cell and is composed of proteins, glycoproteins, and glycolipids that apparently modify the permeability of the vessel by occupying spaces within the wall or via electrostatic attraction or repulsion (Luft 1976). Plasma proteins, especially albumin and orosomucoid, are thought to contribute

483

significantly to maintaining the selective permeability of the endothelium (Michel et al. 1985; Curry 1985; Curry et al. 1987, 1989; Haraldsson and Rippe 1987).

On a morphologic basis, capillary walls may be continuous, fenestrated, or discontinuous (Taylor and Granger 1985; Renkin 1977). Continuous capillaries, which are found in the majority of tissues and organs of the body, are so called because the wall is composed of a continuous endothelial cell layer and basement membrane. They are freely permeable to water and small solutes such as sodium but are relatively impermeable to macromolecules. The passage of smaller plasma proteins, such as albumin (molecular radius 3.5 nm), is restricted less than passage of larger plasma proteins. Fenestrated capillaries have a continuous basement membrane with regions that are covered only by thin endothelial diaphragms or entirely devoid of endothelium. They are found in tissues in which there are large fluxes of water and small solutes such as the glomerulus and intestine. Interestingly, the permeability of fenestrated capillaries to macromolecules is similar to that of continuous capillaries. A net negative charge of the basement membrane of fenestrated capillaries appears to be an important determinant of permeability (Simionescu et al. 1982; Bent-Hansen et al. 1993). Discontinuous capillaries are found in the liver, spleen, bone marrow, and some glands. They have gaps up to 1 μm between endothelial cells with no basement membrane and therefore are freely permeable to protein.

The permeability of the microvascular barrier has been explained by the presence of pores of different sizes (Pappenheimer et al. 1951). Pore sizes often are extrapolated from experimental data regarding fluid and solute fluxes and do not always correlate with morphologic studies such as electron microscopy, implying that they may represent functional rather than anatomic entities. The majority of experimental data suggest two effective pore sizes in the microvascular barrier in most tissues, with a high frequency of small pores that restrict the efflux of macromolecules and a low frequency of large pores through which macromolecules can pass freely (Rippe and Haraldsson 1994).

Rather than a free fluid space, the interstitium actually represents a dynamic environment that may contribute to the permeability characteristics of the microvascular barrier and modify the flow of fluid and macromolecules from the blood vessels to the lymphatics (Aukland and Reed 1993; Bent-Hansen 1991a, 1991b). The interstitium is composed of a collagen framework that contains a gel phase of glycosaminoglycans (of which hyaluronan is the most common), along with protein macromolecules and electrolytes in solution. The relative proportions of these constituents differ widely among organs and tissues, resulting in variations in the permeability and mechanical properties of the interstitium. Glycosaminoglycans are extremely long chains of repeating disaccharide subunits wound into random coils and entangled with each other and the collagen framework. They have molecular weights on the order of 10^7, and each molecule bears many thousand anionic moieties (Aukland and Reed 1993). It has been suggested that this interstitial structure mechanically opposes distention (i.e., edema formation) and resists contraction during dehydration because of repulsion between the anionic moieties (Granger et al. 1984). The interstitial matrix itself is differentially permeable to macromolecules, and a colloid osmotic gradient also can exist from the perimicrovascular space across the interstitium. Although the collagen network and many of the glycosaminoglycans are fixed in the interstitium, hyaluronan may be mobilized and removed via lymphatic drainage, thereby changing the permeability of the interstitium (Aukland and Reed 1993).

▶ Transvascular Fluid Dynamics

Although not stated implicitly in his seminal paper, Starling's hypothesis subsequently was formalized to state simply that the hydrostatic pressure gradient between the capillary and the interstitium ($P_c - P_i$) is equal to the osmotic pressure gradient between the plasma and the interstitium ($\pi_p - \pi_i$). This expression can be expanded to describe fluid flux (J_v) across the microvascular barrier:

Fluid flow = hydrostatic gradient − osmotic gradient

or

$$J_v = (P_c - P_i) - (\pi_p - \pi_i)$$

For a given solute to exert its full osmotic pressure across a membrane, the membrane must be impermeable to the solute in question. If the membrane is partially permeable to the solute molecule, the equilibrium concentration gradient is lower and the solute exerts only part of its potential osmotic pressure. The realization that the microvasculature was only partially impermeable to smaller macromolecules led to the inclusion of the reflection coefficient (σ) in the fluid flux equation (Staverman 1952).

$$J_v = (P_c - P_i) - \sigma(\pi_p - \pi_i)$$

In descriptive terms, the reflection coefficient is the fraction of the total potential osmotic pressure exerted by the solute in question. Conceptually, one also can consider it as the fraction of the solute molecules reflected from the microvascular barrier. If a membrane is completely impermeable, no solute molecules pass through, the concentration gradient is maximal, and the solute exerts its full osmotic pressure (i.e., the reflection coefficient is equal to one). If the membrane is completely permeable to the solute in question, it passes through freely, no concentration difference exists, and no osmotic pressure can be exerted (i.e., the reflection coefficient is zero).

Further research showed that fluid flow from vessels differed among tissues depending on the surface area of the capillary beds in the various organs and the hydraulic conductance (i.e., the ease of fluid flow) through the microvascular barrier. To account for this variability, the fluid flux equation is modified by the filtration coefficient (K_{fc}). This term simply implies that fluid flow is equal to a fraction of the effective hydrostatic and osmotic pressure gradients.

$$J_v = K_{fc}[(P_c - P_i) - \sigma(\pi_p - \pi_i)]$$

Each different constituent of plasma may differ in its rate of efflux from a vessel depending on such factors as its molecular radius, shape, and charge and the permeability of the microvascular barrier to the constituent. The two major groups of molecules with respect to transvascular fluid flux are termed the solvent phase and the solute phase, and expressions were developed to predict the egress of both major groups of molecules from the microvasculature (Pappenheimer 1953; Kedem and Katchalsky 1958; Landis and Pappenheimer 1963; Patlak et al. 1963). The solvent phase is considered to include water and molecules that are not significantly impeded in their passage through the microvascular barrier, whereas the solute flux equation describes the passage of molecules that do not flow freely from the vasculature.

The solvent flow equation remains the same as the previous expression for fluid flow except that the filtration coefficient is subdivided into the hydraulic conductance (L_p) and the membrane surface area (S) and the hydrostatic and osmotic gradients are expressed as ΔP and $\Delta \pi$, respectively:

$$J_v = L_p S(\Delta P - \sigma \Delta \pi)$$

The two major mechanisms of solute flow through the microvascular barrier are convection (i.e., carriage in a bulk flow of fluid) and diffusion (i.e., random motion resulting in net movement of molecules from an area of high concentration to an area of lower concentration) (Rippe and Haraldsson 1994). An analogy to illustrate the two mechanisms would be a wave breaking on a beach. Some of the sodium molecules in the wave are moving away from the beach by diffusion; however, the forward convective flow of the wave carries them in the opposite direction.

The solute flow equation (which is the most relevant expression with respect to intravenous therapy with fluids containing macromolecules) states simply that the rate of solute flux (J_s) is equal to the sum of the convective flow and the diffusional movement:

$$\text{Solute flow } (J_s) = \text{convective flow} + \text{diffusion}$$

Convective flow is equal to the product of fluid flow (J_v), the fractional permeability of the membrane ($1 - \sigma$), and the mean intramembrane solute concentration, $\bar{C}$. Diffusion is equal to the product of the solute permeability (P), the surface area of the microvascular barrier (S), and the solute concentration gradient across the membrane (ΔC). The expression representing macromolecular flux therefore becomes

$$J_s = J_v(1 - \sigma)\bar{C} + PS \Delta C$$

Solute flow = convective flow + diffusion

At normal lymph flow rates, convection has been estimated to account for about 30% of the total flux of albumin into lymph (Renkin et al. 1977). An important point that warrants further emphasis is that the rate of solute efflux is dependent on the rate of solvent efflux. Any condition that increases the rate of fluid flow across a membrane can increase the extravasation of macromolecules. Hence, intravenous fluid therapy with crystalloid or colloid can increase albumin loss into the interstitium (Rieger 1967).

These mathematical expressions give the impression of a constant hydrostatic pressure gradient acting across a single membrane of static and uniform conductivity and permeability (homoporous), with filtration opposed by an osmotic pressure related to a single impermeant solute, the plasma "protein." In fact, the hydrostatic pressure and osmotic pressure gradients vary among different tissues and at different levels of the capillary bed within the same tissue (Renkin 1985; Taylor 1981; Taylor et al. 1994). The total osmotic gradient is a summation of all the impermeant solutes present within plasma, which have unique reflection coefficients and efflux rates (Taylor 1981). Furthermore, the surface area of the capillary bed may change depending on precapillary sphincter activity, and the permeability of the microvascular barrier also can vary physiologically as well as in disease states (Wissig and Charonis 1984; Granger et al. 1984; Parker et al. 1984; Bates and Curry 1996; Yuan et al. 1992).

▶ Normal Starling Forces and the Tissue Safety Factors

Plasma Colloid Osmotic Pressure

Although in popular usage colloid often is interpreted as referring to a macromolecule that cannot pass through a membrane, the strict definition refers to the dispersion in a gas, liquid, or solid medium of atoms or molecules that resist sedimentation, diffusion, and filtration. This definition is in contradistinction to that of crystalloids, which are freely diffusible. Oncotic pressure is defined as the osmotic pressure exerted by colloids in solution (hence it is redundant to use the phrase colloid oncotic pressure). The osmotic pressure exerted by the colloids in plasma is higher than that calculated for an ideal solution. One of the main reasons for this discrepancy is that negatively charged proteins (such as albumin, which has a net negative charge of 17 at physiologic pH) retain cations within the intravascular space by electrostatic attraction (termed the Donnan effect) (Granger et al. 1984). These cations contribute to the effective plasma protein osmotic pressure because osmotic pressure is proportional to the number of molecules present rather than their size. Colloid osmotic pressure (COP) would therefore be the most correct term when referring to the osmotic pressure exerted by plasma proteins and their associated electrolyte molecules. For comparison, the oncotic pressure exerted by an albumin solution of 7 g/dL is 19.8 mm Hg, the in vivo colloid osmotic pressure is 28 mm Hg, and the total osmotic pressure of all plasma solutes is 5400 mm Hg (Granger et al. 1984).

By virtue of its relatively high concentration in the vascular space, albumin usually accounts for 60 to 70% of the plasma COP with globulins making up the remainder (Navar and Narar 1977; Weisberg 1978; Tullis 1977). Interestingly, the variation in COP in dogs may be due more to differences in globulin concentration than to differences in albumin concentration (Navar and Narar 1977; Gabel et al. 1980). Red blood cells and platelets do not contribute significantly to plasma COP (Prather et al. 1968). Serum albumin concentration is determined by the relative rates of synthesis, degradation, and loss from the body and its distribution between the extravascular and interstitial spaces. Albumin synthesis, which is unique to the liver, appears to be regulated, at least in part, by hepatic plasma COP. (Dich et al. 1973; Pietrangelo et al.

1992; Rothschild et al. 1964). Increases of plasma COP independent of albumin concentration, such as in hyperglobulinemia, are associated with reduced serum albumin concentration. (Rothschild et al. 1962, 1965; Bjorneboe and Schwartz 1959). The main site of albumin degradation is uncertain, although the reticuloendothelial system has been suggested. Equations have been derived to estimate plasma COP from plasma protein concentrations (Navar and Narar 1977; Thomas and Brown 1992), but direct measurement is more accurate (Thomas and Brown 1992; Brown et al. 1994; Barclay and Bennett 1987; Weisberg 1968). Colloid osmotic pressures measured in normal dogs and cats are given in Table 23–1.

Interstitial Colloid Osmotic Pressure

It is important to appreciate that, although the microvascular barrier greatly restricts macromolecular flux, capillaries are permeable to protein. Of the total quantity of albumin present in the body, 40% is intravascular and 60% is extravascular (Rothschild et al. 1979). Furthermore, all of the albumin present in plasma circulates through the interstitium every 24 h (Parving and Rasmussen 1973). The interstitial COP varies from tissue to tissue depending on such factors as the permeability of the capillary wall to protein, the rate of transvascular solvent flow, the retention of protein in the interstitial matrix, and the rate of lymphatic clearance of protein. The microvascular barrier of skeletal muscle or subcutaneous tissue is relatively impermeable to protein, whereas the pulmonary capillary endothelium is more permeable with a reflection coefficient to albumin of approximately 0.5 to 0.64 (Parker et al. 1984). Consequently, the normal protein concentration in lymph from skin or skeletal muscle is about 50% of plasma compared with 65% in pulmonary lymph (Parker et al. 1984). Hyaluronan and its associated cations also may contribute to interstitial COP (Aukland and Reed 1993). Because of the volume occupied by the interstitial matrix, interstitial albumin is distributed in a volume that is less than the total interstitial volume. This phenomenon is called the volume exclusion effect, and the "excluded volume" with respect to albumin may be as high as one-half to two-thirds of the total interstitial volume (Weiderhelm and Black 1976; Bert et al. 1982; Parker et al. 1980). Consequently, in a normally hydrated interstitium, much less protein is required to exert a given osmotic pressure and relatively smaller volumes of extravasated fluid result in greater decrements in interstitial COP to maintain the intravascular-to-extravascular COP gradient. Conversely, when the interstitial volume is overexpanded by fluid in edematous states, there is a dramatic increase in the volume available for albumin sequestration (Granger et al. 1984). The increase in interstitial COP that occurs with dehydration acts to restrict mobilization of interstitial fluid (Heir and Wiig 1988).

Intravascular Hydrostatic Pressure

Intravascular hydrostatic pressure is the main force that determines fluid egress from the vasculature. It may vary in different tissues and at different levels within each capillary bed. The normal hydrostatic pressure in the capillary bed is controlled by local myogenic, neurogenic, and humoral modulation of the arterial and venous resistances. Precapillary arteriolar constriction may reduce flow, and therefore hydrostatic pressure, through a capillary bed or shunt flow away from that bed, resulting in changes in the total surface area available for transvascular fluid movement. The hydrostatic pressure within a blood vessel at any particular site depends in part on where resistance to flow occurs, with hydrostatic pressures falling most across the areas of major resistance. In most tissues, the majority of resistance has been attributed to small arterioles, but experimental studies of the lung suggest there may be a significant pressure drop across the pulmonary capillary bed itself (Bhattacharya et al. 1982, 1989; Shepard et al. 1988).

Interstitial Hydrostatic Pressure

As with the other Starling forces, normal interstitial pressure also varies among tissues. Interestingly, in many tissues the resting pressure is slightly negative (subatmospheric), tending to favor rather than oppose fluid filtration from the microvasculature (Wiig and Reed 1987). This finding has been postulated to be due to the molecular structure of the interstitial matrix, such that at normal hydration the biomechanical stresses on the molecules and the repulsion among like electrostatic charges act to expand the interstitium (Aukland and Reed 1993). In encapsulated organs, such as the kidney, normal interstitial pressures are positive. Interstitial pressures can change depending on the functional state of the organ. For example, interstitial pressures in the nonabsorbing intestine are negative to slightly positive, whereas intestinal interstitial pressures are positive in the absorptive state (Granger and Barrowman 1971). As mentioned before, the molecular structure of the interstitium mechanically opposes distention. Conventionally, it is said that one-third of the total body water is found in the extracellular space and that the interstitium constitutes three-fourths of the extracellular space. These figures are averages for the whole body, and the relative sizes of the intravascular and interstitial spaces vary among tissues. Tissues vary in their capacity to accommodate interstitial fluid depending on the size of the interstitial space relative to the total volume of the tissue and the nature of the interstitial matrix itself, especially its distensibility.

TABLE 23–1. Colloid Osmotic Pressure in Normal Dogs and Cats

Species	Colloid Osmotic Pressure, Mean ± SD (mm Hg)	Reference
Canine (plasma)	20.8 ± 1.8	Zweifach and Intaglietta 1971
Canine (plasma)	17.5 ± 3.0	Navar and Narar 1977
Canine (whole blood)	19.9 ± 2.1	Culp et al. 1994
Feline (plasma)	19.8 ± 2.4	Zweifach and Intaglietta 1971
Feline (whole blood)	24.7 ± 3.7	Culp et al. 1994

The distensibility of an organ or tissue is termed its compliance and, depending on the nature of the tissue, the compliance of the interstitium may vary widely. Extreme examples would be tendon (which is relatively noncompliant) and loose subcutaneous connective tissue (which is relatively distensible). The peribronchial accumulation of edema fluid in the lungs is probably due to the higher compliance of this region of the pulmonary interstitium.

An extremely important concept related to the interstitial hydrostatic pressure is that of stress relaxation. In a normally hydrated animal, the interstitium in most tissues is relatively noncompliant. Small increases in volume caused by increased fluid extravasation result in large changes in interstitial hydrostatic pressure that act to oppose further extravasation of fluid and increase lymphatic drainage pressure—two of the tissue safety factors described later (Guyton et al. 1971; Taylor 1990). As the interstitium gradually becomes more distended, it opposes further distention until a critical point is reached (suggested to correspond to the disordering of the interstitial matrix). Abruptly, the resistance to distention falls (i.e., compliance increases) and fluid then can accumulate without a corresponding protective rise in interstitial pressure and lymph flow. At this point, the distended interstitium no longer opposes the movement of fluid and protein, resulting in increased extravasation and self-perpetuation of the edemagenic process. Furthermore, the greatly increased interstitial space provides a large volume for protein sequestration.

Tissue Safety Factors

From the previous discussion, it should be apparent that there are three main ways in which accumulation of fluid in the interstitium can be avoided. First, extravasation of fluid into a relatively nondistensible interstitium results in an increased interstitial pressure that opposes further extravasation. Second, after extravasation of low-protein fluid, the interstitial COP falls because of dilution and washout of protein, thereby maintaining the COP gradient between the intravascular space and the interstitium. Third, because the perimicrovascular interstitium is not compliant, increased interstitial fluid results in an increased driving pressure for lymphatic drainage. These alterations in Starling forces that act to limit interstitial fluid accumulation have been termed the tissue safety factors (Guyton et al. 1971; Taylor 1990). Their relative importance varies depending on the characteristics of the tissue (Aukland and Reed 1993; Chen et al. 1976). In a tissue that is relatively nondistensible (e.g., tendon), an increase in interstitial pressure may be the most important means by which to counteract filtration. In a tissue with moderate distensibility and a relatively impermeable microvascular barrier (e.g., skin), the decrease in interstitial COP assumes more importance in protecting against interstitial fluid accumulation. In a distensible tissue that is quite permeable to protein, (e.g., lung), increased lymph flow appears to be the most important safeguard against interstitial edema (Zarins et al. 1976).

▶ Pharmacokinetics and Pharmacodynamics of Macromolecular Plasma Volume Expanders

Transvascular fluid dynamics are extremely complex. The balance of the hydrostatic and osmotic pressure gradients between the intravascular and interstitial fluid compartments forms the basis for microvascular fluid exchange. This simple concept, however, is belied by the great heterogeneity in Starling forces and transvascular fluid dynamics that exist among and within tissues. The relative importance of the different tissue safety factors also varies among tissues, and the potential for self-regulation of transvascular fluid fluxes often is underestimated. A great deal of emphasis has been placed on the manipulation of individual Starling forces (such as intravascular COP) in isolation rather than addressing the system in its entirety. Maintenance of intravascular volume depends on an intricate and dynamic interaction between the intravascular and interstitial Starling forces and the structure and function of the microvascular barrier, interstitium, and lymphatic system. Infusion of intravenous fluids can change all of the Starling forces, modify the permeability of the microvascular barrier, change the volume and composition of the interstitium, and increase lymphatic flow. Furthermore, the magnitude and relative significance of these changes vary among and within tissues. Consequently, it is a gross and potentially dangerous oversimplification to view the body as the homogeneous sum of its individual parts when contemplating intravenous fluid therapy. From a clinical standpoint, the differences between the lungs and the systemic circulation are of the utmost importance. For example, in a dog with systemic inflammatory response syndrome and aspiration pneumonia causing pulmonary edema by means of increased microvascular permeability, colloid therapy may limit subcutaneous edema at the expense of worsening pulmonary fluid extravasation.

Despite this great heterogeneity, the concept that net fluid extravasation is dependent on the balance between intravascular COP and capillary hydrostatic pressure forms the basis for intravenous colloid therapy (Guyton and Lindsay 1959; Gaar et al. 1987; Kramer et al. 1983; Wareing et al. 1989). By virtue of their larger molecular size, and in the absence of an increase in microvascular permeability, colloid molecules are retained within the vasculature to a greater degree than are crystalloids. Consequently, smaller volumes of colloid result in greater plasma volume expansion compared with crystalloid (Davidson et al. 1990; Shoemaker 1976; Shoemaker et al. 1981), and crystalloid is expected to leak into the interstitium to a greater degree than colloid and cause more interstitial edema (Brown et al. 1995). There is evidence that tissue perfusion is better after volume expansion with colloids than with crystalloids, even when resuscitation is titrated to physiologic end points (Funk and Baldinger 1995).

One hour after infusion of a crystalloid solution, as little as 10% may remain in the intravascular space (Shoemaker et al. 1981). Many factors influence the volume and duration of intravascular expansion associated with artificial colloids, including the species of animal, dose, specific colloid formulation, preinfusion intravascular volume status, and microvascular permeability. These factors may explain the great variability in intravascular persistence and volume expansion observed in published studies. Artificial colloids are polydisperse; that is, they contain molecules that vary in molecular weight. In contrast, in a monodisperse colloid, such as albumin, molecules are all the same size. The artificial colloids have extremely complex pharmacokinetics in part because of this large range of molecular sizes (Klotz and Kroemer 1987). The smaller molecules pass rapidly into the urine and interstitium, whereas the larger molecules remain in circulation and are gradually hydrolyzed by amylase or removed by the monocyte phagocytic system (Thompson et al. 1970). This initial rapid excretion of small, osmotically active molecules followed by a gradual elimination of large molecules results in an exponential decline in intravascular expansion. Manufacturer data sheets can be misleading because they imply that a major proportion of the volume expansion lasts for 24 to 36 h. Estimates of the degree of initial plasma volume expansion for hetastarch and dextran 70 vary from 70 to 170% of the infused volume (Rieger 1967; Lamke and Liljedahl 1976; Gollub et al. 1969; Hempel et al. 1975; Korttila et al. 1984). This value falls to approximately 50% of the infused volume after 6 h. Volume expansion with hydroxyethyl starch declines gradually from 60 to 40% of the infused volume over the next 12 to 18 h, whereas with dextran 70 it falls gradually from 40 to 20% of the infused volume (Thompson et al. 1970). In dogs with hypoalbuminemia of varying causes receiving hydroxyethyl starch, COP was not significantly different from baseline 12 h after infusion (Moore and Garvey 1996). In the author's experience, the duration of volume expansion with artificial colloids can be even shorter, especially with capillary leak syndromes. The relatively short duration of action and high cost of artificial colloids have led some authors to question the cost-effectiveness of colloid infusions in veterinary patients (Wall et al. 1996).

The duration of action of colloids may be expressed in terms of plasma colloid concentrations, plasma COP measurements, or degree of volume expansion. The initial volume of intravascular expansion is due to the COP of the infused colloid, which is determined by the number of molecules, not their size. This is an extremely important concept because the distribution of molecular weights is narrowed after intravenous infusion (Farrow et al. 1970; Ferber et al. 1985). The smaller molecules that are responsible for a large part of the COP and intravascular volume expansion are excreted or extravasated within hours. The concentration (i.e., mass per unit volume) is still high but COP is relatively low, and hence COP and degree of volume expansion tend to fall faster than does the plasma concentration of colloid. Data from an experimental study of euvolemic human volunteers given twice the usual dose of a high-molecular-weight form of hydroxyethyl starch may therefore have little bearing on the effects of commercially available hetastarch in a dog with systemic inflammatory response syndrome in hypodynamic septic shock.

It is important to assess critically the need for colloidal support and the response to therapy. Colloid therapy is not a panacea; rather it is one more group of drugs in the pharmacy with specific indications, contraindications, benefits, and risks. Two meta-analyses have been published that document a higher overall mortality with colloidal volume expansion than with crystalloids (Velanovich 1989; Schierhout and Roberts 1998). The limitations of meta-analysis notwithstanding, subdivision of the population of patients of one study (Velanovich 1989) demonstrates that in trauma patients there was a 12.3% difference in mortality rate in favor of crystalloid therapy, and when data from studies that used nontrauma patients were pooled, there was a 7.8% difference in mortality rate in favor of colloid treatment. Perhaps most importantis the authors' conclusion that colloid therapy was deleterious in patients with sepsis, capillary leak syndrome, and adult respiratory distress syndrome after trauma.

The osmotic effect of macromolecules is due to their number rather than size, and if more than 50% leak into the interstitium there can be a net reduction in intravascular volume as water leaves the intravascular space with colloid. The dilemma therefore becomes determining the magnitude of the increase in permeability (i.e., how big the "gaps" in the microvascular barrier are). Although experimental techniques are available to detect an increase in microvascular permeability (Berthezene et al. 1991; Brigham et al. 1977), they are not currently applicable in a clinical setting. There is a growing body of evidence that hydroxyethyl starches can reduce the increases in microvascular permeability in several capillary leak states (Oz et al. 1995; Chi et al. 1996; Zikria 1994). The optimal molecular mass for this effect appears to be between 100 and 300 kd (Zikria et al. 1989). Unfortunately, there are relatively few molecules in this size range in artificial colloids available in the United States. For example, only 35% of the molecules in hetastarch fall within this optimal size range (Zikria 1994).

The artificial colloids used most commonly in the United States, and the ones that have been studied in most detail, are hetastarch and dextran 70, both of which are available as 6% (6 g/dL) solutions in 0.9% saline. The hydroxyethyl starches are derived from amylopectin (the branched form of plant starch), whereas dextrans are prepared from a macromolecular polysaccharide produced by bacterial fermentation of sucrose. The parent mixtures then are separated into fractions by molecular weight. The hydroxyethyl starches have a much wider range of molecular weights than does dextran 70, and the distribution of molecular weights in the available preparations of hydroxyethyl starch often is underestimated. The package insert states that 80% of molecules fall between 2 and 2500 kd; however, this also means that 20% fall outside this range. An independent analysis found that 85% of Hespan consisted of molecules smaller than 300 kd, 50% consisted of molecules smaller than 100 kd, and molecular masses ranged up to 5000 kd (Zikria 1994). Hydroxyethyl starch with a weight average molecular mass of 100 to 300 kd seems to provide the best compromise between colloid osmotic volume expansion and duration of action (Conhaim et al. 1993). Furthermore, this size distribution has less effect on coagulation (Treib et al. 1997b) and is best for reducing the increases in permeability present in vascular leak states (Zikria 1994).

To reduce intravascular hydrolysis of hydroxyethyl starch by amylase, the amylopectin is hydroxyethylated at carbons 2, 3, and 6. The number of hydroxyethyl groups per glucose unit is defined as the molar substitution ratio, and the pattern of substitution varies depending on the synthetic process. Substitution at the 2 carbon position is more effective in reducing intravascular hydrolysis than hydroxyethylation at the other positions (Treib et al. 1995). Hydroxyethyl starches therefore are characterized by their weight average molecular weight, substitution ratio, and C-2/C-6 hydroxyethylation ratio (Treib et al. 1997a). Two forms of high-molecular-weight hydroxyethyl starch are available in the United States, hetastarch 450/0.7 (Hespan, DuPont Pharmaceuticals) and the hydroxyethyl starch currently marketed by Abbott Laboratories (North Chicago, IL), which has a weight average molecular weight of 700,000, a molar substitution of 0.75, and a high C-2/C-6 ratio. Pentastarch is a hydroxyethyl starch with a narrower range of molecular weights that currently is approved for leukapheresis.

The recommended dosage for both hydroxyethyl starch and dextran is 20 mL/kg/day. Although higher dosages have been used without apparent side effects, (Moore and Garvey 1996; Smiley and Garvey 1994) the deleterious effects on coagulation occur at and above this dosage. It should also be borne in mind that 20 mL/kg represents one-quarter of a dog's blood volume, and if repeated doses are required to maintain perfusion, the underlying reason should be aggressively pursued. At the time of writing, the average wholesale prices for these colloids were $52.30 for 500 mL of hetastarch and $24.25 for 500 mL of dextran 70, whereas lactated Ringer's solution was $1.43 for 500 mL. These solutions contain no bacteriostat and therefore are intended for single-dose usage.

Albumin has a molecular weight of approximately 69,000 and a molecular radius of 3.5 nm. It is a monodisperse colloid (i.e., all albumin molecules are the same size). In addition to its role in maintaining plasma COP, it carries a wide range of substances such as bilirubin, fatty acids, metals and other ions, hormones, and drugs (Rothschild et al. 1988). Albumin most commonly is given to small animal patients as stored or fresh frozen plasma, stored whole blood, or fresh whole blood. Albumin equilibrates with the interstitial space more rapidly and to a greater extent than artificial colloids, and relatively large volumes must be given to achieve a sustained rise in plasma COP. When considering chronic albumin supplementation, as opposed to acute volume expansion with blood products, the amount of albumin required can be estimated using an equation that corrects for the expected volume of distribution across the intravascular and interstitial spaces (Hardin et al. 1986).

$$\text{Albumin deficit (g)} = 10 \times [\text{desired [albumin] (g/dL)} - \text{patient [albumin] (g/dL)}] \times (\text{body weight [kg]} \times 0.3)$$

To increase serum albumin concentration from 1.5 to 2.5 g/dL in a 20-kg dog,

$$\text{Albumin deficit} = 10 \times (2.5 - 1.5) \times 20 \times 0.3 = 60 \text{ g}$$

This is equivalent to 2 L of plasma or 4 L of fresh whole blood!

▶ Colloid Therapy in Pulmonary Disease

The majority of pulmonary diseases result in accumulation of excess fluid in the interstitium alone or in the interstitium and alveoli. This increase in extravascular lung water is synonymous with pulmonary edema. The lung is relatively resistant to the edemagenic effects of hypoproteinemia (Zarins et al. 1978), and the two most important mechanisms by which pulmonary edema may occur are an increase in pulmonary hydrostatic pressure and increase in pulmonary microvascular permeability (Staub 1984). High-pressure edema may be secondary to left-sided heart failure or volume overload, whereas increased permeability edema may be caused by pneumonia, sepsis, toxic lung injury, or pancreatitis. In some clinical settings, the pathogenesis of pulmonary edema may be unclear or include both components (e.g., neurogenic and reexpansion edema).

The pulmonary endothelium is relatively permeable to protein compared with other tissues, and albumin (Vaughan et al. 1979) and hetastarch (Korent et al. 1997) equilibrate more rapidly with the interstitial space even in normal lung. Consequently, the effective COP gradient that can be generated between the intravascular space and pulmonary interstitium is lower than that in other tissues. The lung must therefore rely more on increased lymph flow than interstitial COP dilution to protect against pulmonary edema (Staub 1984). Certain types of lung injury, such as pneumonia or chemical injury, further increase the permeability of the capillary endothelium to protein. When one considers the Starling equation, it becomes obvious that capillary hydrostatic pressure becomes the major determinant of edema formation. Smaller increases in capillary hydrostatic pressure result in much greater fluid extravasation when the endothelium is damaged than when it remains intact. This finding clearly explains clinical and experimental studies that show that colloid therapy significantly worsens pulmonary edema caused by increased microvascular permeability (Holcroft et al. 1979). If the alveolar epithelium also is damaged, interstitial edema can rapidly progress to alveolar flooding.

Absorption of water, solutes, and protein occurs via different mechanisms and at vastly different rates. Resorption of sodium-containing alveolar fluid occurs mainly via active transport by the alveolar epithelium, most likely via a sodium-potassium pump with glucose cotransport, which is stimulated by β-adrenergic agonists (Sakuma et al. 1994). Fluid absorption occurs against the colloid osmotic gradient, which increases as fluid is reabsorbed and protein remains behind. Protein is cleared from the alveoli at a very low rate (Matthay et al. 1985), which is one of the reasons for the protracted resolution often seen with edema caused by increased permeability.

Colloid therapy may worsen pulmonary edema if the

increase in endothelial permeability is such that the majority of colloid molecules can pass through the pulmonary capillary endothelium (Holcroft et al. 1977). This is particularly true if a significant increase in pulmonary capillary pressure occurs, as is more likely with colloid infusion. Considering the extremely slow clearance of macromolecules from the alveolar space, this increase in edema may be life threatening. On the other hand, if the increase in permeability is insufficient to allow loss of colloid into the interstitium, prudent colloid therapy can reduce extravascular lung water. It therefore is important to evaluate critically the patient's response to a test infusion of colloid. An increase in COP should be titrated to avoid an increase in extravascular lung water or pulmonary capillary wedge pressure or, at worst, a decrease in arterial oxygen concentration. When using colloids in the patient with a systemic vascular leak state, and in the absence of hemorrhage, failure to retain colloid in the intravascular space for an appropriate time suggests that extravascular leakage of colloid is worsening, not helping, hypovolemia and edema. If arterial oxygenation worsens after colloid therapy in an animal with pulmonary edema caused by altered permeability, one must consider the possibility that the colloid is contributing to the pulmonary edema.

The use of colloids with high-pressure pulmonary edema is controversial because of their greater propensity for volume overload. Colloid therapy therefore should be used with extreme caution to avoid increases in pulmonary capillary hydrostatic pressure. Existing therapies for heart failure are very effective, and colloid support in the patient with left-sided heart failure should be used only in a critical care environment with invasive monitoring capabilities. Increased left atrial pressure secondary to left-sided heart failure results in increased pulmonary capillary pressure and increased fluid extravasation into the pulmonary interstitium (Guyton and Lindsay 1959). Lymph flow in the lung increases to protect against interstitial fluid accumulation (Zarins et al. 1978), but as extravasation increases, fluid begins to accumulate in the interstitium. In the alveoli, where gas exchange occurs, the capillary endothelial cell is closely apposed to the alveolar epithelial cell and the perimicrovascular interstitium is relatively noncompliant. In contrast, the peribronchovascular interstitial tissue is more compliant, and fluid tends to accumulate as peribronchovascular edema cuffs, thereby protecting gas exchange (Conhaim et al. 1986, 1989). Eventually, edema fluid distends all parts of the pulmonary interstitium and ultimately fills the airspaces of the lung. Current theory suggests that, because the alveolar membrane is so impermeable to solutes, alveolar filling does not occur by fluid flow through the epithelium but rather fluid spills into the airspaces at the junction of the alveolar and airway epithelia (Staub 1983). In the absence of increases in permeability, maintenance of intravascular COP via colloid administration can be protective against cardiogenic pulmonary edema (Wareing et al. 1989). Furosemide also increases COP and, contrary to popular belief, it does not appear to reduce plasma volume (da Luz et al. 1975; Schuster et al. 1984). Because of the opposing effects of intravascular hydrostatic pressure and COP, monitoring the gradient between pulmonary artery occlusion pressure and COP has been suggested in the management of pulmonary edema (da Luz et al. 1975; Rackow et al. 1977, 1982).

▶ Chronic Hypoproteinemia

The effective COP acting to retain fluid within the intravascular space is the net difference between the intravascular COP and the interstitial COP. As intravascular COP falls, fluid with a lower COP passes from the vasculature and dilutes the interstitial protein concentration such that interstitial COP also falls. Consequently, the gradient between intravascular and interstitial COP is preserved. This effect means that a low plasma COP per se does not necessitate colloid therapy in the absence of clinical signs such as hypovolemia or edema. Indeed, people with a hereditary form of complete albumin deficiency have plasma COP that still is half of normal because of increased globulin concentrations, and affected individuals exhibit minimal peripheral edema (Bennhold 1960; Dammacco et al. 1980). Also, there appear to be no serious clinical signs in autosomal recessive hereditary albumin deficiency in rats (Nagase et al. 1979). Interestingly, affected rats exhibited marked hypercholesterolemia.

In the author's clinical experience and in experimental studies (Zarins et al. 1978), animals with severe hypoproteinemia (COP < 11 mm Hg) may exhibit peripheral edema but rarely develop pulmonary edema. In dogs with hypoalbuminemia, hydroxyethyl starch has been shown to result in clinical improvement of peripheral edema or ascites (Smiley and Garvey 1994). The role of albumin in maintaining the selective permeability of the microvascular barrier to macromolecules (Michel et al. 1985; Curry et al. 1987) provides a rationale for the prophylactic use of albumin or artifical colloid. It is most important to diagnose and treat the underlying cause of hypoproteinemia rather than administer palliative colloid therapy. Furthermore, if there are large ongoing losses, colloid support may not be effective (Moore and Garvey 1996).

▶ Treatment Complications and Side Effects

The debate about whether or not artificial colloids cause abnormalities in coagulation is largely redundant because all of the commonly used artificial colloids can cause abnormal coagulation. The important question is whether or not these coagulopathies are clinically relevant. Despite many studies supporting a lack of clinically relevant bleeding, there also is a large amount of clinical and experimental evidence documenting serious, potentially life-threatening bleeding after administration of hydroxyethyl starch and dextran (Villarino et al. 1992; Baldassarre and Vincent 1997; Boldt et al. 1993; Cope et al. 1997; Treib et al. 1997c). This apparently conflicting evidence implies that coagulation abnormalities are clinically relevant only in *some* cases. The effects on coagulation appear to be directly related to the intravascular concentration of artificial colloid (Treib et al. 1997c). Higher plasma concentrations of colloid may occur after larger doses, repeated administration, or reduced intravascular degradation.

Large colloid molecules have a greater effect on coagulation than do small colloid molecules (Treib et al. 1997b). With repeated administration, the small colloid molecules are constantly excreted and the relative concentration of larger molecules increases. This fact explains why many studies reporting clinically relevant bleeding refer to patients who received repeated doses of colloid over a period of days.

The exact mechanism of action by which coagulation is affected is still not fully understood. The most repeatable findings are reductions in the concentrations of factor VIII and von Willebrand's factor greater than expected by dilution, and weakened clot formation (Gollub and Schaefer 1968; Gollub et al. 1967; Aberg et al. 1977, 1978, 1979; Jones et al. 1997). As a result of these findings, it seems reasonable to supplement clotting factors in animals at risk by use of fresh frozen plasma. In addition, desmopressin has been shown to increase factor VIII:C activity after hydroxyethyl starch infusion and should be considered as adjunctive therapy along with fresh frozen plasma administration (Conroy et al. 1996). Colloid molecules may impair the action of endothelial adhesion molecules, thereby reducing endothelial release of von Willebrand's factor (Collis et al. 1994). This observation also raises the possibility that colloid-induced reduction of adhesion molecule interaction may reduce neutrophil adhesion in sepsis (Collis et al. 1994) and explain the higher neutrophil counts observed after dextran 70 infusion in patients with endotoxic shock (Modig 1988).

Colloids are retained within the vascular system to a greater extent than are crystalloids, and there is a greater likelihood of absolute or relative volume overload with injudicious administration of colloids. Most clinicians are more familiar with crystalloid than with colloid infusion rates, and a helpful method to ensure a safe colloid infusion rate is to estimate the equivalent crystalloid infusion rate. Approximately 20 to 25% of crystalloid remains within the intravascular space 1 h after infusion, compared with 100% of the volume of infused colloid; therefore multiplying the colloid infusion rate by four allows one to conceptualize the volume expansion effects of the colloid in terms of an equivalent crystalloid volume. Although this approach can be helpful in limiting excessive infusion rates, animals with cardiac or pulmonary disease or oliguria warrant direct monitoring of central venous pressure.

The low-molecular-weight dextrans such as dextran 40 have been reported to cause acute renal failure (Mailloux et al. 1967; Ferraboli et al. 1997). Glomerular filtration of a high concentration of small dextran molecules is postulated to cause obstruction of the renal tubules or osmotic nephrosis (Mailloux et al. 1967; Ferraboli et al. 1997). Colloids should be used with caution in patients with oliguric or anuric renal failure because the kidneys are the major route of excretion for all artificial colloids. Nevertheless, colloids likely provide the most effective means of intravascular volume expansion in patients with capillary leak syndrome and oliguria related to hypovolemia and hypotension.

Anaphylactic or anaphylactoid reactions have been reported with use of dextrans, hydroxyethyl starches, and gelatins (Ring 1985), but the incidence of serious complications is extremely low (Ring and Messmer 1977). Hydroxyethyl starch was associated with pruritus in up to 33% of patients treated with long-term infusions (Gall et al. 1996). Deposits of hydroxyethyl starch in cutaneous nerves (Metze et al. 1997) and histiocytic skin infiltrates (Cox and Popple 1996) were thought to be responsible. Interestingly, pruritus also has been reported after infusion of lactated Ringer's solution (Bothner et al. 1998). Several studies have raised concerns about the potential effects of plasma substitutes on reticuloendothelial function (Schildt et al. 1975). Decreased concentrations of the opsonic plasma factor fibronectin have been reported with use of hydroxyethyl starch (Treib et al. 1996) and gelatins (Brodin et al. 1984).

▶ Laboratory Tests and Interpretation, Clinical Evaluation, and Monitoring

Refractometry does not accurately reflect the concentration of synthetic colloids (Bumpus et al. 1998). The forms of hydroxyethyl starch and dextran 70 available in the United States yield refractometric total solids concentrations of 4.5 g/dL. As plasma volume is replaced by artificial colloid, the measured refractometric concentration of total solids approaches that of the artificial colloid. Consequently, administering artificial colloid to an animal with an initial total solids concentration greater than 4.5 g/dL reduces the measured total solids, whereas administering artificial colloid to an animal with an initial refractometric total solids concentration less than 4.5 g/dL increases the measured total solids toward 4.5 g/dL. Failure to appreciate the effect of artificial colloid on refractometric total solids can cause the clinician to misinterpret the decrease in total solids concentration as an indication for more colloid. Assays for determination of serum colloid concentrations are not readily available, and therapy with artificial colloids is best monitored by direct measurement of COP using a membrane osmometer. The clinician should anticipate the dilutional effect caused by the effective intravascular expansion arising from colloid infusion. Packed cell volume, albumin concentration, and serum potassium concentration are most affected. After administration of hydroxyethyl starch, serum amylase concentration may be increased 200 to 250% of normal because of its binding to hydroxyethyl starch and reduced excretion (Boon et al. 1976; Kohler et al. 1977; Mishler and Durr 1979). Hydroxyethyl starch also can produce predictable but potentially misleading results in blood typing and crossmatching (Daniels et al. 1982).

REFERENCES

Aberg M, Arfors KE, and Bergentz SE: Effect of dextran on factor VIII and thrombus stability in humans. Significance of varying infusion rates. *Acta Chir Scand* 143:417–419, 1977.

Aberg M, Hedner U, and Bergentz SE: Effect of dextran 70 on factor VIII and platelet function in von Willebrand's disease. *Thromb Res* 12:629–634, 1978.

Aberg M, Hedner U, and Bergentz SE: Effect of dextran on factor

VIII (antihemophilic factor) and platelet function. *Ann Surg* 189:243–247, 1979.

Aukland K and Reed RK: Interstitial-lymphatic mechanisms in the control of extracellular fluid volume. *Physiol Rev* 73:1–78, 1993.

Baldassarre S and Vincent JL: Coagulopathy induced by hydroxyethyl starch. *Anesth Analg* 84:451–453, 1997.

Barclay SA and Bennett ED: The direct measurement of colloid osmotic pressure is superior to colloid osmotic pressure derived from albumin or total protein. *Intensive Care Med* 13:114–118, 1987.

Bates DO and Curry FE: Vascular endothelial growth factor increases hydraulic conductivity of isolated perfused microvessels. *Am J Physiol* 271:H2520–H2528, 1996.

Bennhold H, Klaus D, Scheurlen PG: Volume regulation and renal function in analbuminemia. *Lancet* 2:1169–1170, 1960.

Bent-Hansen L: Initial plasma disappearance and tissue uptake of ^{131}I-albumin in normal rabbits. *Microvasc Res* 41:345–356, 1991a.

Bent-Hansen L: Whole body capillary exchange of albumin. *Acta Physiol Scand Suppl* 603:5–10, 1991b.

Bent-Hansen L, Feldt-Rasmussen B, Kverneland A, et al.: Plasma disappearance of glycated and non-glycated albumin in type 1 (insulin-dependent) diabetes mellitus: Evidence for charge dependent alterations of the plasma to lymph pathway. *Diabetologia* 36:361–363, 1993.

Bert JL, Mathieson JM, and Pearce RH: The exclusion of human serum albumin by human dermal collagenous fibres and within human dermis. *Biochem J* 201:395–403, 1982.

Berthezene Y, Vexler V, Jerome H, et al.: Differentiation of capillary leak and hydrostatic pulmonary edema with a macromolecular MR imaging contrast agent. *Radiology* 181:773–777, 1991.

Bhattacharya J, Nanjo S, and Staub NC: Factors affecting lung microvascular pressure. *Ann N Y Acad Sci* 384:107–114, 1982.

Bhattacharya S, Glucksberg MR, and Bhattacharya J: Measurement of lung microvascular pressure in the intact anesthetized rabbit by the micropuncture technique. *Circ Res* 64:167–172, 1989.

Bjorneboe M and Schwartz M: Investigations concerning the changes in serum proteins during immunization: The cause of hypoalbuminemia with high gamma globulin levels. *J Exp Med* 110:259–270, 1959.

Boldt J, Knothe C, Zickmann B, et al.: Influence of different intravascular volume therapies on platelet function in patients undergoing cardiopulmonary bypass. *Anesth Analg* 76:1185–1190, 1993.

Boon JC, Jesch F, Ring J, et al.: Intravascular persistence of hydroxyethyl starch in man. *Eur Surg Res* 8:497–503, 1976.

Bothner U, Georgieff M, and Vogt NH: Assessment of the safety and tolerance of 6% hydroxyethyl starch (200/0.5) solution: A randomized, controlled epidemiology study. *Anesth Analg* 86:850–855, 1998.

Brigham KL, Harris TR, and Owen PJ: [^{14}C]Urea and [^{14}C] sucrose as permeability indicators in histamine pulmonary edema. *J Appl Physiol* 43:99–101, 1977.

Brodin B, Hesselvik F, and von Schenck H: Decrease of plasma fibronectin concentration following infusion of a gelatin-based plasma substitute in man. *Scand J Clin Lab Invest* 44:529–533, 1984.

Brown RH, Zerhouni EA, and Mitzner W: Visualization of airway obstruction in vivo during pulmonary vascular engorgement and edema. *J Appl Physiol* 78:1070–1078, 1995.

Brown SA, Dusza K, and Boehmer J: Comparison of measured and calculated values for colloid osmotic pressure in hospitalized animals. *Am J Vet Res* 55:910–915, 1994.

Bumpus SE, Haskins SC, and Kass PH: Effect of synthetic colloids on refractometric readings of total solids. *J Vet Emerg Crit Care* 8(1):21–26, 1998.

Chen HI, Granger HJ, and Taylor AE: Interaction of capillary, interstitial, and lymphatic forces in the canine hindpaw. *Circ Res* 39:245–254, 1976.

Chi OZ, Lu X, Wei HM, et al.: Hydroxyethyl starch solution attenuates blood-brain barrier disruption caused by intracarotid injection of hyperosmolar mannitol in rats. *Anesth Analg* 83:336–341, 1996.

Collis RE, Collins PW, Gutteridge CN, et al.: The effect of hydroxyethyl starch and other plasma volume substitutes on endothelial cell activation; an in vitro study. *Intensive Care Med* 20:37–41, 1994.

Concannon KT: Colloid oncotic pressure and the clinical use of colloidal solutions. *J Vet Emerg Crit Care* 3:49–62, 1993.

Conhaim RL, Lai-Fook SJ, and Staub NC: Sequence of perivascular liquid accumulation in liquid-inflated dog lung lobes. *J Appl Physiol* 60:513–520, 1986.

Conhaim RL, Lai-Fook SJ, and Eaton A: Sequence of interstitial liquid accumulation in liquid-inflated sheep lung lobes. *J Appl Physiol* 66:2659–2666, 1989.

Conhaim RL, Rosenfeld DJ, Schreiber MA, et al.: Effects of intravenous pentafraction on lung and soft tissue liquid exchange in hypoproteinemic sheep. *Am J Physiol* 265:H1536–H1543, 1993.

Conroy JM, Fishman RL, Reeves ST, et al.: The effects of desmopressin and 6% hydroxyethyl starch on factor VII:C. *Anesth Analg* 83:804–807, 1996.

Cope JT, Banks D, Mauney MC, et al.: Intraoperative hetastarch infusion impairs hemostasis after cardiac operations. *Ann Thorac Surg* 63:78–82, 1997.

Cox NH and Popple AW: Persistent erythema and pruritus, with a confluent histiocytic skin infiltrate, following the use of a hydroxyethylstarch plasma expander. *Br J Dermatol* 134:353–357, 1996.

Culp AM, Clay ME, Baylor IA, et al.: Colloid osmotic pressure (COP) and total solids (TS) measurement in normal dogs and cats (abstract). *Fourth International Veterinary Emergency and Critical Care Symposium,* San Antonio, p. 705, 1994.

Curry FE: Effect of albumin on the structure of the molecular filter at the capillary wall. *Fed Proc* 44:2610–2613, 1985.

Curry FE, Michel CC, and Phillips ME: Effect of albumin on the osmotic pressure exerted by myoglobin across capillary walls in frog mesentery. *J Physiol* 387:69–82, 1987.

Curry FE, Rutledge JC, and Lenz JF: Modulation of microvessel wall charge by plasma glycoprotein orosomucoid. *Am J Physiol* 257:H1354–H1359, 1989.

da Luz P, Shubin H, Weil MH, et al.: Pulmonary edema related to changes in colloid osmotic and pulmonary artery wedge pressure in patients after acute myocardial infarction. *Circulation* 51:350–357, 1975.

Dammacco F, Miglietta A, D'Addabbo A, et al.: Analbuminemia: Report of a case and review of the literature. *Vox Sang* 39:153–161, 1980.

Daniels MJ, Strauss RG, and Smith-Floss AM: Effects of hydroxyethyl starch on erythrocyte typing and blood crossmatching. *Transfusion* 22:226–228, 1982.

Dawidson IJ, Willms C, Sandor ZF, et al.: Lactated Ringer's solution versus 3% albumin for resuscitation of a lethal intestinal ischemic shock in rats. *Crit Care Med* 18:60–66, 1990.

Dich J, Hansen SE, and Thieden HID: Effect of albumin concentration and colloid osmotic pressure on albumin synthesis in the perfused rat liver. *Acta Physiol Scand* 89:352–358, 1973.

Falk JL, Rackow EC, and Weil MH: Colloid and crystalloid fluid resuscitation. In Shoemaker WC and Ayres S (eds): *Textbook of Critical Care.* Philadelphia, WB Saunders Co., pp. 1055–1073, 1989.

Farrow SP, Hall M, and Ricketts CR: Changes in the molecular composition of circulating hydroxyethyl starch. *Br J Pharmacol* 38:725–730, 1970.

Ferber HP, Nitsch E, and Forster H: Studies on hydroxyethyl starch. Part II: Changes of the molecular weight distribution for hydroxyethyl starch types 450/0.7, 450/0.5, 450/0.3, 300/0.4, 200/0.7, 200/0.5, and 200/0.1 after infusion in serum and urine of volunteers. *Arzneimittelforschung* 35:615–622, 1985.

Ferraboli R, Malheiro PS, Abdulkader RC, et al.: Anuric acute renal failure caused by dextran 40 administration. *Ren Fail* 19:303–306, 1997.

Funk W and Baldinger V: Microcirculatory perfusion during volume therapy. A comparative study using crystalloid or colloid in awake animals. *Anesthesiology* 82:975–982, 1995.

Gaar KAJ, Taylor AE, Owens LJ, et al.: Effect of capillary pressure and plasma protein on development of pulmonary edema. *Am J Physiol* 213:79–82, 1967.

Gabel JC, Scott RL, Adair TH, et al.: Errors in calculated oncotic pressure of dog plasma. *Am J Physiol* 239:H810–H812, 1980.

Gall H, Schultz KD, Boehncke WH, et al.: Clinical and pathophysiological aspects of hydroxyethyl starch–induced pruritus: Evaluation of 96 cases. *Dermatology* 192:222–226, 1996.

Gollub S and Schaefer C: Structural alteration in canine fibrin produced by colloid plasma expanders. *Surg Gynecol Obstet* 127:783–793, 1968.

Gollub S, Schaefer C, and Squitieri A: The bleeding tendency associated with plasma expanders. *Surg Gynecol Obstet* 124:1203–1211, 1967.

Gollub S, Kangwalklai K, and Schaefer C: Treatment of experimental hemorrhage with colloid-crystalloid mixtures. *J Surg Res* 9:311–317, 1969.

Granger DN and Barrowman JA: Gastrointestinal and liver edema. In Staub NC and Taylor AE (eds): *Edema*. New York, Raven Press, pp. 615–656, 1984.

Granger HJ, Laine GA, Barnes GE, et al.: Dynamics and control of transmicrovascular fluid exchange. In Staub NC and Taylor AE (eds): *Edema*. New York, Raven Press, pp. 189–228, 1984.

Guyton AC and Lindsay NW: Effect of elevated left atrial pressure and decreased plasma protein concentration on the development of pulmonary edema. *Circ Res* 7:649–657, 1959.

Guyton AC, Granger HJ, and Taylor AE: Interstitial fluid pressure. *Physiol Rev* 51:527–563, 1971.

Haraldsson B and Rippe B: Orosomucoid as one of the serum components contributing to normal capillary permselectivity in rat skeletal muscle. *Acta Physiol Scand* 129:127–135, 1987.

Hardin TC, Page CP, and Schwesinger WH: Rapid replacement of serum albumin in patients receiving total parenteral nutrition. *Surg Gynecol Obstet* 163:359–362, 1986.

Heir S and Wiig H: Subcutaneous interstitial fluid colloid osmotic pressure in dehydrated rats. *Acta Physiol Scand* 133:365–371, 1988.

Hempel V, Metzger G, Unseld H, et al.: The influence of hydroxyethyl starch solutions on circulation and on kidney function in hypovolaemic patients. *Anaesthesist* 24:198–201, 1975.

Holcroft JW, Trunkey DD, and Carpenter MA: Sepsis in the baboon: Factors affecting resuscitation and pulmonary edema in animals resuscitated with Ringer's lactate versus Plasmanate. *J Trauma* 17:600–610, 1977.

Holcroft JW, Trunkey DD, and Carpenter MA: Extravasation of albumin in tissues of normal and septic baboons and sheep. *J Surg Res* 26:341–347, 1979.

Jones PA, Tomasic M, and Gentry PA: Oncotic, hemodilutional, and hemostatic effects of isotonic saline and hydroxyethyl starch solutions in clinically normal ponies. *Am J Vet Res* 58:541–548, 1997.

Kedem O and Katchalsky A: Thermodynamic analysis of the permeability of biological membranes to non-electrolytes. *Biochim Biophys Acta* 27:229–246, 1958.

Kirby R and Rudloff E: The critical need for colloids: maintaining fluid balance. *Compend Contin Educ Pract Vet* 19:705–718, 1997.

Klotz U and Kroemer H: Clinical pharmacokinetic considerations in the use of plasma expanders. *Clin Pharmacokinet* 12:123–135, 1987.

Kohler H, Kirch W, and Horstmann HJ: Hydroxyethyl starch–induced macroamylasemia. *Int J Clin Pharmacol Biopharm* 15:428–431, 1977.

Korent VA, Conhaim RL, McGrath AM, et al.: Molecular distribution of hetastarch in plasma and lung lymph of unanesthetized sheep. *Am J Respir Crit Care Med* 155:1302–1308, 1997.

Korttila K, Grohn P, Gordin A, et al.: Effect of hydroxyethyl starch and dextran on plasma volume and blood hemostasis and coagulation. *J Clin Pharmacol* 24:273–282, 1984.

Kramer GC, Harms BA, Bodai BI, et al.: Effects of hypoproteinemia and increased vascular pressure on lung fluid balance in sheep. *J Appl Physiol* 55:1514–1522, 1983.

Lamke LO and Liljedahl SO: Plasma volume changes after infusion of various plasma expanders. *Resuscitation* 5:93–102, 1976.

Landis EM and Pappenheimer JR: Exchange of substances through the capillary walls. In Hamilton WF and Dow P (eds): *Handbook of Physiology*, Vol. 2. Baltimore, Williams & Wilkins, p. 961, 1963.

Luft JH: The structure and properties of the cell surface coat. *Int Rev Cytol* 45:291–382, 1976.

Mailloux L, Swartz CD, Capizzi R, et al.: Acute renal failure after administration of low-molecular weight dextran. *N Engl J Med* 277:1113–1118, 1967.

Mathews KA: The various types of parenteral fluids and their indications. *Vet Clin North Am Small Anim Pract* 28:483–513, 1998.

Matthay MA, Berthiaume Y, and Staub NC: Long-term clearance of liquid and protein from the lungs of unanesthetized sheep. *J Appl Physiol* 59:928–934, 1985.

Metze D, Reimann S, Szepfalusi Z, et al.: Persistent pruritus after hydroxyethyl starch infusion therapy: A result of long-term storage in cutaneous nerves. *Br J Dermatol* 136:553–559, 1997.

Michel CC, Phillips ME, and Turner MR: The effects of native and modified bovine serum albumin on the permeability of frog mesenteric capillaries. *J Physiol (Lond)* 360:333–346, 1985.

Mishler JM: Synthetic plasma volume expanders: Their pharmacology, safety, and clinical efficacy. *Clin Haematol* 13:75–92, 1984.

Mishler JM and Durr HK: Macroamylasaemia following the infusion of low molecular weight hydroxyethyl starch in man. *Eur Surg Res* 11:217–222, 1979.

Modig J: Beneficial effects of dextran 70 versus Ringer's acetate on pulmonary function, hemodynamics and survival in a porcine endotoxin shock model. *Resuscitation* 16:1–12, 1988.

Moore LE and Garvey MS: The effect of hetastarch on serum colloid oncotic pressure in hypoalbuminemic dogs. *J Vet Intern Med* 10:300–303, 1996.

Nagase S, Shimamune K, and Shumiya S: Albumin-deficient rat mutant. *Science* 205:590–591, 1979.

Navar PD and Narar LG: Relationship between colloid osmotic pressure and plasma protein concentration in the dog. *Am J Physiol* 233:H295–H298, 1977.

Oz MC, FitzPatrick MF, Zikria BA, et al.: Attenuation of microvascular permeability dysfunction in postischemic striated muscle by hydroxyethyl starch. *Microvasc Res* 50:71–79, 1995.

Pappenheimer JR: Passage of molecules through capillary walls. *Physiol Rev* 33:387–423, 1953.

Pappenheimer JR, Renkin EM, and Borrero LM: Filtration, diffusion and molecular sieving through peripheral capillary membranes. A contribution to the pore theory of capillary permeability. *Am J Physiol* 167:13–46, 1951.

Parker JC, Falgout HJ, Grimbert FA, et al.: The effect of increased vascular pressure on albumin-excluded volume and lymph flow in the dog lung. *Circ Res* 47:866–875, 1980.

Parker JC, Perry MA, and Taylor AE: Permeability of the microvascular barrier. In Staub NC and Taylor AE (eds): *Edema*. New York, Raven Press, pp. 143–187, 1984.

Parving HH and Rasmussen SM: Transcapillary escape rate of albumin and plasma volume in short- and long-term juvenile diabetics. *Scand J Clin Lab Invest* 32:81–87, 1973.

Patlak CS, Goldstein DA, and Hoffman JF: The flow of solute and solvent across a two membrane system. *J Theor Biol* 5:426–442, 1963.

Pietrangelo A, Panduro A, Chowdhury JR, et al.: Albumin gene expression is down-regulated by albumin or macromolecule infusion in the rat. *J Clin Invest* 89:1755–1760, 1992.

Prather JW, Gaar KA, and Guyton AC: Direct continuous recording of plasma colloid osmotic pressure of whole blood. *J Appl Physiol* 24:602–605, 1968.

Rackow EC, Fein IA, and Leppo J: Colloid osmotic pressure as a prognostic indicator of pulmonary edema and mortality in the critically ill. *Chest* 72:709–713, 1977.

Rackow EC, Fein IA, and Siegel J: The relationship of the colloid osmotic–pulmonary artery wedge pressure gradient to pulmonary edema and mortality in critically ill patients. *Chest* 82:433–437, 1982.

Renkin EM: Multiple pathways of capillary permeability. *Circ Res* 41:735–743, 1977.

Renkin EM: B. W. Zweifach Award lecture: Regulation of the microcirculation. *Microvasc Res* 30:251–263, 1985.

Renkin EM, Joyner WL, Sloop CH, et al.: Influence of venous pressure on plasma-lymph transport in the dog's paw: Convective and dissipative mechanisms. *Microvasc Res* 14:191–204, 1977.

Rieger A: Blood volume and plasma protein. 3. Changes in blood volume and plasma proteins after bleeding and immediate substitution with Macrodex, Rheomacrodex and Physiogel in the splenectomized dog. *Acta Chir Scand Suppl* 379:22–38, 1967.

Ring J: Anaphylactoid reactions to plasma substitutes. *Int Anesthesiol Clin* 23:67–95, 1985.

Ring J and Messmer K: Incidence and severity of anaphylactoid reactions to colloid volume substitutes. *Lancet* 1:466–469, 1977.

Rippe B and Haraldsson B: Transport of macromolecules across microvascular walls: The two pore theory. *Physiol Rev* 74:163–219, 1994.

Roberts JS and Bratton SL: Colloid volume expanders. Problems, pitfalls and possibilities. *Drugs* 55:621–630, 1998.

Rothschild MA, Oratz M, Franklin EC, et al.: The effect of hypergammaglobulinemia on albumin metabolism in hyperimmunized rabbits studied with albumin I^{131}. *J Clin Invest* 41:1564–1571, 1962.

Rothschild MA, Oratz M, Evans C, et al.: Alterations in albumin metabolism following serum and albumin infusions. *J Clin Invest* 43:1874–1880, 1964.

Rothschild MA, Oratz M, Mongelli J, et al.: Albumin metabolism in rabbits during gamma globulin infusions. *J Lab Clin Med* 66:733–740, 1965.

Rothschild MA, Oratz M, and Schreiber SS: Extravascular albumin. *N Engl J Med* 301:497–498, 1979.

Rothschild MA, Oratz M, and Schreiber SS: Serum albumin. *Hepatology* 8:385–401, 1988.

Rudloff E and Kirby R: The critical need for colloids: Selecting the right colloid. *Compend Contin Educ Pract Vet* 19:811–826, 1997.

Rudloff E and Kirby R: The critical need for colloids: Administering colloids effectively. *Compend Contin Educ Pract Vet* 20:27–43, 1998a.

Rudloff E and Kirby R: Fluid therapy. Crystalloids and colloids. *Vet Clin North Am Small Anim Pract* 28:297–328, 1998b.

Sakuma T, Okaniwa G, Nakada T, et al.: Alveolar fluid clearance in the resected human lung. *Am J Respir Crit Care Med* 150:305–310, 1994.

Schierhout G and Roberts I: Fluid resuscitation with colloid or crystalloid solutions in critically ill patients: A systematic review of randomised trials. *Br Med J* 316:961–964, 1998.

Schildt B, Bouveng R, and Sollenberg M: Plasma substitute induced impairment of the reticuloendothelial system function. *Acta Chir Scand* 141:7–13, 1975.

Schuster CJ, Weil MH, Besso J, et al.: Blood volume following diuresis induced by furosemide. *Am J Med* 76:585–592, 1984.

Shepard JM, Gropper MA, Nicolaysen G, et al.: Lung microvascular pressure profile measured by micropuncture in anesthetized dogs. *J Appl Physiol* 64:874–879, 1988.

Shoemaker WC: Comparison of the relative effectiveness of whole blood transfusions and various types of fluid therapy in resuscitation. *Crit Care Med* 4:71–78, 1976.

Shoemaker WC, Schluchter M, Hopkins JA, et al.: Comparison of the relative effectiveness of colloids and crystalloids in emergency resuscitation. *Am J Surg* 142:73–84, 1981.

Simionescu M, Simionescu N, and Palade GE: Preferential distribution of anionic sites on the basement membrane and the abluminal aspect of the endothelium in fenestrated capillaries. *J Cell Biol* 95:425–434, 1982.

Smiley LE: The use of hetastarch for plasma expansion. *Probl Vet Med* 4:652–667, 1992.

Smiley LE and Garvey MS: The use of hetastarch as adjunct therapy in 26 dogs with hypoalbuminemia: A phase two clinical trial. *J Vet Intern Med* 8:195–202, 1994.

Starling EH: On the absorption of fluid from the connective tissue spaces. *J Physiol (Lond)* 19:312–326, 1896.

Staub NC: Alveolar flooding and clearance. *Am Rev Respir Dis* 127:S44–S51, 1983.

Staub NC: Pulmonary edema. In Staub NC and Taylor AE (eds): *Edema.* New York, Raven Press, pp. 117–142, 1984.

Staub NC and Taylor AE: *Edema.* New York, Raven Press, 1984.

Staverman AJ: Non-equilibrium thermodynamics of membrane processes. *Trans Faraday Soc* 48:176–185, 1952.

Taylor AE: Capillary fluid filtration: Starling forces and lymph flow. *Circ Res* 49:557–575, 1981.

Taylor AE: The lymphatic edema safety factor: The role of edema dependent lymphatic factors (EDLF). *Lymphology* 23:111–123, 1990.

Taylor AE and Granger DN: Exchange of macromolecules across the microcirculation. In Renkin EM and Michel CC (eds): *Handbook of Physiology: Microcirculation.* Bethesda, MD, American Physiological Society, p. 462, 1985.

Taylor AE, Moore T, and Khimenko P: Microcirculatory exchange of fluid and protein and development of the third space. In Zikria BA, Oz MO, and Carlson RW (eds): *Reperfusion Injuries and Clinical Capillary Leak Syndrome.* Armonk, NY, Futura Publishing Co., pp. 59–92, 1994.

Thomas LA and Brown SA: Relationship between colloid osmotic pressure and plasma protein concentration in cattle, horses, dogs, and cats. *Am J Vet Res* 53:2241–2243, 1992.

Thompson WL, Fukushima T, Rutherford RB, et al.: Intravascular persistence, tissue storage, and excretion of hydroxyethyl starch. *Surg Gynecol Obstet* 131:965–972, 1970.

Treib J, Haass A, Pindur G, et al.: HES 200/0.5 is not HES 200/0.5. Influence of the C2/C6 hydroxyethylation ratio of hydroxyethyl starch (HES) on hemorheology, coagulation and elimination kinetics. *Thromb Haemost* 74:1452–1456, 1995.

Treib J, Haass A, Pindur G, et al.: Decrease of fibronectin following repeated infusion of highly substituted hydroxyethyl starch. *Infusionsther Transfusionsmed* 23:71–75, 1996.

Treib J, Haass A, Pindur G, et al.: A more differentiated classification of hydroxyethyl starches is necessary. *Intensive Care Med* 23:709–710, 1997a.

Treib J, Haass A, Pindur G, et al.: Avoiding an impairment of factor VIII:C by using hydroxyethyl starch with a low in vivo molecular weight. *Anesth Analg* 84:1391, 1997b.

Treib J, Haass A, and Pindur G: Coagulation disorders caused by hydroxyethyl starch. *Thromb Haemost* 78:974–983, 1997c.

Tullis JL: Albumin. 1. Background and use. *JAMA* 237:355–360, 1977.

Vaughan TRJ, Erdmann AJ, Brigham KL, et al.: Equilibration of intravascular albumin with lung lymph in unanesthetized sheep. *Lymphology* 12:217–223, 1979.

Velanovich V: Crystalloid versus colloid fluid resuscitation: A meta-analysis of mortality. *Surgery* 105:65–71, 1989.

Villarino ME, Gordon SM, Valdon C, et al.: A cluster of severe postoperative bleeding following open heart surgery. *Infect Control Hosp Epidemiol* 13:282–287, 1992.

Wall PL, Nelson LM, and Guthmiller LA: Cost effectiveness of use of a solution of 6% dextran 70 in young calves with severe diarrhea. *J Am Vet Med Assoc* 209:1714–1715, 1996.

Wareing TH, Gruber MA, Brigham KL, et al.: Increased plasma oncotic pressure inhibits pulmonary fluid transport when pulmonary pressures are elevated. *J Surg Res* 46:29–34, 1989.

Weiderhelm CA and Black LL: Osmotic interaction of plasma proteins with interstitial macromolecules. *Am J Physiol* 231:638–641, 1976.

Weisberg HF: Osmotic pressure of the serum proteins. *Ann Clin Lab Sci* 8:155–164, 1978.

Wiig H and Reed RK: Volume-pressure relationship (compliance) of interstitium in dog skin and muscle. *Am J Physiol* 253:H291–H298, 1987.

Wissig SL and Charonis AS: Capillary ultrastructure. In Staub NC and Taylor AE (eds): *Edema*. New York, Raven Press, pp. 117–142, 1984.

Yuan Y, Granger HJ, Zawieja DC, et al.: Flow modulates coronary venular permeability by a nitric oxide–related mechanism. *Am J Physiol* 263:H641–H646, 1992.

Zarins CK, Rice CL, Smith DE, et al.: Role of lympathics in preventing hypooncotic pulmonary edema. *Surg Forum* 27:257–259, 1976.

Zarins CK, Rice CL, Peters RM, et al.: Lymph and pulmonary response to isobaric reduction in plasma oncotic pressure in baboons. *Circ Res* 43:925–930, 1978.

Zikria BA: A biophysical approach: sealing of capillary leak by intravenous biodegradable macromolecules. In Zikria BA, Oz MO, and Carlson RW (eds): *Reperfusion Injuries and Clinical Capillary Leak Syndrome*. Armonk, NY, Futura Publishing Co., pp. 547–600, 1994.

Zikria BA, King TC, Stanford J, et al.: A biophysical approach to capillary permeability. *Surgery* 105:625–631, 1989.

Zweifach BW and Intaglietta M: Measurement of blood plasma colloid osmotic pressure. II. Comparative study of different species. *Microvasc Res* 3:83–88, 1971.

CHAPTER 24

Hypertonic Fluid Therapy

ERIC R. SCHERTEL   TODD A. TOBIAS

Hypertonic saline solutions were first used as a treatment for Asiatic cholera. In 1909, Rogers reported a dramatic decrease in the mortality of patients at the Calcutta General Hospital with use of 1.5% NaCl to treat patients in the collapsed stage of cholera. In 1917, there were several reports of the clinical and experimental use of hypertonic solutions. Bainbridge and Trevan (1917) reported that 2.1% NaCl was more effective than other solutions in treating shock experimentally induced in dogs by administration of adrenaline. In the same year, Marshall advocated use of 2.1% NaCl to treat shock in human patients and Cannon recommended 4% $NaHCO_3$. Mann supported Cannon's work the following year by suggesting that hypertonic salt solutions were of value in treating shock and that alkaline saline solutions were preferable. Penfield, who has commonly been credited with the first reported use of hypertonic NaCl solutions, did not publish his work with gum acacia and hypertonic sodium bicarbonate until 1919.

In one of the earliest recorded uses of extremely hypertonic NaCl solutions, Danowski and colleagues (1946) compared 5% NaCl, normal saline (0.9% NaCl), and 5% dextrose for treatment of experimental salt depletion shock. Administration of 5% NaCl returned measurements of hemodynamic and oxygen transport parameters and plasma volume to control values. The volume of hypertonic saline required to produce these effects was a fraction of that necessary for normal saline to produce similar effects. The dextrose solution was without significant benefit. Baue and coworkers (1967) compared equimolar 5.2% NaCl and 7.5% $NaHCO_3$ in hemorrhaged dogs and found no significant difference in the resuscitative effects of these two solutions.

In 1980, Velasco and colleagues reported that a small volume (4 mL/kg) of 7% NaCl resuscitated dogs subjected to controlled hemorrhage and resulted in 100% survival. Mean arterial pressure, cardiac output, and acid-base status were returned nearly to control values within minutes after administration of the hypertonic solution. In a control group, an equal volume of 0.9% NaCl resulted in neither resuscitation nor survival. The contrast in terms of volume between the 4 mL/kg of 7% NaCl needed for resuscitation and the 120 mL/kg of 0.9% NaCl commonly considered necessary under similar clinical conditions is readily apparent. The efficacy and economy of the hypertonic solution drew immediate attention, particularly for its potential use in the field management of trauma victims and its relative ease and speed of administration.

An interesting aspect of Velasco's study was the finding that significant plasma volume expansion, based on Evans blue indicator dilution, did not occur. These results contradicted previous findings and findings in conscious sheep. Administration of 7% NaCl at 4 mL/kg to sheep after moderate hemorrhage resulted in resuscitative effects similar to those observed by Velasco and colleagues (Nakayama et al. 1984). However, the hemodynamic improvement seen in the sheep was found to be the result of plasma volume expansion. These findings have resulted in some controversy regarding the mechanisms of action of hypertonic fluids and suggested possible species variation in the response to hypertonic saline.

In 1980, 7% NaCl was used to treat human patients in shock who were refractory to conventional fluid therapy (de Felippe et al. 1980). The patients responded to the treatment without complications, but the study was not well controlled. In 1983, the first controlled clinical study conducted in the United States was reported. Hypertonic sodium lactate (514 mOsm/L) was compared with lactated Ringer's solution for fluid therapy in operations of the abdominal aorta (Shackford et al. 1983). The patients treated with hypertonic sodium lactate required 50% less fluid than the group treated with lactated Ringer's solution to maintain similar cardiac and urine outputs. Postoperatively, patients treated with the hypertonic solution had reduced intrapulmonary shunting (i.e., improved pulmonary function), lower interstitial fluid pressure, and less clinical evidence of edema and were ambulatory sooner. The results suggested that the overall recovery of patients treated with the hypertonic solution was a function of the solution used or the smaller volume of fluid administered.

By the early 1980s, experimental studies of animals and clinical studies of humans had clearly established the great potential of hypertonic saline solutions for both hospital and field use and a compelling need for further investigation. The experimental studies, however, had not defined the primary mechanism of action of hypertonic saline solutions. Plasma volume expansion was thought to play a key role in the resuscitative effects of hypertonic saline, but a proposed vagal nerve–mediated reflex still required verification and explanation.

▶ Mechanisms of Action

Plasma Volume Expansion

Plasma volume expansion after hypertonic saline administration was first demonstrated in 1946 (Danowski et al. 1946; Winkler et al. 1946). In experiments involving dogs in hypovolemic shock, the plasma volume expansion and resuscitative effects of small volumes (16 mL/kg) of 5% NaCl were equivalent to those of large volumes (135 mL/kg) of 0.9% NaCl (Danowski et al. 1946). The average net plasma volume expansion was 7.7 mL/kg. Thus, the study of Velasco and coworkers (1980), in which plasma volume expansion was not observed, was at odds with previous work. However, Velasco and colleagues helped to resolve the controversy by their subsequent finding that administration of 7% NaCl at 5 mL/kg to hemorrhaged dogs expanded plasma volume by approximately 20 mL/kg (Rocha e Silva et al. 1990; Velasco et al. 1989). Similar degrees of plasma volume expansion have been observed by other investigators studying 7% NaCl in dogs (Schertel et al. 1990), horses (Schmall et al. 1990), and pigs (Wade et al. 1989).

A mathematical model of fluid compartments based on thermodynamic transport equations and physiologic data predicted immediate shifts of water into the plasma from red blood cells and endothelium and then from the interstitium and tissue cells after hypertonic saline infusion (Mazzoni et al. 1988). The increase in blood volume was predicted to be transient with hyperosmotic solutions but to occur in a fraction of the time when compared with the blood volume expansion that occurs when isotonic fluids are administered at the same infusion rate. The experimental studies performed in anesthetized rabbits supported the model (Mazzoni et al. 1988). Findings in large animal species have been consistent in that peak vascular volume expansion occurred by the end of the infusion period (i.e., within 5 min) (Mazzoni et al. 1988; Schertel et al. 1990). Peak improvements in arterial blood pressure, cardiac output, and oxygen delivery also occurred at this time (Smith et al. 1985; Tobias et al. 1993; Velasco et al. 1980).

The observation that adding a synthetic colloid (e.g., dextran 70) to 7% NaCl prolonged the resuscitative effect (Smith et al. 1985) further supports the concept of volume expansion as a primary mechanism of action for hypertonic solutions. Colloid solutions (including plasma) expand and stabilize blood volume by increasing plasma oncotic pressure. Administration of 4 mL/kg of 7% NaCl in 6% dextran 70 to hemorrhaged sheep resulted in cardiac output and mean arterial pressure increases that were better sustained than those obtained with 6% dextran 70 or 7% NaCl alone. The improved efficacy of combined hypertonic saline–dextran solutions also has been reported in studies carried out in hemorrhaged dogs (Velasco et al. 1989) and pigs (Maningas et al. 1989; Wade et al. 1989). The combination of 6% hetastarch (another synthetic colloid) with 7% NaCl produced a response in hemorrhaged sheep nearly equivalent to that observed with the hypertonic saline–dextran combination (Kramer et al. 1989b). The difference was attributed to the higher osmotic pressure of 6% dextran.

Lung Vagal Reflex

Controversy over the mechanisms of action of hypertonic saline began in 1981, when it was reported that the resuscitative effects of 7% NaCl in dogs were dependent on stimulation of a pulmonary reflex that traveled in the vagus nerves (Lopes et al. 1981). Three lines of evidence ultimately were presented to support this concept. The first was that hypertonic saline infused into the postpulmonary circulation (i.e., left atrium or aorta) did not result in resuscitation, whereas infusion of the same volume into the prepulmonary circulation (i.e., peripheral veins, right atrium, or pulmonary artery) resulted in resuscitation (Lopes et al. 1981). The second line of evidence supporting this concept was the demonstration that vagotomy performed immediately before administration of hypertonic saline prevented recovery of mean arterial pressure, cardiac output, and related cardiorespiratory parameters (Lopes et al. 1981). When these results were interpreted in light of the need for prepulmonary infusion, it was concluded that increased osmolality induced a vagal-mediated reflex responsible for resuscitation. In a study providing the third line of evidence supporting a vagal reflex, 7% NaCl was infused into the pulmonary artery of either a denervated or innervated lung lobe of dogs (Younes et al. 1985). When hypertonic saline was infused into the denervated lung, mean arterial pressure did not recover to the same extent, suggesting that lung innervation participated in the resuscitative effects of hypertonic saline.

In another study examining the vagal reflex mechanism, hypertonic saline was found to restore mean circulatory filling pressure* in hemorrhaged dogs (Lopes et al. 1986). When vagotomy was performed, mean circulatory filling pressure was not restored. The investigators interpreted this finding as meaning that hypertonic saline administration induced venoconstriction and a decrease in vascular capacitance through a vagal nerve–mediated reflex. In yet another study, the increase in cardiac output induced by hypertonic saline was accompanied by marked increases in renal and mesenteric blood flow and a limited increase in femoral blood flow (Rocha e Silva et al. 1986). Vagotomy attenuated the increase in cardiac output and reversed the effects on organ blood flow. The investigators concluded that the observed pattern of blood flow distribution in the dog was a result of a hypertonic saline–stimulated vagal reflex.

Hands and colleagues (1988) first questioned the interpretation of the data supporting a vagal reflex. In a

---

*Mean circulatory filling pressure is the pressure in the circulatory system when the heart is stopped and the arterial and venous pressures equilibrate. This measurement reflects the capacitance of the venous system and blood volume. Venous vasomotor tone is one determinant of venous capacitance.

study carried out in sheep, hypertonic saline was infused into systemic arterial (postpulmonary) and systemic venous (prepulmonary) circulations and identical resuscitative effects were observed. The study contradicted previous work demonstrating the need for prepulmonary infusion (Lopes et al. 1981). Hands and colleagues (1988) proposed that vagotomy altered the resuscitative effects of hypertonic saline by ablation of neural pathways from the cardiopulmonary region that may be involved in protective cardiovascular reflexes.

In a study directly addressing the role of the vagus in hemorrhagic shock, vagotomy performed during hemorrhagic shock in dogs resulted in an immediate decline in arterial pressure and cardiac output (Schertel et al. 1991). The deterioration in hemodynamics after vagotomy was significantly greater than that which occurred in animals subjected only to hemorrhagic shock. Survival at 240 min after hemorrhage and vagotomy was significantly reduced compared with that of dogs subjected only to hemorrhage. Furthermore, vagotomy attenuated the resuscitative effects (mean arterial pressure and cardiac output response) of isotonic fluid administration. The results clearly demonstrate the important role of vagal innervation in circulatory control during hypovolemia.

The effects of hypertonic saline on the mechanical properties of the systemic circulation were examined in hypovolemic dogs using a right heart bypass preparation (Schertel et al. 1990). Hypertonic saline administration did not alter the mechanical properties of the venous bed, implying that venoconstriction did not occur as a result of the direct or indirect (reflex) effects of hypertonic saline. The increase in venous return observed was attributed to plasma volume expansion. The study provided direct evidence for the mechanism of plasma volume expansion but was unable to substantiate the venoconstriction theory.

The claim that hypertonic saline produces a reflex-mediated redistribution of cardiac output to favor increased splanchnic and renal blood flow at the expense of femoral flow also has been challenged (Kreimeier et al. 1990; Maningas 1987; Schertel et al. 1991). In hemorrhaged conscious pigs, the distribution of cardiac output to major vascular beds did not differ between isotonic and hypertonic solutions (Maningas 1987), implying that a reflex mechanism was not involved. Anesthetized dogs subjected to traumatic-hemorrhagic hypotension and treated with a small volume of 7% NaCl were found to have markedly improved cardiac output (Kreimeier et al. 1990). Blood flow to the kidneys and intestinal viscera did not recover to baseline values in these animals, but skeletal muscle blood flow increased to above baseline. These results are in direct conflict with previous findings in hemorrhaged dogs in which blood flow increased in the renal and splanchnic vascular beds to a greater extent than in the femoral bed after infusion of isotonic saline (Rocha e Silve et al. 1986). The fact that vagotomy prevented this increase in renal and splanchnic flows after isotonic saline provided clear evidence that the results of previous studies might have been misinterpreted. The vagus nerve appeared to be an important participant in the circulatory control mechanisms operative during hemorrhage.

The third line of evidence supporting a hypertonic saline–induced reflex has also been disputed. In a study of hemorrhaged dogs (Allen et al. 1992), no difference was observed in hemodynamics when hypertonic saline was administered into either the innervated or denervated pulmonary circulation.

In conclusion, the studies using denervation of the vagus to prove involvement of a hypertonic saline–induced reflex mechanism were probably misinterpreted. Vagal nerve traffic appears to be crucial to circulatory control during stresses of the cardiovascular system but is not essential to the resuscitative mechanism of hypertonic saline.

Inotropic Effects

Several investigators have suggested that the improved myocardial performance observed after hypertonic saline infusion may be a direct effect of the solutions on the heart (Rochae Silva et al. 1987; Velasco et al. 1980). These claims were based on increased left ventricular dP/dt_{max},* cardiac output, and stroke work after hypertonic saline administration. However, in vitro studies of isolated hearts and papillary muscle have suggested that hypertonic saline may have negative inotropic effects (Brown et al. 1990; Goethals et al. 1975; Kawata et al. 1983). The latter results were supported by subsequent studies in anesthetized dogs, in which hypertonic saline was found to have negative inotropic effects (Constable et al. 1994; Liang and Hood 1978; Newell et al. 1980). Hypertonic saline may bring about its overall positive effect on left ventricular performance by increased adrenergic activity through catecholamine release (Liang and Hood 1978) or by improved coronary blood flow and oxygen delivery to the myocardium.

Oxygen Delivery

Optimizing oxygen delivery has been considered by many investigators and clinicians to be the ultimate goal of shock resuscitation (Shoemaker et al. 1990). The ability of hypertonic solutions to improve oxygen delivery has been inferred from studies demonstrating improvement in cardiac output, a main determinant of oxygen delivery. However, all crystalloids (including hypertonic saline) produce some hemodilution when used for blood volume replacement (Kramer et al. 1986; Smith et al. 1985). Hemodilution reduces oxygen-carrying capacity—the other main determinant of oxygen delivery. Despite the effects of hemodilution, small volumes of 7% NaCl administered after severe hemorrhage have been found to return oxygen delivery and oxygen consumption almost to control values (Chudnofsky et al. 1989; Hannon et al. 1989). In a study of hemorrhagic shock in pigs, oxygen delivery and consumption were found to be significantly greater and mortality less when 7% NaCl in 6% dextran

---

*Left ventricular dP/dt_{max} is the maximal rate of change of pressure with respect to time and is considered to be an index of contractility.

70 was administered as compared with equal volumes of 0.9% NaCl (Chudnofsky et al. 1989).

Not all studies have found that hypertonic saline provides better oxygen transport than other crystalloid and colloid solutions. Administration of a small volume of 7% saline in 6% hydroxyethyl starch did not increase oxygen delivery and meet oxygen demand as effectively as four times that volume of 6% hydroxyethyl starch (Reinhart et al. 1989). However, the latter study emphasized the need for standardizing resuscitation end points in order to provide a sensible method for comparing the efficacies of various resuscitation regimens. Perhaps the best method for comparing effects of crystalloid therapy on oxygen transport is to resuscitate the animal to a target cardiac output. If cardiac output is controlled as the resuscitative end point, the influence of the treatment in question on other parameters of oxygen delivery and consumption can be better evaluated. Oxygen delivery and consumption differed little when cardiac output was used as the resuscitative end point and 7% NaCl in 6% dextran 70 was compared with 0.9% NaCl in studies of conscious sheep and anesthetized dogs (Kramer et al. 1986; Tobias et al. 1993). Despite this, the time required for resuscitation and the volume of fluid needed to maintain cardiac output are much less for hypertonic saline–dextran solutions than for isotonic solutions (Tobias et al. 1993).

Immunomodulatory Effects

Hypertonic saline and associated plasma hypertonicity have been found to have immunomodulatory effects that may protect organs from oxidative injury and enhance cell-mediated immune function. Junger and colleagues (1994) demonstrated that T-cell proliferation in vitro was enhanced by increasing plasma hypertonicity, and Coimbra and colleagues (1996) found that T-cell suppression associated with hemorrhagic shock was reversed when hypertonic saline was used as the resuscitative fluid. In an animal model of hemorrhage and intraabdominal sepsis, there was lower mortality in animals treated with hypertonic saline than in animals resuscitated with lactated Ringer's solution (Coimbra et al. 1997). The lungs and livers of the animals receiving hypertonic saline had markedly less organ injury as assessed by histopathologic examination. In a study of hemorrhaged mice, hypertonic saline–treated animals had less lung injury than those treated with lactated Ringer's solution (Angle et al. 1998). The myeloperoxidase activity (a measure of neutrophil number and activity) of the lung was significantly greater in the animals treated with lactated Ringer's solution. Neutrophil numbers in the bronchoalveolar lavage fluid were less in the animals treated with hypertonic saline and basal H_2O_2 production was significantly greater in those treated with lactated Ringer's solution. The results of these studies strongly support a direct or indirect immunomodulatory action of hypertonic saline solutions. Although these studies need further verification, the results are consistent with the often reported ability of hypertonic saline to limit lung and cerebral fluid accumulation in various forms of shock and organ injury.

▶ Actions and Indications in Various Forms of Shock

Hemorrhagic Shock

Shock caused by acute blood loss is a primary indication for hypertonic saline therapy. The majority of the reports cited earlier were from studies of animal models of hemorrhagic shock. Hemorrhagic shock is clearly the form of shock in which the greatest experimental and clinical experience has been obtained and reported to date. The experimental studies of animals and clinical studies of human patients have demonstrated that hypertonic saline and hypertonic saline–synthetic colloid solutions are superior to equal volume isotonic solutions for resuscitation in hemorrhagic shock. When these resuscitative regimens have been compared in terms of equivalent plasma volume expansion, the differences have been minimized. However, hypertonic solutions generally result in faster recovery of hemodynamic variables. There may also be value in the ability of hypertonic solutions to produce hemodynamic effects equivalent to those of larger volumes of isotonic fluid while limiting the total volume of free water administered. The latter effects may prove beneficial in patients with lung or head injury and other conditions that may be exacerbated by fluid excess.

Traumatic Shock

Traumatic shock also may be considered an indication for hypertonic saline solution therapy. Clinical studies of veterinary (Schertel et al. 1996) and human (Holcroft et al. 1987, 1989; Maningas et al. 1989) patients suffering from blunt or penetrating trauma have supported the use of hypertonic fluids. In a prospective, randomized, "blinded" study in which 7% NaCl in 6% dextran 70 was compared with lactated Ringer's solution in canine trauma patients, the hypertonic saline–dextran solution was found to return hemodynamic parameters to baseline more rapidly than lactated Ringer's solution (Schertel et al. 1996). The hypertonic solution also limited the total volume of fluid administered. The latter effect has been demonstrated to diminish the potentially detrimental effects of excessive water administration, such as interstitial edema (Shackford et al. 1983). The smaller volume of fluid associated with hypertonic saline resuscitation also reduces the overall time demand on veterinary staff for management of fluid administration. The time demand on staff is primarily an issue with larger dogs because of the large volumes of fluid required and the time expended monitoring and changing fluid bags. However, careful monitoring of fluid administration in smaller animals also is necessary to avoid overhydration.

The osmotic forces and resuscitative effects of small volumes of hypertonic saline have focused attention on issues of fluid balance within the vascular, interstitial, and intracellular fluid spaces. Edema of the brain and edema of the lung are important examples of tissue fluid accumulation that occur commonly in shock states and especially in traumatic shock. Intracranial pressure (ICP) decreases during hemorrhage and increases above baseline values after conventional fluid therapy. Increased ICP may contribute to cerebral edema by altering fluid balance within the microvasculature of the brain. Small-volume 7% NaCl treatment of hemorrhagic shock in dogs prevented the increase in ICP that occurred with equivalent resuscitation using lactated Ringer's solution (Prough et al. 1985). In another study of hemorrhagic shock in dogs, 3% NaCl prevented the increase of ICP that occurred with infusion of 0.9% NaCl and 10% dextran 40 (Gunnar et al. 1986). These studies demonstrated that hypertonic NaCl solution use in hemorrhagic shock may limit increases in ICP and associated detrimental effects.

In a model of traumatic brain injury in rabbits, infusion of lactated Ringer's solution caused greater increases in ICP and brain water content than equivalent resuscitation with mildly hypertonic lactated Ringer's solutions (469 mOsm/kg) (Zornow et al. 1989). In studies using an epidural balloon to simulate the space-occupying lesion that commonly occurs with head injury and intracranial hemorrhage, increases in ICP were less severe in dogs (Gunnar et al. 1988) and pigs (Ducey et al. 1989) when 3% and 6% NaCl solutions were compared with 0.9% NaCl, dextran 40, hetastarch, and whole blood. In rats subjected to hemorrhage and mechanical brain injury, brain water content in normal brain was lower after 6.5% NaCl infusion as compared with lactated Ringer's solution but not in the injured brain (Wisner et al. 1990). Somatosensory evoked potentials, measured in hemorrhaged pigs, recovered better with 6% hetastarch than with 7% NaCl in 6% dextran 70 and 0.9% NaCl (Ducey et al. 1990). The diminished recovery of this measure of neurologic function was attributed to the vasodilatory effects of hypertonic saline and lower cerebral perfusion pressures. Overall, these results suggest that hypertonic saline solutions may limit the increase in ICP that occurs after aggressive fluid therapy in shock and that cerebral perfusion pressure may be better maintained by hypertonic solutions in the presence of space-occupying lesions (e.g., subdural hematomas). Fluid accumulation in the central nervous system, however, may not be limited by hypertonic saline when direct trauma to the brain has occurred.

In anesthetized sheep subjected to severe hemorrhage, administration of 3% NaCl in a volume sufficient to return hemodynamic parameters to baseline values had little influence on cardiopulmonary function or the accumulation of extravascular lung water (Layon et al. 1987). Systemic and pulmonary lymph flow increased in a similar manner when either mildly hypertonic saline solution (1.2%) or lactated Ringer's solution was administered to chronically instrumented sheep subjected to moderate hemorrhage (Nerlich et al. 1983). However, the pulmonary hypertension observed with lactated Ringer's treatment was not seen in animals treated with hypertonic saline. In normovolemic or hypovolemic guinea pigs, respiratory system mechanics, as assessed by passive elastance and airway resistance, were not altered significantly by either hypertonic (7%) or isotonic saline solutions (Martins et al. 1988). In a canine model of lung injury produced by oleic acid infusion, 7% NaCl infusion resulted in a mild increase in pulmonary shunt, suggesting a worsening pulmonary condition (Johnson et al. 1985). However, the increase in pulmonary shunt was more than compensated for by the increase in cardiac output, oxygen delivery, and tissue oxygen consumption that occurred as a result of hypertonic saline infusion. Hence, the influence of hypertonic solutions on normal respiratory system function and mechanics appears to be similar to that of conventional fluid therapy. The safety of this form of fluid therapy in the presence of lung injury has not been clearly determined and warrants further investigation.

Septic and Endotoxemic Shock

Treatment of septic shock related to cholera was the first reported application of hypertonic saline. Interest in this form of therapy waned as the use of isotonic saline and glucose solutions became more popular. There has been renewed interest, however, in the use of these solutions for the treatment of septic and endotoxic shock.

In an experimental study comparing use of 4% NaCl and 0.9% NaCl in severe endotoxic shock in dogs, intravascular pressures were returned to normal with both solutions, but cardiac output, stroke volume, and oxygen consumption were significantly higher in dogs treated with hypertonic saline (Luypaert et al. 1986). When small-volume 3.4% NaCl was compared with an equivalent sodium load as lactated Ringer's solution in dogs, there were few differences in terms of hemodynamic effects (Mullins and Hudgens 1987). The net fluid gain, however, was significantly less in the animals treated with hypertonic saline, possibly explaining the observation that there was less hindpaw lymph production. The significance of the latter finding is that hypertonic fluids may limit interstitial fluid accumulation and the detrimental effects of tissue edema that occur with isotonic fluid administration. In another study performed in endotoxic dogs, 7% NaCl in 6% dextran 70 resulted in equivalent resuscitation with less volume when compared with 0.9% NaCl but did not provide significant benefit in terms of oxygen transport–related variables (Weeren et al. 1994). In a contrasting study, administration of 7% NaCl in 6% hetastarch to dogs in endotoxic shock provided only transient hemodynamic improvement when compared with equal volumes of isotonic saline in 6% hetastarch (Armistead et al. 1989). Thus, the evidence that hypertonic saline is superior to isotonic saline for resuscitation in septic and endotoxic shock is not conclusive.

Although no optimal solution for resuscitation in endotoxic or septic shock has been identified (Prough and Johnston 1989), mildly hypertonic solutions (e.g., 1.2–3% NaCl) may have greater utility than concentrated saline solutions (e.g., 7% NaCl) for treatment of these conditions. Patients in endotoxic and septic shock commonly are dehydrated and administration of 7% NaCl may complicate preexisting hypernatremia and hyperosmolality. Hypoproteinemia is another common feature of endotoxemia and sepsis that may affect selection of the type of fluid for resuscitation. The hemodilution that occurs with isotonic crystalloid therapy may aggravate hypoproteinemia. As a result, synthetic colloid therapy has been recommended in order to stabilize vascular volume in these patients. Thus, the combination of hypertonic saline and synthetic colloids ultimately may prove valuable in these forms of shock. In summary, care must be exercised in the selection of a hypertonic saline solution for patients with endotoxemic or septic shock. When hypertonic saline solutions are chosen, midly hypertonic solutions, such as 1.8 to 3% NaCl (600–1800 mOsm/L), may be more appropriate. Colloid solutions often are indicated in these forms of shock and may be combined with the hypertonic solution or given separately.

Gastric Dilatation-Volvulus–Induced Shock

Shock caused by gastric dilatation-volvulus (GDV) is a common problem in small animal veterinary practice and is primarily a result of volume maldistribution. Administration of large volumes of isotonic fluid has been the conventional form of fluid therapy. In a study of dogs with experimental GDV-induced shock (Allen et al. 1991), 7% NaCl in 6% dextran 70 administered at a dosage of 5 mL/kg was compared with 0.9% saline administered at 60 mL/kg. Both initial treatments were followed by maintenance administration of isotonic saline (20 mL/kg/h). Both treatments returned cardiac output and blood pressure to control values during the first hour of treatment. In subsequent hours, however, cardiac output and oxygen delivery declined in the group treated with isotonic saline and remained significantly lower than in the group treated with the hypertonic saline–dextran solution despite maintenance fluid therapy. The improvement in cardiac output in dogs treated with hypertonic saline–dextran was attributed to higher heart rate, increased myocardial performance, and lower systemic vascular resistance. The effect of the hypertonic fluid on oxygen delivery was attributed to increased cardiac output and higher hematocrit. In a subsequent prospective clinical study of canine patients with GDV-induced shock, administration of hypertonic saline–dextran solution rapidly restored cardiorespiratory function in a manner equivalent to administration of large volumes of lactated Ringer's solution (Schertel et al. 1997). The dogs receiving hypertonic saline–dextran required less total fluid to resuscitate them, thus making the treatment regimen more efficient.

On the basis of the clinical and experimental studies of dogs (Allen et al. 1991; Schertel et al. 1997), 7% NaCl in 6% dextran 70 is an efficacious mode of fluid therapy for GDV-induced shock. This form of therapy has the potential for rapidly resuscitating patients with GDV and providing stable hemodynamics and oxygen delivery. A resuscitative dose of the hypertonic solution can be delivered within 5 to 10 min, whereas isotonic solutions require up to 60 min to provide the volume of fluid necessary for equivalent effects.

Burn Shock

Mildly hypertonic fluids (600 mOsm/L) have been used for several decades to treat burn shock and burn-associated fluid and electrolyte deficits (Monato et al. 1973). The tremendous sodium deficit that may develop in burn shock has been attributed to an intracellular accumulation of sodium and sodium loss at the burn site. Mildly hypertonic (1.8%) sodium lactate solutions have been found to meet the tremendous sodium needs characteristic of the burn patient but involve less net free-water administration than isotonic fluids (Monafo et al. 1973). Mortality rates were reported to be lower in clinical studies of burn patients treated with mildly hypertonic fluid (1.8%) (Monafo et al. 1973). In an experimental study of burn injury in guinea pigs, the optimal fluid therapy for maintaining normal cardiac function was 7% NaCl in 6% dextran 70 followed by isotonic fluid therapy (Horton et al. 1990). In a burn study in dogs, hypertonic sodium lactate (1.8%) therapy limited net free-water gain and produced natriuresis while providing resuscitative effects similar to those of isotonic fluids (Moylan et al. 1973). In rats with 40% body surface area burns, however, 7% NaCl was not successful in improving hemodynamic parameters (Onarheim et al. 1989a). The reason for this disparate finding is not clear. The lack of response may have been due to a slow rate of infusion and limited plasma volume expansion or to the greater hypertonicity of the solution studied.

Although uncommon in small animal practice, burn shock and hypovolemia related to thermal injury are indications for hypertonic saline therapy. The 7% NaCl solutions may be too concentrated for use in burn shock and may not provide sufficient water to replace losses (Horton et al. 1990; Onarheim et al. 1989a, 1989b). The hypertonic saline solutions used most commonly have been those with an osmolality of 600 mOsm/L (1.8%) (Caldwill and Bowser 1979; Gunn et al. 1989; Monato 1970; Monato et al. 1973). These solutions replace the tremendous sodium and water losses that occur, yet limit the volume of water administered when compared with isotonic fluids. Administration of less total free water may limit tissue edema, a common complication in burn patients. Clinical management of thermal injury in the dog must be guided by serial determinations of serum electrolyte concentrations regardless of the form of fluid therapy employed.

Shock in Acute Pancreatitis

In an experimental study of acute bile-induced pancreatitis in dogs, 7% NaCl in 6% dextran 70 was compared with lactated Ringer's solution (Horton et al. 1989). The hypertonic saline–dextran solution was given as a 4 mL/kg bolus in one group of dogs and followed by lactated Ringer's solution at a rate sufficient to maintain cardiac output and mean arterial pressure at control values. Lactated Ringer's solution was administered to the second group to achieve the same resuscitative end points. Pulmonary hypertension related to an increase in pulmonary vascular resistance occurred in the dogs treated with lactated Ringer's solution and was associated with increased lung water content. The hypertonic saline–dextran group had significantly less hemodilution and as a direct result greater oxygen delivery than the lactated Ringer's group. Cardiac function was found to be better in the hypertonic solution group. Clinical use of hypertonic solutions in canine patients with acute pancreatitis has not been reported.

▶ Administration
Route

Hypertonic saline solutions with osmolalities as high as 2400 mOsm/L have been infused safely through peripheral and central venous catheters in numerous species including dogs, cats, and humans and through peripheral arterial catheters in sheep (Hands et al. 1988). Histologic examination of sites where 7% NaCl had been infused showed only mild inflammatory changes in the area of vessel puncture and no intimal vascular changes, suggesting that injury to the vascular wall at the site of infusion did not occur (Hands et al. 1988). Hypertonic saline also has been administered by the intraosseous route in dogs (Okrasinski et al. 1992) and sheep (Kramer et al. 1989a). Transient lameness was associated with intraosseous administration of hypertonic saline in dogs. In sheep, histologic sections of sternal bone marrow 2 weeks after infusion showed evidence of local fibrinous change consistent with repair. Different sites of infusion do not appear to alter the resuscitative effects of hypertonic saline except in the dog, in which a difference was observed for intravenous and intraarterial infusions (Kramer et al. 1989a). Intraarterial injection, however, is not recommended in clinical patients.

Dosage

The dosage of hypertonic solutions differs with the percent concentration and formulation of the solution and the severity of the fluid deficit. Dosages for 7% NaCl and 7% NaCl in 6% dextran 70 are best defined. The dosage of 7% NaCl (2400 mOsm/L) required to return hemodynamic parameters nearly to control values in moderate to severe hemorrhagic shock is approximately 4 to 6 mL/kg. This dosage also has been used effectively to treat traumatic and GDV-induced shock. The largest reported dosages of these solutions in hemorrhaged dogs averaged 10 mL/kg (Tobias et al. 1993). This dosage produced a mean serum sodium concentration of 167 mEq/L when measured immediately after infusion. The recommended method of administering 7% NaCl (with or without dextran 70) is to infuse an initial dosage of 2 to 6 mL/kg. The dosage selected should be based on the severity of the shock state and fluid deficit. Dosages of 2 mL/kg may be repeated on the basis of the patient's response. When the total dosage equals 6 to 8 mL/kg, serum sodium concentration should be measured before additional hypertonic fluid is given. Seven percent NaCl in 6% dextran 70 may be administered at a similar dosage. When hypertonic saline is not formulated with dextran, 6% dextran 70 may be administered separately at a dosage of 4 to 6 mL/kg.

Mildly hypertonic solutions must be administered in greater volume than 7% NaCl solution because of their lower sodium concentration. Approximately 40 mL/kg of a 1.4% sodium lactate solution was required to return hemodynamic parameters to control levels in hemorrhaged pigs (Peters et al. 1986). In hemorrhaged sheep, 3% NaCl at 39 mL/kg returned hemodynamic parameters to control values for 60 min but resulted in a peak serum sodium concentration of 183 mEq/L. In dogs in experimental endotoxic shock, 3% NaCl at 12 mL/kg produced resuscitation similar to that achieved with 100 mL/kg of isotonic lactated Ringer's solution, but serum sodium concentrations were not reported (Mullins and Hudgens 1987). In two clinical studies of human patients, resuscitation of surgical hypovolemia to equivalent hemodynamic end points required 61 mL/kg of 1.5% sodium lactate and 128 mL/kg of lactated Ringer's solution (Shackford et al. 1983, 1987). The mean serum sodium concentration in patients of the latter studies peaked at 154 mEq/L. Estimated safe dosages for hypertonic saline solutions of varying percent concentrations are presented in Table 24-1. These estimates are based on experimental and clinical data for animals and humans with normal serum sodium concentrations before treatment.

Hypertonic saline solutions should not be used as the only form of fluid therapy in patients in shock. After initial administration of hypertonic fluids, isotonic fluids should be administered for several hours to ensure stable plasma volume expansion. The dosage of isotonic solutions most commonly employed is 20 mL/kg/h. The patient's response to treatment should be considered in determining the dosage of subsequent fluids and other treatments. Clinical monitoring of the shock state (see Chapter 20) should be used to guide additional fluid administration and other ancillary therapy.

Type of Solution

Various formulations of hypertonic solutions have been investigated in experimental and clinical studies. Hypertonic sodium lactate and acetate solutions have resuscitative effects similar to those of sodium chloride solutions of similar osmolality (Rocha e Silva et al. 1987; Smith et al. 1985). The advantage of lactate- and acetate-containing solutions is the ability of the body to metabolize these substances and produce bicarbonate. The bicarbonate produced acts as a buffer for the metabolic acidosis of shock. Mildly hypertonic sodium lactate solutions have

TABLE 24-1. Estimated Safe Dosages for Hypertonic Saline Solutions

	NaCl (%)					
	1.2	2.4	3	4	5	7
Approximate osmolality (mOsm/kg)	400	800	1000	1400	1800	2400
Maximum dosage range (mL/kg)	40–60	20–30	15–20	10–14	6–10	4–8
Maximum infusion rate (mL/kg)	2	2	2	2	1	1
Manufacturers	NA	NA	Baxter, Braun-McGaw, various others	NA	Abbott, Baxter, Braun-McGaw, various others	Butler, Vedco

been studied in human patients in a hospital setting (Shackford et al. 1983, 1987). The solutions in these studies were a combination of sodium lactate and sodium chloride, with lactate constituting less than 50% of the anionic components of the solution. The benefit of providing a metabolizable anion in hypertonic solutions has not been demonstrated, despite its theoretical advantages.

Commercially available hypertonic fluid products are listed in Table 24–1. Currently, these products are limited to sodium chloride solutions. Many of the solutions discussed in this chapter were formulated by the investigators, hospital pharmacies, or as experimental solutions by various manufacturers of parenteral solutions. A 7% NaCl solution is commercially available in 500-mL plastic vials (Butler, Columbus, OH). The addition of 60 mL of 23.4% NaCl (LyphoMed, Rosemont, IL) to a 500-mL bag of 5% NaCl (Baxter Healthcare, Chicago, IL) produces a 7% NaCl solution. To make up 7% NaCl in 6% dextran 70, 33.0 g of anhydrous NaCl is added to a 500-mL bag of 6% Gentran 70 in 0.9% NaCl (Baxter Healthcare, Chicago, IL). This is accomplished by placing half of the crystals into the barrel of a 35-mL syringe and withdrawing in a sterile manner an adequate volume of the Gentran solution to dissolve the crystals. This solution then is injected back into the bag through a 0.22-μm filter. The remaining crystals are treated similarly. The shelf life of such a solution is estimated to be 3 months from the time of compounding.

Rate

The rate of infusion of hypertonic solutions is of critical importance (see Table 24–1). Infusion of 7% NaCl at rates in excess of 1 mL/kg/min results in vagally mediated hypotension and bradycardia (Schertel et al. 1985). These effects usually are transient and resolve with slowing of the infusion rate but could be deleterious in a critical patient. This maximum rate of infusion still allows administration of a dosage of 5 mL/kg over 5 min. Five percent sodium chloride solution also should be infused at this slow rate (i.e., ≤1 mL/kg/min). The mildly hypertonic (≤3% NaCl) solutions can be administered safely at a rate of 2 mL/kg/min. This is the conventional rate of administration of isotonic fluids to shock patients. All patients must be carefully monitored during infusion for evidence of adverse responses. The systemic arterial pressure and electrocardiogram are the most important parameters to monitor during infusion.

▶ Precautions and Contraindications

Electrolyte and Osmolality Disturbances

Disturbances of electrolyte concentration and osmolality probably are the most common problems associated with hypertonic saline solution administration. As such, these problems also are natural contraindications for the use of hypertonic saline solutions. Animals in shock related to hemorrhage, trauma, or GDV that are otherwise normal are unlikely to have preexisting electrolyte or osmolality abnormalities. Therefore, hypertonic saline may be used for these animals without previous knowledge of electrolyte concentrations and osmolality with minimal risk. The status of electrolyte concentrations and osmolality should be evaluated before treatment of patients with other medical problems with hypertonic solutions.

Hypernatremia is a direct result of hypertonic saline administration. Serum sodium concentrations above the normal range (140 to 155 mEq/L) but less than 165 mEq/L appear to be well tolerated by dogs, awake sheep (Hands et al. 1988), and humans (Holcroft et al. 1987, 1989). Serum osmolality rises proportionally with serum sodium concentration after administration of hypertonic saline solution. Serum osmolality has approached 360 mOsm/kg in human patients (Holcroft et al. 1987) and awake sheep (Hands et al. 1988) without untoward effects. Thus, the hypernatremia and hyperosmolality resulting from bolus administration of an appropriate dosage of hypertonic saline are unlikely to have adverse effects. Evidence of preexisting hypernatremia or hyperosmolality should be considered a contraindication for use of hypertonic saline. Dehydration may be accompanied by hypernatremia and hyperosmolality and is a contraindication for use of hypertonic solutions.

Administration of hypertonic saline solutions to hemorrhaged animals may cause hypokalemia (Nakayama et al. 1984; Smith et al. 1985; Tobias et al. 1993). Serum potassium concentration has been found to decrease by approximately 1 to 2 mEq/L after a standard dosage (4–5 mL/kg) of 7% NaCl for treatment of severe hemorrhage (see Table 24–1). However, this change is not unique to resuscitation with hypertonic solutions. There is evidence that aggressive 0.9% NaCl therapy brings about similar changes in serum potassium concentration (Tobias et al. 1993). Regardless of the form of fluid therapy, hypokalemia has been associated with serious cardiovascular system complications. As a result, serum potassium concentrations should be evaluated before and after hypertonic saline therapy. Preexisting hypokalemia is an indication for aggressive potassium replacement therapy.

Cardiovascular Effects

Hypertonic saline solutions infused rapidly into the venous circulation produce hypotension, bradycardia, bronchoconstriction, and rapid shallow breathing (Schertel et al. 1985). Slow administration, therefore, is strongly recommended (discussed earlier; see Table 24–1). The mechanism of the cardiopulmonary response involves, in part, a vagally mediated pulmonary reflex. This reflex is responsible for a centrally mediated decrease in sympathetic nervous system activity and increase in parasympathetic nervous system activity (Mancia et al. 1976). Anticholinergic drugs, such as atropine, block the bradycardia of the parasympathetic component of the reflex but do not prevent all the untoward effects of overzealous infusion rates. Inotropic support in the form of epinephrine may be necessary to maintain arterial pressure and cardiac function. Slowing the rate of infusion, however, generally is adequate to reverse these reflex-mediated effects.

Hemostasis and Related Concerns

One major concern in prehospital use of hypertonic saline has been the potential of hypertonic saline to cause rehemorrhaging in trauma patients. Rehemorrhaging refers to blood loss that occurs because of the breakdown of ill-formed clots at the site of a previous vascular injury and blood loss. Rehemorrhaging is thought to result from a sudden increase in cardiac output and systemic arterial pressure. Rehemorrhaging is not unique to hypertonic saline administration and may occur during any therapy that rapidly increases cardiac output and arterial pressure. It has not been associated with isotonic fluid administration in the prehospital setting because the volume commonly administered does not produce sufficient hemodynamic changes. Experimental evidence suggests that infusion of small-volume 7% NaCl in the presence of major vascular injury leads to increased blood loss and mortality (Gross et al. 1988, 1989, 1990). Rehemorrhaging has not been a problem in studies of prehospital hypertonic saline use in human trauma victims (Gross et al. 1988, 1989, 1990; Holcroft et al. 1987, 1989; Maningas et al. 1989), but the theoretical concern remains.

A concern related to rehemorrhaging is the effect of hypertonic saline solutions on coagulation and platelet function. In an in vitro study of human blood, serial dilution of plasma with hypertonic saline resulted in a deterioration of coagulation and platelet aggregation (Reed et al. 1991). Thus, hypertonic saline does exhibit anticoagulant activity, but this effect was observed at serum osmolalities much higher than those that occur with normal dosages of hypertonic saline. There have been no reported occurrences of coagulation defects as a complication of hypertonic saline use.

Dextrans are known to inhibit platelet function and also may inhibit coagulation mechanisms. These effects have not been observed in clinical studies of hypertonic saline–dextran combinations (Holcroft et al. 1987, 1989), nor have they been observed by us during clinical and laboratory use of dextrans in dogs. Hypertonic saline and saline-dextran combinations should be used with caution in clinical patients when coagulopathies, thrombocytopenia, or platelet dysfunction has been identified or is suspected.

Injuries to vessels, perivascular tissues, and blood components (e.g., red blood cells) have concerned investigators studying the clinical applications of hypertonic solutions. As discussed earlier, 7% NaCl does not have significant detrimental effects on the vessel wall at the site of injection. When hypertonic saline solutions have been inadvertently infused into perivascular tissues, the tissues were found to be resistant to osmotic injury (Eaglstein 1990). Hemolysis has been reported to occur with use of extremely hypertonic saline solutions (e.g., 23% NaCl) (Rocha Silva et al. 1990), but not with commonly employed hypertonic saline solutions (see Table 24–1).

▶ Summary

Hypertonic saline solutions are highly efficacious alternatives to conventional isotonic fluids for resuscitation in several different forms of shock in animals. When hypertonic saline solutions are combined with synthetic colloids, their efficacy may be superior to that of isotonic solutions because of the ability of colloids to stabilize the vascular volume expansion of the hypertonic solution. Hypertonic saline solutions may have other advantages over isotonic fluids. Hypertonic solutions generally produce more rapid recovery of hemodynamic parameters when compared with isotonic solutions. Hypertonic solutions also limit the free water administered, reducing edema formation and possibly limiting fluid accumulation in the lung and brain. Veterinary practice often demands a simple, convenient, and effective form of resuscitative fluid therapy, underscoring another advantage of hypertonic saline solutions. Because technical assistance in veterinary medicine often is limited and the demands on the time of the practicing veterinarian are great, use of hypertonic saline or saline-dextran solutions may reduce the amount of time necessary for administration of a resuscitative dose of fluids.

Shock related to hemorrhage, trauma, or GDV is a clear indication for use of 7% NaCl or hypertonic saline–dextran combinations. These concentrated solutions may not be as efficacious or safe in other forms of shock, particularly those in which dehydration and electrolyte abnormalities are more common. Mildly hypertonic (≤3%) solutions may be preferred in septic, endotoxic, or burn shock, especially when laboratory results are not available before treatment. Hypertonic solutions should never be administered as the sole form of fluid therapy but should be supplemented with maintenance infusions of isotonic fluids. Regardless of the clinical setting or disease state being treated, the veterinary clinician choosing to use hypertonic fluids must be well informed about the advantages and disadvantages of this form of therapy.

REFERENCES

Allen, DA, Schertel ER, Muir WW, and Valentine AK: Hypertonic saline/dextran resuscitation of dogs with experimentally induced gastric dilation-volvulus shock. *Am J Vet Res* 52:92–96, 1991.

Allen DA, Schertel ER, Schmall LM, and Muir WW: Lung innervation and the hemodynamic response to 7% NaCl in hypovolemic dogs. *Circ Shock* 38:189–194, 1992.

Angle N, Hoyt DB, Coimbra R, et al.: Hypertonic saline resuscitation diminishes lung injury by suppressing neutrophil activation after hemorrhagic shock. *Shock* 9:164–170, 1998.

Armistead CW, Vincent J, Preiser J, et al.: Hypertonic saline solution–hetastarch for fluid resuscitation in experimental septic shock. *Anesth Analg* 69:714–720, 1989.

Bainbridge FA and Trevan JW: Memorandum upon surgical shock and some allied conditions. Great Britain Medical Research Committee, 1917.

Baue AE, Tragus ET, and Parkins WM: A comparison of isotonic and hypertonic solutions and blood on blood flow and oxygen consumption in the initial treatment of hemorrhagic shock. *J Trauma* 7:743–756, 1967.

Brown JM, Grosso MA, and Moore EE: Hypertonic saline and dextran: Impact on cardiac function in the isolated rat heart. *J Trauma* 30:646–651, 1990.

Caldwell FT and Bowser BH: Critical evaluation of hypertonic and hypotonic solutions to resuscitate severely burned children: A prospective study. *Ann Surg* 189:546–552, 1979.

Cannon WB: The physiological factors concerned in surgical shock. *Boston Med Surg J* 176:859–867, 1917.

Chudnofsky CR, Dronen SC, Syverud SA, et al.: Intravenous fluid therapy in the prehospital management of hemorrhagic shock:

Improved outcome with hypertonic saline/6% dextran 70 in a swine model. *Am J Emerg Med* 7:357–363, 1989.

Coimbra R, Junger WG, Hoyt DB, et al.: Hypertonic saline resuscitation restores hemorrhage induced immunosuppression by decreasing prostaglandin E_2 and interleukin 4 production. *J Surg Res* 64:203–209, 1996.

Coimbra R, Hoyt DB, Junger WG, et al.: Hypertonic saline resuscitation decreases susceptibility to sepsis after hemorrhagic shock. *J Trauma* 42:602–607, 1997.

Constable PD, Muir WW, and Binkley PF: Hypertonic saline is a negative inotropic agent in normovolemic dogs. *Am J Physiol* 267:H667–H677, 1994.

Danowski TS, Winkler AW, and Elkinton JR: The treatment of shock due to salt depletion; comparison of the hemodynamic effects of isotonic saline, of hypertonic saline, and of isotonic glucose solutions. *J Clin Invest* 25:130–138, 1946.

de Felippe J, Timoner J, Velasco IT, et al.: Treatment of refractory hypovolaemic shock by 7.5% sodium chloride injections. *Lancet* 2:1002–1004, 1980.

Ducey JP, Mozingo DW, Lamiell JM, et al.: A comparison of the cerebral and cardiovascular effects of complete resuscitation with isotonic and hypertonic saline, hetastarch, and whole blood following hemorrhage. *J Trauma* 29:1510–1518, 1989.

Ducey JP, Lamiell JM, and Gueller GE: Cerebral electrophysiologic effects of resuscitation with hypertonic saline-dextran after hemorrhage. *Crit Care Med* 18:744–749, 1990.

Eaglstein WH: Inadvertent intracutaneous injection with hypertonic saline (23.45%) in two patients without complication. *J Dermatol Surg Oncol* 16:878–879, 1990.

Goethals MA, Adele SM, and Brutsaert DL: Contractility in mammalian heart muscle: Calcium and osmolality. *Circ Res* 36:27–33, 1975.

Gross D, Landau EH, Assalia A, and Krausz MM: Is hypertonic saline resuscitation safe in 'uncontrolled' hemorrhagic shock? *J Trauma* 28:751–756, 1988.

Gross D, Landau EH, Klin B, and Krausz MM: Quantitative measurement of bleeding following hypertonic saline therapy in 'uncontrolled' hemorrhagic shock. *J Trauma* 29:79–83, 1989.

Gross D, Landau E, Klin B, and Krausz M: Treatment of uncontrolled hemorrhagic shock with hypertonic saline solution. *Surg Gynecol Obstet* 170:106–112, 1990.

Gunn ML, Hansbrough JF, Davis JW, et al.: Prospective, randomized trial of hypertonic sodium lactate versus lactated Ringer's solution for burn shock resuscitation. *J Trauma* 29:1261–1267, 1989.

Gunnar W, Jonasson O, Merlotti G, et al.: Head injury and hemorrhagic shock: Studies of the blood brain barrier and intracranial pressure after resuscitation with normal saline solution, 3% saline solution, and dextran-40. *Surgery* 103:398–407, 1988.

Gunnar WP, Merlotti GJ, Barrett J, and Jonasson O: Resuscitation from hemorrhagic shock: Alterations of the intracranial pressure after normal saline, 3% saline, and dextran-40. *Ann Surg* 204:686–692, 1986.

Hands R, Holcroft JW, Perron PR, and Kramer GC: Comparison of peripheral and central infusions of 7.5% NaCl/6% dextran 70. *Surgery* 103:684–689, 1988.

Hannon JP, Wade CE, Bossone CA, et al.: Oxygen delivery and demand in conscious pigs subjected to fixed-volume hemorrhage and resuscitated with 7.5% NaCl in 6% dextran. *Circ Shock* 29:205–217, 1989.

Holcroft JW, Vassar MJ, Turner JE, et al.: 3% NaCl and 7.5% NaCl/dextran 70 in the resuscitation of severely injured patients. *Ann Surg* 206:279–288, 1987.

Holcroft JW, Vassar MJ, Perry CA, et al.: Use of a 7.5% NaCl/6% dextran 70 solution in the resuscitation of injured patients in the emergency room. *Prog Clin Biol Res* 299:331–338, 1989.

Horton JW, Dunn CW, Burnweit CA, and Walker PB: Hypertonic saline–dextran resuscitation of acute canine bile-induced pancreatitis. *Am J Surg* 158:48–56, 1989.

Horton JW, White J, and Baxter CR: Hypertonic saline dextran resuscitation of thermal injury. *Ann Surg* 211:301–311, 1990.

Johnston W, Alford P, Prough D, et al.: Cardiopulmonary effects of hypertonic saline in canine oleic acid–induced pulmonary edema. *Crit Care Med* 13:814–817, 1985.

Junger WG, Liu FC, Loomis WH, and Hoyt DB: Hypertonic saline enhances cellular immune function. *Circ Shock* 42:190–196, 1994.

Kawata H, Ohba M, Hatae J, and Kishi M: A study on the mechanism of twitch potentiation by hypertonic solution in the frog atrial muscle. *J Mol Cell Cardiol* 15:281–293, 1983.

Kramer GC, Perron PR, Lindsey DC, et al.: Small-volume resuscitation with hypertonic saline dextran solution. *Surgery* 100:239–246, 1986.

Kramer GC, Walsh JC, Hands RD, et al.: Resuscitation of hemorrhage with intraosseous infusion of hypertonic saline/dextran. *Braz J Med Biol Res* 22:283–286, 1989a.

Kramer GC, Walsh JC, Perron PR, et al.: Comparison of hypertonic saline/dextran versus hypertonic saline/hetastarch for resuscitation of hypovolemia. *Braz J Med Biol Res* 22:279–282, 1989b.

Kreimeier U, Bruckner UB, Niemczyk S, and Messmer K: Hyperosmotic saline dextran for resuscitation from traumatic-hemorrhagic hypotension: Effect on regional blood flow. *Circ Shock* 32:83–99, 1990.

Layon J, Duncan D, Gallagher TJ, and Banner MJ: Hypertonic saline as a resuscitation solution in hemorrhagic shock: Effects on extravascular lung water and cardiopulmonary function. *Anesth Analg* 66:154–158, 1987.

Liang CS and Hood WB Jr: Mechanism of cardiac output response to hypertonic sodium chloride infusion in dogs. *Am J Physiol* 235:H18–H22, 1978.

Lopes O, Pontieri V, Rocha e Silva M, and Velasco I: Hyperosmotic NaCl and severe hemorrhagic shock: Role of the innervated lung. *Am J Physiol* 241:H883–H890, 1981.

Lopes OU, Velasco IT, Guertzenstein PG, et al.: Hypertonic sodium chloride restores mean circulatory filling pressure in severely hypovolemic dogs. *Hypertension* 8:I195–I199, 1986.

Luypaert P, Vincent J, Domb M, et al.: Fluid resuscitation with hypertonic saline in endotoxic shock. *Circ Shock* 20:311–320, 1986.

Mancia G, Shepherd JT, and Donald DE: Interplay among carotid sinus, cardiopulmonary, and carotid body reflexes in dogs. *Am J Physiol* 230:19–24, 1976.

Maningas PA: Resuscitation with 7.5% NaCl in 6% dextran-70 during hemorrhagic shock in swine: Effects on organ blood flow. *Crit Care Med* 15:1121–1126, 1987.

Maningas PA, Mattox KL, Pepe PE, et al.: Hypertonic saline–dextran solutions for the prehospital management of traumatic hypotension. *Am J Surg* 157:528–534, 1989.

Mann FC: Further experimental study of surgical shock. *JAMA* 71:1184–1188, 1918.

Marshall G: Mentioned in memorandum upon surgical shock and some allied conditions. *Br Med J* 1:381–383, 1917.

Martins MA, Younes RN, Lin CA, et al.: Hypovolemic shock resuscitation with hyperosmotic 7.5% NaCl: Effects on respiratory system mechanics. *Circ Shock* 26:147–155, 1988.

Mazzoni MC, Borgstrom P, Arfors KE, and Intaglietta M: Dynamic fluid redistribution in hyperosmotic resuscitation of hypovolemic hemorrhage. *Am J Physiol* 255:H629–H637, 1988.

Monafo WW: The treatment of burn shock by the intravenous and oral administration of hypertonic lactated saline solution. *J Trauma* 10:575–586, 1970.

Monafo WW, Chuntrasakul C, and Ayvazian VH: Hypertonic sodium solutions in the treatment of burn shock. *Am J Surg* 126:778–783, 1973.

Moylan JA, Reckler JM, and Mason AD: Resuscitation with hypertonic lactate saline in thermal injury. *Am J Surg* 125:580–584, 1973.

Mullins RJ and Hudgens RW: Hypertonic saline resuscitates dogs in endotoxin shock. *J Surg Res* 43:37–44, 1987.

Nakayama S-I, Sibley L, Gunther RA, et al.: Small-volume resuscitation with hypertonic saline (2,400 mOsm/liter) during hemorrhagic shock. *Circ Shock* 13:149–159, 1984.

Nerlich M, Gunther R, and Demling RH: Resuscitation from hemorrhagic shock with hypertonic saline or lactated Ringer's (effect on the pulmonary and systemic microcirculations). *Circ Shock* 10:179–188, 1983.

Newell JD, Higgins CB, Kelley MJ, et al.: The influence of hyperosmolality on left ventricular contractile state: Disparate effects of nonionic and ionic solutions. *Invest Radiol* 15:363–370, 1980.

Okrasinski EB, Krahwinkel DJ, and Sanders WL: Treatment of dogs in hemorrhagic shock by intraosseous infusion of hypertonic saline and dextran. *Vet Surg* 21:20–24, 1992.

Onarheim H, Lund T, and Reed R: Thermal skin injury: I. Acute hemodynamic effects of fluid resuscitation with lactated Ringer's, plasma, and hypertonic saline (2,400 mosmol/l) in the rat. *Circ Shock* 27:13–24, 1989a.

Onarheim H, Lund T, and Reed R: Thermal skin injury: II. Effects on edema formation and albumin extravasation of fluid resuscitation with lactated Ringer's, plasma, and hypertonic saline (2,400 mosmol/l) in the rat. *Circ Shock* 27:25–37, 1989b.

Penfield WG: The treatment of severe and progressive hemorrhage by intravenous injections. *Am J Physiol* 48:121–132, 1919.

Peters RM, Shackford SR, Hogan JS, and Cologne JB: Comparison of isotonic and hypertonic fluids in resuscitation from hypovolemic shock. *Surg Gynecol Obstet* 163:219–224, 1986.

Prough D and Johnston W: Fluid resuscitation in septic shock: No solution yet. *Anest Analg* 69:699–704, 1989.

Prough DS, Johnson JC, Poole GV Jr, et al.: Effects on intracranial pressure of resuscitation from hemorrhagic shock with hypertonic saline versus lactated Ringer's solution. *Crit Care Med* 13:407–411, 1985.

Reed RL II, Johnston TD, Chen Y, and Fischer RP: Hypertonic saline alters plasma clotting times and platelet aggregation. *J Trauma* 31:8–14, 1991.

Reinhart K, Rudolph T, Bredle DL, and Cain SM: O_2 uptake in bled dogs after resuscitation with hypertonic saline of hydroxyethylstarch. *Am J Physiol* 257:H238–H243, 1989.

Rocha e Silva M, Negraes GA, Soares AM, et al.: Hypertonic resuscitation from severe hemorrhagic shock: Patterns of regional circulation. *Circ Shock* 19:165–175, 1986.

Rocha e Silva M, Velasco IT, Nogueirira da Silva RI, et al.: Hyperosmotic sodium salts reverse severe hemorragic shock: Other solutes do not. *Am J Physiol* 253:H751–H762, 1987.

Rocha e Silva M, Velasco I, and Porfirio M: Hypertonic saline resuscitation: Saturated salt-dextran solutions are equally effective, but induce hemolysis in dogs. *Crit Care Med* 18:203–207, 1990.

Rogers L: The treatment of cholera by injections of hypertonic saline solutions with a simple and rapid method of intra-abdominal administration. *Philipp J Sci* 4:99–105, 1909.

Schertel ER, Schneider DA, Zissimos AG, et al.: Cardiopulmonary reflexes induced by osmolality changes in the airways and pulmonary vasculature. *Fed Proc* 44:835, 1985.

Schertel ER, Valentine AK, Rademakers AM, and Muir WW: Influence of 7% NaCl on the mechanical properties of the systemic circulation in the hypovolemic dog. *Circ Shock* 31:203–214, 1990.

Schertel ER, Valentine AK, Schmall LM, et al.: Vagotomy alters the hemodynamic response of dogs in hemorrhagic shock. *Circ Shock* 34:393–397, 1991.

Schertel ER, Allen DA, Muir WW, and Hansen BA: Evaluation of a hypertonic sodium chloride/dextran solution for treatment of traumatic shock in dogs. *J Am Vet Med Assoc* 208:366–370, 1996.

Schertel ER, Allen DA, Muir WW, et al.: Evaluation of a hypertonic saline–dextran solution for treatment of dogs with shock induced by gastric dilatation-volvulus. *J Am Vet Med Assoc* 210:226–230, 1997.

Schmall LM, Muir WW, and Robertson JT: Haemodynamic effects of small volume hypertonic saline in experimentally induced haemorrhagic shock. *Equine Vet J* 22:273–277, 1990.

Shackford SR, Sise MJ, Fridlund PH, et al.: Hypertonic sodium lactate versus lactated Ringer's solution for intravenous fluid therapy in operations on the abdominal aorta. *Surgery* 94:41–51, 1983.

Shackford SR, Fortlage DA, Peters RM, et al.: Serum osmolar and electrolyte changes associated with large infusions of hypertonic sodium lactate for intravascular volume expansion of patients undergoing aortic reconstruction. *Surg Gynecol Obstet* 164:127–136, 1987.

Shoemaker W, Kram H, and Appel P: Therapy of shock based on pathophysiology, monitoring, and outcome prediction. *Crit Care Med* 18:S19–S25, 1990.

Smith GJ, Kramer GC, Perron P, et al.: A comparison of several hypertonic solutions for resuscitation of bled sheep. *J Surg Res* 39:517–528, 1985.

Tobias TA, Schertel ER, Schmall LM, et al.: Comparative effects of 7.5% NaCl in 6% dextran 70 and 0.9% NaCl on cardiorespiratory parameters after cardiac output–controlled resuscitation from canine hemorrhagic shock. *Circ Shock* 39:139–146, 1993.

Velasco IT, Pontieri V, Rocha e Silva M, and Lopes OU: Hyperosmotic NaCl and severe hemorrhagic shock. *Am J Physiol* 239:H664–H673, 1980.

Velasco IT, Rocha e Silva M, Oliveira MA, et al.: Hypertonic and hyperoncotic resuscitation from severe hemorrhagic shock in dogs: A comparative study. *Crit Care Med* 17:261–264, 1989.

Wade CE, Hannon JP, Bossone CA, et al.: Resuscitation of conscious pigs following hemorrhage: Comparative efficacy of small-volume resuscitation. *Circ Shock* 29:193–204, 1989.

Weeren FR, Tobias TA, Schertel ER, et al.: Comparative effects of 7% NaCl in 6% dextran 70 and 0.9% NaCl on oxygen transport in endotoxemic dogs. *Shock* 2:1–7, 1994.

Winkler AW, Danowski TS, and Elkinton JR: The role of colloid and of saline in the treatment of shock. *J Clin Invest* 25:220–225, 1946.

Wisner D, Schuster L, and Quinn C: Hypertonic saline resuscitation of head injury: Effects on cerebral water content. *Trauma* 30:75–78, 1990.

Younes R, Aun F, Tomida R, and Birolini D: The role of lung innervation in the hemodynamic response to hypertonic sodium chloride solutions in hemorrhagic shock. *Surgery* 98:900–906, 1985.

Zornow MH, Scheller MS, and Shackford SR: Effect of a hypertonic lactated Ringer's solution on intracranial pressure and cerebral water content in a model of traumatic brain injury. *J Trauma* 29:484–488, 1989.

CHAPTER 25

Peritoneal Dialysis

DENNIS J. CHEW STEPHEN P. DiBARTOLA M. SUSAN CRISP

Dialysis is the transfer of water and solute from one compartment to another across a semipermeable membrane. This process is governed by diffusion, convection, and ultrafiltration (Parker et al. 1972; Henderson 1979; Maher 1980; Parker 1980; Thornhill 1981; Rudnick et al. 1987; Carter et al. 1989; Nolph 1991).

Diffusion is the random thermal movement of molecules from a region of high activity or concentration to one of low activity or concentration (Maher 1980). The term osmosis refers to the diffusion of water from an area of high activity for water molecules (i.e., low solute concentration) to one of low activity for water molecules (i.e., high solute concentration). Equilibrium is reached when further osmosis is prevented by development of an equal but opposing hydrostatic force on the other side of the semipermeable membrane.

The processes of solute diffusion and osmosis ultimately equalize the concentrations of solute and water on both sides of the membrane, provided the membrane is permeable to both water and the solute in question and sufficient time is allowed for equilibration. Diffusion occurs for each solute and water according to the individual concentration gradients for these substances across the membrane (Rudnick et al. 1987). The rate of diffusion of solute into the fluid compartment that initially contained the lower solute concentration progressively decreases as the solute concentration in that compartment increases. The rate of diffusion of solute into the compartment containing the initially low solute concentration can be increased by stirring the fluid in that compartment or by draining it and adding fresh solute-free fluid. Increasing the temperature of the fluid in either compartment also increases diffusion by increasing random thermal molecular motion.

Convection refers to the transfer of solute that occurs when a solution containing a permeant solute moves en masse across a semipermeable membrane in response to favorable osmotic or hydrostatic pressure gradients. This type of solute transfer has been called *solute drag* because of the frictional forces involved (Henderson 1966; Henderson and Nolph 1969; Nolph 1991). Convection allows additional solute to be transferred beyond that moving by diffusion down a favorable concentration gradient. The removal of solutes by convection does not occur in direct proportion to their individual concentrations in the compartment because of the sieving effect that occurs as charged and uncharged particles of different sizes and shapes attempt to move across a semipermeable membrane under the influence of bulk fluid flow (Rudnick et al. 1987; Nolph 1991).

Ultrafiltration refers to the movement of water across a semipermeable membrane as a result of favorable osmotic or hydrostatic gradients. In hemodialysis, ultrafiltration is accomplished by altering the hydrostatic gradient across the membrane of the artificial kidney. Effective ultrafiltration can occur during peritoneal dialysis only by manipulating the osmotic gradient (i.e., by changing the tonicity of the dialysis fluid).

The peritoneum is the semipermeable membrane between the fluid of the peritoneal cavity and that of the extracellular compartment. This barrier includes the capillary endothelium, basement membrane, and peritoneal mesothelium (see later). Water and solute may move from extracellular fluid to the peritoneal cavity or vice versa. Normally, there is little fluid in the peritoneal cavity. The technique of peritoneal dialysis takes advantage of the fact that fluid can be introduced easily into the peritoneal cavity. The fluid instilled into the peritoneal cavity is referred to as the *dialysate*. The cycle consisting of fluid infusion into the peritoneal cavity (i.e., *inflow*), fluid *dwell* time within the peritoneal cavity, and drainage of effluent fluid from the peritoneal cavity (i.e., *outflow*) is referred to as an *exchange*. Clinical peritoneal dialysis includes a prescription for the volume and chemical composition of the dialysate as well as the time to be allowed for inflow, dwell, and outflow. The direction and magnitude of solute and water transfer can be manipulated to the patient's advantage by modifying the dialysis prescription. The five steps of peritoneal dialysis are summarized in Table 25–1.

TABLE 25–1. The Five Steps of Peritoneal Dialysis

1. Dialysate preparation
2. Infusion (inflow) of dialysate (<5 min)
3. Dwell time (45 min–4 h)
4. Drainage (outflow) of dialysate (5–15 min)
5. Serial monitoring of the patient (see Table 25–18)

TABLE 25–2. Some Substances That Accumulate in Uremia

Acute-phase proteins (e.g., β_2-microglobulin)
Amino acids
Ammonia
Bacterial products (e.g., aliphatic amines, aromatic amines, indoles, skatoles, polyamines)
Carbohydrate derivatives (e.g., *myo*-inositol, mannitol, sorbitol)
Enzymes (e.g., renin, ribonuclease, lysozyme)
Guanidino compounds (e.g., creatinine, guanidinosuccinic acid, guanidinoacetic acid, creatine, guanidine, methylguanidine, urea)
Hippurates
Hormones (e.g., insulin, glucagon, parathyroid hormone, gastrin, growth hormone, atrial natriuretic factor)
Inorganic anions (e.g., phosphate, sulfate, cyanate)
Intermediary metabolites (e.g., lactate, pyruvate)
"Middle molecules" (molecular weight 500–5000)
Nucleic acid metabolites (e.g., uric acid, nucleotides, pyridines)
Oxalates
Trace elements

The usual objective of peritoneal dialysis is the transfer of undesirable solutes from the blood of a uremic patient into the dialysate solution as a substitute for the impaired excretory function of the native kidneys. Blood concentrations of urea nitrogen, creatinine, and phosphorus are used to monitor the effectiveness of dialysis, but many other potentially toxic solutes in uremic patients also may be removed during dialysis (Table 25–2). Solutes also may be transferred from dialysate to extracellular fluid, as commonly occurs with bicarbonate or its precursors (e.g., lactate) and calcium. Transfer of other solutes (e.g., glucose, potassium) can occur and may not be desirable or beneficial to the patient under some circumstances. Water can either be removed from or added to extracellular fluid, depending on the dialysis method employed. The peritoneal clearance of a solute may be calculated as $C_D Q_D / C_P$ where

C_D = concentration of solute in effluent dialysate at the end of the exchange

Q_D = effluent dialysate volume/dwell time

C_P = plasma concentration of solute at midpoint of exchange

The clinician must realize, however, that dialysis does not replace the failed endocrine and metabolic functions of the kidneys. Factors affecting the peritoneal clearance of solutes are listed in Table 25–3 and methods that may be employed to increase the clearance of solutes are listed in Table 25–4.

Peritoneal dialysis is the most practical form of dialysis

TABLE 25–3. Factors Affecting Peritoneal Clearance

Molecular size	Intercellular channel size
Molecular charge	Dialysate flow rate (volume/time)
Protein binding	Dialysate composition
Peritoneal blood flow	Dialysate temperature
Surface area available	

TABLE 25–4. Factors That May Improve Peritoneal Clearance

Increasing dialysate volume*
Decreasing dwell time to 30 or 45 min
Increasing temperature of dialysate to slightly above body temperature
Using hypertonic dialysate (e.g., 2.5 or 4.25% glucose)
Consider use of vasodilator drugs

*Overdistention of the abdomen with dialysate produces excessive hydrostatic pressure and impairs transfer of solute into dialysate (infusion volume should be ≤ 40 mL/kg).

for veterinary patients. Hemodialysis is available at some referral centers, but the high cost and technical expertise required have limited its use in veterinary medicine (Gourley et al. 1973; Dhein 1981; Thornhill 1984a; DiBartola et al. 1985; Cowgill and Langston 1996; Langston et al. 1997; Mashita et al. 1997). Hemodialysis is more efficient than peritoneal dialysis in the removal of low-molecular-weight substances from blood, but it is less efficient in the removal of so-called middle molecules (molecular weight 500 to 5000) (Rudnick et al. 1987), which may be important in some manifestations of uremia. Peritoneal dialysis and hemodialysis are compared in Table 25–5 and hemodialysis is discussed in detail in Chapter 26.

Peritoneal dialysis has been described as available in some form to every veterinarian (Parker et al. 1972) but this procedure is labor intensive. Dialysis can be employed successfully in private practice, but most veterinarians prefer to refer animals in need of dialysis to centers with technical expertise in dialysis and 24-h critical care facilities. Unfortunately, dialysis in clinical veterinary medicine often is not considered until the patient is near death. Peritoneal dialysis may be more rewarding as a therapeutic tool if instituted earlier in the clinical course of dogs and cats with severe acute intrinsic renal failure, especially those with oligoanuria.

▶ Types of Peritoneal Dialysis

Dialysis can be characterized both by the flow pattern of the dialysate and by the time period over which dialysis

TABLE 25–5. Comparison of Peritoneal Dialysis and Hemodialysis

	Peritoneal Dialysis	Hemodialysis
Cost	+ +	+ + + +
Expertise/equipment	+	+ + + +
Efficiency	+ +	+ + + +
Removal of middle molecules	+ + + +	+
Removal of toxins	+ +	+ + + +
Risk of peritonitis	+ +	—
Risk of hypothermia	+	—
Risk of hypotension	—	+
Use in coagulopathy	+	—
Use in small patients	+	—

TABLE 25-6. Indications for Acute Peritoneal Dialysis
Acute intrinsic renal failure awaiting surgical catheter placement
Acute overhydration
Severe acute hyperkalemia, metabolic acidosis
Acute decompensation of chronic renal failure
Dialyzable toxin or drug (e.g., ethylene glycol intoxication <24 h after ingestion; barbiturates)
Hypercalcemia
Hypothermia
Hyperthermia
Peritonitis

TABLE 25-7. Indications for Long-Term Peritoneal Dialysis
Established acute intrinsic renal failure with potentially reversible renal lesions
Renal failure of uncertain etiology while awaiting renal biopsy results
Early hydronephrosis
Severe chronic hyperkalemia, metabolic acidosis
Chronic overhydration

occurs (Rudnick et al. 1987; Twardowski 1989; Nolph 1991). During *continuous-flow* dialysis or *peritoneal lavage*, dialysate is administered by continuous infusion through one catheter while simultaneously being drained by gravity through another catheter. This technique is not commonly used. *Intermittent peritoneal dialysis* occurs when dialysate is infused and allowed to dwell for a variable period of time before drainage. Intermittent peritoneal dialysis entails a series of successive exchanges followed by a period during which no dialysis is occurring. During *continuous peritoneal dialysis*, dialysate is always present within the peritoneal cavity except for a short period after drainage of effluent dialysate and before infusion of fresh dialysate (Thornhill 1981; Twardowski 1989). This technique is often called *chronic ambulatory peritoneal dialysis* (CAPD) and is described in more detail later. Dwell time during chronic continuous dialysis usually is 4 to 10 h (Twardowski 1989), whereas dwell time may be less than 1 h during acute continuous dialysis. In *tidal peritoneal dialysis,* a reservoir of dialysate is maintained in the peritoneal cavity at all times and a portion of this fluid is drained periodically and fresh fluid introduced. This technique is considered a hybrid of intermittent and continuous dialysis (Twardowski 1989) and may have advantages over either technique alone. Tidal peritoneal dialysis has not been evaluated in veterinary patients.

Acute peritoneal dialysis usually is used for 1 to 4 days to maintain a patient with an underlying disease process that can be managed and corrected over a short period of time. Chronic peritoneal dialysis is used for 4 to 30 days in animals with conditions that require a longer time for successful management and recovery of renal function. In many human patients, CAPD provides lifelong maintenance of renal function or provides support until renal transplantation can be performed. CAPD rarely has been attempted in veterinary medicine (Thornhill et al. 1984). The indications for acute and chronic peritoneal dialysis are listed in Tables 25-6 and 25-7 and are discussed in the following sections.

▶ Experimental Peritoneal Dialysis in Dogs

After bilateral nephrectomy, experimental dogs survived 2 to 5 days without treatment (Grollman et al. 1951). Survival reached 5 days when a low-protein, low-salt diet was fed. Continuous peritoneal irrigation and drainage through separate catheters for 20 h/day at rates of 25 to 35 mL/min in 15 bilaterally nephrectomized dogs decreased blood urea nitrogen (BUN) concentration from 100–250 mg/dL to 20–50 mg/dL (Seligman et al. 1946). Subsequently, continuous peritoneal lavage was performed for 8 to 10 h each day for maintenance. Three dogs in this study survived 6, 9, and 13 days, respectively, and death was attributed to infection rather than inadequate control of uremia. Survival times of 30 to 70 days were achieved when two daily exchanges with hypertonic dialysate were performed in bilaterally nephrectomized dogs using an intermittent technique (Grollman et al. 1951). In this study, dialysis was accomplished by repeated needle punctures using 17-gauge needles, and dialysate was allowed to remain in the peritoneal cavity for at least 3 h. Serum creatinine concentrations were 4.7 to 9.7 mg/dL, BUN concentrations 58 to 93 mg/dL, and serum phosphorus concentrations 6.0 to 9.0 mg/dL, whereas serum sodium, potassium, chloride, and bicarbonate concentrations were nearly normal after dialysis. Nearly normal serum creatinine and BUN concentrations could be maintained by performing 8 to 16 exchanges per day.

Equilibration for urea and potassium in dialysate was 90% complete by 40 min and 98% complete by 60 min in a model of uremia induced by bilateral ureteral ligation in dogs (Parker et al. 1972; Parker 1980) (Fig. 25-1). In contrast, 2 h was required for urea equilibration in another experimental study in dogs (Grollman et al. 1951).

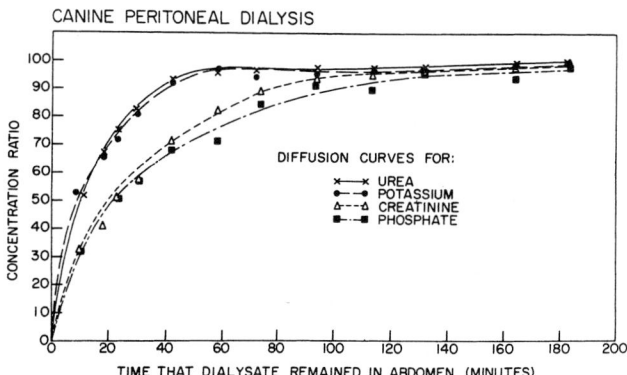

FIGURE 25-1. Equilibrium for urea, potassium, creatinine, and phosphate during peritoneal dialysis in dogs. Urea and potassium diffused rapidly and reached 85% of equilibrium in 40 min, whereas creatinine and phosphate were only 65% equilibrated. The flattening shapes of diffusion curves indicate that equilibration periods (dwell times) of 40 min or less were most efficient. (From Kirk RW: *Current Veterinary Therapy VII.* Philadelphia, WB Saunders Co., p. 1107, 1980.)

Equilibration for creatinine and phosphorus was 65% complete at 40 min and 80% complete at 60 min, and complete equilibration did not occur until after 2 h (Parker et al. 1972; Parker 1980). The longer time required for equilibration of creatinine and phosphorus was attributed to the larger molecular size of these solutes. A dwell time of 40 to 60 min was recommended for optimal solute removal, because the most rapid diffusion of these solutes occurred within the first 30 min. It was possible to decrease BUN concentration from 250 to 100 mg/dL and serum creatinine concentration from 15 to 6 mg/dL by the end of seven consecutive hourly exchanges and to reduce serum potassium concentration from approximately 8.0 mEq/L to less than 5.0 mEq/L after five hourly exchanges, using the Parker dialysis cannula (see later). A dwell time of 30 to 60 min and at least four consecutive exchanges were considered necessary for significant improvement of the metabolic condition of anuric dogs in these studies (Parker et al. 1972; Parker 1980).

Five bilaterally nephrectomized dogs underwent peritoneal dialysis using the column disc catheter (see later) and survived 37 to 83 days (mean, 54 days) with maintenance of BUN concentrations at 70 to 90 mg/dL, serum creatinine concentrations at 5 to 10 mg/dL, and serum phosphorus concentrations at 6 to 9 mg/dL (without use of intestinal phosphorus-binding agents). Three exchanges of 2 L each were performed daily and the dextrose concentration of the dialysate was varied to prevent hypotension or weight gain. Dialysate effluent volume was greater than infusion volume when dwell time was ≤10 h for both 1.5 and 4.5% dextrose-containing dialysate solutions. Dialysate effluent volume was less than that infused when dwell times of 12 to 16 h were employed. Protein loss in dialysate increased with longer dwell times and averaged 5 g/day with the 1.5% dextrose-containing solutions and 7.5 g/day with the 4.5% dextrose-containing solutions (Rubin et al. 1983).

Blood urea nitrogen concentration was maintained at 80 to 90 mg/dL and serum creatinine concentration at 8 to 9 mg/dL in one bilaterally nephrectomized dog maintained for 51 days with CAPD using the column disc catheter and three to four exchanges per day (Simmons et al. 1980). Chronic ambulatory peritoneal dialysis employing the column disc catheter resulted in survival of a bilaterally nephrectomized dog for 54 days in another study (Thornhill et al. 1984). Six exchanges per day were required to maintain a BUN concentration of 26 to 53 mg/dL, a serum creatinine concentration of 3.4 to 7.0 mg/dL, and a serum phosphorus concentration of 2.7 to 6.4 mg/dL (with use of intestinal phosphorus-binding agents).

Chronic ambulatory peritoneal dialysis employing the column disc catheter and four daily exchanges of dialysate resulted in survival of two dogs for 49 and 67 days, respectively, after bilateral ureteral ligation (Wells et al. 1985). The BUN concentration was maintained at 20 to 70 mg/dL and serum creatinine concentration at 4 to 8 mg/dL. In this study, addition of specific amino acids (DL-serine, L-lysine, DL-alanine) to the dialysate solution reduced daily losses of amino acids and protein into the dialysate.

The effects of dextrose in dialysate were studied in four bilaterally nephrectomized dogs during CAPD with the column disc catheter (Johnson et al. 1983). Five daily exchanges of either 1.5 or 4.5% dextrose in Dianeal (Baxter Healthcare, Deerfield, IL) were performed. Dialysate osmolality progressively decreased over an 8-h period for both 1.5 and 4.5% solutions. This effect was attributed to dilution of glucose in the dialysate by osmotically mediated ultrafiltration of water and to absorption of glucose from the dialysate. Ultrafiltration almost ceased when dialysate osmolality approached that of serum. The glucose concentration and osmolality sharply declined in the 4.5% dextrose–containing dialysate during the first 2 to 3 h, whereas the observed changes were more gradual in the 1.5% dextrose–containing solution. Four exchanges using 1.5% dextrose solution with a 4-h dwell time and one exchange of 4.5% dextrose solution with an 8-h dwell time were estimated to provide 457 kcal (absorbed from the dialysate solution) and 1134 mL of ultrafiltrate (added to the dialysate solution) (Johnson et al. 1983). In another study of dogs, glucose disappeared from the dialysate over 2 to 6 h, depending on the original concentration of dextrose in the dialysate solution (1, 2, or 3%) (Grollman et al. 1951).

▶ Clinical Experience with Peritoneal Dialysis in Veterinary Medicine

The first clinical report of dialysis in uremic dogs described the use of intermittent peritoneal dialysis (Kirk 1957). Treatment involved a dwell time of 2 h during two to three daily exchanges using 400 to 2000 mL of dialysate. Dialysate was infused through 16- or 18-gauge needles and drained with 13-gauge, 3-in. needles with additional perforations. Another clinical report of peritoneal dialysis in uremic dogs described the successful use of 12-gauge, 1.5-in. needles for infusion and drainage. The needle was kept in place throughout the exchange and was inserted 5 to 8 cm caudal and to the right of the umbilicus. In this study, 700 to 1500 mL of dialysate solution was infused for a dwell time of 30 min during one or two daily exchanges (Jackson 1964). In these reports, dialysis usually was continued for 3 to 4 days. Most of the treated dogs had acute renal failure, but prerenal azotemia was not ruled out. It is unlikely that these dogs would have experienced such rapid and complete resolution of their azotemia after so few exchanges each day if the underlying renal lesions had been severe.

A dog with nonoliguric acute intrinsic renal failure (AIRF) caused by ethylene glycol poisoning was dialyzed for 5 days using the column disc catheter (Fox et al. 1987). Exchanges were performed every 2 h for the first 36 h and then three times per day for the next 3½ days. The BUN concentration decreased from approximately 200 to 90 mg/dL and serum creatinine concentration from 9.0 to 6.0 mg/dL after the first day of hourly exchanges. A dog with oliguric AIRF associated with hypoadrenocorticism was supported by 21 consecutive hourly exchanges using 1.5 L of dialysate solution per exchange via the column disc catheter (Thornhill et al. 1980). The BUN concentration decreased from 188 to 106 mg/dL, serum creatinine concentration from 12.0 to 9.4 mg/dL, and serum phosphorus concentration from 15.0 to 12.2 mg/dL.

The use of CAPD has been described in a small dog (8 kg) in which a single 2-L bag of dialysate was used for multiple small-volume exchanges of 250 mL each for four consecutive exchanges each day (Carter et al. 1989). The peritoneal effluent was drained back into the original reservoir bag, effectively diluting the uremic toxins. Dialysate is not wasted in this technique, and there is less chance for bacterial contamination because dialysate bags are changed less frequently. Pleural dialysis with chronically indwelling thoracic catheters was used successfully as an alternative to peritoneal dialysis in two dogs for 7 and 25 days, respectively (Shahar and Holmberg 1985).

The use of peritoneal dialysis in a teaching hospital setting was reviewed for 25 dogs and 2 cats (Crisp et al. 1989). The column disc catheter was used in 15 patients, whereas a variety of chest tubes and improvised catheters were used in the remaining animals. In this study, the most common indication for dialysis was AIRF, and 6 to 24 daily exchanges were performed using an approximate dialysate volume of 40 mL/kg. Median values for serum creatinine concentration decreased by 28 to 64%, whereas those for BUN decreased by 36 to 75% after 1.5 to 3.0 days of dialysis.

▶ Factors Affecting Peritoneal Dialysis

Intrinsic characteristics of the peritoneum and the solutes of interest, composition of the dialysate, and the method employed for dialysis all interact to determine the efficiency of solute and water clearance (see Table 25-3). Solute and water transport across the peritoneum can be altered by bacterial or chemical peritonitis, changes in vascular or interstitial hydrostatic pressure, and the systemic or local administration of hormones or drugs. Molecular size, charge, shape, and extent of protein binding all influence the kinetics of peritoneal dialysis. High-molecular-weight substances are not as readily cleared as those with lower molecular weights. Also, charged particles are not handled in the same way as those without charge. Highly protein-bound solutes are not as readily removed during peritoneal dialysis as are those that are not extensively bound to plasma proteins (Parker et al. 1972; Thornhill 1981; Rudnick et al. 1987; Nolph 1991) Methods that may be used to improve peritoneal clearance of solutes are listed in Table 25-4.

▶ The Peritoneum: Barriers to Diffusion and Ultrafiltration

The peritoneum is a continuous membrane that covers the internal abdominal organs (visceral peritoneum) and the abdominal wall (parietal peritoneum) and forms the mesentery (Rubin et al. 1986; Nolph 1991). The surface area of the peritoneum is very large. The area available for solute and water exchange, however, is relatively small because exchange occurs only across the peritoneal capillaries and possibly across terminal arterioles (Nolph 1991). It has been estimated that less than 0.2% of the peritoneal surface area has functional capacity for exchange. Blood flow in peritoneal vessels far exceeds the maximal clearance for small solutes (e.g., urea) during peritoneal dialysis, suggesting that diffusion barriers are more important than solute delivery in limiting clearance (Rudnick et al. 1987; Nolph 1991). Peritoneal blood flow may become limiting during peritoneal dialysis when severe hypotensive shock is present (Kliger 1981; Rudnick et al. 1987; Nolph 1991). Omentectomy, mesenterectomy, and abdominal evisceration did not alter acute peritoneal dialysis dynamics for glucose, urea, or insulin in an experimental study in dogs (Rubin et al. 1986). The portion of the peritoneal membrane essential for dialysis remains uncertain, but the parietal peritoneum is a likely candidate on the basis of this study.

The role of lymphatics in peritoneal dialysis has received little attention, but they could be important if lymphatic drainage is substantial. Peritoneal lymphatics are responsible for the isosmotic absorption of fluid, macromolecules, cells, bacteria, and other particles (Mactier et al. 1987; Mactier and Khanna 1989). Reduced ultrafiltration and solute clearance during CAPD in some human patients has been attributed to excessive lymphatic absorption (Mactier et al. 1987). End lymphatics in the diaphragm (stomata) are responsible for most of the lymphatic drainage from the peritoneal cavity, whereas omental and mesenteric lymphatics make minor contributions. Unlike peritoneal capillaries, lymphatics bring about one-way return of fluid to the circulation. Increased peritoneal lymphatic flow can occur with increased intraperitoneal hydrostatic pressure (overfilling), with exaggerated diaphragmatic movements (hyperventilation), and after chemical peritonitis. Lymphatic contractility is increased by several mediators of inflammation that may be present in peritonitis (Mactier et al. 1987).

Diffusion and ultrafiltration from the peritoneal capillaries to peritoneal fluid are opposed by layers of fluid within the capillary lumen, capillary endothelial cells, capillary basement membrane, interstitium, mesothelial cells, and peritoneal cavity (Rudnick et al. 1987; Mactier and Khanna 1989; Nolph 1991). Transport of water and solute across endothelial or mesothelial cells may occur via vesicles, intercellular junctions, or transcytoplasmic routes. The interstitium represents the longest component of distance for solute and water to traverse during movement from blood to peritoneal fluid and poses a barrier of extracellular fluid, connective tissue, lymphatics, and both gel-phase and free-phase mucopolysaccharides.

Transport across the peritoneum can be described by a "three-pore" model (Flessner 1997). The interstitium and mesothelium behave as if they had very large pores (more than 15 to 20 nm and possibly as wide as 50 to 100 nm), but the anatomic basis for these pores is not known. Only the largest macromolecules (e.g., hyaluronic acid) are impeded by these large pores and they allow proteins to pass through unimpeded. Water moves across this barrier by hydrostatic pressure, and it accounts for approximately 5 to 7% of total pore surface area. The interendothelial clefts between the capillary endothelial cells constitute the second level of pores in the peritoneal barrier. These pores are approximately 4 to 6 nm wide and restrict the passage of proteins but allow the diffusion of lower molecular weight solutes such as glucose and creatinine. These pores constitute 90 to 93% of total pore surface area, and water passes through this component of the peritoneal barrier by classical Starling forces (i.e., hydrostatic and osmotic pressure differences). The capillary endothelium also contains water channels that are less than 0.8 nm in diameter and through which water passes by osmosis (Pannekeet and Krediet 1996; Flessner 1997). These channels constitute only 1 to 2% of the total pore surface area but they account for 40% of osmotic water flow. The aquaporin water channel AQP-CHIP has been identified in peritoneal endothelial cells and presumably represents the molecular basis for these water channels (Pannekeet et al. 1996).

Mesothelial cells are covered with microvilli, which greatly increase surface area. Fluid trapped between microvilli prevents friction between surfaces but also may promote stagnation of fluid and impair solute exchange during dialysis. The role of microvilli during peritoneal dialysis has not been clarified, and microvilli may play an important role if transcellular fluid movement is more important than intercellular movement (Nolph 1991). Surfactant properties of the mesothelial cell surface repel fluid and favor one-way movement of fluid from capillaries into the peritoneal cavity (Mactier and Khanna 1989).

Peritonitis may alter peritoneal blood flow, effective peritoneal surface area, or peritoneal permeability. Peritonitis also can result in the loss of mesothelial microvilli and increase the diameter of intercellular gaps (Nolph 1991). In human patients, chronic peritoneal dialysis during peritonitis increases the clearance of urea and creatinine, increases glucose absorption from dialysate, increases protein loss into dialysate, and impairs effluent drainage (Rubin et al. 1981). Peritoneal dialysis during acute bacterial or chemical peritonitis in normal dogs did not alter the clearance of urea or potassium, but protein loss into the dialysate increased (Meengs et al. 1970). Thus, peritonitis probably does not reduce clearance of uremic solutes during peritoneal dialysis. The nature of the peritoneal membrane and the efficiency of peritoneal dialysis in dogs may change with age. Puppies younger than 1 month old exhibited greater peritoneal membrane permeability and increased functional peritoneal membrane surface area relative to body weight when compared with adult dogs (Elzouki et al. 1981).

▶ Composition of Dialysate

Solute and water transport across the peritoneum is dependent on the composition of the dialysate solution to which the peritoneum is exposed (Zelman et al. 1977). Hypertonic dialysate is much more efficient than isotonic dialysate in removal of uremic solutes (Henderson 1966; Henderson and Nolph 1969; Brown et al. 1978a). Sodium and its attendant anions along with dextrose account for most of the osmolality of dialysate. During dialysis, the osmolality of dialysate is altered by varying the concentration of dextrose in the dialysate solution from a minimum of 1.5% to a maximum of 4.25% (Table 25–8). Hypertonic dialysate increases solute clearance by a combination of solute drag during ultrafiltration (i.e., convection), capillary vasodilatation, increased pore diameter (Thornhill 1981), and dehydration of the peritoneal interstitium with consequent alteration of interstitial aqueous channels (Nolph 1991). Increased solute clearance after use of 4.25% dextrose–containing dialysate may persist during subsequent exchanges with dialysate containing 1.5% dextrose or with hypotonic dialysate (Henderson and Nolph 1969; Zelman et al. 1977; Brown et al. 1978b). Repeated exchanges using 4.25% dextrose–containing dialysate can cause severe dehydration (Zelman et al. 1977; Brown et al. 1978b). Consequently, alternating dialysate containing 4.25% dextrose with that containing 1.5% dextrose dialysate has been recommended (Brown et al. 1978b) as a method to increase dialysis efficiency without causing dehydration. The composition of commercial dialysate is compared with lactated Ringer's solution with 1.5% dextrose in Table 25–9.

Long-term exposure of the peritoneum to conventional dialysis solutions may be harmful to the peritoneum and ultimately may lead to impaired ultrafiltration and peritoneal fibrosis. Factors contributing to these adverse effects include low pH, high lactate concentration, high

TABLE 25–8. Comparison of Dianeal PD-1* Dialysate Composition with Three Different Concentrations of Glucose

	1.5% Dextrose	2.5% Dextrose	4.25% Dextrose
Sodium (mEq/L)	132	132	132
Calcium (mEq/L)	3.5	3.5	3.5
Magnesium (mEq/L)	1.5	1.5	1.5
Potassium (mEq/L)	0	0	0
Chloride (mEq/L)	102	102	102
Lactate (mEq/L)	35	35	35
Glucose (g/L)	15	25	42.5
Osmolality (mOsm/kg)	357	413	510

*PD-1 is available in 500, 1000, 1500, 2000, 3000, and 5000 mL bags (Baxter Healthcare, Deerfield, IL 60015). PD-2 is also available with 3.5% dextrose (2500 mL size only).

TABLE 25–9. Comparison of Commercially Available Dialysis Solutions (Dianeal PD-1 and PD-2 with 1.5% Dextrose)* with Lactated Ringer's Solution with 1.5% Dextrose

	PD-1	PD-2	LRS With 1.5% Dextrose
Sodium (mEq/L)	132	132	130
Calcium (mEq/L)	3.5	3.5	3.0
Magnesium (mEq/L)	1.5	0.5	0
Potassium (mEq/L)	0	0	4.0
Chloride (mEq/L)	102	96	109
Lactate (mEq/L)	35	40	28
Glucose (g/L)	15	15	15
Osmolality (mOsm/kg)	357	355	357

*PD-1 is available in 500, 1000, 1500, 2000, 3000, and 5000 mL bags. PD-2 is available in 250, 500, 750, 1000, 1500, 2000, 2500, 3000, and 5000 mL bags (Dianeal, Baxter Healthcare, Deerfield, IL 60015).

glucose concentration, and high osmolality of the dialysate (Cancarini 1997; Gokal 1997; Krediet 1998). Prolonged exposure of the peritoneal interstitium to glucose results in glycosylation and cross-linking of proteins, deposition of type IV collagen, and eventually increased thickness and rigidity of the peritoneal diffusion barrier (Krediet 1998). Hyperglycemia, hypertriglyceridemia, obesity, and inappetence are other adverse effects encountered in human patients receiving CAPD (Hain and Kessel 1987; Nolph 1991). In addition, the osmotic effect of glucose is short lived because of its rapid absorption across the peritoneum. These problems have led to attempts to identify alternative osmotic agents for use in peritoneal dialysis (Vanholder and Lameire 1996; Krediet et al. 1997).

Icodextrin is a glucose polymer containing glucose molecules connected by α-1,4 linkages. The peritoneum is impermeable to glucose polymers, resulting in a prolonged ultrafiltration effect of 8 to 16 h (Mistry and Gokal 1996; Faller 1998; Peers and Gokal 1998). This osmotic effect is enhanced by the fact that amylase is not found in the peritoneal cavity. Icodextrin, however, is slowly absorbed by lymphatics and metabolized to maltose by amylase at other sites in the body. Most icodextrin molecules contain 2 to 300 glucose residues and few contain less than 10 residues (Peers and Gokal 1998). The large size of the icodextrin molecule results in a colloid osmotic effect that facilitates ultrafiltration without the need for high osmotic pressure. The osmolality of a 7.5% icodextrin solution is 277 mOsm/kg.

Amino acid solutions have been used as alternative osmotic agents and to provide nutritional support for human patients receiving CAPD in whom protein losses in dialysate typically are high (8 to 15 g/day) (Jones 1995; Faller 1996, 1998). A 1.1% solution of amino acids (Nutrineal) used once a day represents the best compromise between nutritional support and aggravation of azotemia and metabolic acidosis that can occur with use of a 2% amino acid solution. Between 60 and 90% of the administered amino acids are absorbed across the peritoneum and contribute to normalization of plasma essential and nonessential amino acid profiles, positive nitrogen balance, and increased serum albumin concentration. Serum potassium and phosphorus concentrations decrease in patients treated with amino acid solutions, a finding that also indicates the presence of an anabolic state. A 1% solution of amino acids has an osmolality of 365 mOsm/kg. Such a solution does not adversely affect the transport characteristics of the peritoneum and provides an ultrafiltration effect equivalent to that of a 1.5% glucose solution. Nutrineal has a pH of 6.7 and contains 40 mEq/L lactate as a buffer to counter the tendency of amino acid solutions to contribute to metabolic acidosis. Serum bicarbonate concentrations tend to remain stable in human patients treated with this solution.

Alkali precursors are added to commercial dialysate solutions to combat metabolic acidosis (Feriani 1996). Bicarbonate-containing solutions are more biocompatible than solutions containing lactate and do not adversely affect the peritoneum. Such solutions, however, are associated with technical limitations because of the potential for calcium and magnesium carbonate precipitation. Consequently, lactate still is the alkali precursor used in most dialysate solutions. These solutions require a low pH (5.2 to 6.2) to prevent the caramelization of glucose that occurs during heat sterilization at higher pH. Unfortunately, solutions containing both high lactate concentration and low pH cause intracellular acidosis and are injurious to the peritoneium. Lactate concentrations in dialysate of 35 to 45 mEq/L usually are adequate to correct uremic acidosis in human dialysis patients (Nolph 1991). Acetate no longer is used as an alkali precursor in dialysate because its use has been associated with vasodilatation, hyperpermeability, and eventually loss of ultrafiltration and peritoneal sclerosis. Although use of a bicarbonate-containing solution would be ideal, technical problems remain with the production and delivery of such solutions. Proportioning systems, addition of bicarbonate to acidic solutions, double-chamber bags that allow separation of bicarbonate from calcium and magnesium, and addition of stabilizing agents (e.g., glycylglycine) have been evaluated for facilitating bicarbonate delivery. At present, lactate remains the primary source of alkali for conventional dialysate solutions. Dialysate solutions containing alkali precursors are designed for chronic correction of metabolic acidosis and should not be relied upon for rapid correction of acidosis or correction of severe metabolic acidosis. Systemic administration of alkali is necessary in these instances.

▶ Management of Azotemia Before Dialysis

Death before dialysis may be due to the severe metabolic derangements of uremia (e.g., hyperkalemia, metabolic acidosis), dehydration, iatrogenic overhydration by overzealous fluid therapy, infection, and malnutrition (Chew 1985). An attempt should be made to improve renal blood flow, glomerular filtration rate (GFR), and renal tubular flow rate by conventional medical therapy before considering dialysis. Dialysis may not be necessary if azotemia, hyperkalemia, metabolic acidosis, fluid imbalance, and uremic symptoms can be reduced sufficiently by conventional therapy. Reduced GFR and consequent accumulation of uremic solutes can result from a variety of prerenal, intrarenal, and postrenal factors that may not be obvious on initial examination of the animal. Reduced renal perfusion (prerenal azotemia) commonly contributes to azotemia, either alone or in combination with intrarenal or postrenal factors. Fluid therapy in patients with renal failure is discussed in Chapter 19.

▶ Indications for Peritoneal Dialysis

The primary candidates for peritoneal dialysis are animals with AIRF, those with acutely decompensated chronic renal failure, and those with postrenal azotemia unable to undergo immediate surgical correction. Tube cystostomy drainage is preferable in the acute management of urethral obstruction before surgical correction. Dialysis is instituted whenever severe clinical signs and laboratory abnormalities of uremia cannot be managed by medical or

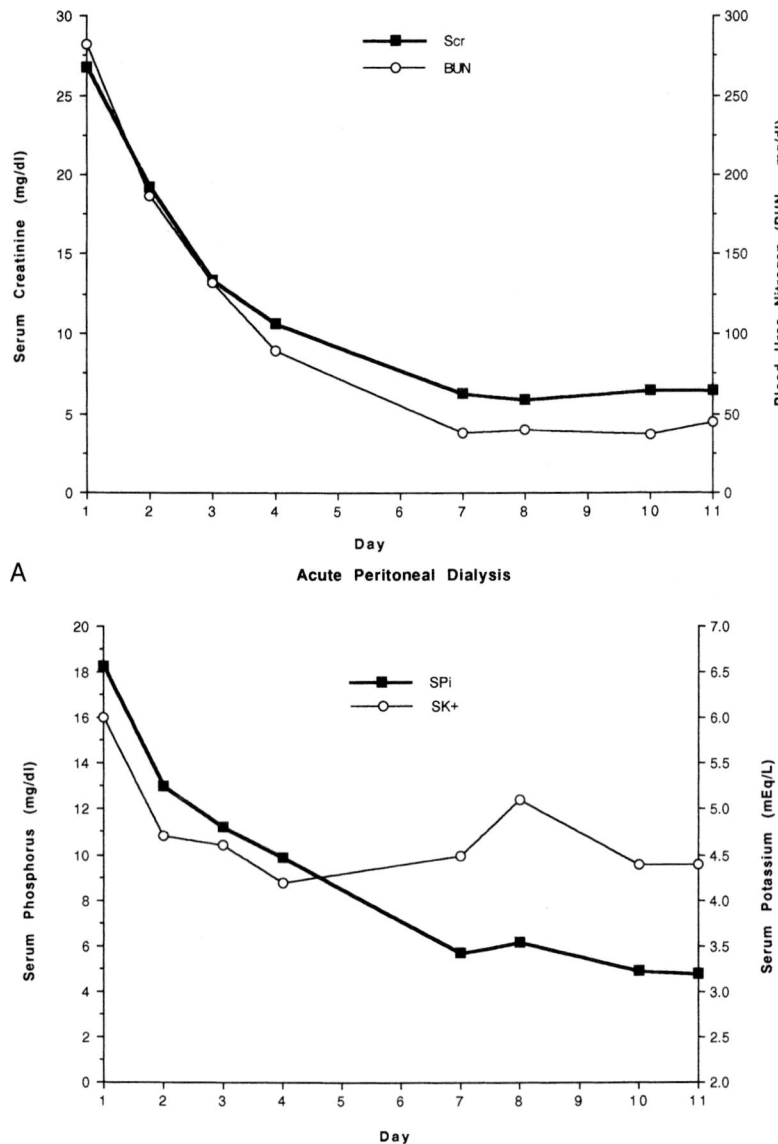

FIGURE 25-2. Effects of acute and chronic dialysis on serum urea, creatinine, potassium, and phosphate concentrations in a dog. (A and B) Acute peritoneal dialysis.

surgical means alone. Peritoneal dialysis is recommended when the underlying renal lesion is potentially reversible (e.g., AIRF) or when amelioration of uremic clinical signs is likely to improve the patient's future quality of life without dialysis. Unfortunately, it may not be obvious from a clinical standpoint whether or not the underlying renal lesion is reversible at the time dialysis must be instituted to maintain life. Thus, the animal may undergo peritoneal dialysis while awaiting the results of renal biopsy. The indications for dialysis are listed in Tables 25–6 and 25–7.

Peritoneal dialysis is not indicated for the treatment of prerenal azotemia, nor is it indicated for the long-term management of chronic renal failure in animals with underlying irreversible renal lesions. Some animals with chronic renal failure may benefit from several days of peritoneal dialysis to reduce uremic signs so that clinical recompensation can occur, but this approach is not often attempted.

Aggressive medical therapy (see Chapter 19) is continued until it is clear that further improvement in renal function will not occur without dialysis. Clinical signs, urine output, and results of hematology and serum biochemistry must be considered together when making the decision to begin dialysis or euthanatize the animal. Dialysis should not be instituted solely on the basis of the magnitude of azotemia. A rapid increase in BUN or serum creatinine concentration (regardless of the magnitude of azotemia), severe oliguria or anuria, overhydration, hyperkalemia, hypernatremia, hyperphosphatemia, hypocalcemia, and metabolic acidosis despite aggressive medical treatment are indications to begin dialysis in an animal with a potentially reversible renal disease. Using conventional medical therapy, it is difficult to manage normally hydrated animals with clinical signs of uremia, BUN concentrations above 100 mg/dL, and serum creatinine concentrations above 10 mg/dL. Dialysis is unlikely to be beneficial in animals with moderate azotemia be-

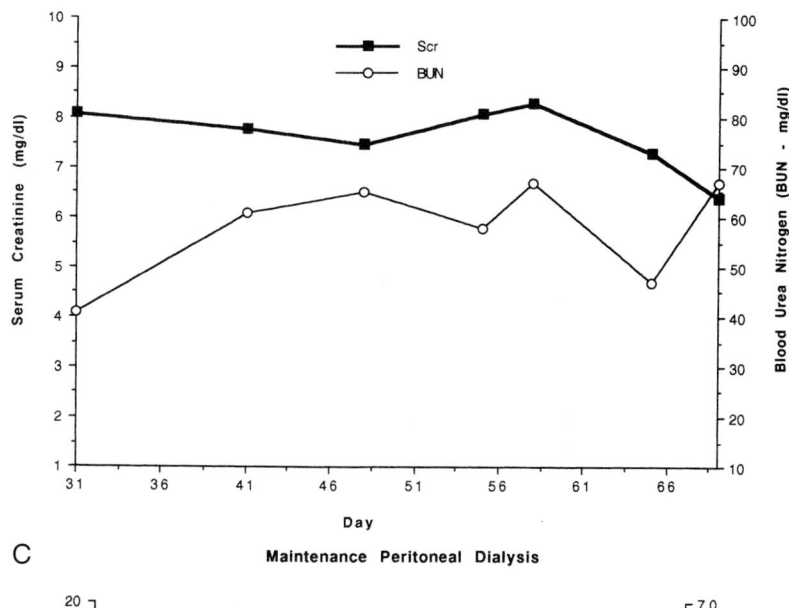

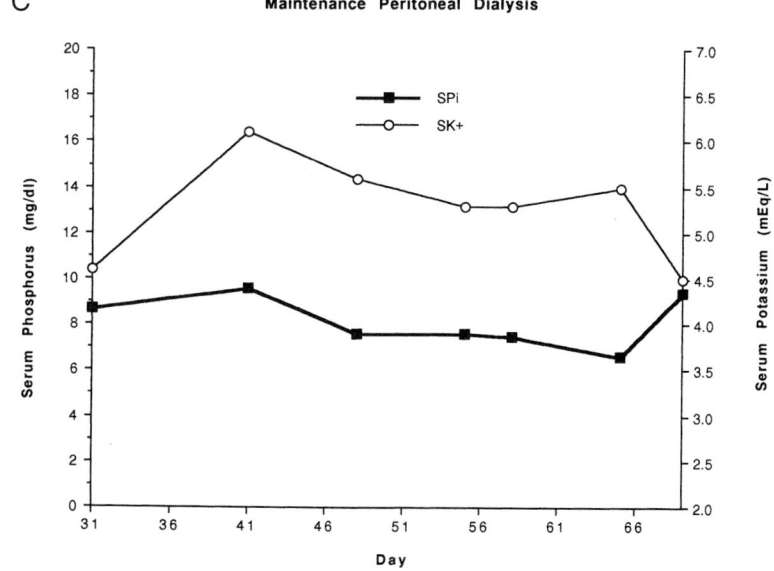

FIGURE 25-2. *Continued* (*C* and *D*) Maintenance peritoneal dialysis.

cause BUN concentrations of 40 to 80 mg/dL and serum creatinine concentrations of 4 to 7 mg/dL are the expected result of dialysis with current CAPD techniques (Fig. 25–2A to D).

Peritoneal dialysis has been most successful for both short- and long-term management of dogs and cats when a column disc catheter has been placed (see following procedure). Acute dialysis using intermittent needle puncture for two to four exchanges per day over 2 to 3 days may help alleviate uremic signs if a dialysis catheter is not available. This approach may allow recompensation in some animals with chronic renal failure or may be a temporary solution for an animal awaiting chronic peritoneal dialysis with a surgically placed catheter. Peritoneal dialysis using repeated needle punctures for longer periods of time is difficult because of trauma to the patient, time commitment, and mechanical difficulties with this technique.

Rare indications for acute peritoneal dialysis include hypothermia (Reuler 1978; Welton et al. 1978), hyperthermia (Nolph 1991), hypercalcemic crisis (Hamilton et al. 1980; Nolph 1991), and dialyzable intoxication such as with barbiturates or early ethylene glycol poisoning (Vale et al. 1976). Occasionally, life-threatening overhydration unresponsive to diuretic therapy can be managed by several exchanges of hypertonic dialysate.

▶ Techniques of Peritoneal Dialysis

Strict aseptic technique is imperative with any type of peritoneal dialysis (Thornhill 1981; Copley 1987). This includes presurgical scrubbing of the site and sterile surgical technique during catheter placement as well as the use of sterile gloves, application of disinfectants, and aseptic handling of dialysate, catheters, and fluid lines during dialysis.

Alcohols are the preferred class of chemical for disinfection of dialysis connections because of their broad range of antimicrobial activity, their activity in the presence of organic matter, and their rapid evaporation (Werner 1988). Chlorhexidine and the iodophores may be inadequate for disinfection in the dialysis environment, and both types of product occasionally have been observed to be contaminated with bacteria. In addition, chlorhexidine is predominantly bacteriostatic, whereas iodophores have limited effectiveness against *Staphylococcus aureus* and are inactivated by blood and glucose (Werner 1988).

▶ Access to the Peritoneal Cavity

It has been said that "the catheter is both the heart and the Achilles heel of peritoneal dialysis" (Cowgill 1995). The catheter used for peritoneal dialysis is vital for delivery and removal of dialysate and yet is the element of the therapeutic process most susceptible to mechanical difficulty and failure. Several types of catheters, cannulas, and needles are available for performing peritoneal dialysis. Selection of a particular catheter depends on the anticipated duration of dialysis and the number of daily exchanges required to manage the patient's uremia. Animals with severe adhesions along the midline or those with ileus require a surgically placed catheter.

Acute Access: Percutaneous Peritoneal Dialysis

Acute (temporary) dialysis can be carried out simply by intermittent abdominal punctures using large-gauge needles for infusion and drainage of dialysate. To infuse dialysate, an 18- or 20-gauge needle is introduced along the ventral midline 2 cm caudal to the umbilicus. Adequate drainage of dialysate may require a 16-, 14-, or 12-gauge needle or a plastic cannula. Distention of the abdomen by the previous infusion of dialysate minimizes the possibility of trauma to abdominal viscera during subsequent needle puncture for drainage. A sterile intravenous extension set and empty collection bag are attached to the drainage needle during outflow. Trauma from multiple punctures and difficulty obtaining adequate outflow of dialysate limit the long-term usefulness of this technique. To minimize trauma, large-gauge needles or plastic cannulas may be secured in place during each dwell period. Obstruction of dialysate outflow is common with this technique and frequent postural adjustments or repeated punctures often are necessary to promote continued drainage of effluent dialysate. Hydropulsion with dialysate or mechanical dislodgement of obstructing material using a small-gauge urinary catheter introduced through the puncture needle or cannula also may be helpful.

Peritoneal lavage (continuous peritoneal dialysis) may be used as an alternative to intermittent needle puncture. A sterile 14 Fr feeding tube (Brunswick sterile disposable feeding tube and urethral catheter, Sherwood Medical Instruments, St. Louis, MO) is placed percutaneously in the flank for infusion of dialysate. One or more outflow drains are placed inside a fenestrated Penrose drain and then inserted into the ventral abdomen (tube or sump Shirley wound drain, ANPRO, HN Anderson Products, Oyster Bay, NY). This approach constitutes an open drainage system and infection can be a serious complication (Parks 1974).

A catheter commercially available for peritoneal dialysis in human patients (Trocath, McGraw Laboratories, Division of American Hospital Supply, Glendale, CA) is composed of a stiff plastic tube with multiple fenestrations placed over an internal stylet to facilitate introduction. The main advantage of this catheter is that it can be placed percutaneously using only local anesthesia. It is difficult, however, to obtain a good seal at the point of entry, and this may lead to leakage of dialysate or infection. Except for its anchor site, this catheter floats free in the abdominal cavity, and omental migration with obstruction of the small fenestrations in the catheter is a commonly encountered problem. In dogs, this type of catheter often becomes obstructed during the first week of chronic dialysis (Thornhill 1981).

Before placing the catheter, the abdomen is distended by infusion of warmed dialysate solution via needle puncture to decrease the possibility of injury to abdominal viscera. A small scalpel incision is made through the skin and subcutaneous tissues and the catheter and stylet are inserted into the abdomen. After passage through the abdominal wall, the stylet is retracted slightly before advancing the catheter caudally to a position near the urinary bladder.

The Cohen acute pediatric peritoneal dialysis catheter system (Cook Incorporated, Bloomington, IN) consists of a flexible fenestrated tube and wire stylet. Local anesthetic (2% lidocaine) is injected at the site of catheter placement (2 cm caudal to the umbilicus and just to one side of the midline), and the urinary bladder is emptied before catheter placement. After pulling the skin back to allow a subcutaneous tunnel, the introducer needle is placed and the stylet is threaded through the introducer needle. The needle is removed, leaving the stylet in place, and the catheter is threaded over the stylet, twisting slightly to facilitate passage of the catheter through the peritoneum. The stylet is removed after it is determined that all catheter fenestrations lie within the abdomen and a purse-string suture is placed at the entry site. The catheter is secured and a sterile bandage applied. Although designed for acute access, this catheter system has been employed successfully in dogs for as long as 30 days (GM Kauffman, personal communication, 1990).

Long-Term Access: Surgically Placed Catheters

The Parker peritoneal dialysis cannula (CPA Vet, Marysville, CA) consists of a trocar, guide tube, stainless steel needle, and silicone rubber dialysis cannula (Fig. 25–3). This catheter is positioned in the abdomen in a bowed fashion ventral to the bladder and anchored at both flanks. It can be placed using local anesthesia in severely uremic animals. Leakage of dialysate is minimal because of the dorsal flank location of the catheter's exit site. A Dacron cuff on the catheter is positioned at the level of the body wall to minimize the possibility of ascending infection. Using this catheter, chronic dialysis in dogs successfully

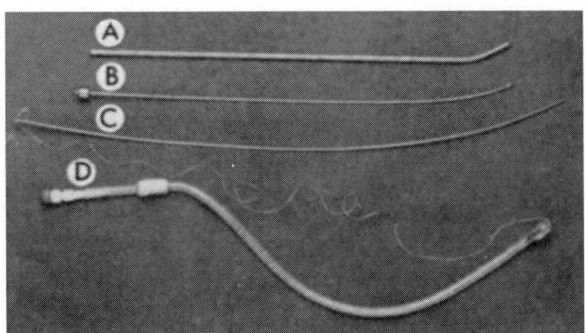

FIGURE 25–3. The Parker peritoneal dialysis cannula. From top to bottom, the stainless steel needle guide *(A)*, the trochar *(B)*, the stainless steel needle (armed with Vetafil suture) *(C)*, and the silicone rubber cannula *(D)*. The cannula is closed with a tapered plastic adapter and a B–D diaphragm cap Luer-Lok plug. (From Kirk RW: *Current Veterinary Therapy VII*. Philadelphia, WB Saunders Co., p. 1108, 1980.)

reduced accumulated uremic solutes and effluent dialysate was rapidly and effectively drained from the abdomen (Parker et al. 1972; Parker 1980).

The column disc catheter (previously manufactured as Vet Cath, Physio-Control, Redmond, WA and Life Cath, Quinton Instrument Co., Seattle, WA) has been used for chronic peritoneal dialysis in small animals because of its relative freedom from obstruction and ability to drain effluent dialysate rapidly (Thornhill 1981). This catheter is made of silicone and consists of a single tube opening between two parallel discs separated by numerous pillars (Fig. 25–4A and B). The main advantages of this catheter are excellent effluent drainage and minimal leakage of dialysate. The pillars aid in prevention of catheter outflow occlusion by omentum, fibrin, and abdominal organs. The disc catheter is secured against the abdominal wall and two Dacron cuffs on the catheter allow fibrous tissue growth and prevent ascending bacterial migration.

The column disc catheter can be placed under local anesthesia through a small incision if the animal is severely depressed or moribund. General anesthesia, however, is recommended for ideal catheter placement (Birchard et al. 1988). This surgical procedure combines catheter placement from within the abdominal cavity, partial omentectomy, and renal biopsy. Partial omentectomy enhances the success of dialysis by preventing omental occlusion of the catheter and improving outflow of effluent dialysate (Birchard et al. 1988; Carter et al. 1989). A renal biopsy should be obtained for all animals undergoing chronic peritoneal dialysis to establish a diagnosis, facilitate treatment, and formulate a prognosis.

A wedge biopsy of the left kidney is obtained through a left paramedian incision at the time of catheter placement. The caudal two-thirds of the omentum is removed unless peritonitis is present or the animal has recently undergone intestinal surgery. Instead of omentectomy, an omentopexy is performed in the latter instances. The disc of the catheter is placed just cranial to the pelvic brim, and its tubing is pulled through a stab incision in the abdominal wall 2 to 3 cm cranial to the pelvic brim. The disc of the catheter is pulled flush with the parietal peritoneum, and the Dacron cuff closest to the disc is positioned in the abdominal musculature. A purse-string suture is placed around the catheter tubing in the rectus fascia, and the tubing is tunneled subcutaneously 6 to 8 cm cranially before exiting the skin via a ventral midline stab incision. The second Dacron cuff is positioned in the subcutaneous tissue, which is then meticulously closed in a simple, continuous pattern using absorbable suture material (e.g., Vicryl, Dexon) to eliminate dead space. The skin is closed routinely with Vetafil or monofilament nylon. The technique for surgical placement of this catheter is depicted in Figure 25–5A to D and summarized in Table 25–10.

The dialysis catheter is flushed several times with heparinized saline at the time of placement to prevent obstruction by blood clots (Fig. 25–6). The abdomen then is lavaged to remove fibrin clots that might occlude the dialysis catheter. Heparinized lactated Ringer's solution or heparinized dialysate should be instilled into the abdominal cavity and proper drainage capability verified at the time of closure. A residual volume of 10 to 20 mL/kg heparinized peritoneal fluid should remain to minimize the risk of clotting in the dialysis catheter. If possible, dialysis is delayed for 12 to 24 h after catheter placement to enable a tight seal to develop at the catheter exit site. Dialysis may be started sooner if necessary because of severe uremia or hyperkalemia.

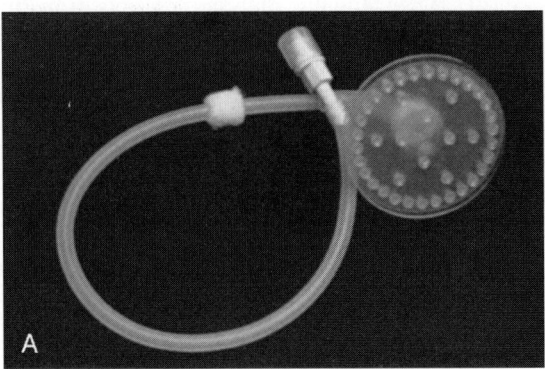
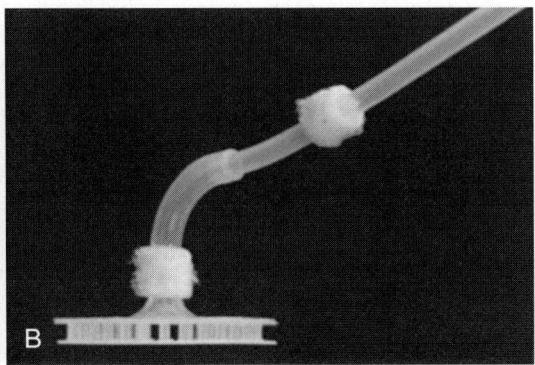

FIGURE 25–4. *(A)* Purdue column disc peritoneal dialysis catheter. *(B)* The disc portion of the catheter is two Silastic sheets separated by 1-cm-tall pillars. Also note two Dacron cuffs on the tubing. (From Birchard SJ, Chew DJ, Crisp MS et al.: Modified technique for placement of a column disc peritoneal dialysis catheter. *J Am Anim Hosp Assoc* 24:664, 1988.)

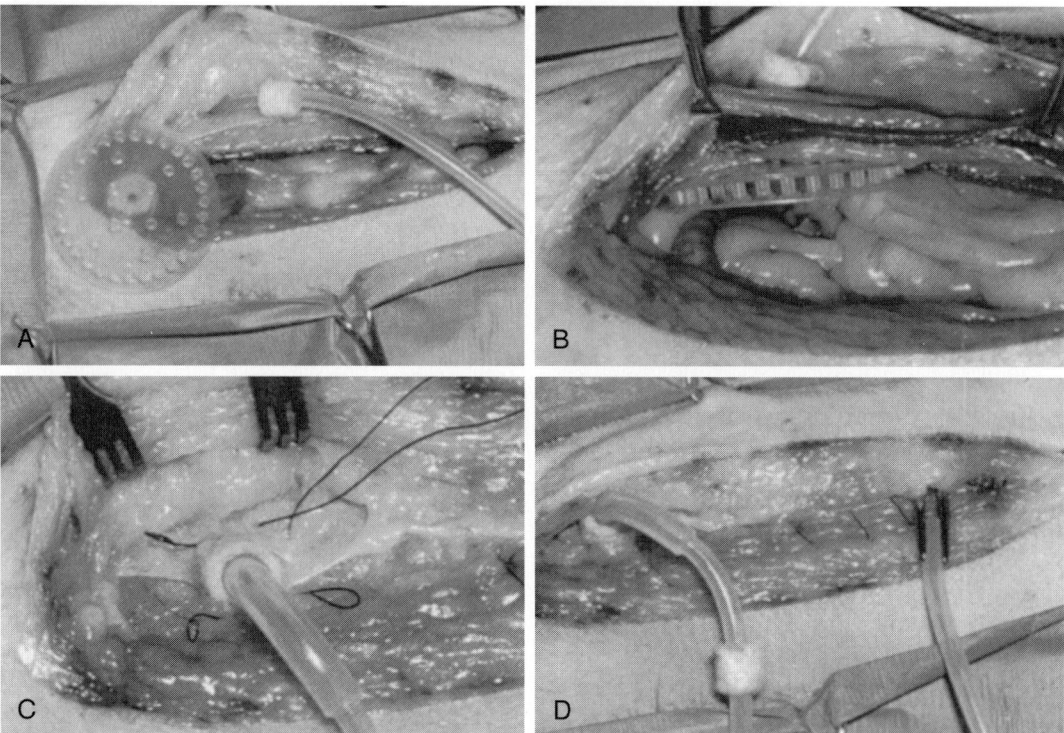

FIGURE 25-5. (A) Left paramedian approach to the abdomen. Tubing has been placed through a stab incision in the abdominal wall. (B) The disc portion of the catheter should be flush with the ventral abdominal wall. The Dacron cuff closest to the disc is at the level of the abdominal musculature. (C) A purse-string suture in the fascia is placed around the tubing to prevent leakage of dialysate. (D) A stab incision through skin and subcutaneous tissue is made cranially and the tubing pulled to the exterior with forceps. The Dacron cuff farthest from the disc is buried subcutaneously. (From Birchard SJ, Chew DJ, Crisp MS et al.: Modified technique for placement of a column disc peritoneal dialysis catheter. J Am Anim Hosp Assoc 24:665, 1988.)

The Vet Cath and Life Cath column disc catheters are no longer commercially available. A new silicone catheter composed of a transabdominal tube with two Dacron cuffs connected by a T shape to a transverse cylinder that contains eight 1-mm-wide fluted openings (grooves) instead of side holes has been developed (Ash Advantage peritoneal dialysis catheter, Fig. 25-7A and B). These grooves provide minimal resistance for fluid transfer while avoiding omental attachment. The T-fluted catheter allowed successful peritoneal dialysis in 17 dogs for 7 to 60 days without evidence of omental obstruction. (Ash and Janle 1993; Dzyban et al. 1999) By comparison, Tenckhoff's catheters used in control dogs became completely obstructed in 2 to 4 days because of omental attachment to the side holes.

▶ Selection and Preparation of Dialysate

Dialysate typically is formulated to approximate the electrolyte composition of normal extracellular fluid (Rudnick et al. 1987). Ideally, dialysate composition should be tailored to the needs of the individual patient for sodium, chloride, potassium, and alkali. The concentration gradient between blood and dialysate determines which solutes are removed from or added to the patient's blood. A large concentration gradient from blood to dialysate favors solute removal, whereas a large concentration gradient from dialysate to blood favors uptake of solute by the patient. The composition of dialysate should be such that there is no concentration gradient between blood and dialysate for solutes that are not to be removed from or added to the body.

Commercial Dialysate

Commercially available dialysate solutions designed for use in human patients work well in dogs and cats (see

TABLE 25-10. **Surgical Placement of the Column Disc Catheter**

1. Left paramedian approach
2. Omentectomy (caudal two-thirds of omentum)
3. Place catheter as far caudal as possible (just cranial to the brim of the pelvis)
4. Secure first Dacron cuff with a purse-string suture at exit in ventral abdominal wall
5. Bury second Dacron cuff in subcutaneous tissue
6. Catheter should exit skin 6–8 cm cranial
7. Catheter should be flushed with 20–30 mL heparinized saline before closure

Data from: Birchard SJ, Chew DJ, Crisp MS et al.: Modified technique for placement of a column disc peritoneal dialysis catheter. J Am Anim Hosp Assoc 24:663–666, 1988.

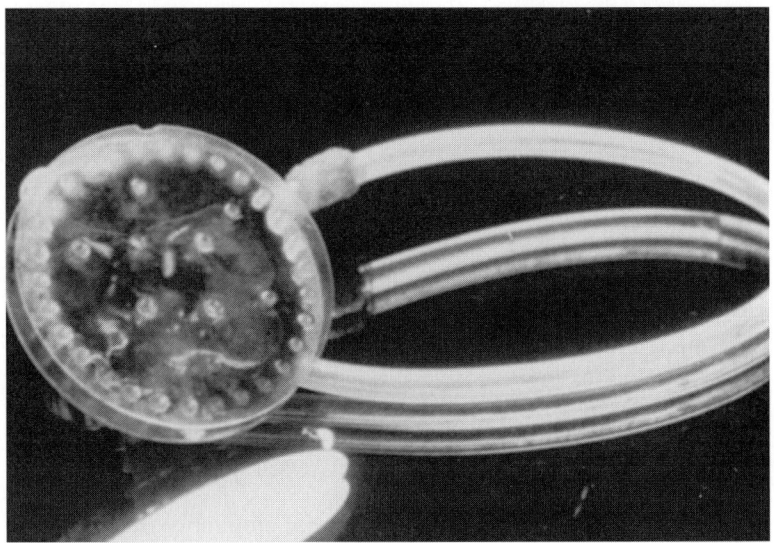

FIGURE 25-6. Obstruction of column disc catheter by clotted blood.

Tables 25–8 and 25–9). These solutions approximate the electrolyte composition of normal extracellular fluid and contain dextrose at concentrations of 1.5, 2.5, or 4.25%. Dialysate containing 1.5% dextrose is used most commonly, but solutions containing 2.5 or 4.25% dextrose may be required to remove water by ultrafiltration and correct overhydration or when effluent dialysate volume is inadequate because of severe hyperosmolality of the patient's extracellular fluid. Hypernatremia may occur during peritoneal dialysis because of ultrafiltration of solute-free water. Consequently, it may be advantageous to select dialysate solutions that contain lower sodium concentrations than plasma during the course of dialysis.

Improvised Dialysate Solution

As an alternative to commercially available peritoneal dialysis solutions, dialysate may be improvised using lactated Ringer's solution, 0.45% NaCl, or 0.9% NaCl as a starting solution that can be tailored to the individual needs of the patient. Commercial dialysate solutions generally are preferred, however, because alteration of the dialysate with additives introduces the possibility of formulation errors and increases the risk of bacterial contamination during preparation. All homemade dialysate solutions require the addition of glucose. To achieve a 1.5% dextrose solution, 30 mL of 50% dextrose is added to each liter of dialysate solution. To achieve a 2.5% dextrose solution, 50 mL of 50% dextrose is added. To achieve a 4.25% dextrose solution, 85 mL of 50% dextrose is added (see Table 25–8).

MAGNESIUM

If anorexia persists, magnesium should be added to homemade dialysate solutions after the first few days of dialysis. To achieve a concentration of 1.5 mEq/L, 71.5 mg of $MgCl_2$ is added to 1 L of dialysate. Magnesium chloride may not be readily available as a sterile commercial solution. Consequently, $MgCl_2$ may be dissolved in dextrose and passed through an appropriate Millipore filter to achieve sterility before addition to dialysate.

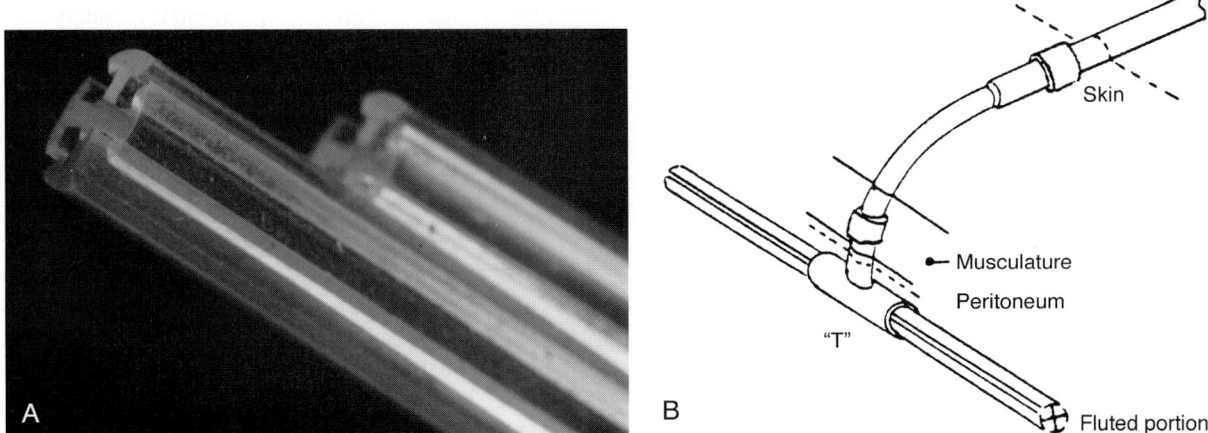

FIGURE 25-7. (A) Photograph of the Ash Advantage T-fluted peritoneal dialysis catheter. (B) Diagram showing design and placement of the Ash Advantage T-fluted peritoneal dialysis catheter. (B from Ash SR and Janle EM: T-fluted peritoneal dialysis catheter. *Adv Peritoneal Dial* 9:223, 1993.)

SODIUM BICARBONATE

As a source of alkali, NaHCO$_3$ should be added to homemade dialysate solution improvised from 0.45 or 0.9% NaCl to achieve a final HCO$_3^-$ concentration of 30 to 45 mEq/L. Lactated Ringer's solution contains lactate as an alkali equivalent at a concentration of 28 mEq/L, and NaHCO$_3$ should not be added to lactated Ringer's solution because of the potential for precipitation of magnesium or calcium carbonate.

HEPARIN

Heparin is added to both commercial and homemade dialysate solutions just before infusion at a concentration of 1000 U per liter of final dialysate solution to decrease the possibility of clot formation and outflow obstruction.

ANTIBIOTICS

There is no advantage to using prophylactic antibiotics in the dialysate to prevent bacterial peritonitis, but antibiotics should be added to dialysate if peritonitis is diagnosed (see later).

POTASSIUM

Commercial dialysate solutions for use in CAPD usually do not contain potassium (see Table 25–9). Potassium-free dialysate is ideal for the treatment of hyperkalemia during initial dialysis and may be continued during maintenance dialysis for animals that are able to eat or those receiving enteral nutritional support. Hypokalemia, however, can develop during aggressive dialysis with potassium-free dialysate, especially when hourly exchanges are performed or when more than four exchanges are performed per day in an anorexic animal. In these instances, it is necessary to add potassium to parenterally administered fluids or to the dialysate solution. Potassium chloride can be added to potassium-free solutions to achieve a final potassium concentration of 4 mEq/L. This may prevent hypokalemia in animals that are not eating after the first 24 to 48 h of aggressive dialysis. The amount of KCl added to dialysate varies and depends on the severity of the hypokalemia and the number of daily exchanges performed, but as much as 10 to 20 mEq/L can be added to dialysate to correct hypokalemia if necessary. Potassium should be added to dialysate solutions cautiously to avoid development of hyperkalemia, and serum potassium concentration should be monitored frequently whenever dialysate solution is supplemented with potassium.

CALCIUM

Calcium-free commercial dialysate solutions are not available. In patients with hypercalcemia or in those with severe hyperphosphatemia, it may be advisable initially to use a homemade dialysate solution free of calcium (e.g., 0.9% NaCl) with added glucose.

Warming Dialysate

Dialysate solution should be warmed before infusion when exchanges are to be performed frequently (every 1–3 h). Dialysate may be warmed to slightly above normal body temperature to promote vasodilatation and enhance solute transfer (Parker et al. 1972). Warming of dialysate

TABLE 25–11. Dialysate Preparation

1. Collect materials needed (e.g., bag of dialysate, 50% dextrose, alcohol, syringes, needles).
2. Wash hands and wear sterile surgical gloves.
3. Wipe all injection ports with alcohol before using.
4. Add 1000 U heparin per liter of dialysate.
5. If using lactated Ringer's solution, add 30 mL 50% dextrose per liter (for a 1.5% dextrose solution).
6. Add other medications as required.
7. Attach label to bag indicating all added medications.
8. Warm dialysate to slightly above body temperature.
9. Invert bag several times to mix before beginning infusion.

before infusion is less important with longer dwell times because heat dissipation occurs (Nolph 1991). Warming of dialysate solution before infusion is recommended for all hypothermic animals. Administration of cold dialysate should be avoided to prevent vasoconstriction of peritoneal vessels. Plastic bags of dialysate solution can be warmed in a microwave oven for a few minutes until warm to the touch, but care must be taken to be sure that the solution has been uniformly warmed (i.e., the contents of the bag should be mixed by inverting the bag several times). Hot water baths can be used, but bacterial contamination may be a problem with this approach (Nolph 1991). Preparation of dialysate is summarized in Table 25–11.

▶ Infusion of Dialysate (Inflow)

Rapid infusion of dialysate by gravity flow at rates of 200 to 300 mL/min is well tolerated by animals (Parker et al. 1972; Thornhill 1981). Infusion volumes of 250, 500, 750, 1000, or 2000 mL often are chosen to approximate a dosage of 40 mL/kg body weight (Thornhill 1981). Normally, inflow of dialysate should require less than 5 to 10 min. The abdomen should be palpably distended after dialysate infusion to ensure maximal contact of fluid with peritoneal surfaces (Robson et al. 1978). The abdomen should not be distended to the point that ventilatory excursions are reduced or the patient experiences discomfort. Infusion of an excessive volume of dialysate is undesirable because it enhances peritoneal capillary and lymphatic uptake of fluid and solute as a consequence of increased hydrostatic pressure in the peritoneal cavity and may reduce peritoneal membrane permeability by reducing pore size (Thornhill 1981). Dialysate should be drained immediately if dyspnea occurs during infusion. Dialysate volume also should be decreased when substantial subcutaneous leakage of infused dialysate occurs.

Commercial dialysate (Dianeal) is available in many package sizes ranging from 250 mL to 5 L (see Table 25–9). After inflow and dwell are completed, the empty dialysate bag is used to collect effluent dialysate using the same administration set. The bag of effluent dialysate then is discarded, and a bag of fresh dialysate solution is attached to the infusion line. When only a portion of the bag is to be infused, it is advisable to infuse dialysate solution through one line of a Y-connector system (e.g., a three-way stopcock with appropriate IV extension sets) and drain effluent dialysate into a sterile empty bag via another administration set. After drainage of effluent dialysate by this method, additional fresh dialysate solution can be infused from the original bag, thus minimizing waste of dialysate and reducing the risk of contamination by decreasing the number of times bags must be changed. Use of the Y-connector system also facilitates maintenance of aseptic technique during peritoneal dialysis (Lane et al. 1992).

It is difficult to deliver a small volume of dialysate accurately by estimating the fluid level in a plastic bag. More accurate delivery can be achieved by serially weighing the bag on a gram scale during dialysis (1 g of fluid = 1 mL). For example, 100 mL of dialysate has been infused from a 1-L bag when the weight of the bag has decreased by 100 g. For animals weighing less than 5 kg, a Buretrol reservoir positioned between the dialysate bag and inflow line can be used to measure small infusion volumes (≤150 mL) accurately before inflow into the patient.

▶ Dwell Time for Dialysate Solution

The prescribed dwell time for dialysate is based on the urgency of the need to correct the metabolic abnormalities of uremia. Animals with life-threatening disturbances, such as hyperkalemia and metabolic acidosis, may require hourly exchanges until stabilization is achieved. Animals with AIRF may require 12 to 48 consecutive hourly exchanges before a marked reduction in azotemia and hyperphosphatemia can be demonstrated. Frequent exchanges allow greater efficiency in the removal of uremic solutes because a favorable concentration gradient for diffusion of solutes into dialysate is maintained by frequent replacement of effluent dialysate with fresh dialysate solution. Gentle palpation of the abdomen during the dwell period may help mix stagnant dialysate with fresh solution and facilitate diffusion when a maximal rate of solute transfer is considered essential. After the initial stabilization of the uremic patient, dwell time gradually is increased to 4 to 8 h (three to six daily exchanges) during maintenance chronic dialysis. Dialysate dwell time is summarized in Table 25–12.

▶ Drainage of Effluent Dialysate (Outflow)

Dialysate is drained from the abdomen by gravity flow, usually during 15 min after an appropriate dwell time (Thornhill 1981). Whenever the entire bag of dialysate is infused into the patient during one exchange, effluent

TABLE 25-12. Summary of Dialysate Dwell Time

1. Initial dwell time: 45 min.
2. As uremia resolves, dwell time is extended (90, 120, 180, 240 min).
3. If patient is debilitated, allow dialysate bag to hang from drip stand.
4. If patient is ambulatory, tape dialysate bag to patient's belly wrap and cover.

TABLE 25-13. Causes of Catheter Failure

Improper placement
Loss of siphon effect (e.g., connection to a vacuum, clamps not open)
Kinking of fluid lines or catheter
Outflow obstruction of column disc (e.g., omentum, blood clots)
Peritonitis

dialysate should be drained into the same bag during outflow so that the risk of bacterial contamination is minimized. Excessively rapid drainage of effluent dialysate and rapid decompression of the abdomen may be painful for some dogs (Parker et al. 1972) but this seems to be rare. The volume of effluent dialysate retrieved during the first few exchanges may be less than the volume infused because of absorption of some fluid by dehydrated patients or sequestration of fluid in the abdomen. Effluent volume should match or exceed the volume infused during subsequent hourly exchanges with 1.5% dextrose solutions. Records should be kept of the volume of dialysate infused and the volume of effluent dialysate retrieved for each exchange period, and the patient's cumulative balance should be monitored (see later).

During hourly exchanges, prolonged outflow times (>15 min) and failure to retrieve 90% or more of the infused dialysate usually indicate a mechanical problem with drainage. First, all inflow and outflow lines and the accessible portion of the dialysis catheter itself should be inspected for kinks. The animal should be repositioned as necessary to enhance drainage. Several postural changes should be attempted (e.g., left and right lateral recumbency, raising the animal's forelimbs or hindquarters). Lastly, the dialysis catheter is flushed with heparinized saline to remove any occluding blood clots, fibrin strands, or omentum. All of these procedures must be carried out using proper sterile technique. Uncommonly, persistent obstruction necessitates replacement of the catheter. Causes of catheter failure are listed in Table 25–13.

Occasionally, reduced effluent volume is a result of increased peritoneal absorption of fluid. This can occur with marked dehydration (low capillary hydrostatic pressure), increased plasma osmolality, or increased plasma protein concentration (increased oncotic pressure) so that fluid absorption into vessels is favored. Concurrent IV fluid therapy restores adequate capillary hydrostatic pressure and reduces oncotic pressure in peritoneal vessels, whereas increasing osmolality of the dialysate solution (e.g., 2.5 or 4.25% dextrose) establishes an osmotic gradient that favors ultrafiltration. Peritonitis also results in reduced recovery of effluent dialysate because of enhanced absorption of glucose and water.

▶ Complications

The complications of dialysis are summarized in Table 25–14. Most of these complications can be managed successfully. Hypoalbuminemia and dialysate retention (including that caused by mechanical obstruction of the catheter) are the most common complications observed in dogs and cats treated by peritoneal dialysis (Crisp et al. 1989). Dialysate retention, catheter obstruction (Fig.

TABLE 25–14. **Frequency of Complications During Dialysis in Dogs and Cats**

Complication	Percentage Affected
Hypoalbuminemia	41
Dialysate retention, catheter obstruction	30
Peritonitis	22
Hypochloremia	22
Subcutaneous leakage of dialysate	22
Limb edema	19
Hypokalemia	19
Hyponatremia	19
Hypomagnesemia	15*
Hyperkalemia	11

From: Crisp MS, Chew DJ, DiBartola SP et al.: Peritoneal dialysis in dogs and cats: 27 cases (1976–1987). *J Am Vet Med Assoc* 195:1262–1266, 1989.
*Serum magnesium concentration measured in 4 of 27 animals.

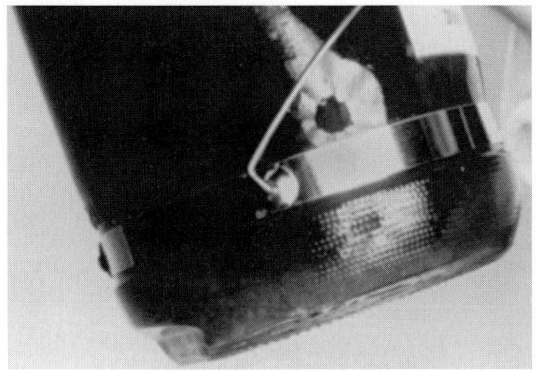

FIGURE 25–9. Turbidity of effluent dialysate caused by peritonitis.

25–8), and subcutaneous leakage of dialysate are less common with the modified surgical technique of column disc catheter placement (see earlier). Loss of body protein into effluent dialysate during numerous exchanges leads to development of hypoalbuminemia, the severity of which may be magnified by the presence of peritonitis.

Peritonitis

Bacteria may colonize the peritoneal cavity if they ascend through or around the dialysis catheter (Copley 1987; Werner 1988). Also, the low pH and high osmolality of dialysate solution may interfere with the phagocytic function of neutrophils (Nolph 1991).

Effluent dialysate may be blood tinged for 1 to 2 days after catheter placement. The gross appearance of the effluent dialysate should be monitored on a daily basis, because turbidity may be an early indicator of peritonitis (Fig. 25–9). Cytologic evaluation (including Gram's stain) and bacteriologic culture (anaerobic and aerobic) should be obtained whenever the effluent appears turbid. In the absence of turbidity, cytologic evaluation and Gram's staining of effluent dialysate two to three times per week may allow early detection of peritonitis. Normal effluent contains less than 50 white blood cells per microliter, and most of these are mononuclear cells. Turbidity of the effluent caused by bacterial peritonitis is associated with white blood cell counts above 100 to 200/μL and most of the cells observed on cytology are neutrophils (Thornhill 1983, 1984b). Weekly bacteriologic culture of effluent is recommended for monitoring of the patient, even in the absence of clinical signs or effluent turbidity.

Millipore filtration of effluent dialysate and bacteriologic culture of the filter membrane have been advocated to increase the likelihood of isolating small numbers of bacteria that may be responsible for peritonitis. With this technique, 60 mL of effluent dialysate is suctioned through a 0.2-μm filter, and the filter is placed on a blood agar plate for bacterial isolation. This technique is useful for isolating bacteria after antibacterial therapy and is superior to either direct agar plating or broth isolation using effluent dialysate (Thornhill 1983).

The use of a once-daily dilute iodine solution flush is recommended to prevent bacterial peritonitis during the first 5 days after catheter placement. This technique also is useful when breaks in sterile technique occur during

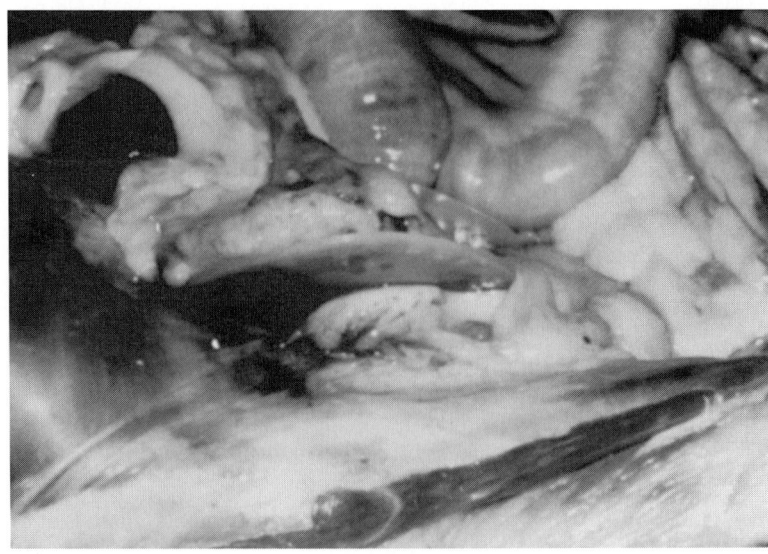

FIGURE 25–8. Obstruction of column disc catheter by omentum.

preparation, inflow, or outflow of dialysate. Iodine in combination with water forms hypiodous acid, which is microbicidal (Thornhill 1981). Routine addition of antibiotics to the dialysate solution as a prophylactic measure is not recommended during this period.

The following protocol is recommended for the iodine flush (Table 25–15): Effluent dialysate is drained from the abdomen and 0.9% NaCl (40 mL/kg up to a total volume of 1 L) is instilled and then immediately drained from the abdomen to remove dextrose, because dextrose converts iodine to inactive iodide. Next, 0.2 mL of a 2% iodine USP solution is added to 1 L of 0.9% NaCl. Povidine-iodine should not be substituted for USP iodine, because povidine may be associated with toxicity (Lagarde and Balton 1978). The iodine-containing 0.9% NaCl solution is infused, allowed to dwell for 4 min, drained, and dialysis is resumed. If bacterial peritonitis is suspected, iodine flushes are performed twice daily or the volume of 2% iodine USP added to 0.9% NaCl is doubled (0.4 vs. 0.2 mL/L) and iodine flushes are continued once daily. If control of peritonitis is not achieved within 24 h, iodine flushes are discontinued and antibiotics are added to the dialysate (Thornhill 1983).

Lethargy, anorexia, fever, abdominal pain, diarrhea, and vomiting are clinical signs that may be observed in animals with bacterial peritonitis. Gram-positive organisms predominated in some studies of peritonitis during dialysis in dogs (Thornhill 1983, 1984b) but gram-negative organisms predominated in another report (Crisp et al. 1989). Treatment with broad-spectrum antibiotics should be instituted after a diagnosis of peritonitis is made, and antimicrobial therapy is adjusted as necessary when the results of bacterial susceptibility tests become available. Conventional systemic administration of antimicrobial agents may not result in therapeutic concentrations of antibiotics in peritoneal fluid. Consequently, a portion of the daily dose of antimicrobial should be added to the dialysate solution.

Initially, cephalothin is recommended for empirical treatment of peritonitis while waiting for the results of bacterial cultures. Aminoglycosides have been recommended for treatment of gram-negative or polymicrobic peritonitis (Thornhill 1983, 1984b) but these drugs should be used only when absolutely necessary (e.g., life-threatening sepsis, culture results indicating no reasonable alternative drug) because of their potential for causing additional renal injury. Systemic concentrations of cephalothin in the therapeutic range can be achieved rapidly by peritoneal administration alone. A cephalothin dosage of 250 mg per 2-L bag of dialysate solution has been recommended during chronic maintenance dialysis

TABLE 25–15. Saline–Saline Plus Iodine Flush

1. Rapidly inflow 0.9% NaCl (no glucose).
2. Outflow immediately (no dwell).
3. Inflow 0.9% NaCl containing 0.2 mL iodine USP per liter.
4. Allow to dwell for 4 min.
5. Drain.
6. Resume dialysis.
7. Repeat procedure daily.

TABLE 25–16. Avoidance of Peritonitis

Strict adherence to aseptic technique
Daily saline–saline plus iodine flush
Maintenance of a closed system
Use of Y-connector system with three-way stopcock to direct inflow and outflow of dialysate
Disinfection of all fluid line connections when changing lines
Daily sterile dressing change
Keep animal clean and dry
Monitor appearance of effluent dialysate and submit for bacteriologic culture as needed

(Thornhill 1983, 1984b). If aminoglycosides are to be used, one loading dose of gentamicin or tobramycin is recommended at 4 mg/kg intramuscularly (IM) followed by a dosage of 10 mg per 2-L bag of dialysate solution to maintain systemic therapeutic concentrations (Thornhill 1983, 1984b). Other drugs can be added to the dialysate solution, and the following recommendations have been extrapolated from human medicine: penicillin G (50,000 U/L), ampicillin (50 mg/L), cloxacillin (100 mg/L), ticarcillin (100 mg/L), vancomycin (30 mg/L), amikacin (50 mg/L), clindamycin (50 mg/L), and trimethoprim-sulfadiazine (25 and 5 mg/L). Heparin should not be mixed with penicillin, vancomycin, or aminoglycosides (Thornhill 1983, 1984b).

Occasionally, peritonitis may not respond to these management recommendations. Removal of the peritoneal dialysis catheter and replacement with a new catheter may be required if peritonitis is not responsive to medical therapy. Nonresponsive peritonitis can be severe enough to cause death or warrant euthanasia. Measures to be used to avoid peritonitis are summarized in Table 25–16.

Other complications that have been reported during peritoneal dialysis in dogs include peritonitis associated with *Candida albicans* in one dog (Seligman et al. 1946) and pleural effusion in another dog (Carter et al. 1989). Pleural effusion after peritoneal dialysis has been observed in human patients (Lorentz 1979; Rudnick et al. 1979) and may be the result of movement of dialysate across the diaphragm via lymphatics. In one report, overhydration of the patient was reported to be the most common complication of peritoneal dialysis (Dzyban et al., in press, 2000). Overhydration was recognized by weight gain, increased central venous pressure, and impaired recovery of effluent dialysate. Use of hypertonic dialysate to promote ultrafiltration was recommended in overhydrated dialysis patients.

▶ Evaluating the Effectiveness of Dialysis

Record Keeping

Accurate record keeping is important during peritoneal dialysis to document exchange volumes and the patient's weight. Careful recording allows the clinician to assess the patient's hydration status and prevent progressive overhydration or dehydration. The patient's weight should

TABLE 25-17. Sample Flowchart for Monitoring Peritoneal Dialysis

Clinician: _____
Date: _____ ICU Day # _____
Weight: _____ lbs/kg _____ AM
Weight: _____ lbs/kg _____ PM

Dialysate Type:

Diagnosis:
Comments:

Exchange Number	Inflow: Time Start	Time Finish	Volume (mL)	Outflow: Time Start	Time Finish	Volume (mL)	Net Balance: (mL) Exchange/ Cumulative	IV Fluids: (mL) Exchange/ Cumulative	Urine: (mL) Exchange/ Cumulative	Medications Added:
1										
2										
3										
4										
5										
6										
7										
8										
9										

be obtained at least twice daily using the same scale and after the animal's bladder has been emptied. The inflow, dwell, and outflow times, as well as the volume of dialysate infused and drained, should be accurately recorded for each exchange. The net fluid balance of the patient includes the net flux of dialysate solution (inflow minus outflow), any IV fluid infused during the exchange period, and any urine produced (Table 25-17). Net fluid balance is calculated both for the individual exchange period and on a cumulative basis. The goal is to have a net fluid balance of zero when the volume of IV fluid administered and urine output have been considered.

If the patient has a positive fluid balance (i.e., less dialysate drained than infused and weight gain) and mechanical obstruction has been ruled out, it is necessary to alter the composition of dialysate by increasing its osmolality (i.e., increase the glucose concentration). If the patient has a negative fluid balance (i.e., more dialysate drained than infused and weight loss), it is necessary either to increase the IV infusion of fluid or to decrease dialysate osmolality (i.e., decrease the glucose concentration). Increasing dwell time also reduces effluent volume. Serial measurement of hematocrit and total plasma protein concentration provides additional useful information about the animal's hydration status. A sample flow sheet for peritoneal dialysis is presented in Table 25-17.

Laboratory Evaluation

Laboratory parameters that should be followed on a serial basis in patients undergoing peritoneal dialysis include BUN and serum creatinine concentrations, serum electrolyte (sodium, potassium, chloride, calcium, phosphorus) concentrations, and blood gas analysis (Table 25-18). Resolution of severe hyperkalemia, azotemia, and metabolic acidosis is mandatory for the patient's survival. Vomiting and decreased activity, strength, appetite, and sociability are other facets of uremia that can be improved or successfully managed with peritoneal dialysis in dogs and cats. Improved renal function (increased GFR, decreased serum creatinine or BUN concentrations) and resolution of underlying renal lesions as dialysis is withdrawn represent the final goals of dialysis therapy.

The serum concentrations of uremic solutes (e.g., urea, creatinine, phosphorus) reflect their clearance from extracellular fluid into dialysate, the rate of new solute generation, and solute redistribution from intracellular to

TABLE 25-18. Monitoring of the Patient

Time inflow begun (each exchange)
Time inflow completed (each exchange)
Dialysate volume infused (each exchange)
Time outflow begun (each exchange)
Time outflow completed (each exchange)
Effluent dialysate retrieved (each exchange)
Net balance per exchange and cumulative (each exchange)
Patient weight (twice daily using same scale)
Hematocrit/total plasma proteins (twice daily)
Serum chemistry (daily)*
Monitor effluent dialysate for infection (daily)

*Including BUN, creatinine, calcium, phosphorus, sodium, potassium, chloride, total CO_2.

extracellular fluid. It is common to see a rebound increase in BUN and serum creatinine concentrations shortly after interrupting acute dialysis. This effect is attributed to redistribution of uremic solutes from intracellular to extracellular fluid. Peritoneal dialysis is a cumulative process, and only a portion of the total body uremic solute load is removed during each exchange. Animals that are in a markedly catabolic state generate urea at a higher rate than animals in nitrogen balance. This effect has not been studied in dogs or cats undergoing dialysis in a clinical setting.

The magnitude of azotemia considered successful or appropriate during chronic peritoneal dialysis is a matter of debate. Survival is the first priority, followed by improvement of the animal's sense of well-being and establishment of oral nutrient intake. Individual animals, however, tolerate the same level of azotemia differently. For example, one dog with a serum creatinine concentration of 7.0 mg/dL may show few clinical signs and maintain a good appetite, whereas another dog with the same serum creatinine concentration may exhibit severe clinical signs (e.g., anorexia, lethargy, vomiting). Thus, dialysis must be individually tailored to alleviate the clinical manifestations of uremia. It remains to be determined whether there is a level of azotemia (and, hence, retention of uremic solutes) above which renal repair is hindered and below which recovery is facilitated. During dialysis, most dogs improve dramatically when BUN concentration falls below 90 mg/dL and serum creatinine concentration falls below 9 mg/dL. Maintenance regimens of CAPD usually do not result in complete correction of hyperphosphatemia. Intestinal phosphorus-binding agents usually are necessary along with provision of a low-phosphorus, low-protein diet to maintain normal serum phosphorus concentration.

Animals with severe azotemia in the maintenance phase of AIRF have a poor prognosis for return of normal renal structure and function, with or without dialysis. This may be a consequence of inadequate control of the uremic environment despite improvement in the animal's clinical condition and reduction in the concentrations of uremic solutes by dialysis. Insufficient numbers of dogs and cats with AIRF treated by peritoneal dialysis have been evaluated to determine whether more aggressive dialysis to control uremic solute accumulation would enhance resolution of underlying renal lesions and improve renal function and survival.

Peritoneal dialysis usually is performed on critically ill uremic animals. Dialysis may result in dramatic reductions in uremic solute concentrations and in resolution of disturbances of fluid, electrolyte, and acid-base balance. Parenteral fluid therapy, however, must be continued for several days until adequate control of the uremic environment has been achieved by dialysis. Parenteral fluid therapy may not be necessary during maintenance dialysis if the patient is able to sustain normal oral nutrient and fluid intake.

▶ Ending Dialysis

Ideally, peritoneal dialysis is continued until renal function returns to normal or until there is sufficient resumption of renal excretory function that the patient can survive without dialysis. In almost all instances, euthanasia is warranted if it becomes apparent that renal function cannot return to the extent that the animal can have a reasonable quality of life without dialysis. This decision is made only after serial evaluation of serum biochemistry results and renal histopathology. Dialysis is discontinued if the patient's quality of life is not improved to an acceptable degree after several days of mechanically successful peritoneal dialysis. Patients considered for euthanasia include those that do not improve biochemically, those in which uremic clinical signs (e.g., anorexia, lethargy, vomiting) do not improve despite successful reduction of azotemia, and those with intractable peritonitis.

REFERENCES

Ash SR and Janle EM: T-fluted peritoneal dialysis catheter. *Adv Peritoneal Dial* 9:223–226, 1993.

Birchard SJ, Chew DJ, Crisp MS, et al.: Modified technique for placement of a column disc peritoneal dialysis catheter. *J Am Anim Hosp Assoc* 24:663–666, 1988.

Brown EA, Kliger AS, and Finkelstein FO: Peritoneal dialysis clearances, a practical approach to the measurement of small and middle-molecule clearances. *Nephron* 21:310–316, 1978a.

Brown EA, Kliger AS, Goffinet J, et al.: Effect of hypertonic dialysate and vasodilators on peritoneal dialysis clearances in the rat. *Kidney Int* 13:271–277, 1978b.

Cancarini GC: The future of peritoneal dialysis: problems and hopes. *Nephrol Dial Transplant* 12:84–88, 1997.

Carter LJ, Wingfield WE, and Allen TA: Clinical experience with peritoneal dialysis in small animals. *Compend Cont Educ Pract Vet* 11:1335–1343, 1989.

Chew DJ: Urogenital emergencies. In Sherding RG (ed): *Medical Emergencies.* New York, Churchill Livingstone, pp. 187–212, 1985.

Copley JB: Prevention of peritoneal dialysis catheter-related infections. *Am J Kidney Dis* 10:401–407, 1987.

Cowgill LD: Application of peritoneal dialysis and hemodialysis in the management of renal failure. In Osborne CA and Fingo DR (eds): *Canine and Feline Nephrology and Urology.* Baltimore, Williams & Wilkins, pp. 573–596, 1995.

Cowgill LD and Langston CE: Role of hemodialysis in the management of dogs and cats with renal failure. *Vet Clin North Am* 26:1347–1378, 1996.

Crisp MS, Chew DJ, DiBartola SP, et al.: Peritoneal dialysis: 27 cases (1976–1987). *J Am Vet Med Assoc* 195:1262–1266, 1989.

Dhein CR: Hemodialysis in the dog. *Compend Contin Educ Pract Vet* 3:1031–1045, 1981.

DiBartola SP, Chew DJ, Tarr MJ, et al.: Hemodialysis of a dog with acute renal failure. *J Am Vet Med Assoc* 186:1323–1326, 1985.

Dzyban LA, Labato MA, and Ross LA: CVT Update: Peritoneal dialysis. In Bonagura JD (ed): *Kirk's Current Veterinary Therapy XIII.* Philadelphia, WB Saunders Co., pp. 859–861, 1999.

Dzyban LA, Ross LA, Labato MA, et al.: Peritoneal dialysis: A tool in veterinary critical care. *J Vet Emerg Crit Care,* in press, 2000.

Elzouki AY, Gruskin AB, Baluarte HJ, et al.: Developmental aspects of peritoneal dialysis kinetics in dogs. *Pediatr Res* 15:853–858, 1981.

Faller B: Amino acid-based peritoneal dialysis solution. *Kidney Int* 50:S81–S85, 1996.

Faller B: New peritoneal dialysis techniques and their evaluation. *Adv Nephrol* 27:189–221, 1998.

Feriani M: Buffers: Bicarbonate, lactate and pyruvate. *Kidney Int* 50:S75–S80, 1996.

Flessner MF: The peritoneal dialysis system: Importance of each component. *Perit Dial Int* 17:S91–S97, 1997.

Fox LE, Grauer GF, Dubielzig RR, et al.: Reversal of ethylene glycol–induced nephrotoxicosis in a dog. *J Am Vet Med Assoc* 191:1433–1435, 1987.

Gokal R: New strategies for peritoneal dialysis fluids. *Nephrol Dial Transplant* 12:74–77, 1997.

Gourley IM, Parker HR, Bell RL, et al.: Responses of nephrectomized dogs during hemodialysis. *Am J Vet Res* 34:1421–1425, 1973.

Grollman A, Turner LB, and McLean JA: Intermittent peritoneal lavage in nephrectomized dogs and its application to the human being. *Arch Intern Med* 87:379–390, 1951.

Hain H and Kessel M: Aspects of new solutions for peritoneal dialysis. *Nephrol Dial Transplant* 2:67–72, 1987.

Hamilton JW, Lasrich M, and Hirszel P: Peritoneal dialysis in the treatment of severe hypercalcemia. *J Dial* 4:129–138, 1980.

Henderson LW: Peritoneal ultrafiltration dialysis: Enhanced urea transfer using hypertonic peritoneal dialysis fluid. *J Clin Invest* 45:950–955, 1966.

Henderson LW: Hemodialysis. In Earley LE and Gottschalk CW (eds): *Strauss and Welt's Diseases of the Kidney*. Boston, Little, Brown & Co., pp. 421–462, 1979.

Henderson LW and Nolph KD: Altered permeability of the peritoneal membrane after using hypertonic peritoneal dialysis fluid. *J Clin Invest* 48:992–1001, 1969.

Jackson RF: The use of peritoneal dialysis in the treatment of uremia in dogs. *Vet Rec* 76:1481–1486, 1964.

Johnson RC, Bock F, Knab W, et al.: A model for study of the kinetics of continuous ambulatory peritoneal dialysis (CAPD). *Trans Am Soc Artif Intern Organs* 29:67–70, 1983.

Jones MR: Intraperitoneal amino acids: A therapy whose time has come? *Peritoneal Dial Int* 15:S67–S74, 1995.

Kirk RW: Peritoneal lavage in uremia in dogs. *J Am Vet Med Assoc* 131:101–103, 1957.

Kliger AS: Current concepts in peritoneal dialysis. *Nephron* 27:209–214, 1981.

Krediet RT: Advances in peritoneal dialysis: Towards improved efficacy and safety. *Blood Purif* 16:1–14, 1998.

Krediet RT, Douma CE, Pannekeet MH, et al.: Impact of different dialysis solutions on solute and water transport. *Perit Dial Int* 17:S17–S26, 1997.

Lagarde MC and Balton JS: Intraperitoneal povidone-iodine in experimental peritonitis. *Ann Surg* 187:613–619, 1978.

Lane IF, Carter LJ, and Lappin MR: Peritoneal dialysis: An update on methods and usefulness. In Kirk RW and Bonagura JD (eds): *Kirk's Current Veterinary Therapy XI*. Philadelphia, WB Saunders Co., pp. 865–870, 1992.

Langston CE, Cowgill LD, and Spano JA: Applications and outcome of hemodialysis in cats: A review of 29 cases. *J Vet Intern Med* 11:348–355, 1997.

Lorentz WB: Acute hydrothorax during peritoneal dialysis. *Pediatrics* 94:417–419, 1979.

Mactier RA and Khanna R: Absorption of fluid and solutes from the peritoneal cavity, theoretic and therapeutic implications and applications. *Trans Am Soc Artif Intern Organs* 35:122–131, 1989.

Mactier RA, Khanna R, and Twardowski ZJ: Role of peritoneal cavity lymphatic absorption in peritoneal dialysis. *Kidney Int* 32:165–172, 1987.

Maher JF: Peritoneal transport rates: Mechanisms, limitations, and methods for augmentation. *Kidney Int* 18:S117–S120, 1980.

Mashita T, Yasuda J, Iijima M, et al.: Short-term hemodialysis in dogs and cats with total uretic obstruction. *Jpn J Vet Res* 45:59–65, 1997.

Meengs W, Greene JA, and Weller JM: Peritoneal clearance of urea and potassium and protein removal during acute peritonitis in dogs. *J Lab Clin Med* 76:903–906, 1970.

Mistry CD and Gokal R: Optimal use of gluose polymer (icodextrin) in peritoneal dialysis. *Perit Dial Int* 16:S104–S108, 1996.

Nolph KD: Peritoneal dialysis. In Brenner BM and Rector FC (eds): *The Kidney*. Philadelphia, WB Saunders Co., pp. 2299–2335, 1991.

Pannekeet MM, Mulder JB, Weening JJ, et al.: Demonstration of aquaporin-CHIP in peritoneal tissue of uremic and CAPD patients. *Perit Dial Int* 16:S54–S57, 1996.

Pannekeet MMH and Krediet RT: Water channels in the peritoneum. *Perit Dial Int* 16:225–229, 1996.

Parker HR: Current status of peritoneal dialysis. In Kirk RW (ed): *Current Veterinary Therapy VII*. Philadelphia, WB Saunders Co., pp. 1106–1111, 1980.

Parker HR, Gourley IM, and Bell RL: Current developments in peritoneal and hemodialysis. Gaines 22nd Veterinary Symposium, Stillwater, OK, pp. 3–15, 1972.

Parks J: Peritoneal lavage. *J Am Vet Med Assoc* 165:148–149, 1974.

Peers E and Gokal R: Icodextrin provides long dwell peritoneal dialysis and maintenance of intraperitoneal volume. *Artif Organs* 22:8–12, 1998.

Reuler JB: Peritoneal dialysis in the management of hypothermia. *JAMA* 240:2289–2290, 1978.

Robson M, Oreopoulos DG, Izatt S, et al.: Influence of exchange volume and dialysate flow rate on solute clearance in peritoneal dialysis. *Kidney Int* 14:486–490, 1978.

Rubin J, McFarland S, Hellems EW, et al.: Peritoneal dialysis during peritonitis. *Kidney Int* 19:460–464, 1981.

Rubin J, Jones Q, Quillen E, et al.: A model of longterm peritoneal dialysis in the dog. *Nephron* 35:259–263, 1983.

Rubin J, Jones Q, Planch A, et al.: The importance of the abdominal viscera to peritoneal dialysis in the dog. *Am J Med Sci* 292:203–208, 1986.

Rudnick MR, Cohen RM, Gordon A, et al.: Fluid-electrolyte complications of dialysis. In Maxwell MH, Kleeman CR, and Narins RG (eds): *Clinical Disorders of Fluid and Electrolyte Metabolism*. New York, McGraw-Hill Book Co., pp. 1053–1103, 1987.

Rudnick MR, Coyle JF, Beck LH, et al.: Acute massive hydrothorax complicating peritoneal dialysis, report of 2 cases and a review of the literature. *Clin Nephrol* 12:38–44, 1979.

Seligman AM, Frank HA, and Fine J: Treatment of experimental uremia by means of peritoneal irrigation. *J Clin Invest* 25:211–219, 1946.

Shahar R and Holmberg DL: Pleural dialysis in the management of acute renal failure in two dogs. *J Am Vet Med Assoc* 187:952–954, 1985.

Simmons EE, Lockard BS, Moncrief JW, et al.: Experience with continuous ambulatory peritoneal dialysis and maintenance of a surgically anephric dog. *Southwest Vet* 33:129–135, 1980.

Thornhill JA: Peritoneal dialysis in the dog and cat: An update. *Compend Contin Educ Pract Vet* 3:20–34, 1981.

Thornhill JA: Peritonitis associated with peritoneal dialysis: Diagnosis and treatment. *J Am Vet Med Assoc* 182:721–724, 1983.

Thornhill JA: Hemodialysis. In Bovee KC (ed): *Canine Nephrology*. Media, PA, Harwal, pp. 755–802, 1984a.

Thornhill JA: Therapeutic strategies involving antimicrobial treatment of small animals with peritonitis. *J Am Vet Med Assoc* 185:1181–1184, 1984b.

Thornhill JA, Ash SR, Dhein CR, et al.: Peritoneal dialysis with the Purdue column disc catheter. *Minn Vet* 20:27–33, 1980.

Thornhill JA, Hartman J, Boon GD, et al.: Support of an anephric dog for 54 days with ambulatory peritoneal dialysis and a newly designed peritoneal catheter. *Am J Vet Res* 45:161–182, 1984.

Twardowski ZJ: Peritoneal dialysis current technology and techniques. *Postgrad Med* 85:161–182, 1989.

Vale JA, Widdop B, and Bluett NH: Ethylene glycol poisoning. *Postgrad Med* 52:598–602, 1976.

Vanholder RC and Lameire NH: Osmotic agents in peritoneal dialysis. *Kidney Int* 50:S86–S91, 1996.

Wells IC, Durr MP, Grabner BJ, et al.: Experimental study of chronic ambulatory peritoneal dialysis. *Clin Physiol Biochem* 3:8–15, 1985.

Welton DE, Mattox KL, Miller RR, et al.: Treatment of profound hypothermia. *JAMA* 240:2291–2292, 1978.

Werner HP: Disinfectants in dialysis: Dangers, drawbacks and disinformation. *Nephron* 49:1–8, 1988.

Zelman A, Gisser D, and Whittman PJ: Augmentation of peritoneal dialysis efficiency with programmed hyper/hyposmotic dialysates. *Trans Am Soc Artif Intern Organs* 23:203–209, 1977.

CHAPTER 26

Hemodialysis

LARRY D. COWGILL   DENISE A. ELLIOTT

Hemodialysis is a therapeutic procedure that integrates the physical principles of diffusion, convection, and ultrafiltration to correct the volume, electrolyte, and acid-base disorders and toxicities associated with uremia. Hemodialysis is similar conceptually to peritoneal dialysis (familiar to most veterinarians) except that an artificial membrane replaces the peritoneal lining as an exchange surface. Blood is interposed directly with the dialysate across the membrane, and the dialytic process occurs outside the animal's body. Solutes and water transfer across the artificial membrane along diffusive and hydrostatic gradients between plasma water and the dialysate in a hemodialyzer. During dialysis, waste solutes and excess water are removed from the animal in a manner analogous to their excretion by healthy kidneys.

Of the 260,000 human patients with end-stage renal disease in the United States, 214,000 receive maintenance dialysis. Approximately 86% of these patients receive hemodialysis compared with various forms of peritoneal dialysis (Renal Data System 1997). The application of dialytic therapies and especially hemodialysis has been limited in veterinary practice by lack of expertise and the technical aspects of dialysis delivery. In the past 5 to 8 years, these constraints have lessened with the evolution of modern dialysis equipment and procedures better suited to dogs and cats. These changes have heightened the interest in, applications of, and utilization of hemodialysis in veterinary therapeutics (Cowgill 1995a; Cowgill and Langston 1996; Cowgill and Maretzki 1995).

▶ Historical Perspective and Current Applications

The conception of modern hemodialysis can be traced to the discovery of the "osmotic membrane" by Thomas Graham in 1854 (Drukker 1989). Hemodialysis was first performed in experimental dogs in 1913 by Abel, Rowntree, and Turner and now has returned to clinical application in the species in which the technology was inaugurated. Veterinary application of hemodialysis was described first by Butler in 1968, but these early efforts were foiled by technical difficulties that have largely been resolved. Parker and colleagues (Parker et al. 1972; Gourley et al. 1973) extended these pioneering techniques using single-pass dialysate systems and silicone-Teflon arteriovenous shunts for vascular access. Clinical application of hemodialysis for uremic dogs was reported in the early 1980s (Cowgill 1980; Dhein 1981; Thornhill 1984), and the feasibility of hemodialysis in cats was demonstrated in the 1990s with the availability of neonatal dialyzers, dialysis catheters, and blood tubing sets (Cowgill and Langston 1996; Langston et al. 1997). Currently, there are four veterinary hemodialysis centers in the United States, and the outlook for expansion of this therapy is promising (see Appendix).

The principal application of hemodialysis is for the supportive management of acute and chronic renal failure. Conventional therapies cannot approach the efficacy, efficiency, and clinical benefits of hemodialysis for these conditions. Hemodialysis should be instituted when the morbidity or pending mortality associated with severe uremia cannot be alleviated by conservative therapies.

Acute Renal Failure

Acute renal failure is the most common indication for hemodialysis in dogs and cats (Cowgill 1995a; Cowgill and Langston 1996; Cowgill and Maretzki 1995). Without dialysis, animals with severe acute renal failure generally die from complications of uremia before renal repair can be achieved. Hemodialysis extends the life expectancy of these animals and provides the potential for recovery to occur. Selection of patients has been predicted on the subjective criteria predicting the likelihood for repair of the renal damage and return of adequate renal function. However, these criteria are inadequate and must be redefined for patients receiving hemodialysis. Whereas 3 to 4 weeks have been benchmark intervals to define reversible from irreversible renal failure in the past, with dialytic support the time for such decisions extends to 4 to 6 months.

Dialysis should be initiated when the clinical consequences of the azotemia, fluid, electrolyte, and acid-base disturbances cannot be managed with medical therapy. Animals with severe oliguria or anuria in which an effective diuresis cannot be maintained with replacement fluids, osmotic or chemical diuretics, and renal vasodilators should be transferred immediately to a referral center where dialysis can be performed. Further attempts with conservative therapies generally are unproductive, result in deterioration of the animal's condition, delay the start of dialysis, and predispose the animal to life-threatening hypervolemia.

Chronic Renal Failure

The use of hemodialysis in animals with end-stage renal disease is considerably less than its use in acute uremia, despite its prevalent use to manage human patients with chronic renal failure (Renal Data System 1997; Pastan 1998). Improved dialysis equipment and techniques, the increased sophistication of veterinary practice and pet owners, and the development of medical adjuncts for the management of chronic renal failure have extended the use of intermittent hemodialysis for the management of chronic renal failure in animals. The efficacy of medical approaches for the treatment of chronic uremia becomes limited as the serum creatinine concentration exceeds 7 mg/dL, and the clinical manifestations of uremia become overt as the blood urea nitrogen (BUN) concentration exceeds 90 to 100 mg/dL. At this stage of disease, some form of renal replacement therapy is necessary to ameliorate the azotemia, electrolyte and acid-base disorders, nutritional deficiencies, and systemic hypertension complicating chronic renal failure. Intermittent hemodialysis is required indefinitely for animals with end-stage renal disease; however, many pet owners desire short periods of dialytic support to adjust to the inevitable outcome of the animal's disease.

Finite periods of hemodialysis may be indicated for the preoperative management of animals awaiting renal transplantation. Many candidates for renal transplantation have overt nutritional deficiencies, anemia, and metabolic disorders that would preclude successful transplantation. Hemodialysis facilitates the conditioning of these animals otherwise unsuitable or at attendant risk for the surgery. Postoperatively, hemodialysis is used during periods of delayed graft function, acute rejection, or pyelonephritis to stabilize the animal until the episode has resolved.

Acute Intoxications and Fluid Overloads

Dialysis is uniquely suited for the management of acute poisoning when the toxin is not bound to plasma proteins and is dialyzable (Garella 1988; Garella and Lorch 1993). Rapid elimination of a toxin and its metabolites from the body ameliorates or prevents its harmful effects. Hemodialysis is particularly effective for antifreeze poisoning and advantageous over treatment with alcohol or 4-methylpyrazole, which delay the metabolism of ethylene glycol without facilitating its removal from the body. Timely and aggressive hemodialysis can eliminate ethylene glycol and its metabolites from animals before development of renal damage (Fig 26-1). Oliguric animals have an impaired ability to excrete ethylene glycol and its metabolites and may have sustained toxic concentrations as late as 7 days after exposure despite appropriate administration of either alcohol or 4-methylpyrazole. Institution of hemodialysis at these delayed times eliminates the residual toxins and precludes ongoing renal injury.

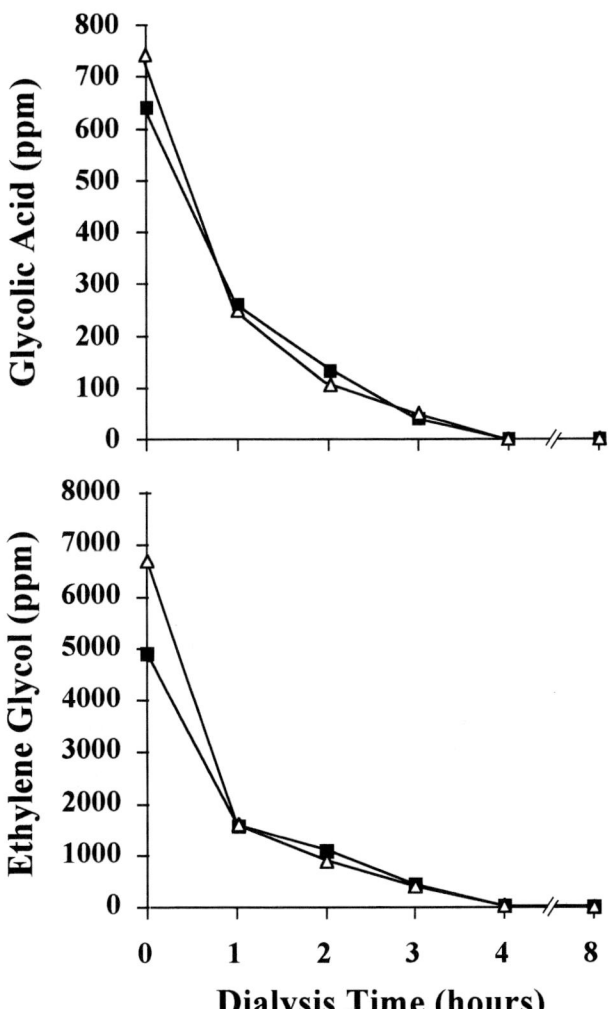

FIGURE 26-1. Changes in serum glycolic acid and ethylene glycol concentrations in two dogs treated with hemodialysis after simultaneous exposure to antifreeze 4 to 6 h before presentation. Despite the extremely high initial concentrations of these toxicants, both dogs recovered uneventfully with no evident renal injury after a single dialysis treatment.

Overhydration (associated systemic hypertension, ascites, peripheral and pulmonary edema, pleural effusion, and congestive heart failure) are common complications of aggressive fluid therapy in animals with acute uremia. Animals with end-stage renal disease may have insufficient excretory ability to eliminate intravenous or subcutaneous fluid treatments, oral fluid supplements, or dietary water. These excessive fluid loads can be removed readily by the ultrafiltration capability of hemodialysis. Ultrafiltration is indicated for animals with iatrogenic overhydration, life-threatening pulmonary edema, or congestive heart failure and for animals with limited excretory capacity receiving therapies requiring delivery of large volumes of fluid.

▶ Physical Principles of Hemodialysis

Hemodialysis is a process whereby the composition of blood is altered by exposure to a contrived solution, the dialysate, across a semipermeable membrane. A semipermeable membrane can be conceptualized as a limiting sheet perforated by pores. Water and low-molecular-weight solutes can pass readily through the membrane pores, but the movement of larger solutes, plasma proteins, and the cellular components of blood is limited by pore size. The passage of solutes through the membrane occurs by either diffusion or ultrafiltration (convection) (Sargent and Gotch 1989).

The movement of solutes by diffusion results from their random thermal motion in solution. A low-molecular-weight solute collides randomly with the semipermeable membrane. If the solute encounters a membrane pore of appropriate size, it can pass to the opposite side of the membrane. A solute is as likely to move in one direction as the other. If the concentration of solute (e.g., urea) on one side of the membrane is higher than its concentration on the opposite side, more random solute movement is likely to occur on the side of the higher solute concentration yielding net movement down the concentration gradient of the solute. If adequate time is allowed, the solute concentrations on both sides of the membrane equalize, the gradient is abolished, and filtration equilibrium is achieved. At filtration equilibrium, there is no further change in composition of the respective solutions (Van Stone and Daugirdas 1994). To prevent filtration equilibrium and maximize diffusion during hemodialysis, blood and dialysate are continuously replenished to maintain the diffusion gradients.

The rate of solute diffusion is determined collectively by the concentration gradient for the solute, the velocity of kinetic motion, and the permeability of the semipermeable membrane. The higher the molecular weight of the solute, the lower its kinetic motion and the slower its transport. Small solutes such as urea (60 daltons) diffuse faster than larger solutes such as creatinine (113 daltons), and the plasma concentration of urea decreases faster than that of larger solutes during the course of dialysis (Mujais and Schmidt 1995). The permeability of the membrane is determined by the thickness of the membrane, its effective surface area, and the number, size, and shape of the pores or diffusion channels (Mujais and Schmidt 1995). Resistance to solute transport is high if the membrane is thick, if the number of pores is low, or if the pores are small. Membrane resistance also is increased by unstirred layers of fluid on either side of the membrane, which decrease the effective concentration gradient at the membrane surface. The unstirred layer is dissipated by the flow rate of dialysate and blood and by the dialyzer design.

The second mechanism of solute movement across a semipermeable membrane is convective transport associated with ultrafiltration. Ultrafiltration occurs when water is driven through the membrane by hydrostatic or osmotic pressure (Henderson 1989). Flow occurs from the solution at higher pressure to the solution at lower pressure. Diffusible solutes dissolved in the water then are swept through the membrane by solvent drag. Unlike diffusive transport, convective transport does not require a concentration gradient across the membrane to achieve solute transfer. The transmembrane hydrostatic pressure gradient between the blood and dialysate compartments and the hydraulic permeability and surface area of the membrane determine the rate of ultrafiltration and solute transfer. During hemodialysis, the blood pump generates a positive pressure in the blood compartment of the dialyzer, and a vacuum pump creates a negative pressure in the dialysate compartment to establish transmembrane pressure. Ultrafiltration thus is controlled by adjusting the transmembrane pressure by changing the positive pressure in the blood compartment or, more commonly, by altering the negative pressure in the dialysate compartment. The permeability of dialysis membranes to water varies with the thickness and pore size of the membrane. The hydraulic permeability of a hemodialyzer is rated by its ultrafiltration coefficient, K_{uf}, defined as milliliters of fluid transferred per hour across the dialyzer per mm Hg transmembrane pressure. A minimum transmembrane pressure of 25 mm Hg is required for ultrafiltration to occur because the oncotic pressure of plasma proteins favors fluid reabsorption and opposes ultrafiltration (Mujais and Schmidt 1995). Convective transport may make a significant additional contribution to diffusive transport, especially for removal of large solutes when highly permeable membranes are used.

Vital electrolytes are preserved by formulating their dialysate concentrations to be equivalent to their corresponding concentrations in plasma so as to create filtration equilibrium and no net solute transfer. Solutes depleted from the animal by renal failure (e.g., bicarbonate) may be replenished by formulating a higher concentration of these solutes in dialysate than in blood.

▶ Hemodialysis Techniques for Dogs and Cats

The techniques for performing hemodialysis in animal patients have been adopted conceptually from those used in dialysis of humans. The delivery of hemodialysis is a technically and professionally demanding process that requires (1) high-volume vascular access; (2) a hemodialyzer or artificial kidney; (3) an extracorporeal blood circuit to deliver blood to the hemodialyzer and return blood to the patient; (4) a dialysis delivery system to formulate and deliver the dialysate, control blood flow in the extracorporeal circuit, deliver anticoagulant, and monitor the integrity and safety of the entire dialysis process; (5) physiologic monitoring equipment; (6) a source of purified water; and (7) a specifically trained and dedicated nursing and professional staff (Cowgill and Langston 1996).

Vascular Access

Vascular access is the crux and the curse of hemodialysis. It is required for regular and reproducible delivery of large volumes of blood to and from the body and hemodialyzer. Transcutaneous (double-lumen) venous dialysis catheters have become mainstays for both acute and chronic dialysis in animals. Immediate or short-term vascular access, as required for ethylene glycol intoxication or critically ill animals, can be achieved with polyurethane

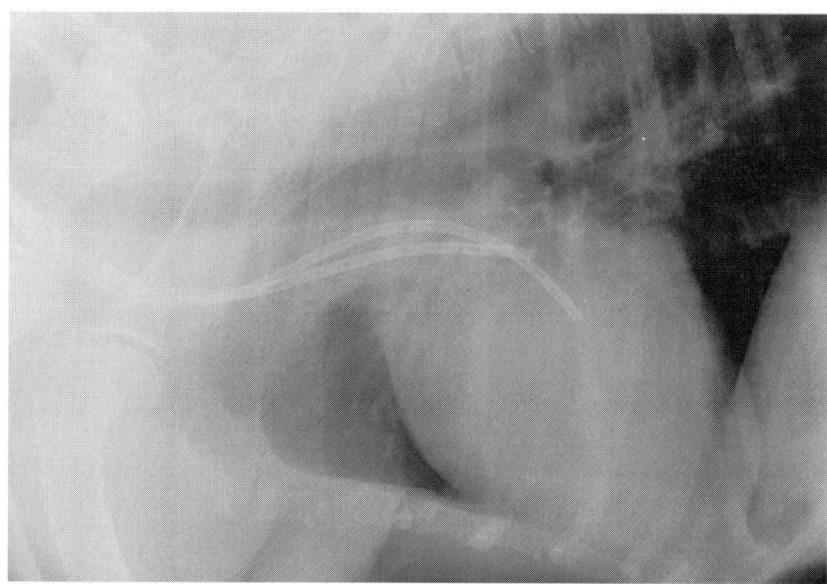

FIGURE 26-2. Lateral thoracic radiograph illustrating transcutaneous Tesio twin single-lumen catheters positioned in the right atrium for hemodialysis in a dog.

or silicone catheters* placed percutaneously using local analgesia. These temporary catheters are appropriate for courses of hemodialysis lasting less than 1 week. If more extended dialysis is required, a permanent catheter often can be replaced percutaneously in the same vascular site.

Long-term or semipermanent vascular access is accomplished with silicone double-lumen or twin-lumen dialysis catheters placed by either percutaneous or simple surgical techniques. Although seemingly less invasive, percutaneous placement techniques are rarely quicker and often promote more vascular damage and hemorrhage than a direct surgical cutdown and venotomy. With either technique, the catheter is advanced to the right atrium or cranial vena cava (Fig. 26–2). The extravascular portion of the catheter is tunneled subcutaneously to exit the skin in the cranial cervical area of the neck. A subcutaneous Dacron cuff on permanent catheters helps stabilize their position, helps prevent accidental displacement from the vessel, and impairs extension of local infection. Permanent dialysis catheters are available in a variety of cross-sectional areas, lengths, and geometric shapes to accommodate differences in the size and shape of the animal, flow characteristics of the vessel, and thrombogenicity. The Quinton Instrument PermCath† has been used most consistently for hemodialysis in dogs. The PermCath is available in lengths from 28 to 46 cm and diameters from 4.9 to 5.9 mm. The external jugular vein in cats generally is too small to permit percutaneous placement, but 8 Fr, 18-cm neonatal dialysis catheters‡ can be inserted through a transverse venotomy in the external jugular vein. Frequently, the jugular vein in cats is smaller than these neonatal catheters and surgical placement can be difficult. The Tesio catheter° with twin vascular segments represents a departure from conventional catheter geometry but appears advantageous compared with side-by-side or coaxial double-lumen designs for prolonged serviceability, reduced thrombogenicity, enhanced flow characteristics, reduced recirculation, reduced risk of infection, and more flexible replacement characteristics (see Fig. 26–2) (Tesio et al. 1994; Prabhu et al. 1997).

Between dialysis sessions, each lumen of the catheter is filled with heparin† (500–1000 U/mL in cats, 1000–2500 U/mL in dogs) to prevent intraluminal thrombosis. Heparin slowly diffuses from the ports of the catheter, which predisposes the patient to systemic heparinization and bleeding if the concentration of heparin in the catheter is too high for the size of the animal. Aspirin is administered at 1 to 5 mg/kg once daily (dogs) or every 48 h (cats) to prevent intravascular thrombosis around the catheter. Transcutaneous venous catheters can remain serviceable for many months if properly maintained.

Hemodialysis catheters must be replaced if they become physically damaged, recurrently occluded, infected, or fail to provide adequate blood flow. It is preferable to place the new catheter in the opposite jugular vein rather than in the previous access site. Temporary polyurethane catheters are less flexible than silicone catheters and are prone to kinking and physical damage but often can be replaced with a permanent catheter over a guide wire without additional surgery. Dialysis catheters must be used only for dialysis procedures and handled only by dialysis personnel to prevent inadvertent injection of the heparin lock or bacterial contamination. They are the "lifeline" for dialysis patients and should never be used for any other purpose as a convenience.

Arteriovenous fistulas and grafts are surgically constructed subcutaneous anastomoses created from native

---

*Mahurkar dual-lumen catheter, Quinton Instrument Co., Seattle, WA; Flexicon II, Vas-Cath, Mississauga, Ontario, Canada; Hemo-Cath silicone double-lumen catheter, MedComp, Harleysville, PA.

†PermCath dual-lumen catheters, Quinton Instrument Co., Seattle, WA.

‡Pediatric Hemo-Cath (diameter 8 Fr; length 18 cm), MedComp, Harleysville, PA.

°Bio-Flex Tesio catheter, MedComp, Harleysville, PA.

†Heparin sodium injection, Organon, West Orange, NJ.

vessels or synthetic vascular materials, respectively. Both interconnect a peripheral artery (usually the radial artery) and a peripheral vein (cephalic vein) and are the access of choice for human patients with chronic renal failure (Brescia et al. 1989; Berkoben and Schwab 1995). When fully serviceable, they provide a large subcutaneous channel with a natural endothelial lining that is penetrated with percutaneous needles. Neither arteriovenous fistulas nor grafts have been used for routine dialysis in dogs and cats, but they will evolve as long-term maintenance hemodialysis becomes commonplace for animals with chronic renal failure.

Artificial Kidneys (Hemodialyzers)

The artificial kidney shares many characteristics with the native kidneys it replaces. Modern hemodialyzers have a high capacity to remove solutes of both low (<300 daltons) and middle (300 to 5000 daltons) molecular mass from the blood while selectively retaining plasma proteins and the cellular components of blood. The hemodialyzer must regulate water removal independently of solute flux and must be sterile, nontoxic, and free of adverse biologic interactions with the patient (Walton and Cheung 1995; Hoenich et al. 1989). Modern hemodialyzers are compact, disposable, efficient, and reliable and may be tailored to the size, biologic compatibility, and excretory requirements of individual patients (Hoenich et al. 1989). Hemodialyzers are classified as hollow fiber or parallel plate according to the physical characteristics and arrangement of the membrane material used in their construction.

The hollow fiber design is used most commonly in North America for dialysis of human patients and is used exclusively for hemodialysis of companion animals in the United States. In hollow fiber dialyzers, blood is directed through the lumens of bundled small-diameter capillary fibers (similar to soda straws) while the dialysate is distributed around the fiber bundle in a countercurrent direction. This design provides a large ratio of surface area to blood volume and low blood flow resistance. The thinness and porosity of the fiber wall allow efficient solute diffusion, yet it is sufficiently rigid to accommodate high transmembrane pressures for ultrafiltration of water. Hollow fiber dialyzers have effective surface areas between 0.22 and 2.5 m². Pediatric hollow fiber dialyzers have blood compartment volumes between 18 and 60 mL, making them well suited for dialysis of veterinary patients.

The performance and biocompatibility of hemodialyzers are determined by the composition of the membrane material. Conventional (cellulosic) dialyzers are composed of chemically modified cellulose membranes (cuprophan, regenerated cellulose, cellulose acetate, cellulose triacetate, hemophan) (Hoenich et al. 1989). Conventional dialyzers have good diffusion characteristics for low-molecular-weight solutes but are less effective for the middle molecules preferentially removed by convection associated with ultrafiltration. In general, cellulosic dialyzers have lower ultrafiltration coefficients and are more bioreactive than synthetic membrane dialyzers. (Hoenich et al. 1989).

High-efficiency and high-flux dialyzers have synthetic polymer membranes (polycarbonate, polyacrylonitrile, polysulfone) that have superior diffusion and ultrafiltration characteristics, greater mechanical strength, lower thrombogenicity, and better biocompatibility than cellulosic dialyzers (Walton and Cheung 1995; Hoenich et al. 1989; Woffindin and Hoenich 1988; Ward et al. 1993). High-flux dialyzers permit shortened treatment intervals and improved removal of fluid, solute, and middle molecules but are more costly than conventional dialyzers and must be reused several times to be cost effective.

Despite the benefits of synthetic membranes, cellulosic dialyzers have remained the standard for dialysis of animals because of their low cost, disposability, and adequate solute removal and ultrafiltration characteristics. Hemophan-based cellulosic dialyzers provide better solute removal and ultrafiltration characteristics, reduced heparin requirements, and improved biocompatibility compared with other cellulosic materials. Their performance compares favorably with that of many synthetic polymer membranes yet they retain single-use economy (Ward et al. 1993; Falkenhagen et al. 1987; Cases et al. 1997; Hoenich et al. 1995; Schaefer et al. 1987; Lucchi et al. 1989).

Extracorporeal Circuit

The extracorporeal circuit is the route of the patient's blood during hemodialysis (Fig. 26–3). For safe dialysis,

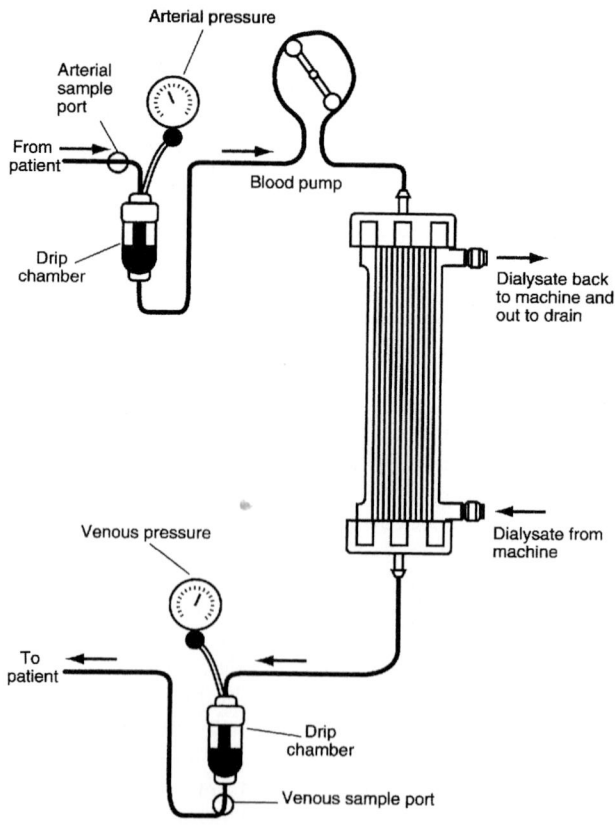

FIGURE 26–3. Illustration of the extracorporeal blood path used for hemodialysis. The blood and dialysate flow in opposite (countercurrent) directions in the hemodialyzer. (From Burrows-Hudson S and Hudson MV: Module IV hemodialysis devices. In *Core Curriculum for the Dialysis Technician.* Thousand Oaks, CA, Medical Media Publishing, p. 34, 1992.)

the extracorporeal path must be monitored for blood leaks, disconnected or kinked tubing, and clots or air in the blood path. These dangers are detected by sensors in response to changes in segmental pressure in the circuit. The sensors send an alarm to the delivery system when conditions are unsafe, and blood flow is discontinued until the conditions have been corrected.

The small size of animal patients requires that the inclusive volume of the extracorporeal circuit be minimized with use of neonatal and pediatric blood tubing sets and hemodialyzers. The extracorporeal circuit should contain less than 10% of the patient's blood volume unless the circuit is primed with compatible blood or volume expanders (Fine and Tejani 1994). A pediatric blood circuit (including the hemodialyzer) contains 100 to 130 mL of blood and safely accommodates dogs larger than 14 kg. The volume of neonatal blood circuits is 50 to 65 mL and is appropriate for dogs larger than 7 kg. For cats and small dogs weighing between 2.5 and 7.0 kg, a 60-mL extracorporeal circuit represents 17 to 33% of the animal's total blood volume and imposes risks of hypotension and hypovolemia throughout the dialysis session. These animals can be dialyzed safely by priming the extracorporeal circuit with a 3 to 6% dextran 70 solution.*

Dialysis Delivery Systems

The dialysis delivery system (the hemodialysis machine) is a complex, microprocessor-controlled machine that integrates, monitors, and controls the delivery of the hemodialysis treatment to the patient. Minimally, the dialysis delivery system formulates the dialysate from concentrated salt and bicarbonate solutions; monitors the dialysate composition, temperature, and pH; and regulates extracorporeal blood flow, delivery of anticoagulant, and the rate of ultrafiltration. The sophistication of the delivery system determines the type of dialytic therapy that can be provided. The dialysate proportioning system mixes a concentrated solute solution with highly purified water to generate a diluted dialysate solution of proper composition. Older systems produce a fixed-ratio dilution (e.g., 1:35) in which the composition of the preformed concentrate determines the final dialysate composition. More sophisticated proportioning systems use variable-ratio dilutions that permit moderate adjustment and modeling of dialysate composition throughout the treatment. The proportioning system also monitors the composition of the dialysate by measuring its conductivity and pH to ensure that it remains within safe tolerances. Internal alarms are activated if any alteration of conductivity, pH, or temperature or blood leaks are detected, and the dialysate is diverted (bypassed) away from the dialyzer to protect the patient until the abnormality is corrected.

Bicarbonate is the most appropriate buffer replacement for the dialysate solutions, but its instability and precipitation with calcium and magnesium in solution prompted the use of acetate for base-generating equivalents in commercial dialysate. The high acetate load delivered by an acetate-based dialysate to small or critically ill animals can induce vasodilatation, reduced myocardial contractility, hypotension, and hemodynamic instability (Ward 1995; Ledebo 1993). Hypoxemia, hypoventilation, nausea, vomiting, and fatigue also may be recognized (Cowgill 1995a; Cowgill and Maretzki 1995). To prevent these effects, bicarbonate-based dialysate became the current industry standard with the advent of high-flux dialyzers. The production of bicarbonate-based dialysate requires separate proportioning systems for the bicarbonate concentrate and the concentrate for other solutes. To prevent precipitation of calcium and magnesium with the bicarbonate, the interim solutions are mixed when appropriately diluted to form the final solution. All dialysis in cats has been performed with bicarbonate-based dialysate, as hemodynamic concerns related to the relatively large extracorporeal volume would be exacerbated by acetate.

Purified Water System

The most abundant component of dialysate is water. During a single dialysis session, the animal's blood is exposed to approximately 150 L of water. The magnitude of this exposure requires that the water used to generate the dialysate be chemically pure. Minute traces of routine impurities, water treatment chemicals (fluorine, chloramine), herbicides, bacteria, viruses, or endotoxins that are safe in drinking water constitute a formidable risk to dialysis patients. Supply water must be processed sequentially with particulate filters, carbon sorbents for organic solutes, water softeners to reduce excessive minerals, and deionization beds to remove inorganic cations and anions. Reverse osmosis is used as a final treatment to remove residual contaminants. The supply plumbing must be maintained free from bacterial and chemical contamination and leachable contaminants so that the purified water is not altered en route to the delivery system.

Ultrafiltration Control Systems

The ultrafiltration control system regulates the rate and volume of ultrafiltration during dialysis. Newer dialysis machines have precise volumetric measuring systems in which the desired volume or rate of ultrafiltration is programmed at the start of the dialysis session and fluid removal is automatically and accurately regulated throughout the treatment. Ultrafiltration controllers are essential for small animal dialysis to prevent subtle or undetected fluctuations in transmembrane pressure from inducing volume depletion or hypotension.

Miscellaneous Monitoring Equipment

A variety of monitoring equipment is required for safety during hemodialysis and to monitor trends in critically ill animals. Hypotension is an ever present concern during hemodialysis, and blood pressure must be monitored at regular intervals. It is preferable to have both indirect Doppler and oscillometric blood pressure monitors available to obviate inconsistencies of blood pressure measurement in animals.

Predialysis coagulation time must be determined to prescribe the initial dose of heparin to anticoagulate the animal. Subsequent coagulation times help regulate ongoing heparin requirements during the treatment to prevent

---

*6% Gentran 70, Baxter Healthcare Corp., Deerfield, IL.

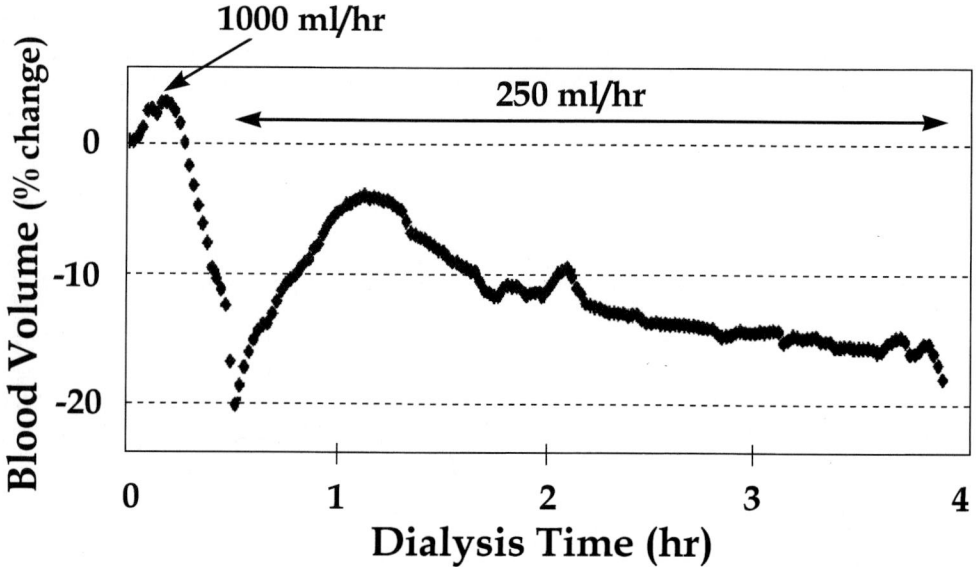

FIGURE 26-4. Percent change in blood volume determined by in-line blood volume profiling during ultrafiltration. The rapid drop in blood volume during the initial 30 min of dialysis was caused by excessive ultrafiltration (1000 mL/h) and promoted a hypotensive event as blood volume decreased by 20%. Decreasing the rate of ultrafiltration to 250 mL/h permitted intravascular volume to refill and blood pressure to normalize. The lower rate of fluid removal better regulated intravascular volume and maintained normal blood pressure. (From Cowgill LD and Langston CE: Role of hemodialysis in the management of dogs and cats with renal failure. *Vet Clin North Am Small Anim Pract* 26:1347–1378, 1996.)

spontaneous bleeding or clotting in the dialyzer. Activated clotting time* or partial thromboplastin time† can be measured by automated devices with small blood samples to facilitate heparin management.

Intravascular volume is an effective predictor of fluid balance and hemodynamic stability in patients predisposed to hypotension or undergoing ultrafiltration (Fig. 26–4) (Steuer et al. 1993, 1996). Changes in vascular volume can be evaluated with in-line blood volume profiling equipment‡ that simultaneously monitors hematocrit and oxygen saturation during the treatment. Bioimpedance analysis is a noninvasive technique that measures real-time changes in total body water and intracellular and extracellular fluid volume (De Lorenzo et al. 1997; Matthie et al. 1998). A bioimpedance spectrometer§ facilitates the management of human patients and animals during periods of dynamic fluid change associated with ultrafiltration or fluid administration (Fig. 26–5) (Jaffrin et al. 1996; Fisch and Spiegel 1996; Jabara and Mehta 1995). Bioimpedance analysis also estimates sequential changes in body cell mass, fat-free mass, and percent body fat as measures of nutritional adequacy or deficiency during the course of an animal's management (Fig. 26–6).

▶ Use of Hemodialysis to Correct Uremic Toxicity

Renal failure often is called *uremic toxicity* because it resembles an intoxication by retained metabolic waste products that the damaged kidneys have failed to excrete from the body (Bergstrom 1989). To some extent, this analogy is valid because many clinical manifestations of renal failure are alleviated by the nonspecific removal of low-molecular-weight solutes from body fluids with dialysis (Table 26–1) (May and Mitch 1996). Despite the similarities to an intoxication, no single solute has been shown to account for the stereotypic clinical signs of uremia (May and Mitch 1996). To the contrary, hundreds of solutes of various sizes accumulate in body fluids with the onset of renal failure; however, only a few have been shown to mimic or reproduce particular aspects of the uremic syndrome. It is likely that the signs of uremia result from the interactive effects of multiple solutes that individually have limited inherent toxicity.

There is an empirical link between the appearance of uremic signs and the accumulation of nitrogenous end products of protein (or amino acid) oxidation (Cotton et al. 1979; Cotton and Knochel 1985). Urea is the nitrogenous metabolite retained to the greatest extent in renal

TABLE 26-1. **Clinical Signs Associated with Azotemia in Animals**

Uremic oral odor	Hypothermia
Anorexia	Immune suppression
Bleeding abnormalities	Cardiac arrhythmia
Nausea and vomiting	Polyneuropathies
Diarrhea	Uremic pneumonitis
Glossitis	Uremic pericarditis
Oral ulceration	Hyperglycemia
Gastritis, gastric ulceration	Neuromuscular irritability
Seizures	Weakness, fatigue
Central nervous system depression	

---

*Automated coagulation timer, HemoTec, Englewood, CO.
†Endpoint, Edison Institute, Edison, NJ.
‡Crit-Line, In-Line Diagnostics, Riverdale, UT.
§Hydra ECF-ICF bioimpedance spectrometer, Xitron Technologies, San Diego, CA.

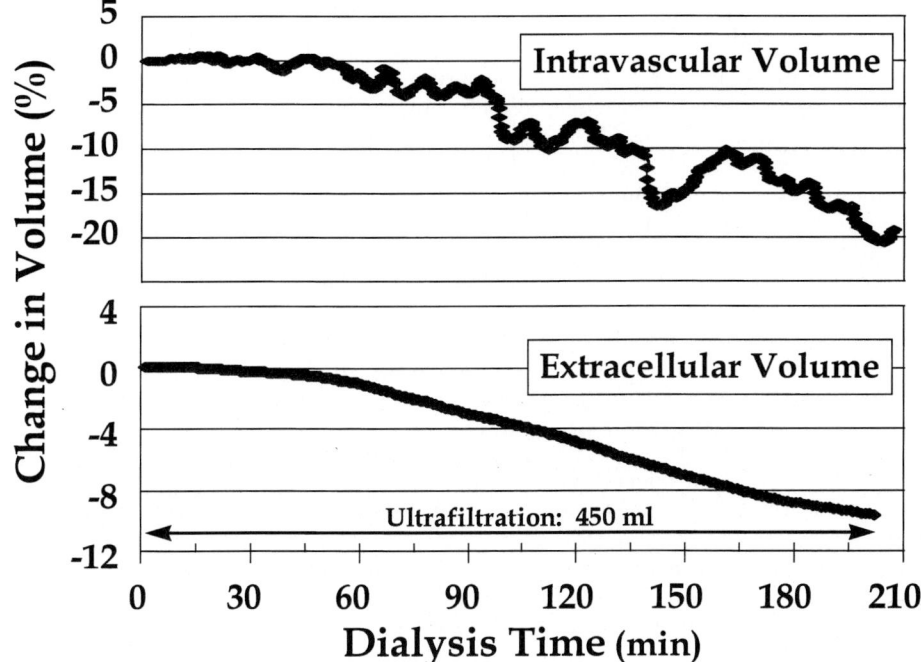

FIGURE 26–5. Percent changes in intravascular and extracellular fluid volume in a 20-kg dog undergoing ultrafiltration during a hemodialysis session. Changes in intravascular volume were measured with in-line blood volume profiling using a Crit-Line blood volume monitor. Extracellular fluid volume was measured with a Xitron Hydra bioimpedance spectrometer.

failure, but it contributes to the nausea, vomiting, stomatitis, malaise, hypothermia, and bleeding tendency characteristic of renal failure only at very high serum concentrations (greater than 170 mg/dL) (Johnson et al. 1972; Grollman and Grollman 1959). Clearly, the symptoms of the azotemia must be attributed to other nitrogenous compounds, protein carbamylations, redirected metabolic pathways, or other small molecular solutes. Despite its minor contributions to the signs of uremia, removal of urea correlates with clinical improvement and decreased morbidity and mortality of renal failure (Gotch and Sargent 1985; Owen et al. 1993; Collins et al. 1994; Lowrie et al. 1981; Held et al. 1996; Parker et al. 1994). As a result, urea has become the surrogate index for all putative low-molecular-weight uremia toxins, and the dialytic removal of urea is used both to prescribe the "dose" of dialysis delivered to the patient and to monitor the efficiency and adequacy of dialytic therapy (Sargent and Gotch 1989; Lowrie et al. 1981; Parker et al. 1994; Hakim 1990; Hakim et al. 1994; Depner 1991; NKF-DOQI 1997; Gotch 1995).

The rapid and often profound accumulation of uremia toxins in animals with acute renal failure prevents the acclimation and compensations that are characteristic of animals with chronic uremia. The clinical expression of uremia typically is more severe in patients with acute renal failure, and correction of the azotemia becomes a therapeutic priority to alleviate these clinical signs.

The diffusive removal of urea and other low-molecular-weight solutes is exceptionally efficient in animals because of the small size (and distribution volume) of dogs and cats relative to the surface area and clearance capabil-

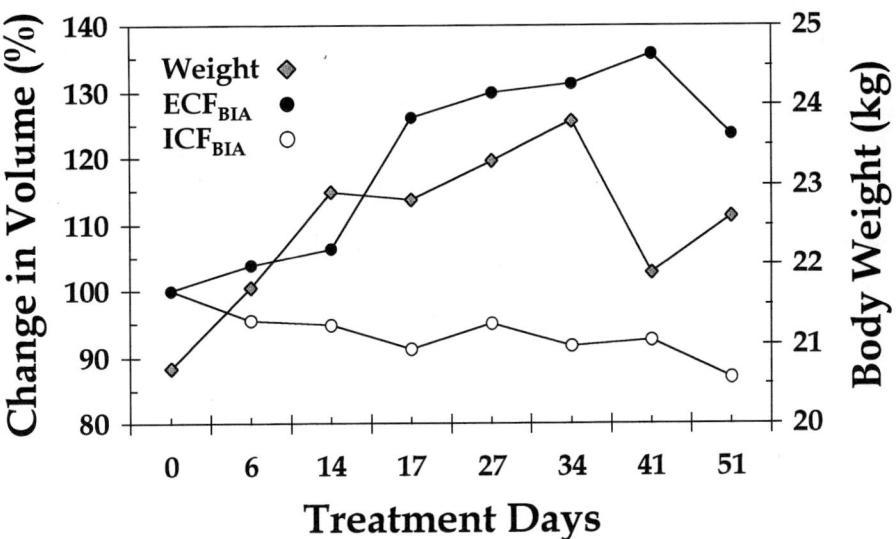

FIGURE 26–6. Sequential bioimpedance analysis measurements in a dog with end-stage renal disease maintained with hemodialysis. The data document that the progressive increase in body weight (shaded diamonds) corresponds to an increase in extracellular fluid volume (ECF_{BIA}, filled circles) associated with the development of peripheral edema and ascites. Concurrently there is a progressive decline in intracellular fluid volume (ICF_{BIA}, open circles) that corresponds to loss of lean body mass not predicted by the change in body weight.

ities of the hemodialyzer. There are clinical limits to the rate at which these solutes can be removed (see dialysis disequilibrium syndrome later), but the serum concentrations of urea and creatinine generally are normal by the end of the dialysis session. With cessation of dialysis, the concentration of urea (and other solutes) increases until a new steady state is achieved or until the next dialysis session. During dialysis, the change in urea concentration (assuming urea generation is negligible) is influenced by the size of the animal, the rate of blood and dialysate flow through the dialyzer, the diffusive characteristics and surface area of the dialyzer, the rate of ultrafiltration, and the length of the dialysis session according to the relationship

$$C = C_0 e^{-(K_r + K_d)t/V}$$

where C is the urea concentration at time t, C_0 is the predialysis concentration of urea, e is the exponential, t is the dialysis time, V is the total body water volume of the animal (proportional to body weight), K_d is the urea clearance of the dialyzer (including dialyzer blood and dialysate flow rates, surface area, diffusive characteristics of the membrane material, and volume of ultrafiltration), and K_r is the residual renal urea clearance of the animal.

The efficacy of the dialysis treatment can be controlled by appropriate prescription of blood flow rate, dialysate flow rate, type and surface area of the hemodialyzer, rate of ultrafiltration, and length of the dialysis session to accommodate the size of the animal and the degree of azotemia.

After dialysis, the increase in urea concentration is determined by urea generation from dietary nitrogen and endogenous protein catabolism and residual renal function. The higher the dietary protein intake, the more catabolic the patient, and the lower the residual renal function, the steeper is the subsequent increase in urea concentration. Urea returns to a steady-state concentration determined by its production and renal excretion unless interrupted by an intervening dialysis treatment. The more frequently and effectively a patient is dialyzed, the lower are the peak predialysis and time-averaged urea concentrations and presumably the exposure to urea and other uremia toxins.

The dialysis prescription for animals has been derived empirically without attempts to justify or standardize dialysis therapy. In contrast, in human medicine numerous outcome studies have correlated dialysis dose with therapeutic outcome, patient morbidity, and mortality (Gotch and Sargent 1985; Owen et al. 1993; Collins et al. 1994; Lowrie et al. 1981; Held et al. 1996; Parker et al. 1994; Hakim 1990; Hakim et al. 1994). Minimum standards have been defined recently, and monitoring practices to assess the overall adequacy of hemodialysis have been established (NKF-DOQI 1997).

The most empirical assessment of dialysis efficacy is based on predialysis serum urea concentration or the change in urea concentration during dialysis treatment. This simplistic approach does not provide an adequate or accurate assessment of the multifactorial variables that influence urea and other uremic solutes. The state of hydration, nutrition, catabolism, and residual renal function influence serum urea concentration without predicting the adequacy of the hemodialysis prescription. In cats, body weight and dialyzer selection are fairly uniform, so the volume of blood processed during the treatment serves as a useful estimate of dialysis dose (Fig. 26–7) (Langston et al. 1997).

Quantitation of urea removal during the dialysis session provides a more critical assessment of the efficacy of an individual treatment. Urea is the designated uremia solute because its molecular size mimics that of other small toxins. It is readily dialyzed, distributes in total body water, and constitutes the major catabolic waste of protein metabolism (Sargent and Gotch 1989; Johnson et al. 1972; NKF-DOQI 1997; Gotch 1995). Also, urea is linked metabolically and kinetically to exogenous and endogenous protein metabolism and can be used to predict dietary intake and the catabolic status of the animal (Sargent and Gotch 1989; Johnson et al. 1972; Gotch 1995).

The most commonly utilized measure of urea removal is the parameter Kt/V. This is a kinetically modeled index reflecting the fractional clearance of urea from its distri-

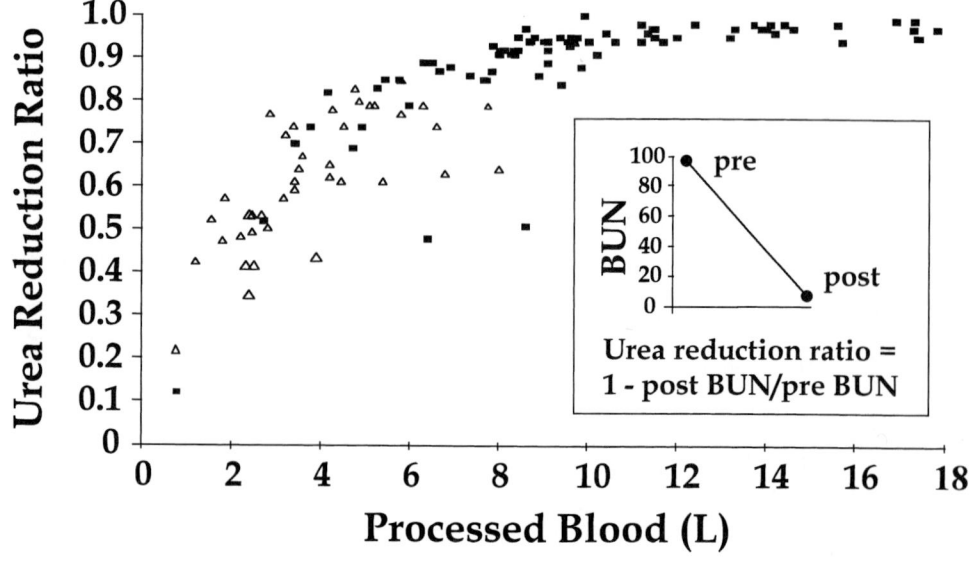

FIGURE 26–7. Correlation between the volume of blood processed and the urea reduction ratio (URR) as indices of the efficacy of individual hemodialysis treatments in cats. Each symbol represents a single dialysis treatment ($n = 149$). Open diamonds depict an initial or second treatment of lower intensity; filled squares represent the third or greater treatment. The insert describes the formula for the URR. (From Cowgill LD and Langston CE: Role of hemodialysis in the management of dogs and cats with renal failure. Vet Clin North Am Small Anim Pract 26:1347–1378, 1996.)

bution volume during a single dialysis session. In this index, K is the urea clearance of the dialyzer (mL/min), t is the time of dialysis (min), and V is the volume of urea distribution (L), which approximates total body water (Sargent and Gotch 1989; Gotch and Sargent 1985; Depner 1991; NKF-DOQI 1997; Gotch 1995). Conventionally, Kt/V is computed with sophisticated mass balance algorithms using input parameters including predialysis, postdialysis and predialysis BUN measurements and body weights for 2 consecutive dialysis sessions, treatment time, the interval between consecutive treatments, the effective urea clearance of the hemodialyzer, and the residual urea clearance of the patient. The higher the Kt/V value, the greater the dose of dialysis and efficacy of the dialysis treatment. Kt/V has been shown to correlate with the morbidity and mortality of dialysis patients and is a standard index to predict adequacy of the dialysis prescription (Gotch and Sargent 1985; Owen et al. 1993; Held et al. 1996; Charra et al. 1992). Kt/V values between 1.2 to 1.4 are considered adequate hemodialysis doses in human patients, but conventional dialysis prescriptions in animals often result in Kt/V values between 2.5 to 3.0, reflecting highly effective dialysis treatment (Cowgill and Langston 1996).

The urea reduction ratio (URR) is an alternative to but less rigorous predictor of dialysis delivery than conventional urea kinetics but has shown good correlation with Kt/V and outcome predictions (see Fig 26–7) (Owen et al. 1993; Held et al. 1996; Daugirdas 1995; Depner 1993). URR is defined as [1 − (postdialysis BUN/predialysis BUN)]. As can be seen in Figure 26–7, the more intense the dialysis prescription (liters of blood dialyzed) the greater the urea removal. A URR between 0.65 and 0.70 is considered adequate for human patients, but it is typical to obtain a URR between 0.85 and 0.95 in animal patients with standard dialysis prescriptions (Cowgill and Langston 1996; Langston et al. 1997; NKF-DOQI 1997).

For initial dialysis treatments in severely uremic animals (BUN > 150 mg/dL), a moderate dialysis prescription resulting in a URR between 0.25 and 0.4 is necessary to prevent dialysis disequilibrium syndrome. Unlike Kt/V, the URR fails to account for the contributions of convective solute removal associated with ultrafiltration and urea generation during the dialysis session. Hence, URR underestimates the actual delivery of dialysis (amount of urea removed) although corrections can be applied to the calculation to account for these influences (Depner 1993; Sherman et al. 1995). URR is a reliable and useful index for monitoring dialysis prescription and dialysis delivery, but it does not permit assessment of the nutritional aspects of urea metabolism.

Neither Kt/V nor URR provides useful predictions of the long-term adequacy of the dialysis prescription, because they ignore the frequency of dialysis and other factors (nutritional adequacy, dietary nitrogen, and catabolic state) that influence urea metabolism. The long-term effects of dialysis and ancillary contributions to urea metabolism over multiple dialysis treatments can be evaluated by using the time average urea concentration (TAC). Time average urea is a kinetically modeled value that reflects the effective exposure of the patient to urea (and presumably unmeasured nitrogenous uremia toxins) over successive dialysis treatments (Cowgill and Maretzki 1995; Cowgill 1995a; Depner 1991). The higher the TAC, the greater the toxicity and clinical expression of uremia. TAC is influenced by the delivery of individual dialysis treatments, the dialysis schedule, and nondialysis influences on urea metabolism. It provides a more global perspective on treatment adequacy than dialysis dose alone. As an example, a dog with no residual renal function can be maintained with a mean predialysis BUN concentration <70 mg/dL and a TAC <40 mg/dL with a high-efficiency (Kt/V = 2.59) thrice-weekly dialysis schedule. A twice-weekly schedule with the same dialysis prescription results in a less satisfactory predialysis BUN of 98 mg/dL and TAC of 54 mg/dL (Cowgill 1995a). In general, a lower TAC and predialysis BUN portend greater clinical benefits, but the combined prescription and frequency should produce at minimum a predialysis BUN <90 mg/dL and a TAC ≤60 mg/dL over the week.

The hemodialysis prescription must be formulated to meet the specific needs of the individual animal and differs with the severity of the azotemia and whether the renal failure is acute or chronic. Severe azotemia should be corrected expeditiously, but its resolution often is constrained by the physiologic tolerance of the animal to rapid changes in serum urea concentration. The dialysis prescription (dialyzer surface area, blood flow rate, dialysis time) must be tempered to avoid dialysis disequilibrium. Animals with chronic renal failure generally tolerate initial dialysis sessions better than animals with acute renal failure, but after two or three dialysis sessions a more effective and aggressive prescription can be provided.

Hemodialysis Prescription for Acute Renal Failure

For acute renal failure, a conventional hollow fiber dialyzer with a surface area between 0.6 and 1.0 m² and a priming volume of approximately 50 mL is appropriate for dogs more than 10 kg in body weight.* For the initial hemodialysis treatment, a dialyzer with a smaller surface area (0.2 to 0.5 m²) may be chosen specifically to reduce the intensity of the treatment and risk of dialysis disequilibrium if the predialysis BUN is ≥ 150 mg/dL. For cats and dogs weighing less than 5 kg, a dialyzer with a surface area between 0.2 and 0.3 m² and a priming volume of less than 20 mL is well tolerated.† Use of synthetic membrane dialyzers may lessen morbidity and improve survival in human patients with acute renal failure. There have been no comparisons of cellulosic and synthetic membrane dialyzers for animal patients, but anecdotal experience with cellulosic materials has shown Hemophan to be less thrombogenic and more biocompatible than Cuprophan dialysis membranes.

Extracorporeal blood flow for initial treatments should be restricted to 1 to 3 mL/kg/min in animals with BUN concentrations >180 mg/dL and 3 to 5 mL/kg/min in

---

*Cobe Centrysystem 200 HG or 400 HG, COBE Laboratories, Lakewood, CO.
†Cobe Centrysystem 100 HG, COBE Laboratories, Lakewood CO.

animals with predialysis BUN concentrations between 100 and 180 mg/dL to prevent an excessive rate of urea clearance and dialysis disequilibrium. By the second or third session, blood flow rate can be increased cautiously to 10 to 20 mL/kg/min for high-efficiency dialysis. For severely uremic cats or small dogs with BUN concentrations >250 mg/dL, "extended-slow" treatment sessions (5 to 8 or more hours) using total blood flow rates no greater than 2 mL/kg/min provide a more gradual and better tolerated reduction of the azotemia. A URR no greater than 0.1 or 0.2 per hour should be targeted (Fig. 26-8).

Dialysis time for the initial sessions should be limited to 60 to 120 min unless extended-slow treatments are warranted. Blood flow rate and dialysis time largely determine the intensity of the dialysis treatment. These parameters should be selected to achieve a urea reduction ratio no greater than 0.4. When the predialysis BUN is <120 mg/dL, dialysis time for both dogs and cats can be extended to 180 to 300 min concurrently with faster blood flow to achieve a urea reduction ratio greater than 0.9.

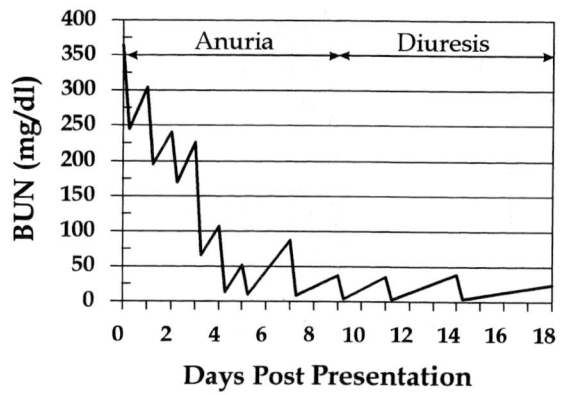

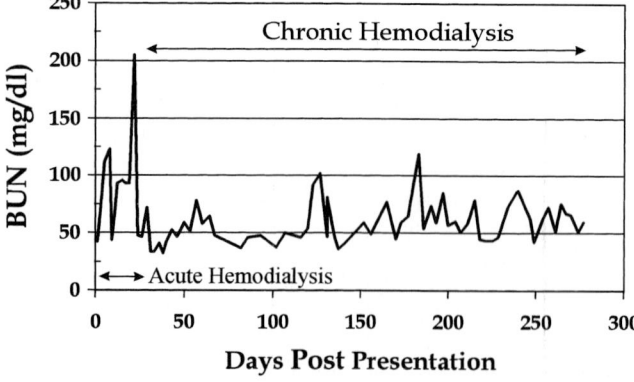

FIGURE 26-8. (Top) Pre- and postdialysis BUN concentrations in a dog presented with acute renal failure secondary to leptospirosis. The severe azotemia was cautiously controlled in the first 3 days of treatment and then maintained during the remaining 6 days that the dog was anuric. With the onset of diuresis renal function improved and dialysis was discontinued on day 14. (Bottom) Predialysis BUN concentrations in a dog with essentially no residual renal function undergoing acute and subsequent long-term hemodialysis after ethylene glycol poisoning. Hemodialysis was performed three times weekly for the first 125 days of treatment and twice weekly thereafter. With few exceptions, the predialysis BUN remained <90 mg/dL. This dog survived nearly 16 months with intermittent hemodialysis with good quality of life.

Dialysate composition suitable for acute uremia is sodium, 145 mmol/L (dogs), 150 mmol/L (cats); potassium, 0.0 to 3.0 mmol/L; bicarbonate, 25 to 35 mmol/L; chloride, 99 to 112 mmol/L (dogs), 112 to 122 mmol/L (cats); calcium, 3.0 mmol/L; magnesium, 1.0 mmol/L; dextrose 200 mg/dL. Dialysate flow is conventionally 500 mL/min but can be reduced if required for initial treatments. If the delivery system permits variable proportioning, a modeled dialysate with a sodium concentration of 155 mmol/L for the initial 20% of the session, 150 mmol/L for the next 40% of the session, and 145 mmol/L for the remainder of the session has been effective in dogs to minimize dialysis disequilibrium and hypotension. For cats, sodium modeling using sodium concentrations of 160, 155, and 150 mmol/L, respectively, have been recommended (Cowgill and Langston 1996; Langston et al. 1997).

Hemodialysis effectively resolves the azotemia and clinical consequences of acute renal failure. The azotemia usually is controlled after two to four dialysis treatments, and subsequently these animals can be treated on an outpatient basis until sufficient renal function has been reestablished to discontinue dialysis. The prognosis for recovery is influenced by the severity of the initial azotemia, the underlying renal injury, and comorbid conditions associated with multiple organ failure. Infectious conditions such as pyelonephritis and leptospirosis and ischemic injury may resolve with 3 to 4 weeks of dialytic support. On the other hand, ethylene glycol intoxication may require months of hemodialysis before renal repair is sufficient to discontinue treatment. It is important not to base the prognosis for recovery on arbitrary criteria associated with conventional therapy. Time-honored perceptions of reversible and irreversible acute renal failure must be revised with the advent of hemodialysis. Before 1995, animals that did not recover within 4 weeks with dialytic support were not expected to recover and usually were euthanized. Some animals maintained with dialysis for extended periods (3 to 9 months) ultimately (and sometimes spontaneously) recover sufficient renal function to be managed with conventional medical therapy. These animals may demonstrate continued improvement of renal function for up to 15 months after the initial renal injury. Animals with severe azotemia, prolonged oliguria or anuria, and profound clinical signs should be considered to have a legitimate expectation to recover sufficient renal function if supported for an appropriate time with hemodialysis.

Hemodialysis Prescription for Chronic Renal Failure

Hemodialysis is clearly indicated, effective, and affords a good quality of life for animals with end-stage renal disease. How much hemodialysis is necessary to control uremia adequately is a topic of considerable controversy in human nephrology. Adequacy standards for animals with chronic renal failure await future definition, but intensive hemodialysis provided every 2 to 4 days can supplement residual excretory capacity and facilitate the management of end-stage renal disease. The dialysis prescription is formulated to reduce the azotemia maximally during each session. Animals with severe end-stage renal disease or decompensated chronic renal failure should be treated with an acute dialysis prescription for initial sessions until the predialysis BUN is <100 mg/dL (see earlier section on hemodialysis prescription for acute renal failure). Thereafter, high-efficiency dialysis schedules are well tolerated. The dialysis prescription should promote a predialysis BUN <90 mg/dL, a postdialysis BUN <10 mg/dL, and a time-averaged BUN <60 mg/dL over the interdialysis interval (see Fig. 26–8).

The choice of dialyzer and dialysate composition generally is the same as for acute dialysis sessions. Blood flow rates can be increased cautiously to 15 to 25 mL/kg/min and the dialysis time lengthened to 240 to 300 min for maximum urea removal. The temptation to reduce dialysis time with the availability of increased dialysis efficiency should be avoided. Three treatments per week is a traditional schedule for human patients and is used for animal patients whose serum creatinine concentrations are >8 mg/dL. Twice-weekly dialysis is the minimum effective schedule and still benefits animals with serum creatinine concentrations between 5 and 8 mg/dL. There is little indication to initiate chronic dialysis therapy in animals with serum creatinine concentrations <5 mg/dL. Therapeutic efforts should be directed toward aggressive medical management (Polzin et al. 1995; Polzin and Osborne 1995).

Animals supported with chronic hemodialysis still must be supplemented with medical therapy to manage the nutritional deficiencies, anemia, mineral disturbances, acidosis, and hypertension associated with severe renal failure (Polzin et al. 1995; Polzin and Osborne 1995; Cowgill 1995b). The prolonged survival of animals supported with hemodialysis fosters expression of complications of chronic renal failure rarely identified in animal patients. Hyperkalemia, fluid retention, renal osteodystrophy, and refractory hypertension become important clinical features.

Presurgical Support for Renal Transplantation

Renal transplantation is a more economical and effective long-term solution to severe uremia resulting from acute ethylene glycol intoxication, bilateral ureteral obstruction, or end-stage renal disease in cats. However, a variable course of dialysis often is required to correct the uremia associated with these conditions and to reduce the treatment risks of anesthesia and surgery. Hemodialysis also broadens the available pool of animals with chronic renal failure that would otherwise be unsuitable for transplantation because of the severity of their uremia and risk for surgery (Cowgill 1995a; Cowgill and Langston 1996). As renal transplantation becomes available for dogs, combined availability of these renal replacement services will become increasingly necessary.

▶ Use of Hemodialysis to Correct Disorders of Fluid Balance

Animals with oliguric or anuric forms of acute renal failure are not able to excrete administered fluid loads and are predisposed to life-threatening hypervolemia that is difficult to correct. Aggressive fluid administration frequently promotes hypervolemia and circulatory overload manifested by chemosis, pleural effusion, peripheral or pulmonary edema, congestive heart failure, and hypertension, and, once established, overhydration may not resolve with cessation of fluids and diuretic administration. Similarly, animals with chronic end-stage renal disease may develop fluid overload if ingestion of sodium and water exceeds renal excretory capacity. Even the water content of canned food may exceed urine output in animals with minimal renal function.

A judgment about the volume of fluid to be removed and rate of ultrafiltration must be made for each dialysis prescription for the degree of overhydration based on clinical findings (e.g., blood pressure, presence of edema, pulmonary congestion) and the deviation of body weight from the animal's *ideal dry body weight* Ideal dry body weight is an arbitrary value determined as the body weight at which further fluid removal produces hypotension or signs of hypovolemia. It is estimated from evaluation of previous postdialysis body weights when blood pressure was controlled and there was no demonstrated fluid accumulation. The rate and volume of ultrafiltration are contingent upon the hemodynamic stability of the animal. Available hemodialyzers have the capacity to remove fluid from the vascular space much faster than its redistribution from the interstitium and intracellular compartments. This imbalance predisposes the animal to hypovolemia, circulatory collapse, and hypotension (Baldamus and Pollok 1989). Ultrafiltration must be carefully regulated in small animals by dialysis delivery systems with ultrafiltration controllers. Small errors in the amount or rate of fluid removal could result in depletion of a significant percentage of intravascular volume. Slow rates of ultrafiltration at 5 to 10 mL/kg/h generally are tolerated. The safety of increased rates must be based on the animal's vital signs and fluid monitoring equipment (see Fig. 26–4). Profiling the rate of ultrafiltration during the dialysis session is feasible with some dialysis systems. Ultrafiltration profiling coordinates the timing of ultrafiltration with periods of greatest hemodynamic stability at the end of the session. Sodium modeling techniques also can be used to offset the hypovolemic and hypotensive effects of aggressive ultrafiltration. During sodium modeling, high dialysate sodium concentrations temporarily increase serum sodium and expand intravascular fluid volume by enhancing the redistribution of fluid from the interstitium and intracellular compartments. Fluid is ultimately mobilized from regions of excess without significant compromise of intravascular volume.

The deleterious effects of excessive fluid removal, hypotension, and circulatory collapse can be detected by regular assessment of heart rate and blood pressure using indirect Doppler ultrasound or oscillometry (Crowe and Spreng 1995; Bodey et al. 1994). The real-time influence of ultrafiltration on blood volume can be assessed continuously with an in-line hematocrit monitor (Steuer et al. 1993; Katzarski 1996). This monitoring device simplifies the adjustment of fluid removal to acceptable reductions of intravascular volume, thus maximizing the rate of safe ultrafiltration (see Fig. 26–4). Adverse changes in blood volume can be determined in advance of changes in heart rate or blood pressure to forecast impending hemodynamic crises in sufficient time to intervene. Bioelectrical impedance analysis also can be used to monitor total body water, ideal dry weight, and real-time changes in extracellular fluid volume (see Fig. 26–5) (De Lorenzo et al. 1997; Matthie et al. 1998; Jaffrin et al. 1996; Fisch and Spiegel 1996).

Animals with life-threatening fluid overload and severe azotemia are at risk for excessive urea removal if treated with a long dialysis session to resolve the fluid complications (Rosa et al. 1981). These animals can be safely managed by prescribing *ultrafiltration without hemodialysis* after the azotemia has been appropriately treated. With this technique, dialysate is diverted away from the hemodialyzer but blood flow and transmembrane pressure are maintained to extend the ultrafiltration session. This allows slower and more complete fluid removal without producing excessive hemodialysis. Ultrafiltration can be used to treat other conditions of refractory circulatory overload including congestive heart failure, pulmonary edema, or malignant hypertension. Ultrafiltration enables continued administration of necessary blood products, drugs, and alimentation solutions in oliguric animals that could not otherwise tolerate these high-volume therapies.

▶ Use of Hemodialysis to Correct Electrolyte Imbalances

Serum electrolyte concentrations can be adjusted to any appropriate value by the diffusive properties of the dialyzer with proper formulation of dialysate composition. Hyperkalemia is a common electrolyte disturbance that causes cardiovascular instability and death in uremic animals. The toxicity of hyperkalemia is intensified by coexistent acidosis, hypocalcemia, or hyponatremia that may accompany renal failure. Hyperkalemia is most commonly associated with acute renal failure, but serum potassium concentrations between 6 and 9 mEq/L also are consistent findings in animals with severe chronic renal failure maintained with hemodialysis. Medical treatments to alleviate hyperkalemia merely shift extracellular potassium to intracellular pools or antagonize its neuromuscular toxicity (DiBartola 1992). In contrast, hemodialysis corrects the hyperkalemia and removes the excess potassium from extracellular and intracellular pools. A standard dialysate potassium concentration of 3 mmol/L can be used for most animals with acute or chronic renal failure. For very short dialysis sessions (<120 min) serum potassium concentration may not be corrected completely with standard dialysate, and dialysate formulated with zero potassium should be used. The bulk of body potassium is compartmentalized in intracellular pools. Its transfer to the extracellular space is variable and may not equal its transfer from ECF into the dialysate. As a result, animals may have postdialysis hypokalemia and rebound hyperkalemia within hours because of delayed equilibrium from intracellular pools. Daily dialysis may be required until the bulk of the potassium load is alleviated. Animals with persistent predialysis hyperkalemia require elimination of potassium-rich diets and potassium-containing fluids and dialysis with a 0 to 1 mmol/L potassium dialysate.

Modern dialysis delivery systems provide variable sodium proportioning to formulate the dialysate with a sodium concentration ranging from 125 to 160 mmol/L. The sodium concentration of a modeled dialysate also can be programmed to change in user-defined patterns throughout the dialysis session to achieve defined changes in serum sodium concentration or to correct abnormalities in predialysis sodium concentration. Hyponatremia caused by excessive vomiting, diarrhea, diuretic administration, sodium-deficient fluid administration, or free-water ingestion can be treated by programming the dialysate sodium concentration to increase in single-step or variable increments to the desired postdialysis concentration. Hypernatremia resulting from free-water loss or excessive bicarbonate or hypertonic saline administration may be difficult or inappropriate to correct with additional fluid administration but can be normalized in progressive or incremented steps by adjusting the dialysate sodium below the serum concentration. The rate of reduction can be regulated precisely without concern about overcorrection.

▶ Use of Hemodialysis to Correct Acid-Base Disorders

Impairment of both glomerular filtration and tubular function results in retention of hydrogen ions and production of a high-anion-gap metabolic acidosis. Hydrogen ions are present at too low a concentration for the accumulated acid burden to be disposed of by dialysis alone (Ward 1995). Alternatively, the acid load can be buffered by bicarbonate supplied in the dialysate. By formulating buffers (acetate or bicarbonate) in the dialysate to concentrations greater than those in plasma, its diffusive transfer results in accrual of new buffer by the patient to replenish preexisting deficits in body buffer stores. The amount of base transferred depends on the dialysate buffer concentration, choice of dialyzer, and the blood and dialysate flow rates.

Conventional delivery systems provide variable bicarbonate proportioning to permit formulation of dialysate with bicarbonate concentrations ranging from 25 to 35 mmol/L. A lower bicarbonate concentration is chosen for animals with severe metabolic acidosis in which rapid correction of serum bicarbonate concentration might predispose to dialysis disequilibrium or paradoxical cerebral acidosis (Arieff et al. 1978; Andrew 1991; Arieff 1994). A lower bicarbonate concentration also should be selected for animals with predialysis metabolic alkalosis. The bicarbonate concentration of the dialysate also can be altered throughout the dialysis session to achieve programmed changes in serum bicarbonate concentration.

For maintenance hemodialysis treatments, a dialysate bicarbonate concentration of 30 mmol/L produces postdialysis serum bicarbonate concentrations of approximately 25 mmol/L. A dialysate concentration of 35 mmol/L yields greater accrual of buffer but often is associated with persistent panting during the treatment.

▶ Use of Hemodialysis to Correct Disorders of Mineral Balance

Mineral imbalances including hyperphosphatemia, hypercalcemia, and hypocalcemia are common features of acute or chronic renal failure. Hyperphosphatemia participates in the development of secondary hyperparathyroidism and soft tissue mineralization (Bricker 1972; Brown et al. 1991; Slatopolsky and Delmez 1995). Correspondingly, normalization of serum phosphate concentration is a therapeutic priority (Polzin et al. 1995; Polzin and Osborne 1995; Delmez and Slatopolsky 1992). The dialysance of phosphate is considerably less than that of either urea or creatinine. In addition, the interstitial pool of phosphate is vast, compartmentalized, and poorly exchangeable with the serum pool so the amount of phosphate eliminated from the body during an individual dialysis treatment is small compared with the overall phosphate burden (Delmez and Slatopolsky 1992).

Dialysate contains no phosphate, and during a routine hemodialysis treatment, the serum phosphate concentration can be reduced to 15 to 20% of its predialysis value. Transient hypophosphatemia is common at the end of dialysis but is not associated with clinical sequelae and resolves rapidly after the treatment. Hemodialysis is a useful adjunct for phosphate management, but adequate control of hyperphosphatemia in animals with chronic renal failure requires concurrent treatment with phosphate-restricted diets and phosphate-binding agents (Polzin et al. 1995; Polzin and Osborne 1995; Delmez and Slatopolsky 1992).

Serum calcium concentrations vary in animals depending on the nature of the renal failure. Animals with acute renal failure or acute decompensation of underlying chronic renal failure may have profound hypocalcemia secondary to the sudden hyperphosphatemia or the underlying etiology of the uremia (e.g., antifreeze intoxication, pancreatitis). Animals with chronic renal failure tend to have increased total serum calcium concentrations as renal function declines (Kruger et al. 1996). Serum ionized calcium concentrations may be normal or low, reflecting increased complexed calcium, which may be physiologically inactive. Conventional dialysate formulations used for animal dialysis contain 3 mmol/L calcium, which approximates the serum calcium concentration achieved at the end of the dialysis treatment whether the predialysis calcium concentration is low or high. The normalization of serum calcium concentration after dialysis generally is transient if the cause of the calcium imbalance is not corrected.

▶ Use of Hemodialysis in Acute Intoxications

Hemodialysis should be considered an alternative to conservative therapy for moderate or severe intoxications when initial therapy has been delayed or there is no specific antidote. Dialysis hastens elimination of the toxin or its metabolites according to their diffusibility, molecular size, concentration in extracellular fluid, distribution pool, and degree of protein binding (Garella 1988). Hemodialysis is indicated for the treatment of poisoning with ethylene glycol, methanol, salicylate, lithium, ethanol, phenobarbital, acetaminophen, theophylline, aminoglycosides, tricyclic antidepressants, and possibly metaldehyde (Garella 1988). Hemodialysis secondarily corrects the acid-base and electrolyte abnormalities that may accompany some intoxications (e.g., ethylene glycol, salicylate). Selection criteria for the institution of hemodialysis in acute poisoning are listed in Table 26–2. Hemodialysis should be initiated when conventional treatments are deemed to be ineffective and continued until the concentration of the toxin has decreased to an acceptable level and the clinical toxicity has disappeared. Dialysis treatments should be continued for prolonged periods for toxins with delayed toxicity (e.g., paraquat) and low blood concentrations.

Ethylene glycol (antifreeze) poisoning is one of the most common intoxications encountered in companion animal practice. Clinical signs develop within minutes and progress from lethargy, nausea, vomiting, dehydration, agitation, and depression to convulsions, coma, and death. Severe metabolic acidosis and hypocalcemia often accompany the intoxication (Thrall et al. 1995). In later stages of the intoxication (12 to 24 h), hypertension, cardiopulmonary failure, and acute oliguric renal failure dominate the clinical presentation. The goals for hemodialysis are to eliminate ethylene glycol and its metabolites from the animal as quickly as possible and to correct the accompanying fluid, electrolyte, and acid-base disorders and associated uremia. Even at a late stage, high blood concentrations of ethylene glycol and its metabolites can be identified. For suspected cases, hemodialysis should be initiated without delay to ensure elimination of the toxin from the animal regardless of previous antidotal therapy or the absence of clinical signs. If the animal needs to be transported to a distant dialysis center, an initial dose of ethanol or 4-methylpyrazole should be administered, and supportive therapy should be provided for dehydration and metabolic acidosis (Thrall et al. 1995). The dialysis session should be intensive to maximize the rate and amount of toxin removed. For acute poisoning, all the toxins and clinical signs can be eliminated with a single dialysis treatment (see Fig. 26–1). For nonazotemic animals in which one or two dialysis treatments are anticipated, a temporary dialysis catheter can be placed quickly, provides adequate blood flow, and is less costly and easily removed. The largest hemodialyzer compatible with the

TABLE 26–2. Selection Criteria for Use of Hemodialysis in Acute Poisoning

Strong history or known exposure to a potentially lethal and dialyzable toxin
Impaired route of excretion of the toxin (i.e., renal)
Persistence of a significant blood toxin concentration
Persistent absorption and metabolic conversion of toxin or metabolites
Failure of conventional medical therapy to alleviate the toxicity
Rapid clinical deterioration
Lack of an effective medical antidote
Ethylene glycol intoxication

extracorporeal volume requirement of the animal should be used to maximize diffusive removal of the toxins. Rapid blood flow rates between 15 and 25 mL/kg/min generally are tolerated during the first treatment. A standard dialysate flow between 500 and 600 mL/min is used. A dialysate formulated with 3 to 4 mmol/L potassium, 25 mmol/L bicarbonate, and a physiologic sodium concentration is appropriate unless specific electrolyte, acid-base, or hemodynamic disorders are present. Sodium modeling and ultrafiltration are not required in euvolemic animals. Ultrafiltration can be used in animals with pulmonary edema or congestive heart failure secondary to the toxin or fluid administration. Ultrafiltration, however is minimally effective for pulmonary effusions secondary to respiratory distress syndrome or uremic pneumonitis associated with antifreeze poisoning. Simultaneous fluid administration and balanced ultrafiltration can increase toxin removal by convection without net alterations in fluid balance.

In uremic animals the goals for toxin removal are constrained by the requirement to prevent dialysis disequilibrium (see dialysis disequilibrium syndrome later) secondary to the rapid removal of urea, and dialysis must be delivered carefully to accommodate all of the patient's needs. A permanent dialysis catheter should be placed initially if it is anticipated that hemodialysis will be required for more than 10 days to support the associated renal failure. If the BUN concentration is <125 mg/dL, an intensive treatment as used for toxin removal in nonuremic animals is suitable. For animals with BUN concentrations >125 mg/dL, a prescription tailored to acute uremia is more appropriate (see preceeding section on hemodialysis prescription for acute renal failure). Multiple daily dialysis sessions of short duration to achieve a URR ≤0.4 should be scheduled until the predialysis BUN concentration is <125 mg/dL. Alternatively, a slow and prolonged session of 6 to more than 12 h and designed to produce a URR of 0.05 to 0.1 per hour can achieve safe urea reduction and more rapid toxin removal. The remainder of the dialysis prescription should be formulated to the specific complications of uremia, fluid volume status, and hemodynamic stability. Mannitol* should be administered at 0.5 to 1.0 g/kg intravenously 45 to 60 min after starting dialysis in both mildly and severely azotemic animals to prevent manifestations of dialysis disequilibrium.

▶ Complications of Hemodialysis

Hemodialysis is a technically complex therapy applied to patients with profound physiologic and metabolic derangements. Therapeutic complications can be anticipated from both the technical aspects of the process and the dramatic corrections of homeostasis that result from therapy. It is often difficult to distinguish whether adverse events are due to the uremia per se or its treatment. The frequency and intensity of these events diminish as the patient adapts to dialysis and the uremia is controlled.

---

*Mannitol injection USP, Abbott Laboratories, North Chicago, IL.

Technical Complications

Technical complications arise from inappropriate or unsafe dialysate proportioning, overheating the dialysate, hemolysis caused by the blood pump, undetected ultrafiltration, air embolism, blood leakage into the dialysate, or blood losses from leaks or clotting in the extracorporeal path. These complications ostensibly have been eliminated by the sophistication, intrinsic safeguards, internal sensors, and integrated microprocessor systems designed into modern dialysis delivery systems. The purity of water provided by conventional water treatment systems also has minimized exposure to chemical contaminants that pose immediate or long-term health risks during hemodialysis. The evolution of dialyzer design and delivery technology has established hemodialysis as a safe and readily applicable therapy for animals. Temptations to initiate a hemodialysis program with obsolete, discarded, or surplus equipment based on outdated technology should be abandoned solely on the basis of the technical risks such an approach might pose.

Vascular Access

Tunneled transcutaneous venous catheters represent a formidable advance in vascular access compared with the arteriovenous shunts they replaced, but they remain the most predictable, problematic, and serious source of dialysis-related complications. Double-lumen hemodialysis catheters are large-diameter, inherently stiff appliances subject to intermittent contact with the right atrium or vena cava and positional interference with blood flow. Positional effects can be managed temporarily by decreasing the speed of the blood pump, constraining the position of the animal, or reversing the connections of the catheter and blood lines. These compromises are a nuisance for the treatment and influence the comfort and adequacy of the delivered dialysis.

Thrombosis within the access and major vessels is one of the most frequent complications of animal dialysis and a major factor limiting its adequate delivery. The incidence of catheter-associated thrombosis has not been defined precisely but appears to be higher in dogs and cats than in human patients, suggesting differences in their respective coagulation mechanisms or catheter interactions. Thrombosis within the lumen of the catheter is infrequent and readily managed by careful thromboaspiration, disruption with a wire, or instillation of fibrinolytic agents (urokinase or streptokinase) into the catheter lumen. Fibrin sheaths or clots surrounding the catheter in the vascular space or the right atrium are more common, problematic, and difficult to correct. These thrombi obstruct the ports of the catheter or seal the lumen of the vessel, restricting delivery of blood to the dialyzer (Fig. 26–9). Pulmonary vein thromboembolism resulting from dislodged clots in the cranial vena cava or right atrium is uncommon but can cause acute respiratory dysfunction or pneumothorax, which may be life threatening. Central thrombi in the cranial vena cava or right atrium cause facial and cervical edema that may impair respiration and induce pleural effusion. Long-standing deep vein or right atrial thrombi ultimately organize and are covered by

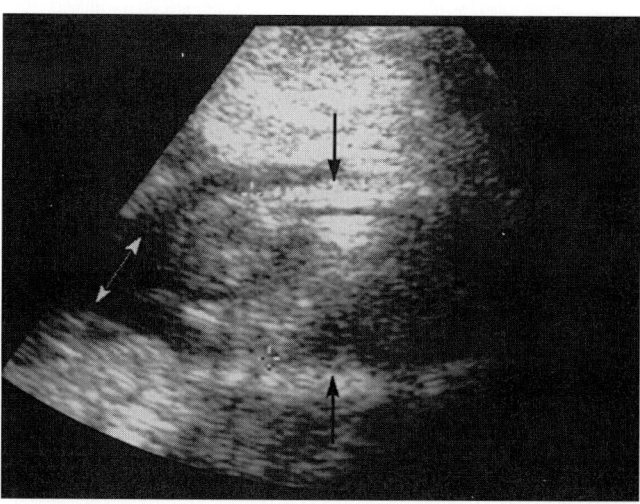

FIGURE 26-9. Ultrasound image of cranial vena cava (double white arrow) illustrating a large intraluminal thrombus (black arrows) surrounding a transcutaneous twin-lumen hemodialysis catheter. Color-flow Doppler image demonstrated only minimal blood flow around the thrombus.

endothelium. Attempts to dissolve thromboemboli using urokinase, streptokinase, or tissue plasminogen activator are variably successful in people but virtually futile in dogs and cats.

Infection associated with the dialysis catheter is infrequent, but the catheter requires meticulous attention and care. The catheter exit site should be cleansed with antiseptic soap during each dialysis session. Application of a disinfectant-soaked dressing (0.2% chlorhexidine solution*) to the catheter exit site during dialysis sessions helps seal the exit site and reduce superficial skin infections. Any discharge or exudate from the exit site should be cultured to document the infection and determine the appropriate antimicrobial therapy. Superficial skin infections should be managed aggressively with antibiotics until the inflammation is resolved. Infection of the cutaneous tunnel or the Dacron cuff and catheter-induced bacteremia or endocarditis are uncommon but should be treated aggressively with appropriate antibiotics. If the fever or bacteremia is not resolved within 48 to 72 h, the catheter should be removed and appropriate antibiotics administered on the basis of blood or catheter tip cultures and continued until the infection is resolved. A new catheter should be placed in a different vessel if possible.

Hypotension

Hypotension is an anticipated but generally transient and clinically insignificant complication of hemodialysis (Langston et al. 1997). Blood pressure should be monitored at 15- to 30-min intervals throughout the dialysis session. The susceptibility to hypotensive events is influenced by body size, hydration status, the severity of uremia, the presence of concurrent cardiac disease or comorbid conditions (e.g., hemorrhage, anemia, sepsis, pancreatitis), and current medications (e.g., antihypertensives, diuretics). Rarely, animals experience hypotension as a biocom-

---

*Chlorhexidine diacetate (Nolvasan solution), Fort Dodge Laboratories, Fort Dodge, IA.

patibility reaction to cellulosic dialysis membranes or after exposure to pyrogens in the dialysate or blood circuit. For cats and small dogs, the volume of the extracorporeal circuit may approach 35% of intravascular volume and represents a significant "steal" from cardiac output. The rapid removal of plasma solutes in the early stages of a dialysis treatment diminishes intravascular volume and opposes "refilling" of fluid from the extravascular space. Sodium modeling prescriptions counteract this osmotic drain and promote fluid movement from the interstitium into the vascular compartment to blunt this initial hypovolemia (Stewart and Fleming 1974; Raja 1996). Priming the extracorporeal volume with dextran solutions helps to maintain or bolster intravascular volume in small animals. Excessive or rapid ultrafiltration of fluid from the vascular compartment faster than it can be replenished from the extravascular reserves can cause hypovolemia and transient hypotension (see Fig. 26–4). These events can be avoided or ameliorated by administering modest volumes of fluid and slowing the rate of ultrafiltration. Dialysis-induced hypotension also responds quickly to modest fluid supplementation, which transiently refills vascular volume while fluid from the extravascular space is mobilized. Supplementation of fluids to maintain adequate blood pressure, however, is counterproductive for animals that are fluid overloaded and require ultrafiltration.

Neurologic Complications

Dialysis disequilibrium syndrome is a serious neurologic condition induced by rapid dialysis of animals with severe azotemia. The pathogenesis of dialysis disequilibrium is poorly understood but culminates in the development of cerebral edema. The disproportionate mobilization of urea and buffering of hydrogen ions in extracellular and intravascular fluid relative to cerebrospinal fluid cause an interposed osmotic gradient and influx of water into the brain, an increase in cerebrospinal fluid pressure, cerebral edema, and paradoxical cerebral acidosis (Arieff 1982; Arieff et al. 1973; Kennedy et al. 1962; Funder and Wieth 1967). Paradoxical cerebral acidosis in turn exacerbates the osmotic gradient by induction of "idiogenic osmoles" within the brain, causing further brain swelling (Rosa et al. 1981; Arieff et al. 1978; Andrew 1991; Arieff 1994).

Dialysis disequilibrium is most serious in cats and small dogs during initial dialysis treatments when azotemia and metabolic acidosis are most severe. Signs including tremors, restlessness, disorientation, vocalization, amaurosis, seizures, and coma may develop during the dialysis session or up to 24 h after hemodialysis. When not properly managed, cerebral edema may progress to death resulting from respiratory arrest or compression or herniation of the cerebellum or brain stem (Fig. 26–10). In dogs, dialysis disequilibrium commences with restlessness and vocalization before the onset of seizures or coma, providing ample opportunity to intervene. Cats, on the other hand, often progress rapidly from a normal appearance to coma without warning.

Treatment of dialysis disequilibrium consists of slowing or discontinuing the hemodialysis treatment and administering an intravenous bolus of mannitol (0.5 to 1.0 g/kg) to increase plasma osmolality and dissipate the os-

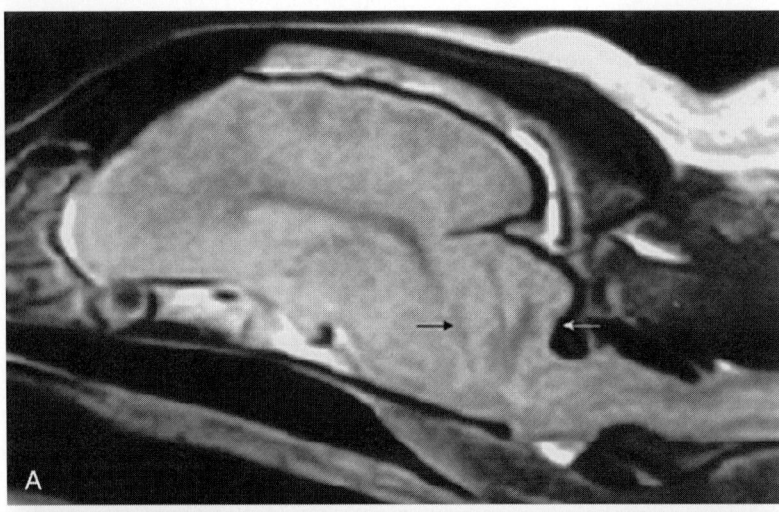
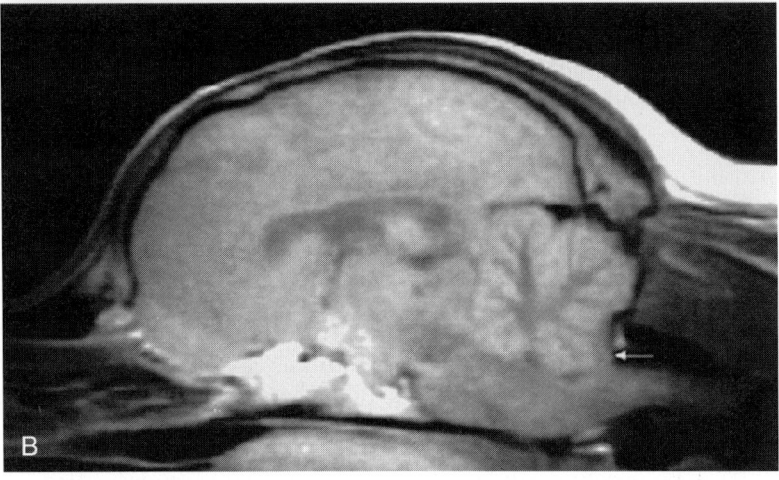

FIGURE 26-10. *(A)* Sagittal magnetic resonance image of a cat brain after acute respiratory arrest during hemodialysis. There is evidence of severe cerebral edema producing distortion and lateral compression of the cerebellum (arrows) consistent with acute dialysis disequilibrium syndrome. *(B)* Sagittal magnetic resonance image of the brain of a dog suffering acute respiratory arrest and dialysis disequilibrium syndrome. The image depicts moderate cerebral edema and ventral herniation of the cerebellum (arrow) and brain stem.

motic gradient. Diazepam* is used as required to control seizures (Cowgill and Langston 1996). Animals with preexisting neurologic disease, BUN concentrations >125 mg/dL, severe metabolic acidosis, or body weights <5 kg are at highest risk. For high-risk animals the efficiency of the dialysis treatment should be reduced by selecting a smaller hemodialyzer, using minimum blood flow rates, lowering the dialysate flow rate, reversing dialysate flow in the hemodialyzer, and lowering the dialysate bicarbonate concentration to better match that of the patient. These steps reduce the rate of solute removal and development of osmotic disequilibrium. Mannitol can be administered prophylactically at 0.5 to 1.0 g/kg IV at 30 to 60 min from the start of dialysis. Mild signs usually dissipate immediately with mannitol administration, whereas severe signs may require multiple doses of mannitol and 24 to 48 h of supportive care before resolution. Respiratory arrest caused by cerebral edema and brain stem compression requires ventilatory support until the edema resolves, but the prognosis for recovery is poor.

Respiratory

Mild to moderate hypoxemia develops during dialysis in both human and animal patients (DeBroe 1994). The

---

*Diazepam Injection, USP, Schein Pharmaceutical, Inc., Norham Park, NJ.

effect is maximal within 30 to 60 min of the start of dialysis and resolves within 120 min after discontinuing the treatment. Activation of the alternative complement pathway by contact of blood with the dialyzer membrane causes leukocyte and platelet aggregation in the pulmonary microvasculature, which interferes with oxygen diffusion. The effect is more pronounced with cellulosic than with more biocompatible synthetic membrane dialyzers (Woffindin and Hoenich 1988; DeBroe 1994; Hakim and Lowie 1982; Kolb et al. 1990). Acetate-based dialysate causes hypoventilation resulting from loss of carbon dioxide into the dialysate, which exacerbates the hypoxemia. This effect is not seen with bicarbonate-based dialysate (DeBroe 1994).

Pulmonary thromboembolism caused by platelet aggregation and thrombus formation induced by the catheter can cause acute onset of mild to severe dyspnea during or between dialysis treatments. Other causes of hypoxemia including fluid overload, pulmonary edema, and uremic pneumonitis are related directly to the uremia. Uremic pneumonitis is a form of respiratory distress syndrome in which uremia toxins alter the permeability of pulmonary capillaries and promote leakage of a high-protein effusion into alveoli and pulmonary interstitium (Bleyl et al. 1981). Radiographically, uremic pneumonitis appears as an interstitial or mixed interstitial and alveolar pattern, but it is frequently overshadowed by concurrent pulmonary edema. Ultrafiltration helps to resolve fluid overload and pulmonary edema but is ineffective in correcting uremic pneumonitis. Adequate dialysis is used to resolve the azotemia perpetuating the condition, but established cases are difficult to rectify, and the prognosis for recovery is grave even with ventilatory support.

Hematologic

Decreases in white blood cell and platelet counts occur routinely during dialysis and are related to membrane biocompatibility reactions (Heierli et al. 1988; Levett et al. 1986). Contact of blood with the hemodialysis membrane activates the alternative complement pathway, causing a decrease in total hemolytic complement and development of reactive C3 and C5 fragments (Woffindin and Hoenich 1988; Falkenhagen et al. 1987; Hoenich et al. 1995; Bingel et al. 1989). This reaction proceeds within minutes of starting dialysis, is maximal at 15 to 30 min, and resolves within hours as a result of down-regulation of the complement system. Binding of complement to the dialysis membrane activates leukocytes and platelets as they circulate through the dialyzer, causing neutropenia and thrombocytopenia as these cells aggregate in the pulmonary vasculature (Walton and Cheung 1995; Woffindin and Hoenich 1988; Falkenhagen et al. 1987; Hoenich et al. 1995; DeBroe 1994; Kolb et al. 1990; Heierli et al. 1988; Levett et al. 1986). These transient changes in leukocytes have no overt clinical significance, but complement activation may induce chills, mild discomfort, and hypoxemia. Cellulosic dialysis membranes are consistently less biocompatible than synthetic membranes (Woffindin and Hoenich 1988; Falkenhagen et al. 1987; Hoenich et al. 1995; Bingel et al. 1989). However, the substituted cellulosic membrane Hemophan, conventionally used for animal dialysis, is more biocompatible than other cellulosic membranes, approaching the biocompatibility of synthetic polymer membranes (Woffindin and Hoenich 1988; Ward et al. 1993; Falkenhagen et al. 1987; Hoenich et al. 1995; Lucchi et al. 1989).

Anemia in dialyzed animals is a persistent problem related to decreased erythropoiesis and blood loss during the treatment (Cowgill 1995a, 1995b). Blood losses caused by clotting in the dialyzer should be minimized by carefully managed heparinization and careful rinse-back techniques at the end of the treatment. Repeated diagnostic blood sampling, bleeding resulting from excessive heparinization and platelet dysfunction, and gastrointestinal hemorrhage contribute to the blood loss. Hemolysis could be due to improper adjustment of the blood pump, excessive pressures in the extracorporeal circuit, or impurities (e.g., copper, aluminum, zinc, nitrates, formaldehyde), overheating, or hypotonicity of the dialysate. All blood loss is significant in uremic animals that require routine treatment with recombinant human erythropoietin* and periodic blood transfusion (Cowgill 1995b).

Gastrointestinal

Anorexia, nausea, and vomiting are common complications of uremia but also may develop during a dialysis session as a result of hypotension and diversion of blood from the gastrointestinal tract, biocompatibility reactions, or contaminants in the dialysate. Dialysis disequilibrium also can cause centrally mediated nausea and vomiting. The use of slow blood flow at the start of dialysis treatments with gradual increases to the prescribed rate minimizes these signs and the patient's discomfort.

▶ Conclusions

Hemodialysis is a technically feasible, safe, efficacious, and indispensable therapy for both dogs and cats with life-threatening renal failure. Its complexity and limited applications restrict widespread employment of hemodialysis in veterinary practice. However, there is no alternative therapy for animals with severe uremia, refractory oliguria, or hypervolemia. The increased awareness and acceptance of dialysis by primary care veterinarians, increased sophistication of specialty veterinary practice and academic centers, increased training of veterinary internists with interest in and knowledge of nephrology, and increased demand by pet owners for this service promise its further expansion and availability on a regional basis.

REFERENCES

Abel JJ, Rowntree LC, Turner BB: On the removal of diffusible substances from the circulating blood by means of dialysis. *Trans Assoc Am Physiol* 28:41, 1913.

Andrew RD: Seizure and acute osmotic change: Clinical and neurophysiological aspects. *J Neurol Sci* 101:7–18, 1991.

Arieff AI: Dialysis disequilibrium syndrome: current concepts on pathogenesis. *Controv Nephrol* 4:367, 1982.

Arieff A: Dialysis disequilibrium syndrome: Current concepts on pathogenesis and prevention. *Kidney Int* 45:629–635, 1994.

Arieff AI, Massry SG, Barrientos A, Kleeman CR: Brain water and electrolyte metabolism in uremia: effects of slow and rapid hemodialysis. *Kidney Int* 4:177–187, 1973.

Arieff AI, Lazarowitz VC, Guisado R: Experimental dialysis disequilibrium syndrome: Prevention with glycerol. *Kidney Int* 14:270, 1978.

Baldamus CA, Pollok M: Ultrafiltration and hemofiltration: practical applications. In Maher JF (ed): *Replacement of Renal Function by Dialysis: A Textbook of Dialysis*, 3rd ed. Dordrecht, Kluwer Academic Publishers, pp. 327–346, 1989.

Bergstrom J: Toxicity of uremia: Physiopathology and clinical signs. *Contrib Nephrol* 71:1–9, 1989.

Berkoben MS, Schwab SJ: Vascular access for hemodialysis. In Nissenson AR, Fine RN, Gentile DE (eds): Clinical Dialysis, 3rd ed. Norwalk, CT, Appleton & Lange, pp. 26–45, 1995.

Bingel M, Arndt W, Schulze M, et al: Comparative study of C5a plasma levels with different hemodialysis membranes using an enzyme-linked immunosorbent assay. *Nephron* 51:320–324, 1989.

Bleyl U, Sander E, Schindler T: The pathology and biology of uremic pneumonitis. *Intensive Care Med* 7:193–202, 1981.

Bodey AR, Young LE, Bartram DH, et al.: A comparison of direct and indirect (oscillometric) measurements of arterial blood pressure in anaesthetised dogs, using tail and limb cuffs. *Res Vet Sci* 57:265–269, 1994.

Brescia MJ, Cimino JE, Appel K, et al.: Chronic hemodialysis using venipuncture and a surgically created arteriovenous fistula. *N Engl J Med* 275:1089–1092, 1989.

Bricker N: On the pathogenesis of the uremic state: An exposition of the trade-off hypothesis. *N Engl J Med* 286:1093–1099, 1972.

Brown SA, Crowell WA, Barsanti JA, et al.: Beneficial effects of

---

*Epogen, Amgen, Thousand Oaks, CA.

dietary mineral restriction in dogs with marked reduction of functional renal mass. *J Am Soc Nephrol* 1:1169–1179, 1991.

Butler HC: Advanced therapy for renal failure. *Proceedings of the 35th Annual Meeting of the American Animal Hospital Association,* Las Vegas, pp. 174–182, 1968.

Cases A, Reverter JC, Escolar G, et al.: In vivo evaluation of platelet activation by different cellulosic membranes. *Artif Organs* 21:330–334, 1997.

Charra B, Calemard E, Ruffet M, et al.: Survival as an index of adequacy of dialysis. *Kidney Int* 41:1286–1291, 1992.

Collins AJ, Ma JZ, Umen A, et al.: Urea index and other predictors of hemodialysis in patient survival. *Am J Kidney Dis* 23:272–282, 1994.

Cotton JR, Knochel JP: Correction of uremic cellular injury with a protein-restricted, amino acid–supplemented diet. *Am J Kidney Dis* 5:233–236, 1985.

Cotton JR, Woodard T, Carter NW, Knochel JP: Resting skeletal muscle membrane potential as an index of uremic toxicity. *J Clin Invest* 63:501–506, 1979.

Cowgill LD: Current status of veterinary hemodialysis. In Kirk RW (ed): *Current Veterinary Therapy VII. Small Animal Practice.* Philadelphia, WB Saunders Co., pp. 1111–1113, 1980.

Cowgill, LD: Application of peritoneal dialysis and hemodialysis in the management of renal failure. In Osborne CA, Finco DR (eds): *Canine and Feline Nephrology and Urology.* Baltimore, Williams & Wilkins, pp. 573–596, 1995a.

Cowgill LD: Medical management of the anemia of chronic renal failure. In Osborne CA, Finco DR (eds): *Canine and Feline Nephrology and Urology.* Baltimore, Williams & Wilkins, pp. 539–554, 1995b.

Cowgill LD, Langston CE: Role of hemodialysis in the management of dogs and cats with renal failure. *Vet Clin North Amer* 26:1347–1378, 1996.

Cowgill LD, Maretzki CH: CVT update: veterinary applications of hemodialysis. In Bonagura JD, Kirk RW (eds): *Kirk's Current Veterinary Therapy XII. Small Animal Practice.* Philadelphia, WB Saunders Co., pp. 975–977, 1995.

Crowe DT, Spreng DE: Doppler assessment of blood flow and pressure in surgical and critical care patients. In Bonagura JD, Kirk RW (eds): *Kirk's Current Veterinary Therapy XII. Small Animal Practice.* Philadelphia, WB Saunders Co., pp. 113–117, 1995.

Daugirdas JT: Simplified equations for monitoring Kt/V, PCRn, eKtV, and ePCRn. *Adv Ren Replace Ther* 2:295–304, 1995.

DeBroe ME: Haemodialysis-induced hypoxaemia. *Nephrol Dial Transplant* 9:173–175, 1994.

Delmez JA, Slatopolsky E: Hyperphosphatemia: Its consequences and treatment in patients with chronic renal disease. *Am J Kidney Dis* 19:303–317, 1992.

De Lorenzo A, Andreoli A, Matthie J, et al: Predicting body cell mass with bioimpedance by using theoretical methods: A technological review. *J Appl Physiol* 82:1542–1558, 1997.

Depner TA: Urea modeling: introduction. In *Prescribing Hemodialysis: A Guide to Urea Modeling.* Boston, Kluwer Academic Publishers, pp.39–64, 1991.

Depner TA: Estimation of Kt/V from the URR for varying levels of dialytic weight loss: A bedside graphic aid. *Semin Dial* 6:242, 1993.

Dhein CRM: Hemodialysis in the dog. *Compend Contin Educ* 3:1031–1045, 1981.

DiBartola SP, De Morais HSA: Disorders of potassium: hypokalemia and hyperkalemia. In DiBartola SP (ed): *Fluid Therapy in Small Animal Practice.* Philadelphia, WB Saunders Co., pp. 89–115, 1992.

Drukker W: Haemodialysis: A historical review. In Maher JF (ed): *Replacement of Renal Function by Dialysis: A Textbook of Dialysis,* 3rd ed. Dordrecht, Kluwer Academic Publishers, pp. 20–86, 1989.

Falkenhagen D, Bosch T, Brown GS, et al.: A clinical study on different cellulosic dialysis membranes. *Nephrol Dial Transplant* 2:537–545, 1987.

Fine RN, Tejani A: Dialysis in infants and children. In Daugirdas JT, Ing TS (eds): *Handbook of Dialysis,* 2nd ed. Boston, Little, Brown, pp. 553–568, 1994.

Fisch BJ, Spiegel DM: Assessment of excess fluid distribution in chronic hemodialysis patients using bioimpedance spectroscopy. *Kidney Int* 49:1105–1109, 1996.

Funder J, Wieth JO: Changes in cerebrospinal fluid composition following hemodialysis. *Scand J Clin Lab Invest* 19:301–312, 1967.

Garella S: Extracorporeal techniques in the treatment of exogenous intoxications. *Kid Int* 33:735–754, 1988.

Garella S, Lorch JA: Hemodialysis and hemoperfusion for poisoning. *AKF Nephrol Lett* 10:1–19, 1993.

Gotch FA: Kinetic modeling in hemodialysis. In Nissenson AR, Fine RN, Gentile DE (eds): *Clinical Dialysis,* 3rd ed. Norwalk, Appleton & Lange, pp. 156–188, 1995.

Gotch FA, Sargent JA: A mechanistic analysis of the National Cooperative Dialysis Study (NCDS). *Kidney Int* 28:526–534, 1985.

Gourley IM, Parker HR, Bell RL, et al.: Responses of nephrectomized dogs during hemodialysis. *Am J Vet Res* 34:1421–1425, 1973.

Grollman EF, Grollman A: Toxicity of urea and its role in the pathogenesis of uremia. *J Clin Invest* 38:749–754, 1959.

Hakim RM: Assessing the adequacy of dialysis. *Kidney Int* 37:822–832, 1990.

Hakim RM, Lowrie EG: Hemodialysis-associated neutropenia and hypoxemia: The effect of dialyzer membrane materials. *Nephron* 32:32–39, 1982.

Hakim RM, Breyer J, Ismail N, et al.: Effects of dose of dialysis on morbidity and mortality. *Am J Kidney Dis* 23:661–669, 1994.

Heierli C, Markert M, Lambert PH, et al.: On the mechanisms of haemodialysis-induced neutropenia: A study with five new and re-used membranes. *Nephrol Dial Transplant* 3:773–783, 1988.

Held PJ, Port FK, Wolfe RA, et al.: The dose of hemodialysis and patient mortality. *Kidney Int* 50:550–556, 1996.

Henderson LW: Biophysics of ultrafiltration and hemofiltration. In Maher JF (ed): *Replacement of Renal Function by Dialysis: A Textbook of Dialysis,* 3rd ed. Dordrecht, Kluwer Academic Publishers, pp. 300–326, 1989.

Hoenich NA, Woffindin C, Ward MK: Dialyzers. In Maher JF (ed): *Replacement of Renal Function by Dialysis: A Textbook of Dialysis,* 3rd ed. Dordrecht, Kluwer Academic Publishers, pp. 144–180, 1989.

Hoenich NA, Woffindin C, Mathews JN, Vienken J: Biocompatibility of membranes used in the treatment of renal failure. *Biomaterials* 16:587–592, 1995.

Jabara AE, Mehta RL: Determination of fluid shifts during chronic hemodialysis using bioimpedance spectroscopy and an in-line hematocrit monitor. *ASAIO J* 41:M682–M687, 1995.

Jaffrin MY, Maasrani M, Boudailliez B, et al.: Extracellular and intracellular fluid volume monitoring during dialysis by multifrequency impedancemetry. *ASAIO J* 42:M533–M538, 1996.

Johnson WJ, Hagge WW, Wagoner RD, et al.: Effects of urea loading in patients with far-advanced renal failure. *Mayo Clin Proc* 47:21–29, 1972.

Katzarski KS: Monitoring of blood volume during haemodialysis treatment of acute renal and multiple organ failures. *Nephrol Dial Transplant* 11:20–23, 1996.

Kennedy AC, Linton AL, Easton JC: Urea levels in cerebrospinal fluid after haemodialysis. *Lancet* 1:410–411, 1962.

Kolb G, Hoffken H, Muller T, et al.: Kinetics of pulmonary leukocyte sequestration in man during hemodialysis with different membrane-types. *Int J Artif Organs* 13:729–736, 1990.

Kruger JM, Osborne CA, Nachreiner RF, Refsal KR: Hypercalcemia

and renal failure. *Vet Clin North Am Small Anim Pract* 26:1417–1445, 1996.
Langston CE, Cowgill LD, Spano JA: Applications and outcome of hemodialysis in cats: A review of 29 cases. *J Vet Intern Med* 11:348–355, 1997.
Ledebo I: Bicarbonate in high-efficiency hemodialysis. *Cont Issues Nephrol* 27:9–25, 1993.
Levett DL, Woffindin C, Bird AG, et al.: Complement activation in haemodialysis: A comparison of new and re-used dialysers. *Int J Artif Organs* 9:97–104, 1986.
Lowrie EG, Laird NM, Parker TF, Sargent JA: Effect of hemodialysis prescription on patient morbidity: Report from the National Cooperative Dialysis Study. *N Engl J Med* 305:1176–1180, 1981.
Lucchi L, Bonucchi D, Acerbi MA, et al.: Improved biocompatibility by modified cellulosic membranes: The case of hemophan. *Artif Organs* 13:417–421, 1989.
Matthie J, Zarowitz B, De Lorenzo, et al.: Analytic assessment of the various bioimpedance methods used to estimate body water. *J Appl Physiol* 84:1801–1816, 1998.
May RC, Mitch WE: Pathophysiology of uremia. In Brenner BM (ed): *The Kidney*, 5th ed. Philadelphia, WB Saunders Co., pp. 2148–2169, 1996.
Mujais SK, Schmidt B: Operating characteristics of hollow fiber dialyzers. In Nissenson AR, Fine RN, Gentile DE (eds): *Clinical Dialysis*, 3rd ed. Norwalk, Appleton & Lange, pp. 77–92, 1995.
NKF-DOQI clinical practice guidelines for hemodialysis adequacy. *Am J Kidney Dis* 30:S15–S66, 1997.
Owen WF, Lew NL, Liu Y, et al.: The urea reduction ratio and serum albumin concentration as predictors of mortality in patients undergoing hemodialysis. *N Engl J Med* 329:1001–1006, 1993.
Parker HR, Gourley IM, Bell RL: Current developments in peritoneal and hemodialysis. *Proceedings of the 22nd Gaines Veterinary Symposium*, Stillwater, pp. 3–15, 1972.
Parker T, Husni L, Huang W, et al.: Survival of hemodialysis patients in the United States is improved with greater quantity of dialysis. *Am J Kidney Dis* 23:670–680, 1994.
Pastan S: Dialysis therapy. *N Engl J Med* 338:1428–1437, 1998.
Polzin DJ, Osborne CA: Conservative medical management of chronic renal failure. In Osborne CA, Finco DR (eds): Canine and Feline Nephrology and Urology. Baltimore, Williams & Wilkins, pp. 508–538, 1995.
Polzin DJ, Osborne CA, Bartges JW, et al.: Chronic renal failure. In Ettinger SJ, Feldman ED (eds): *Textbook of Veterinary Internal Medicine. Diseases of the Dog and Cat*, 4th ed, Vol 2. Philadelphia, WB Saunders Co., pp. 1734–1760, 1995.
Prabhu PN, Kerns SR, Sabatelli FW, et al.: Long-term performance and complications of the Tesio twin catheter system for hemodialysis. *Am J Kidney Dis* 30:213–218, 1997.
Raja RM: Sodium profiling in elderly haemodialysis patients. *Nephrol Dial Transplant* 11:42–45, 1996.
Renal Data System: *USRDS 1997 Annual Data Report*. Bethesda, MD, National Institute of Diabetes and Digestive and Kidney Diseases, 1997.
Rosa AA, Shideman J, McHugh R, et al.: The importance of osmolality fall and ultrafiltration rate on hemodialysis side effects. *Nephron* 27:134–41, 1981.
Sargent JA, Gotch FA: Principles and biophysics of dialysis. In Maher JF (ed): *Replacement of Renal Function by Dialysis: A Textbook of Dialysis*, 3rd ed. Dordrecht, Kluwer Academic Publishers, pp. 87–143, 1989.
Schaefer RM, Horl WH, Kokot K, Heidland A: Enhanced biocompatibility with a new cellulosic membrane: Cuprophan versus hemophan. *Blood Purif* 5:262–267, 1987.
Sherman RA, Cody RP, Rogers ME, Solanchick JC: Accuracy of the urea reduction ration in predicting dialysis delivery. *Kidney Int* 47:319–321, 1995.
Slatopolsky E, Delmez JA: Pathogenesis of secondary hyperparathyroidism. *Miner Electrolyte Metab* 21:55–62, 1995.
Steuer RR, Harris DH, Conis JM: A new optical technique for monitoring hematocrit and circulating blood volume: Its application in renal dialysis. *Dial Transplant* 22:260–265, 1993.
Steuer RR, Leypoldt JK, Cheung AK, et al.: Reducing symptoms during hemodialysis by continuously monitoring the hematocrit. *Am J Kidney Dis* 27:525–532, 1996.
Stewart WK, Fleming LW: Blood pressure control during maintenance heamodialysis with isonatric (high sodium) dialysate. *Postgrad Med J* 50:260–264, 1974.
Tesio F, De Baz H, Panarello G, et al.: Double catheterization of the internal jugular vein for hemodialysis: Indications, techniques, and clinical results. *Artif Organs* 18:301–304, 1994.
Thornhill JA: Hemodialysis. In Bovee KC (ed): *Canine Nephrology*. Harwal, Media, PA, pp. 755–802, 1984.
Thrall MA, Grauer GF, Dial SM: Antifreeze poisoning. In Bonagura JD, Kirk RW (eds): *Kirk's Current Veterinary Therapy XII. Small Animal Practice*. Philadelphia, WB Saunders, Co. pp. 232–237, 1995.
Van Stone JC, Daugirdas JT: Physiological principles. In Daugirdas JT, Ing TS (eds): *Handbook of Dialysis*, 2nd ed. Boston, Little, Brown, pp. 13–29, 1994.
Walton DF, Cheung AK: Membrane biocompatibility. In Nissenson AR, Fine RN, Gentile DE (eds): *Clinical Dialysis*, 3rd ed. Norwalk, Appleton & Lange, pp. 93–120, 1995.
Ward RA: Acid-base homeostasis in dialysis patients. In Nissenson AR, Fine RN, Gentile DE (eds): *Clinical Dialysis*, 3rd ed. Norwalk, Appleton & Lange, pp. 495–517, 1995.
Ward RA, Schaefer RM, Falkenhagen D, et al.: Biocompatibility of a new high-permeability modified cellulose membrane for haemodialysis. *Nephrol Dial Transplant* 8:47–53, 1993.
Woffindin C, Hoenich NA: Blood-membrane interactions during haemodialysis with cellulose and synthetic membranes. *Biomaterials* 9:53–57, 1988.

Appendix to Chapter 26
Regional Hemodialysis Referral Centers

Companion Animal Hemodialysis Unit, Veterinary Medical Teaching Hospital, University of California-Davis, Davis, CA 95616. Phone: 530 752-1393.

The Animal Medical Center, 510 East 62nd Street, New York, NY 10021. Phone: 212 838-8100.

Veterinary Referral Associates, Inc., 15021 Dufief Mill Road, Gaithersburg, MD 20878. Phone: 301 340-3224.

Veterinary Clinical Center, Michigan State University, East Lansing, MI 48824. Phone: 517 347-5034.

APPENDIX

Clinical Cases

STEPHEN P. DiBARTOLA HELIO AUTRAN DE MORAIS

This appendix consists of 34 clinical cases derived primarily from the medical records of the Ohio State University Veterinary Teaching Hospital. The cases demonstrate application of the principles discussed earlier in the book, and wherever possible reference is made to individual chapters for further reading. Each case consists of a brief history and physical findings followed by laboratory findings and diagnosis; then the interpretation of the laboratory findings is discussed at length. Finally, the treatment and outcome are summarized. Formulas and rules required for evaluation of the cases are summarized in the following tables for quick reference.

Case 1 (Table App–8)

Signalment. 2-year-old intact male Doberman pinscher, 27 kg

Chief Complaint. Seizures

History. The dog normally lived outdoors but was placed in a garage to protect him from recent cold weather. The next morning, the owners found the dog trembling, standing with an arched back, and stumbling when he attempted to walk. A generalized seizure followed. The dog was anorexic but extremely thirsty before the onset of seizures and had urinated several times. He also vomited several times in the past 24 h, and the vomitus contained salt granules from a bag of water softener that the dog had chewed open, as well as fragments of plasterboard dry-wall material.

Physical Examination. The dog was having a seizure at presentation, and the examination was conducted after intravenous administration of diazepam. The dog's temperature was 106°F. The dog was thin and 5–7% dehydrated. Mucous membranes were bright red and dry, and capillary refill time was under 1 s. The eyes were sunken in their sockets. There were no abnormalities on abdominal palpation, and the bladder was small.

Ancillary Findings. Blood lead concentration was 18 µg/dL.

Diagnosis. Salt poisoning

Interpretation. The clinical findings for this dog resemble those reported in dogs that received water containing 10% NaCl as a result of a defective water softener (Hughes and Sokolowski 1978). These signs included progressive ataxia, seizures, prostration, and death. Clinical signs are due to osmotic movement of water out of brain cells. A rapid decrease in brain volume may cause rupture of small cerebral vessels and focal hemorrhage. The severity of clinical signs is related more to the rapidity of onset of hypernatremia than to its magnitude. The entire clinical course in this dog was less than 48 h. In all likelihood, the dog's brain did not have sufficient time to protect itself from hyperosmolality by development of idiogenic osmoles.

Treatment. At presentation, several doses of diazepam and phenobarbital were administered in an attempt to stop the dog's seizures. An intravenous infusion of lactated Ringer's solution was begun while awaiting laboratory results, and approximately 500 mL was adminis-

TABLE APP–1. Compensatory Response in Simple Acid-Base Disturbances in Dogs*

Metabolic acidosis	For each 1 mEq/L decrease in [HCO_3^-] P_{CO_2} decreases 0.7 mm Hg
Metabolic alkalosis	For each 1 mEq/L increase in [HCO_3^-] P_{CO_2} increases 0.7 mm Hg
Acute respiratory acidosis	For each 1 mm Hg increase in P_{CO_2} [HCO_3^-] increases 0.15 mEq/L
Chronic respiratory acidosis	For each 1 mm Hg increase in P_{CO_2} [HCO_3^-] increases 0.35 mEq/L
Acute respiratory alkalosis	For each 1 mm Hg decrease in P_{CO_2} [HCO_3^-] decreases 0.25 mEq/L
Chronic respiratory alkalosis	For each 1 mm Hg decrease in P_{CO_2} [HCO_3^-] decreases 0.55 mEq/L

*See Chapter 12.

TABLE APP–2. **Normal Mean Values for Venous and Arterial Blood Gases in Dogs**

Site of Collection: Sample	Carotid Artery Arterial	Pulmonary Artery Mixed Venous	Jugular Vein Venous	Cephalic Vein Venous	Unit
pH	7.395	7.361	7.352	7.360	
P_{O_2}	102.1	53.1	55.0	58.4	mm Hg
P_{CO_2}	36.8	43.1	42.1	43.0	mm Hg
HCO_3^-	21.4	23.0	22.1	23.0	mEq/L
Total CO_2	22.4	24.1	23.2	24.1	mEq/L
Base excess	−1.8	−1.1	−2.0	−1.2	mEq/L

Source: From Ilkiw JE, Rose RJ, and Martin ICA: A comparison of simultaneously collected arterial, mixed venous, jugular venous, and cephalic venous blood samples in the assessment of blood gas and acid base status in the dog. *J Vet Intern Med* 5:294–298, 1991.

*Note that venous P_{CO_2} values are approximately 5–6 mm Hg higher than arterial values.

tered during the first hour of hospitalization. After return of the laboratory results, fluids were changed to 0.45% NaCl in 2.5% dextrose administered over the next 8 h. An infusion of 5% dextrose in water was begun approximately 10 h after admission. An attempt was made to reduce serum sodium concentration slowly by beginning with 0.45% NaCl in 2.5% dextrose followed by 5% dextrose in water. Ideally, serum sodium concentration should be lowered at a rate of 2 mEq/L/h or less over the first 48 h. Adjunctive therapy may include administration of furosemide to promote natriuresis and chloruresis.

Outcome. The dog died within 24 h of admission to the hospital. At necropsy, moderately severe meningoencephalitis, characterized by accumulation of lymphocytes and macrophages, was observed. There was moderate encephalomalacia with glial cell pyknosis and neuronal degeneration.

Case 2 (DiBartola et al. 1994) (Tables App–9, App–10)

Signalment. 6-year-old intact male mixed-breed dog, 5 kg

Chief Complaint. Seizures

History. The dog had been obtained from an animal shelter 4 months before admission and had been kept as an experimental animal in a laboratory animal facility. The dog was not currently being used in any research project and was reportedly normally active, but its appetite varied greatly. On the day of admission, the animal caretaker observed that the dog staggered and then seizured shortly after feeding. The dog was treated with lactated Ringer's solution and hydrocortisone sodium succinate and was referred for further evaluation.

Physical Examination. The dog was dehydrated, emaciated, lethargic, and slightly hypothermic (99.7°F).

There was gingivitis, moderate dental tartar, and the ears contained a brownish-black dark exudate. Head bobbing, muscular tremors, and generalized muscular rigidity of the trunk were observed.

Ancillary Findings. Thoracic and abdominal radiographs on day 1 were unremarkable. Fundic examination was normal. Neurologic examination on day 2 showed head tremors, hypermetria, mild generalized weakness, ataxia, impaired conscious proprioception in the pelvic limbs, positional nystagmus, and hyperreflexic patellar myotatic reflexes. The pupils were dilated and poorly responsive to light. The dog bumped into objects but followed cotton balls tossed by its field of vision. It was concluded that the dog had widespread cerebral and cerebellar disease with dementia. The hypernatremia was thought to be secondary to underlying central nervous system disease. Adrenocorticotropic hormone (ACTH) and thyroid-stimulating hormone (TSH) stimulation tests performed on day 6 were normal. Computed tomography of the head on day 30 showed dilated lateral ventricles compatible with hydrocephalus. Cytologic analysis of cerebrospinal fluid was normal, and an electroencephalogram showed moderate intermittent slow-wave activity compatible with metabolic disease.

Diagnosis. Hydrocephalus; hypodipsia; essential hypernatremia

Interpretation. Hypernatremia in this dog was thought to be due to primary hypodipsia resulting from underlying neurologic disease, the residual effect of which appeared to be hydrocephalus. The dog maintained a slightly higher than normal serum sodium concentration, both when drinking water voluntarily (162 ± 10 mEq/L, range 154–201 mEq/L) and when water was added to the food (158 ± 6 mEq/L, range 150–168 mEq/L). Essential hypernatremia appears to represent insensitivity of the

TABLE APP–3. **Calculation of Alveolar-Arterial Oxygen Difference***

$$(A-a)D_{O_2} = (150 - 1.25\ Pa_{CO_2}) - Pa_{O_2}$$
Normal < 25 mm Hg

*See Chapter 11 for further information.

TABLE APP–4. **Anion and Osmolal Gaps**

Anion gap = $([Na^+] + [K^+]) - ([Cl^-] + [HCO_3^-])$
Normal anion gap = 12–25 mEq/L
Osmolal gap = P_{OSM} (measured) − P_{OSM} (calculated)
Normal osmolal gap = 0–10 mOsm/kg
P_{OSM} (measured) is determined by freezing-point depression osmometry
P_{OSM} (calculated) = $2\ [Na^+]$ + BUN/2.8 + glucose/18

TABLE APP-5. Formulas Used in Application of the Nontraditional Approach to Acid-Base Disturbances

Inorganic strong-ion difference, $[SID]_i = [Na^+] - [Cl^-]$
ΔUnmeasured anions = Base excess $- (\Delta FW + \Delta Cl + \Delta Albumin)$*

For Dogs
$[Cl^-]_{corrected} = [Cl^-] \times (146/[Na^+])$
ΔFree water $= 0.25([Na^+] - 146)$
ΔChloride $= 110 - [Cl^-]_{corrected}$
ΔAlbumin $= 3.7(3.1 - [Albumin])$ or, ΔProtein $= 3.0(6.4 - [Protein])$

For Cats
$[Cl^-]_{corrected} = [Cl^-] \times (156/[Na^+])$
ΔFree water $= 0.25([Na^-] - 156)$
ΔChloride $= 120 - [Cl^-]_{corrected}$
ΔAlbumin $= 3.7(3.1 - [Albumin])$ or, ΔProtein $= 3.0(7.2 - [Protein])$

*This equation assumes that the weak-acid component of plasma is made up entirely of proteins. Consequently, phosphates are included in this derived value for unmeasured anions. The resulting error is minimal when serum phosphorus concentration is normal but can become substantial whenever hyperphosphatemia is present.

TABLE APP-7. Serum Biochemistry Values for Dogs and Cats*

Substance	Dog	Cat	Units
CO_2	21	19	mEq/L
Calcium	10	9	mg/dL
Phosphorus	4	4	mg/dL
Sodium	146	156	mEq/L
Potassium	4	4	mEq/L
Chloride	110	120	mEq/L
Total proteins	6.4	7.2	g/dL
Albumin	3.1	3.1	g/dL
BUN	8–25	15–35	mg/dL
Creatinine	<1.2	<1.8	mg/dL
Glucose	70–120	70–120	mg/dL

*These values are intended as guidelines only for use with this appendix. Laboratories performing these tests on dogs and cats have their own established normal ranges that should be consulted when interpreting values for individual patients.

TABLE APP-6. Calculation of Serum Phosphorus Concentration in mEq/L from mg/dL with Correction for Blood pH*

Almost all serum phosphorus is in the form of orthophosphate. Orthophosphoric acid is governed by the following set of equilibria:

$$H_3PO_4 \rightleftharpoons H_2PO_4^- + H^+ \rightleftharpoons HPO_4^{2-} + H^+ \rightleftharpoons PO_4^{3-} + H^+$$
$$pK_a\ 2.0 \qquad pK_a\ 6.8 \qquad pK_a\ 12.4$$

At the normal pH of extracellular fluid, H_2PO_4 and PO_4^{3-} are present in negligible amounts (see Appendix 1 in Chapter 7). Thus, plasma inorganic phosphorus is largely a mixture of $H_2PO_4^-$ and HPO_4^{2-}. The ratio of

$$HPO_4^{2-}/H_2PO_4^- = 10^{(pH - 6.8)}$$

At a pH of 7.4

$$HPO_4^{2-}/H_2PO_4^- = 10^{(7.4 - 6.8)} = 10^{(0.6)} = 4$$

and there is four times as much HPO_4^{2-} as $H_2PO_4^-$.

Serum phosphorus concentration in mg/dL is converted to mmol/L by multiplying by 10 and dividing by 31 (the atomic weight of phosphorus). If serum phosphorus concentration is 4 mg/dL:

$$4.0(10)/31 = 1.29\ mmol/L$$

At pH 7.4, 80% of the phosphorus is in the divalent (HPO_4^{2-}) form. Thus,

$$0.8 \times 1.29 = 1.03\ mmol/L$$

To convert to mEq/L

$$1.03\ mmol/L \times 2\ mEq/mmol = 2.06\ mEq/L$$

The remaining 20% of phosphorus is in the monovalent ($H_2PO_4^-$) form. Thus,

$$0.2 \times 1.29 = 0.26\ mmol/L$$

To convert this to mEq/L

$$0.26\ mmol/L \times 1\ mEq/mmol = 0.26\ mEq/L$$

The total phosphorus concentration in mEq/L is

$$2.06 + 0.26 = 2.32\ mEq/L$$

Source: Adapted from Gabow PA: Disorders associated with an altered anion gap. Kidney Int 27:472–483, 1985.

*See Chapter 7 for additional information.

hypothalamic osmoreceptors, so that volume depletion becomes the primary stimulus for antidiuretic hormone (ADH) release. See Chapter 3 for more information on this subject.

Defective function of the osmoreceptors can be demonstrated by hypertonic saline infusion. Administration of hypertonic saline increases plasma osmolality while causing volume expansion, so that the osmoreceptors are stimulated but the volume receptors are inhibited. In normal individuals, the response to hyperosmolality takes precedence, and ADH release leads to a decrease in urine volume and an increase in urine osmolality. In patients with essential hypernatremia, the osmoreceptors are defective and the response to volume takes precedence, so that ADH release is inhibited by volume expansion and urine volume increases while urine osmolality decreases. The latter type of response was observed in this dog after administration of hypertonic saline (see earlier).

Primary hypodipsia has been reported in young female miniature schnauzer dogs (Crawford et al. 1984; Hoskins and Rothschmitt 1984). Affected schnauzer dogs

TABLE APP-8. Laboratory Findings

Laboratory Test	0 h	2 h	11 h	Unit
Hematocrit	53	52	42	%
Plasma proteins	6.6	5.4	5.3	g/dL
Urine specific gravity	1.063			
CO_2	20			mEq/L
Calcium	10.0			mg/dL
Phosphorus	4.0			mg/dL
Sodium	177	165	158	mEq/L
Potassium	4.4	3.6	4.0	mEq/L
Chloride	153	136	138	mEq/L
Total protein	5.9			g/dL
Albumin	3.4			g/dL
BUN	41			mg/dL
Creatinine	1.4			mg/dL
Glucose	119			mg/dL
Osmolality	373			mOsm/kg

TABLE APP-9. Laboratory Findings

Laboratory Test	Day 1	Day 2	Day 3	Day 4	Day 12	Unit
Hematocrit	32			25		%
Plasma proteins	8.6			6.6		g/dL
Urine specific gravity	1.037			1.020		
CO_2	28		17	24	26	mEq/L
Calcium	10.1		9.3	10.0	10.3	mg/dL
Phosphorus	6.3		5.4	4.4	4.5	mg/dL
Sodium	201	172	162	160	161	mEq/L
Potassium	5.0	4.2	4.2	4.3	4.8	mEq/L
Chloride	161	138	130	123	117	mEq/L
Total protein	6.7		5.7	5.7	6.2	g/dL
Albumin	3.0		2.5	2.5	2.8	g/dL
BUN	100		29	19	14	mg/dL
Creatinine	1.0		0.9	0.9	0.8	mg/dL
Glucose	72		72	72	85	mg/dL
Osmolality	456	358	319	316	317	mOsm/kg

TABLE APP-10. Hypertonic Saline Infusion Study*

Time (min)	Urine Volume (mL)	U_{osm} (mOsm/kg)	USG	Na^+ (mEq/L)	K^+ (mEq/L)	P_{osm} (mOsm/kg)
0	28	1492	1.042	154	4.1	311
15	39	559	1.012	163	3.6	333
30	64	386	1.006	171	3.8	348
60	165	395	1.006	183	4.0	366
90	126	482	1.007	179	4.0	358
120	71	511	1.008	178	3.8	359
150	78	499	1.008	176	3.8	358
180	70	512	1.009	174	3.5	351
210	55	534	1.009	175	3.5	350
240	44	532	1.009	170	3.5	350
480	40	658	1.013	171	3.5	348
1440	ND	ND	ND	168	4.2	340

*Conditions of study: 20 mL/kg water given orally at 0 min; 400 mL 2.5% NaCl infused IV from 0–60 min; weight at 0 min: 7.5 kg; weight at 1440 min: 7.0 kg; vomited three times between 30 and 90 min.

See Figure App–1.

ND = not determined.

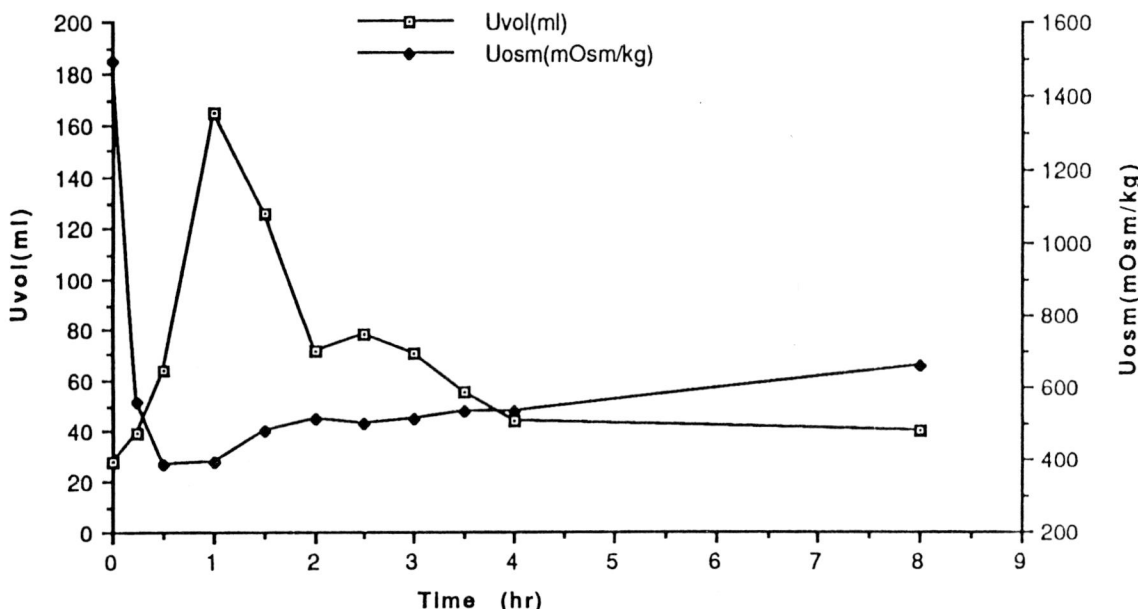

FIGURE APP-1. Urine volume (mL, left vertical axis) and urine osmolality (mOsm/kg, right vertical axis) during hypertonic saline infusion in a dog with essential hypernatremia.

have normal pituitary function and respond favorably to addition of water to their food. They appear to have a form of essential hypernatremia and show the typical response to hypertonic saline infusion described above.

Treatment. On days 1–4, the dog was treated with intravenous 0.45% NaCl with 2.5% dextrose. The dog urinated several times and began to eat on day 2. The dog was gradually weaned from intravenous fluids and allowed to eat and drink on its own.

Outcome. The dog was donated and remained in the hospital for 6 months. During this time, its voluntary water intake ranged from 9 to 43 mL/kg/day (mean, 23 ± 10 mL/kg/day). Normal water consumption in dogs ranges from 20 to 90 mL/kg/day. Water was added to the dog's food to ensure adequate water intake. The dog's serum sodium concentration ranged from 154 to 201 mEq/L (mean, 160 ± 10 mEq/L) during its hospitalization.

After 6 months, the dog was euthanized. On necropsy, there was hydrocephalus with moderate dilatation of the lateral ventricles and mild dilatation of the third ventricle. There was atrophy of the septum pellucidum and fornix, and these changes were thought to be due to destruction of these structures by increased pressure within the ventricular system. Histologically, there was neuraxonal dystrophy of the cuneate nuclei with large eosinophilic spheroids adjacent to neuronal cell bodies. The latter lesion was severe and may have contributed to the observed ataxia. There was no myelinolysis and thus no evidence of excessively rapid correction of hypernatremia. The cause of the observed lesions was unknown.

Case 3 (Simpson et al. 1994) (Table App–11)

Signalment. 3.5-year-old intact male dachshund, 8 kg

Chief Complaint. Anorexia, edema, abdominal distention

History. The owner reported that anorexia, lethargy, edema, and abdominal distention followed ingestion of Baker's chocolate 10 days before admission. The dog had vomited three to four times and passed several dark stools 2 days after ingestion of the chocolate. Abdominal distention, subcutaneous edema, and lethargy developed over the next 8 days. The owner insisted that the dog had been normal before eating the chocolate. The referring veterinarian treated the dog with antibiotics and gave two 25-mg doses of furosemide over a 3-day period.

Physical Examination. The dog was tachypneic (60/min) and hypothermic (99°F). Hepatomegaly and ascites were noted on abdominal palpation. Subcutaneous edema was present in the ventral cervical, thoracic, and abdominal regions. There was bilateral jugular venous distention, and femoral pulses were slightly weak. Increased bronchovesicular sounds (but no murmurs) were heard on thoracic auscultation.

Ancillary Findings. Thoracic radiographs showed severe, generalized cardiomegaly with enlargement of the caudal vena cava. Abdominal radiographs demonstrated hepatomegaly and ascites. Echocardiography showed severe dilatation of the right atrium, right ventricle, and tricuspid valve annulus. Tricuspid regurgitation was observed with color flow Doppler echocardiography. The valve was widely patent during systole, and this probably accounted for the lack of systolic murmur.

Diagnosis. Right-sided congestive heart failure

Interpretation. This dog had severe right-sided congestive heart failure because of a rare condition, right ventricular dysplasia. The severe hyponatremia resulted from free-water retention caused by activation of the renin-angiotensin-aldosterone system and nonosmotic stimulation of ADH release related to perceived volume depletion in the kidneys and central nervous system, re-

TABLE APP-11.	Laboratory Findings			
Laboratory Test	Day 1	Day 3 (AM)	Day 3 (PM)	Unit
Hematocrit	45	41		%
Plasma proteins	6.2	6.4		g/dL
Urine specific gravity	1.023			
Urine glucose	negative			
CO_2	16	23		mEq/L
Calcium	9.3	8.9		mg/dL
Phosphorus	6.3	4.9		mg/dL
Sodium	123	120	121	mEq/L
Potassium	5.8	4.0	3.3	mEq/L
Chloride	91	82		mEq/L
Total protein	5.1	5.2		g/dL
Albumin	2.7	2.7		g/dL
BUN	89	57		mg/dL
Creatinine	1.3	0.9		mg/dL
Glucose	207	192		mg/dL

spectively. Hyponatremia is commonly observed in patients with advanced right-sided or generalized heart failure. Hypochloremia was due to the dilutional effect of free-water retention ($[Cl^-]_{corrected}$ = 108 mEq/L). The mildly decreased CO_2 on admission suggests dilutional acidosis, also caused by free-water retention. The azotemia in this dog probably was prerenal in origin, resulting from reduced renal perfusion. The somewhat low urine specific gravity on admission may have reflected the effect of prior furosemide therapy on the urinary concentrating mechanism. The mild hyperkalemia probably resulted from impaired urinary excretion of potassium as a result of decreased renal perfusion and reduced distal tubular flow rate. The mild reduction in serum protein concentration may have been dilutional in origin or may have resulted from increased loss of protein via the gastrointestinal tract because of increased hydrostatic pressure in the splanchnic circulation. The hyperglycemia resulted from stress and endogenous release of glucocorticoids. The electrolyte and acid-base disturbances encountered in patients with heart failure are discussed further in Chapter 18.

Treatment. The dog initially was treated with furosemide 18 mg intravenously (IV) and 18 mg intramuscularly (IM), with subsequent IV doses every 6 h. Fluid therapy consisted of 0.45% NaCl with 2.5% dextrose administered IV at a rate of 2 mL/kg/h (370 mL/day) in an attempt to resolve prerenal azotemia and prevent further dehydration. Digoxin 0.08 mg per os (PO: orally) twice a day (q12h) also was begun. When hyperkalemia resolved, Aldactazide (spironolactone and hydrochlorothiazide) 25 mg PO q24h was begun. Furosemide was decreased to 18 mg q8h.

Outcome. On day 2, the dog was improved and there was partial resolution of edema and ascites. Intravenous fluids were discontinued. The dog was drinking water voluntarily at this time. On day 3, a dopamine infusion at 2 µg/kg/min in 0.45% NaCl with 2.5% dextrose with 28 mEq KCl per liter was begun. The owners elected euthanasia on day 4. At necropsy, the right ventricle was extremely dilated and the right ventricular free wall was very thin. No valvular changes were observed in the tricuspid valve, and this observation ruled out a diagnosis of tricuspid dysplasia. Other necropsy findings included edema of subcutaneous tissues, hepatomegaly, and pleural effusion. These findings were consistent with the diagnosis of right-sided congestive heart failure. The role of chocolate ingestion in this case remains unknown.

The use of loop and thiazide diuretics in this dog was not helpful in correcting the electrolyte disturbances, and thiazides may even contribute to free-water retention and aggravate hyponatremia. Partial water restriction may have increased serum sodium concentration, but this also may have worsened prerenal azotemia. The appropriate crystalloid solution to use in this dog is uncertain. The choice of 0.45% NaCl with 2.5% dextrose was made over 0.9% NaCl because of concern about sodium retention due to activation of the renin-angiotensin-aldosterone system. On the other hand, the concentration of sodium in 0.45% NaCl with 2.5% dextrose (77 mEq/L) would be expected to worsen hyponatremia in a patient with nonosmotic stimulation of ADH release. The ideal therapy in this case would increase cardiac output, thus correcting the perception of volume depletion in the periphery. This was attempted using digoxin and dopamine. Another approach would have been the judicious use of an angiotensin-converting enzyme inhibitor (e.g., enalapril) in an attempt to block activation of the renin-angiotensin-aldosterone system and its role in sodium retention. Enalapril was not used in this dog because of concern that right ventricular failure would prevent any significant increase in cardiac output in response to arterial vasodilatation and left ventricular afterload reduction.

Case 4 (Table App–12)

Signalment. 5-year-old spayed female mixed-breed dog, 11 kg

Chief Complaint. Vomiting

History. The dog had been vomiting two to three times per day over the 2–3 weeks before admission. The dog's appetite was fair, and vomiting occurred 3–4 h after feeding. The owner felt the dog also had lost weight in the past 2–3 weeks and seemed lethargic and weak. No diarrhea was observed, and the dog was still drinking water. The dog's water consumption before the onset of illness may have been increased from normal. Urinations decreased since the onset of illness. There was no known exposure to toxins or foreign bodies, and the dog was not receiving any medications.

Physical Examination. The dog was weak, hypothermic (98.7°F), bradycardic (52/min), and approximately 5–7% dehydrated. Mucous membranes were pink, but capillary refill time was prolonged and peripheral pulses were weak. There were no abnormalities on abdominal palpation.

Ancillary Findings. At presentation, an electrocardiogram showed a slow sinoventricular rhythm with T-wave amplitude exceeding R-wave amplitude and no discernible P waves. Plasma cortisol concentrations were lower than 1.0 µg/dL before and 1 h after administration

TABLE APP-12. **Laboratory Findings**

Laboratory Test	Day 1	Day 2	Day 29	Day 57	Unit
Hematocrit	46				%
Plasma proteins	7.4				g/dL
White blood cells	15,700				/µL
Segmented neutrophils	7,222				/µL
Lymphocytes	5,338				/µL
Monocytes	1,256				/µL
Eosinophils	1,884				/µL
Urine specific gravity	1.021				
CO_2	11.0	18.5	18.0	18.0	mEq/L
Calcium	11.9	8.5	10.8	11.3	mg/dL
Phosphorus	21.0	4.3	5.1	4.8	mg/dL
Sodium	126	148	132	148	mEq/L
Potassium	10.4	4.3	5.4	5.4	mEq/L
Chloride	92	120	100	111	mEq/L
Total protein	7.2	5.2	7.5	8.3	g/dL
Albumin	3.1	2.1	3.6	4.0	g/dL
BUN	114	17	22	19	mg/dL
Creatinine	6.6	0.9	0.9	0.9	mg/dL
Glucose	55.	94	110	113	mg/dL

of cosyntropin (synthetic adrenocorticotropic hormone, ACTH). Fecal flotation was negative.

Diagnosis. Hypoadrenocorticism

Interpretation. This dog was presented for evaluation of vomiting and weakness. These complaints are nonspecific but are common in dogs with hypoadrenocorticism. The presence of bradycardia (due to hyperkalemia) despite other evidence of hypovolemic shock (e.g., poor capillary refill, weak pulses) is suggestive of hypoadrenocorticism. The severe hyponatremia and hyperkalemia (Na/K ratio of 12:1) in the absence of urinary tract obstruction or anuric renal failure also are suggestive, and the results of the ACTH stimulation test were conclusive.

The low total CO_2 concentration (equivalent to bicarbonate concentration on an aerobically handled specimen) suggests the presence of metabolic acidosis due to the lack of aldosterone effect on H^+ secretion in the distal nephron and lactic acidosis due to reduced tissue perfusion. The presence of azotemia and hyperphosphatemia with low urine specific gravity may cause confusion, and a presumptive diagnosis of renal failure may be made. Less than maximal urine concentration is common at presentation in dogs with hypoadrenocorticism, despite a lack of intrinsic renal disease. This presumably is due to renal medullary solute washout caused by prolonged urinary loss of NaCl. After rehydration, renal function almost always returns to normal in dogs with hypoadrenocorticism.

Hypoadrenocorticism has been considered in the differential diagnosis of hypoglycemia. This dog had a blood glucose concentration of 55 mg/dL at presentation and required dextrose supplementation of its fluids. In one review of dogs with hypoadrenocorticism, however, hyperglycemia actually was more common than hypoglycemia (Willard et al. 1982). Mild hypercalcemia was observed in this dog at presentation and has been reported in dogs with hypoadrenocorticism. Proposed mechanisms for hypercalcemia include hyperproteinemia due to dehydration and hemoconcentration, lack of restraining effect of glucocorticoids on gastrointestinal absorption of calcium, increased parathyroid gland activity, and increased renal tubular reabsorption of calcium (Peterson and Feinman 1982). Mild hypercalcemia in this dog was probably due to dehydration.

The leukogram in dogs with hypoadrenocorticism typically shows normal numbers of lymphocytes and eosinophils despite severe stress. In this dog, lymphocytosis and increased numbers of eosinophils were observed.

Treatment. An intravenous infusion of 0.9% NaCl with 2.5% dextrose was begun. Fifteen mEq $NaHCO_3$ was given IV and 1 mg deoxycorticosterone acetate (DOCA) was given IM. Approximately 30 min later, another 15 mEq $NaHCO_3$ was given IV. After completion of the ACTH stimulation test, hydrocortisone sodium succinate 50 mg subcutaneously (SQ) q8h was begun. On day 2, fluids were changed to lactated Ringer's solution with 2.5% dextrose. On day 3, parenteral hydrocortisone and DOCA were discontinued and treatment was begun with 0.2 mg fludrocortisone PO q24h.

Outcome. On day 2, the dog was much improved. Its heart rate was 144/min and it ate readily. Serum sodium and potassium concentrations were 149 mEq/L and 4.1 mEq/L, respectively, on days 4 and 5. The dog was released from the hospital on day 6. At reevaluation on day 29, serum sodium concentration had decreased slightly and serum potassium concentration had increased. The dosage of fludrocortisone was increased to 0.3 mg PO q24h. This dog was treated medically over the next 8 years. Prednisone 5 mg PO q24h was added after approximately 1 year, and the dosage of fludrocortisone required a gradual increase to 0.7 mg PO q24h over 8 years. The dog was euthanized when it developed paraparesis at 13 years of age.

Case 5 (Tables App–13, App–14, App–15)

Signalment. 11-year-old male unilaterally cryptorchid miniature schnauzer dog, 11 kg

Chief Complaint. Urethral calculi, probable ruptured bladder

History. The dog was presented to the referring veterinarian for stranguria. The bladder was enlarged, and radiographs showed a urethral stone in the ischial area. Under anesthesia, the stone was retropulsed into the bladder, and the dog was treated with a calculolytic diet (Prescription Diet S/D) and antibiotics. One month later, there was no change in the appearance of the stone, and 2 weeks later a cystotomy was performed, and the dog was castrated. No cystic calculi were found at surgery. Postoperative radiographs showed two stones in the region of the prostate, but a urinary catheter could be passed easily. Four days after surgery, the dog was lethargic and began to vomit repeatedly. The dog was straining to urinate but only dribbling. It was dehydrated and experienced pain on abdominal palpation. Radiographs showed decreased abdominal detail, and paracentesis

TABLE APP–13. **Laboratory Findings**

Laboratory Test	Day 1	Day 2	Day 3	Day 65	Unit
Hematocrit	52				%
Plasma proteins	9.6				g/dL
Urine specific gravity	1.011				
CO_2	16			22	mEq/L
Calcium	9.8			10.8	mg/dL
Phosphorus	22.3			3.4	mg/dL
Sodium	139	169	170	150	mEq/L
Potassium	6.0	3.6	4.2	4.4	mEq/L
Chloride	90			115	mEq/L
Total protein	8.6			6.5	g/dL
Albumin	3.1			3.1	g/dL
BUN	201			21	mg/dL
Creatinine	10.5	3.6	1.9	1.5	mg/dL
Glucose	142			92	mg/dL

yielded free peritoneal fluid. The dog was referred for probable ruptured bladder.

Physical Examination. The dog was lethargic and 5–7% dehydrated. It was very tense and experienced pain on abdominal palpation.

Ancillary Findings. There was no bacterial growth on fluid obtained by paracentesis from the abdomen. Urine obtained by catheterization yielded fewer than 100 colony-forming units (CFU)/mL of *Escherichia coli*. The creatinine concentration of the abdominal fluid was 21.2 mg/dL, and the serum concentration was 10.6 mg/dL. Radiographs of the abdomen on day 2 showed poor abdominal detail, and the bladder could not be identified. Two stones were observed in the urethra distal to the ischial arch and proximal to the os penis. Ultrasound examination confirmed the presence of free fluid in the abdomen, and the bladder was identified. The stones removed at surgery (see later) were calcium oxalate on quantitative analysis.

Diagnosis. Ruptured bladder; urethral calculi

Interpretation. The hyponatremia, hypochloremia, hyperkalemia, azotemia, hyperphosphatemia, and metabolic acidosis observed in this dog at presentation were due to uroabdomen that occurred as a result of urethral obstruction by calculi and urine leakage from the site of the previous cystotomy. These abnormalities occur as urine is reabsorbed from the peritoneal cavity into extracellular fluid. The metabolic changes that occur with uroabdomen have been described in experimental dogs (Burrows and Bovee 1974). The hyponatremia and hypochloremia develop at least in part because urine normally contains much lower sodium and chloride concentrations than does extracellular fluid.

The increased hematocrit and plasma protein concentration at admission resulted from dehydration and hemoconcentration. The high blood glucose concentration may be attributed to stress. The low urine specific gravity is compatible with obstructive uropathy.

On admission, blood gas analysis showed a mixed acid-base disturbance characterized by metabolic acidosis due to ruptured bladder and respiratory alkalosis presumably due to hyperventilation secondary to abdominal pain. If the disturbance were a simple metabolic acidosis, the expected P_{CO_2} would be $37 - 0.7 (21 - 14.2) = 32.3$ mm Hg, and this value is more than 2–3 mm Hg higher than the observed P_{CO_2} of 25.9 mm Hg. On day 2, metabolic acidosis had resolved.

The $[SID]_i$ was 49 mEq/L, and the anion gap 39 mEq/L in this dog on day 1. The occurrence of a high $[SID]_i$ and high anion gap in a patient with normal plasma protein concentration indicates the presence of hypochloremic alkalosis and organic acidosis.

The dog's metabolic acidosis was due to hyperphosphatemia (-12.8 mEq/L) and accumulation of organic anions, such as lactic acid (-10.5 mEq/L), resulting in ΔUnmeasured anions of -23.3 mEq/L. There was an opposing hypochloremic alkalosis contributing $+16.0$ mEq/L to the measured base excess of -9.1 mEq/L. Thus, a triple disorder was present on day 1: metabolic acidosis due to hyperphosphatemia and accumulation of organic acids, hypochloremic metabolic alkalosis due to vomiting, and respiratory alkalosis. See Chapter 10 for more information.

Treatment. On day 1, the dog was treated with intravenous 0.9% NaCl and cephalothin 250 mg IV q6h was begun. A urinary catheter was placed, and urine output monitored. On day 2, fluids were changed to lactated Ringer's solution, with 26 mEq KCl added per liter.

Outcome. At surgery on day 2, the abdomen contained 300–400 mL free fluid, and urine was observed to be leaking from the previous cystotomy site, which appeared partially necrotic. The urethral stones were retropulsed from the urethra into the bladder and removed. The bladder wall defect was repaired. On day 3, fluids were changed to 0.45% NaCl with 20 mEq KCl per liter and the dog was switched to oral cephalexin 250 mg PO q6h. On day 4, fluids were tapered and the dog was released from the hospital on day 6. The dog was doing well when reevaluated on day 65.

TABLE APP–14. **Blood Gas Analysis**

Sample	Day 1 Arterial	Day 2 Arterial	Unit
pH	7.342	7.434	
P_{O_2}	94	85	mm Hg
P_{CO_2}	25.9	34.4	mm Hg
HCO_3^-	14.2	23.3	mEq/L
Total CO_2	15.0	24.3	mEq/L
Base excess	-9.1	$+0.2$	mEq/L

TABLE APP–15.

ΔFree water	-1.8 mEq/L
ΔChloride	$+16.0$ mEq/L
ΔAlbumin	0 mEq/L
ΔUnmeasured anions	-23.3 mEq/L*
Base excess	-9.1 mEq/L

*Includes ΔPhosphate $= -12.8$ mEq/L.

Case 6 (Tables App–16, App–17)

Signalment. 7-year-old spayed female mixed-breed dog, 18 kg

Chief Complaint. Diarrhea

History. The dog was lethargic, anorexic, and had passed liquid brown diarrhea for the past 7–10 days. Increased water consumption and possibly increased urinations also were observed by the owner. There was no blood or mucus in the feces, and the dog did not strain to defecate. The dog was passing five to six stools per day. The owner felt that the dog experienced profound weight loss during the past 2 weeks, and the medical record documented that the dog weighed 24 kg when examined 4 years previously.

Physical Examination. The dog was thin, 7–10% dehydrated, and had a dry unkempt haircoat. No pain was experienced and no masses were detected on abdominal palpation.

Ancillary Findings. Abdominal radiographs showed a fluid-filled colon but no other abnormalities. Thoracic radiographs showed severe microcardia and decreased pulmonary vascular size. Resting cortisol concentration was 22.0 µg/dL, and plasma cortisol concentration was 26.2 µg/dL 2 h after ACTH administration. A fecal flotation revealed *Trichuris vulpis*. A fecal culture was negative for *Salmonella*.

Diagnosis. Hypoadrenocorticism-like syndrome associated with *T. vulpis* infection

Interpretation. A syndrome with clinical and laboratory features resembling hypoadrenocorticism has been observed in dogs with gastrointestinal disease caused by trichuriasis, salmonellosis, and perforated duodenal ulcer (DiBartola et al. 1985; Malik et al. 1990). These animals develop hyponatremia and hyperkalemia with Na/K ratios that often are 20:1 or less. They rapidly develop hypokalemia if they are treated with mineralocorticoids.

Blood gas analysis indicated metabolic acidosis due to diarrhea and hypovolemia with reduced tissue perfusion with a greater than expected compensatory respiratory alkalosis. The normal expected compensation would have been $37 - 0.7 (21 - 8.2) = 28$ mm Hg. The observed P_{CO_2} of 19.1 mm Hg suggests the presence of a mixed acid-base disturbance (primary metabolic acidosis and primary respiratory alkalosis). Sepsis is a common cause of primary respiratory alkalosis and may have contributed to the mixed acid-base disturbance in this dog.

The high cortisol concentrations before and after ACTH stimulation are typical of hypoadrenocorticism-like syndrome in dogs with gastrointestinal disease and probably represent maximal adrenal stimulation by the stress of the underlying disease process. These results rule out a diagnosis of hypoadrenocorticism (see Case 4). The hyponatremia is due to gastrointestinal losses and is exacerbated by continued drinking and nonosmotic stimulation of ADH release in response to volume depletion. The hyperkalemia may be related in part to metabolic acidosis, but decreased urinary excretion of potassium caused by reduced distal renal tubular flow rate probably is the most important cause.

The azotemia and hyperphosphatemia at presentation were prerenal in nature as evidenced by their resolution over the following 2 weeks. The high BUN/creatinine ratio at admission (31:1) is compatible with reduced tubular flow rate and prerenal azotemia. The leukogram differential and marked hyperglycemia at presentation were the result of stress-induced endogenous release of glucocorticoids. Hemoconcentration at admission masked underlying hypoproteinemia due to protein and blood loss through the gastrointestinal tract.

Treatment. A saline solution (0.9%) was administered IV at a rate of 100 mL/h for the first hour and then at 75 mL/h, and 20 mEq $NaHCO_3$ was administered IV. Hydrocortisone sodium succinate (20 mg) was administered IV after completion of the ACTH stimulation test. Treatment with 280 mg trimethoprim-sulfadiazine SQ q12h was begun. In the evening, 25 g dextrose, 50 mEq $NaHCO_3$, and 5 mEq KCl were added per liter of 0.9% NaCl. After 24 h, 50 g dextrose and 20 mEq KCl were added per liter of 0.9% NaCl. Fluid therapy was tapered and discontinued by day 4.

Outcome. The dog vomited several times and had watery brown diarrhea with straining during the first 24

TABLE APP–16. **Laboratory Findings**

Laboratory Test	Day 1	Day 4	Day 13	Unit
Hematocrit	55	39		%
Plasma proteins	7.3	5.0		g/dL
White blood cells	61,000			/µL
Bands	600			/µL
Segmented neutrophils	54,900			/µL
Lymphocytes	600			/µL
Monocytes	4,900			/µL
Eosinophils	0			/µL
Platelets	326,000			/µL
Urine specific gravity	1.023			
Urine glucose/ketones	negative			
CO_2	8	19	20	mEq/L
Calcium	10.5	8.1	10.5	mg/dL
Phosphorus	10.7	2.0	3.4	mg/dL
Sodium	115	137	151	mEq/L
Potassium	6.3	3.5	4.2	mEq/L
Chloride	80	104	115	mEq/L
Total protein	6.5	4.1	5.5	g/dL
Albumin	3.3	2.0	2.5	g/dL
BUN	107	14	24	mg/dL
Creatinine	3.4	1.5	1.1	mg/dL
Glucose	319	114	111	mg/dL

TABLE APP–17. **Blood Gas Analysis**

Sample	Day 1 Arterial	4 h Later Venous	Unit
pH	7.237	7.307	
P_{O_2}	103	46	mm Hg
P_{CO_2}	19.1	24.8	mm Hg
HCO_3^-	8.2	12.5	mEq/L
Total CO_2	8.8	13.2	mEq/L
Base excess	−16.3	−11.3	mEq/L

h of therapy. Within 24 h, the dog was more alert but still lethargic and weak. After 72 h, the dog was alert and responsive but still had diarrhea. Panacur was administered for trichuriasis. By day 4, the stools had a consistency of pudding, and the dog had a good appetite. The dog was released from the hospital on day 5 and weighed 19 kg at that time. At a checkup 1 week after discharge, the dog was doing very well at home and weighed 21 kg.

Case 7 (Table App–18)

Signalment. 13-year-old spayed female silky terrier, 4 kg

Chief Complaint. Dyspnea due to pleural effusion

History. The dog developed a cough 6 weeks before admission, and pleural effusion was diagnosed by the referring veterinarian 3 weeks before admission. A chest tube was placed, and 350 mL serosanguineous fluid was removed over a 1-week period before referral. The fluid removed from the chest had become progressively more hemorrhagic during this time. The dog was lethargic and anorexic but continued to drink water. Dyspnea and coughing were observed whenever pleural fluid accumulated. The dog had been treated with antimicrobials (amoxicillin, trimethoprim-sulfadiazine, cefadroxil), corticosteroids (triamcinolone, dexamethasone) and furosemide. There was no history of trauma.

Physical Examination. The dog was lethargic and 5–7% dehydrated. The heart sounds were muffled and lung sounds were increased dorsally. Respiratory rate was increased (76/min).

Ancillary Findings. Thoracic radiographs showed pleural effusion and possible collapse or neoplasia of the left caudal lung lobe. The chest tube was noted to be directed caudally and dorsally. On cytologic evaluation, the pleural fluid was determined to be a serosanguineous modified transudate containing nondegenerate neutrophils. No neoplastic cells or etiologic agents were noted. Bacteriologic culture of the pleural fluid yielded small numbers of *Pseudomonas aeruginosa* sensitive only to aminoglycoside antibiotics.

Diagnosis. Pleural effusion of undetermined cause (probable lung lobe torsion or neoplasm)

Interpretation. The hyponatremia and hyperkalemia are probably the result of third-space loss of sodium due to repeated thoracocentesis and decreased urinary excretion of potassium. The hyponatremia could have been exacerbated by continued drinking and nonosmotic stimulation of ADH release in response to volume depletion. These electrolyte changes have been reported in dogs with experimental and naturally occurring chylothorax that have been subjected to repeated thoracocentesis (Willard et al. 1991). Recognition of this association and its differentiation from hypoadrenocorticism are clinically important for proper care of the patient.

In this dog, the underlying cause of the hemorrhagic pleural effusion may have been a bleeding pulmonary neoplasm. The hemogram indicates a regenerative anemia with mild hypoproteinemia compatible with ongoing blood loss. The leukogram and hyperglycemia are compatible with the effects of stress and exogenously administered glucocorticoids.

The mild azotemia and hyperphosphatemia probably were prerenal in origin, and prior administration of glucocorticoids and furosemide may have interfered with urinary concentrating ability. Decreased urinary excretion of potassium could have resulted from decreased distal renal tubular flow rate. Reduced tubular flow rate and prerenal azotemia are supported by the high BUN/creatinine ratio of almost 40:1. These principles are discussed further in Chapters 2, 3, and 5.

Treatment. The dog was treated with amoxicillin-clavulanic acid 125 mg PO q12h (pending culture results) and received an infusion of 0.9% NaCl at a rate equal to twice maintenance needs.

Outcome. The chest tube was aspirated after 6 h of hospitalization, and 140 mL of hemorrhagic fluid was removed. At this time, the dog's mucous membranes were pale, its hematocrit was 16%, and its plasma proteins were 4.2 g/dL. These findings suggested ongoing hemorrhage into the pleural space. The dog experienced cardiac arrest, and attempts at resuscitation were unsuccessful. Request for necropsy was declined.

Case 8 (Tables App–19, App–20)

Signalment. 8-year-old spayed female mixed-breed dog, 23 kg

Chief Complaint. Recent development of jaundice after acute pancreatitis

History. The dog developed fever, anorexia, lethargy, and vomiting 48–72 h after eating raw bacon. Serum

TABLE APP–18. Laboratory Findings

Laboratory Test	Day 1	Unit
Hematocrit	25	%
Plasma proteins	6.0	g/dL
Reticulocytes	572,400	/µL
Red cell morphology	polychromasia, anisocytosis	
White blood cells	27,200	/µL
Bands	3,000	/µL
Segmented neutrophils	22,300	/µL
Monocytes	1,400	/µL
Nucleated red cells	500	/µL
Platelets	149,000	/µL
Urine specific gravity	1.017	
CO_2	16.0	mEq/L
Calcium	10.3	mg/dL
Phosphorus	9.8	mg/dL
Sodium	125	mEq/L
Potassium	7.7	mEq/L
Chloride	96	mEq/L
Total protein	4.9	g/dL
Albumin	2.5	g/dL
BUN	54	mg/dL
Creatinine	1.4	mg/dL
Glucose	172	mg/dL

TABLE APP–19. **Laboratory Findings**

Laboratory Test	Day 1	Unit
Hematocrit	41	%
Plasma proteins	6.0	g/dL
White blood cells	41,600	/µL
Bands	2,500	/µL
Segmented neutrophils	37,900	/µL
Lymphocytes	800	/µL
Monocytes	400	/µL
Platelets	157,000	/µL
CO_2	15	mEq/L
Calcium	9.4	mg/dL
Phosphorus	6.2	mg/dL
Sodium	128	mEq/L
Potassium	5.0	mEq/L
Chloride	100	mEq/L
Total protein	5.6	g/dL
Albumin	2.0	g/dL
BUN	18	mg/dL
Creatinine	1.0	mg/dL
Glucose	126	mg/dL
Bilirubin	6.9	mg/dL
Alkaline phosphatase	2,860	IU/L
Alanine aminotransferase	269	IU/L
Amylase	876	IU/L
Lipase	754	IU/L

lipase concentration was increased, and a tentative diagnosis of acute pancreatitis was made. The dog was treated with intravenous lactated Ringer's solution and cephalosporin antibiotics. Jaundice was first observed 4–5 days after the onset of acute pancreatitis. Corticosteroids were added to the treatment regimen. The dog continued to deteriorate over the next 10 days and was referred.

Physical Examination. The dog was 5–7% dehydrated, lethargic, and had icteric mucous membranes on physical examination. No abdominal pain or masses were detected on abdominal palpation.

Ancillary Findings. Abdominal radiographs showed loss of abdominal detail, presumably due to peritoneal effusion. A 4 × 5 cm soft tissue mass was suspected in the cranial abdomen. Abdominal ultrasonography confirmed the presence of peritoneal effusion and showed that the gallbladder was enlarged and the common bile duct dilated. A 3 × 3 cm echogenic mass was observed in the region of the proximal duodenum. Cytologic analysis of the peritoneal fluid showed many neutrophils and macrophages, extracellular and intracellular yellow-brown

TABLE APP–20 **Blood Gas Analysis**

Sample	Venous	Unit
pH	7.272	
P_{O_2}	45	mm Hg
P_{CO_2}	33.6	mm Hg
HCO_3^-	15.6	mEq/L
Total CO_2	16.7	mEq/L
Base excess	−9.5	mEq/L

pigment compatible with bilirubin, but no etiologic agents. The bilirubin concentration of the fluid was 17.0 mg/dL. Bacteriologic culture of the fluid yielded no growth.

Diagnosis. Acute pancreatitis, pancreatic abscess, or pancreatic neoplasia with posthepatic bile duct obstruction and bile peritonitis

Interpretation. Blood gas analysis indicated the presence of simple metabolic acidosis with normal respiratory compensation. The observed P_{CO_2} of 33.6 mm Hg was nearly identical to the calculated expected value of 37 − 0.7 (21 − 15.6), or approximately 33 mm Hg.

The hyponatremia and hypochloremia are due to third-space loss of these electrolytes caused by peritoneal effusion and impairment of renal water excretion by nonosmotic stimulation of ADH release in response to volume depletion. Adequate renal function and urinary potassium loss presumably prevented development of hyperkalemia.

The hyperbilirubinemia and increased alkaline phosphatase activity are compatible with posthepatic biliary obstruction caused by pancreatitis or pancreatic neoplasia. The leukocytosis with left shift is compatible with the presence of pancreatitis and bile peritonitis.

Treatment. The dog initially was treated with 0.45% NaCl in 2.5% dextrose and 20 mEq KCl per liter at a rate equal to 1.5 × maintenance, cephalothin 500 mg IV q8h, heparin 500 U SQ q8h, and vitamin K_1 8 mg SQ q8h When the serum electrolytes returned, fluids were changed to 0.9% NaCl with 20 mEq KCl per liter, and amikacin 115 mg IV q8h was added to the treatment regimen.

Outcome. A peritoneal drain was placed, and more than 2 L of yellow-brown fluid was removed from the abdomen over a 12-h period. An exploratory laparotomy was performed, and severe necrotizing pancreatitis and bile peritonitis were present, but no rupture of the biliary system could be demonstrated. The dog was euthanized at surgery because of the poor prognosis.

Case 9 (Tables App–21, App–22)

Signalment. 10-year-old castrated male domestic shorthair cat, 6 kg

Chief Complaint. Abdominal distention

History. The cat was presented for lethargy and abdominal distention that had developed over the past 7–10 days. Appetite had been poor over the past several months, and the feces had been formed but soft during the past month. No vomiting had been observed, and urinations were normal.

Physical Examination. The cat was lethargic and the abdomen was very distended, suggesting the presence of peritoneal effusion.

Ancillary Findings. Abdominal radiographs showed loss of visceral detail compatible with marked peritoneal effusion. There were several mineralized densities of vary-

TABLE APP-21. **Laboratory Findings**

Laboratory Test	Day 1	Unit
Hematocrit	31	%
Plasma proteins	7.3	g/dL
Urine specific gravity	1.037	
CO_2	16	mEq/L
Calcium	9.0	mg/dL
Phosphorus	6.9	mg/dL
Sodium	135	mEq/L
Potassium	7.0	mEq/L
Chloride	105	mEq/L
Total protein	5.8	g/dL
Albumin	2.5	g/dL
BUN	29	mg/dL
Creatinine	1.8	mg/dL
Glucose	158	mg/dL

ing sizes throughout the cranial abdomen, suggestive of carcinomatosis. Thoracic radiographs were unremarkable. Abdominal ultrasound examination confirmed the presence of peritoneal effusion. The resting cortisol concentration was 5.7 µg/dL, and it was 8.2 µg/dL 2 h after ACTH administration. The urea and creatinine concentrations of the peritoneal fluid were 28 mg/dL and 1.3 mg/dL, respectively. Abdominal paracentesis yielded serosanguineous fluid. Cytologic evaluation of the fluid indicated that it was a modified transudate with nondegenerate neutrophils, macrophages, and lymphocytes. No etiologic agents or neoplastic cells were noted. An FeLV ELISA was negative. Electrocardiography and echocardiography were normal.

Diagnosis. Peritoneal effusion of unknown cause, suspect carcinomatosis

Interpretation. Blood gas analysis indicates presence of metabolic acidosis without respiratory compensation. In the presence of normal respiratory compensation, a dog would have been expected to have a P_{CO_2} of approximately 34 mm Hg. There is some evidence, however, that cats do not adapt to metabolic acidosis as dogs and humans do. The reason for this lack of compensation is unknown. The acidosis in this cat primarily was dilutional in nature.

The hyponatremia was attributed to third-space loss of sodium and dilution of extracellular sodium concentration by continued drinking and nonosmotic stimulation of ADH release secondary to volume depletion. The hyperkalemia was attributed to decreased urinary excretion of potassium due to reduced distal tubular flow rate secondary to volume depletion. An ACTH stimulation test ruled out the possibility of hypoadrenocorticism as a cause for the electrolyte disturbances. The normal urea and creatinine concentrations of the peritoneal fluid ruled out uroabdomen as a cause. Hyponatremia and hyperkalemia have been reported in dogs with pleural effusion (e.g., chylothorax) (Willard et al. 1991).

Mild hypoproteinemia may have been due to loss of protein in the peritoneal effusion (fluid protein concentration was 3.7 g/dL), and mild hyperglycemia was attributed to the effect of endogenous glucocorticoids released in response to the stress of the disease process.

Treatment. The cat received lactated Ringer's solution subcutaneously during the course of its medical evaluation. At exploratory laparotomy, omental and mesenteric carcinomatosis were found.

Outcome. The cat was euthanized at the time of surgery. At necropsy, the origin of the carcinomatosis was found to be a colonic adenocarcinoma. Osteoid metaplasia was observed in the stroma of the neoplastic nodules and, presumably, accounted for the mineralization observed radiographically.

Case 10 (Tables App-23, App-24)

Signalment. 2-year-old castrated male domestic shorthair cat, 4 kg

Chief Complaint. Collapsed, unresponsive

History. The cat was kept outdoors and was poorly observed by the owner. Three days before admission the owner had noted that the cat was lethargic and partially anorexic. On the day of admission, the owner found the cat recumbent and unresponsive. The owner was not aware of the cat's urinary habits.

Physical Examination. The cat was recumbent and unresponsive to painful stimuli. There was bilateral mydriasis, and the pupils were poorly responsive to light. The cat was bradycardic (60/min), hypothermic (<94°F), and 12–15% dehydrated. Mucous membranes were dry but pink, and capillary refill time was prolonged. Abdominal palpation revealed an extremely large, turgid bladder that could not be expressed manually.

Ancillary Findings. An electrocardiogram obtained 2 h after admission and relief of obstruction showed a normal sinus rhythm with a heart rate of 120/min.

Diagnosis. Prolonged urethral obstruction

Interpretation. This cat presented with dehydration, metabolic acidosis, hyperkalemia, hypochloremia, hyperphosphatemia, hypocalcemia, and azotemia caused by prolonged urethral obstruction. Similar laboratory findings have been observed in cats with experimentally induced urethral obstruction (Finco and Cornelius 1977).

Blood gas analysis (5 min after $NaHCO_3$ administration) indicated the presence of a mixed disturbance characterized by metabolic acidosis due to postrenal uremia and respiratory acidosis due to impaired ventilation re-

TABLE APP-22. **Blood Gas Analysis**

Sample	Venous	Unit
pH	7.248	
P_{O_2}	26	mm Hg
P_{CO_2}	38.4	mm Hg
HCO_3^-	16.9	mEq/L
Total CO_2	18.1	mEq/L
Base excess	−9.1	mEq/L

TABLE APP–23. **Laboratory Findings**

Laboratory Test	0 h	3 h	72 h	96 h	Units
Hematocrit	42				%
Plasma proteins	9.1				g/dL
Urine specific gravity		1.014 (Obtained after relief of obstruction)			
CO_2	13		23		mEq/L
Calcium	7.2	4.9	9.0		mg/dL
Phosphorus	21.6		4.6		mg/dL
Sodium	151	160	154	157	mEq/L
Potassium	11.1	6.2	2.8	4.0	mEq/L
Chloride	95	112	113	114	mEq/L
Albumin	3.1		2.5		g/dL
BUN	322	205	20		mg/dL
Creatinine	16.5		2.1		mg/dL
Glucose	120		158		mg/dL

sulting from the semicomatose condition of the cat. There is some evidence that otherwise normal cats do not compensate for metabolic acidosis to the same extent as dogs and humans do. Even if this is true, the observed P_{CO_2} of 47.2 mm Hg is higher than normal and suggests a complicating respiratory acidosis. Administration of sodium bicarbonate presumably contributed to the hypercapnia observed in this cat. The presence of an additive mixed disorder also explains why the venous blood pH was so low (7.215).

Measurement of urine volume after relief of the obstruction demonstrated profound postobstructive diuresis during the first 2 days. Serial measurement of serum electrolyte concentrations demonstrated rapid resolution of hyperkalemia after relief of the obstruction and parenteral fluid therapy, development of hypokalemia during postobstructive diuresis, and resolution of hypokalemia with potassium supplementation of fluids and return of urine production to normal. These principles are discussed further in Chapter 5.

Treatment. Obstruction was relieved with an open-end polypropylene catheter by retrograde flushing of the urethra with saline, and the bladder was emptied of urine. Intravenous infusion of 0.9% NaCl was begun at 90 mL/kg/h for the first 2 h and the rate of infusion was then reduced. Sodium bicarbonate (20 mEq) was administered IV over 5 min. The cat was placed in the intensive care unit on a water-circulating heating pad. Fluid therapy was continued at insensible needs (16 mL/4 h) plus a volume equal to the urine production of the preceding 4 h ("ins and outs"). Fluid therapy was changed to lactated Ringer's solution after 12 h, and 20 mEq KCl was added per liter of lactated Ringer's after 48 h.

Outcome. During the first 48 h, the cat's urine production was 50–125 mL/h (normal, 6–12 mL/h). After 24 h, the cat was alert, and its appetite returned after 48 h. Urine production decreased to 7–12 mL/h during hospital day 3. Urinary and intravenous catheters were removed on hospital day 4. During hospital day 5, the cat's bladder remained large but was easily expressed by manual palpation. On hospital day 6, the cat was urinating normally, and its bladder remained small. The cat was discharged from the hospital, and the owner was given instructions about the medical management of feline lower urinary tract disease.

Case 11 (Table App–25)

Signalment. 8-year-old castrated male Himalayan cat, 5 kg

Chief Complaint. Severe dyspnea

History. The cat developed severe respiratory distress 1 week before admission. Treatment by the referring veterinarian included amoxicillin–clavulanic acid, furosemide, and aminophylline.

Physical Examination. The cat was lethargic, weak, and moderately dehydrated. Increased lung sounds and a gallop rhythm were heard on thoracic auscultation, but no murmurs were detected. He had weak femoral pulses.

Ancillary Findings. Thoracic radiographs on day 1 showed moderate to severe cardiomegaly with prominence of the pulmonary vasculature. Echocardiography was compatible with dilated cardiomyopathy. Serum thyroxine concentration was normal.

Diagnosis. Dilated cardiomyopathy

Interpretation. The leukocytosis with mature neutrophilia and hyperglycemia were attributed to stress. The mild azotemia was thought to be prerenal in origin (i.e., due to dehydration). The urine specific gravity was only 1.022, but the cat had been treated with furosemide, which may have interfered with urinary concentrating ability.

The increased total CO_2 concentration was attributed to hypochloremic alkalosis ($[SID]_i$ = 44 mEq/L) and probably was caused by prior furosemide administration. The combination of hypochloremia, hyponatremia, and hypokalemia may occur in animals with gastric vomiting or, as probably occurred in this cat, in patients that have been treated with loop diuretics. On day 6, the total CO_2 concentration was even higher, and this was attributed to a combination of hypochloremic alkalosis ($[SID]_i$ = 44 mEq/L), hypoproteinemic alkalosis, and resolution of the mild dilutional acidosis present on day 1.

Sodium concentration decreased, whereas potassium concentration increased on day 3. Hyponatremia with hyperkalemia may occur in hypoaldosteronism, in animals with third-space loss of fluid, or after treatment with angiotensin-converting enzyme inhibitors (e.g., captopril,

TABLE APP–24. **Blood Gas Analysis (5 min after receiving 20 mEq NaHCO₃ IV)**

Sample	Venous	Unit
pH	7.215	
P_{O_2}	47.4	mm Hg
P_{CO_2}	47.2	mm Hg
HCO_3^-	18.6	mEq/L
Total CO_2	20.3	mEq/L
Base excess	−8.8	mEq/L

TABLE APP–25. Laboratory Findings

Laboratory Test	Day 1	Day 3	Day 4	Day 6	Unit
Hematocrit	31				%
Plasma proteins	7.7				g/dL
White blood cells	26,900				/µL
Segmented neutrophils	24,700				/µL
Lymphocytes	1,600				/µL
Monocytes	500				/µL
Urine specific gravity	1.022				
CO_2	28			31	mEq/L
Calcium	9.5			9.3	mg/dL
Phosphorus	5.2			3.5	mg/dL
Sodium	142	137	151	157	mEq/L
Potassium	3.1	6.6	3.9	3.8	mEq/L
Chloride	98			113	mEq/L
Total protein	6.6			5.5	g/dL
Albumin	3.1			2.5	g/dL
BUN	59			28	mg/dL
Creatinine	1.8			1.5	mg/dL
Glucose	178			92	mg/dL

enalapril). The dosage of enalapril in this cat was decreased to 0.625 mg PO q24h on day 3, and the serum sodium and potassium concentrations normalized on the following day (day 4).

Treatment. On day 1, the cat was placed in an O_2 cage (FiO_2 = 40%), and furosemide (6.25 mg q24h), enalapril (0.625 mg q12h), digoxin (0.03 mg q48 h), taurine (250 mg q8h), and subcutaneous fluids were administered. Nitroglycerin ointment was used on days 6 and 7, and milrinone was administered on day 7.

Outcome. The cat responded well to treatment and did not have additional problems after release from the hospital.

Case 12 (Table App–26)

Signalment. 3-year-old castrated male domestic shorthair cat, 3 kg

Chief Complaint. Severe muscular weakness

History. The cat had developed severe rear limb and neck muscle weakness in the 5 days before admission. It had been anorexic and lethargic for the past week. At presentation, the cat could not hold its head up. Intermittent weakness and polydipsia had been observed by the owner over the previous 3 months. The cat had always been fed one brand of "low ash" cat food, promoted for its ability to acidify the urine and prevent feline lower urinary tract disease.

Physical Examination. The cat was hypothermic (99.8°F), thin, lethargic, and 5–7% dehydrated. On abdominal palpation, the kidneys were small, firm, and irregular. The cat held its head in a ventroflexed position. Fleas and flea dirt were observed.

Ancillary Findings. Urine culture yielded no growth. Renal ultrasonography showed cortical hyperechogenicity in both kidneys.

Diagnosis. Hypokalemic nephropathy

Interpretation. In this cat, anemia; azotemia; hyperphosphatemia; low urine specific gravity; and small, firm, irregular kidneys on abdominal palpation were indicative of chronic renal failure. The magnitude of the anemia was probably masked by dehydration as evidenced by hyperproteinemia. The markedly high fractional excretion of potassium (FE_K = 52.7%; normal, <24%) in the presence of marked hypokalemia (2.5 mEq/L) was inappropriate and identified the kidneys as the avenue of potassium loss. The muscular weakness was attributed to hypokalemia. The low CO_2 (13 mEq/L) at presentation suggested chronic metabolic acidosis as a contributing factor in development of potassium depletion.

Metabolic acidosis and hypokalemia resolved with fluid therapy and oral potassium supplementation, and renal function stabilized but did not return to normal. The FE_K gradually decreased during the course of treatment, despite ongoing oral potassium supplementation.

TABLE APP–26. Laboratory Findings

Laboratory Test	Day 1	Day 27	Day 122	Unit
Hematocrit	30			%
Plasma proteins	9.0			g/dL
Urine specific gravity	1.017			
CO_2	13	19	21	mEq/L
Calcium	10.7	9.9	11.0	mg/dL
Phosphorus	9.6	2.9	4.0	mg/dL
Sodium	153	156	155	mEq/L
Potassium	2.5	4.2	4.6	mEq/L
Chloride	116	119	117	mEq/L
Total protein	8.0	7.0	7.2	g/dL
Albumin	3.8	3.3	3.5	g/dL
BUN	102	54	39	mg/dL
Creatinine	4.5	2.8	2.2	mg/dL
Glucose	114	111	104	mg/dL
FE_K	52.7	37.9	16.4	%

Hypokalemic nephropathy characterized by chronic tubulointerstitial nephritis has been described in cats fed diets marginally low in potassium and with high acid content (Dow et al. 1987; DiBartola et al. 1993). These principles are discussed further in Chapter 5.

Treatment. The cat was given lactated Ringer's solution containing an additional 30 mEq/L KCl subcutaneously, and treatment was begun with oral potassium gluconate (Kaon) 5.3 mEq q12h.

Outcome. The cat improved with parenteral fluid therapy and oral potassium supplementation and was discharged from the hospital on day 4. Instructions were given to administer 2.7 mEq potassium gluconate PO q12h. The diet was changed to Prescription Diet Feline K/D. The cat was reevaluated several times over the following year and the dosage of potassium gluconate was varied between 2.5 and 3.5 mEq PO q12h. Serum creatinine concentration stabilized at approximately 2 mg/dL and BUN at approximately 40 mg/dL. During this time, $Al(OH)_3$ (Amphojel) was administered as a phosphorus binder.

Case 13 (Tables App–27, App–28)

Signalment. 8-year-old spayed female miniature schnauzer, 9 kg

Chief Complaint. Polyuria, polydipsia

History. The owner had noticed increased water consumption and urinations over the several weeks before admission. Appetite was normal, and no vomiting or diarrhea had been observed.

Physical Examination. The dog was 5–7% dehydrated, and there was a grade III/VI left apical systolic murmur on thoracic auscultation. There was severe dental tartar and periodontal disease. There were several small masses in the skin.

Ancillary Findings. A renal biopsy performed on day 8 showed mild tubular vacuolization in the renal cortex. Blood pressure determined by femoral arterial catheterization on day 50 was 205/85 mm Hg, with a mean value of 130 mm Hg.

Diagnosis. Hyperaldosteronism due to adrenal cortical carcinoma

Interpretation. This dog had hypokalemia due to primary hyperaldosteronism caused by a functional adrenocortical carcinoma. Mineralocorticoid excess is an uncommon cause of urinary potassium loss and hypokalemia in dogs and cats (Feldman and Nelson 1996; Reine et al. 1999). Increased secretion of aldosterone causes sodium retention, volume expansion with mild hypertension, potassium depletion and hypokalemia, and metabolic alkalosis. Stimulation of distal nephron Na-H and Na-K exchange by excess mineralocorticoids probably is the most important pathophysiologic mechanism in this disease.

The marked hypokalemia and increased urinary potassium loss in this dog were due to stimulation of distal nephron Na-K exchange by excess mineralocorticoids. Potassium depletion and hypokalemia lead to functional and morphologic changes in the kidney. The occurrence of polyuria and polydipsia in potassium depletion has psychogenic and nephrogenic components. Decreased responsiveness of the collecting ducts to ADH is related to decreased medullary tonicity, increased medullary blood flow, and impaired cyclic adenosine monophosphate (cAMP) generation in response to ADH. Potassium depletion and hypokalemia may have caused the polyuria and polydipsia observed in this dog.

The blood gas analysis indicates the presence of mild metabolic alkalosis. Enhanced Na-H exchange in the distal nephron due to excess mineralocorticoids may be responsible for this mild metabolic alkalosis.

Treatment. On its initial hospitalization (days 1–11), the dog was given parenteral fluid therapy with potassium supplementation and was discharged on oral potassium (Kay Ciel) supplementation.

Outcome. On day 152, the owner reported that the dog had persistent polyuria and polydipsia but otherwise had been doing well until recently. In the past 2 days, however, the dog had vomited several times and become anorexic. Water consumption and urinations decreased during this time, and the dog was straining to urinate. On day 154, pyuria and an *Escherichia coli* urinary tract infection were identified, and antibiotics were prescribed.

TABLE APP–27. Laboratory Findings

Laboratory Test	Day 1	Day 151	Day 318	Unit
Hematocrit	54	48	39	%
Plasma proteins	7.1	7.0	5.2	g/dL
Urine specific gravity	1.003	1.011	1.003	
CO_2	NA	NA	NA	mEq/L
Calcium	10.5	9.9	8.8	mg/dL
Phosphorus	4.7	5.5	3.6	mg/dL
Sodium	144	142	140	mEq/L
Potassium	2.8	2.6	4.7	mEq/L
Chloride	102	102	110	mEq/L
Albumin	NA	NA	NA	g/dL
BUN	14	18	10	mg/dL
Creatinine	1.2	1.8	0.6	mg/dL
Glucose	104	100	85	mg/dL

NA = not available.

TABLE APP–28. Arterial Blood Gas Analysis and Serum Electrolytes

	Day 42	Day 50	Day 176	Unit
pH	7.470	7.439	7.478	
Po_2	66.0	70.2	80.6	mm Hg
Pco_2	38.1	38.8	38.5	mm Hg
HCO_3^-	26.9	25.6	27.8	mEq/L
Total CO_2	28.0	26.8	29.0	mEq/L
Base excess	+4.5	+2.5	+4.5	mEq/L
Sodium	144	138		mEq/L
Potassium	3.2	2.9		mEq/L
Chloride	106	106		mEq/L

On follow-up 3 weeks later (day 176), polyuria and polydipsia were still present, stranguria had returned again, pyuria was present on urinalysis, and *Pseudomonas aeruginosa* was cultured from the urine. At this time, the dog was dehydrated, and azotemia (BUN 120 mg/dL, creatinine 4.3 mg/dL) was present. Hyponatremia (134 mEq/L), hypokalemia (2.4 mEq/L), and hypochloremia (89 mEq/L) were present. The prerenal azotemia and electrolyte abnormalities resolved with fluid therapy over the next 3 days. Antibiotics again were prescribed for the urinary tract infection, and a follow-up urine culture 2 weeks later yielded no growth. Over the next 5 months the dog remained nonazotemic, and serum electrolyte concentrations were maintained as follows: sodium 138–150 mEq/L, potassium 3.0–5.0 mEq/L, chloride 100–115 mEq/L, with parenteral fluid therapy and oral potassium supplementation as necessary.

The dog was euthanized and necropsied on day 326. The liver was enlarged and contained several gray nodules of various sizes, and similar nodules of various sizes (up to 1 cm) were present in the omentum. The left adrenal gland was effaced by a 5.5-cm mass. There was an old infarct in the right kidney, which was smaller and more nodular than the left kidney. The right ventricle of the heart was dilated, and both the mitral and tricuspid valves were thickened. The sternal lymph node was enlarged.

Histologically, the neoplasm was an adrenal cortical carcinoma arising in the left adrenal gland. It had metastasized to the liver, omentum, and sternal lymph node. There was mild to moderate cortical interstitial fibrosis in the kidneys, and the right kidney contained a mature infarct. The lesions in the atrioventricular valves represented endocardiosis.

Case 14 (Table App–29)

Signalment. 6-year-old castrated male Old English sheepdog, 29 kg

Chief Complaint. Polyuria, polydipsia

History. The owner observed increased water consumption and urinations in the dog over the past several weeks. Within the past 2 weeks the dog became anorexic, lethargic, and water consumption decreased.

Physical Examination. The dog was lethargic and had mild peripheral lymphadenopathy, including submandibular, prescapular, popliteal, and superficial inguinal lymph nodes. The spleen was enlarged on abdominal palpation.

Ancillary Findings. On day 1, thoracic radiographs showed an enlarged sternal lymph node, and abdominal radiographs showed splenomegaly. A coagulation profile on day 2 was normal except for mild thrombocytopenia (129,000/µL). A lymph node aspirate on day 3 indicated lymphosarcoma. A renal biopsy on day 3 showed mineralization of tubular basement membranes compatible with hypercalcemic nephropathy. A bone marrow aspirate on day 3 showed erythroid hypoplasia and increased numbers of plasma cells. Serum calcium concentrations in this dog are presented in Figure App–2.

Diagnosis. Lymphosarcoma; hypercalcemia of malignancy; hypercalcemic nephropathy

Interpretation. The decreases in hematocrit and plasma protein concentration over the first day indicate rehydration. The hyposthenuria at presentation (USG 1.006) reflected the effect of hypercalcemia on urinary concentrating ability. Fluid therapy with 0.9% NaCl had a modest effect on serum calcium concentration, decreasing it from 15.2 to 13.9 mg/dL. Addition of furosemide resulted in a further decrease in serum calcium concentration to 12.6 mg/dL. Within 24 h of beginning chemotherapy with prednisone and vincristine, however, serum calcium concentration had declined to 8.6 mg/dL. Serum phosphorus concentration was in the low-normal range at presentation, presumably due to the mass law effect and soft tissue mineralization. The increased serum creatinine concentration presumably reflected hypercalcemic nephropathy. The differential diagnosis and treatment of hypercalcemia are discussed further in Chapter 6.

Treatment. On days 1 and 2, the dog was given 1.5 L 0.9% NaCl with 2.5% dextrose. On day 2, 50 mg furosemide PO q12h was started. On day 3, fluids were

TABLE APP–29. Laboratory Findings

Laboratory Test	Day 1	Day 2	Day 3	Day 4	Day 5	Day 6	Day 8	Day 11	Unit
Hematocrit	52	43							%
Plasma proteins	7.0	6.5							g/dL
Urine specific gravity	1.006								
CO_2	24	22							mEq/L
Calcium	15.2	13.9	13.4	12.6	8.6	9.4	9.3	10.3	mg/dL
Phosphorus	3.0	2.5	4.2	3.2	5.2	3.3			mg/dL
Sodium	159		159	154	146	154			mEq/L
Potassium	3.7		3.9	4.2	3.7	4.2			mEq/L
Chloride	117		116	112	105	113			mEq/L
Total protein			6.3						g/dL
Albumin			2.8						g/dL
BUN	24								mg/dL
Creatinine	2.1	2.2				1.4	1.5		mg/dL
Glucose	135	115							mg/dL

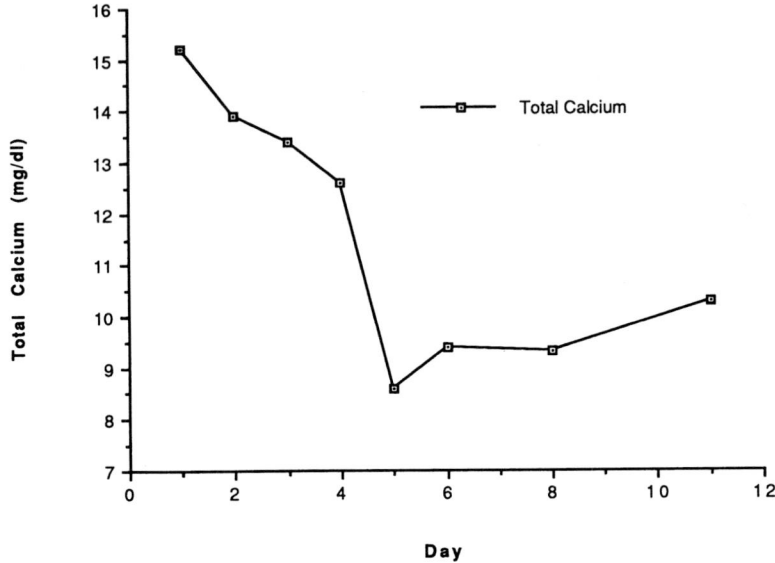

FIGURE APP-2. Serum total calcium concentrations over an 11-day period in a dog with hypercalcemia of malignancy caused by lymphosarcoma.

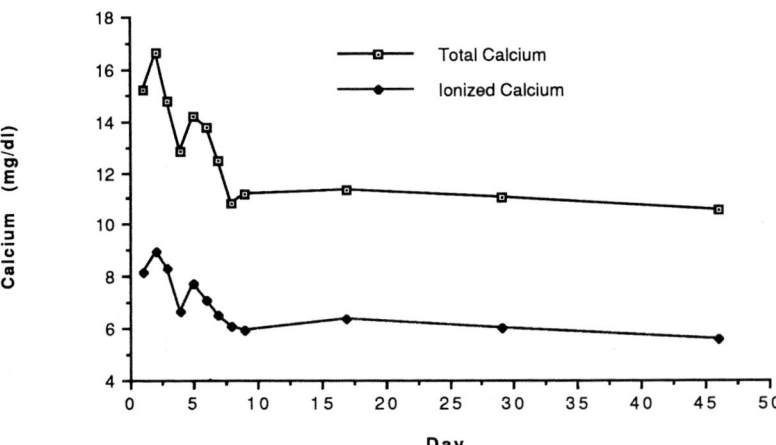

FIGURE APP-3. Serum total and ionized calcium concentrations over a 46-day period from a dog that had ingested a cholecalciferol-containing rat poison.

TABLE APP-30. **Laboratory Findings**

Laboratory Test	Day 1	Day 3	Day 5	Day 8	Day 17	Unit
Hematocrit	49					%
Plasma proteins	7.5					g/dL
Urine specific gravity	1.009					
CO_2	24	25	23	20	25	mEq/L
Calcium	15.7	14.8	13.9	10.9	11.8	mg/dL
Phosphorus	3.8	3.2	2.3	2.0	4.1	mg/dL
Sodium	155	150	150	149	158	mEq/L
Potassium	3.9	3.3	2.9	2.3	4.5	mEq/L
Chloride	114	106	111	109	111	mEq/L
Total protein	6.7	6.1	6.0	5.2	5.5	g/dL
Albumin	3.3	3.0	3.0	2.6	2.7	g/dL
BUN	36	30	15	19	30	mg/dL
Creatinine	1.0	0.9	0.8	0.8	1.0	mg/dL
Glucose	106	134	156	155	105	mg/dL

changed to lactated Ringer's solution 1.5 L/day. On day 4, prednisone 35 mg PO q12h was started. Vincristine (0.875 mg) was given IV on days 4 and 11. Fluids were decreased to 1 L of lactated Ringer's solution per day on day 5. Cyclophosphamide 50 mg PO was given on days 7–10. The dog was released from the hospital with COP (cyclophosphamide-vincristine-prednisone) chemotherapy.

Outcome. The dog improved clinically by day 5, and lymph nodes were noted to be much smaller in size. Approximately 1 month after release, the dog seemed normal to the owner.

Case 15 (Tables App–30, App–31)

Signalment. 3-year-old intact female miniature poodle dog, 3 kg

Chief Complaint. Ingested rat poison

History. The dog ate one package of Quintox, a cholecalciferol-containing rat poison, 6 days before admission. Anorexia, lethargy, and vomiting had been noted during the 6 days before admission. The dog was initially treated with vitamin K for suspected warfarin poisoning. When it was realized that the dog had ingested a cholecalciferol-containing rat poison, serum calcium concentration was measured and found to be 19.3 mg/dL. At that time, the dog was treated with intravenous 0.9% NaCl, 12.5 mg furosemide, and 5 mg prednisone and referred for further evaluation and treatment.

Physical Examination. The dog was weak, tachycardic, and excitable on physical examination.

Ancillary Findings. An electrocardiogram on day 1 showed sinus tachycardia (200/min) with shortening of the QT interval, possibly secondary to hypercalcemia.

Diagnosis. Hypercalcemia due to cholecalciferol (vitamin D_3) toxicity

Interpretation. Hypercalcemia caused by cholecalciferol intoxication may cause severe acute renal failure. Fortunately, this dog received aggressive therapy and did not develop overt renal failure. The decreased urine specific gravity at admission may have reflected the effect of hypercalcemia on urinary concentrating ability or previous therapy by the referring veterinarian (0.9% NaCl, furosemide, prednisone).

Aggressive therapy with 0.9% NaCl contributed to mild hypernatremia. Marked hypokalemia resulted from diuresis with potassium-free parenteral fluids (0.9% NaCl) and frequent administration of furosemide. Management of hypokalemia during concurrent administration of furosemide required aggressive potassium supplementation of parenteral fluids.

The effects of cholecalciferol can last several weeks. This persistent effect was emphasized by the reappearance of hypercalcemia on day 5 after the dog was fed. Recommendation should be made to feed affected animals a low-calcium diet during recovery from cholecalciferol toxicosis. In this dog, use of a low-calcium diet (Prescription Diet S/D) did not prevent postprandial hypercalcemia.

Prednisone therapy is used to antagonize the effects of vitamin D on gastrointestinal absorption of calcium. Glucocorticoid therapy may have contributed to the mild hyperglycemia noted in this dog during its hospitalization.

TABLE APP-31. **Serum Total and Ionized Calcium Concentrations in a Dog That Had Ingested a Cholecalciferol-Containing Rat Poison**

Day	Total Calcium (mg/dL)	Ionized Calcium (mg/dL)
1	15.2	8.15
2	16.6	8.93
3	14.8	8.28
4	12.8	6.66
5	14.2	7.74
6	13.8	7.07
7	12.5	6.53
8	10.8	6.11
9	11.2	5.91
17	11.3	6.40
29	11.0	5.98
46	10.5	5.56

Phosphorus binders are recommended to lower serum phosphorus concentration and minimize soft tissue mineralization when animals with cholecalciferol intoxication have renal failure and hyperphosphatemia. Such therapy was not required in this dog.

The cause for the lingual necrosis (see later) is unclear. It is an occasional complication of severe uremia, which was not present in this dog. Vitamin D intoxication may have contributed in some other way to the observed lingual necrosis.

Treatment. On day 1, the dog was treated with intravenous 0.9% NaCl at 1.5 times calculated maintenance needs, 7 mg furosemide IV q6h, and 7.5 mg prednisolone SQ q12h. On day 2, glucocorticoid therapy was changed to 10 mg prednisone PO q12h, and the remaining therapy was not changed. On day 3, 10 mEq KCl was added per liter of 0.9% NaCl. On day 4, 0.9% NaCl was increased to 2.5 times calculated maintenance, and a low-calcium diet was begun (Prescription Diet S/D). After feeding on day 4, serum calcium concentration on day 5 was observed to be increased. On days 5–7, potassium supplementation of 0.9% NaCl was increased to 20 mEq KCl per liter, and other treatments were continued as before. Hypokalemia persisted, and on day 8 potassium supplementation of 0.9% NaCl was increased to 60 mEq KCl per liter and the infusion rate reduced to calculated maintenance needs. Furosemide was decreased to 7 mg SQ q12h. Also on day 8, necrosis of the rostral portion of the tongue was first observed. On day 9, the dog was released from the hospital with prednisone 5 mg PO q12h with recommendation for a low-calcium diet.

For serum calcium concentrations, see Figure App–3.

Outcome. The dog was evaluated several times over the next 2 months and progressed well. A small rostral portion of the tongue sloughed, but healing of the remainder of the tongue was uneventful and there was no residual difficulty in prehension.

Case 16 (Tables App–32, App–33)

Signalment. 9-year-old castrated male beagle dog, 23 kg

Chief Complaint. Hypercalcemia

TABLE APP–32. Laboratory Findings

Laboratory Test	Day 1	Day 3	Day 10	Unit
Hematocrit	46			%
Plasma proteins	7.0			g/dL
CO_2	25	23	22	mEq/L
Calcium	16.6	13.8	8.1	mg/dL
Phosphorus	2.3	2.5	6.0	mg/dL
Sodium	159	153	147	mEq/L
Potassium	4.7	4.6	5.4	mEq/L
Chloride	123	115	109	mEq/L
Total protein	6.0	5.7	6.4	g/dL
Albumin	2.6	2.8	2.6	g/dL
BUN	7	<5	14	mg/dL
Creatinine	0.9	0.7	0.8	mg/dL
Glucose	97	93	105	mg/dL

TABLE APP–33. Serum Total and Ionized Calcium Concentrations

Day	Total Calcium (mg/dL)	Ionized Calcium (mg/dL)
1	17.6	8.86
2	16.6	8.96
3	13.8	8.29
4	14.3	7.33
5	10.2	6.43
6	11.9	6.25
7	9.1	5.05
8	8.3	4.07
9	7.6	3.76
10	8.1	3.83
11	8.9	4.45

History. Approximately 4 months before admission, the dog was presented to the referring veterinarian for decreased appetite and lethargy. No cause for these abnormalities was detected. Approximately 1 week before admission, the referring veterinarian diagnosed cystic calculi and performed a cystotomy to remove the stones. Four days before admission, the dog was presented for anorexia, decreased water consumption, and lethargy. Serum biochemistry testing showed a serum calcium concentration of 20 mg/dL. The dog was treated with IV 0.9% NaCl and referred for evaluation of hypercalcemia.

Physical Examination. The dog was lethargic and approximately 5–7% dehydrated. There was a 1-cm soft subcutaneous mass at the thoracic inlet and mild submandibular lymphadenopathy.

Ancillary Findings. A needle aspirate of the mass at the thoracic inlet yielded fat consistent with a diagnosis of lipoma. Thoracic and abdominal radiographs were unremarkable. A coagulation profile on day 2 was normal. Serum parathyroid hormone (PTH) concentration was 63 pmol/L (normal: 2–13 pmol/L). Surgical exploration of the cervical region was performed on day 3 and showed enlargement of both thyroid glands. There was a 1-cm black nodule in the left thyroid gland and a 1.5-cm white

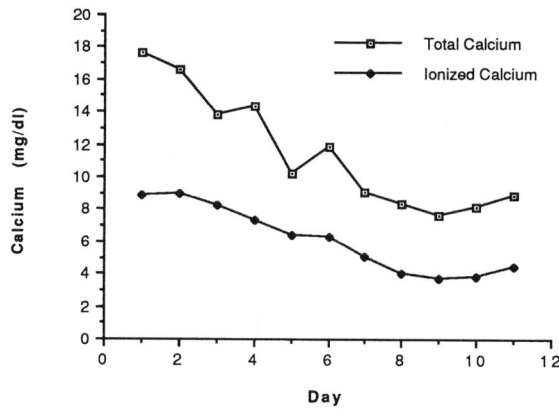

FIGURE APP–4. Serum total and ionized calcium concentrations over an 11-day period from a dog with primary hyperparathyroidism due to a parathyroid adenoma.

mass in the capsule of the right thyroid gland. No extracapsular parathyroid gland could be identified on the right side. Bilateral thyroidectomy was performed, removing both masses but keeping the left external parathyroid gland intact. On histopathology, the left thyroid mass was a follicular thyroid carcinoma, whereas the right-sided mass was a parathyroid adenoma. The sugical margins of both tumors were free of neoplastic cells. A bone marrow aspirate on day 6 showed no cytologic abnormalities.

Diagnosis. Primary hyperparathyroidism due to parathyroid adenoma; thyroid carcinoma

Interpretation. This dog had severe hypercalcemia due to primary hyperparathyroidism caused by a parathyroid adenoma. Primary hyperparathyroidism was confirmed by increased serum concentration of PTH. The accompanying thyroid carcinoma was an unexpected finding. Clinical signs similar to those observed in this dog (e.g., anorexia, lethargy, weakness) have been reported in other dogs with primary hyperparathyroidism due to parathyroid adenoma (Berger and Feldman 1987). Polyuria and polydipsia are also commonly observed, and hypercalcemic nephropathy may occur. Calcium phosphate or calcium oxalate stones may develop in dogs with primary hyperparathyroidism (Klausner et al. 1987). This dog had no evidence of impaired renal function but did have a history of cystic calculi.

The mild hypernatremia and hyperchloremia observed on days 1 and 3 probably were due to administration of 0.9% NaCl. These changes resolved after discontinuation of fluid therapy on day 8. The severe hypercalcemia and mild hypophosphatemia observed in this dog are typical of primary hyperparathyroidism. Hypocalcemia may develop postoperatively due to previous suppression of the contralateral parathyroid gland and usually occurs 2–6 days after surgery. Serum calcium concentration reached its nadir in this dog on day 9 (postoperative day 6), and muscle tremors were noted on days 5–7. Postoperative hypocalcemia may be treated with oral vitamin D and calcium supplementation. This dog received calcitriol and calcium carbonate beginning on day 8. Care must be taken to avoid development of hypercalcemia as the contralateral parathyroid glands resume normal function.

Treatment. During the first 7 days of hospitalization, the dog was given an IV infusion of 0.9% NaCl with 20 mEq KCl added per liter at a rate equal to twice calculated maintenance needs. Slight muscle tremors were observed on days 5–7, but appetite was good. Fluid therapy was discontinued, and the muscle tremors disappeared on day 8. Calcium carbonate 2400 mg PO q8h and calcitriol approximately 40 ng PO q8h were started on day 8.

For serum calcium concentrations, see Figure App–4.

Outcome. The dog was released from the hospital on day 11. The dosage of calcitriol was decreased to q12h, and the calcium carbonate was continued as before. The referring veterinarian was to monitor the dog's serum calcium concentration and adjust the dosage of the calcitriol and calcium carbonate to avoid recurrence of hypercalcemia as the remaining suppressed parathyroid gland resumed activity. The follicular thyroid carcinoma in this dog was diagnosed early in its course as a result of the clinical signs of hypercalcemia and primary hyperparathyroidism. This may result in a more favorable prognosis, and the referring veterinarian was to monitor the dog for recurrence of the thyroid carcinoma.

Case 17 (Table App–34)

Signalment. 11-year-old intact female miniature poodle, 11 kg

Chief Complaint. Polydipsia, polyuria

History. The dog developed increased water consumption, urinations, lethargy, and weakness in the pelvic limbs during the 3 weeks before admission. Appetite was still present, but it was decreased from normal. There was no vomiting or diarrhea. The last heat cycle was 7 months before admission.

Physical Examination. The haircoat was thin, and numerous comedones were observed. There were increased bronchovesicular sounds on thoracic auscultation, and on rectal examination there was a small, firm, nonpainful mass in the region of the right anal sac.

Ancillary Findings. Thoracic radiographs on day 2 showed mineralization of main stem and intermediate

TABLE APP–34. Laboratory Findings

Laboratory Test	Day 1	Day 4	Day 6	Day 9	Day 11	Day 14	Unit
Hematocrit	37						%
Plasma proteins	7.2						g/dL
Urine specific gravity	1.009						
CO_2	16.0	13.0	14.0	23.5	20.0	17.0	mEq/L
Calcium	15.8	13.0	10.1	10.8	9.5	8.9	mg/dL
Phosphorus	5.7	5.9	5.8	4.7	5.0	6.8	mg/dL
Sodium	149	150	157	166	149	153	mEq/L
Potassium	3.9	3.9	3.7	3.9	3.5	3.4	mEq/L
Chloride	116	119	126	125	126	109	mEq/L
Albumin	3.1	3.5	2.8	2.3	2.1	2.3	g/dL
BUN	61	44	49	41	29	49	mg/dL
Creatinine	2.8	3.5	3.6	3.8	3.7	3.9	mg/dL
Glucose	141	152	91	135	205	120	mg/dL

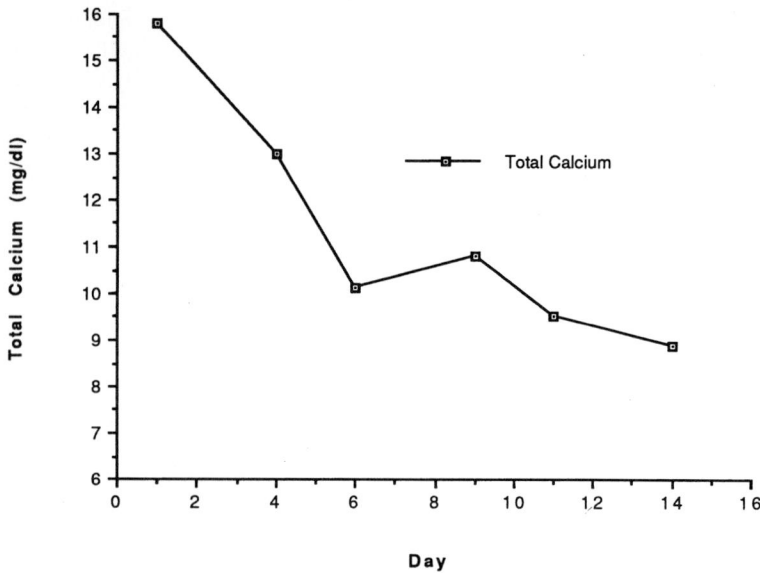

FIGURE APP-5. Serum total calcium concentrations over a 2-week period in a dog with hypercalcemia of malignancy caused by an apocrine gland adenocarcinoma of the anal sac.

bronchi. Abdominal radiographs were normal. Skeletal survey radiographs showed no bony lesions. Serum calcium concentrations in this dog are presented in Figure App–5.

Diagnosis. Apocrine gland adenocarcinoma of the anal sac; hypercalcemia of malignancy

Interpretation. This dog had hypercalcemia secondary to apocrine gland adenocarcinoma of the anal sac. This tumor occurs predominantly in older female dogs. Polyuria, polydipsia, weakness, and anorexia often are the first signs recognized by the owners, and the primary tumor can be very small at presentation. This neoplasm often metastasizes to the internal iliac lymph nodes, and metastasis often is heralded by recurrence of hypercalcemia. Hypercalcemia of malignancy is discussed further in Chapter 6.

The low urine specific gravity and azotemia in this dog may have been due to hypercalcemic nephropathy. Mild azotemia persisted after removal of the tumor and resolution of hypercalcemia, suggesting residual renal damage from hypercalcemia. Hypercalcemia resolved slightly with 0.9% NaCl diuresis, but complete correction of hypercalcemia followed surgical resection of the tumor.

The reduction in CO_2 observed on days 4 and 6 may have reflected the acidifying effect of the high chloride concentration of 0.9% NaCl (154 mEq/L). This also was reflected in a progressive increase in serum chloride concentration during saline diuresis. The hyperchloremia did not resolve when lactated Ringer's and ultimately 0.45% NaCl with 2.5% dextrose were substituted for 0.9% NaCl but eventually resolved after discontinuation of fluid therapy on day 13. The progressive increase in serum sodium concentration also may have resulted from therapy with 0.9% NaCl, but it did not improve after substitution of lactated Ringer's and required substitution of 0.45% NaCl with 2.5% dextrose before returning to within the normal range. The mild hyperglycemia at presentation may have been due to endogenous glucocorticoid release, and that observed on days 9 and 11 probably was due to the 2.5% dextrose in 0.45% NaCl. Hyperglycemia resolved with discontinuation of fluid therapy on day 13. It is surprising and unexplained why more severe hypokalemia did not develop in this dog over its hospital course. Hypokalemia would have been expected considering that the animal was anorexic, vomiting, and given potassium-free fluids at a rate sufficient to induce diuresis.

Treatment. The perirectal mass was removed surgically on day 4. Postoperatively, the dog was observed closely for signs of hypocalcemia (e.g., restlessness, muscle fasciculations, seizures) with orders to give 1–5 mL 10% calcium gluconate IV as needed. Clinical signs of hypocalcemia did not develop postoperatively.

Fluid therapy consisted of 750 mL per day of 0.9% NaCl administered IV on days 2–5. On days 6–8, fluid therapy consisted of lactated Ringer's solution, 750 mL per day. On days 9–12, fluid therapy consisted of 0.45% NaCl with 2.5% dextrose, 750 mL per day. Fluids were discontinued on day 13. Follow-up combination chemotherapy (e.g., 5-fluorouracil, cyclophosphamide, and doxorubicin) might have been considered in this case as additional therapy in an attempt to improve survival time.

Outcome. The animal vomited intermittently and was anorexic from days 5–8. Vomiting resolved, and the animal began to eat on day 10. The animal was released from the hospital on day 15. The owner did not return the dog to the hospital for follow-up, but telephone conversations indicated that the dog did well after release for several months, despite the lack of follow-up chemotherapy.

Case 18 (Sherding et al. 1980) (Tables App–35, App–36)

Signalment. 5-year-old female Irish wolfhound, 54 kg

Chief Complaint. Acute collapse

History. In the 3 weeks before admission, anorexia, weight loss, polyuria, and polydipsia had been observed by the owner. The dog experienced several bouts charac-

TABLE APP–35. **Laboratory Findings**

Laboratory Test	Day 1	Unit
Hematocrit	56	%
Plasma proteins	6.3	g/dL
Urine specific gravity	1.019	
CO_2	NA	mEq/L
Calcium	4.3	mg/dL
Magnesium	1.8	mg/dL
Phosphorus	6.3	mg/dL
Sodium	152	mEq/L
Potassium	4.1	mEq/L
Chloride	115	mEq/L
Total protein	5.6	g/dL
Albumin	2.9	g/dL
BUN	11	mg/dL
Creatinine	0.8	mg/dL
Glucose	108	mg/dL

NA = not available

terized by tachypnea, disorientation, aggressive personality change, and a stiff, stilted gait characterized by generalized shaking in all four limbs when she attempted to walk. The dog was normal between these bouts, but muscle spasms had been observed on occasion while she was sleeping. On the day of admission, the dog developed tachypnea, severe muscle tremors, and acute collapse.

Physical Examination. The temperature was 105.2°F, the pulses 180/min, and there was severe tachypnea (panting). The dog was very thin. The gait was ataxic and spastic, and there were severe muscle tremors. The heart could not be heard due to the muscle tremors.

Ancillary Findings. An electrocardiogram and thoracic radiographs were normal. Serum immunoreactive parathyroid hormone concentration was decreased. The clinical course of this dog is represented in Figure App–6 (Sherding et al. 1980).

Diagnosis. Primary hypoparathyroidism

Interpretation. The blood gas analysis indicates the presence of a primary respiratory alkalosis with compensatory metabolic acidosis. The expected bicarbonate concentration is $21 - 0.55 (37 - 25.4) = 14.6$ mEq/L. The observed bicarbonate concentration is 15.9 mEq/L and, because this value falls within 2–3 mEq/L of the predicted concentration, a simple acid-base disturbance is diagnosed. Respiratory alkalosis in this dog was attributed to fever and panting. Chronic respiratory alkalosis is the

TABLE APP–36. **Blood Gas Analysis**

Sample	Arterial	Unit
pH	7.430	
P_{O_2}	92.3	mm Hg
P_{CO_2}	25.4	mm Hg
HCO_3^-	15.9	mEq/L
Total CO_2	16.7	mEq/L
Base excess	−5.1	mEq/L

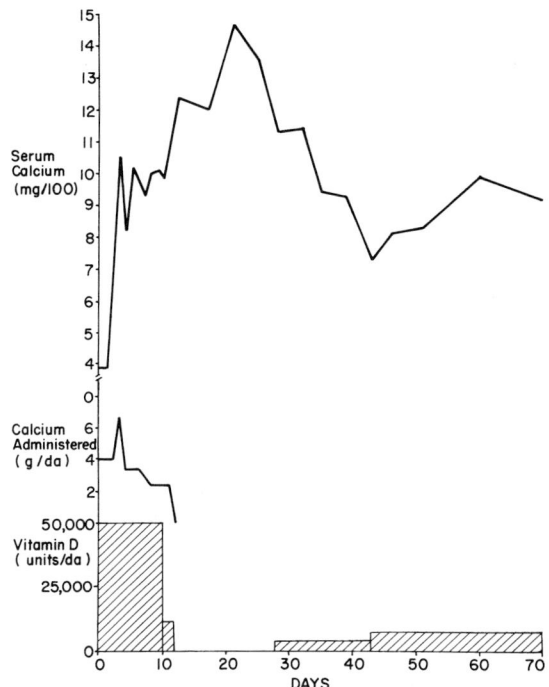

FIGURE APP–6. Serum total calcium concentrations and oral doses of calcium (g/day) and vitamin D (U/day) over a 70-day period in a dog with primary hypoparathyroidism due to lymphoplasmacytic parathyroiditis. (From Sherding RG, Meuten DJ, Chew DJ, et al.: Primary hypoparathyroidism in the dog. *J Am Vet Med Assoc* 176:439–444, 1980.)

only acid-base disturbance in which the compensated pH often falls within the normal range (see Chapter 12).

The profound hypocalcemia was responsible for the observed muscle tremors, which in turn led to hyperthermia and hyperventilation. Mild hyperphosphatemia is commonly observed in dogs with primary hypoparathyroidism (Sherding et al. 1980). The normal albumin concentration ruled out hypoalbuminemia as a cause of hypocalcemia. The normal magnesium concentration ruled out hypomagnesemia as a cause of the muscular tremors. The cause of polydipsia and secondary polyuria in primary hypoparathyroidism is unknown, but they may be psychogenic in origin, based on the other behavioral aberrations that have been observed. Development of polyuria and polydipsia during treatment of primary hypoparathyroidism should lead the clinician to suspect the complication of hypercalcemia, as occurred in this dog during the course of treatment (see under Outcome).

Treatment. Initially, the dog was treated with an intravenous infusion of lactated Ringer's solution (2 L/day) with 1 g calcium gluconate added to each 500 mL of lactated Ringer's solution. Oral administration of vitamin D also was started. On day 4, oral ergocalciferol (vitamin D_2, 50,000 U q24h) and oral calcium lactate (1 g q8h) were started. Fluid therapy was tapered and discontinued on day 7. The dosage of vitamin D gradually was increased until the dog's serum calcium concentration entered the normal range on day 12 (9.4 mg/dL).

Outcome. There was much improvement over the first 4 days, but the dog's gait remained spastic. The dog was walking normally by day 6. Surgical exploration of the parathyroid glands was performed on day 10, and the histologic diagnosis was lymphoplasmacytic parathyroiditis. At follow-up on day 20, the dog had polydipsia, polyuria, and nocturia. Serum calcium concentration was 14.6 mg/dL, and there was mild azotemia (BUN 44 mg/dL, creatinine 1.5 mg/dL) attributed to hypercalcemic nephropathy. Over the next year, the dosages of vitamin D_2 and calcium lactate were adjusted periodically and the dog's serum calcium concentration maintained between 7.0 and 12.3 mg/dL. Polyuria and polydipsia resolved with the correction of hypercalcemia.

Case 19 (Table App–37)

Signalment. 7-year-old intact male Yorkshire terrier, 3 kg

Chief Complaint. Abdominal distention

History. The owner had observed abdominal distention during the 1 month before admission. Intermittent diarrhea (once every 3 days) had been present over the past several months. During the past few weeks, intermittent vomiting also had occurred. The dog's appetite remained normal.

Physical Examination. The dog was thin and had marked abdominal distention, attributed to ascites. Dental tartar and a grade I–II/VI left basilar systolic murmur also were detected.

Ancillary Findings. Thoracic radiographs were normal, but abdominal radiographs indicated the presence of peritoneal effusion. Fluid obtained from the abdomen by paracentesis was clear and colorless and had a protein concentration under 2.5 g/dL. On cytologic examination, it contained very few cells and was interpreted to be a transudate. A fecal flotation was negative. Liver and small-intestine biopsies were obtained at exploratory laparotomy on day 50. The liver was normal, and biopsies of the jejunum and ileum showed lymphangiectasia.

Diagnosis. Protein-losing enteropathy due to lymphangiectasia; hypocalcemia due to hypoproteinemia

TABLE APP–37. Laboratory Findings

Laboratory Test	Day 1	Day 40	Unit
Hematocrit	42	45	%
Plasma proteins	3.1	3.0	g/dL
Urine specific gravity	1.048	1.052	
Urine protein	25	25	mg/dL
CO_2	20	25	mEq/L
Calcium	6.4	6.6	mg/dL
Phosphorus	3.4	3.9	mg/dL
Sodium	148	144	mEq/L
Potassium	4.8	5.2	mEq/L
Chloride	122	117	mEq/L
Total protein	2.8	2.5	g/dL
Albumin	1.1	0.9	g/dL
BUN	19	26	mg/dL
Creatinine	0.6	0.6	mg/dL
Glucose	104	90	mg/dL

Interpretation. This dog had asymptomatic hypocalcemia as a result of severe hypoproteinemia caused by lymphangiectasia. All plasma proteins are lost in the feces in protein-losing enteropathy, leading to decreased concentrations of both albumin and globulins. Approximately 45% of total serum calcium concentration is bound to proteins, predominantly albumin. Thus, although the protein-bound fraction is markedly reduced by hypoalbuminemia, the ionized fraction of calcium presumably is normal. A formula has been devised to correct serum calcium concentration for hypoalbuminemia in dogs (Meuten et al. 1980). According to this formula: corrected calcium = calcium − albumin + 3.5. Using this formula on days 1 and 40 yielded corrected serum total calcium concentrations of 8.8 and 9.2 mg/dL, respectively. These values were normal, suggesting that the ionized calcium concentration in this dog was normal. The relationship between serum albumin or protein concentration and serum calcium concentration is not as strong in cats, and a reliable formula for correction has not been established (Flanders et al. 1989). See Chapter 6 for further discussion of these principles.

The cause of the mild hyperchloremia in this dog on day 1 (122 mEq/L) was not clear. It is possible that the dog had a hyperchloremic metabolic acidosis ($[SID]_i = 26$ mEq/L) due to intermittent diarrhea and that this acid-base disturbance was equally opposed by hypoproteinemic alkalosis, resulting in the observed normal total CO_2 concentration of 20 mEq/L. Hyperchloremia was less marked on day 40 (117 mEq/L), but hypoalbuminemia was worse (0.9 g/dL). This allowed the hypoproteinemic alkalosis to be unmasked somewhat, as suggested by the increase in total CO_2 concentration (25 mEq/L). See Chapter 10 for a discussion of the principles leading to these conclusions.

Treatment. During its first hospitalization, the dog was treated with a low-fat diet (Prescription Diet R/D) and medium-chain triglyceride oil. The dog was released with these medications on day 12.

Outcome. Clinically, the dog did well for approximately 1 month. At that time, appetite was decreased, and abdominal distention and vomiting recurred. No diarrhea was observed during this time. The dog was returned to the hospital on day 40 for reevaluation and biopsy. The dog was released from the hospital again on day 56 receiving Prescription Diet R/D, medium-chain triglyceride oil, prednisolone 2.5 mg PO q12h, and furosemide 6.25 mg PO q12h.

Case 20 (Tables App–38, App–39)

Signalment. 16-year-old spayed female domestic shorthair cat, 4 kg

Chief Complaint. Polyuria, polydipsia, polyphagia, increased activity

History. Over the past several months, the owner had noted increased food and water consumption, increased urinations, and increased level of physical activity in this previously sedentary older cat.

TABLE APP-38. **Laboratory Findings**

Laboratory Test	Day 1	Day 7	Day 16	Day 73	Unit
Hematocrit	33	28			%
Plasma proteins	7.4	7.5			g/dL
Urine specific gravity	1.012				
CO_2	13	16	19	23	mEq/L
Calcium	9.3	9.6	13.1	12.8	mg/dL
Phosphorus	5.6	5.4	6.1	4.3	mg/dL
Sodium	158	154	150	154	mEq/L
Potassium	3.5	3.8	4.2	4.1	mEq/L
Chloride	123	114	116	118	mEq/L
Total protein	7.5	7.0	7.5	7.9	g/dL
Albumin	3.2	2.8	3.0	3.1	g/dL
BUN	58	40	51	72	mg/dL
Creatinine	3.0	2.1	3.1	3.9	mg/dL
Glucose	104	122	93	90	mg/dL
Thyroxine	3.4			0.7	µg/dL

Physical Examination. The cat was thin, and the haircoat was dry and unkempt. There was a II–III/VI left apical systolic murmur on thoracic auscultation, and the kidneys were firm and smaller than normal on abdominal palpation. A right-sided thyroid nodule was palpated in the neck.

Ancillary Findings. Histology of the excised thyroid gland showed microfollicular thyroid adenoma.

Diagnosis. Hyperthyroidism; chronic renal failure; postoperative hypocalcemia

Interpretation. This cat presented for clinical signs resulting from hyperthyroidism and underlying chronic renal failure. The azotemia, low urine specific gravity, and small, firm kidneys on abdominal palpation are indicative of the underlying chronic renal disease. The presence of systemic nonthyroidal illness (chronic renal disease) in this cat most likely explains the normal serum T_4 concentration on day 1 (McLoughlin et al. 1993; DiBartola and Brown 2000).

Hypocalcemia after thyroidectomy may result from reversible or irreversible traumatic impairment of blood supply to the parathyroid glands during surgery. Hypocalcemia is most likely to develop within 1–4 days of thyroidectomy. Thus, clinical signs and serum calcium concentration should be monitored for 4–7 days after surgery.

TABLE APP-39. **Serum Total and Ionized Calcium Concentrations**

Day	Time	Total Calcium (mg/dL)	Ionized Calcium (mg/dL)
3	AM	8.0	4.71
4	AM	7.2	4.07
4	PM	6.5	NA
5	AM	9.8	5.44
6	AM	10.7	6.05
7	AM	8.6	4.95
8	AM	8.1	4.81
10	AM	10.6	5.67

NA = not available

Clinical signs of hypocalcemia include restlessness, muscle fasciculations, tetany, and seizures. Iatrogenic hypoparathyroidism usually lasts several days but may be permanent in some cats if the parathyroid glands have sustained irreversible damage. Approximately 48 h after surgery, this cat developed transient symptomatic hypocalcemia that was managed by parenteral administration of calcium gluconate followed by oral administration of dihydrotachysterol (vitamin D_2) and calcium carbonate. In this case, therapy was complicated by development of hypercalcemia, which ultimately was managed by adjusting the dosage of vitamin D_2 and calcium carbonate. The vitamin D_2 eventually was discontinued, but the calcium carbonate was continued as a phosphorus-binding agent in treatment of the cat's chronic renal failure.

For serum calcium concentrations, see Figure App-7.

Treatment. Bilateral thyroidectomy was performed on day 2. On days 2 and 3, fluid therapy consisted of intravenous lactated Ringer's solution supplemented with KCl to provide a total of 32 mEq potassium per liter at 1.5 times calculated maintenance needs. L-Thyroxine (0.1 mg) PO q24h also was given. The cat vomited several times during the first few days postoperatively but was released from the hospital on day 4. Extreme caution must be taken when treating hyperthyroidism in cats with chronic renal failure. Resolution of hyperthyroidism often results in deterioration of renal function (DiBartola and Brown 2000).

Outcome. The cat developed muscle spasms progressing to tetany on the evening of day 4 (approximately 60 h after surgery). The cat was readmitted to the intensive care unit and given 5 mL of 10% calcium gluconate (46.5 mg, or 2.3 mEq, calcium) and placed on 0.9% NaCl with 40 mL of 10% calcium gluconate (372 mg, or 18.4 mEq, calcium) and 28 mEq KCl per liter at 1.5 times calculated maintenance needs. Also, 0.2 mg dihydrotachysterol (vitamin D_2) PO q24h was begun.

On day 6, calcium gluconate supplementation of fluids was decreased to 20 mL of a 10% solution (186 mg, or 9.2 mEq, calcium) per liter of 0.9% NaCl. On day 7, calcium gluconate supplementation of parenteral fluids was discontinued, dihydrotachysterol was decreased to 0.1

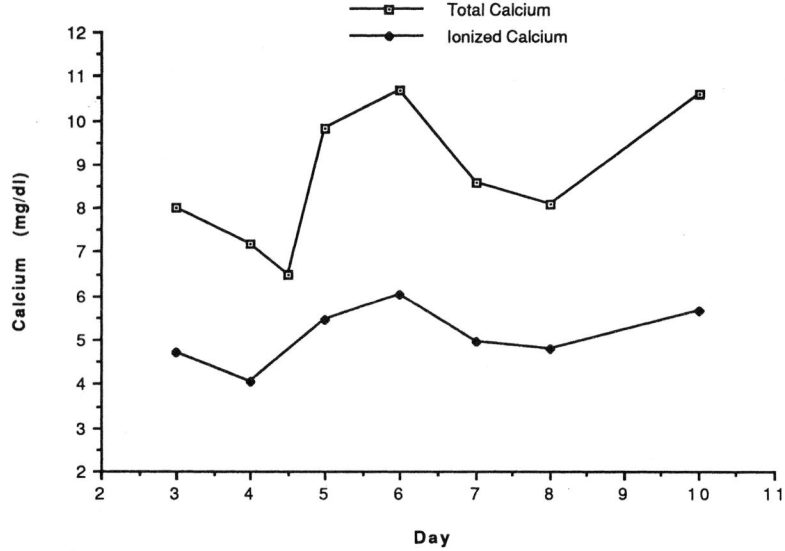

FIGURE APP-7. Serum total and ionized calcium concentrations over a 10-day period in a cat with iatrogenic hypocalcemia following thyroidectomy for treatment of hyperthyroidism.

mg PO q24h, and cimetidine 20 mg IV q12h was added. The cat began to eat again on day 7. On day 8, Tums (calcium carbonate) 125 mg PO q12h was begun as a calcium supplement and phosphorus-binding agent.

At reevaluation on day 16, treatment consisted of 0.05 mg dihydrotachysterol PO q48h, 125 mg Tums PO q48h, and potassium gluconate supplementation. The cat was treated conservatively for chronic renal failure for the following 6 months.

Case 21 (Tables App–40, App–41)

Signalment. 8-year-old castrated male domestic shorthair cat, 4 kg

Chief Complaint. Vomiting

History. The cat was diagnosed as having diabetes mellitus 3 years before admission and until recently had been controlled well with 5 U neutral protamine Hagedorn (NPH) insulin SQ once daily. One month before admission, the owner observed weight loss, decreased appetite, and lethargy. Insulin therapy was changed from NPH to protamine zinc insulin (PZI) 1 week before admission. There was initial improvement in appetite but vomiting began after 4 days of PZI insulin. The cat was treated at the local emergency clinic with regular insulin (2 U IV followed by 3 U SQ for two additional doses) and IV fluids (0.9% NaCl with 28 mEq KCl per liter).

Physical Examination. The cat was hypothermic (96.8°F), thin, had pale mucous membranes, and was approximately 10% dehydrated.

Ancillary Findings. Ultrasound examination on day 2 showed dilatation of the gallbladder, cystic bile duct, and common bile duct, suggestive of extrahepatic biliary

TABLE APP–40. **Laboratory Findings**

Laboratory Test	Day 1	Day 3	Day 7	Day 365	Unit
Hematocrit	41	16	17	28	%
Plasma proteins	9.5	6.6	5.7	8.6	g/dL
	Icteric	*Hemolysis*			
Urine specific gravity	1.042			1.035	
Urine glucose	4+			2+	
Urine ketones	1+			neg	
CO_2	9	17	18	16	mEq/L
Calcium	10.7	8.4	8.2	10.1	mg/dL
Phosphorus	1.7	0.9	4.0	5.5	mg/dL
Sodium	161	147	151	153	mEq/L
Potassium	3.3	4.4	4.8	5.5	mEq/L
Chloride	113	125	125	113	mEq/L
Total protein	7.9	4.9	4.7	7.9	g/dL
Albumin	3.6	3.2	2.0	3.6	g/dL
BUN	42	13	15	26	mg/dL
Creatinine	3.0	1.7	1.6	1.7	mg/dL
Glucose	372	351	101	305	mg/dL
Amylase	717	702	979		U/L
Lipase	15	32	6		U/L

TABLE APP–41. **Blood Gas Analysis**

Sample	Day 1 Venous	8 h Later Venous	Unit
pH	7.145	7.283	
P_{O_2}	38	35	mm Hg
P_{CO_2}	37.2	36.4	mm Hg
HCO_3^-	13	17.4	mEq/L
Total CO_2	14.1	18.5	mEq/L
Base excess	−14.6	−7.9	mEq/L

obstruction due possibly to pancreatitis. The pancreas, however, could not be visualized. Acute pancreatitis was supported by increased serum lipase concentration on day 3.

Diagnosis. Diabetic ketoacidosis; acute pancreatitis; hemolysis due to hypophosphatemia

Interpretation. Severe hypophosphatemia developed in this cat during treatment of ketoacidosis with insulin and was associated with development of hemolysis and severe anemia on day 3. Hemolysis results from reduction of red cell ATP and usually is not observed until serum phosphorus concentration decreases to approximately 1.0 mg/dL. Hypophosphatemia responded to supplementation of parenteral fluids with sodium phosphate. Hypophosphatemia is discussed further in Chapter 7.

Blood gas analysis on day 1 showed severe metabolic acidosis. Venous pH was dangerously low (7.145) despite an HCO_3^- concentration of 13 mEq/L because there was no apparent respiratory compensation (P_{CO_2} = 37.2 mm Hg). There is some evidence that cats with metabolic acidosis do not compensate to the extent observed in human beings and dogs, and caution should be exercised in concluding that a mixed acid-base disturbance is present (i.e., mixed metabolic and respiratory acidosis). Until more information is available, respiratory acidosis should be diagnosed in cats only if the P_{CO_2} is increased above normal. The high $[SID]_i$ (48 mEq/L) and history of vomiting suggest that this cat actually may have had a mixed metabolic acidosis and metabolic alkalosis.

Mild prerenal azotemia in this cat resolved with fluid therapy, and hypokalemia was corrected by supplementation of fluids with KCl. Diligent potassium supplementation is especially important in diabetic patients with hypokalemia because insulin administration results in translocation of potassium into cells. Treatment of hypokalemia is discussed in Chapter 5. The mild hypocalcemia observed during fluid therapy on day 3 may have been related to hypoalbuminemia, but supplementation of fluids with sodium phosphate also may have contributed (i.e., soft tissue precipitation of calcium phosphate). Acute pancreatitis is difficult to diagnose in cats (Kitchell et al. 1986) but was suspected in this cat based on the increase in serum lipase concentration on day 3 and evidence of extrahepatic biliary obstruction on ultrasound examination. Measurement of trypsin-like immunoreactivity may be helpful in the diagnosis of pancreatitis in cats (Bruner et al. 1997). Pancreatitis also could have contributed to hypoalbuminemia and hypocalcemia in this cat.

Treatment. Initial treatment consisted of intravenous infusion of 0.45% NaCl with 40 mEq KCl and 10 mEq $NaHCO_3$ per liter, and the cat was placed on a water-circulating heating pad. Regular insulin therapy was begun with 2 U SQ q6h. Parenteral fluids were supplemented with 2.5% dextrose whenever blood glucose concentration decreased to 100 mg/dL or below. Sodium phosphate (0.01–0.03 mmol/kg/h) was added to fluids on day 3, and two transfusions of whole blood were administered. Hemoglobinuria was observed after the second transfusion. A third transfusion was given on day 4, and the insulin dosage was increased to 3 U SQ q6h.

Outcome. The cat improved over hospital days 5–7 and was discharged on day 8. Two weeks after discharge (day 21), the cat became anorexic and lethargic. Fever (104.4°F) was found on physical examination. The cat was treated with lactated Ringer's solution given SQ, regular insulin, and cephalothin. The cat was released from the hospital on day 26 receiving cefadroxil and PZI insulin.

In the year after initial presentation, the cat experienced two episodes of anorexia, vomiting, and ketoacidosis. One of these episodes was associated with recurrence of hypophosphatemia. The cat was eating well and gaining weight 1 year after admission (see laboratory data in the preceding table). The cat was treated for 2 more years, during which time it experienced one episode of feline lower urinary tract disease with urethral obstruction and one episode of suspected acute pancreatitis or cholangiohepatitis. The cat was euthanized 3 years after initial presentation.

Case 22 (Table App–42)

Signalment. 10-year-old spayed female Scottish terrier, 10 kg

Chief Complaint. Peripheral lymphadenopathy

History. The owners noticed masses in the neck approximately 2 weeks before admission. No other abnormalities had been observed, and the dog's appetite was normal. The referring veterinarian performed a biopsy, and a diagnosis of lymphosarcoma was made. The dog was referred for treatment.

Physical Examination. The dog had generalized peripheral lymphadenopathy, including the submandibular, prescapular, axillary, inguinal, and popliteal lymph nodes.

Ancillary Findings. A low-dose dexamethasone suppression test was normal and ruled out hyperadrenocorticism as a cause for the increased serum alkaline phosphatase concentration.

Diagnosis. Lymphosarcoma; acute tumor lysis syndrome

Interpretation. This dog was presented for multicentric lymphosarcoma. The high alkaline phosphatase concentration and hypoglycemia on day 1 suggested the possibility of neoplastic involvement of the liver. The low urine specific gravity on day 56 probably was the result of prednisone therapy. The development of hypoproteinemia on day 105 was further evidence of serious hepatic involvement. Acute tumor lysis syndrome developed ter-

TABLE APP-42. Laboratory Findings

Laboratory Test	Day 1	Day 56	Day 105	Day 106	Unit
Hematocrit	38	33	33	30	%
Plasma proteins	6.9	8.0	5.2	5.5	g/dL
Urine specific gravity	1.021	1.011			
CO_2	22	23	20	13	mEq/L
Calcium	11.5	10.9	11.3	10.0	mg/dL
Phosphorus	5.4	3.9	2.4	9.7	mg/dL
Sodium	152	151	142	143	mEq/L
Potassium	4.5	4.7	4.7	6.6	mEq/L
Chloride	111	109	110	111	mEq/L
Total protein	6.0	7.5	4.3	4.2	g/dL
Albumin	2.9	4.2	2.3	2.1	g/dL
BUN	14	11	14	62	mg/dL
Creatinine	0.8	0.8	0.8	2.8	mg/dL
Glucose	57	89	95	11	mg/dL
Alkaline phosphatase	1544	3541	2744	2593	IU/L

minally during rescue chemotherapy with doxorubicin and dacarbazine. The development of tumor lysis syndrome was heralded by the sudden onset of azotemia, hyperphosphatemia, metabolic acidosis, and hyperkalemia on day 106. Severe hypoglycemia occurred terminally and may have resulted from severe neoplastic involvement of the liver and sepsis. Acute tumor lysis syndrome is uncommon in small animal medicine, but large tumor cell burdens (as observed in this dog at necropsy) may predispose patients to its occurrence. Acute tumor lysis syndrome is described further in Chapter 7.

Treatment. On day 1, the dog was begun on a chemotherapy protocol consisting of cyclophosphamide, vincristine, cytosine arabinoside, and prednisone. Three weeks after beginning chemotherapy, peripheral lymphadenopathy remained, and the dosages of cyclophosphamide, vincristine, and prednisone were increased. A second course of cytosine arabinoside and one dose of L-asparaginase were administered. On day 56, the dog appeared to be in remission, and maintenance chemotherapy was begun (chlorambucil, methotrexate, prednisone). The dog relapsed on day 105, and rescue therapy with doxorubicin and dacarbazine was begun on the morning of day 106.

Outcome. The dog's initial response to chemotherapy was poor, but remission eventually was achieved and the dog began maintenance chemotherapy on day 56. By day 105, lymphadenopathy had returned. Thoracic radiographs showed a widened mediastinum, sternal and tracheobronchial lymphadenopathy, and interstitial and peribronchial pulmonary infiltrates. Shortly after beginning rescue therapy on day 106, the dog developed dyspnea and was placed in 40% oxygen. Repeated thoracic radiographs showed no change from those obtained 24 h earlier, and additional laboratory work was obtained (see day 106 above). The dog died later on day 106. At necropsy, lymphosarcoma involved the lymph nodes, bone marrow, corticomedullary junctions of the kidneys, lungs, and liver. Over 50% of the histologic section of liver was effaced by neoplastic lymphocytes arising in the periportal areas.

Case 23 (Tables App–43, App–44)

Signalment. 6-month-old male mixed-breed dog, 16 kg

Chief Complaint. Vomiting, semicomatose

History. The dog seemed normal 1 day before admission. On the day of admission, the owner found the dog recumbent in the yard and vomiting. The owner had changed the antifreeze in his car and poured the old antifreeze in the yard by the fence. The dog was unvaccinated.

Physical Examination. The dog was semicomatose, 5–7% dehydrated, and hypothermic (98.8°F). The mucous membranes were injected, and the pupils miotic bilaterally.

TABLE APP-43. Laboratory Findings

Laboratory Test	Day 1	Unit
Hematocrit	55	%
Plasma proteins	8.5	g/dL
Urine specific gravity	1.012	
Urine glucose	1000	mg/dL
Sediment	many "hippurate" crystals	
CO_2	6.0	mEq/L
Calcium	10.8	mg/dL
Phosphorus	11.7	mg/dL
Sodium	169	mEq/L
Potassium	4.7	mEq/L
Chloride	111	mEq/L
Total protein	7.6	g/dL
Albumin	3.3	g/dL
BUN	63	mg/dL
Creatinine	3.0	mg/dL
Glucose	136	mg/dL
Measured osmolality	435	mOsm/kg
Calculated osmolality	368	mOsm/kg
Osmolal gap	67	mOsm/kg (normal: <10 mOsm/kg)
Anion gap	56	mEq/L (normal: 12–25 mEq/L)

TABLE APP–44. **Blood Gas Analysis**

Sample	Arterial	Unit
pH	7.173	
P_{O_2}	66.3	mm Hg
P_{CO_2}	18.9	mm Hg
HCO_3^-	6.6	mEq/L
Total CO_2	7.2	mEq/L
Base excess	−19.5	mEq/L

Ancillary Findings. None

Diagnosis. Ethylene glycol intoxication

Interpretation. This dog demonstrates the typical laboratory features of early ethylene glycol intoxication. Hemoconcentration was evidenced by the increased hematocrit and plasma protein concentration. Low urine specific gravity, azotemia, and hyperphosphatemia indicated emerging renal failure. The hyperglycemia probably was due to glucocorticoid-induced stress and the peripheral antagonism of insulin characteristic of uremia. Glucosuria represented renal proximal tubular damage. Most dogs with acute renal failure due to ethylene glycol intoxication become severely oliguric or anuric. If this dog was anuric, the normal serum potassium concentration suggests that the clinical course of the disease was shorter than 48–72 h. The presence of so-called hippurate (actually calcium oxalate monohydrate) crystals in the urine also is typical of early ethylene glycol intoxication. The high anion and osmolal gaps resulted from the accumulation of the anionic metabolites of ethylene glycol (glycolate, glyoxylate, and oxalate) after titration of extracellular fluid HCO_3^-. The hypernatremia probably resulted from vomiting in the absence of oral intake of fluids. See Chapter 10 for more information about ethylene glycol intoxication.

This dog had a marked normochloremic (high-anion-gap) metabolic acidosis, which was confirmed by arterial blood gas analysis. The observed P_{CO_2} of 18.9 mm Hg is considerably lower than the predicted value of $37 - 0.7 (21 - 6.6) = 26.9$ mm Hg. The alveolar-arterial oxygen gradient in this dog was 60.1 mm Hg (normal: <25 mm Hg). Arterial hypoxemia and increased alveolar-arterial oxygen gradient in this dog may have been due to pulmonary edema. The discrepancy between the observed and predicted P_{CO_2} values may have resulted from a mixed acid-base disturbance (i.e., normochloremic or high-anion-gap metabolic acidosis and respiratory alkalosis). The concept of the alveolar-arterial oxygen gradient is discussed further in Chapter 11. Ethylene glycol can cause cardiopulmonary complications, and the presence of pulmonary edema at necropsy argues for the presence of a mixed acid-base disturbance.

The high $[SID]_i$ (58 mEq/L) and high anion gap (56 mEq/L) in this dog indicate the concurrent presence of hypochloremic alkalosis caused by vomiting and organic acidosis caused by the accumulation of ethylene glycol metabolites. The hypernatremia (169 mEq/L) was attributed to vomiting and inadequate oral intake of water due to the comatose condition of the animal. This free-water deficit resulted in a seemingly normal serum chloride concentration of 111 mEq/L and masked the underlying hypochloremia ($[Cl^-]_{corrected} = 96$ mEq/L). In summary, the mixed acid-base disorder in this dog actually represents a triple disorder (i.e., hypochloremic metabolic alkalosis, organic metabolic acidosis, and respiratory alkalosis). Mixed acid-base disorders are discussed in Chapter 12.

Treatment. No treatment was attempted. The treatment of ethylene glycol intoxication is discussed in Chapter 10.

Outcome. The owners elected euthanasia because of the grave prognosis. At necropsy, severe pulmonary edema was present, and the kidneys were pale and swollen on their cut surface. Renal histopathology showed multifocal tubular epithelial necrosis with numerous oxalate crystals.

Case 24 (Tables App–45, App–46, App–47)

Signalment. 3-year-old female mixed-breed dog, 25 kg

Chief Complaint. Collapse

History. The dog worked as a guard dog at an auto-wrecking company and was observed to drink discarded antifreeze 4 days before admission on day 1. The owner reported that the dog vomited soon after drinking the antifreeze. The dog was somewhat lethargic the next day but was not observed the following day. The dog was found collapsed on the third day after it drank the antifreeze. The owner had not observed any urinations since the dog drank the antifreeze. The referring veterinarian treated the dog with 2.5 L 0.9% NaCl and 500 mL 5% dextrose in water. Furosemide and $NaHCO_3$ were administered, and the dog was referred for possible dialysis. Muscular twitching and excitability were observed when the dog was handled and she had a generalized seizure at presentation.

Physical Examination. The dog was recumbent, 10% dehydrated, hypothermic (99°F), bradycardic (72/min), and tachypneic (92/min) on presentation. She had weak pulses, dark mucous membranes, and melena was observed. Only 2 mL of urine could be obtained from the bladder by catheterization.

Ancillary Findings. Renal biopsy showed acute tubular necrosis with numerous intratubular oxalate crystals.

Diagnosis. Anuric acute renal failure due to ethylene glycol intoxication; symptomatic hypocalcemia and hyperkalemia

Interpretation. This dog presented with severe anuric renal failure 4 days after having ingested ethylene glycol. The muscular twitching, excitability, and seizure probably were due to severe hypocalcemia. Presumably, calcium oxalate deposition in tissues and soft tissue mineralization due to deposition of calcium phosphate as a result of the mass law effect and severe hyperphosphatemia (Ca × P = constant) caused the severe hypocalcemia. The severe azotemia and hyperphosphatemia are

TABLE APP-45. Laboratory Findings

Laboratory Test	Day 1	Day 2	Unit
Hematocrit	44	27	%
Plasma proteins	6.8	5.6	g/dL
Urine specific gravity	1.015		
Urine glucose	250		mg/dL
Urine protein	1000		mg/dL
CO_2	12.0	9.5	mEq/L
Ionized calcium	2.5	2.1	mg/dL
Total calcium	4.8	5.6	mg/dL
Phosphorus	26.7	27.9	mg/dL
Sodium	144	145	mEq/L
Potassium	6.8	7.7	mEq/L
Chloride	98	96	mEq/L
Total protein	5.2	4.8	g/dL
Albumin	2.5	2.4	g/dL
BUN	366	510	mg/dL
Creatinine	13.8	15.3	mg/dL
Glucose	140	245	mg/dL
Measured osmolality	436	486	mOsm/kg
Calculated osmolality	427	486	mOsm/kg
Osmolal gap	9	0	mOsm/kg
Anion gap	41	47	mEq/L

due to marked reduction in glomerular filtration rate. Administration of parenteral fluids and acute diffuse pulmonary hemorrhage contributed to the decrease in serum protein concentration and hematocrit during hospitalization. The hyperglycemia at presentation was due to a combination of endogenous glucocorticoid release due to stress and peripheral antagonism of insulin characteristic of the uremic environment. The aggravation of hyperglycemia on day 2 probably resulted from administration of dextrose-containing fluids. The normal osmolal gap is not unusual several days after ingestion of ethylene glycol (Grauer et al. 1984). Compare these findings with those of Case 23, in which there was less time between ingestion of ethylene glycol and presentation to the hospital.

Evaluation of blood gas data on day 1 shows metabolic acidosis with respiratory compensation and arterial hypoxemia. This conclusion is based on the fact that the predicted P_{CO_2} is $37 - 0.7(21 - 14.8) = 32.7$ mm Hg and this value is within 2–3 mm Hg of the observed P_{CO_2} of 31.8 mm Hg. On day 2, there is a mixed metabolic acidosis and respiratory alkalosis, with a normal pH of 7.403 and arterial hypoxemia. The predicted P_{CO_2} at this time is $37 - 0.7(21 - 14.2) = 32.2$ mm Hg, and the observed P_{CO_2} of 22.6 mm Hg is more than 2–3 mm Hg lower than the predicted value, indicating a mixed disorder. Hyperventilation due to pulmonary pathology (see necropsy results) presumably was responsible for the respiratory alkalosis. The presence of pulmonary disease also was supported by the increased values for (A-a) D_{O_2} on days 1 and 2 (normal, <25 mm Hg).

The low serum chloride concentration in this dog suggests a more complex acid-base disturbance. The increased $[SID]_i$ of 46 and 49 mEq/L (normal: approximately 36 mEq/L) concurrently with an increased anion gap (41 and 47 mEq/L) and relatively normal plasma protein concentration suggests coexistence of a high-anion-gap metabolic acidosis and hypochloremic metabolic alkalosis. On day 1, a mixed disorder characterized by metabolic acidosis and metabolic alkalosis is present. On day 2, a triple disorder characterized by metabolic acidosis, metabolic alkalosis, and respiratory alkalosis is present. Using the nontraditional approach:

TABLE APP-46. Blood Gas Analysis

Sample	Day 1 Arterial	Day 2 Arterial	Unit
pH	7.271	7.403	
P_{O_2}	59	50	mm Hg
P_{CO_2}	31.8	22.6	mm Hg
HCO_3^-	14.8	14.2	mEq/L
Total CO_2	15.7	14.9	mEq/L
Base excess	−10.3	−7.7	mEq/L
(A-a) D_{O_2}	51.2	71.7	mm Hg

TABLE APP-47. Nontraditional Acid-Base Analysis

Analysis	Day 1	Day 2	Unit
ΔFree water	−0.5	−0.2	mEq/L
ΔChloride	+10.6	+13.3	mEq/L
ΔAlbumin	+2.2	+2.6	mEq/L
ΔUnmeasured anions*	−22.6	−23.4	mEq/L
Base excess	−10.3	−7.7	mEq/L
*Includes ΔPhosphate	−15.0	−16.2	mEq/L

This analysis indicates +10.6 and +13.3 mEq/L contributions to base excess due to hypochloremic alkalosis on days 1 and 2. There was no history of severe vomiting in this dog, but vomiting could contribute to hypochloremic alkalosis. The dog was treated with furosemide by the referring veterinarian and this also could have contributed to the hypochloremia. The calculated effects of ΔFree water and ΔAlbumin are relatively mild and not clinically significant. The values for ΔUnmeasured anions of −22.6 and −23.4 mEq/L, however, are clinically significant. The calculations used in the nontraditional approach assume that the weak-acid component of plasma consists entirely of protein. Consequently, phosphates appear in the derived values for ΔUnmeasured anions (see Chapter 10). In this uremic dog, phosphates contributed −15.0 and −16.2 mEq/L to the calculated values for ΔUnmeasured anions on days 1 and 2. The remaining unmeasured anions consisted of retained uremic solutes and metabolites of ethylene glycol. In summary, this dog's metabolic acid-base disturbance was a combination of organic acidosis due to uremia and accumulation of ethylene glycol metabolites, hyperphosphatemic acidosis due to uremia, and hypochloremic alkalosis.

Treatment. On admission the dog was given 40 mEq $NaHCO_3$ IV slowly, and 40 mEq $NaHCO_3$ was added to 500 mL 5% dextrose in water and administered over the next 12 h. Doses of 2 mL 10% calcium gluconate and 5 mg diazepam were given to control muscular twitching and short seizures over the first 12 h. Cimetidine 130 mg SQ q12h was also begun.

Outcome. On day 2, the dog was still trembling and tachypneic. A renal biopsy was performed, and a catheter was placed for peritoneal dialysis, but the dog died shortly after these procedures. At necropsy, there was severe diffuse pulmonary alveolar hemorrhage and acute tubular necrosis with widespread calcium oxalate deposition.

Case 25 (Tables App–48, App–49)

Signalment. 9-year-old intact male German shepherd dog, 27 kg

Chief Complaint. Weight loss, polydipsia, lethargy, anorexia

History. The owner reported that the dog had been lethargic and anorexic for the 5 days before admission. The dog also had lost weight in the past few weeks and had difficulty getting up in the hindquarters. Water consumption during that time had been increased, but urinations were not observed.

Physical Examination. The dog was thin and lethargic. There were increased inspiratory bronchovesicular sounds on thoracic auscultation, and an abdominal component to respiration was noted.

Ancillary Findings. Abdominal radiographs on day 1 were unremarkable. On neurologic examination on day 3, the dog demonstrated generalized weakness (worse in the pelvic limbs) with a swaying gait and crossing over of the pelvic limbs while walking. Knuckling of both the forelimbs and hindlimbs was noted during walking, and conscious proprioception was slow in all four limbs. Cranial nerve examination was unremarkable. Deep tendon reflexes were decreased in the pelvic limbs, and crossed extension was present. Diffuse muscle atrophy was noted. The suspected diagnosis was degenerative myelopathy.

Diagnosis. Diabetic ketoacidosis; degenerative myelopathy

Interpretation. This dog had severe diabetic ketoacidosis at presentation and concurrent degenerative my-

TABLE APP–48. Laboratory Findings

Laboratory Test	Day 1	Day 3	Day 8	Unit
Hematocrit	33		22	%
Plasma proteins	9.4		8.5	g/dL
Urine specific gravity	1.023			
Urine glucose	2000			mg/dL
Urine ketones	3+			
CO_2	4.0	20	21	mEq/L
Calcium	9.0	8.0	9.6	mg/dL
Phosphorus	6.7	1.9	5.1	mg/dL
Sodium	141	154	144	mEq/L
Potassium	4.5	5.8	5.5	mEq/L
Chloride	97	110	101	mEq/L
Total protein	7.1	5.8	5.5	g/dL
Albumin	2.7	2.2	2.4	g/dL
BUN	43	73	59	mg/dL
Creatinine	3.2	4.6	2.7	mg/dL
Glucose	855	275	870	mg/dL
Anion gap	44.5	29.8	27.5	mEq/L

TABLE APP–49. Blood Gas Analysis

Sample	Day 1 Arterial	Unit
pH	7.017	
P_{O_2}	73	mm Hg
P_{CO_2}	19.0	mm Hg
HCO_3^-	4.9	mEq/L
Total CO_2	5.5	mEq/L
Base excess	−23.9	mEq/L
(A-a) D_{O_2}	53.3	mm Hg

elopathy. The anemia may have been due to chronic renal disease, and its severity initially was masked by hemoconcentration. The urine specific gravity of 1.023 is lower than expected in a dehydrated dog. This is a result of solute diuresis due to glucosuria and ketonuria, and underlying renal disease (as evidenced by persistent mild azotemia) also may have contributed to the low urine specific gravity. Asymptomatic hypophosphatemia developed on day 3, presumably due to insulin therapy (see Chapter 7). The reason for development of mild hyperkalemia on day 3 is unclear, but it may have been related to overzealous supplementation of parenteral fluids with KCl in the face of underlying renal disease during the first 2 days of hospitalization.

Blood gas analysis on day 1 indicated presence of a high-anion-gap metabolic acidosis. The predicted P_{CO_2} is $37 − 0.7 (21 − 4.9) = 25.7$ mm Hg, suggesting the possibility of a mixed disorder with metabolic acidosis and respiratory alkalosis. The (A-a) D_{O_2} is increased (53.3 mm Hg; normal: <25 mm Hg), supporting the presence of underlying pulmonary disease and primary respiratory alkalosis. Respiratory acid-base disturbances are discussed in Chapter 11.

Application of the nontraditional or Stewart approach indicates that this dog had a $[Cl^-]_{corrected}$ of 100 mEq/L and a ΔCl of $110 − 100$, or $+10.0$ mEq/L. This suggests a concurrent hypochloremic alkalosis that has partially offset the severe metabolic acidosis caused by ketone accumulation. This conclusion is supported by the presence of a high $[SID]_i$ (44 mEq/L) concurrently with a high anion gap (44.5 mEq/L) on day 1 despite relatively normal serum albumin and protein concentrations. The history does not reveal any obvious cause for this underlying disturbance. The ΔFree water (-1.2 mEq/L) and ΔAlbumin ($+1.5$ mEq/L) on day 1 have not contributed to the acid-base disturbance to any significant extent.

Treatment. The dog initially was treated with 4 L of lactated Ringer's solution with 34 mEq KCl added per liter over the first 24 h. The dog also was given 20 mEq $NaHCO_3$ IV after the blood gas results returned from the laboratory. Six units of regular insulin were administered IM hourly until blood glucose concentration reached approximately 250 mg/dL. After that time, the dog was treated with 7 U of regular insulin IM q8h. On day 2, fluids were changed to 2 L per day of 0.45% NaCl and 2.5% dextrose with 28 mEq KCl added per liter. Five units of regular insulin were administered IM q8h, and the animal was fed a small amount at the time of insulin administration. On day 3, the fluid volume was increased to 3 L 0.45% NaCl and 2.5% dextrose with 14 mEq KCl added per liter. The owners could not afford continued treatment in the hospital and took the dog home on therapy with NPH insulin SQ q24h on day 3.

Outcome. The dog was reevaluated on day 8 and was eating well but was still weak in the hindquarters. There had been no vomiting, but increased urinations and water consumption were observed. The daily dosage of NPH insulin had ranged from 12 to 24 U.

Case 26 (DiBartola and Leonard 1982)
(Tables App–50, App–51, App–52)

Signalment. 8-year-old spayed female German shepherd dog, 29 kg

Chief Complaint. Polyuria, polydipsia

History. The dog had developed increased water consumption and increased urinations over the 1–2 years before admission and occasionally urinated in the house. The dog also had a history of pruritic skin disease over the past 6 years and had received glucocorticoid injections every 2 months. No parenteral glucocorticoids had been administered in the 6 months before admission. There was no history of diarrhea or use of drugs including urinary acidifiers (e.g., NH_4Cl) or carbonic anhydrase inhibitors. The dog's appetite and attitude were considered normal by the owner.

Physical Examination. The coat was dry and scaling, and there were small crusts at the margins of both ears. A large bladder was noted on abdominal palpation.

Ancillary Findings. During its initial hospitalization, the dog drank 117–214 mL/kg/day (normal: <100 mL/kg/day), confirming polydipsia. A urine culture yielded no growth. Abdominal radiographs were normal except for mild splenomegaly. Resting plasma cortisol concentration was 3.2 μg/dL, and it was 12.6 μg/dL 2 h after administration of 40 U ACTH gel IM. Endogenous creatinine clearance was determined on days 7, 125, and 189, and values of 2.57, 2.26, and 2.08 mL/min/kg, respectively, were obtained (normal: 2–5 mL/min/kg). A water deprivation test was performed on day 42. Before beginning water deprivation, urine specific gravity was 1.008 (U_{osm} = 244 mOsm/kg). After 28 h, the dog had lost 5% of its body weight, and urine specific gravity was 1.017 (U_{osm} = 510 mOsm/kg). Four hours after 5 U of repositol ADH IM, urine specific gravity increased further to 1.020 (U_{osm} = 591 mOsm/kg). An NH_4Cl challenge test was performed on day 45 (see Table App–52). Excretory urography showed normal renal size and structure but mild left hydroureter. A renal biopsy specimen on day 51 was normal by routine light microscopy.

Diagnosis. Distal renal tubular acidosis (RTA); renal glucosuria; impaired urinary concentrating ability

Interpretation. The presence of hyperchloremic (serum chloride concentration 122–124 mEq/L) metabolic acidosis and normal anion gap (12–13 mEq/L) in the absence of any history of diarrhea or administration of urinary acidifiers or carbonic anhydrase inhibitors in this dog was suggestive of RTA. The simultaneous occurrence

TABLE APP–50. Laboratory Findings

Laboratory Test	Day 1	Day 7	Day 191	Unit
Hematocrit	38		48	%
Plasma proteins	6.8		6.6	g/dL
Urine specific gravity	1.005	1.010	1.012	
Urine pH	7.5	8.0	8.0	
Urine glucose	500	112	20	mg/dL
Calcium	9.5	10.0	10.4	mg/dL
Phosphorus	4.4	6.0	4.5	mg/dL
Sodium	136	140	154	mEq/L
Potassium	4.0	3.8	4.8	mEq/L
Chloride	124	122	122	mEq/L
Total protein	6.8	6.8	6.6	g/dL
BUN	9	12	15	mg/dL
Creatinine	0.8	0.9	1.0	mg/dL
Glucose	99	111	79	mg/dL

TABLE APP–51. Arterial Blood Gas Analysis and Serum Electrolytes

	Day 2	Day 7	Day 45*	Day 58†	Unit
pH	7.219	7.199	7.136	7.343	
P_{O_2}	94.8	87.6	109.9	108.9	mm Hg
P_{CO_2}	19.5	24.8	22.3	26.1	mm Hg
HCO_3^-	7.8	9.4	7.3	13.9	mEq/L
Total CO_2	8.4	10.2	8.0	14.7	mEq/L
Base excess	−18.5	−16.0	−20.0	−9.0	mEq/L
Sodium	139	140			mEq/L
Potassium	4.1	3.8			mEq/L
Chloride	122	122			mEq/L
Anion gap	13.3	12.4			mEq/L

	Day 116‡	Day 123§	Day 152‖	Day 202	Unit
pH	7.189	7.202	7.208	7.285	
P_{O_2}	109.8	101.7	75.6	106.5	mm Hg
P_{CO_2}	24.1	24.5	31.3	27.9	mm Hg
HCO_3^-	9.0	9.5	12.3	13.1	mEq/L
Total CO_2	9.8	10.2	13.3	14.0	mEq/L
Base excess	−17.8	−17.0	−14.0	−11.5	mEq/L

*Day of NH_4Cl challenge test.
†After 975 mg $NaHCO_3$ PO q8h for 1 week (1.2 mEq/kg/day).
‡After 1625 mg $NaHCO_3$ PO q8h for 38 days (2 mEq/kg/day).
§After 2275 mg $NaHCO_3$ PO q8h for 17 days (2.8 mEq/kg/day).
‖After 3250 mg $NaHCO_3$ PO q8h for 18 days (4 mEq/kg/day).

TABLE APP–52. Ammonium Chloride Challenge Test*

Time	Urine pH	Arterial pH	P_{CO_2} (mm Hg)	$[HCO_3^-]$ (mEq/L)
11:00	7.46	7.136	22.3	7.3
12:00	7.60	7.161	20.5	7.1
13:00	7.70			
14:00	7.57			
15:00	7.64			
16:00	7.64			
17:00	7.52			

*0.1 g/kg NH_4Cl PO at 9:00.

of severe metabolic acidosis with urine pH above 7.0 suggested a diagnosis of distal RTA. This was confirmed by the NH_4Cl challenge test. The resistance to increasing dosages of $NaHCO_3$, however, was not typical of distal RTA in humans. In human patients with distal RTA, administration of an amount of $NaHCO_3$ sufficient to titrate daily endogenous acid production (approximately 1–3 mEq/kg/day in humans) normally is sufficient to control acidosis. This is in contrast to human patients with proximal RTA, in whom large amounts of alkali must be administered due to the renal wasting of bicarbonate that occurs whenever serum bicarbonate concentration is increased to within the normal range. Renal tubular acidosis is discussed further in Chapter 10.

The renal glucosuria in this dog indicated the presence of proximal tubular dysfunction as well as distal RTA. The polyuria and polydipsia appeared to be the result of defective urinary concentrating ability, which also could not be explained as a result of distal RTA alone. Thus, this dog appeared to have multiple abnormalities of renal function, despite normal glomerular filtration rate, based on repeatedly normal values for endogenous creatinine clearance.

Evaluation of the blood gas data in this dog shows that a more liberal compensation rule of a 1.1 mm Hg decrease in P_{CO_2} for each 1 mEq/L decrease in HCO_3^- successfully predicts the observed P_{CO_2} within 2–3 mm Hg on all occasions but one (day 152). On that day, the observed P_{CO_2} is predicted better by the compensation rule of a 0.7 mm Hg decrease in P_{CO_2} for each 1 mEq/L decrease in HCO_3^-. It is most likely that this dog had a simple hyperchloremic metabolic acidosis with very efficient respiratory compensation. Nothing in the clinical findings suggested concurrent respiratory alkalosis as a separate acid-base disturbance. The rules for compensation presented in this book are based on mean values obtained in experimental dogs under a wide variety of different conditions (de Morais and DiBartola 1991) and serve only as guidelines. Presumably, this dog had exceptional ability to compensate for its metabolic acidosis by alveolar hyperventilation.

The mild hyponatremia noted on day 1 may have been related to marked polydipsia, which may have had some psychogenic component. This possibility is supported by the hyposthenuria (urine specific gravity 1.005) and low BUN concentration (9 mg/dL) observed on day 1. The gradual increase in serum sodium concentration to 154 mEq/L may have been related to a decrease in water consumption and treatment with large amounts of $NaHCO_3$.

Treatment. The dog showed some initial response to 975 mg $NaHCO_3$ PO q8h (1.2 mEq/kg/day) on day 58 but became unresponsive to progressive increases in the dosage of $NaHCO_3$ (see Table App–51).

Outcome. The dog had stable glomerular function based on normal values for endogenous creatinine clearance over a 7-month period. The dog was active and ate well during this time. The dog was donated on day 89. The dog was euthanized on day 230, and there were no additional findings at necropsy.

Case 27 (Tables App–53, App–54)

Signalment. 1-year-old female Labrador retriever, 19 kg

Chief Complaint. Vomiting

History. Intermittent vomiting, unrelated to eating, had occurred one to three times per day for the past 3 weeks. The vomitus contained digested blood and white frothy material. The dog's appetite had been poor to absent for the past 3–4 weeks, but she continued to drink water. The dog also had lost weight during the past month. The feces were soft with mucus and occasionally black in appearance. There was no known exposure to drugs, toxins, or foreign bodies.

Physical Findings. The dog was thin, lethargic, and 7–10% dehydrated. Mucous membranes were pale pink. No abnormalities were detected on abdominal palpation.

Ancillary Findings. Thickened gastric rugal folds were observed on abdominal radiography. Upper gastrointestinal endoscopy showed diffuse gastric mucosal thickening and partial pyloric outflow obstruction. Digested blood and blood clots were present in the lumen of the stomach. At exploratory laparotomy on day 2, a pyloric mass was found, and the regional lymph nodes were enlarged. A partial resection of the mass was performed.

Diagnosis. The histologic diagnosis was zygomycosis (phycomycosis).

Interpretation. This dog had marked hypochloremic metabolic alkalosis due to vomiting of stomach contents. Disproportionate loss of chloride and volume depletion were caused by vomiting and led to enhanced renal reabsorption of HCO_3^- and Na^+ in exchange for K^+ due to the relative lack of Cl^-. This led to development of metabolic alkalosis and a potassium deficit.

The compensatory respiratory response was as expected, assuming a 0.7 mm Hg increment in P_{CO_2} for each 1 mEq/L increase in $[HCO_3^-]$. Assuming a normal venous P_{CO_2} of 37 mm Hg and normal $[HCO_3^-]$ of 21 mEq/L, the expected compensatory P_{CO_2} would be 0.7 (40.1 − 21) + 37 = 50.4 mm Hg. The observed P_{CO_2}

TABLE APP–53. Laboratory Findings

Laboratory Test	Day 1	Day 6	6 Months Later	Unit
Hematocrit	32	28	41	%
Plasma proteins	8.5	5.6	6.0	g/dL
Urine specific gravity	1.033			
CO_2	40	26	21	mEq/L
Calcium	10.8	9.3	10.2	mg/dL
Phosphorus	7.2	4.2	4.3	mg/dL
Sodium	125	143	151	mEq/L
Potassium	3.6	5.0	4.2	mEq/L
Chloride	64	111	115	mEq/L
Total proteins	8.0	5.0	5.5	g/dL
Albumin	3.3	2.4	2.3	g/dL
BUN	48	5	12	mg/dL
Creatinine	1.4	1.0	0.9	mg/dL
Glucose	141	101	92	mg/dL

TABLE APP-54. Blood Gas Analysis

Sample	Venous	Unit
pH	7.494	
P_{O_2}	29	mm Hg
P_{CO_2}	51.6	mm Hg
HCO_3^-	40.1	mEq/L
Total CO_2	41.7	mEq/L
Base excess	+15.0	mEq/L

was 51.6 mm Hg, and because this value differs from the predicted value by less than 2–3 mm Hg, a diagnosis of simple hypochloremic metabolic alkalosis with compensatory respiratory acidosis was made (i.e., a mixed disorder was not present). Provision of chloride as 0.9% NaCl is the critical factor in resolution of hypochloremic metabolic alkalosis. Cimetidine may decrease gastric HCl secretion and be a useful adjunctive treatment.

Marked hyponatremia developed as a result of volume depletion, continued consumption of water, and impaired water excretion caused by nonosmotic stimulation of ADH release. The sodium concentration of gastric fluid is low and vomiting per se probably contributed little to the hyponatremia. Mild hypokalemia is present due to anorexia, loss of potassium in the vomitus, and ongoing urinary loss of potassium caused by secondary hyperaldosteronism. Hyperaldosteronism resulted from volume depletion and contributed to development of the potassium deficit and perpetuation of the alkalosis by stimulation of Na-H and Na-K exchange in the distal nephron. See Chapters 3, 4, 5, and 10 for further discussion of these principles.

The observed mild azotemia and hyperphosphatemia were prerenal in origin. Blood loss through the gastrointestinal tract contributed to the observed anemia and hypoproteinemia, both of which were partially masked at presentation by dehydration and hemoconcentration. The mild hyperglycemia presumably was stress induced.

Treatment. Initially, 0.9% NaCl with 30 mEq/L KCl was administered intravenously, and the dog was treated with cimetidine. Fluid therapy with 0.9% NaCl with KCl supplementation was continued after surgery. On hospital day 4, fluid therapy was changed to lactated Ringer's solution with 2.5% dextrose and 40 mEq KCl/L based on serial evaluation of serum electrolyte concentrations.

Outcome. The dog improved postoperatively, and vomiting resolved on the seventh hospital day. The dog was released on the 9th hospital day on cimetidine, metoclopramide, ferrous sulfate, and ketoconazole. One month later, antifungal chemotherapy was changed to itraconazole.

Case 28 (Tables App–55, App–56)

Signalment. 3-year-old female Labrador retriever

Chief Complaint. Vomiting

TABLE APP-55. Laboratory Findings

Laboratory Test	Day 1	Day 3	Unit
Hematocrit	47		%
Plasma proteins	6.4		g/dL
CO_2	34		mEq/L
Calcium	9.7		mg/dL
Phosphorus	4.1		mg/dL
Sodium	135	145	mEq/L
Potassium	2.3	4.4	mEq/L
Chloride	89	112	mEq/L
Total proteins	5.7		g/dL
Albumin	2.9		g/dL
BUN	8		mg/dL
Creatinine	1.0		mg/dL
Glucose	113		mg/dL

History. The dog had been vomiting food and water for the past 2 weeks. During this time, the appetite also was decreased and the dog had been lethargic. She continued to drink and her urinations were normal.

Physical Examination. The dog was lethargic and 7–10% dehydrated, but there were no abnormalities detected on abdominal palpation.

Ancillary Findings. Abdominal radiographs showed gaseous distention of the small intestine in the cranial abdomen.

Diagnosis. Suspected small-intestinal obstruction; possible foreign body

Interpretation. This dog had moderately severe hypochloremic metabolic alkalosis and marked hypokalemia due to vomiting caused by small-intestinal obstruction. Disproportionate loss of chloride and volume depletion led to enhanced renal reabsorption of sodium. The kidneys have reabsorbed Na^+ and HCO_3^- in the proximal tubules and Na^+ in exchange for K^+ in the distal tubules because of the relative lack of Cl^-. This led to development of metabolic alkalosis and a potassium deficit. Normal respiratory compensation for metabolic alkalosis is predicted to result in a P_{CO_2} of $37 + 0.7 (31.1 - 21) = 44$ mm Hg. The observed P_{CO_2} was 39.3 mm Hg and, because this value is more than 2–3 mm Hg below what was expected, a mixed-acid base disturbance (primary metabolic alkalosis and primary respiratory alkalosis) should be considered. This less than average respiratory compensation explains why the dog's blood pH was so

TABLE APP-56. Blood Gas Analysis

Sample	Arterial	Unit
pH	7.502	
P_{O_2}	83	mm Hg
P_{CO_2}	39.3	mm Hg
HCO_3^-	31.1	mEq/L
Total CO_2	32.3	mEq/L
Base excess	+8.0	mEq/L
(A-a) D_{O_2}	17.9	mm Hg

high (7.502). In human patients, the respiratory response to metabolic alkalosis may be less efficient than the response to metabolic acidosis. Some authors suggest that any increase in Pco_2 may represent evidence of a compensatory response, and a mixed disorder should not be diagnosed unless the Pco_2 is less than normal (Narins and Emmett 1980). There was no suggestion of any underlying disease process in this dog that could account for primary respiratory alkalosis, and it is probable that the dog had a simple but partially compensated metabolic alkalosis. When the observed findings do not match the expected findings, the clinical findings must be considered carefully. In this dog, there were no clinical findings to suggest underlying pulmonary disease ((A-a) Do_2 gradient = 17.9 mm Hg).

Hyponatremia developed as a result of volume depletion, continued drinking, and nonosmotic stimulation of ADH release. Loss of potassium in the vomitus, anorexia, ongoing urinary losses of potassium, and enhanced Na-K exchange in the distal nephron due to a relative lack of Cl^- contributed to the potassium deficit. Provision of chloride as 0.9% NaCl is the critical factor in resolving hypochloremic metabolic alkalosis. Supplementation of the fluids with KCl also facilitates resolution of the potassium deficit. Cimetidine may be helpful in reducing gastric acid secretion. See Chapters 3, 4, 5, and 10 for further discussion of these principles.

Treatment. The dog was treated with 0.9% NaCl containing 60 mEq/L KCl and administered intravenously at a rate equal to 1.5 times maintenance needs. Cimetidine 300 mg IV q8h also was administered. An exploratory laparotomy was performed on hospital day 2, and obstruction of the proximal jejunum by a corn cob fragment was found. The foreign body was removed by enterotomy.

Outcome. Fluid therapy was changed to lactated Ringer's solution at a rate equal to maintenance needs after metabolic alkalosis and hypokalemia had been resolved. Cimetidine was continued, and cephalothin was begun. The dog was released from the hospital on day 6.

Case 29 (Table App–57)

Signalment. 14-year-old spayed female cockapoo dog, 6 kg

Chief Complaint. Anorexia, vomiting

History. Approximately 3 months before admission, the dog was evaluated for coughing by another veterinarian. A diagnosis of cardiac disease was made, and treatment with furosemide was begun. The owner had been administering the furosemide daily since that time. Approximately 10 days before admission, the dog became anorexic and began vomiting. Vomiting occurred as many as three times per day and consisted of yellowish fluid with white flecks. Water consumption also had decreased in the past week. The owner discontinued the furosemide 2 days before admission.

Physical Examination. The dog was dehydrated and lethargic on physical examination. There was a grade II/VI right-sided systolic heart murmur, lenticular sclerosis in both eyes, moderately severe dental tartar, and mild submandibular lymphadenopathy. A cough was easily elicited by tracheal palpation. Both patellas luxated medially.

Ancillary Findings. On day 1, thoracic radiographs were unremarkable, and abdominal radiographs showed small kidneys. Urine culture showed no growth of bacteria. Serum amylase and lipase concentrations on day 2 were normal, and fecal flotation was negative. On day 2, abdominal ultrasound examination showed that the kidneys were small, hyperechoic, and had poor corticomedullary distinction compatible with chronic renal disease. Cardiac ultrasound examination showed normal cardiac contractility. Blood pressure on day 6 was normal.

Diagnosis. Chronic renal failure, tracheal collapse, mild tricuspid valve endocardiosis. Prerenal azotemia, dehydration, metabolic alkalosis, and hypokalemia due to furosemide therapy, vomiting, anorexia, and decreased water consumption.

Interpretation. This dog had mild tricuspid endocardiosis, early chronic renal failure, and tracheal collapse. The tracheal collapse most likely was responsible for the dog's cough, because the heart appeared normal on ultrasound examination. Dehydration, prerenal azotemia, metabolic alkalosis, and hypokalemia developed when anorexia and vomiting were superimposed on long-standing furosemide therapy and underlying chronic renal disease.

TABLE APP–57. Laboratory Findings

Laboratory Test	Day 1	Day 3	Day 6	Day 114	Unit
Hematocrit	39	33			%
Plasma proteins	8.6	7.0			g/dL
Urine specific gravity	1.010				
CO_2	32	20	17	22	mEq/L
Calcium	11.7	11.4	10.6	10.4	mg/dL
Phosphorus	6.9	5.4	6.6	4.4	mg/dL
Sodium	153	154	138	155	mEq/L
Potassium	2.9	5.1	4.4	4.4	mEq/L
Chloride	96	115	106	116	mEq/L
Total protein	7.2	5.8	5.6	6.9	g/dL
Albumin	2.7	2.2	2.5	2.9	g/dL
BUN	132	78	54	46	mg/dL
Creatinine	5.8	4.7	5.0	2.4	mg/dL
Glucose	108	82	102	109	mg/dL

At presentation, dehydration masked the presence of mild anemia. The increased plasma protein concentration and mild hypercalcemia at presentation also reflect dehydration. It is likely that this dog's urinary concentrating ability was impaired by its underlying chronic renal disease. Prior furosemide therapy, however, prevented any conclusion about the significance of the dog's dilute urine in the face of azotemia. Serial serum biochemical evaluation indicated that the dog's initial azotemia had both prerenal and renal components. The abdominal radiographic and ultrasonographic findings supported a diagnosis of chronic renal disease.

Metabolic alkalosis and hypokalemia in this dog resulted from a disproportionate loss of chloride due to both vomiting and long-term furosemide therapy. Volume depletion and sodium avidity in the presence of chloride depletion contributed to the metabolic alkalosis and hypokalemia. Provision of chloride is the most important factor in resolution of these abnormalities. These principles are discussed further in Chapter 10. When the metabolic alkalosis was discovered, this dog's fluid therapy was changed from lactated Ringer's solution with added KCl to 0.45% NaCl and 2.5% dextrose with added KCl. Rather than using 0.9% NaCl, 0.45% NaCl with 2.5% dextrose was chosen because the dog's serum sodium concentration was relatively high. Use of 0.45% NaCl and 2.5% dextrose probably contributed to development of very mild hyponatremia on day 6. What actually incited this dog's vomiting remains unclear.

Treatment. On admission, the dog was treated with IV lactated Ringer's solution with 20 mEq KCl added per liter at a rate equal to 1.5 times calculated maintenance needs. When the admission serum potassium concentration was determined to be 2.9 mEq/L, potassium supplementation of the parenteral fluids temporarily was increased to 60 mEq KCl per liter. Cimetidine 30 mg IV q12h also was started. On day 2, fluids were changed to 0.45% NaCl and 2.5% dextrose with 20 mEq KCl per liter at a rate equal to twice calculated maintenance needs. The same fluid prescription was continued on days 3–4. Potassium supplementation was decreased to 12 mEq KCl per liter of 0.45% NaCl and 2.5% dextrose on days 5–6.

Outcome. The dog vomited intermittently on days 1–3. After this time, the vomiting resolved, and the dog began to eat on day 5. The dog was released from the hospital on conservative medical management for chronic renal failure on day 6. The dog was seen for reevaluation several times during the next 4 months.

Case 30 (Tables App–58, App–59)

Signalment. 2-year-old intact female Great Dane, 54 kg

Chief Complaint. Paresis

History. The dog had been missing for 2 days. She was normal when she disappeared. On the third day after she disappeared, the owner found the dog lying by the side of the road. She could walk but was ataxic. One day later, her appetite was decreased and she could no longer walk.

Physical Examination. The dog was alert and nervous. A few puncture wounds were noted on the left side of the face. Neurologic examination disclosed diffuse lower motor neuron tetraparesis. Mentation, cranial nerve examination, and pain sensation were normal.

Ancillary Findings. Electromyography on day 4 showed many positive sharp waves in all muscles tested, compatible with denervation related to diffuse lower motor neuron disease. Abdominal radiographs on day 2 were normal. Thoracic radiographs on day 3 showed right-sided cardiomegaly. A microfilaria test was negative. Thoracic radiographs taken on day 6 were unchanged from those taken previously.

Diagnosis. Polyradiculoneuritis (coonhound paralysis)

Interpretation. This dog developed respiratory paralysis secondary to severe polyradiculoneuritis. The laboratory results obtained on admission were relatively normal. The mild hypernatremia, hyperchloremia, and increased plasma protein concentrations may have reflected a water deficit due to decreased water consumption ($[Cl^-]_{corrected}$ = 110 mEq/L). The mild hyperglycemia probably reflected endogenous glucocorticoid release due to stress.

On day 3, respiratory paralysis resulted in development of acute respiratory acidosis. The HCO_3^- predicted for acute respiratory acidosis was: $21 + 0.15(45.7 - 37) = 22.3$ mEq/L, and the observed HCO_3^- was 22.9 mEq/L. At that time, the dog was placed in an O_2 cage with 40% O_2. At 14:20, the O_2 cage had not been helpful, and acute respiratory acidosis was more severe. The predicted HCO_3^- was: $21 + 0.15(59.4 - 37) = 24.4$ mEq/L, which coincides exactly with the observed HCO_3^-. Arterial hypoxemia persisted. At 18:00, blood gas analysis was done after a tracheostomy had been performed, and the dog was being mechanically ventilated with 60% O_2. Blood gases at that time were nearly normal, but the arterial P_{O_2} of 219.1 mm Hg was less than expected for a dog breathing 60% O_2. The rule of thumb is that the P_{O_2} should be approximately five times the F_{IO_2}, or 300 mm Hg in this instance. At 8:00 on day 4, the dog developed

TABLE APP–58. Laboratory Findings

Laboratory Test	Day 1	Unit
Hematocrit	43	%
Plasma proteins	7.4	g/dL
Urine specific gravity	1.043	
CO_2	22.0	mEq/L
Calcium	9.7	mg/dL
Phosphorus	4.0	mg/dL
Sodium	155	mEq/L
Potassium	4.3	mEq/L
Chloride	117	mEq/L
BUN	12	mg/dL
Creatinine	1.1	mg/dL
Glucose	120	mg/dL

TABLE APP–59. Blood Gas Analysis

Sample	Day 3 10:30* Arterial	Day 3 14:20† Arterial	Day 3 18:00‡ Arterial	Day 4 8:00‡ Arterial	Unit
pH	7.323	7.232	7.359	7.465	
Po_2	56.7	53.2	219.1	270.8	mm Hg
Pco_2	45.7	59.4	33.6	25.6	mm Hg
HCO_3^-	22.9	24.4	18.2	17.7	mEq/L
Total CO_2	24.5	26.2	19.2	18.6	mEq/L
Base excess	−2.8	−3.9	−5.6	−3.1	mEq/L
(A-a) Do_2	36				mm Hg

*Room air (21% O_2).
†Oxygen cage (40% O_2).
‡With tracheostomy and mechanical ventilation (60% O_2).

acute respiratory alkalosis, presumably from overzealous mechanical ventilation. The predicted HCO_3^- was 21 − 0.25 (37 − 25.6) = 18.2 mEq/L, which was within 2 mEq/L of the observed value of 17.7 mEq/L. The arterial Po_2 at that time (270.8 mm Hg) was closer to the expected value of approximately 300 mm Hg. Other than the slight increase in (A-a) Do_2 on day 3, there were no clinical findings suggestive of underlying pulmonary pathology. This was supported by the necropsy findings (see below). Respiratory acid-base disorders are discussed in Chapter 11.

Treatment. Initially, the dog was treated by diligent nursing care (hand feeding, hand watering, frequent turning, keeping the animal clean and dry). On day 2, the dog could hardly hold its head up. On day 3, she was weaker, and there was marked abdominal breathing with minimal movement of intercostal muscles. The animal was placed in a 40% O_2 cage with minimal to no beneficial effect (see preceding blood gas analysis). A tracheostomy was performed, and the dog was placed on a mechanical ventilator with 60% O_2 at 8–12 breaths/min. On day 4, the dog was alert, but there was no change in its tetraparesis or respiratory paralysis. The dog become anorexic on day 5 and was treated with lactated Ringer's solution, 2 L per day IV.

Outcome. The dog became progressively worse and died on day 6. At necropsy, no microscopic lesions were observed in the brain or spinal cord, but the ventral roots were not examined. There were no lesions in other organs except for mild right atrial and ventricular dilatation of undetermined cause.

Case 31 (Tables App–60, App–61)

Signalment. 4-year-old male Yorkshire terrier, 6 kg

Chief Complaint. Seizures

History. The dog had experienced respiratory arrest after receiving xylazine and ketamine for routine castration. During recovery from anesthesia, the dog began to seizure. It did not respond to diazepam administration and was anesthetized with pentobarbital. At that time, the dog was referred for further evaluation.

Physical Examination. The dog was unresponsive and slightly hypothermic (98.1°F).

Ancillary Findings. Thoracic radiographs on day 1 showed mild cardiomegaly. Blood ammonia concentration on day 1 was mildly increased (59.1 μmol/L), but bile acid concentration on day 6 was normal (9.3 μmol/L).

Diagnosis. Respiratory arrest after xylazine and ketamine administration

Interpretation. Blood gas analysis on day 1 showed mild acute respiratory acidosis. The expected $[HCO_3^-]$ was 21 + 0.15 (44.6 − 37) = 22.1 mEq/L, which is within 2–3 mm Hg of the observed value of 23.4 mEq/L. Respiratory acidosis with a normal (A-a) Do_2 gradient in a patient breathing room air at sea level suggests hypoventilation as the cause of respiratory acidosis. It was likely in this dog that the acute respiratory acidosis was due to depression of central nervous system respiratory centers as a result of pentobarbital anesthesia.

Hypochloremia is a normal compensatory response to chronic respiratory acidosis, but this response usually is not observed in acute respiratory acidosis. This dog did have hypochloremia at presentation (serum chloride concentration, 100 mEq/L). The high $[SID]_i$ (52 mEq/L) and high anion gap (33 mEq/L) suggest that hypochloremic metabolic alkalosis and organic acidosis of similar but

TABLE APP–60. Laboratory Findings

Laboratory Test	Day 1	Unit
Hematocrit	37	%
Plasma proteins	6.7	g/dL
Urine specific gravity	1.048	
CO_2	23	mEq/L
Calcium	10	mg/dL
Phosphorus	4.0	mg/dL
Sodium	152	mEq/L
Potassium	3.6	mEq/L
Chloride	100	mEq/L
Total protein	5.9	g/dL
Albumin	3.1	g/dL
BUN	13	mg/dL
Creatinine	0.8	mg/dL
Glucose	105	mg/dL

TABLE APP–61. Blood Gas Analysis

Sample	Day 1 Arterial	Day 2 Arterial	Day 2 Central Venous	Unit
pH	7.325	7.390	7.337	
Po_2	83	90	29	mm Hg
Pco_2	44.6	39.7	51.5	mm Hg
HCO_3^-	23.4	24.2	27.9	mEq/L
Total CO_2	24.7	25.4	29.4	mEq/L
Base excess	−2.1	0	+1.7	mEq/L
(A-a) Do_2	11.2	10.4		mm Hg

opposing magnitudes occurred simultaneously in this dog, resulting in a relatively normal [HCO_3^-]. A specific cause for the hypochloremia and mild hypernatremia could not be found. The organic acidosis may have been due to lactic acidosis, because this animal was neither uremic nor ketoacidotic. The low Po_2 in the central venous sample obtained on day 2 also supports this conclusion. Respiratory acid-base disorders are discussed in Chapter 11.

Treatment. On day 1, the dog was placed on a water-circulating heating pad, observed for seizures, and given intravenous lactated Ringer's solution with 28 mEq/L KCl. The dog was given furosemide on admission for possible pulmonary edema and treated with antibiotics. On day 2, antibiotics and furosemide were discontinued, and the dog was given lactulose and neomycin because of concern about the possibility of an underlying portosystemic shunt. These medications were discontinued when the bile acid concentration results were obtained.

Outcome. The dog improved dramatically during its hospitalization, and was released on day 6. He was normal at the time of release.

Case 32 (Tables App–62, App–63)

Signalment. 10-year-old male Australian terrier, 44 kg

Chief Complaint. Chronic cough

History. The dog suffered smoke inhalation 4 years before admission and had a chronic dry cough since that time. The cough had increased in frequency and become moist in the 10 days before admission. The owner also reported that the dog's appetite had decreased recently.

Physical Examination. The dog was obese and was panting. There were increased bronchovesicular sounds on thoracic auscultation.

Ancillary Findings. Thoracic radiographs on day 1 showed increased interstitial and peribronchial markings and generalized cardiomegaly. Cytologic evaluation of a tracheal wash showed mucopurulent inflammation. *Pasteurella multocida* and *Klebsiella* sp. were cultured from the tracheal wash, whereas hemolytic *Escherichia coli* was cultured from the urine.

Diagnosis. Smoke inhalation; bacterial pneumonia; bacterial urinary tract infection

TABLE APP–62. Laboratory Findings

Laboratory Test	Day 1	Unit
Hematocrit	46	%
Plasma proteins	8.6	g/dL
White blood cells	22,200	/μL
Bands	2,200	/μL
Segmented neutrophils	17,300	/μL
Lymphocytes	900	/μL
Monocytes	1,800	/μL
Urine specific gravity	1.042	
Urine protein	100	mg/dL
Urine sediment	many leukocytes	/hpf*
	20–25 erythrocytes	/hpf
CO_2	22	mEq/L
Calcium	10.3	mg/dL
Phosphorus	4.0	mg/dL
Sodium	147	mEq/L
Potassium	3.2	mEq/L
Chloride	109	mEq/L
Total protein	7.2	g/dL
Albumin	2.5	g/dL
BUN	15	mg/dL
Creatinine	1.3	mg/dL
Glucose	100	mg/dL

*hpf = high-power field.

Interpretation. The leukocytosis with neutrophilia and left shift was probably due to bacterial pneumonia. The active sediment on urinalysis was thought to be due to urinary tract infection, which was confirmed by bacterial culture of the urine. The increased plasma protein concentration presumably resulted from a combination of dehydration and inflammation (lungs and urinary tract). The mild hypokalemia was unexplained but may have resulted from anorexia. The slightly increased serum creatinine concentration (1.3 mg/dL) in the presence of a high urine specific gravity (1.042) was due to prerenal factors (i.e., dehydration). Presumably, an increase in BUN did not occur because of the anorexia.

Blood gas analysis indicated chronic respiratory alkalosis. The expected [HCO_3^-] is 21 − 0.55 (37 − 26.4) = 15.2 mEq/L, which is within 2 mEq/L of the observed value of 16.3 mEq/L. The dog also had hypoxemia and an increased arterial-alveolar O_2 difference of 51 mm Hg (normal: <25 mm Hg). The combination of hypoxemia, chronic respiratory alkalosis, and increased (A-a) Do_2 probably was caused by ventilation-perfusion mismatch, but a right-to-left shunt could result in similar findings.

TABLE APP–63. Blood Gas Analysis

Sample	Arterial	Unit
pH	7.395	
Po_2	66	mm Hg
Pco_2	26.4	mm Hg
HCO_3^-	16.3	mEq/L
Total CO_2	17.0	mEq/L
Base excess	−6.2	mEq/L
(A-a) Do_2	51	mm Hg

Pulmonary fibrosis secondary to smoke inhalation and secondary bacterial pneumonia were judged to be responsible for these findings. The radiographic findings also supported this conclusion. Chronic respiratory alkalosis is the only simple acid-base disorder in which compensation results in a normal blood pH. Respiratory acid-base disorders are discussed in Chapter 11.

Treatment. The dog was treated with aminophylline and trimethoprim-sulfadiazine.

Outcome. The dog improved over the following days. Trimethoprim-sulfadiazine was discontinued after 14 days, but the aminophylline was continued.

Case 33 (Tables App–64, App–65)

Signalment. 9-year-old spayed female mixed-breed dog, 11 kg

Chief Complaint. Dyspnea

History. The owner observed that the dog had developed labored breathing characterized by shortness of breath over the 4 weeks before presentation. During that time, there also was a history of lethargy, anorexia, weight loss, and intermittent vomiting. No coughing was observed by the owner. The dog had been treated with furosemide by the referring veterinarian for possible pulmonary edema.

Physical Examination. The dog was 5–7% dehydrated and dyspneic. There were increased bronchovesicular lung sounds and end-inspiratory, early-expiratory crackles on thoracic auscultation.

Ancillary Findings. Thoracic radiographs showed a diffuse increase in interstitial pulmonary density suggestive of poor lung expansion. A lung biopsy showed widespread pulmonary interstitial and subpleural fibrosis.

Diagnosis. Pulmonary fibrosis

Interpretation. The increased hematocrit, increased total protein and albumin concentrations, and mildly increased serum creatinine concentration probably reflected hemoconcentration. It also is possible that the mild increase in hematocrit was due to chronic hypoxemia. The normal BUN concentration in the face of a mild increase in serum creatinine concentration may have been due to chronic anorexia. Hypokalemia was thought to be due to anorexia, weight loss, vomiting, and previous furosemide administration.

Blood gas analysis showed a mixed disorder characterized by metabolic alkalosis and respiratory alkalosis with hypoxemia and increased (A-a) Do_2 of 55.6 mm Hg (normal: <25 mm Hg). If a simple chronic respiratory alkalosis were present, the expected $[HCO_3^-]$ would have been $21 - 0.55 (37 - 27.5) = 15.8$ mEq/L. The observed value of 22 mEq/L suggested the presence of concurrent metabolic alkalosis. The metabolic alkalosis was due to hypochloremia ($[SID]_i = 47$ mEq/L) and, presumably, was the result of previous vomiting and furosemide administration.

The association of hypoxemia with respiratory alkalosis was suggestive of primary pulmonary disease. The increased (A-a) Do_2 indicated diffusion impairment, ventilation-perfusion mismatch, or a right-to-left shunt as potential causes for the hypoxemia and hypocapnia. The increase in Po_2 after administration of 100% O_2 on day 5 excluded right-to-left shunt as a cause of hypoxemia, and the failure of Po_2 to increase after administration of 40% O_2 argued against diffusion impairment as a cause for the hypoxemia. The hypercapnia ($Pco_2 = 48.2$ mm Hg) on day 5 presumably was due to hypoventilation associated with anesthesia for thoracotomy and lung biopsy.

In pulmonary fibrosis, the lungs become stiff, resulting in reduced pulmonary compliance and a restrictive ventilatory defect. Total lung capacity is decreased, reflected by a flattening of the diaphragm and poor lung expansion observed on the thoracic radiographs. An increase in respiratory rate (possibly mediated by the juxtacapillary receptors) develops to compensate for the decrease in the total lung capacity. Patients with pulmonary fibrosis usually have chronic respiratory alkalosis and mild hypoxemia with increased (A-a) Do_2, as observed in this dog. These concepts are discussed further in Chapter 11.

Treatment. The dog was rehydrated by parenteral fluid therapy and furosemide was discontinued. Serum electrolyte concentrations returned to normal on day 3.

Outcome. The dog was released from the hospital receiving prednisone. The dyspnea became progressively worse despite glucocorticoid therapy, and the dog died several weeks after discharge.

TABLE APP–64. Laboratory Findings

Laboratory Test	Day 1	Day 3	Unit
Hematocrit	57		%
Plasma proteins	7.5		g/dL
CO_2	23	22	mEq/L
Calcium	10.9	9.8	mg/dL
Phosphorus	3.3	2.3	mg/dL
Sodium	149	149	mEq/L
Potassium	3.2	4.1	mEq/L
Chloride	102	112	mEq/L
Total proteins	7.1	5.8	g/dL
Albumin	3.4	2.8	g/dL
BUN	22	16	mg/dL
Creatinine	1.9	1.6	mg/dL
Glucose	129	80	mg/dL

TABLE APP–65. Blood Gas Analysis

Sample	Day 1 Arterial	Day 5 Arterial	Day 6 Arterial	Unit
Fio_2	21	100	40	%
pH	7.507	7.309	7.394	
Po_2	60	379	50	mm Hg
Pco_2	27.5	48.2	32	mm Hg
HCO_3^-	22	24.4	19.7	mEq/L
Base excess	+0.8	−1.7	−3.5	mEq/L
(A-a) Do_2	55.6			mm Hg

Case 34 (Table App–66)

Signalment. 6-month-old intact male mixed-breed dog, 15 kg

Chief Complaint. Hit by a car

History. The dog had been hit by a car approximately 45 min before presentation and was bleeding from the nose and mouth. There was no prior history of illness, and vaccinations had been administered at 9 weeks of age.

Physical Examination. The dog was hyperthermic (106.8°F), tachycardic (226/min), and panting. The femoral pulses were weak, and the dog was bleeding from its nose. There was bilateral miosis, and the dog was semicomatose, but there were no other abnormalities on neurologic examination.

Ancillary Findings. Skull radiographs showed multiple maxillary fractures and increased soft-tissue density in the nasal passages compatible with hemorrhage. Thoracic radiographs showed a diffuse increase in interstitial density indicative of pulmonary contusions and microcardia compatible with hypovolemic shock.

Diagnosis. Skull fractures, pulmonary contusions, hypovolemic shock, and probable cerebral edema associated with head trauma

Interpretation. At admission, blood gas analysis showed a mixed acid-base disorder consisting of primary metabolic acidosis due to shock and reduced tissue perfusion complicated by primary respiratory alkalosis due to hyperventilation, presumably induced by pain. The observed blood pH was nearly normal, but both the bicarbonate concentration and P_{CO_2} were very low. If the primary problem were metabolic acidosis with normal respiratory compensation, we would expect the P_{CO_2} to be $37 - 0.7(21 - 10.3) = 29.5$ mm Hg. The observed P_{CO_2} is 17.5 mm Hg, which is more than 2–3 mm Hg below the calculated value. Therefore, a mixed acid-base disorder (metabolic acidosis and respiratory alkalosis) is diagnosed. The presence of two opposing acid-base disturbances (metabolic acidosis and respiratory alkalosis) explains why the observed pH is nearly normal. This case demonstrates that a normal blood pH does not always imply normal acid-base balance. The dog's acid-base balance had returned nearly to normal by the following day, as evidenced by the venous sample obtained 24 h after admission. These principles are discussed further in Chapter 12.

Treatment. The dog was treated with 500 mg hydrocortisone sodium succinate and rapid infusion of lactated Ringer's solution. Dexamethasone 1.5 mg subcutaneously q8h and cimetidine 150 mg subcutaneously q8h also were administered.

Outcome. Within 24 h, the dog was much more alert and responsive. The epistaxis had resolved, and the pupils were normal-sized and responsive to light. The dog was able to walk but appeared to be in pain. Within 48 h, the dog was walking normally and eating. It was released from the hospital after 72 h.

REFERENCES

Berger B and Feldman EC: Primary hyperparathyroidism in dogs: 21 cases (1976–1986). J Am Vet Med Assoc 191:350–356, 1987.

Bruner JM, Steiner JM, Williams DA, et al: High feline trypsin-like immunoreactivity in a cat with pancreatitis and hepatic lipidosis. J Am Vet Med Assoc 210(12):1757–1760, 1997.

Burrows CF and Bovee KC: Metabolic changes due to experimentally-induced rupture of the canine urinary bladder. Am J Vet Res 35:1083–1088, 1974.

Crawford MA, Kittleson MD, and Fink GD: Hypernatremia and adipsia in a dog. J Am Vet Med Assoc 184:818–821, 1984.

de Morais HS and DiBartola SP: Ventilatory and metabolic compensation in dogs with acid-base disturbances: A review. J Vet Emerg Crit Care 1(2):39–49, 1991.

DiBartola SP and Leonard PO: Renal tubular acidosis in a dog. J Am Vet Med Assoc 180(1):70–72, 1982.

DiBartola SP, Johnson SE, Davenport DJ, et al.: Clinicopathologic findings resembling hypoadrenocorticism in dogs with primary gastrointestinal disease. J Am Vet Med Assoc 187:60–63, 1985.

DiBartola SP, Buffington CA, Chew DJ, et al: Development of chronic renal disease in cats fed a commercial diet. J Am Vet Med Assoc 202(5):744–751, 1993.

DiBartola SP, Johnson SE, Johnson GC, et al: Hypodipsic hypernatremia in a dog with defective osmoregulation of antidiuretic hormone. J Am Vet Med Assoc 204(6):922–925, 1994.

DiBartola SP and Brown SA: The kidney and hyperthyroidism. In Bonagura JD: *Kirk's Current Veterinary Therapy XIII.* Philadelphia, WB Saunders Co., pp. 337–339, 2000.

Dow SW, Fettman MJ, LeCouteur RA, et al.: Potassium depletion in cats: Renal and dietary influences. J Am Vet Med Assoc 191:1569–1575, 1987.

Feldman EC and Nelson RW: Hyperadrenocorticism (Cushing's syndrome). In Feldman EC and Nelson RW: *Canine and Feline Endocrinology and Reproduction,* 2nd ed., Philadelphia, WB Saunders Co., p. 262, 1996.

Finco DR and Cornelius LM: Characterization and treatment of water, electrolyte, and acid-base imbalances of induced urethral obstruction in the cat. Am J Vet Res 38:823–830, 1977.

Flanders JA, Scarlett JM, and Blue JT: Adjustment of total serum calcium concentration for binding to albumin and protein in cats. J Am Vet Med Assoc 194:1609–1611, 1989.

Grauer GF, Thrall MA, Henre BA, et al.: Early clinicopathologic findings in dogs ingesting ethylene glycol. Am J Vet Res 45:2229–2303, 1984.

Hoskins JD and Rothschmitt J: Hypernatremic thirst deficiency in a dog. Vet Med 79:489–491, 1984.

Hughes DE and Sokolowski JH: Sodium chloride poisoning in the dog. Canine Pract 5:28–31, 1978.

Ilkiw JE, Rose RJ, and Martin ICA: A comparison of simultaneously collected arterial, mixed venous, jugular venous, and cephalic venous blood samples in the assessment of blood gas and acid base status in the dog. J Vet Intern Med 5:294–298, 1991.

TABLE APP–66. Blood Gas Analysis

Sample	Day 1 Arterial	Day 2 Venous	Unit
pH	7.383	7.367	
P_{O_2}	102	40	mm Hg
P_{CO_2}	17.2	33.4	mm Hg
HCO_3^-	10.3	19.3	mEq/L
Total CO_2	10.9	20.4	mEq/L
Base excess	−11.2	−4.4	mEq/L

Kitchell BE, Strombeck DR, Cullen J, et al.: Clinical and pathologic changes in experimentally induced pancreatitis in cats. *Am J Vet Res* 47:1170–1173, 1986.

Klausner JS, O'Leary TP, and Osborne CA: Calcium urolithiasis in two dogs with parathyroid adenomas. *J Am Vet Med Assoc* 191:1423–1426, 1987.

Malik R, Hunt GB, Hinchliffe JM, et al.: Severe whipworm infection in the dog. *J Small Anim Pract* 31:185–188, 1990.

McLoughlin MA, DiBartola SP, Birchard SJ, et al.: Influence of systemic non-thyroidal illness on serum concentrations of thyroxine in hyperthyroid cats. *J Am Anim Hosp Assoc* 29:227–234, 1993.

Meuten DJ, Chew DJ, Kociba GJ, et al.: Relationship of serum total calcium to albumin and total proteins in dogs. *J Am Vet Med Assoc* 180:63–67, 1980.

Narins RG and Emmett M: Simple and mixed acid-base disorders: A practical approach. *Medicine (Baltimore)* 59:161–187, 1980.

Peterson ME and Feinman JM: Hypercalcemia associated with hypoadrenocorticism in 16 dogs. *J Am Vet Med Assoc* 181:802–804, 1982.

Reine NJ, Hohenhaus AE, Peterson ME, Patnaik AK: Deoxycorticosterone-secreting adrenocortical carcinoma in a dog. *J Vet Intern Med* 13:386–390, 1999.

Sherding RG, Meuten DJ, Chew DJ, et al.: Primary hypoparathyroidism in the dog. *J Am Vet Med Assoc* 176:439–444, 1980.

Simpson KW, Bonagura JD, and Eaton KA: Right ventricular cardiomyopathy in a dog. *J Vet Intern Med* 8(4):306–309, 1994.

Willard MD, Schall WD, McCaw DE, et al.: Canine hypoadrenocorticism: Report of 37 cases and review of 39 previously reported cases. *J Am Vet Med Assoc* 180:59–62, 1982.

Willard MD, Fossum TW, Torrance A, et al.: Hyponatremia and hyperkalemia associated with idiopathic or experimentally induced chylothorax in four dogs. *J Am Vet Med Assoc* 199:353–358, 1991.

Index

Note: Page numbers in *italics* indicate figures; page numbers followed by t indicate tables.

A

(A–a) O$_2$ gradient (alveolar-arterial oxygen difference), *242*, 242–243, 243t, 250, 549t
Abbocath-T catheter, 283t
Abdominal compartment syndrome, perioperative management of, 313
Abdominal distention, due to carcinomatosis, 558–559, 559t
 due to congestive heart failure, 552–553, 553t
 due to protein-losing enteropathy, 570, 570t
Abdominal effusion. See *Ascites*.
Abdominocentesis, for ascites, 365, *366*
ABP (arterial blood pressure), control of, 387, *388*, 389t
 in shock, 444
Absorption, of water and electrolytes, 330–335, *330–335*
A-Cath catheter, 283t
ACD (anticoagulant/citrate/dextrose), for donated blood, 456t
ACE inhibitors. See *Angiotensin-converting enzyme (ACE) inhibitors*.
Acepromazine, effects of, 316
 for congestive heart failure, 399
Acetate, in dialysate, 513
Acetated polyionic solutions, compatibility of, with other IV products, 311t
 during anesthesia and surgery, 320, *321*
 physicochemical properties of, 320
Acetazolamide, metabolic acidosis due to, 216–217
 renal effects of, 394, *395*, 395t
Acetest, in diabetic ketoacidosis, 220
Acetylcholine, in control of absorption and secretion, 335
Acetylsalicylic acid, salicylate intoxication due to, 220
Acid(s), defined, 189
 fixed, 189, 195–196
 hypersecretion of, 338
 in dissociation equilibrium equation, 190
 net excretion of, 205
 nonvolatile, 189, 195–196
 volatile, 189, 195–196
Acid load, acute, body buffer response to, 211, *212*
 renal response to, 212
 respiratory response to, 211–212
Acid pump, in stomach, 330

Acid-base balance, acidity in, 189
 anion gap in, 200–202, 201t
 bicarbonate–carbonic acid system in, 192–193
 body buffers in, 193–194, *194*, 194t
 buffering in, 190–192, *192*
 chloride and, 74–76
 external hydrogen ion balance in, 204
 isohydric principle in, 192, 192t
 law of mass action in, 190
 pH in, 189–190, *190*, 191t
 potassium and, 85–86, 93, 207–208
 renal regulation of, 205–207, *205–208*
 whole-body regulation of, 204–205
 with vomiting and diarrhea, 338
Acid-base disorders, 189–208
 blood gas measurement in, 196–200, *198*, 200t
 compensatory (secondary, adaptive) responses in, 195, 195t, 196, 196t, *197*, 252t, 548t
  in mixed disorders, 253
  metabolic, 243–244, *244*, *245*, 252
  respiratory, 196t, 251–252
 hemodialysis for, 540
 in congestive heart failure, 398
 in liver disease, 354
  treatment of, 362–363
 metabolic, 195, 211–236. See also *Metabolic acidosis; Metabolic alkalosis*.
 mixed. See *Mixed acid-base disorders*.
 nontraditional approach to, 202–204, 203t, 204t, 550t
 physiologic lines of defense in, 194–195
 primary, 195, 195t
 respiratory, 195. See also *Respiratory acidosis; Respiratory alkalosis*.
 simple, 195–196, 251
 terminology for, 195
 with gastric dilatation-volvulus, 339
Acid-base maps, 196, *197*
Acid-base status, in various diseases, 268t
Acidemia, defined, 196, 251
Acidity, 189
 titratable, 194, 205, 206
Acidosis, defined, 196, 251
 dilutional, 217
 lactic. See *Lactic acidosis*.
 metabolic. See *Metabolic acidosis*.
 paradoxical CNS, 221
 renal tubular. See *Renal tubular acidosis (RTA)*.

Acidosis *(Continued)*
 respiratory. See *Respiratory acidosis*.
 uremic, 221–222, 416
Acromegaly, hyperphosphatemia due to, 170
 polyuria and polydipsia due to, 66t
ACTH (adrenocorticotropic hormone) stimulation test, for hypoadrenocorticism, 382
Active transport, primary, 34
 secondary, 34–35
Activity coefficient, 189
Acute intrinsic renal failure (AIRF). See *Renal failure, acute*.
Acute renal failure (ARF). See *Renal failure, acute*.
Adaptive responses, in acid-base disorders. See *Compensatory responses*.
Addison's disease, 381. See also *Hypoadrenocorticism*.
Additive solutions, 270, 272–273
 for donated blood, 456t
 labels for, 275, *275*
Adenocarcinoma, apocrine gland, case study of, 567–568, 567t, *568*
 hypercalcemia due to, 131–132, *133*, *134*
 parathyroid gland, hypercalcemia due to, 134–136
Adenoma, parathyroid, case study of, *566*, 566–567, 567t
 hypercalcemia due to, 134–136
ADH. See *Antidiuretic hormone (ADH)*.
Adrenocortical carcinoma, case study of, 562–563, 562t
Adrenocortical insufficiency. See *Hypoadrenocorticism*.
Adrenocorticotropic hormone (ACTH) stimulation test, for hypoadrenocorticism, 382
Adsol, for donated blood, 456t
AG. See *Anion gap (AG)*.
Aging, perioperative management with, 313
Air embolism, 298
 due to transfusion, 459
AIRF (acute intrinsic renal failure). See *Renal failure, acute*.
"Alabama rot," 454
Albumin, and colloid oncotic pressure, 436
 and colloid osmotic pressure, 485–486
 buffering by, 194
 dosage of, 489
 for ascites, 366

589

Albumin *(Continued)*
  for hypoproteinemia, 490
  in liver disease, 363–364
  in malnutrition, 467
  metabolism of, 343–345, *344*
Aldosterone, in congestive heart failure, 393
  in liver disease, 350
  in metabolic alkalosis, 228
  in potassium excretion, 88, 89–90, 91–93
  in sodium balance, 47, 49, 50t
Aldosterone antagonists, for congestive heart failure, 400
  renal effects of, 395t
Alkalemia, and hepatic encephalopathy, 358t
  defined, 196, 251
Alkali, administration of, metabolic alkalosis due to, 231
Alkali precursors, in dialysate, 513
Alkaline picrate reaction, 30
Alkaline tide, 330
Alkalinizing agent, for hypercalcemia, 141t, 142–143
Alkalosis, defined, 196, 251
  hypochloremic, 75–76
  metabolic. See *Metabolic alkalosis*.
  "refeeding," 235
  respiratory. See *Respiratory alkalosis*.
Allergic reactions, to dextrans, 321, 491
  to gelatin solutions, 324, 491
  to hetastarch, 323, 491
  to plasma protein, 324, 325
  to synthetic colloids, in liver disease, 364
Alpha$_1$ antagonists, effects of, 316
Alpha intercalated cells, potassium transport in, 87, *88*
Aluminum, and hypercalcemia, 129
Aluminum carbonate, for hyperphosphatemia, 170
Aluminum hydroxide, for hyperphosphatemia, 170
  for hypervitaminosis D, 145
Alveolar ventilation, in metabolic acidosis, 211
  in metabolic alkalosis, 228, *229*
  in respiratory acidosis, 246
  in respiratory alkalosis, 247
  Pco$_2$ and, 241–242
Alveolar-arterial oxygen difference ([A−a] O$_2$ gradient), *242*, 242–243, 243t, 250, 549t
Amikacin, for peritonitis, 523
  for shock, 441
Amiloride, renal effects of, 394, 394t, *395*, 395t
Amino acids, aromatic, and hepatic encephalopathy, 357t
  cationic, metabolic acidosis due to, 217
  in dialysate, 513
  in parenteral nutrition, 469–470, 473
  tubular reabsorption of, 36
Aminoglycosides, for peritonitis, 523
  for shock, 441
Amlodipine, for congestive heart failure, 401
Ammonia, and hepatic encephalopathy, 357t, 358–359
  detoxification of, 345, *346*, 346
Ammoniagenesis, in hypokalemia, 94–95, 353
  in metabolic alkalosis, 228
  serum potassium concentration and, 346
Ammonium (NH$_4^+$), excretion of, 207, *207*, *208*
  in uremic acidosis, 222
Ammonium chloride (NH$_4$Cl), metabolic acidosis due to, 217
Ammonium chloride (NH$_4$Cl) tolerance test, 215
Ammonium salts, excretion of, 205

Ampicillin, for peritonitis, 523
  metabolic alkalosis due to, 235
Amputation, catheter, 298
Anal sac adenocarcinoma, case study of, 567–568, 567t, *568*
  hypercalcemia due to, 131–132, *133*, *134*
Analgesia, for shock, 434, 440–441, 441t
Anaphylactic shock, 432
Anaphylactoid reactions, to dextrans, 321, 491
  to hetastarch, 323, 491
Anemia, in renal failure, 421–422
  perioperative management of, *308*, 308–309
  with hemodialysis, 545
Anesthesia, blood samples during, 318
  compatibility of IV solutions during, 311t
  effects of, 316–317
  fluid therapy during, 307
  for catheter placement, 285
  regional, 317
  vascular access for, 316
  with aging, 313
  with anemia, *308*, 308–309
  with hypercalcemia, 310
  with hyperkalemia, 310
  with hypernatremia, 309
  with hyperosmolality, 310
  with hyperthyroidism, 316
  with hypocalcemia, 310
  with hypoglycemia, 310–311
  with hypokalemia, 310
  with hyponatremia, 309
  with hypoproteinemia, 309
  with hypothyroidism, 316
  with increased intracranial pressure, 313
  with increased intraocular pressure, 313
  with metabolic acidosis, 311, 311t
  with metabolic alkalosis, 312
  with peripheral edema, 312
  with peritoneal fluid, 313
  with pleural fluid, 312
  with polycythemia, 309
  with pregnancy, 313
  with pulmonary edema, 312
  with renal disease, 315
Angiocath radiopaque Teflon catheter, *282*, 283t
Angiotensin II, and extracellular fluid volume, 40
  and glomerular filtration rate, 29
  in congestive heart failure, 393
  in sodium balance, 49–50, 50t
Angiotensin receptor blockers, renal effects of, 393, 394t
Angiotensin-converting enzyme (ACE) inhibitors, for congestive heart failure, 399–400, 401
  hyperkalemia due to, 102
  renal effects of, 393, 394t, *395*, 396
Animal Blood Bank, 452t
Anion(s), as additives to crystalloid solutions, 272
  concentrations of, 200–201, 201t
  defined, 3
  strong, 202
  unmeasured, 13, *13*
  weak, 202
Anion gap (AG), 13, *13*, 200–202, 201t
  calculation of, 13, 201, 549t
  defined, 201
  in acid-base evaluation, 202–203, 204t
  in IgG multiple myeloma, 201–202
  in lactic acidosis, 223
  in metabolic acidosis, 74–75, 201
    increased, 213t, *214*, 217–226, *218*, *219*, 222t, 256t, 257–258

Anion gap (AG) *(Continued)*
  normal, 213–217, 213t, *214*, 214t, *215*, 216t
  in metabolic alkalosis, 230
  in mixed acid-base disorders, 253, 254t
  normal, 549t
Anorexia, 467
  fluid therapy for, 268t
  with chronic renal failure, 581–582, 581t
  with congestive heart failure, 552–553, 553t
  with diabetic ketoacidosis, 577–578, 577t
  with hepatic encephalopathy, 358t
ANP. See *Atrial natriuretic peptide (ANP)*.
Antacids, hypophosphatemia due to, 166
Antiarrhythmic agents, for shock, 440
Antibiotic-coated catheters, 284
Antibiotics, for shock, 441
  in dialysate, 520
Anticoagulant solutions, for donated blood, 456, 456t
Anticoagulant/citrate/dextrose (ACD), for donated blood, 456t
Antidiuretic hormone (ADH), and glomerular filtration rate, 29
  and urinary free water, 16
  anesthesia effect on, 316
  chemical structure of, *50*
  for central diabetes insipidus, 55
  in congestive heart failure, 393, 397
  in free-water excretion, 350
  in hypernatremia, 53–55
  in potassium balance, 89
  in urinary concentrating mechanism, 37–38
  in water balance, 50, 50–51, *51*
  stimuli for release of, 51, *51*
  syndrome of inappropriate secretion of, hyponatremia due to, 63
Antidiuretic hormone (ADH) testing, exogenous, 70, 70t
Antifreeze ingestion, case studies of, 574–577t, 574t–576t
  hemodialysis for, 529, *529*, 541–542
  hypocalcemia due to, 150
  metabolic acidosis due to, 217–220, *218*, *219*
  peritoneal dialysis for, 510–511
Antiseptic agents, for catheter placement, 286
Antizol (methylpyrazole), for ethylene glycol ingestion, 219
Anuria, defined, 412
Apocrine gland adenocarcinoma, case study of, 567–568, 567t, *568*
  hypercalcemia due to, 131–132, *133*, *134*
Aqueous vasopressin test, 70, 70t
ARF (acute renal failure). See *Renal failure, acute*.
Arginine, metabolic acidosis due to, 217
Arginine vasopressin (AVP). See *Antidiuretic hormone (ADH)*.
Argyle Intramedicut intravenous catheter, 283t
Argyle Medicut intravenous catheter, *282*, 283t
Aromatic amino acids, and hepatic encephalopathy, 357t
Arrhythmias, due to dopamine, 420–421
  due to hypercalcemia, 140
  due to hypokalemia, 94
  due to magnesium deficiency, 179, 181
  due to shock, 440
  magnesium for, 183, 184, *184*
Arrow radial artery catheterization set, *282*, *282*, 283t
Arrow Twin Cath catheter, 283
Arterial blood pressure (ABP), control of, 387, *388*, 389t

Arterial blood pressure (ABP) *(Continued)*
   in shock, 444
Arterial blood samples, 198, 199
Arterial vasodilatation hypothesis, of ascites, 360–361, *361*
Arteriovenous fistulas, for hemodialysis, 531–532
Ascites, assessment of, 361
   classic underfilling hypothesis of, 360
   hyponatremia due to, 63
   in liver disease, 349–350, 360–361, *361*
     treatment of, 362, 365–366, *366*
   measurement of, 318
   overflow theory of, 360
   pathophysiology of, 360–361, *361*
   peripheral arterial vasodilatation hypothesis of, 360–361, *361*
   treatment of, 362, 365–366, *366*
   with hypoalbuminemia, 347
Ash Advantage T-fluted peritoneal dialysis catheter, 518, *519*
Aspirin, for transfusion reactions, 460t
   renal effects of, 396–397
   salicylate intoxication due to, 220
   with hemodialysis, 531
Asthma, magnesium for, 183
Atomic weight, 3, 3t
Atrial natriuretic peptide (ANP), for renal failure, 421
   in congestive heart failure, 393
   in sodium balance, 50, 50t
Auricular arteries, catheterization of, 318
Autonomic nervous system, and glomerular filtration rate, 29
Autoregulation, of renal blood flow, *31*, 31–32
Autoregulatory escape, 431
Autotransfusion, 308
   for hemorrhagic shock, 436
Avogadro's law, 4
AVP (arginine vasopressin). See *Antidiuretic hormone (ADH)*.
Azium. See *Dexamethasone (Azium)*.
Azotemia, and hepatic encephalopathy, 358t
   before dialysis, 513
   clinical signs of, 534t
   due to hypercalcemia, 139
   during peritoneal dialysis, 525
   in congestive heart failure, 399, 399t
   in hypoadrenocorticism, 381
   in renal failure, 411–412

B

Babesiosis, mixed acid-base disturbances with, 255
Bandaging, of intravenous catheters, 295–296
Baroreceptors, hepatic, 350
Bartter's syndrome, 96
Baruria, 46
Basal energy requirement (BER), 20, 275–276, *277*
Basal fluid needs, 14–15, 20–21
Base, 190
Base deficit, 197
Base excess (BE), 197, 202
Basolateral membranes, 33
Benazepril, for congestive heart failure, 400
   renal effects of, 394–395
Benzodiazepines, endogenous, and hepatic encephalopathy, 357t
BER (basal energy requirement), 20, 275–276, *277*
Beta blockers, for congestive heart failure, 400
   hyperkalemia due to, 102
Betadine (povidone-iodine), for catheter placement, 286

Bicarbonate (HCO_3^-). See also *Sodium bicarbonate ($NaHCO_3$)*.
   after hypercapnia, 234
     acute, 244, *244*
     chronic, 244–245, *245*
   alkali administration and, 231
   as buffer in extracellular fluid, 193–194
   in acid-base evaluation, 200, 202, 204
   in anion gap, 201
   in diabetic ketoacidosis, 220, 221
   in dialysate, for hemodialysis, 540
     for peritoneal dialysis, 513, 533
   in gastric fluid loss, 231–232
   in intestine, 333, 334
   in metabolic alkalosis, 227–231
   in pancreas, 332
   in respiratory acidosis, 245
   in respiratory alkalosis, 247
   in stomach, 330
   in uremic acidosis, 221–222
   in venous *vs*. arterial blood, 241
   Pco_2 and, 243
   reabsorption of, 34, *34*, 205, *205*, *206*
     in proximal renal tubular acidosis, 215
   regeneration of new, 205, *205*, *206*
   standard, 196–197
Bicarbonate–carbonic acid system, 192–193
Bile, formation, composition, and flow of, 342–343, 342t, *343*
Bile acids, 342
   and hepatic encephalopathy, 357t
Bile ducts, normal physiology of, 342–343, 342t, *343*
Bile peritonitis, 367
Bile salts, 342
Bisphosphonates, for hypercalcemia, 141t, 144
Bladder, ruptured, case study of, 554–555, 555t
Blastomycosis, hypercalcemia due to, 137
Bleeding. See *Hemorrhage*.
Bleeding disorders. See *Coagulopathies*.
Blood, administration of, 456–458
   anticoagulants and preservatives for, 456, 456t
   compatibility of, with other IV products, 311t
   sources of, 451, 452t, 453
   whole. See *Whole blood*.
Blood banks, 452t, 453
Blood components, 451–453, *453*
Blood composition, changes in, *308*, 308–312, 311t
   monitoring of, 318
Blood donation, autologous, 308
Blood donors, blood typing of, 454–455, 455t, *461*
   collection of blood from, 455–456, 456t
   crossmatching of, 460–461, 460t, *461*, 461t
   for cats, 454–455, 454t
   for dogs, 453–454, 454t
   health maintenance of, 455
   screening of, 455
   selection of, 453–455
   sources of, 453
Blood flow, renal. See *Renal blood flow (RBF)*.
Blood gases, in acid-base disorders, 253
   in liver disease, 354–355, *355*
   in shock, 445
   interpretation of data on, 199–200
   measurement of, 196–200, *198*, 200t
   normal values for, 199, 200t, 549t
   sample collection and handling of, 198–199
Blood loss, perioperative management of, 307–308

Blood pressure, and shock, 428, 444
   arterial, control of, 387, *388*, 389t
     in shock, 444
   central venous. See *Central venous pressure (CVP)*.
   in hypocapnia, 248
   systolic, in monitoring fluid therapy, 317
   wedge. See *Pulmonary capillary wedge pressure (PCWP)*.
   with hemodialysis, 533, *534*
Blood products, for congestive heart failure, 403
   for shock, 436, 442–443
   immunogenicity of, 451
   in renal failure, 421–422
   sources of, 451, 452t, 453
Blood samples, in monitoring fluid therapy, 318
Blood substitute, 461–462
Blood transfusion. See *Transfusion(s)*.
Blood typing, 454–455, 454t, 461, *461*
Blood urea nitrogen (BUN), in congestive heart failure, 397, 399
   in liver disease, 351, 352, *353*
   in malnutrition, 467
   in renal failure, 411–412, 422
   with hemodialysis, for renal failure, 537–539, *538*
   with peritoneal dialysis, 509, *509*, 514–515, 524–525
Blood volume, 5–6, 6t
   changes in, 307–308
     monitoring of, 317–318
   effective circulating, 12, 47–48
   in heart failure, 387, 389t
   in hemodialysis, 534, *534*, 535
Body buffers, 193–194, *194*, 194t
   response to acute acid load by, 211, *212*
Body condition score, 466–467
Body fluid(s). See also *Extracellular fluid (ECF); Intracellular fluid (ICF)*.
   electroneutrality and anion gap in, 13, *13*
   homeostasis (zero balance) of, *14*, 14–15, 15t
   osmolal gap in, 14, 14t
   solutes in. See *Solute(s)*.
   water intake and, *18*, 18–20, 18t–20t, *19*
   water losses and, 15–18, 15t, *16*, 17t, 18t
   water requirements and, 20–21, 21t
Body fluid compartments, exchange of water between, 10–13, *11*, 12t, *13*
   volume measurements for, 5–9, 6t–8t, *9*
Body weight. See *Weight*.
Bone, as source of buffer, 193
   calcitriol effects on, 120
   calcium release from, 109–110
   response of, to parathyroid hormone, 115
Bone biopsy, 125
Bone marrow aspiration, 125
Bone metastases, hypercalcemia due to, 133–134
Bone resorption inhibitors, for hypercalcemia, 141t, 143–144
Bowman's capsule, 27
Bowman's space, 27
Bradycardia, in hypoadrenocorticism, 381
Bubble detector, in-line, *300*
"Buddies for Life," 452t
Buffer(s), 190
   bicarbonate as, 193–194
   body, 193–194, *194*, 194t
   intracellular, 194, *194*, 194t
   nonbicarbonate, 194, *194*, 194t
   phosphates as, 194
   proteins as, 194, *194*, 194t

Buffer curve, 191–192, *192*
Buffer response, acute, to metabolic alkalosis, 228, *228*
Buffering, 190–192, *192*, 192t
  in respiratory acid-base disorders, 244, *244*
Bumetanide, renal effects of, 394, *395*, 395t
BUN. See *Blood urea nitrogen (BUN)*.
Buprenorphine, for congestive heart failure, 399
  for pancreatitis, 340
  for shock, 441, 441t
Buretrol system, 275, *276*
Burette, valveless, *299*
Burn shock, hypertonic solutions for, 501
Butorphanol, effects of, 316
  for blood donation, 456
  for congestive heart failure, 399
  for shock, 440–441, 441t
Butterfly catheter, 283t

C

Ca^{2+}. See *Calcium (Ca^{2+})*.
Cachexia, 467
$CaCl_2$. See *Calcium chloride ($CaCl_2$)*.
Calcidiol, 117, *118*
  serum concentration of, 121t, 125
Calciferol. See *Vitamin D*.
Calcitonin, 120
  for hypercalcemia, 141t, 143–144
Calcitriol, 40–41, 117
  actions of, 119–120
  and parathyroid hormone, 111–112, *113*, 120
  for hypocalcemia, 152t, 153
  in calcium homeostasis, 108, *109*, 110, 120–121
  in phosphate absorption, 164
  serum concentration of, 121t, 125
  synthesis of, *118*, 119
Calcium (Ca^{2+}), and parathyroid hormone, 111, 112–113, *113*, 114–116
  distribution of, *110*, 110–111
  extracellular, 110, *110*
  in dialysate, 520
  in renal failure, 415–416
  in threshold cell membrane potential, *84*, 85
  intracellular, 110–111
  normal physiology of, 108–111, *109*, *110*
  serum concentration of, 110, *110*
    fractionated, 123–124
    ionized, 121t, 122–124
    normal, 121–124, 121t
    total, 121–122, 121t
  uses of, 108
  with transfusion, 325
Calcium acetate, for hyperphosphatemia, 170, 171
Calcium balance, disorders of. See *Hypercalcemia; Hypocalcemia*.
Calcium carbonate, for hyperphosphatemia, 171
  for hypocalcemia, 152t, 153
  for uremic acidosis, 222
Calcium channel blocker, for hypercalcemia, 145
Calcium chloride ($CaCl_2$), 10%, 271t
  for hypermagnesemia, 184
  for hypocalcemia, 152t
  for transfusion reactions, 460t
Calcium citrate, for hyperphosphatemia, 171
Calcium gluconate, for ethylene glycol ingestion, 218
  for hyperkalemia, 103, 103t
  for hypermagnesemia, 184
  for hypoadrenocorticism, 383

Calcium gluconate (*Continued*)
  for hypocalcemia, 151, 152, 152t
  for transfusion reactions, 460t
Calcium homeostasis, 108–110, *109*
Calcium lactate, for hypocalcemia, 152t
Calcium metabolism, calcitriol in, 119
Calcium oxalate crystals, from ethylene glycol ingestion, 218, *219*
Calcium salts, for hypocalcemia, 151–153, 152t
Calcium oxalate urolithiasis, hypercalcemia with, 137, 140
Calciuretics, for hypercalcemia, 141t, 142
Calculi, urethral, case study of, 554–555, 555t
Caloric needs, maintenance, 20
Calories, daily requirements for, 266, 266t, 267
Cancer, hypercalcemia associated with, 129–134, *131–134*
Cannulation. See *Catheterization*.
CAPD (chronic ambulatory peritoneal dialysis), 509, 510, 511
Capillaries, continuous, 484
  discontinuous, 484
  fenestrated, 484
Capillary blood samples, 199
Capillary endothelium, of glomerulus, 27, *27*
Capillary hydrostatic pressure, 12, 13, *13*
Capillary oncotic pressure, 13, *13*
Capillary refill time, in monitoring fluid therapy, 317
Captopril, renal effects of, 394t
Carbenicillin, metabolic alkalosis due to, 235
Carbicarb, for lactic acidosis, 225–226
Carbohydrates, and water intake, 20, 20t
Carbon dioxide (CO_2), and chloride shift, 241, *241*
  buffering of, 244, *244*
  partial pressure of. See *Partial pressure of carbon dioxide (PCO_2)*.
  solubility coefficient of, 192
Carbon dioxide (CO_2) combining power, 196
Carbon dioxide (CO_2) content, total, 196
  in acid-base evaluation, 200, 204
Carbon dioxide (CO_2) tension. See *Partial pressure of carbon dioxide (PCO_2)*.
Carbon dioxide (CO_2) titration curves, whole blood vs. whole body, 197, *198*
Carbonic acid, 192–193
Carbonic anhydrase, 192
Carbonic anhydrase inhibitors, metabolic acidosis due to, 216–217
  renal effects of, 394, *395*, 395t
Carcinoma, adrenocortical, case study of, 562–563, 562t
  parathyroid gland, hypercalcemia due to, 134–136
  thyroid, case study of, 566, 566–567, 567t
Carcinomatosis, peritoneal effusion due to, 558–559, 559t
Cardiac arrest, lactic acidosis due to, 224
  mixed acid-base disorders in, 256
Cardiac output, and arterial blood pressure, 387, *388*, 389t
  and central venous pressure, 301
  anesthesia effect on, 316
  in anemia, 308
  in congestive heart failure, 406
  in hypocapnia, 248
  in monitoring fluid therapy, 317–318
  in shock, 428, 429
  monitoring of, 444
Cardiogenic shock, 431, 432, 433–434
  fluid therapy for, 439
Cardiomyopathy, dilated, case study of, 560–561, 561t

Cardiopulmonary resuscitation (CPR), lactic acidosis during, 224
  mixed acid-base disturbances with, 255
Cardiovascular disease, perioperative management of, 313–314
Cardiovascular drugs, and renal function, 393–397, 394t, *395*, 395t
Cardiovascular effects, of congestive heart failure, 389, 390t
  of dopamine, 420–421
  of hypercalcemia, 140
  of hyperkalemia, 97, *99*
  of hypertonic solutions, 503
  of hypokalemia, 94
  of liver disease, 357
  of magnesium deficiency, 179, 181
  of metabolic acidosis, 212–213
Cardiovascular support, for shock, 439–440
Catabolism, and hepatic encephalopathy, 358t, 359
Catecholamines, in sodium balance, 49, 50t
  renal effects of, 394t
Catheter(s), antibiotic-coated, 284
  composition of, 284, 284t
  cut-down, *282*
  damage to, 285
  for hemodialysis, 530–531, *531*
    complications of, 542–543, *543*
  for parenteral nutrition, 476–477
    complications of, 477–478
  for peritoneal dialysis, causes of failure of, 521t
    peritonitis due to, 522, 522–523, 523t
    placement of, 516–518, *517–519*, 518t
  heparinization of, 296
  maintenance of, 296
  over-the-needle, *282*, 282–284, 283t
    placement of, 287–288, *288–289*
  placement of, 285–296
    bandaging in, 295–296
    percutaneous access procedures for, 286–293
    skin preparation for, 285–286
    vascular access procedures for, 293–295
  removal of, 296
  site selection for, 284–285
  through-the-needle, *282*, 283t, 284
    placement of, 288–293, *290–292*
  types of, *282*, 282–284, 283t
  winged needle, *282*, *282*, 283t
    placement of, 286–287, *287*
Catheterization, 285–296
  central venous, 285
  percutaneous, 286–293
  peripheral vein, 285
  pulmonary, 404, *405*
  site selection for, 284–285
  skin preparation for, 285–286
  urinary tract infection with, 318
  vascular access procedures for, 293–295
Cation(s), concentrations of, 200–201, 201t
  defined, 3
  strong, 202
  unmeasured, 13, *13*
Cationic amino acids, metabolic acidosis due to, 217
Cell membrane, 24–25
Cell membrane potential, resting, 24, 83–84
  hypocalcemia and, 230, *230*
  potassium in, 24, 83–84
  threshold, *84*, 84–85
Central diabetes insipidus (CDI), hypernatremia due to, 54–55
  polyuria and polydipsia due to, 66t
Central nervous system (CNS), paradoxical acidosis of, 221

INDEX

Central vein infusion, of parenteral nutrition, 477
Central venous catheterization, 285
Central venous pressure (CVP), defined, 300–301
　factors affecting, 301
　in congestive heart failure, 404, 405, 406
　　right-sided, 314
　in monitoring fluid therapy, 278, 278–279, 300–305, 301–304, 304t, 317
　in renal failure, 412
　in shock, 443–444
　interpretation of, 303–305, 304t
　measurement of, 302–303, 302–304, 405, 406
　normal, 278
Centrasil catheter, 283t
Cephalic vein, for vascular access, 273, 285
Cephalothin, for peritonitis, 523
Cerebral edema, 309
　in hepatic encephalopathy, 359–360
　with hemodialysis, 543–544, 544
　with hypertonic fluid therapy, 499–500
Cestrum diurnum, vitamin D toxicity due to, 136
Chemical activity, 189
Chemical concentration, 189
Chemoreceptor(s), in alveolar ventilation, 242
Chemoreceptor trigger zone (CTZ), in vomiting, 335–336, 336
CHF. See *Congestive heart failure (CHF)*.
Children, oral rehydration solutions for, 339
Chlorhexidine gluconate (Hibiclens, Solvahex), for catheter placement, 286
Chloride (Cl^-), and acid-base balance, 74–76, 202–203, 204t, 233, 234
　for gastric fluid loss, 233
　in chronic hypercapnia, 244
　in congestive heart failure, 396, 398
　in intestine, 333, 334, 335, 335
　in metabolic alkalosis, 228, 235
　in pancreas, 332
　in renal failure, 413
　in stomach, 330
　in various body fluids, 73, 73t
　metabolism of, 73–74
Chloride concentration, corrected, 76–77, 77t
　intracellular, 73
　plasma, 73
　with fluid therapy, 272
Chloride disorders. See *Hyperchloremia; Hypochloremia*.
Chloride shift, 241, 241
Chlorothiazide, for diabetes insipidus, 56
Chlorpromazine, effects of, 316
Chlorpropamide, for central diabetes insipidus, 55
Chlorthalidone, renal effects of, 395t
Cholecalciferol, 40, 117
　excess, 136–137
Cholecalciferol toxicity, case study of, 564, 565–566, 566t
Cholecystokinin, and pancreatic juice, 332, 332
Chronic ambulatory peritoneal dialysis (CAPD), 509, 510, 511
Chronic renal failure (CRF). See *Renal failure, chronic*.
Cimetidine, for metabolic alkalosis, 235
Circulation, in heart failure, 388–392, 390t, 391, 392
　normal, 387–389, 388, 389t
Cirrhosis, ascites in, 349–350
　blood gas abnormalities in, 354–355, 355
　hyponatremia due to, 63

Cirrhosis (Continued)
　with hypoalbuminemia, 347, 348
Citrate, in blood products, 325
Citrate loading, hemorrhage due to, 365
Citrate metabolism, in liver disease, 356–357
Citrate phosphate dextrose adenine (CPDA-1), for donated blood, 456t
Cl^-. See *Chloride (Cl^-)*.
^{36}Cl dilution studies, 8
Classic underfilling hypothesis, of ascites, 360
Clearance, renal, 26–27
Clear-cath catheter, 283t
Clindamycin, for peritonitis, 523
Clodronate, for hypercalcemia, 141t, 144
Cloxacillin, for peritonitis, 523
CNS (central nervous system), paradoxical acidosis of, 221
CO_2. See *Carbon dioxide (CO_2)*.
Coagulopathies, in liver disease, 364–365
　perioperative management of, 314–315
　with colloid therapy, 490–491
　with dextrans, 321–323
　with gelatin solutions, 324
　with hetastarch, 269, 323
　with synthetic colloids, in liver disease, 364
Coccidioidomycosis, hypercalcemia due to, 137
Collapse, due to ethylene glycol ingestion, 575–577, 576t
　due to primary hypoparathyroidism, 568–570, 569, 569t
　due to urethral obstruction, 559–560, 560t
Collecting duct(s), functions of, 26
　in urinary concentrating mechanism, 37–38, 37t
　in water balance, 51–52
　potassium transport in, 87, 88
　sodium resorption in, 47, 48
Collecting tubules, chloride transport in, 74
Colloid(s), 269, 483–491
　complications and side effects of, 490–491
　contraindications to, 488
　dosage for, 489
　duration of action of, 488
　during anesthesia and surgery, 321–326, 322t
　evaluation and monitoring of, 490–491
　for ascites, 366
　for chronic hypoproteinemia, 490
　for peritonitis, 368
　hypertonic solution and, 500–501
　in liver disease, 363–364
　in pulmonary disease, 489–490
　pharmacokinetics and pharmacodynamics of, 487–489
　physicochemical basis for, 483–487, 486t
　physicochemical properties of, 321, 322t
　synthetic (artificial), 321, 322t, 488–489
　　in liver disease, 364
　volume expansion with, 488, 491
Colloid oncotic pressure (COP), 436, 437
　monitoring of, 443
Colloid osmotic pressure (COP), and duration of action, 488
　in hypoproteinemia, 490
　in pulmonary edema, 489, 490
　interstitial, 486
　normal, 486, 486t
　plasma, 485–486
Colon, absorption and secretion of water by, 332, 333, 334–335, 335
　chloride reabsorption in, 74
Column disc peritoneal dialysis catheter, 517, 517–519, 518t
Coma, hyperosmolar diabetic, 380–381

Compensatory responses, 195, 195t, 196, 196t, 197, 252t, 548t
　in mixed acid-base disorders, 253
　metabolic, 243–244, 244, 245, 252
　respiratory, 196t, 251–252
Compliance, 487
Compounding, of total nutrient admixture, 474–476, 475t, 476
Concentration, 189
Congestive heart failure (CHF), 387–406
　acid-base disturbances in, 398
　backward, 390, 391
　biventricular, 391, 392
　cardiovascular adaptations in, 389, 390t
　causes of, 389, 390t
　circulation in, 388–392, 390t, 391, 392
　defined, 387
　fluid accumulation in, 389–390, 391, 391, 392
　fluid therapy in, 268t, 401–406
　　indications for, 401
　　parenteral solutions for, 402–403
　forward, 390
　hemodynamic consequences of, 389–391, 390t, 391
　hyponatremia due to, 63
　left-sided, 391, 392
　monitoring of, 403–406, 404t, 405, 406
　neurohormonal adaptations in, 389, 390t
　perioperative management of, 314
　plasma volume in, 387, 389t
　renal function in, 389, 390t, 392–393, 399, 399t
　　cardiovascular drugs and, 393–397, 395, 395t
　right-sided, 391, 392
　　case study of, 552–553, 553t
　　central venous pressure in, 314
　serum biochemical abnormalities in, 396, 397, 397–399, 399t
　　management of, 403
　serum proteins in, 398
　sodium retention in, 391–393
　therapy of, 399–401
　ventricular function curves in, 390–391, 392
Connecting segment, functions of, 26
　sodium resorption in, 47
Constant-field equation, 24–25, 84
Constipation, and hepatic encephalopathy, 358t, 359
Convection, 507
Convective flow, 485
Convulsions. See *Seizures*.
Coonhound paralysis, case study of, 582–583, 582t, 583t
COP. See *Colloid oncotic pressure (COP); Colloid osmotic pressure (COP)*.
Cortical collecting duct, functions of, 26
　in urinary concentrating mechanism, 37, 37t
Cotransport, 34
Cough, due to pneumonia, 584–585, 584t
　due to tricuspid endocardiosis, 581
Countercurrent exchange, 39
Countercurrent multiplication, 36–37, 38
Countertransport, 34
CPAP, renal function with, 317
CPDA-1 (citrate phosphate dextrose adenine), for donated blood, 456t
CPR (cardiopulmonary resuscitation), lactic acidosis during, 224
　mixed acid-base disturbances with, 255
Creatine kinase, in malnutrition, 467
Creatine synthesis, in liver disease, 351–352, 352, 353

Creatinine, serum concentrations of, in congestive heart failure, 397, 399
  with peritoneal dialysis, 509, 510, 514–515, 524–525
Creatinine clearance, 30
  endogenous, 67
  in liver disease, 351–352, 352, 353
  in renal failure, 411–412
CRF (chronic renal failure). See *Renal failure, chronic.*
Crossmatching, 460–461, 460t, *461*, 461t
Cryoprecipitate, 452–453
  preoperative infusion of, 314
Crystalloids, 269–273
  additives to, 270
  choice of, 270–271
  defined, 269
  during anesthesia and surgery, 319–321, *321*
  electrolyte composition of, 269, 270, *270*, 271t, 272t
  for shock, 434t, 435–436, 438
  hypertonic. See *Hypertonic solutions.*
  maintenance, 269
  potassium supplementation of, 270, 271t
  replacement, 269
  sodium contents of, 402
  types of, 269–270
CTZ (chemoreceptor trigger zone), in vomiting, 335–336, *336*
Cushing's syndrome, metabolic alkalosis in, 235
Cutaneous and renal glomerular vasculopathy, 454
Cut-down catheter, 282
Cut-down procedure, elective, 294
  emergency, 293–294
CVP. See *Central venous pressure (CVP).*
Cytokines, in shock, 429, 433

D

DA-1 receptor(s), 419–420
DA-1 receptor agonists, 420–421
DA-2 receptor(s), 419–420
DCA (dichloroacetate), for lactic acidosis, 225
DEA (dog erythrocyte antigen), 454, 454t, 461
1-Deamino-8-D-arginine vasopressin (DDAVP, desmopressin), chemical structure of, *50*
  for central diabetes insipidus, 55
  for liver disease, 365
Dehydration, and hepatic encephalopathy, 358t
  defined, 265
  fluid therapy for, 268t
  hypotonic, 46, *47*
  in hypercalcemia, 126, 139, 142
  in various diseases, 268t
  in water deprivation test, 69
  laboratory findings in, 268, 269t
  perioperative management of, 312
  physical findings in, 267–268, 269t
  types of, 46, *47*, 265
Desmopressin. See *1-Deamino-8-D-arginine vasopressin (DDAVP, desmopressin).*
Desoxycorticosterone pivalate (Percorten-V), for hypoadrenocorticism, 382
Dexamethasone (Azium), for hypercalcemia, 141t
  for hypoadrenocorticism, 382
Dexamethasone sodium phosphate (Azium-SP), for hypoadrenocorticism, 382
  for shock, 441
  for transfusion reactions, 460t
Dextrans, 269
  allergic reactions to, 321, 491

Dextrans *(Continued)*
  compatibility of, with other IV products, 311t
  dosage for, 489
  during anesthesia and surgery, 321–323
  for ascites, 366
  for shock, 437
  hemostasis with, 321–323
  in liver disease, 364
  Normosol-R plus, 272t
  physicochemical properties of, 321, 322t, 437, 488
  renal failure with, 323, 491
Dextrose, 2.5%, in 0.45% NaCl, 271t
  in half-strength ionic solution, during anesthesia and surgery, 321
  in Ringer's lactated solution, 271t
  5%, 269–270, *270*, 271t
    compatibility of, with other IV products, 311t
    during anesthesia and surgery, 320–321
    in 0.45% NaCl, 271t
    in 0.9% NaCl, 271t
    in Ringer's lactated solution, *270*, 271t
    Normosol-M in, 271t
    Plasma-Lyte M in, 271t
  10%, 271t
    for hypoadrenocorticism, 383
  20%, for renal failure, 417
  50%, 271t
    for hyperkalemia, 103, 103t
  in dialysate, 510, 512, 512t
  in total nutrient admixture, 472–473
Dextrose solutions, 472–473
Dextrose-to-lipid ratio, 472–473
DHA (docosahexaenoic acid), for congestive heart failure, 400
DHT (dihydrotachysterol), for hypocalcemia, 152t, 153
Diabetes, hyperglycemic hyperosmolar nonketotic, 380–381
Diabetes insipidus (DI), central (pituitary), hypernatremia due to, 54–55
  polyuria and polydipsia due to, 66t
  nephrogenic, 55–56, 56t
    hypernatremia due to, 55–56, 56t
  perioperative management of, 315
  polyuria and polydipsia due to, 66t
Diabetes mellitus (DM), fluid therapy for, 268t
  hyperchloremia in, 80
  hyperkalemia in, 98–99
  hyponatremia with hyperosmolality in, 61
  hypophosphatemia in, 166
  mixed acid-base disorders with, 257
  perioperative management of, 311, 315
  polyuria and polydipsia in, 66t
  with pancreatitis, 340
Diabetic coma, hyperosmolar, 380–381
Diabetic ketoacidosis (DKA), 220–221, 375–380
  bicarbonate administration for, 221, 379–380
  case studies of, 572–573, 572t, 573t, 577–578, 577t
  fluid therapy for, 221, 376–377
  hyperchloremia with, 80
  hypophosphatemia with, 166
  insulin therapy for, 221, 377–378
  pathophysiology of, 220–221, 375–376
  perioperative management of, 311
  phosphorus supplementation for, 379
  potassium supplementation for, 378–379, 379t
  treatment of, 221, 376–380

Dialysate, commercial, 518–519
  defined, 507
  dextrose in, 510, 512, 512t
  drainage of, 521
  dwell time for, 507, 521, 521t
  for hemodialysis, 533
    in metabolic acidosis, 540
    in mineral imbalances, 541
    in renal failure, 538
  improvised, 519–520
  infusion of, 520–521
  selection and preparation of, 518–520, 520t
  warming of, 520
Dialysis, defined, 507
  hemo-. See *Hemodialysis.*
  peritoneal. See *Peritoneal dialysis.*
Dialysis disequilibrium syndrome, 543–544, *544*
Dianeal, 512t, 520
Diarrhea, due to *Trichuris vulpis*, 556–557, 556t
  fluid and electrolyte abnormalities in, 337–338
  fluid therapy for, 268t, 338–339
  metabolic acidosis due to, 213–214, 214t, *215*, 337
  mixed acid-base disturbances due to, 255–256, 258
  osmotic, 337
  pathomechanisms of, 336–337
  secretory, 336–337
Diazepam, for blood donation, 456
DIC (disseminated intravascular coagulation), perioperative management of, 315
Dichloroacetate (DCA), for lactic acidosis, 225
Diet. See also *Nutrition.*
  and water intake, *18*, 18–20, 18t, *19*
  assessment of, 470
  for ascites, 365
  for congestive heart failure, 400, 402
  for hepatic encephalopathy, 359, 360t
  for hyperphosphatemia, 170
  for hypervitaminosis D, 145
  hypocalcemia due to, 150
  hypophosphatemia due to, 165–166
  magnesium in, 175, 176
  phosphorus in, 164
Diffusion, barriers to, 511–512
  defined, 507
  facilitated, 34
  passive, 34
  rate of, 507
Diffusion impairment, (A–a) O_2 gradient with, 243
Diffusion trapping, 220
Digitalis glycosides, renal effects of, 394t, 396
Digoxin, for congestive heart failure, 400, 553
  renal effects of, 394t, 396
Dihydrotachysterol (DHT), for hypocalcemia, 152t, 153
1,25-Dihydroxyvitamin D_3. See *Calcitriol.*
24,25-Dihydroxyvitamin D_3, 117
Dilated cardiomyopathy, case study of, 560–561, 561t
Diltiazem, for congestive heart failure, 400
  for hypercalcemia, 145
Dilution studies, of fluid volumes, 5–9, 6t–9t
  of solutes, *9*, 9–10, 10t
Dilutional acidosis, 217
Dimethydisulfide, and hepatic encephalopathy, 357t
Diphenhydramine, for transfusion reactions, 460t
Disseminated intravascular coagulation (DIC), perioperative management of, 315

Dissociation constant (K_a), 190
Dissociation equilibrium equation, 190
Dissociative drugs, effects of, 316
Distal tubule, chloride transport in, 74
    functions of, 26
    potassium transport in, 87, 88
    sodium resorption in, 47, 48
Distributive shock, 432
Disuse osteoporosis, hypercalcemia due to, 138
Diuresis, 46
    postobstructive, polyuria and polydipsia due to, 66t
Diuretics, and potassium excretion, 90
    and renal function, 393–396, 394t, 395, 395t
    for ascites, 365
    for congestive heart failure, 400–401
    for hypercalcemia, 141t, 142
    for hyperkalemia, 103, 103t
    for hypocalcemia, 153
    for renal failure, 416, 417–421
    hyperkalemia due to, 102
    hypokalemia due to, 96, 397–398
    hyponatremia due to, 63
    impairment of ammonia detoxification by, 346
    metabolic alkalosis due to, 223–234
    mixed acid-base disorders due to, 257
DKA. See *Diabetic ketoacidosis (DKA)*.
DM. See *Diabetes mellitus (DM)*.
Dobutamine, for congestive heart failure, 399
    for shock, 439
    renal effects of, 394t
Docosahexaenoic acid (DHA), for congestive heart failure, 400
Dog erythrocyte antigen (DEA), 454, 454t, 461
Donnan effect, 485
Dopamine hydrochloride (Intropin), cardiovascular effects of, 420–421
    dilution of, 420
    drug interactions with, 420
    for congestive heart failure, 399
    for hypokalemia and renal failure, 415
    for pancreatitis, 341
    for renal failure, 417, 418–421
    for shock, 439–440
    rate of infusion of, 420
    renal effects of, 394t, 419
    renal-dose, 419, 420
    with furosemide, 421
Dopamine receptor(s), 418–419
Dopamine receptor agonists, 419–420
Dorsal pedal artery, blood samples from, 318
Drinking, water intake from, 18–19, 19, 19t. See also *Hypodipsia; Polydipsia*.
Drip chamber, in-line, 299
Drip rate, 274, 299
Drip sensor, 299, 300
Drug(s), and hepatic encephalopathy, 358t, 359
    hypercalcemia due to, 137
    hyperchloremia due to, 80
    hyperkalemia due to, 102
    hyponatremia due to, 64
    polyuria and polydipsia due to, 66t
    with total nutrient admixture, 474, 474t
Drug metabolism, nutrition and, 465–466
Dwell time, for dialysate, 507, 521, 521t
Dyspnea, due to dilated cardiomyopathy, 560–561, 561t
    due to pleural effusion, 557, 557t
    due to pulmonary fibrosis, 585, 585t

E

Ear veins, for catheter placement, 285
Eastern Veterinary Blood Bank, 452t
Ecadotril, renal effects of, 394t
ECF. See *Extracellular fluid (ECF)*.
ECG. See *Electrocardiogram (ECG)*.
Eclampsia, hypocalcemia due to, 148, 150–151
    magnesium for, 183
Edema, cerebral, 309
    in hepatic encephalopathy, 359–360
    with hemodialysis, 543–544, 544
    with hypertonic fluid therapy, 499–500
    fluid therapy with, 362
    peripheral, measurement of, 318
        perioperative management of, 312
    pulmonary, colloid therapy in, 489–490
        in congestive heart failure, 389–390, 391, 391, 392
        management of, 400–401
        mixed acid-base disturbances with, 255, 256
        perioperative management of, 312
    subcutaneous, hyponatremia due to, 63, 67
        in congestive heart failure, 389–390, 391, 552–553, 553t
EDP (end-diastolic pressure), and central venous pressure, 301, 301, 302
EDTA, for hypercalcemia, 141t, 144
EDV (end-diastolic volume), and central venous pressure, 301, 301–302, 302
Effective circulating blood volume, 12, 47–48
EG ingestion. See *Ethylene glycol (EG) ingestion*.
EHDP-Didronel, for hypercalcemia, 141t
Eicosapentaenoic acid (EPA), for congestive heart failure, 400
Elastomeric hydrogel catheters, 284, 284t
Electrocardiogram (ECG), in monitoring fluid therapy, 318
    in renal failure, 414
    of dopamine infusion, 420
    with hyperkalemia, 97, 99
    with hypokalemia, 94
    with magnesium deficiency, 181
Electrochemical equivalence, 3–4
Electrolyte(s). See also specific electrolytes, e.g., *Sodium (Na^+)*.
    absorption and secretion of, 330–335, 330–335
    daily requirements for, 267
    in commercially available fluids, 271t
    in crystalloid solutions, 269, 270, 270, 271t, 272t
    in intestinal fluid, 213, 214t, 215
    in total nutrient admixture, 473–474
    plasma concentrations of, 9, 9–10, 10t
Electrolyte abnormalities. See also specific abnormalities, e.g., *Hyperkalemia*.
    hemodialysis for, 540
    in congestive heart failure, 396, 397, 397–399, 399t
        management of, 403
    in renal failure, 413–416
    with hypertonic solutions, 503
Electrolyte balance, in various diseases, 268t
Electrolyte solutions, 473
Electroneutrality, 3, 9, 12, 13, 13
Embolism, air, 298
    due to transfusion, 459
    catheter, 298
    due to transfusion, 459
Enalapril, for congestive heart failure, 399, 400
    renal effects of, 393, 394t, 395, 396
Encephalopathy, hepatic. See *Hepatic encephalopathy (HE)*.
End-diastolic pressure (EDP), and central venous pressure, 301, 301, 302
End-diastolic volume (EDV), and central venous pressure, 301, 301–302, 302
Endocrine disorders, fluid therapy in, 375–384
    perioperative management of, 315–316
Endocrine functions, of kidney, 39–41
Endogenous creatinine clearance, 67
Endopeptidase inhibitors, neutral, renal effects of, 394t
Endotoxic shock, due to transfusion, 459
    fluid therapy for, 268t, 338
    hypertonic solutions for, 500–501
Energy expenditure, maintenance, 20
Energy requirements, 468–469
    basal, 20
    maintenance, 20, 269, 275–276
    resting, 469–470
Energy solutions, 472–473
Enteral feeding, 471
    with parenteral nutrition, 478
Enteropathy, protein-losing, case study of, 570, 570t
    fluid therapy for, 339
    hypoalbuminemia in, 347–348
EPA (eicosapentaenoic acid), for congestive heart failure, 400
Epinephrine, for shock, 440
    in potassium balance, 85
Epithelia, leaky, 33
    tight, 33
EPO (erythropoietin), production of, 40
Epsom salt (magnesium sulfate), for magnesium depletion, 182–183
Equivalent weight, 4
Ergocalciferol, 117
    excess, 136–137
    for hypocalcemia, 152t, 153
Erythrocyte(s), in malnutrition, 467
    magnesium concentrations of, 177
    sodium and potassium concentrations of, 90–91, 91t
    spleen as reservoir for, 5–6
Erythrocyte volume, 5–6, 6t
Erythropoietin (EPO), production of, 40
Ethacrynic acid, renal effects of, 394, 395, 395t
Ethanol, for ethylene glycol ingestion, 218–219
Ethyl alcohol, for catheter placement, 286
Ethylene glycol (EG) ingestion, case studies of, 574–577, 574t–576t
    hemodialysis for, 529, 529, 541–542, 541t
    hypocalcemia due to, 150
    metabolic acidosis due to, 217–220, 218, 219
    peritoneal dialysis for, 510–511
Etidronate, for hypercalcemia, 144
Etomidate, effects of, 317
Euglycemia, in liver disease, 362
Evaporative losses, 16–18, 17t, 18t
Exercise, fluid therapy for, 268t
    hyperkalemia due to, 99–100
    mixed acid-base disturbances with, 255
Exogenous antidiuretic hormone testing, 70, 70t
Exsanguination, 298
Extracellular fluid (ECF), bicarbonate as buffer in, 193–194
    calcium concentration in, 110, 110
    defined, 5
    osmolality of, 11
    potassium concentration in, 83, 85
    sodium concentration in, 83

Extracellular fluid (ECF) (Continued)
   solute concentrations in, 9, 9, 10t
   water and solute losses from, 12, 12t
Extracellular fluid (ECF) compartment,
   subcompartments of, 8–9, 9
   water exchange between intracellular fluid
      compartment and, 10–12, 11, 12t
Extracellular fluid volume (ECFV), 5–9,
   6t–8t, 9
   and renal bicarbonate reabsorption, 206
   renin-angiotensin system and, 40
Extracellular fluid (ECF) volume deficit, with
   hypochloremic alkalosis, 75
   with hypotonic fluid loss, 56, 56, 57
   with pure water loss, 53, 55
Extracellular fluid volume (ECFV) depletion,
   in metabolic alkalosis, 228
Extracellular fluid (ECF) volume gain, in
   hyponatremia with volume depletion, 62,
   62
   with gain of impermeant solute, 57, 58
Extracorporeal circuit, 532, 532–533
Extravasation, 296
E-Z Set infusion set, 282, 283t

F

Facilitated diffusion, 34
Factitious hyponatremia, 60–61, 61
Famotidine, for metabolic alkalosis, 235
Fanconi's syndrome, 215–216
   hypophosphatemia due to, 166
Fat(s), and water intake, 20, 20t
Fat stores, 467
Fatty acids, and hepatic encephalopathy, 357t
   in colon, 334–335
Feces, water loss in, 15, 16
Feeding method, assessment of, 470
FE_K (fractional excretion of potassium), 91
Feline immunodeficiency virus (FIV), in
   blood donors, 455
Feline infectious peritonitis (FIP), in blood
   donors, 455
Feline leukemia virus (FeLV), in blood
   donors, 455
Feline lower urinary tract disease (FLUTD),
   19
Felodipine, for renal failure, 421
Femoral arterial catheter, 318
Femoral artery samples, 198
Femoral vein catheter, 285
Fenoldopam, 419, 420
FEP Teflon (fluoroethylenepropylene)
   catheters, 284, 284t
FE_{Pi} (fractional excretion of phosphate), 171
Ferrocyanide dilution studies, 7–8
Fetus, parathyroid hormone–related protein
   in, 117
Fick principle, 32
Filtration coefficient, 484
Filtration fraction, 32
FIP (feline infectious peritonitis), in blood
   donors, 455
FIV (feline immunodeficiency virus), in blood
   donors, 455
Fixed acid, 189, 194–195
Flash-Cath catheter, 283t
Flow connectors, multiple-port, 298–299
Flow regulators, in-line, 299, 299, 301
Fluid(s). See also Water entries.
   changes in composition of, 308, 308–312,
      311t
      monitoring of, 318
   changes in distribution of, 312–313
      monitoring of, 318–319
   changes in volume of, 307–308
      monitoring of, 317–318

Fluid(s) (Continued)
   colloid. See Colloid(s).
   crystalloid. See Crystalloids.
   temperature of, 316
   types of, 268–273, 270, 271t, 272t
   unbalanced, 269
Fluid administration, rate of, 274–275, 275,
   276, 299
   routes of, 273–274, 281
   sets and connection devices for, 298–300,
      299–301
Fluid balance, 265–266, 266t, 267
   in gastrointestinal tract, 330, 331
Fluid deficit, 275
Fluid depletion. See Hypovolemia.
Fluid dwell time, for dialysate, 507, 521, 521t
Fluid dynamics, transvascular, 484–485
Fluid flux equation, 484–485
Fluid infusion pumps, 275, 276, 299, 300
   for blood transfusion, 457
Fluid losses, contemporary (ongoing), 277,
   277t
   history of, 266, 268t
   hypertonic, 12, 12t
   hypotonic, 12, 12t
      classification of, 57
      hypernatremia due to, 53t, 54, 56, 56–57,
         57, 59
   isotonic, 12, 12t
   physical examination for, 267–268, 269t
   sensible and insensible, 276, 277t
   sources of, 266
Fluid needs, basal, 14–15, 20–21
   maintenance, 14–15, 20–21
Fluid overload. See Hypervolemia.
Fluid push, in renal failure, 416–417
Fluid rate controller, electronic, 299, 299, 301
Fluid requirement, maintenance, 14–15,
   20–21, 275, 276–277, 277t
Fluid therapy, amount of fluid in, 275–278,
   277, 277t
   combination, for shock, 438–439, 439t
   complications of, 279
   components of, 275–277, 277, 277t
   discontinuation of, 279
   during anesthesia, 307
   failure to achieve rehydration with, 277–
      278
   fluid balance and, 265–266, 266t, 267
   for adrenocortical insufficiency, 382–383
   for anorexia, 268t
   for congestive heart failure, 268t, 401–406,
      404t, 405
   for dehydration, 268t
   for diabetes mellitus, 268t
   for diabetic ketoacidosis, 376–377
   for diarrhea, 268t, 338–339
   for endocrine and metabolic disorders,
      375–384
   for exercise, 268t
   for gastric dilatation, 339
   for heatstroke, 268t, 384
   for hyperadrenocorticism, 268t
   for hypercalcemia, 142
   for hyperosmolar diabetic coma, 380–381
   for hypervitaminosis D, 145
   for hypoadrenocorticism, 268t, 382–383
   for hypoglycemia, 383
   for liver disease, 361–366, 366
   for pancreatitis, 339–341
   for protein-losing enteropathy, 339
   for renal failure, 268t, 410–425
   for shock, endotoxic, 268t
      hemorrhagic, 268t
   for small-bowel obstruction, 341–342

Fluid therapy (Continued)
   for starvation, 268t
   for stress, 268t
   for urethral obstruction, 268t
   for volvulus, 339
   for vomiting, 268t, 338–339
   history taking for, 266, 268t
   hyperchloremia due to, 80
   hypertonic, 496–504
   indications for, 265–268
   intraoperative management of, 274, 319–
      326, 321, 322t
   laboratory findings for, 268, 269t
   monitoring of, 278, 278–279, 299–305,
      300–304, 304t
      perioperative, 317–319
   physical examination for, 267–268, 269t
   polyuria due to, 66t
   postoperative management of, 326
   preoperative management of, 307–319
   rate of administration for, 274–275, 275,
      276, 299
   routes for, 273–274, 281
   types of fluids for, 268–273, 270, 271t, 272t
   with ascites, 362
   with edema, 362
   with macromolecular plasma volume expanders, 483–491
Fluid volume, in congestive heart failure, 402
   in hemodialysis, 534, 534, 535
Fluoroethylenepropylene (FEP Teflon)
   catheters, 284, 284t
FLUTD (feline lower urinary tract disease),
   19
Food. See also Diet.
   water in, 18, 18, 18t, 19
Food deprivation, 468
Food intake, assessment of, 470
Formate-chloride exchange mechanism, 74
Fractional excretion of phosphate (FE_{Pi}), 171
Fractional excretion of potassium (FE_K), 91
Frank-Starling curve, 278, 278, 302, 302
Free-water excretion, impaired, in liver
   disease, 350–351
Furosemide (Lasix), adverse effects of, 418
   for ascites, 365
   for congestive heart failure, 399, 400–401,
      403, 553
   for ethylene glycol ingestion, 218
   for hypercalcemia, 141t, 142t
   for hypervitaminosis D, 145
   for renal failure, 417, 418
   for transfusion reactions, 460t
   hypokalemia due to, 96
   renal effects of, 394, 394t, 395, 395t, 396
   with dopamine, 421

G

Gamma-aminobutyric acid (GABA), and
   hepatic encephalopathy, 357t
Gastric acid hypersecretion, 338
Gastric acid secretion, 330, 331
Gastric dilatation, 339
Gastric dilatation-volvulus (GDV), 339
   mixed acid-base disturbances with, 254,
      255, 256, 257, 258
   shock due to, hypertonic solutions for, 501
Gastric fluid loss, metabolic alkalosis due to,
   231–233, 232–234
Gastric lavage, for salicylate intoxication, 220
Gastrinoma, diarrhea due to, 337
Gastroenteritis, metabolic acidosis due to,
   213–214, 214t, 215
Gastrointestinal effects, of hemodialysis, 545
   of hypercalcemia, 140

Gastrointestinal hemorrhage, and hepatic encephalopathy, 358t
Gastrointestinal losses, hyponatremia due to, 62, 63
Gastrointestinal tract (GIT), inflammation of, 335
　management of disorders of, 338–342
　normal physiology of, 330–335, 330–335
　pathophysiology of, 335–338, 336
　water balance in, 330, 331
GDV. See *Gastric dilatation-volvulus (GDV)*.
Gelatin solutions, allergic reactions to, 324, 491
　during anesthesia and surgery, 324
　for shock, 437
　physicochemical properties of, 322t, 324
Gelifundol (oxypolygelatin), for shock, 437
　physicochemical properties of, 322t, 324, 437
Gelofusine (succinylated gelatin), physicochemical properties of, 322t, 324
Gentamicin, for peritonitis, 523
GFR. See *Glomerular filtration rate (GFR)*.
GI. See *Gastrointestinal* entries.
GIT. See *Gastrointestinal tract (GIT)*.
Glaucoma, perioperative management of, 313
Globulins, and colloid osmotic pressure, 485
　buffering by, 194
　metabolism of, 345, 345
Glomerular basement membrane, 27, 27
Glomerular filtration, 27–29, 27–30, 29t
Glomerular filtration rate (GFR), and potassium excretion, 102
　autoregulation of renal blood flow and, 31, 31–32
　defined, 28
　determinants of, 28–30, 29, 29t
　dopamine and, 419–421
　in hypercalcemia, 139
　in liver disease, 352
　in renal failure, 411
　in sodium balance, 49
　measurement of, 30
　single-nephron, 28
Glomerulotubular balance, 49
Glomerulus, charge selectivity of, 28, 28
　functions of, 26
　morphology of, 27, 27–28, 28
　size selectivity of, 28
Glucocorticoids, for hypercalcemia, 141t, 143, 143t
　for hypoadrenocorticism, 382
　for shock, 441–442
　for transfusion reactions, 460t
Gluconeogenesis, 223, 468
Glucose, blood concentration of, 468
　for hyperkalemia, 103
　for hypoadrenocorticism, 382–383
　renal transport of, 35–36, 36
Glucose phosphate, for hypophosphatemia, 167
Glucose polymers, in oral rehydration solutions, 339
Glucose production, in diabetic ketoacidosis, 376
Glucose utilization, in diabetic ketoacidosis, 376
Glucosuria, renal, polyuria and polydipsia due to, 66t
Glutamine, and hepatic encephalopathy, 357t
Glutamine cycle, 345–346, 346
Glycocalyx, 483
Glycogenolysis, 468
Glycoaldehyde, from ethylene glycol ingestion, 218

Glycolic acid, from ethylene glycol ingestion, 218
Glycosaminoglycans, 484
Glyoxylic acid, from ethylene glycol ingestion, 218
Goldman-Hodgkin-Katz constant-field equation, 24–25, 84
Grafts, for hemodialysis, 531–532
Granulomatous disease, hypercalcemia due to, 137
Greyhounds, as blood donors, 454
　lactic acidosis in, 224

H

H^+. See *Hydrogen ion(s) (H^+)*.
Haemaccel (urea-linked gelatin), physicochemical properties of, 322t, 324
Hair loss, due to magnesium deficiency, 181
Hartmann's solution. See *Lactated Ringer's solution (LRS)*.
HBOCs (hemoglobin-based oxygen carriers), 461–462
　for shock, 437–438, 442–443
HCO_3^-. See *Bicarbonate (HCO_3^-)*.
HE. See *Hepatic encephalopathy (HE)*.
Head trauma, shock with, 446
Heart failure. See *Congestive heart failure (CHF)*.
Heart rate, in monitoring fluid therapy, 317
Heatstroke, 383–384
　fluid therapy for, 268t, 384
　mixed acid-base disturbances with, 255
　pathophysiology of, 383–384
Hematocrit, critical value for, 308, 308, 309
　in dehydration, 268, 269t
Hematologic complications, of hemodialysis, 545
Hematologic malignancies, hypercalcemia due to, 132–133
Hemodialysis, 528–545
　anemia due to, 545
　artificial kidneys (hemodialyzers) for, 532
　complications of, 542–545, 543, 544
　delivery systems for, 533
　dialysate for, 533
　　in renal failure, 538
　dialysis disequilibrium syndrome due to, 543–544, 544
　extracorporeal circuit for, 532, 532–533
　for acid-base disorders, 540
　for acute intoxication (poisoning), 529, 529, 541–542, 541t
　for azotemia, 537–539
　for electrolyte imbalances, 540
　for fluid overloads, 529, 539–540
　for hypercalcemia, 144–145
　for hyperkalemia, 103
　for mineral imbalances, 541
　for renal failure, 534–539, 534t, 536
　　acute, 528–529, 537–538, 538
　　chronic, 529, 538–539
　for renal transplantation, 529, 539
　gastrointestinal disorders due to, 545
　hematologic disorders due to, 545
　historical perspective on, 528
　hypotension due to, 535, 534, 543
　hypoxemia due to, 544–545
　machine for, 533
　monitoring equipment for, 533–534, 534, 535
　peritoneal dialysis vs., 508, 508t, 528
　physical principles of, 529–530
　purified water system for, 533
　regional referral centers for, 547
　ultrafiltration control systems for, 533
　ultrafiltration without, 540

Hemodialysis *(Continued)*
　vascular access for, 530–532, 531
　complications involving, 542–543, 543
Hemodialyzers, 532
Hemodynamic consequences, of congestive heart failure, 389–391, 390t, 391
Hemoglobin, buffering by, 194
　in malnutrition, 467
Hemoglobin solutions, during anesthesia and surgery, 326
　for shock, 437–438
Hemoglobin-based oxygen carriers (HBOCs), 461–462
　for shock, 437–438, 442–443
Hemolymphatic malignancies, hyperphosphatemia due to, 167–168
Hemolysis, and hepatic encephalopathy, 358t
　due to hypophosphatemia, 165
Hemopet, 452t
Hemorrhage, due to citrate loading, 365
　resuscitation-induced, 445
Hemorrhagic shock, 431, 432
　autotransfusion for, 436
　blood products for, 442
　fluid therapy for, 268t
　hypernatremia due to, 59
　hypertonic solutions for, 499
Hemostasis, with dextrans, 321–323
　with gelatin solutions, 324
　with hetastarch, 269, 323
　with hypertonic solutions, 503–504
　with synthetic colloids, in liver disease, 364
Henderson equation, 193, 200
Henderson-Hasselbalch equation, 174, 190, 193, 202
Henle's loop. See *Loop of Henle*.
Heparin, for donated blood, 456t
　for pancreatitis, 341
　hyperkalemia due to, 102
　in hemodialysis, 531, 533–534
　in peritoneal dialysis, 520
Heparinization, of catheters, 296
Hepatic baroreceptors, 350
Hepatic disease. See *Liver disease*.
Hepatic encephalopathy (HE), 357–360
　causes of, 357–359, 357t, 358, 358t
　euglycemia in, 362
　nutritional support for, 362
　treatment of, 359–360, 360t
Hepatic lipidosis (HL), 351, 351, 362
Hepatobiliary system, normal physiology of, 342–346, 342t, 343–346
　pathophysiology of, 347–361
Hepatocyte, 342
Hepatorenal syndrome, 349, 349, 349t
Hetastarch. See *Hydroxyethyl starch (HES, hetastarch)*.
HHM (humoral hypercalcemia of malignancy), 116, 127, 129–132, 131–134, 145
HHND (hyperglycemic hyperosmolar nonketotic diabetes), 380–381
Hibiclens (chlorhexidine gluconate), for catheter placement, 286
Hickey-Hare test, 69
Histidine, imidazole group of, 194, 194
　metabolic acidosis due to, 217
Histoplasmosis, hypercalcemia due to, 137
H^+-K^+-ATPase (hydrogen-potassium adenosine triphosphatase), in stomach, 330
HL (hepatic lipidosis), 351, 351, 362
HLS (hypoadrenocorticism-like syndrome), case study of, 556–557, 556t
　mixed acid-base disturbances with, 253, 255, 256

Homeostasis, 12, *14*, 14–15, 15t
Humoral hypercalcemia of malignancy (HHM), 116, *127*, 129–132, *131–134*, 145
Hydralazine, for congestive heart failure, 399, 401
 renal effects of, 394t
Hydration deficit, 275, 277t
Hydrochlorothiazide, for congestive heart failure, 401
 for diabetes insipidus, 56
 renal effects of, 393, 395t
Hydrocortisone sodium succinate (Solu-Cortef), for hypoadrenocorticism, 382
Hydrogen ion(s) (H^+), 189
 and pH, 189–190, *190*, 191t
 in buffering, 190
 in respiratory acidosis, 245
 in stomach, 330
 P_{CO_2} and, 243
 renal tubular excretion of, 205
Hydrogen ion (H^+) balance, and potassium excretion, 90
 external, 204
Hydrogen-potassium adenosine triphosphatase (H^+-K^+-ATPase), in stomach, 330
Hydrostatic pressure, 12–13, *13*
 in renal circulation, 31
 interstitial, 486–487
 intravascular, 486
25-Hydroxycholecalciferol, 40
Hydroxyethyl starch (HES, hetastarch), 269
 allergic reactions to, 323, 364, 491
 and NaCl, 439, 439t
 coagulopathies with, 269, 323
 compatibility of, with other IV products, 311t
 dosage for, 489
 during anesthesia and surgery, 323
 for hypoproteinemia, 490
 for liver disease, 364
 for shock, 437
 monitoring of, 491
 physicochemical properties of, 269, 322t, 437, 488–489
 volume expansion with, 488
25-Hydroxyvitamin D_3, 117, *118*
 serum concentration of, 121t, 125
25-Hydroxyvitamin D_3 toxicity, 136–137
Hyperadrenocorticism, fluid therapy for, 268t
 hypophosphatemia due to, 166
 metabolic alkalosis due to, 235
 mixed acid-base disorders due to, 257
 perioperative management of, 315
 polyuria and polydipsia due to, 66t
Hyperaldosteronism, case study of, 562–563, 562t
 hypernatremia due to, 58
 hypokalemia due to, 96
 hyporeninemic, renal tubular acidosis in, 216
 primary, metabolic alkalosis in, 234–235
Hyperammonemia, and hepatic encephalopathy, 357t, 358–359
 due to diuretics, 346
Hypercalcemia, 125–145
 cancer-associated, 129–134, *131–134*
 cell membrane potential with, *84*, 85
 clinical signs of, 138–140, 138t
 complications of, 151–152
 defined, 125
 differential diagnosis of, 126, 126t
 due to aluminum, 129
 due to anal sac adenocarcinoma, 131–132, *133*, *134*

Hypercalcemia (Continued)
 due to bone metastases, 133–134
 due to cholecalciferol toxicity, *564*, 565–566, 566t
 due to chronic renal failure, 128–129, *130*
 due to dehydration, 126
 due to granulomatous disease, 137
 due to hematologic malignancies, 132–133
 due to hyperparathyroidism, 134–136, *566*, 566–567, 567t
 due to hypervitaminosis D, 136–137
 due to hypoadrenocorticism, 126–128, 141, 381
 due to lymphoma, 130–131, *132*, *133*
 due to multiple myeloma, 133
 due to renal failure, 415–416
 effects of, on other organs, 140
 follow-up of, 151–152
 hemodialysis for, 541
 humoral, of malignancy, 116, *127*, 129–132, *131–134*
 idiopathic, 137–138
 mechanisms of, 125–126, *127*
 nonpathologic, 126–129, 126t
 normal homeostatic response to, 121
 of malignancy, due to apocrine gland adenocarcinoma, 567–568, 567t, *568*
  due to lymphosarcoma, 563–565, 563t
  humoral, 116, *127*, 129–132, *131–134*
  parathyroid hormone in, 129
  parathyroid hormone–related protein in, 129, 130, 131, *131*, 132, *133*
 pathologic (consequential), 126t, 129–138
 perioperative management of, 310
 polyuria and polydipsia due to, 66t
 renal effects of, 139–140
 steroid-sensitive causes of, 143, 143t
 toxicity of, 138–140, 138t
 transient (inconsequential), 126, 126t
 treatment of, 140–145, 140t, 141t, 143t
 uncommon causes of, 138
Hypercalcemic nephropathy, case study of, 563–565, 563t
Hypercalciuria, 154
Hypercapnia, adaptive response to, acute, 244, *244*
 chronic, 244–245, *245*
 and alveolar ventilation, 242
 in metabolic alkalosis, 229
 in respiratory acidosis, 245–247
 metabolic alkalosis after, 234
 primary, 245–247, 252
Hyperchloremia, artifactual, 77, *77*
 corrected, *77*, 79, 79–80, 79t
 pseudo-, 79
Hyperemia, due to magnesium deficiency, 181
Hyperglobulinemia, 345
Hyperglycemia, in diabetic ketoacidosis, 376
 perioperative management of, 311
 with parenteral nutrition, 472–473
Hyperglycemic hyperosmolar nonketotic diabetes (HHND), 380–381
Hyperkalemia, 97–103
 and renal bicarbonate reabsorption, 206
 causes of, 97–102, 100t, *102*
 cell membrane potential with, *84*, 84
 clinical and laboratory features of, 97, *99*, *101*
 due to congestive heart failure, 397, 403
 due to hypoadrenocorticism, 100, 381, 382–383
 due to renal failure, 413
 due to transfusion, 459, 460
 hemodialysis for, 540

Hyperkalemia (Continued)
 metabolic acidosis with, 86, 208
 perioperative management of, 310
 pseudo-, 91, 100t
 treatment of, 102–103, 103t
Hypermagnesemia, 184
 and parathyroid hormone secretion, 112
 in renal failure, 416
Hypernatremia, 52–59
 case study of, 549–552, 550t, 551t, *552*
 causes of, 53, 53t
 clinical approach to, 52–58, *54*
 clinical signs of, 58
 due to gain of impermeant solute, 53t, *54*, 57–58, *58*, 59
 due to hypotonic fluid loss, 53t, *54*, 56, 56–57, *57*, 59
 due to pure water loss, 53–56, 53t, *54*, 55, 56t, 58–59
 due to renal failure, 413
 hemodialysis for, 540
 hypodipsic, 53–54
 perioperative management of, 309
 serum sodium concentration in, 46
 treatment of, 58–59
 with hypertonic solutions, 503
Hyperosmolality, hyponatremia with, 60t, 61
 perioperative management of, 310
 with hypertonic solutions, 503
Hyperosmolar diabetic coma, 380–381
Hyperosmotic solution, 45
Hyperparathyroidism, hypophosphatemia due to, 166
 primary, calcium transport in, *127*
  case study of, *566*, 566–567, 567t
  hypercalcemia due to, 134–136
 renal secondary, hyperphosphatemia due to, 169
 tertiary, 129
Hyperphosphatemia, 167–171
 and hypocalcemia, 167
 and parathyroid hormone secretion, 112
 causes of, 167–170, 169t
 clinical effects of, 167
 hemodialysis for, 541
 in renal failure, 415
 treatment of, 170–171
Hyperproteinemia, perioperative management of, 309
Hypersthenuria, 46
Hypertension, due to hypercalcemia, 140
Hyperthyroidism, case study of, 570–572, 571t, *572*
 perioperative management of, 316
 polyuria and polydipsia due to, 66t
Hypertonic dehydration, 46, *47*
Hypertonic fluid, loss of, 12, 12t
Hypertonic solutions, 496–504
 and colloids, 500–501
 cardiovascular effects of, 503
 contraindications to, 503–504
 defined, 46
 dosage of, 502, 502t
 during anesthesia and surgery, 321
 electrolyte and osmolality disturbances with, 503
 for shock, 438, 499–501
 hemostasis with, 503–504
 immunomodulatory effects of, 499
 inotropic effects of, 498
 lung vagal reflex with, 497–498
 mechanisms of action of, 497–499
 oxygen delivery with, 498–499
 plasma volume expansion with, 496, 497
 precautions with, 503–504

Hypertonic solutions *(Continued)*
  rate of infusion for, 503
  route of administration of, 501–502
  types of, 502–503
Hypertonicity, due to pure water loss, 53, 55
Hypertriglyceridemia, with parenteral nutrition, 473
Hypertrophic osteodystrophy, hypercalcemia due to, 138
Hyperventilation, in metabolic acidosis, 212
Hypervitaminosis D, calcium transport in, *127*
  hypercalcemia due to, 136–137
  treatment of, 141, 145
Hypervolemia, hemodialysis for, 529, 539–540
  hyponatremia with, 60t, 63–64
  perioperative management of, 308
  with colloids, 491
Hypoadrenocorticism, 381–383
  azotemia in, 381
  case study of, 553–554, 554t
  clinical signs of, 381–382
  diagnosis of, 382
  diarrhea due to, 337
  fluid therapy for, 268t, 382–383
  glucocorticoid replacement for, 382
  hypercalcemia in, 126–128, 141, 381
  hyperchloremia in, 80
  hyperkalemia in, 100, 381, 382–383
  hypoglycemia in, 381
  hyponatremia in, 62–63, 381
  laboratory abnormalities in, 381–382
  metabolic acidosis due to, 217, 383
  mineralocorticoid replacement for, 382
  pathophysiology of, 381
  perioperative management of, 315
  polyuria and polydipsia due to, 66t
  treatment of, 382–383
Hypoadrenocorticism-like syndrome (HLS), case study of, 556–557, 556t
  mixed acid-base disturbances with, 253, 255, 256
Hypoalbuminemia, clinical importance of, 347–348, *348*
  defined, 347
  in liver disease, 347, *348*
    treatment of, 363–364
  in pancreatitis, 348
  in protein-losing enteropathy, 347–348
  with hypocalcemia, 147, 347
Hypoaldosteronism, hyperchloremia in, 80
  hyporeninemic, hyperkalemia due to, 102
Hypocalcemia, 145–154
  and parathyroid hormone secretion, 111
  cell membrane potential with, *84*, 85
    resting, 230, *230*
  clinical signs of, 145–147, 146t
  complications of, 151–152
  conditions associated with, 147–150, 147t
  defined, 145
  due to diet, 150
  due to ethylene glycol poisoning, 150
  due to hypoparathyroidism, 148–151
  due to hypoproteinemia, 570, 570t
  due to pancreatitis, 150, 340
  due to phosphate enemas, 150
  due to puerperal tetany (eclampsia), 148, 150–151
  due to renal failure, 415
  due to respiratory alkalosis, 150
  due to thyroidectomy, 570–572, 571t, *572*
  due to transfusion, 459
  due to tumor lysis syndrome, 150
  due to vitamin D deficiency, 150
  follow-up of, 151–152
  hemodialysis for, 541

Hypocalcemia *(Continued)*
  hyperphosphatemia with, 167
  hypoalbuminemia with, 147, 347
  hypomagnesemia with, 180, 181
  normal homeostatic response to, 120–121
  parathyroiditis with, 148
  perioperative management of, 310
  postoperative, 147, 148–149, 151
  renal failure with, 147–148
  seizures due to, 146, 151
  tetany due to, 146, 151
  treatment of, 150–153, 152t
Hypocapnia, adaptive response to, acute, 244, *244*
  chronic, 245
  and alveolar ventilation, 242
  in metabolic acidosis, 212, 217
  in respiratory alkalosis, 247–248
  primary, 247–248, 252
Hypochloremia, artifactual, 77, *77*
  corrected, 77, 77–79, *78*, 78t
  in chronic hypercapnia, 244
  in congestive heart failure, 398, 403
  in renal failure, 413
Hypochloremic alkalosis, 75–76
Hypodipsia, hypernatremia due to, 53–54
  primary, 549–552, 550t, 551t, *552*
Hypoglycemia, and hepatic encephalopathy, 358t, 359
  causes of, 383, 383t
  fluid therapy for, 383
  in hypoadrenocorticism, 381
  in liver disease, 362
  perioperative management of, 310–311
Hypokalemia, 91–97
  and acid-base balance, 93
  and ammoniagenesis, 353
  and hepatic encephalopathy, 358t, 359
  and renal bicarbonate reabsorption, 206
  causes of, 93t, 95–96
  cell membrane potential with, *84*, *84*
  clinical and laboratory features of, 91–95, *92*
  diuretic-induced, 397–398
  effect of, on cardiorespiratory system, 94
    on kidney, 94–95
    on muscle, 93–94
  in congestive heart failure, 397–398, 403
  in diabetic ketoacidosis, 378–379, 379t
  in liver disease, 353
  in renal failure, 413–414
  metabolic acidosis with, 86, 91, 93, 208
  metabolic alkalosis with, 228
  perioperative management of, 309–310
  polyuria and polydipsia due to, 66t
  taurine in, 397
  treatment of, 96–97, 96t, 98t
  with hypertonic solutions, 503
  with hypomagnesemia, 180, 181
Hypokalemic nephropathy, 94–95, 96
  case study of, 561–562, 561t
Hypomagnesemia, 179–183
  and parathyroid hormone secretion, 112
  causes of, 178t, 179, 182
  clinical findings in, 179–181
  criteria for, 179
  in congestive heart failure, 398
  in renal failure, 416
  in sick animals, 181–182
  incidence of, 175
  therapy for, 181–183
Hyponatremia, 59–67
  causes of, 60t
  clinical approach to, 59–65, *60*
  clinical signs of, 65

Hyponatremia *(Continued)*
  dilutional, in liver disease, 350–351
  hemodialysis for, 540
  in congestive heart failure, 397, 402, 403
    case study of, 552–553, 553t
  in hypoadrenocorticism, 62–63, 381
  in renal failure, 413
  perioperative management of, 309
  pseudo- (factitious), 60–61, *61*
  serum sodium concentration in, 46–47
  treatment of, 65–67
  with decreased plasma osmolality, 60t, 61–65
  with hypervolemia, 60t, 63–64
  with hypovolemia, 60t, *62*, 62–63
  with increased plasma osmolality, 60t, 61
  with normal plasma osmolality, 60–61, 60t, *61*
  with normovolemia, 60t, 64–65
Hypoosmolality, hyponatremia with, 60t, 61–65
  perioperative management of, 310
Hypoosmotic solution, 45
Hypoparathyroidism, case study of, 568–570, *569*, 569t
  hyperphosphatemia due to, 170
  hypocalcemia due to, 148–151
  polyuria and polydipsia due to, 66t
  treatment of, 150–151
Hypophosphatemia, 165–167
  and parathyroid hormone secretion, 112
  artifactual, 164
  case study of, 572–573, 572t, 573t
  causes of, 165–167, 165t
  clinical effects of, 165
  in diabetic ketoacidosis, 379
  in liver disease, 353–354
  in renal failure, 415
  treatment of, 167, 168t
Hypoproteinemia, case study of, 570, 570t
  colloids for, 490
  fluid therapy for, 339
  in congestive heart failure, 398
  perioperative management of, 309
Hyporeninemic hypoaldosteronism, hyperkalemia due to, 102
  renal tubular acidosis in, 216
Hyposthenuria, 46
Hypotension, resuscitation with, 445
  with hemodialysis, 533, *534*, 543
Hypothermia, hypophosphatemia due to, 166–167
Hypothyroidism, hyponatremia due to, 65
  perioperative management of, 316
Hypotonic dehydration, 46, *47*
Hypotonic fluid loss(es), 12, 12t
  classification of, 57
  hypernatremia due to, 53t, *54*, *56*, 56–57, *57*, *59*
Hypotonic solution, 46
Hypotonicity, defense against, 52
Hypoventilation, in respiratory acidosis, 246
  (A–a) O_2 gradient with, 242–243
Hypovolemia, and vasopressin release, 51, *51*
  effect of, 12, 12t
  fluid therapy for, 270
  hyponatremia with, 60t, *62*, 62–63
  monitoring of, 317–318
  perioperative management of, 307–308
Hypovolemic shock, 431, 432
  case study of, 586, 586t
  in renal failure, 412
  signs of, 267
Hypoxemia, clinical approach to, 242, *242*
  due to hemodialysis, 544–545

Hypoxemia (Continued)
 (A–a) O₂ gradient with, 242
Hypoxia, in hepatic encephalopathy, 359–360

I

I-Cath catheter, 283t
ICF. See *Intracellular fluid (ICF)* entries.
Icodextrin, in dialysate, 513
ICP. See *Intracranial pressure (ICP)*.
Ideal dry body weight, 539
Idiogenic osmoles, 58
IgG (immunoglobulin G) multiple myeloma, anion gap in, 201–202
Ileum, absorption and secretion of water by, 332, 333, 334, *334*
 chloride reabsorption in, 74
Immune function, blood transfusion and, 325
Immunocompetence, nutrition and, 465
Immunoglobulin G (IgG) multiple myeloma, anion gap in, 201–202
Immunomodulatory effects, of hypertonic solutions, 499
Impermeant solute, hypernatremia due to gain of, 53t, *54*, 57–58, *58*, 59
Increased intracranial pressure, perioperative management of, 313
Increased intraocular pressure, perioperative management of, 313
Infection(s), and hepatic encephalopathy, 358t
 catheter, 297–298
 due to transfusions, 459
 systemic inflammatory response syndrome and septic shock due to, 432–433, 433t
 with hemodialysis, 543
 with parenteral nutrition, 478
 with peritonitis, 366–368, *367*
  due to peritoneal dialysis, 522, 522–523, *523*t
 with renal failure, 424
Inflammation, of gastrointestinal tract, 335
Infusion pumps, 275, *276*, 299, *300*
 for blood transfusion, 457
Inorganic phosphate, 163
 as buffer, 194
Inotropes, for shock, 439–440
Inotropic effects, of hypertonic solutions, 498
"Ins and outs," measurement of, 278, 413
Insulin, continuous IV infusion of, 378
 for diabetic ketoacidosis, 221, 377–378
  fluid therapy before, 376–377
 for hyperkalemia, 103
 for hypoadrenocorticism, 383
 for transfusion reactions, 460t
 in potassium balance, 85
 low-dose IM administration of, 378
 maintenance therapy with, 378
Insulin dilution studies, 7–8
Insulin resistance, in metabolic acidosis, 213
Insulinomas, perioperative management of, 310–311
Insyte catheter, 283t
Interstitial colloid osmotic pressure, 486
Interstitial fluid, solute concentrations in, 9, *9*, 10t
 volume of, 5
Interstitial hydrostatic pressure, 13, 486–487
Interstitial oncotic pressure, 13
Interstitial space, water exchange between plasma and, 12–13, *13*
Intestinal absorption, of magnesium, 176
 of phosphate, 164
 of water, 332–335, *333–335*
Intestinal fluid, electrolyte composition of, 213, 214t, *215*
Intestinal obstruction, 339–341
 case study of, 580–581, 580t

Intestinal rupture, peritonitis due to, 368
Intestinal secretion, of water, 332–335, *333–335*
Intestine, calcitriol effects on, 119–120
Intima catheter, 283t
Intoxication, acute, hemodialysis for, 529, *529*, 541–542, 541t
Intracath intravenous catheter, 282, 283t
Intracellular fluid (ICF), calcium concentration in, 110–111
 osmolality of, 11
 potassium concentration in, 83
 sodium concentration in, 83
 solute concentrations in, 9, *9*, 10t
Intracellular fluid (ICF) compartment, volume of, 5
 water exchange between extracellular fluid compartment and, 10–12, *11*, 12t
Intracellular fluid (ICF) volume deficit, with gain of impermeant solute, 57, *58*
 with hypotonic fluid loss, 56, *57*
 with pure water loss, 53, *55*
Intracellular fluid (ICF) volume depletion, in hyponatremia with volume depletion, 62, *62*
Intracranial pressure (ICP), hypertonic fluid therapy and, 499–500
 increased, perioperative management of, 313
 measurement of, 318
Intrafusor intravenous catheter, 282, 283t
Intrahepatic baroreceptors, 350
Intramedullary route. See *Intraosseous route*.
Intraocular pressure, increased, perioperative management of, 313
 measurement of, 319
Intraoperative management, of fluid therapy, 319–326, *321*, 322t
Intraosseous route, 273–274, 281, 294–295, *295*
 for blood transfusion, 457
 for parenteral nutrition, 477
Intraperitoneal route, 273
Intravascular hydrostatic pressure, 486
Intravenous catheter(s), antibiotic-coated, 284
 composition of, 284, 284t
 cut-down, 282
 damage to, 285
 heparinization of, 296
 maintenance of, 296
 over-the-needle, 282, 282–284, 283t
  placement of, 287–288, *288–289*
 placement of, 285–296
  bandaging in, 295–296
  percutaneous access procedures for, 286–293
  skin preparation for, 285–286
  vascular access procedures for, 293–295
 removal of, 296
 site selection for, 284–285
 through-the-needle, 282, 283t, 284
  placement of, 288–293, *290–292*
 types of, 282, 282–284, 283t
 winged needle, 282, *282*, 283t
  placement of, 286–287, *287*
Intravenous therapy, 273, 281
 complications of, 279, 296–298, *297*
 fluid administration sets and connection devices for, 298–300, *299–301*
 monitoring of, 299–305, *300–304*, 304t
Intropin. See *Dopamine hydrochloride (Intropin)*.
Inulin clearance, 30
Iodine, for catheter placement, 286
Ionic composition, of body water compartments, 9, *9–10*, 10t

Ionization constant, 190
Isoelectric point (pI), 194
Isohydric principle, 192
Isopropyl alcohol, for catheter placement, 286
Isosmotic solution, 45
Isosthenuria, 46
Isotonic dehydration, 46, *47*
Isotonic fluid, loss of, 12, 12t
Isotonic solution, 46

J

Jaundice, due to pancreatitis, 557–558, 558t
Jejunum, absorption and secretion of water by, 332, *333*, 333–334, *334*
 chloride reabsorption in, 73–74
Jelco catheter, 283t
Jelco intermittent injection cap, 299
Jugular vein, blood samples from, 318
 for vascular access, 273, 285
Juxtaglomerular apparatus (JGA), 27, *28*, 32
 in sodium balance, 48

K

K⁺. See *Potassium (K⁺)*.
K_a (dissociation constant), 190
Kappa agonists, effects of, 316
Kayexalate (sodium polystyrene sulfonate), for hyperkalemia, 103, 103t
KCl. See *Potassium chloride (KCl)*.
Ketamine, effects of, 316
 for blood donation, 456
 seizures due to, 583–584, 583t, 584t
Ketoacidosis, diabetic. See *Diabetic ketoacidosis (DKA)*.
Ketogenesis, in diabetic ketoacidosis, 375–376
α-Ketoglutarate, and hepatic encephalopathy, 357t
Ketone bodies, 468
Ketone utilization, in diabetic ketoacidosis, 376
Kidney(s). See also *Renal* entries.
 acid-base regulation by, 205–207, *205–208*
 artificial, 532
 calcitriol effects on, 120
 calcium reabsorption by, 109
 hypercalcemia effects on, 139–140
 hypokalemia effects on, 94–95
 in chloride concentration, 74
 in metabolic acidosis, 212
 in metabolic alkalosis, 229–230
 magnesium regulation by, 176–177
 phosphate handling by, 164–165
 physiology of, 26–41
  blood and plasma flow in, 30–32, *31*
  endocrine functions in, 39–41
  glomerular filtration in, 27–29, *27–30*, 29t
  nephron function in, 26
  renal clearance in, 26–27
  tubular function in, 32–36, *33–36*
  urinary concentrating mechanism in, 36–39, 37t, *38*, *39*
 potassium excretion by, 87–89, *89*
 potassium handling by, 86–90, *87–89*
 sodium balance regulation by, 45t, 47–50, 50t
 sodium handling by, 47, *47*
 water balance regulation by, 45t, 50–52, *50–52*
Kt/V, 536–537

L

Labels, for fluid additives, 275, *275*
 for rate of fluid administration, 275, *275*, 299, *301*
Laboratory findings, in dehydration, 268, 269t

Laboratory findings (Continued)
in monitoring fluid therapy, 278
Lactate, 223
as additive to crystalloid solutions, 272–273
in dialysate, 513
normal plasma concentrations of, 224
Lactate metabolism, in liver disease, 355–356, 356
Lactated Ringer's solution (LRS), 2.5% dextrose in, 271t
5% dextrose in, 271t
compatibility of, with other IV products, 311t, 320
during anesthesia and surgery, 320
electrolyte composition of, 270, 271t, 272t
for hypercalcemia, 142
for metabolic acidosis, 272–273
half-strength, 2.5% dextrose in, 271t
lactate metabolism with, 320
potential disadvantages of, 320
rate of administration of, 274
with cerebral edema, 320
Lactation, magnesium during, 177
Lactic acidosis, 222–226, 222t
causes of, 222–223, 222t
clinical features of, 223–224
D-, 223
defined, 222
due to transfusion, 356
in cardiac arrest and cardiopulmonary resuscitation, 224
in liver disease, 355–356, 356
in racing greyhounds, 224
L-, 223
lymphosarcoma and, 224–225
normal physiology and, 223
pathophysiology of, 223
treatment of, 225–226, 362–363
type A (hypoxic), 222, 222t
type B (nonhypoxic), 222, 222t
Lactulose, for nitrogen intolerance, 362
Landmark catheter, 283t
Lanreotide, for humoral hypercalcemia of malignancy, 145
Lasix. See *Furosemide (Lasix)*.
Law of mass action, 190
Leaky epithelia, 33
Lean body mass, 6–7
Left atrial pressure (LAP), and left-ventricular end-diastolic pressure, 278
Left-sided heart failure, 391, 392
Left-ventricular end-diastolic pressure (LVEDP), 278, 278–279, 301, 301
Lethargy, due to diabetic ketoacidosis, 577–578, 577t
Lidocaine, for catheter placement, 285
for shock, 440
Life Cath column disc catheter, 518
Lingual artery, catheterization of, 318
Lingual veins, blood samples from, 318
Lipid(s), in total nutrient admixture, 472–473
Lipid emulsions, 472–473
Lipidosis, hepatic, 351, 351, 362
Lipolysis, in diabetic ketoacidosis, 375
Lisinopril, for congestive heart failure, 400
renal effects of, 394t
Liver. See also *Hepatic* entries.
albumin synthesis by, 343–345, 344
baroreceptors in, 350
globulin synthesis by, 345, 345
in body fluid and electrolyte balances, 343
nitrogen metabolism by, 345–346, 346
normal physiology of, 342–346, 342t, 343–346
Liver disease, acid-base abnormalities in, 354

Liver disease (Continued)
treatment of, 362–363
aldosterone in, 350
ascites in, 360–361, 361
treatment of, 362, 365–366, 366
bleeding tendencies in, 364–365
blood gas abnormalities in, 354–355, 355
blood urea nitrogen in, 351, 352, 353
cardiovascular changes in, 357
citrate metabolism in, 356–357
colloid administration in, 363–364
creatine synthesis in, 351–352, 352, 353
edema in, 362
euglycemia in, 362
fluid therapy in, 361–366
glomerular filtration rate in, 352
hypoalbuminemia in, 347, 348
treatment of, 363–364
hypokalemia in, 353
hyponatremia in, 63
hypophosphatemia in, 353–354
lactate metabolism and lactic acidosis in, 355–356, 356
treatment of, 362–363
mixed acid-base disturbances in, 255, 257
nutritional considerations in, 361–362
pathophysiology of, 347–361
perioperative management of, 315
polyuria and polydipsia in, 66t, 352
urine specific gravity in, 352, 353
water and sodium disturbances in, 349, 349–351, 349t, 351
water turnover in, 352
Loop diuretics, for congestive heart failure, 401
renal effects of, 393, 394, 394t, 395, 395t
Loop of Henle, functions of, 26
in urinary concentrating mechanism, 36–37, 37t
in water balance, 51
potassium reabsorption in, 87, 87
sodium reabsorption in, 47, 48
Losartan, renal effects of, 393, 394t
LRS. See *Lactated Ringer's solution (LRS)*.
Luminal membranes, 33
Lung vagal reflex, with hypertonic solutions, 497–498
LVEDP (left-ventricular end-diastolic pressure), 278, 278–279, 301, 301
Lymphadenopathy, peripheral, case study of, 573–574, 574t
Lymphangiectasia, protein-losing enteropathy due to, 570, 570t
Lymphatics, in peritoneal dialysis, 511
Lymphoma, hypercalcemia due to, 130–131, 132, 133
Lymphosarcoma, case studies of, 563–565, 563t, 573–574, 574t
hyperphosphatemia due to, 167–168
lactic acidosis due to, 224–225
Lysine, metabolic acidosis due to, 217

M

Macromolecular flux, expression for, 485
Macromolecular plasma volume expanders, 483–491
complications and side effects of, 490–491
evaluation and monitoring of, 490–491
for chronic hypoproteinemia, 490
for pulmonary disease, 489–490
pharmacokinetics and pharmacodynamics of, 487–489
physicochemical basis for effect of, 483–487, 486t
Mag-Carb (magnesium carbonate), for hyperphosphatemia, 170

Mag-Carb (magnesium carbonate) (Continued)
for magnesium depletion, 183
Magnesium, 175–184
absorption of, 176
and parathyroid hormone secretion, 112
as therapeutic agent, 183–184, 184
assessment of, 177–179, 178t
chemistry and biology of, 175–176
dietary intake of, 175, 176, 180
excess, 184
excretion of, 178–179
for magnesium depletion, 182–183
functions of, 176
in congestive heart failure, 398
in dialysate, 519
in renal failure, 416
ionized, 177, 177t
mammary secretion of, during lactation, 177
metabolism of, 175–177
renal regulation of, 176–177
serum concentration of, 177, 177t
sources of, 176
tissue concentration of, 177–178
total body, 175–176
Magnesium carbonate (Mag-Carb), for hyperphosphatemia, 170
for magnesium depletion, 183
Magnesium chloride, for magnesium depletion, 183
Magnesium depletion, 179–183
causes of, 178t, 179, 182
clinical findings in, 179–181
criteria for, 179
in hypocalcemia, 149–150
in sick animals, 181–182
incidence of, 175
therapy for, 181–183
Magnesium gluconate (Magonate), for magnesium depletion, 183
Magnesium oxide (Mag-Ox, Uro-Mag), for magnesium depletion, 183
Magnesium retention test, 178–179
Magnesium salts, for magnesium depletion, 182–183
Magnesium sulfate (Epsom salt), for magnesium depletion, 182–183
Magnesium supplementation, 182–183
Magonate (magnesium gluconate), for magnesium depletion, 183
Mag-Ox (magnesium oxide), for magnesium depletion, 183
Maintenance caloric needs, 20
Maintenance energy expenditure, 20
Maintenance energy requirement (MER), 20, 269, 275–276
Maintenance fluid requirement, 14–15, 20–21, 275, 276–277, 277t
Maintenance solutions, 269
Malignancy, hypercalcemia of, due to apocrine gland adenocarcinoma, 567–568, 567t, 568
due to lymphosarcoma, 563–565, 563t
humoral, 116, 127, 129–132, 131–134, 145
Malnutrition, and drug metabolism, 465–466
and immunocompetence, 465
and tissue synthesis and repair, 465
and wound healing, 465
assessment of, 466–470
clinical importance of, 465–466
food and feeding methods in, 470
nutrients of concern in, 468–470
risk factors for, 467–468

Mannitol, 20%, 271t
  for dialysis disequilibrium syndrome, 544
  for ethylene glycol ingestion, 218
  for renal failure, 417–418
  hyponatremia with hyperosmolality in, 61
Manometer, for CVP measurement, 302, 302–303, 303
Mass action, law of, 190
Measure, units of, 3–5, 3t, 4
Medullary collecting ducts, functions of, 26
  in urinary concentrating mechanism, 37, 37t
Meperidine, effects of, 316
MER (maintenance energy requirement), 20, 269, 275–276
Mercaptans, and hepatic encephalopathy, 357t
Mesangium, of glomerulus, 28
Mesothelial cells, in peritoneal dialysis, 512
Metabolic acid-base disorders, 195, 211–236
Metabolic acidosis, 211–227
  and metabolic alkalosis, 254t, 255–256
  and respiratory acidosis, 256–257, 256t
  and respiratory alkalosis, 254t, 255
  anion gap in, 74–75, 201
    increased, 213t, 214, 217–226, 218, 219, 222t
      in mixed acid-base disorders, 256t, 257–258
    normal, 213–217, 213t, 214, 214t, 215, 216t
  body buffer response to, 211, 212
  cardiovascular function in, 212–213
  causes of, 211, 213, 213t
  chloride in, 74–75, 76
  clinical features of, 212–213
  defined, 195, 195t, 211
  diagnosis of, 213, 213t, 214
  dilutional, 217
  due to ammonium chloride, 217
  due to carbonic anhydrase inhibitors, 216–217
  due to cardiac arrest and CPR, 224
  due to cationic amino acid infusion, 217
  due to congestive heart failure, 398
  due to diabetic ketoacidosis, 220–221
  due to diarrhea, 213–214, 214t, 215, 337
  due to ethylene glycol ingestion, 217–220, 218, 219
  due to hypoadrenocorticism, 217, 383
  due to liver disease, 354
    treatment of, 363
  due to lymphosarcoma, 224–225
  due to renal failure, 416
  due to salicylate intoxication, 220
  due to shock, 442
  hemodialysis for, 540
  hyperchloremic, anion gap and, 74–75, 201, 213, 214
    defined, 211
    disorders associated with, 213t, 217–226, 218, 219, 222t
  hypokalemia in, 86, 91, 93, 208
  in triple acid-base disorder, 258, 258t
  insulin resistance in, 213
  lactic, 222–226, 222t
  normochloremic, anion gap and, 74–75, 201, 213, 214
    disorders associated with, 213–217, 213t, 214t, 215, 216t
  perioperative management of, 311, 311t
  posthypocapnic, 217
  potassium balance in, 86
  potassium excretion in, 90
  renal response to, 212
  renal tubular, 126t, 214–216

Metabolic acidosis (Continued)
  respiratory response to, 211–212, 251, 252
  treatment of, 226–227
  uremic, 221–222
Metabolic alkalosis, 227–236
  acute buffer response to, 228, 228
  and hepatic encephalopathy, 359
  and metabolic acidosis, 254t, 255–256
  and respiratory acidosis, 254–255, 254t
  and respiratory alkalosis, 256t, 257
  causes of, 227, 231–235, 231t
  chloride in, 75–76
  chloride-resistant, 227, 231
    causes of, 231t, 234–235
    treatment of, 236
  chloride-responsive, 227, 231
    causes of, 231–234, 231t, 232–234
    development of, 227–228
    treatment of, 235–236
  classification of, 227
  clinical features of, 230, 230
  defined, 195, 195t, 227
  diagnosis of, 230–231
  due to alkali administration, 231
  due to congestive heart failure, 398
  due to diuretic administration, 233–234
  due to gastric fluid loss, 231–233, 232–234
  due to hyperadrenocorticism, 235
  due to liver disease, 354
    treatment of, 363
  due to penicillin, ampicillin, or carbenicillin, 235
  due to primary hyperaldosteronism, 234–235
  due to vomiting, 336
  hyperkalemia due to, 97–98
  in triple acid-base disorder, 258, 258t
  perioperative management of, 312
  posthypercapnic, 234
  potassium balance in, 86
  potassium excretion in, 88
  "refeeding," 235
  renal response to, 229–230
  respiratory response to, 228–229, 229, 251–252
  response of body to, 228, 228–230, 229
  treatment of, 235–236
Metabolic compensation, 243–244, 244, 245, 252, 252t
Metabolic disorders, fluid therapy in, 375–384
Metabolic processes, respiratory compensation in, 196t, 251–252
Metabolic rate, 468–469
Metabolic water, 20, 20t
Metastases, to bone, hypercalcemia due to, 133–134
Methanethiol, and hepatic encephalopathy, 357t
Methionine, and hepatic encephalopathy, 357t
Methoxamine, for shock, 440
Methoxyflurane, effects of, 317
Methylprednisolone succinate, for transfusion reactions, 460t
Methylpyrazole (Antizol), for ethylene glycol ingestion, 219
Metoclopramide (Reglan), and dopamine, 420
Metolazone, renal effects of, 395
Metronidazole, for nitrogen intolerance, 362
Microcirculation, of respiratory unit, 387–389, 388
Micromineral solutions, 474
Microvascular barrier, 483–484
  fluid flux across, 484–485
Microvilli, in peritoneal dialysis, 512
Midwest Animal Blood Services, 452t

Milliequivalent weight, 4
Millimole (mmol), 3
Milliosmolality, 4
Milliosmolarity, 4
Milliosmoles (mOsm), 4
Milrinone, for congestive heart failure, 401
Mineral(s), in parenteral nutrition, 470, 474
Mineral acidosis, potassium concentration with, 86
  potassium excretion with, 90
Mineral imbalances, hemodialysis for, 541
Mineralocorticoid(s), and potassium excretion, 89–90
Mineralocorticoid excess, hypokalemia due to, 96
Mineralocorticoid replacement, for hypoadrenocorticism, 382
Minicath catheter, 283t
Minicutdown procedure, 293
Miniset catheter, 283t
Mithramycin, for hypercalcemia, 141t, 144
Mitochondrial myopathies, lactic acidosis due to, 222–223
Mitral insufficiency, perioperative management of, 314
Mixed acid-base disorders, 195–196, 251–259
  additive, 251t, 256–258, 256t
  anion gap in, 201
  classification of, 251, 251t
  clinical approach to, 253–254, 253t, 254, 254t
  compensation in, 251–252, 252t, 253
  counterbalancing, 251t, 254–256, 254t
  defined, 251
  treatment for, 258–259
  triple, 251t, 258, 258t
mmol (millimole), 3
MODS (multiple organ dysfunction syndrome), 433
Molar substitution ratio, 489
Mole (mol), 3, 4
Molecular weight, 3, 3t
Monitoring, central venous pressure, 278, 278–279, 300–305, 301–304, 304t
  of changes in composition, 318
  of changes in distribution, 318–319
  of changes in volume, 317–318
  of colloid therapy, 491
  of fluid therapy, 278, 278–279, 299–305, 300–304, 304t
    in renal failure, 422–425
    perioperative, 317–319
  of hemodialysis, 533–534, 534, 535
  of parenteral nutrition, 478–479
  of peritoneal dialysis, 523–525, 524t
  of shock, 443–445
  of transfusion, 457–458
Morphine, effects of, 316
  for congestive heart failure, 399
  for shock, 441, 441t
mOsm (milliosmoles), 4
Mu agonists, effects of, 316
Multiple myeloma, hypercalcemia due to, 133
  IgG, anion gap in, 201–202
  polyuria and polydipsia due to, 66t
Multiple organ dysfunction syndrome (MODS), 433
Muscle wasting, 467
Muscle weakness, due to hyperkalemia, 97
  due to hypokalemia, 93–94
  due to hypokalemic nephropathy, 561–562, 562t
Mycoses, systemic, hypercalcemia due to, 137, 141
Myeloma, multiple, hypercalcemia due to, 133

Myeloma (Continued)
   IgG, anion gap in, 201–202
   polyuria and polydipsia due to, 66t
Myocardial infarction, magnesium in, 179–180, 183–184
Myogenic mechanism, 31

N

Na⁺. See Sodium (Na⁺).
²⁴Na dilution studies, 8
NaCl. See Sodium chloride (NaCl).
NaHCO₃. See Sodium bicarbonate (NaHCO₃).
Nalbuphine, effects of, 316
Nasogastric tube feeding, in renal failure, 422
Neomycin, for nitrogen intolerance, 362
Nephrogenic diabetes insipidus (NDI), 55–56, 56t
   polyuria and polydipsia due to, 66t
Nephron, differential permeability characteristics of segments of, 36–37, 37t
   functions of, 26
Nephropathy, hypercalcemic, case study of, 563–565, 563t
   hypokalemic, 94–95, 96
      case study of, 561–562, 561t
Nephrotic syndrome, hyponatremia due to, 63
Nephrotoxicity, of anesthesia, 317
Nernst equation, 24, 84
Net filtration pressure, 13
Neurohormonal adaptations, to congestive heart failure, 389, 390t
Neurohormonal responses, in shock, 429, 430
Neurologic complications, of hemodialysis, 543–544, 544
Neuromuscular dysfunction, due to magnesium deficiency, 179, 181
Neutral endopeptidase inhibitors, renal effects of, 394t
Neutropenia, with hemodialysis, 545
NH₄⁺. See Ammonium (NH₄⁺).
Nitrogen, metabolism of, 345–346, 346
Nitrogen intolerance, in liver disease, 362
Nitroglycerin paste, for transfusion reactions, 460t
Nitroprusside reagent, in diabetic ketoacidosis, 220
Nodular panniculitis, hypercalcemia due to, 137
Nonvolatile acid, 189, 195–196
No-reflow phenomenon, 446
Norepinephrine, and glomerular filtration rate, 29
   for shock, 440
Normal saline, during anesthesia and surgery, 320
   electrolyte composition of, 270, 271t
Normosol-M, in 5% dextrose, 271t
Normosol-R, 271t, 272t
   plus 2% dextran, 272t
Normovolemia, hyponatremia with, 60t, 64–65
Novalon catheter, 283t
Nutricel, for donated blood, 456t
Nutrineal, 513
Nutrition. See also Diet.
   and drug metabolism, 465–466
   and immunocompetence, 465
   and tissue synthesis and repair, 465
   and wound healing, 465
   parenteral. See Parenteral nutrition (PN).
   total. See Total parenteral nutrition (TPN).
Nutritional assessment, 466–470
Nutritional support. See also Enteral feeding; Parenteral nutrition (PN).
   for hepatic encephalopathy, 359, 360t
   for liver disease, 361–362
   for renal failure, 422

O

Obstructive shock, 432, 434
Octreotide, for humoral hypercalcemia of malignancy, 145
Oliguria, conversion of, 416–421
   defined, 412
   hypercalcemia due to, 138
   hyperkalemia due to, 100
   in monitoring fluid therapy, 278
   in renal failure, 412–413
   perioperative management of, 315
Oncotic pressure, 12–13, 13, 485
Opioids, effects of, 316
   for pancreatitis, 340
   for shock, 434, 440–441, 441t
Oral rehydration solutions (ORSs), 338–339
Oral route, 273
Orthopedic abnormalities, due to magnesium deficiency, 181
Orthophosphate, 163
Orthophosphoric acid, 163
Osm. See Osmole(s) (Osm).
Osmocytes, 58
Osmolal gap, 14, 14t, 45, 549t
Osmolality, defined, 4, 45
   effective, 46
   of extracellular fluid, 11
   of intracellular fluid, 11
   of plasma. See Plasma osmolality.
   of solutions, 270
   of urine, 15–16, 15t, 16t, 38, 46, 46t
      in central diabetes insipidus, 55
Osmolarity, 4, 45
Osmole(s) (Osm), 4
   effective and ineffective, 4, 4–5
   idiogenic, 58
Osmoreceptors, 50
   defective function of, 549–550
Osmoregulation, 45t
Osmosis, 4, 4–5, 507
Osmostat, reset, 64
Osmotic demyelination syndrome, 65
Osmotic diuresis, 46
   in diabetic ketoacidosis, 376
Osmotic pressure, 4, 4–5, 485
   colloid. See Colloid osmotic pressure (COP).
Osteodystrophy, hypertrophic, hypercalcemia due to, 138
Osteolysis, calcium transport in, 127
   hypercalcemia due to, 138
Osteomyelitis, hypercalcemia due to, 138
Osteoporosis, disuse, hypercalcemia due to, 138
Overfeeding, 469
Overflow theory, of ascites, 360
Overhydration, 279
   with peritoneal dialysis, 523
Over-the-needle catheter, 282, 282–284, 283t
   placement of, 287–288, 288–289
Oxalate stones, hypercalcemia with, 137, 140
Oxidative metabolism, 223
Oxygen, partial pressure of. See Partial pressure of oxygen (P_{O_2}).
Oxygen content, in shock, 445
Oxygen delivery, and shock, 428
   in diabetic ketoacidosis, 221
   variables, equations, and normal values for, 429t
   with hypertonic solutions, 498–499
Oxygen gradient, 242, 242–243, 243t, 250, 549t
   in liver disease, 354–355, 355
Oxygen therapy, for congestive heart failure, 399
   for respiratory acidosis, 246, 247
Oxygen transport variables, in shock, 444–445
Oxyglobin, 461–462
   for shock, 438, 442–443
Oxyhemoglobin, during anesthesia and surgery, 326
Oxyhemoglobin dissociation curve, in liver disease, 355
   in metabolic alkalosis, 230
Oxymorphone, effects of, 316
   for shock, 441, 441t
Oxypolygelatin (Vetaplasma, Gelifundol), for shock, 437
   physicochemical properties of, 322t, 324, 437

P

Packed cell volume (PCV), in dehydration, 268, 269t
   in renal failure, 421, 423
   in shock, 442, 443
Packed red blood cells (PRBCs), 452
   during anesthesia and surgery, 325
   for shock, 436
$PaCO_2$, 241, 242
$PaCO_2$, 241–242
Pain, and shock, 433, 440–441, 441t
Pamidronate, for hypercalcemia, 141t, 144
P-aminohippuric acid (PAH) clearance, 32
Pancreas, absorption and secretion of water by, 330–332, 332
Pancreatic juice, ionic composition of, 331–332, 332
Pancreatic peritonitis, 367–368
Pancreatitis, 339–341
   case study of, 557–558, 558t
   hypoalbuminemia due to, 348
   hypocalcemia due to, 150
   shock due to, hypertonic solutions for, 501
Panniculitis, nodular, hypercalcemia due to, 137
Panting, water losses via, 16–18, 18
PaO_2, 250
   difference between PaO_2 and, 250. See also Alveolar-arterial oxygen difference ($[A-a] O_2$ gradient).
   in liver disease, 354–355, 355
Paracellular route, 33
Paracentesis, for ascites, 365, 366
Paradoxical CNS acidosis, 221
Parathyroid gland, calcitriol effects on, 120
Parathyroid gland adenoma, case study of, 566, 566–567, 567t
   hypercalcemia due to, 134–136
Parathyroid gland carcinoma, hypercalcemia due to, 134–136
Parathyroid gland hyperplasia, hypercalcemia due to, 134–136
Parathyroid hormone (PTH), 111–116
   actions of, 114–116
   and phosphate uptake, 36
   calcitriol and, 111–112, 113, 120
   clearance and metabolism of, 113–114, 115
   for hypocalcemia, 151
   in calcium homeostasis, 108, 109, 120–121
   in hypercalcemia, 129
   in hypocalcemia, 148, 149
   in vitamin D synthesis, 118, 119
   mechanism of action of, 116
   receptor for, 116
   serum concentrations of, 121t, 124–125

Parathyroid hormone (PTH) *(Continued)*
  structure of, 111
  synthesis and secretion of, 111–113, *112–114*
Parathyroid hormone–related protein (PTHrP), *116*, 116–117
  in calcium homeostasis, 108, 116
  in humoral hypercalcemia of malignancy, 129, 130, 131, *131*, 132, *133*
  serum concentration of, 121t, 125
Parathyroiditis, with hypocalcemia, 148, 150
Parenteral nutrition (PN), 465–479
  administration of, 476–477
  assessment of patient for, 466–470
  catheter complications in, 477–478
  clinical importance of, 465–466
  combination of enteral and, 478
  compounding in, 474–476, 475t, *476*
  contraindications to, 471
  cost of, 471
  defined, 472–473
  development of plan for, 470–478
  drug additions to, 474, 474t
  indications for, 470–471, 471t
  monitoring of, 478–479
  nutrients of concern in, 468–470
  patient selection for, 470–471, 471t
  products for, 472–474
  risk factors for, 467–468
  total. See *Total parenteral nutrition (TPN)*.
Paresis, due to polyradiculoneuritis, 582–583, 582t, 583t
Parker peritoneal dialysis cannula, 516–517, *517*
Partial pressure of carbon dioxide (P_{CO_2}), alveolar (P_{ACO_2}), 241, 242
  and alveolar ventilation, 241–242
  and renal bicarbonate reabsorption, 206
  arterial (P_{aCO_2}), 241–242
  in acid-base balance, 200, 202, 243
  in metabolic acidosis, 211–212
  in metabolic alkalosis, 228–229
  in respiratory acidosis, 245
  in respiratory alkalosis, 247
  of blood sample, 198–199
  venous, 241
Partial pressure of oxygen (P_{O_2}), alveolar (P_{AO_2}), 250
    difference between P_{aO_2} and, 250. See also *Alveolar-arterial oxygen difference ([A – a] O_2 gradient)*.
    in liver disease, 354–355, *355*
  in mixed venous blood (P_{vO_2}), in shock, 445
  in respiratory acidosis, 246
  inspired (P_{IO_2}), 250
    decreased, (A–a) O_2 gradient with, 243
Passive diffusion, 34
P_{CO_2}. See *Partial pressure of carbon dioxide (P_{CO_2})*.
PCV. See *Packed cell volume (PCV)*.
PCWP. See *Pulmonary capillary wedge pressure (PCWP)*.
PEEP, renal function with, 317
Penicillin, for peritonitis, 523
  metabolic alkalosis due to, 235
Penn Animal Blood Bank, 452t
Pentastarch, 489
  during anesthesia and surgery, 323–324
  for shock, 437
  physicochemical properties of, 322t, 323–324, 437
Pentazocine, effects of, 316
Percorten-V (desoxycorticosterone pivalate), for hypoadrenocorticism, 382

Percutaneous catheterization, 286–293
  over-the needle catheters for, 287–288, *288–289*
  through-the needle catheters for, 288–293, *290–292*
  winged needle catheters for, 286–287, *287*
Percutaneous facilitation procedure, 293
Perfluorocarbon emulsions, for shock, 437–438
Perioperative management, after surgery, 326
  during surgery, 319–326, *321*, 322t
  monitoring fluid therapy in, 317–319
  of access to circulation, 316
  of anemia, *308*, 308–309
  of anesthesia, 316–317
  of cardiovascular disease, 313–314
  of coagulation defects, 314–315
  of dehydration, 312
  of diabetes insipidus, 315
  of diabetes mellitus, 311, 315
  of fluid therapy, 307–326
  of geriatric patients, 313
  of hepatic disease, 315
  of hyperadrenocorticism, 315
  of hypercalcemia, 310
  of hyperglycemia, 311
  of hyperkalemia, 310
  of hypernatremia, 309
  of hyperosmolality, 310
  of hyperproteinemia, 309
  of hyperthyroidism, 316
  of hypervolemia, 308
  of hypoadrenocorticism, 315
  of hypocalcemia, 310
  of hypoglycemia, 310–311
  of hypokalemia, 309–310
  of hyponatremia, 309
  of hypoosmolality, 310
  of hypoproteinemia, 309
  of hypothyroidism, 316
  of hypovolemia, 307–308
  of increased intracranial pressure, 313
  of increased intraocular pressure, 313
  of metabolic acidosis, 311, 311t
  of metabolic alkalosis, 312
  of peripheral edema, 312
  of peritoneal fluid, 313
  of pleural fluid, 312
  of polycythemia, 309
  of pregnancy, 313
  of pulmonary edema, 312
  of renal disease, 315
  thermodynamic considerations in, 316
Peripheral arterial vasodilatation hypothesis, of ascites, 360–361, *361*
Peripheral edema, measurement of, 318
  perioperative management of, 312
Peripheral vein cannulation, 285
Peripheral vein infusion, of parenteral nutrition solution, 477
Peritoneal clearance, of solute, 508, 508t, 511–513, 512t
Peritoneal dialysis, 507–525
  access for, 516–518, *517–519*, 518t
  acute, 509, 509t
  adverse effects of, 512–513
  aseptic technique for, 515–516
  azotemia management before, 513
  blood urea nitrogen with, *509*, 510
  catheter for, causes of failure of, 521t
    peritonitis due to, 522, 522–523, 523t
    placement of, 516–518, *517–519*, 518t
  chronic, 509, 509t
  chronic ambulatory, 509, 510, 511
  clinical experience with, 510–511

Peritoneal dialysis *(Continued)*
  complications of, 521–523, 521t–523t, *522*
  continuous-flow, 509
  creatinine with, *509*, 510
  dialysate for, commercial, 518–519
    composition of, 512–513, 512t
    defined, 507
    dextrose in, 510, 512, 512t
    drainage of, 521
    dwell time for, 507, 521, 521t
    improvised, 519–520
    infusion of, 520–521
    selection and preparation of, 518–520, 520t
    warming of, 520
  evaluation of effectiveness of, 523–525, 524t
  exchange in, 507
  experimental, 509, 509–510
  factors affecting, 508, 508t, 511–513
  for ethylene glycol ingestion, 220
  for hypercalcemia, 141t, 144–145
  for hyperkalemia, 103, 103t
  hemodialysis *vs.*, 508, 508t, 528
  indications for, 509t, 513–515, *514–515*
  inflow in, 507, 520–521
  intermittent, 509, 510
  iodine flush with, 522–523, 523t
  lymphatics in, 511
  mesothelial cells in, 512
  microvilli in, 512
  monitoring of, 523–525, 524t
  objective of, 508, 508t
  outflow in, 507, 521
  overview of, 507, 507t
  percutaneous, 516
  peritoneum in, 507, 511–512
  phosphate with, *509*, 510
  potassium with, *509*, 509
  termination of, 525
  tidal, 509
  types of, 508–509
  urea with, 509, *509*
Peritoneal effusion, case studies of, 557–559, 558t, 559t
  perioperative management of, 313
Peritoneal lavage, 509, 516
Peritoneovenous shunt, for ascites, 365
Peritoneum, structure and function of, 366
  transport across, 507, 511–512
Peritonitis, 366–368, *367*
  bile, 367
  due to peritoneal dialysis, 522, 522–523, 523t
  pancreatic, 367–368
  peritoneal dialysis with, 512
Peritubular capillary factors, in sodium balance, 49
PermCath, 531
Pet food, water in, 18, *18*, 18t, *19*
pH, 189–190, *190*, 191t
  in acid-base disorders, with additive effects, 251t, 256–258
    with neutralizing effects, 251t, 254–256, 254t
  in acid-base evaluation, 200, 202
  in respiratory acidosis, 245
  in treatment of mixed acid-base disorders, 258
  of venous *vs.* arterial blood, 241
  P_{CO_2} and, 243
  urine, in metabolic alkalosis, 230–231
Phenol, and hepatic encephalopathy, 357t
Phosphate(s), as additives, 270
  as buffers, 194, 206

Phosphate(s) *(Continued)*
    in uremic acidosis, 222
    fractional excretion of, 171
    inorganic, 163
    renal uptake of, 36
    with peritoneal dialysis, 509, 510, *514–515*, 524–525
Phosphate binders, 168t
    for hyperphosphatemia, 170–171
        in renal failure, 415
    for hypervitaminosis D, 145
Phosphate enemas, hyperphosphatemia due to, 168
    hypocalcemia due to, 150
Phosphate esters, 163
Phosphate supplementation, 167, 168t
Phospholipids, 163
Phosphorus, and parathyroid hormone secretion, 112
    body stores and distribution of, 163–164
    dietary intake of, 164
    functions of, 163
    in parenteral nutrition, 473
    in renal failure, 415
    intestinal absorption of, 164
    physical chemistry of, 163, 174
    renal handling of, 164–165
    serum concentrations of, calculation of, 550t
        normal, 164
Phosphorus balance, disorders of. See *Hyperphosphatemia; Hypophosphatemia.*
Phosphorus restriction, for hyperphosphatemia, 169–170
Phosphorus supplementation, for diabetic ketoacidosis, 379
Phycomycosis, case study of, 579–580, 579t, 580t
Physical examination, for fluid losses, 267–268, 269t
    for monitoring fluid therapy, 278
pI (isoelectric point), 194
Pimobendan, for congestive heart failure, 401
Pinocytosis, 35, 36
P_{IO_2}, 250
pK_a, 192, 192t
    of weak acid, 206
Plants, vitamin D toxicity due to, 136
Plasma, administration of, 456–458
    compatibility of, with other IV products, 311t
    electrolyte composition of, *270*, 271t
    for liver disease, 363–364
    for pancreatitis, 341
    for peritonitis, 368
    for shock, 436
    fresh, 324
    fresh frozen, 324, 452, *453*
    platelet-rich, 453
    preoperative infusion of, 314
    preparation and use of, 324–325
    solute concentrations in, *9, 9,* 10t
    water exchange between interstitial space and, 12–13, *13*
Plasma colloid osmotic pressure, 485–486
Plasma flow, renal. See *Renal blood flow (RBF).*
Plasma oncotic pressure, 12
Plasma osmolality, 11–12, 45
    and hyponatremia, 60–65, 60t, *61*
    and vasopressin release, 51, *51*
    in central diabetes insipidus, 55
Plasma protein, 324–325
    during anesthesia and surgery, 324–325
    in congestive heart failure, 398

Plasma protein *(Continued)*
    in dehydration, 268, 269t
    in malnutrition, 467, 469–470
    in renal failure, 423
    in shock, 443
    preparation and use of, 324–325
Plasma volume (PV), 5, 6t
    changes in, 307–308
        monitoring of, 317–318
    effective circulating, 12, 47–48
    in heart failure, 387, 389t
    in hemodialysis, 534, *534*, 535
Plasma volume expansion. See *Volume expansion.*
Plasma-Lyte, 271t
Platelet concentrate, 453
Platelet infusion, preoperative, 314–315
Platelet-rich plasma, 453
PLE. See *Protein-losing enteropathy (PLE).*
Pleural effusions, after peritoneal dialysis, 523
    case study of, 557, 557t
    in congestive heart failure, 389–390, 391, *391*
    management of, 400–401
    measurement of, 318
    perioperative management of, 312
PN. See *Parenteral nutrition (PN).*
Pneumonia, case study of, 584–585, 584t
Pneumonitis, uremic, due to hemodialysis, 544–545
P_{O_2}. See *Partial pressure of oxygen (P_{O_2}).*
Podocytes, of glomerulus, 27–28
Poiseuille's law, 274
Poisoning, case study of, *564,* 565–566, 566t
    hemodialysis for, 529, *529,* 541–542, 541t
Polycythemia, perioperative management of, 309
    polyuria and polydipsia due to, 66t
Polydipsia, 67–70
    and hepatic encephalopathy, 358t
    causes of, 66t, 67
    clinical approach to, 67, *68*
    due to apocrine gland adenocarcinoma, 567–568, 567t, *568*
    due to central diabetes insipidus, 55
    due to diabetic ketoacidosis, 570–572, 571t, *572,* 577–578, 577t
    due to hyperaldosteronism, 562–563, 562t
    due to hypokalemia, 94
    due to liver disease, 352
    due to lymphosarcoma, 563–565, 563t
    due to renal failure, 570–572, 571t, *572*
    due to renal tubular acidosis, 578–579, 578t
    laboratory evaluation of, 67–70, 70t
    psychogenic, 55, 64, 66t
    without polyuria, 67
Polyethylene catheters, 284, 284t
Polygelatins, compatibility of, with other IV products, 311t
Polyphagia, due to hyperthyroidism, 570–572, 571t, *572*
Polypropylene catheters, 284, 284t
Polyradiculoneuritis, case study of, 582–583, 582t, 583
Polyurethane catheters, 284, 284t
Polyuria, 67–70
    and hepatic encephalopathy, 358t
    causes of, 66t, 67
    clinical approach to, 67, *68*
    defined, 412
    due to apocrine gland adenocarcinoma, 567–568, 567t, *568*
    due to central diabetes insipidus, 55
    due to diabetic ketoacidosis, 570–572, 571t, *572,* 577–578, 577t

Polyuria *(Continued)*
    due to hyperaldosteronism, 562–563, 562t
    due to hypercalcemia, 139
    due to hypokalemia, 94
    due to liver disease, 352
    due to lymphosarcoma, 563–565, 563t
    due to renal failure, 412–413, 425, 570–572, 571t, *572*
    due to renal tubular acidosis, 578–579, 578t
    laboratory evaluation of, 67–70, 70t
Polyvinyl chloride (PVC) catheters, 284, 284t
Portal hypertension, with hypoalbuminemia, 347
Portosystemic shunting, 350
    hypoglycemia with, 311
Positive-pressure ventilation, renal function with, 317
Postoperative management, of fluid therapy, 326
Potassium (K^+), and acid-base balance, 207–208, 233, *234*
    and ammoniagenesis, 346
    fractional excretion of, 91
    in body fluid compartments, *9, 10,* 10t, 83
    in colon, 334
    in congestive heart failure, *396,* 397–398
    in jejunum, 333–334
    in malnutrition, 467
    in metabolic alkalosis, 228, 229
    in pancreas, 332
    in parenteral nutrition, 473
    in renal failure, 414–415
    in resting cell membrane potential, 24, 83–84
    in stomach, 330
    in threshold cell membrane potential, *84,* 84–85
    renal handling of, 86–90, *87–89*
    serum concentration of, 83, *83*
        acid-base balance and, 85–86
        normal, 90–91, 91t
        with fluid therapy, 272
    total body, 83
    urinary excretion of, 87–89, *89*
        and glomerular filtration rate, *102*
    with peritoneal dialysis, 509, *509,* *514–515,* 520, 524–525
Potassium balance, 85, 85–86, *86*
    and acid-base balance, 85–86, 93
    disorders of. See *Hyperkalemia; Hypokalemia.*
Potassium bicarbonate, for hypokalemia, 98t
Potassium chloride (KCl), 14.9%, 271t
    for congestive heart failure, 402, 403
    for diabetic ketoacidosis, 378–379, 379t
    for hypokalemia, 96–97, 96t, 98t
        in renal failure, 414
    for metabolic alkalosis, 235
    for respiratory acidosis, 247
    in parenteral nutrition, 473
    supplementation of crystalloid solutions with, *270,* 271t
Potassium citrate, for hypokalemia, 98t
Potassium deprivation, 85
Potassium gluconate, for congestive heart failure, 402
    for hypokalemia, 97, 98t
    in renal failure, 414
Potassium gradient, transtubular, 93
Potassium intake, and potassium excretion, 89
Potassium phosphate, for diabetic ketoacidosis, 379
    for hypophosphatemia, 167, 168t
Potassium supplementation, 96–97, 96t, 98t
    for congestive heart failure, 402, 403

Potassium supplementation *(Continued)*
  for diabetic ketoacidosis, 378–379, 379t
  for renal failure, 413, 414
  of crystalloid solutions, 270, 271t
Potassium-sparing diuretics, renal effects of, 394–395, 394t, 395t
Povidone-iodine (Betadine, Xenodine), for catheter placement, 286
Prazosin, renal effects of, 394t
PRBCs. See *Packed red blood cells (PRBCs)*.
Prednisolone sodium succinate (Solu-Delta-Cortef), for hypoadrenocorticism, 382
  for shock, 441
Prednisone, for cholecalciferol toxicity, 565, 566
  for hypercalcemia, 141t, 143
  for hypervitaminosis D, 145
Preeclampsia, magnesium for, 183
Pregnancy, perioperative management with, 313
Premature labor, magnesium for, 183
Premature ventricular complexes (PVCs), due to shock, 440
Preoperative management, of access to circulation, 316
  of anemia, 308, 308–309
  of anesthesia, 316–317
  of cardiovascular disease, 313–314
  of coagulation defects, 314–315
  of dehydration, 312
  of diabetes insipidus, 315
  of diabetes mellitus, 315
  of fluid therapy, 307–319
  of geriatric patients, 313
  of hepatic disease, 315
  of hyperadrenocorticism, 315
  of hypercalcemia, 310
  of hyperglycemia, 311
  of hyperkalemia, 310
  of hypernatremia, 309
  of hyperosmolality, 310
  of hyperproteinemia, 309
  of hyperthyroidism, 316
  of hypervolemia, 308
  of hypoadrenocorticism, 315
  of hypocalcemia, 310
  of hypoglycemia, 310–311
  of hypokalemia, 309–310
  of hyponatremia, 309
  of hypoosmolality, 310
  of hypoproteinemia, 309
  of hypothyroidism, 316
  of hypovolemia, 307–308
  of increased intracranial pressure, 313
  of increased intraocular pressure, 313
  of metabolic acidosis, 311, 311t
  of metabolic alkalosis, 312
  of peripheral edema, 312
  of peritoneal fluid, 313
  of pleural fluid, 312
  of polycythemia, 309
  of pregnancy, 313
  of pulmonary edema, 312
  of renal disease, 315
  thermodynamic considerations in, 316
Preservatives, for donated blood, 456, 456t
  in crystalloid solutions, 273
Pressure natriuresis, in sodium balance, 50
Primary active transport, 34
Procainamide, for shock, 440
Propofol, effects of, 316–317
Propranolol, for congestive heart failure, 400
Prostaglandin(s), and glomerular filtration rate, 29–30
Prostaglandin inhibitors, hyperkalemia due to, 102

Protein(s), and resting energy requirement, 469–470
  and water intake, 20, 20t
  as buffers, 194, *194,* 194t
  dietary, and hepatic encephalopathy, 358t
  in parenteral nutrition, 469–470, 473
  plasma. See *Plasma protein*.
Protein intake, for liver disease, 362
Protein metabolism, 469
Protein solutions, 473
Protein-losing enteropathy (PLE), case study of, 570, 570t
  fluid therapy for, 339
  hypoalbuminemia in, 347–348
Proteolysis, in diabetic ketoacidosis, 375
Proximal tubule(s), functions of, 26
  morphology of, 35, *35*
  reabsorption in, 34, *34*
    of chloride, 74
    of potassium, 86–87
    of sodium, 47, *48*
Pruritus, with hydroxyethyl starch, 491
Pseudohyperchloremia, 79
Pseudohyperkalemia, 91, 100t
Pseudohyponatremia, 60–61, *61*
Psychogenic polydipsia, 55, 64, 66t
PTH. See *Parathyroid hormone (PTH)*.
PTHrP. See *Parathyroid hormone–related protein (PTHrP)*.
Puerperal tetany, 148, 150–151
Pulmonary artery diastolic pressure, *405*
Pulmonary capillary wedge pressure (PCWP), and left-ventricular end-diastolic pressure, 278
  determination of, *405*
  in congestive heart failure, 314, 404–406, *405*
  in monitoring fluid therapy, 317
Pulmonary catheterization, 404, *405*
Pulmonary contusions, shock with, 446
Pulmonary disease, colloid therapy in, 489–490
Pulmonary edema, colloid therapy in, 489–490
  in congestive heart failure, management of, 400–401
  mixed acid-base disturbances with, 255, 256
  perioperative management of, 312
Pulmonary fibrosis, case study of, 585, 585t
Pulmonary thromboembolism, due to hemodialysis, 542, 544
Pulse oximetry, in shock, 445
Pumps, infusion, 275, *276,* 299, *300*
  for blood transfusion, 457
Purdue column disc peritoneal dialysis catheter, 517, *517*
Purpura, posttransfusion, 458–459
PV. See *Plasma volume (PV)*.
PVC (polyvinyl chloride) catheters, 284, 284t
PVCs (premature ventricular complexes), due to shock, 440
Pvo$_2$, in shock, 445
Pyelonephritis, distal renal tubular acidosis with, 216
  polyuria and polydipsia due to, 66t
Pyometra, polyuria and polydipsia due to, 66t
Pyridoxine, for ethylene glycol ingestion, 219
Pyrophosphoric acid, 163
Pyruvate, 223

Q

Quick-Cath catheter, 283t
Quinton Instrument PermCath, 531

R

Radiosulfate dilution studies, 7
Ramipril, renal effects of, 394t
Ranitidine, for metabolic alkalosis, 235
RAP (right atrial pressure), and central venous pressure, 278, 301–302, *302*
RAS (renin-angiotensin system), 40
Rat poison, hyperphosphatemia due to, 169
  ingestion of, *564,* 565–566, 566t
  vitamin D toxicity due to, 136
Rate-consistent pumps, 299, *300*
RBF. See *Renal blood flow (RBF)*.
Reabsorption, renal tubular. See *Renal tubular reabsorption*.
Red blood cells. See *Erythrocyte(s)*.
  packed. See *Packed red blood cells (PRBCs)*.
"Refeeding" alkalosis, 235
Reflection coefficient, 484
Reglan (metoclopramide), and dopamine, 420
Rehemorrhaging, with hypertonic solutions, 503–504
Rehydration, failure to achieve, 277–278
  in renal failure, 412
Renal. See also *Kidney(s)*.
Renal blood flow (RBF), 30–32, *31*
  dopamine and, 419–421
  in hypercalcemia, 139
  in renal failure, 411
Renal clearance, 26–27
Renal compensations, in chronic hypocapnia, 245
  in primary acid-base disorders, 196t
Renal disease, perioperative management of, 315
  with pancreatitis, 340
Renal failure, acute, due to ethylene glycol ingestion, 575–577, 576t
  fluid therapy for, 268t
  hemodialysis for, 528–529, 537–538, *538*
  hypercalcemia due to, 138, 139–140
  hyperphosphatemia due to, 170
  peritoneal dialysis for. See *Peritoneal dialysis*.
  polyuria and polydipsia due to, 66t
  prevalence of, 410
"acute-on-chronic," 410
advanced, hyponatremia due to, 63–64
atrial natriuretic peptide for, 421
calcium transport in, *127*
chronic, case studies of, 570–572, 571t, *572,* 581–582, 581t
  fluid therapy for, 268t
  hemodialysis for, 529, 538–539
  hypercalcemia due to, 128–129, *130*
  hyperkalemia due to, 100
  hyperphosphatemia due to, 169–170
  polyuria and polydipsia due to, 66t
  potassium balance in, 85, *85*
  prevalence of, 410
  with hypocalcemia, 147–148
classification of, 410–411, 410t
clinical signs of, 534t
complications of, 424
diagnostic procedures for, 411t
diuretics for, 416, 417–421
felodipine for, 421
fluid push in, 416–417
fluid therapy during, 268t, 410–425
  conversion from oliguria to nonoliguria in, 416–421
  fluid quality in, 413
  for initial stabilization, 412–422
  for rehydration, 412
  general principles of/goals for, 411–412, 411t

Renal failure *(Continued)*
  indications for, 410–411, 410t, 411t
  monitoring of effects of, 422–425
  outcomes of, 423–424
  route of administration for, 412
  tapering of, 424–425
  urine output and, 412–413
  with blood products, 421–422
  with metabolic abnormalities, 413–416
 hemodialysis for, 534–539, 534t, *536*
 hypercalcemia in, 415–416
 hyperkalemia in, 413
 hypermagnesemia in, 416
 hypernatremia in, 413
 hyperphosphatemia in, 415
 hypocalcemia in, 415
 hypochloremia in, 413
 hypokalemia in, 413–414
 hypomagnesemia in, 416
 hyponatremia in, 413
 hypophosphatemia in, 415
 infections with, 424
 intrinsic (primary), defined, 410
 metabolic acidosis in, 221–222, 416
 mixed acid-base disorders with, 257
 nonoliguric, 410, 410t, 424–425
 nutritional support in, 422
 oliguric, 410, 410t, 412–413, 416–421, 423, 424
 peritoneal dialysis for. See *Peritoneal dialysis.*
 polyuric, 412–413, 425
 urea in, 534–537
 with dextrans, 323, 491
Renal function, anesthesia effect on, 316–317
 in congestive heart failure, 389, 390t, 392–393, 399, 399t
  cardiovascular drugs and, 393–397, *395*, 395t
 with positive-pressure ventilation, 317
Renal function tests, in congestive heart failure, 399
Renal glucosuria, polyuria and polydipsia due to, 66t
Renal plasma flow (RPF). See *Renal blood flow (RBF).*
Renal solute load, 16, 19, 20–21
Renal threshold, 35
Renal transplantation, hemodialysis for, 529, 539
Renal transport, of potassium, 86–87, *87*, 88
 processes of, 34–35
Renal tubular acidosis (RTA), 214–216, 216t
 case study of, 578–579, 578t
 distal (classic, type 1), 214–215, 216t
  hypokalemia with, 95–96
 proximal (type 2), 215–216, 216t
Renal tubular flow rate, in renal failure, 411
Renal tubular function, 32–36, 33–36
Renal tubular reabsorption, 32–34, *34*
 of amino acids, 36
 of bicarbonate, 34, *34*, 205, *205*, 206
  in proximal renal tubular acidosis, 215
 of calcium, 109
 of chloride, 74
 of potassium, 86–87, *87*
 of sodium, 47, *48*
 of urea, 36
Renal tubular secretion, 32–33
Renin, 40
 in congestive heart failure, 393
 in sodium balance, 50t
Renin-angiotensin system (RAS), 40
Reperfusion injury, 446
Replacement requirement, 275, 277t

Replacement solutions, 269
Repositol vasopressin test, 70, 70t
RER (resting energy requirement), 469–470
Reset osmostat, 64
Respiratory acid-base disorders, 195, 241–250
 metabolic compensation in, 243–245, *244, 245*
 overview of, 243–245, *244, 245*
Respiratory acidosis, 245–247
 and metabolic acidosis, 256–257, 256t
 and metabolic alkalosis, 254–255, 254t
 causes of, 246, 246t
 clinical features of, 245–246
 compensatory responses to, acute, 196, 196t, 244, *244*, 252
  chronic, 196, 196t, 244–245, *245*, 252
 defined, 195, 195t, 245
 diagnosis of, 246
 in congestive heart failure, 398
 in liver disease, treatment of, 363
 in triple acid-base disorder, 258, 258t
 pathogenesis of, 245
 potassium balance in, 86
 treatment of, 246–247, *247*
Respiratory alkalosis, 247–248
 and metabolic acidosis, 254t, 255
 and metabolic alkalosis, 256t, 257
 causes of, 247t, 248
 clinical features of, 247–248
 compensatory responses to, acute, 196, 196t, 244, *244*, 252
  chronic, 196, 196t, 244, 244–245, *245*, 252
 defined, 195, 195t, 247
 diagnosis of, 248
 hyperchloremia due to, 80
 hypocalcemia due to, 150
 in congestive heart failure, 398
 in liver disease, 354
  treatment of, 363
 in triple acid-base disorder, 258, 258t
 pathogenesis of, 247
 potassium balance in, 86
 treatment of, 248
Respiratory compensation, 196t, 251–252
Respiratory complications, of hemodialysis, 544–545
Respiratory processes, metabolic compensation in, 243–244, *244, 245*, 252, 252t
Respiratory response, to acute acid load, 211–212
 to metabolic alkalosis, 228–229, *229*
Respiratory system, evaporative losses in, 16–18, 18t
Respiratory unit, microcirculation of, 387–389, *388*
Resting cell membrane potential, 24
 hypocalcemia and, 230, *230*
 potassium in, 24, 83–84
Resting energy requirement (RER), 469–470
Resuscitation, ABC's of, 434
 cardiopulmonary, lactic acidosis during, 224
 mixed acid-base disturbances with, 255
 hemorrhage due to, 445
 hypotensive, 445
 injury after, 445–446
 volume, 435–439
Right atrial pressure (RAP), and central venous pressure, 278, 301–302, *302*
Right ventricular dysplasia, 552–553, 553t
Right-sided heart failure, 391, 392
 case study of, 552–553, 553t
 central venous pressure in, 314
Right-to-left shunt, (A-a) O_2 gradient with, 243, 243t

Ringer's solution, electrolyte composition of, 271t
 lactated, 2.5% dextrose in, 271t
  5% dextrose in, 271t
  compatibility of, with other IV products, 311t, 320
  composition of, 272t
  during anesthesia and surgery, 320
  electrolyte composition of, *270*, 271t
  for hypercalcemia, 142
  for metabolic acidosis, 272–273
 half-strength, 2.5% dextrose in, 271t
  lactate metabolism with, 320
  potential disadvantages of, 320
  rate of administration of, 274
  with cerebral edema, 320
Rodenticides, hyperphosphatemia due to, 169
 ingestion of, *564*, 565–566, 566t
 vitamin D toxicity due to, 136
RPF (renal plasma flow). See *Renal blood flow (RBF).*
RTA. See *Renal tubular acidosis (RTA).*

S

Salicylate intoxication, metabolic acidosis due to, 220
 mixed acid-base disturbances with, 255
Saline, hypertonic. See *Hypertonic solutions.*
 normal. See *Normal saline.*
 physiologic, for hypercalcemia, 141t, 142
Salt, 190
Salt administration, polyuria and polydipsia due to, 66t
Salt depletion, clinical signs of, 12t
Salt poisoning, 57–58
 case study of, 548–549
Saphenous veins, for catheter placement, 285
Saturation of hemoglobin with oxygen (SaO_2), in shock, 445
Schistosomiasis, hypercalcemia due to, 137
Screening, of blood donors, 455
Secondary active transport, 34–35
Secondary responses, in acid-base disorders. See *Compensatory responses.*
Secretin, and pancreatic juice, 332, *332*
Secretion, of water and electrolytes, 330–335, *330–335*
 renal tubular, 32–33
Seizures, due to essential hypernatremia, 50t, 549–552, 551t, *552*
 due to hypocalcemia, 146, 151
 due to magnesium deficiency, 181
 due to salt poisoning, 548–549
 due to xylazine and ketamine administration, 583–584, 583t, 584t
 eclamptic, magnesium for, 183
Semipermeable membrane, 530
Septic peritonitis, 368
Septic shock, 431, 432–433
 antibiotics for, 441
 hypertonic solutions for, 500–501
 mixed acid-base disturbances with, 255, 256
Set-point, for parathyroid hormone secretion, 112–113, *113*
Sevoflurane, effects of, 317
Shock, 428–447
 analgesia for, 434, 440–441, 441t
 anaphylactic, 432
 ancillary supportive therapy for, 439–443
 antiarrhythmic agents for, 440
 antibiotics for, 441
 bicarbonates for, 442
 blood products for, 442–443
 burn, hypertonic solutions for, 501
 cardiogenic, 431, 432, 433–434

608 INDEX

Shock (Continued)
  fluid therapy for, 439
  cardiovascular support for, 439–440
  classification of, 431–434
  clinical signs of, 431
  clinical stages of, 429–431, 431t
  compensatory, 430
    clinical signs of, 431
    fluid therapy for, 446
  decompensatory, early, 430–431
    clinical signs of, 431
    fluid therapy for, 446
    terminal, 431
      clinical signs of, 431
      fluid therapy for, 446–447
  defined, 428
  distributive, 432
  endotoxic, due to transfusion, 459
    fluid therapy for, 268t, 338
    hypertonic solutions for, 500–501
  fluid therapy for, 434–439, 434t
    cardiogenic, 439
    combination, 438–439, 439t
    compensatory, 446
    decompensatory (terminal), 446–447
    early decompensatory, 446
    endotoxic, 268t, 338
    hemorrhagic, 268t
    vascular access for, 435
    with colloids, 434t, 436–438
    with crystalloids, 434t, 435–436, 438
    with head trauma and pulmonary contusions, 446
    with hypertonic solutions, 434t, 438, 499–501
  gastric dilatation-volvulus–induced, hypertonic solutions for, 501
  glucocorticoids for, 441–442
  hemorrhagic, 431, 432
    autotransfusion for, 436
    blood products for, 442
    fluid therapy for, 268t
    hypernatremia due to, 59
    hypertonic solutions for, 499
  hypovolemic, 431, 432
    case study of, 586, 586t
    in renal failure, 412
    signs of, 267
  in acute pancreatitis, hypertonic solutions for, 501
  metabolic acidosis in, 442
  monitoring of, 443–445
  no-reflow phenomenon in, 446
  obstructive, 432, 434
  pain and, 433, 440–441, 441t
  pathophysiology of, 428–429, 429t, 430
  predictors of outcome of, 445
  reperfusion injury in, 446
  resuscitation for, ABC's of, 434
    hemorrhage due to, 445
    hypotensive, 445
    injury after, 445–446
    volume, 435–439
  septic, 431, 432–433
    antibiotics for, 441
    hypertonic solutions for, 500–501
    mixed acid-base disturbances with, 255, 256
  traumatic, 431–432, 433
    hypertonic solutions for, 499–500
  vasogenic, 432
  vicious circle (circulus vitiosus) of, 429, 430
  with head trauma and pulmonary contusions, 446

SIADH (syndrome of inappropriate antidiuretic hormone secretion), hyponatremia due to, 63
SID. See Strong ion difference (SID).
Silicone elastomer (Silastic) catheters, 284, 284t
Single-nephron glomerular filtration rate (SNGFR), 28
Sinorphan, renal effects of, 394t
SIRS. See Systemic inflammatory response syndrome (SIRS).
Skin, evaporative losses in, 16–18, 17t
Skin disorders, due to magnesium deficiency, 181
Skin preparation, for blood donation, 455
  for catheter placement, 285–286
Skin turgor, 267, 317
Small intestine, absorption and secretion of water by, 332, 333, 333–334, 334
Small-bowel obstruction, 339–341
  case study of, 580–581, 580t
SNGFR (single-nephron glomerular filtration rate), 28
Sodium (Na^+), in acid-base analysis, 202–203, 204t
  in body fluid compartments, 9, 9–10, 10t
  in congestive heart failure, 396, 397, 402
  in crystalloid solutions, 402
  in intestine, 333, 334
  in pancreas, 332
  in renal failure, 413
  renal handling of, 47, 48
  renal transport of, 35
  serum concentration of, 46–47
  with fluid therapy, 272
Sodium balance, disorders of. See Hypernatremia; Hyponatremia.
  renal regulation of, 45t, 47–50, 50t
Sodium bicarbonate ($NaHCO_3$), 7.5%, 271t
  8.4%, 271t
  as additive, 270
  compatibility of, with other IV products, 311t
  for cardiac arrest, 224
  for diabetic ketoacidosis, 221, 311, 379–380
  for ethylene glycol ingestion, 218
  for hypercalcemia, 141t, 142–143
  for hyperkalemia, 103
  for hypoadrenocorticism, 383
  for lactic acidosis, 225–226
  for metabolic acidosis, 226–227
  for mixed acid-base disorders, 256, 257
  for respiratory acidosis, 246–247
  for salicylate intoxication, 220
  for shock, 442
  for uremic acidosis, 222, 416
  in dialysate, 520
  metabolic alkalosis due to, 231
Sodium chloride (NaCl), 0.45%, 271t
  2.5% dextrose in, 271t
  5% dextrose in, 271t
  0.9%, 272t
  5% dextrose in, 271t, 272t
  1.2%, 502t
  2.4%, 502t
  3%, 271t, 502, 502t
  4%, 502t
  5%, 496, 502t, 503
  7%. See Sodium chloride (NaCl), hypertonic.
  and hetastarch, 439, 439t
  compatibility of, with other IV products, 311t
  for metabolic alkalosis, 235
  for respiratory acidosis, 247

Sodium chloride (NaCl) (Continued)
  hypertonic, 496
    cardiovascular effects of, 503
    contraindications to, 503–504
    dosage of, 502, 502t
    electrolyte and osmolality disturbances with, 503
    for shock, 499–501
    formulations of, 502–503
    hemostasis with, 503–504
    immunomodulatory effects of, 499
    inotropic effects of, 498
    lung vagal reflex with, 497–498
    mechanisms of action of, 497–499
    oxygen delivery with, 498–499
    plasma volume expansion with, 496, 497
    precautions with, 503–504
    rate of infusion for, 503
    route of administration of, 501–502
  in intestine, 333, 334, 335, 335
Sodium citrate, 3.8%, for donated blood, 456t
Sodium EDTA, for hypercalcemia, 141t, 144
Sodium intake, and potassium excretion, 89
Sodium lactate, hypertonic, 496
Sodium nitroprusside, for congestive heart failure, 399
  renal effects of, 394t
Sodium phosphate, for diabetic ketoacidosis, 379
  for hypercalcemia, 142
  for hypophosphatemia, 167, 168t
Sodium phosphate enemas, hypernatremia due to, 58
Sodium polystyrene sulfonate (Kayexalate), for hyperkalemia, 103, 103t
Sodium restriction, for ascites, 365
  for congestive heart failure, 402
Sodium retention, in congestive heart failure, 391–393
  in liver disease, 349–351
Sodium sulfate, for hypercalcemia, 142
Sodium-chloride (Na^+-Cl^-) cotransporter, 47
Sodium-chloride difference ($[Na^+]$-$[Cl^-]$), in mixed acid-base disorders, 253, 254t
Sodium-hydrogen (Na^+-H^+) antiporter, 47
Sodium-hydrogen (Na^+-H^+) exchangers, in intestine, 333
Sodium-potassium adenosine triphosphatase (Na^+,K^+-ATPase), 47, 83, 91
  in intestine, 333, 334
Sodium-potassium (Na^+,K^+)-ATPase pump, 24–25
Sodium-potassium-chloride (Na^+-K^+-$2Cl^-$) cotransporter, 47
Soft tissue mineralization, due to hypercalcemia, 139
Solubility coefficient of CO_2, 192
Solu-Cortef (hydrocortisone sodium succinate), for hypoadrenocorticism, 382
Solu-Delta-Cortef (prednisolone sodium succinate), for hypoadrenocorticism, 382
  for shock, 441
Solute(s), dietary, 19
  distribution of, 9, 9–10, 10t
  impermeant, hypernatremia due to gain of, 53t, 54, 57–58, 58, 59
  peritoneal clearance of, 508, 508t, 511–513, 512t
  renal load of, 16, 19, 20–21
  renal medullary washout of, polyuria and polydipsia due to, 66t
  total body, 58
  units of measure for, 3–5, 3t, 4
Solute diuresis, 46
Solute drag, 507

Solute flow equation, 485
Solute losses, effect of, 12, 12t
Solute phase, 485
Solution(s), additive, 270, 272–273
    crystalloid, 269–273, *270*, 271t, 272t
    maintenance, 269
    osmolality of, 270
    replacement, 269
Solution administration set, 299
Solvahex (chlorhexidine gluconate), for catheter placement, 286
Solvent drag, 35
    in intestine, 333
Solvent flow equation, 485
Solvent phase, 485
Somatostatin congeners, for humoral hypercalcemia of malignancy, 145
Sovereign indwelling catheter, *282*, 283t
Specific gravity, 46, 46t
    of urine. See *Urine specific gravity (USG)*.
Spironolactone, for ascites, 365
    for congestive heart failure, 400, 401
    hyperkalemia due to, 102
    renal effects of, 393, 394–395, 394t, *395*, 395t
Spleen, as reservoir for erythrocytes, 5–6
Starling curve, *278*, 302
Starling forces, 387–389, *388*, 485–487, 486t
    in sodium balance, 49
Starling's law, 12–13, *13*
Starvation, 468
    fluid therapy for, 268t
Steroids, for hypercalcemia, 141t, 143, 143t
Stomach, absorption and secretion of water by, 330, *331*
Streamline catheter, 283t
Stress, fluid therapy for, 268t
Stress relaxation, 487
Stroke volume (SV), and left-ventricular end-diastolic pressure, *278*, 278
Strong ion difference (SID), 75, 197, 202–204
    apparent and effective, 202–204
    in chronic hypercapnia, 244, *245*
Subcutaneous route, 273, 281
Succinylated gelatin (Gelofusine), physicochemical properties of, 322t, 324
SV (stroke volume), and left-ventricular end-diastolic pressure, *278*, 278
Swan-Ganz pulmonary catheterization, 404, *405*
Sympathetic activity, anesthesia effect on, 316
Syndrome of inappropriate antidiuretic hormone secretion (SIADH), hyponatremia due to, 63
Syringe pumps, *300*
Systemic inflammatory response syndrome (SIRS), 432–433, 433t
    antibiotics for, 441
    fluid therapy for, 436, 437

T

T connector, *299*
TAC (time-averaged concentration), of urea, 537
Tachycardia, in monitoring fluid therapy, 317
Taurine, in hypokalemia, 397
TBS (total body solute), 58
TBW. See *Total body water (TBW)*.
Teflon catheters, 284, 284t
Temperature, of fluids, 316
Tesio catheter, 531
Tetany, due to hypocalcemia, 146, 151
    due to magnesium deficiency, 179
    puerperal, 148, 150–151
Tetrafluoroethylene (TFE Teflon) catheters, 284, 284t

THAM (tromethamine), for lactic acidosis, 226
Thermodynamic considerations, in perioperative period, 316
Thiamine, for ethylene glycol ingestion, 219
Thiamine supplementation, 270
Thiazide diuretics, for congestive heart failure, 401
    for diabetes insipidus, 56
    hypokalemia due to, 96
    hyponatremia due to, 403
    renal effects of, 394, 394t, *395*, 395t
Thiocyanate dilution studies, 7
Thiopental, effects of, 316
Thiosulfate dilution studies, 7
Thirst mechanism, abnormal, hypernatremia due to, 54
Threshold cell membrane potential, *84*, 84–85
Thrombocytopenia, perioperative management of, 314–315
    with hemodialysis, 545
Thromboembolism, mixed acid-base disorders with, 257
    pulmonary, due to hemodialysis, 542, 544
Thrombophlebitis, due to catheter, 297
    with parenteral nutrition, 477–478
Thrombosis, due to catheterization, 285, 297, *297*
    with hemodialysis, 542–543, *543*
Through-the-needle catheter, *282*, 283t, 284
    placement of, 288–293, *290–292*
Thyroid carcinoma, case study of, *566*, 566–567, 567t
Thyroidectomy, hypocalcemia after, 570–572, 571t, *572*
Ticarcillin, for peritonitis, 523
Tight epithelia, 33
Tight junctions, 33
Tiletamine, effects of, 316
Time-averaged concentration (TAC), of urea, 537
Tissue hydrostatic pressure, 12
Tissue oncotic pressure, 12
Tissue perfusion, in shock, 429, *430*
Tissue safety factors, 487
Tissue synthesis and repair, nutrition and, 465
Titratable acidity, 194, 205, 206
Titration curve, 191–192, *192*
TNA. See *Total nutrient admixture (TNA)*.
Tobramycin, for peritonitis, 523
Tocolysis, magnesium for, 183
Tonicity, and osmolality, 5
    defined, 5, 46
    estimation of, 46
    of total body water, *11*, 11–12
Torsemide, renal effects of, 394, *395*, 395t
Total blood volume, 5–6, 6t
Total body solute (TBS), 58
Total body water (TBW), in congestive heart failure, 397
    tonicity of, *11*, 11–12
    volume of, 5–6
Total nutrient admixture (TNA), 471t, 472
    administration of, 476–477
    catheter complications with, 477–478
    compounding of, 474–476, 475t, *476*
    drugs with, 474, 474t
Total parenteral nutrition (TPN). See also *Parenteral nutrition (PN)*.
    hypophosphatemia due to, 165–166
    patient selection for, 471, 471t
    vs. parenteral nutrition, 471–472
Total plasma proteins (TPPs), in dehydration, 268, 269t
    in malnutrition, 467, 469–470

Total plasma proteins (TPPs) *(Continued)*
    in renal failure, 423
    in shock, 443
Transcellular fluid(s), defined, 5
    solute concentrations in, 10
    volume of, 5
Transcellular route, 33
Transepithelial potential difference (TPD), 33, *33*
    and chloride reabsorption, 74
Transfusion(s), 451–462
    administration of, 456–458
    and hepatic encephalopathy, 358t
    and immune function, 325
    autologous, 308
        for hemorrhagic shock, 436
    blood collection for, 455–456, 456t
    blood components for, 451–453, *453*
    blood typing for, 454–455, 454t, 461, *461*
    calcium with, 325
    costs of, 451
    crossmatching for, 460–461, 460t, *461*, 461t
    donor health maintenance for, 455
    donor screening for, 455
    donor selection for, 453–455, 454t
    for anemia, 308–309
    for congestive heart failure, 403
    for hemorrhagic shock, 436, 442
    for liver disease, 364
    for renal failure, 421–422
    indications for, 325
    lactic acidosis due to, 356
    monitoring of, 457–458
    of hemoglobin solutions, 326
    of packed red blood cells, 325
    of plasma protein, 324–325
    of whole blood, 325–326
    rate of, 457
    route of, 457
    sources of blood and blood products for, 451, 452t, 453
    warming of stored blood for, 325–326, 457
Transfusion reactions, 458–461
    acute immunologic (acute hemolytic), 458, 458t
    acute nonimmunologic, 458t, 459
    classification of, 458, 458t
    defined, 458
    delayed immunologic, 458–459, 458t
    delayed nonimmunologic, 458t, 459
    drug therapy for, 459–460, 459t
    evaluation of, 459
    prevention of, 460–461, 460t, *461*, 461t
Transmembrane potential difference, 33, *33*
Transtubular potassium gradient (TTKG), 93
Transtubular potential difference, 33
Transvascular fluid dynamics, 484–485
Traumatic shock, 431–432, 433
    hypertonic solutions for, 499–500
Triamterene, for congestive heart failure, 401
    hyperkalemia due to, 102
    renal effects of, 394, *395*, 395t
Trichuris vulpis, 556–557, 556t
Triiodothyronine, in malnutrition, 468–469
Trimethoprim-sulfamethoxazole, for peritonitis, 523
Triple acid-base disorders, 251t, 258, 258t
Tromethamine (THAM), for lactic acidosis, 226
Tryptophan, and hepatic encephalopathy, 357t
TTKG (transtubular potassium gradient), 93
Tube feeding, 471
    with parenteral nutrition, 478
Tuberculosis, hypercalcemia due to, 137
Tubing, IV extension, 299

Tubular transport maximum, 35
Tubuloglomerular feedback, 31–32
Tumor lysis syndrome, case study of, 573–574, 574t
　hyperphosphatemia due to, 167–168
　hypocalcemia due to, 150
　mixed acid-base disturbances with, 255, 256–257
Twin-Cath catheter, 283t

U

Ulnar artery, catheterization of, 318
Ultrafiltration, 507
　barriers to, 511–512
　in hemodialysis, 530
　without hemodialysis, 540
Ultrafiltration control systems, for hemodialysis, 533
Underfilling hypothesis, of ascites, 360
Units of measure, 3–5, 3t, 4
Urea. See also *Blood urea nitrogen (BUN)*.
　in renal failure, 534–537
　in urinary concentrating mechanism, 39, 39
　time-averaged concentration of, 537
　tubular reabsorption of, 36
　with hemodialysis, 536, 536–537
　with peritoneal dialysis, 509, 509, 514–515, 524–525
Urea cycle, 345–346, 346
Urea reabsorption, vasopressin in, 51
Urea reduction ratio (URR), 536, 537
Urea synthesis, in liver disease, 351, 352, 353
Urea-linked gelatin (Haemaccel), physicochemical properties of, 322t, 324
Uremia. See also *Renal failure*.
　peritoneal dialysis for. See *Peritoneal dialysis*.
　substances that accumulate in, 508, 508t
Uremic acidosis, 221–222, 416
Uremic "crisis," 411
Uremic pneumonitis, due to hemodialysis, 544–545
Uremic toxicity, 534–537
Ureterolithiasis, hypercalcemia with, 137
Urethral calculi, case study of, 554–555, 555t
Urethral obstruction, case study of, 559–560, 560t
　fluid therapy for, 268t
Urinary concentrating mechanism, 36–39, 37t, 38, 39
　in hypercalcemia, 139
Urinary free water, 16
Urinary tract disease, feline lower, 19
Urinary tract infection (UTI), with catheterization, 318
Urinary tract obstruction, partial, polyuria and polydipsia due to, 66t
Urine, magnesium excretion in, 178–179
　normal output of, 67
　potassium excretion in, 87–89, 89
　water loss in, 15–16, 15t, 16
Urine osmolality, 15–16, 15t, 16t, 38, 46, 46t
　in central diabetes insipidus, 55
Urine output, anesthesia effect on, 316
　in monitoring fluid therapy, 278, 299–300, 318
　　during renal failure, 423
　in renal failure, 412–413
　in shock, 444–445
　normal, 412
Urine specific gravity (USG), 46, 46t
　in central diabetes insipidus, 55
　in liver disease, 352, 353
Urine volume, 15–16, 16
Uroabdomen, 367

Urolithiasis, hypercalcemia with, 135, 137, 140
Uro-Mag (magnesium oxide), for magnesium depletion, 183
URR (urea reduction ratio), 536, 537
Urticaria, due to transfusion, 459–460
USG. See *Urine specific gravity (USG)*.
UTI (urinary tract infection), with catheterization, 318

V

Vagal reflex, with hypertonic solutions, 497–498
Valence, 3
Vancomycin, for peritonitis, 523
Vasa recta, 36–37
　in urinary concentrating mechanism, 38–39
Vascular access, for hemodialysis, 530–532, 531
　complications of, 542–543, 543
　perioperative management of, 316
　veins for, 273, 284–285
Vascular resistance, in renal circulation, 31
　systemic, and arterial blood pressure, 387, 388, 389t
Vascular volume. See *Blood volume*.
Vasoactive intestinal polypeptide (VIP), in control of absorption and secretion, 335
Vasoactive intestinal polypeptide–secreting tumors (VIPomas), diarrhea due to, 337–338
Vasoactive mediators, and glomerular filtration rate, 29–30, 29t
Vasodilators, renal effects of, 394t
Vasogenic shock, 432
Vasopressin. See *Antidiuretic hormone (ADH)*.
Vasopressin leak, 64
Vasopressin test, exogenous, 70, 70t
Vasopressors, for shock, 440
VDR (vitamin D receptor), 119
　and parathyroid hormone synthesis and secretion, 113
VDREs (vitamin D response elements), 113
Vein(s), for catheter placement, 273, 284–285
Venocath intravenous catheter, 282, 283t
Venous access, 273, 284–285
　procedures for, 293–295, 295
Venous air embolism, due to transfusion, 459
Venous blood samples, 198, 199
Ventilation-perfusion (V-Q) mismatch, in liver disease, 354–355
　use of $(A-a)$ O_2 gradient in assessment of, 243
Ventilatory response, to metabolic alkalosis, 228–229
Ventricular arrhythmias, due to shock, 440
Ventricular dysplasia, right, 552–553, 553t
Ventricular filling pressures, 404, 405
Ventricular function curves, in congestive heart failure, 390–391, 392
Vet Cath column disc catheter, 517, 518
Vetaplasma (oxypolygelatin), for shock, 437
　physicochemical properties of, 322t, 324, 437
VIP (vasoactive intestinal polypeptide), in control of absorption and secretion, 335
VIPomas (vasoactive intestinal polypeptide-secreting tumors), diarrhea due to, 337–338
Visceral epithelial cells, of glomerulus, 27–28
Vitamin(s), in parenteral nutrition, 470, 474
Vitamin B_1, for liver disease, 362
Vitamin B_{12}, for liver disease, 362
Vitamin D, 117–120
　actions of, 119–120

Vitamin D (Continued)
　activation of, 40–41
　hyperphosphatemia due to, 169
　synthesis of, 117–119, 118
Vitamin D deficiency, hypocalcemia due to, 150
　hypophosphatemia due to, 166
Vitamin D metabolites, 117
　for hypocalcemia, 151–152, 152t, 153
　serum concentrations of, 121t, 125
Vitamin D receptor (VDR), 119
　and parathyroid hormone synthesis and secretion, 113
Vitamin D toxicity, 136–137
Vitamin D_2, 117
　excess, 136–137
　for hypocalcemia, 152t, 153
Vitamin D_3, 40
　excess, 136–137
Vitamin D_3 toxicity, case study of, 564, 565–566, 566t
Vitamin K deficiency, in liver disease, 364–365
Vitamin solutions, 474
Volatile acid, 189, 195–196
Volume control sets, in-line, 299
Volume depletion. See *Hypovolemia*.
Volume exclusion effect, 486
Volume expanders, macromolecular plasma. See *Macromolecular plasma volume expanders*.
Volume expansion, for hypercalcemia, 141t, 142
　for hyperphosphatemia, 170
　in congestive heart failure, 401, 402
　with colloids, 488, 491
　with hypertonic solutions, 496, 497
Volume measurements, for body fluid spaces, 5–9, 6t–8t, 9
Volume overload. See *Hypervolemia*.
Volume regulation, 45t
Volumetric pumps, 299, 300
Volvulus, 339
　with gastric dilatation. See *Gastric dilatation-volvulus (GDV)*.
Vomiting, due to ethylene glycol intoxication, 574–575, 574t, 575t
　due to hypoadrenocorticism, 553–554, 554t
　due to intestinal obstruction, 341, 580–581, 580t
　due to zygomycosis, 579–580, 579t, 580t
　fluid and electrolyte abnormalities due to, 336
　fluid therapy for, 268t, 270–271, 338–339
　in chronic renal failure, 581–582, 581t
　in diabetic ketoacidosis, 572–573, 572t, 573t
　metabolic alkalosis due to, 336
　mixed acid-base disturbances due to, 255–256
　pathomechanisms of, 335–336, 336
von Willebrand's disease, and blood donation, 454
　perioperative management of, 314
V-Q (ventilation-perfusion) mismatch, in liver disease, 354–355
　use of $(A-a)$ O_2 gradient in assessment of, 243

W

Water. See also *Fluid* entries.
　absorption and secretion of, 330–335, 330–335
　daily requirements for, 266, 266t, 267
　exchange of, between body fluid spaces, 10–13, 11, 12t, 13

Water *(Continued)*
  in dialysate, 533
  in food, 18, *18,* 18t, *19*
  ingestion of. See *Water intake.*
  metabolic, 20, 20t
  total body, in congestive heart failure, 397
    tonicity of, *11,* 11–12
    volume of, 5–6
  urinary free, 16
Water balance, in gastrointestinal tract, 330, *331*
  renal regulation of, 45t, 50–52, *50–52*
Water deficit, 59
Water deprivation, clinical signs of, 12t
  effect of, 12, 12t
  gradual, 69
Water deprivation test, 67–69, 70t
  modified, 69
Water diuresis, 46
Water intake, 15t, *18,* 18–20, 18t–20t, *19.* See also *Hypodipsia; Polydipsia.*
  in food-deprived animals, 21, 21t
  normal daily, 67
Water intoxication, 65
Water loss(es), 15–18, 15t, *16,* 17t, 18t
  effect of, 12, 12t

Water loss(es) *(Continued)*
  free, 15
    urinary, 16
  hypernatremia due to, 53–56, 53t, *54, 55, 56t,* 58–59
  insensible, 14, 15
  obligatory, 14, *14,* 15
    urinary and fecal, 15–16, 15t, *16*
  respiratory and cutaneous evaporative, 16–18, 17t, 18t
  salivary, 16
  sensible, 14
  urinary and fecal, 15–16, 15t, *16*
  via panting, 16–18, *18*
Water output, 15t
Water requirements, 20–21, 21t
  basal, 14–15, 20–21
  maintenance, 14–15, 20–21
Water turnover, in liver disease, 352
Weight, and fluid loss, 267–268
  atomic, 3, 3t
  equivalent, 4
  ideal dry body, 539
  in monitoring of intravenous therapy, 299
    during renal failure, 422–423
  milliequivalent, 4

Weight *(Continued)*
  molecular, 3, 3t
Weight loss, in dehydration, 267–268
  in diabetic ketoacidosis, 577–578, 577t
  in malnutrition, 466
Whole blood, 452
  during anesthesia and surgery, 325–326
Whole-blood buffer base, 197–198
Whole-blood volume, 5–6, 6t
Winged needle catheter, 282, *282,* 283t
  placement of, 286–287, *287*
Wound healing, nutrition and, 465

X

Xenodine (povidone-iodine), for catheter placement, 286
Xylazine administration, seizures due to, 583–584, 583t, 584t

Y

YM435, 419–420

Z

Zero balance, *14,* 14–15, 15t
Zygomycosis, case study of, 579–580, 579t, 580t

ISBN 0-7216-7739-8